INTERNATIONAL ENCYCLOPEDIA
OF PHARMACOLOGY AND THERAPEUTICS

Executive Editor: A. C. SARTORELLI, *New Haven*

Section 119

PHARMACOLOGY OF BACTERIAL TOXINS

Some Recent and Forthcoming Volumes

NOTICE TO READERS

Dear Reader

If your library is not already a standing order customer to this series, may we recommend that you place a standing order to receive immediately on publication all new volumes published in this valuable series. Should you find that these volumes no longer serve your needs your order can be cancelled at any time without notice.

The Editors and Publisher will be glad to receive suggestions or outlines of suitable titles for consideration for rapid publication in this series.

ROBERT MAXWELL
Publisher at Pergamon Press

INTERNATIONAL ENCYCLOPEDIA
OF PHARMACOLOGY AND THERAPEUTICS

Section 119

PHARMACOLOGY OF BACTERIAL TOXINS

SECTION EDITORS

F. DORNER
Immuno AG, Orth Donau, Austria

and

J. DREWS
F. Hoffmann-La Roche & Co. Ltd., Basel, Switzerland

PERGAMON PRESS
OXFORD · NEW YORK · BEIJING · FRANKFURT
SÃO PAULO · SYDNEY · TOKYO · TORONTO

U.K.	Pergamon Press, Headington Hill Hall, Oxford OX3 0BW, England
U.S.A.	Pergamon Press, Maxwell House, Fairview Park, Elmsford, New York 10523, U.S.A.
PEOPLE'S REPUBLIC OF CHINA	Pergamon Press, Qianmen Hotel, Beijing, People's Republic of China
FEDERAL REPUBLIC OF GERMANY	Pergamon Press, Hammerweg 6, D-6242 Kronberg, Federal Republic of Germany
BRAZIL	Pergamon Editora, Rua Eça de Queiros, 346, CEP 04011, São Paulo, Brazil
AUSTRALIA	Pergamon Press Australia, P.O. Box 544, Potts Point, N.S.W. 2011, Australia
JAPAN	Pergamon Press, 8th Floor, Matsuoka Central Building, 1-7-1 Nishishinjuku, Shinjuku-ku, Tokyo 160, Japan
CANADA	Pergamon Press Canada, Suite 104, 150 Consumers Road, Willowdale, Ontario M2J 1P9, Canada

First edition 1986

Library of Congress Cataloging in Publication Data
Main entry under title:
Pharmacology of bacterial toxins.
(International encyclopedia of pharmacology and therapeutics; section 119)
"Published as a supplement no. 19 (1985) to the review journal
Pharmacology and therapeutics"—T.p. verso.
1. Bacterial toxins. I. Dorner, F. (Friedrich)
II. Drews, Jürgen, 1933–   III. Pharmacology and therapeutics.
Supplement. IV. Series. [DNLM: 1. Bacterial Toxins—
pharmacodynamics. QV 4 158 section 119]
QP632.B3P47   1985   616'.014   85-12081

British Library Cataloguing in Publication Data
Pharmacology of bacterial toxins.—(International encyclopedia
of pharmacology and therapeutics; section 119)
1. Bacteria, Pathogenic   2. Bacterial toxins
I. Dorner, F.   II. Drews, J.   III. Pharmacology & therapeutics
IV. Series
616'.014   QP632.B3
ISBN 0 08 031988 2

Published as Supplement No. 19 (1986) to the review journal
Pharmacology and Therapeutics. Papers appearing in this volume are
revised, updated versions of papers previously published in the
journal.

Printed in Great Britain by A. Wheaton & Co. Ltd., Exeter

CONTENTS

LIST OF CONTRIBUTORS

Dr. Joseph E. Alouf, Bacterial Antigens Unit, Institut Pasteur, 28 Rue du Dr. Roux, Paris XVe, France.

Dr. J. P. Arbuthnott, University of Dublin, Department of Microbiology, Moyne Institute, Trinity College, Dublin 2, Ireland.

Dr. John G. Bartlett, Johns Hopkins University School of Medicine, Baltimore, Maryland, U.S.A.

Dr. Te-Wen Chang, Tufts University School of Medicine, New England Medical Center Hospital, Department of Medicine, Infectious Diseases Service, 171 Harrison Avenue, Boston, Massachusetts 02111, U.S.A.

Dr. Pedro Cuatrecasas, The Wellcome Research Laboratories, Burroughs Wellcome Company, 3030 Cornwallis Road, Research Triangle Park, NC 27709, U.S.A.

Dr. Arthur Donohue–Rolfe, Division of Geographic Medicine, New England Medical Center Hospital, Clinical Unit of Tufts-New England, Medical Center, 171 Harrison Avenue, Boston Massachusetts 02111, U.S.A.

Dr. Friedrich Dorner, Biomedical Research Center, Immuno AG, Uferstrasse 15, Orth a/d Donau, A-2304, Austria.

Dr. Jürgen Drews, Hoffmann-La Roche & Co. Ltd., Grenzacherstrasse 124, 4002 Basel, Switzerland.

Dr. Herbert L. DuPont, The University of Texas, Medical School at Houston, Program in Infectious Diseases and Clinical Microbiology, Houston Texas 77030, U.S.A.

Dr. Hans Rudolf Ebersold, Swiss Federal Institute of Technology, Institute of Microbiology, Universitätsstrasse 2, CH-8092 Zürich, Switzerland.

Dr. Richard A. Finkelstein, Department of Microbiology, University of Missouri-Columbia, School of Medicine, Columbia Missouri 65212, U.S.A.

Dr. John H. Freer, University of Glasgow, Department of Microbiology, Glasgow, Scotland.

Dr. Chris Galanos, Max-Planck-Institut für Immunobiologie, Postfach 1169, Stübeweg 51, D-78 Freiburg-Zähringen, Germany.

Dr. Sherwood L. Gorbach, Tufts University School of Medicine, New England Medical Center Hospital, Department of Medicine, Infectious Diseases Service, 171 Harrison Avenue, Boston Massachusetts 02111, U.S.A.

Dr. Richard N. Greenberg, Department of Internal Medicine, St. Louis University, School of Medicine, 1325 S Grand Boulevard, St. Louis, Missouri 63104, U.S.A.

Dr. Richard L. Guerrant, Divisions of Geographic Medicine and Infectious Diseases, Department of Medicine, Box No. 485 Medical Center, University of Virginia, Charlottesville, Virginia 22908, U.S.A.

Dr. Kenneth W. Hedlund, Division of Communicable Diseases and Immunology, Walter Reed Army Institute of Research, Washington DC 20307, U.S.A.

Dr. Simon van Heyningen, Department of Biochemistry, University of Edinburgh Medical School, Teviot Place, Edinburgh, Scotland, EH8 9AG.

Dr. Mary Jacewicz, Division of Geographic Medicine, New England Medical Center Hospital, Clinical Unit of Tufts-New England Medical Center, 171 Harrison Avenue, Boston Massachusetts 02111, U.S.A.

Dr. Gerald T. Keusch, Division of Geographic Medicine, New England Medical Center Hospital, Clinical Unit of Tufts-New England Medical Center, 171 Harrison Avenue, Boston Massachusetts 02111, U.S.A.

Dr. Harry LeVine, The Wellcome Research Laboratories, Burroughs Wellcome Company, 3030 Cornwallis Road, Research Triangle Park, North Carolina 27709, U.S.A.

Dr. Asa Ljungh, Department of Clinical Microbiology, Karolinska Hospital, Stockholm, Sweden.

Dr. Otto Lüderitz, Max-Planck-Institut für Immunobiologie, Postfach 1169, Stübeweg 51, D-78 Freiburg-Zähringen, Germany.

Dr. Peter Lüthy, Swiss Federal Institute of Technology, Institute of Microbiology, Universitätsstrasse 2, CH-8092 Zürich, Switzerland.

Dr. Werner K. Maas, Department of Microbiology, New York University Medical Center, School of Medicine, 550 First Avenue, New York, New York 10016, U.S.A.

Dr. James L. McDonel, 814 Cottage Grove Avenue, 96616 South Bend, Indiana, U.S.A.

Dr. Thomas C. Montie, The University of Tennessee, Department of Microbiology, Walters Life Sciences Building, Knoxville Tennessee 37916, U.S.A.

Dr. D. R. Morgan, The University of Texas, Medical School at Houston, Program in Infectious Diseases and Clinical Microbiology, Houston Texas 77030, U.S.A.

Dr. Sjur Olsnes, Norsk Hydro's Institute for Cancer Research, Norwegian Radium Hospital, Montebello Oslo 3, Norway.

Dr. R. Parton, University of Glasgow, Department of Microbiology, Anderson College, 56 Dumbarton Road, Glasgow, Scotland, G11 6NU.

Dr. Johnny W. Peterson, The University of Texas Medical Research, Department of Microbiology, Galveston Texas 77550, U.S.A.

Dr. Alexander Pihl, Norsk Hydro's Institute for Cancer Research, Norwegian Radium Hospital, Montebello Oslo 3, Norway.

Dr. Don W. Powell, Division of Digestive Diseases and Nutrition, Department of Medicine, University of North Carolina, Chapel Hill, North Carolina 27514, U.S.A.

Dr. Ernst Th. Rietschel, Forschungsinstitut Borstel, Institut für experimentelle Biologie und Medizin, Parkallee 1–40, D-2061 Borstel, Germany.

Dr. Donald C. Roberston, Department of Microbiology, University of Kansas, 735 Haworth Hall, Lawrence Kansas 66045, U.S.A.

Dr. Genji Sakaguchi, University of Osaka Prefecture, College of Agriculture, Department of Veterinary Science, 804 Mozu Ume-Machi 4-CHO, Sakai-Shi Osaka 591, Japan.

Dr. Suhas C. Sanyal, Department of Microbiology, Institute of Medical Sciences, Banaras Hindu University, Varanasi-5, India.

Dr. T. K. Satterwhite, The University of Texas, Medical School at Houston, Program in Infectious Diseases and Clinical Microbiology, Houston Texas 77030, U.S.A.

Dr. John Stephen, The University of Birmingham, Department of Microbiology, South West Campus, PO Box 363, Birmingham, B15 2TT.

Dr. N. M. Sullivan, Virginia Polytechnic Institute & the State University, Blacksburg, Virginia.

Professor Yoshifumi Takeda, Department of Bacterial Infection, The Institute of Medical Science, The University of Tokyo, 4–6–1 Shirokanedai, Minato-ku, Tokyo 108, Japan.

Dr. Grace M. Thorne, Tufts University School of Medicine, New England Medical Center Hospital, Department of Medicine, Infectious Diseases Service, 171 Harrison Avenue, Boston MA 02111, U.S.A.

Dr. Peter C. B. Turnbull, Food Hygiene Laboratories, Central Public Health Lab, Colindale Avenue, London, NW9 5HT.

Dr. Tsuyoshi Uchida, Research Institute for Microbial Diseases, Osaka University, Yamada-kami Suita, Osaka 565, Japan.

Dr. Torkel Wadström, Swedish University of Agricultural Science, College of Veterinary Medicine, Department of Bacteriology & Epizootology, Biomedicum, Box 583, S-75123 Uppsala, Sweden

Dr. A. C. Wardlaw, University of Glasgow, Department of Microbiology, Anderson College, 56 Dumbarton Road, Glasgow, Scotland, G11 6NU

Dr. T. D. Wilkins, Virginia Polytechnic Institute & the State University, Blacksburg, Virginia.

Dr. L. V. Wood, The University of Texas, Medical School at Houston, Program in Infectious Diseases and Clinical Microbiology, Houston Texas 77030, U.S.A.

CHAPTER 1

THE ROLE OF TOXINS IN BACTERIAL PATHOGENESIS

JAMES L. McDONEL*, FRIEDRICH DORNER* and JÜRGEN DREWS**

* Immuno AG, Vienna, Austria ** F. Hoffmann-La Roche & Co. AG, Basel, Switzerland

1. INTRODUCTION

Bernheimer (1976) has defined bacterial toxins as a collection of bacterial products whose principal common feature is their capacity to produce injury or to kill when administered in relatively small quantities in living entities. It may be possible to arrive at a more precise definition if one confines the scope to certain groups of well-characterized toxins (see below). However, as the broad collection of reviews in this encyclopedia demonstrates, the diversity of structure, mode of action, predilection, potency, and immunogenicity of the many known bacterial toxins seems to preclude any less general description at this time. Indeed, the field of bacterial toxinology (Toxicology is the study of all substances poisonous to living entities. A subset of toxicology, toxinology, addresses itself only to poisonous substances derived from living organisms. Bacterial toxinology is concerned only with poisonous substances produced by the group of living organisms known as bacteria) appears always to be expanding and becoming more diverse.

The number of different bacterial toxins described since the first 'classical' toxins (diphtheria, tetanus, and botulinum) were discovered nearly a hundred years ago, currently exceeds 150 (Alouf, 1982). In most cases bacterial toxins are relatively high molecular-weight substances in the form of proteins (simple or more complex 'conjugated' forms), peptides, or lipopolysaccharides. However, a few bacterial toxins, such as E. coli ST and Legionella toxin, appear to have molecular weights under 10,000 daltons. The exact degree of characterization, whether physical, chemical, or biological, of the many known toxins varies greatly, and therefore some of the general statements about the class bacterial toxins may change as the degree of understanding increases due to more data becoming available.

In recent years rapid advances in biochemistry, genetics, and physiology have enabled the isolation, purification, and structural characterization of many bacterial toxins, as well as elaboration of their modes of action, genetic coding and regulation of expression, structure-activity relationships, and roles in pathogenesis. These advances have been particularly helpful in increasing our understanding of disease syndromes that involve a previously undefined toxin, more than one toxin, or a combination of bacterial invasion and toxin production. There are numerous examples of incorrect conclusions being drawn about the role of a toxin in a disease syndrome due to observations of systems which have involved impure or otherwise poorly characterized preparations from bacteria. In more classical work, the lack of sufficiently sophisticated tools prevented study in a precise and revealing manner. As the sophistication of technology continues to increase, the relevant application of new methods should continue to increase our understanding of the role of toxins in pathogenesis.

Today the known roles of specific toxins in pathogenesis range from proven beyond a doubt to putative at best. It is interesting to note that in some cases well-characterized toxins have been useful in identifying and/or characterizing suspected, or newly identified ones (i.e., cholera and E. coli enterotoxins). There exist toxins of diverse origins with very similar structure, immunological identity, or mode of action, yet in most cases these toxins can readily be distinguished from one another in terms of their physical or chemical characteristics, the organism of origin, and/or the disease syndrome resulting from their action upon the susceptible host.

The exact role of various toxins in pathogenesis depends to a certain degree upon the complexity of the disease etiology. The easiest roles to define are those in diseases which stem from simple intoxication. Examples are food-borne diseases such as botulism and staphylococcal food poisoning. In both diseases it is not uncommon that live bacterial cells are not present at the time of exposure to the disease-causing agent. The toxin is often produced and excreted by the cells into the food environment, after which unfavorable intrinsic or extrinsic conditions (such as heating of foods for serving) result in complete destruction of viable cells. Sickness results solely from ingestion of a stable toxin. Studies have shown that the complete disease syndrome can be experimentally induced by simple challenge with the toxin alone.

In other disease syndromes, it appears that a single toxin is produced and excreted by bacteria that multiply in the host. Examples are disease due to tetanus toxin, diphtheria toxin, botulinum toxin (wound or infant botulism), plague murine toxin, cholera toxin, and *E. coli* LT or ST. In the case of tetanus, diphtheria, and botulinum toxins, the toxin often spreads throughout the body beyond the locale of the multiplying cells, whereas cholera toxin and *E. coli* LT and ST usually act in the vicinity of the site of cell multiplication. In the case of plague murine toxin, the organism spreads throughout the body, which results in widespread distribution of the toxin as well. Of course, the necessary conditions for multiplication and production of toxin in each of these syndromes must also be met. This can involve, among other things, certain types of tissue damage, breakdown of host defences, presence of suitable receptors for attachment of bacteria, or adequate route of inoculation of the organism.

Ascribing the role of toxins to bacterial pathogenesis becomes much more difficult when the possibility of more than one toxin is involved, and when other processes such as bacterial invasion are also necessary for the development of the disease. For example, more than twenty toxic factors which are produced by Streptococcus species have been described. *C. perfringens* and *B. cereus* are capable of producing a broad spectrum of deleterious compounds as well, including toxins and enzymes that enhance bacterial invasion or survival, or host susceptibility to toxin spread or action. However, there are organisms that are capable of elaborating more than one toxin but that produce a disease whose primary symptoms can be attributed to one agent, or in which the importance of one or more toxins is fairly well defined. Examples are certain diseases due to *C. difficile*, NAG vibrios, Shigella sp., Salmonella sp., and possibly *C. diphtheriae*.

Pertussis is a disease in man that has proven very difficult to mimic in its entirety in an animal model. One primary clinical feature of the disease, the paroxysmal coughing syndrome, develops and can persist for months after the complete disappearance of the organisms. The symptomatology can result from tissue alterations distant from the initial site of infection. Therefore, it is reasonable to assume the involvement of toxin(s) in development of symptoms. Indeed, three toxins from *B. pertussis* have been reasonably well characterized, but so far it has not been possible to delineate the exact contribution of each or any of them to, say, the coughing syndrome. Certain biological activities of the toxins described in animal or cell systems could explain aspects of the basic pathology of the disease in man, but in the absence of a good model system, precise studies are difficult.

Anthrax is a disease whose etiology is clearly multifactorial, and the difficulty in unraveling the role of the various factors has been the topic of long and animated debates. The disease can vary from a localized cutaneous infection in man to a fulminant, systemic infection in cattle, leading to death, which sometimes occurs so quickly that the animals drop dead before overt preliminary symptoms have developed. The exact role of toxin(s) is unclear in this complicated disease syndrome.

In disease due to certain Salmonella and NAG vibrio species, the role of elaborated toxins varies according to whether the organisms remain localized in the gut or become invasive and spread throughout the host. Generally speaking, as the clinical picture and degree of spread become more complicated, the roles of primary and secondary toxins, enzymes, and other virulence factors become more confused and difficult to resolve experimentally. Needless to say, in diseases due to organisms such as Streptococcus and *C. perfringens*, the role of each possible active factor is far from clear. Strep throat, for example, can be characterized by the normal clinical picture resulting from respiratory mucosal inflammation, but the role of toxic factors in longer-term and more serious developments, such as rheumatism and damage to heart tissue, is far more difficult to assess.

With the sophisticated laboratory tools available to modern researchers, it is possible to isolate, purify, and characterize a toxin and define, in relatively precise terms, its molecular mode of action but then be faced with the problem of defining the role or relevance of this information to a clinical presentation. Examples of this situation are the pertussis toxins, toxins of *V. parahaemolyticus*, and enterotoxins from organisms such as *B. cereus* and *S. dysenteriae*. Sometimes a new role in pathogenesis can be suggested for a well-characterized toxin. An example of this is a newly described form of staphylococcal enterotoxin, enterotoxin F, which is suspected by some investigators of being involved in toxic shock syndrome, a role and a disease quite unassociated with the normal intestinal dysfunction induced by staphylococcal enterotoxins. This may be a disease caused by several factors, including a toxin produced under special environmental conditions in the vagina of menstruating women that normally would be produced only under quite different conditions, say, in certain foods. The capacity of several toxigenic organisms to appear in somewhat unlikely places in the body, such as joints, the brain, lungs, and abscesses, also increases the possibility of toxin involvement in pathologies quite different from those normally associated with the causative organism.

Gram negative organisms have endotoxin (lipopolysaccharide) as a major component of their cell walls. When these organisms gain access, through invasion and multiplication, to the susceptible host, a wide range of possible deleterious effects and host responses can result. The exact role of endotoxin in various disease syndromes is not always clear because of possible involvement of other toxins and virulence factors that can mimic or complicate some of the typical activities of the lipid A moiety of the LPS complex. The peptidoglycan of gram positive organisms' cell walls has also been suggested as a possible factor in development of endotoxin-like systemic effects, as well as having the potential to be a potent enhancer of strain virulence (Sparling, 1983).

Aside from specific nomenclature, it is very common that toxins are either named or classified according to their categorical role in pathogenesis. For example, bacterial toxins that exert some deleterious effect and host response exclusively in the small or large intestine are classed as enterotoxins. Members of this group of toxins, which has grown quite large in the past 15 years, elicit alterations in intestinal cell structure or function by a diversity of modes of action, target cell types, receptors, and impacts upon the intestine and host. Another group of toxins, the neurotoxins, act primarily upon the host's nervous system by one means or another. A few other general classes of toxins named for their primary activity are hemolytic, cytolytic, and cytotoxic toxins, as well as toxins that inhibit macromolecular synthesis by some direct mechanism. Once again, the exact mechanism by which one toxin effects, say, cell death, may be quite different from that of another in the same class. Table 1 lists some organisms known to produce toxins in the categories given above. This list is not all-inclusive, and without a doubt the number of toxins and diversity of classes to which they might belong will be ever changing and increasing as research continues in these areas. Alouf (1982) has presented another useful summary of toxins and their structural and functional categories.

It is certain that bacterial toxins play a major role in the pathogenesis of nearly every disease attributable to bacteria. When one includes endotoxin, peptidoglycan, and exoenzymes, which facilitate bacterial penetration of the host defences, in the definition of *toxin*, then it can be said that all bacterial disease develops either directly or indirectly through these substances. As can be seen from the diverse chapters in this volume, our understanding and management of bacterial diseases still not under control will depend directly upon the future isolation and identification of bacterial toxins, as well as on elaboration of the structure, function, genetic origin, role in pathogenesis, and immunity to

TABLE 1. *Bacteria That Produce Characterized Toxins Belonging to General Toxin Classes Based Upon Their Role in Pathogenesis*

ENTEROTOXIN	NEUROTOXIN
V. cholerae	*C. botulinum*
E. coli	*C. tetani*
B. cereus	*S. dysenteriae*
C. perfringens	
Salmonella sp.	CYTOTOXIC, CYTOLYTIC
S. aureus	*Streptococcus* sp.
Shigella sp.	*Staphylococcus* sp.
NAG vibrios	*S. dysenteriae*
A. hydrophila	*A. hydrophila*
	V. parahaemolyticus
HEMOLYTIC	*C. difficile*
Streptococcus sp.	*Legionella* sp.
Staphylococcus sp.	
C. perfringens	DIRECT INHIBITORS, OF
V. parahaemolyticus	MACROMOLECULAR SYNTHESIS
B. cereus	*C. diphtheriae*
A. hydrophila	*B. thuringiensis*
	Y. pestis
	Pseudomonas sp.
ENDOTOXIN	*V. cholerae*
all gram negative bacteria	*E. coli*
EXOENZYMES	
invasive pathogens	

the diseases caused by these agents. Aside from many known or suspected toxins for which this work has yet to be done, new toxins will be discovered, and these will require the same efforts. Nonetheless, the advances made to date are very encouraging compared to the state of the art only 50 years ago.

REFERENCES

ALOUF, J. E. (1982) Bacterial toxins: An outlook. *Toxicon* **20**: 211–16.
BERNHEIMER, A. W. (1976) *Mechanisms in bacterial toxinology*. New York: Wiley.
SPARLING, P. F. (1983) Bacterial virulence and pathogenesis: An overview. *Rev. Infect. Dis.* **5**: S637–46.

CHAPTER 2

GENERAL CHARACTERISTICS: NOMENCLATURE OF MICROBIAL TOXINS

GRACE M. THORNE and SHERWOOD L. GORBACH

Infectious Diseases Service, Department of Medicine,
Tufts-New England Medical Center, Boston, MA 02111, U.S.A.

1. INTRODUCTION

Bacterial toxins were recognized nearly one hundred years ago as the potent substances responsible for such infectious diseases as diphtheria (Loeffler, 1884), tetanus (von Behring and Kitasato, 1890), and botulism (van Ermengen, 1897). The appellation was created in the early studies by coupling the term 'toxin' with the disease name, for example diphtheria-toxin.

The 'term' toxin was first used in the description of the poisonous substance that Roux and Yersin (1888) precipitated from a broth culture of diphtheria bacilli. These workers concluded correctly that this substance was a 'kind of enzyme'. The molecular confirmation of the belief required another eighty years before Honjo *et al.* (1969, 1971) and Gill *et al.* (1969) showed that NAD and EF2 were substrates in a reaction catalyzed by diphtheria toxin.

Since the discovery of these first three toxins, many more have been identified, some have been purified, and for a few, the mode of action has been elucidated. Unfortunately, the role of the vast majority of bacterial toxins in the pathophysiology of a specific disease remains obscure (Tables 1–4). In fact, the list of toxins unequivocally accepted as the agents responsible for the harmful effects of the infecting microorganism is very short, i.e., diphtheria, tetanus, botulinum and cholera toxins; the staphylococcal exfoliating toxin and enterotoxin; and the erythrogenic toxin of *Streptococcus pyogenes*.

The toxins mentioned above are all considered exotoxins. In 1935, Boivin and Mesrobeanu extracted new toxic substances from gram-negative bacteria, the so-called endotoxins. The prefixes exo- and endo- were used originally to describe the differences in apparent cellular location of the toxins, as well as to indicate the gram reaction of the producing bacterial strain. Experimental evidence now indicates that such terminology is inadequate and misleading. Bonventre (1970) has rightly suggested that an effort should be made to discontinue their usage in scientific publications and textbooks.

Since the microbial products historically classified as toxins have been identified as proteins, the term toxin should be restricted to proteins which possess toxic properties in animal models or tissue cultures (Bonventre, 1970; van Heyningen, 1970). Bacterial toxins are usually excreted by actively growing organisms; in some cases the toxin is a product of bacterial cell lysis. In general, protein toxins from different bacterial species have unique and rather specific biological properties and appear to possess distinct mechanisms of action.

The outer membrane of gram-negative bacteria consists of heteropolysaccharide co-valently linked to a lipid region. Traditionally, these substances have been termed 'endotoxin'. In contrast to protein toxins these cell components elicit a variety of biological effects in the host, some of which are toxic: pyrogenicity, abortion, bone marrow necrosis, leucopenia, leucocytosis, hypotension, Shwartzman phenomenon, and death of the animal. Endotoxins can also produce in the host biological effects of metabolic and immunologic consequence. Thus 'endotoxin' is characterized by numerous and diverse biological activities, only a few of which are toxic. These actions have been reviewed by Kabir *et al.*

5

TABLE 1. *Important Bacterial Toxins*

Toxin	Molecular size	Molecular structure	Biological properties	Toxicity LD$_{50}$/test animal	Mode of action	Genetic control
B. anthracis						plasmid
Factor I (edema factor)			Factors I + II edema			
Factor II (protective antigen)	100,000		Factors II + III lethal		adenylate cyclase	?
Factor III (lethal factor)						plasmid
B. thuringiensis	68,000		toxic to lepidopteran insects			plasmid
Bordetella pertussis Islet activating protein					ADP ribosylation	
Diphtheria	62,000	A 21,500 B 38,000	cytotoxic	40 ng/guinea pig	ADP ribosylation of EF 2	bacteriophage
Pasteurella pestis						
A	240,000	polymeric-24,000 m.wt. subunits	lethal	0.5, -0.3 µg/mouse		
B	120,000					
Pseudomonas aeruginosa exotoxin A	66,000	fragments 26,000	lethal necrotic cytotoxic	120 ng/mouse	ADP ribosylation of EF 2	chromosome
Streptococcus pyogenes erythrogenic toxins A, B, C	30,500		pyrogenic scarlet fever rash	3500 µg/kg cynomolgus monkey		bacteriophage
streptolysin O			hemolytic (O labile)			
streptolysin S	12,000–20,000		hemolytic (O stable)			

TABLE 2. *Bacterial Enterotoxins*

Enterotoxins	Molecular size	Molecular structure	Biological properties	Toxicity LD$_{50}$/test animal	Mode of action	Genetic control
B. cereus diarrhoegenic			diarrhoea		stimulates adenylcyclase	unstable
emetic			vomiting			
Cholera toxin	82,000	A$_1$ 21,000 A$_2$ 7,000 B 11,500	enterotoxic cytotonic vascular permeability-skin	5 μg/mouse	ADP ribosylation, stimulation of adenylcyclase	chromosome
E. coli LT toxin	82,000	A$_1$ 21,000 A$_2$ 7,000 B 11,500	enterotoxic cytotonic vascular permeability-skin		ADP ribosylation, stimulation of adenylcyclase	plasmid
ST I toxin	4,400–5,100 (porcine) 1,972 (human) 7,000 (cloned porcine) 1,979 (porcine)		enterotoxic		stimulates guanylate cyclase	plasmid
ST II toxin	5,090		enterotoxic			plasmid
Shiga-like cytotoxin	48,000	A 31,000 B 4,000	lethal cytotoxic enterotoxic			phage plasmid?
Shigella Shiga toxin	68,000	A$_1$ 27,500 A$_2$ 3,000 B 4,000	lethal cytotoxic enterotoxic	1 μg/mouse	inhibits protein, DNA synthesis by inactivation of 60S ribosomal subunit	
Staph. aureus A, B, C$_1$, C$_2$, D, E	28,000–35,000		vomiting			

TABLE 3. *Nonenteric Toxins of Staphylococcus aureus*

Toxin	Molecular size	Molecular structure	Biological properties	Toxicity LD_{50}/test animal	Mode of action	Genetic control
Alpha	28,000	polymeric	hemolytic cytotoxic cytolytic neurotoxic demonecrotic contraction of mammalian smooth muscle	1 μg/mouse	inhibits cAMP dependent protein kinase	chromosome plasmid (?)
Beta	30,000		cytotoxic hemolytic (hot-cold)		sphingomyelinase C	
Delta	2,977	single chain	cytolytic hemolytic		transmembrane "pore"	
Exfoliative A toxin B toxin	23,500–33,000 23,500–33,000		Nikolsky sign (humans, infant mice, infants)	0.5 μg/newborn mouse		chromosome plasmid
Gamma		Component I 29,000 Component II 26,000 (synergistic)	hemolytic cytotoxic	50 μg/guinea pig		
Leucocidin (Panton–Valentine)		F (fast) 32,000 S (slow) 38,000 (synergistic)	leukocytic		production of ion channel in cell membrane	

TABLE 4. *Clostridial Toxins*

Toxins	Molecular size	Molecular structure	Biological properties	Toxicity	Mode of action	Genetic control
Cl. botulinum A, B, C$_1$, C$_2$, D, E, F, G	120,000–155,000	H ~ 100,000 L ~ 50,000	neurotoxic paralytic	1.2×10^6 guinea pig LD$_{50}$/1 mg	acts presynaptically to block release of acetylcholine from nerve terminals	bacteriophage type C, D
Cl. difficile toxin A	240,000		lethal, cytotoxic enterotoxic in rabbit loops	0.26 µg LD$_{50}$/mouse		
toxin B			lethal, cytotoxic	4.4 µg LD$_{50}$/mouse		
Cl. novyi α-toxin	70,000–340,000		necrotizing, lethal	50,000 mouse LD$_{50}$/mg	lecithinase	
β-toxin			necrotizing, hemolytic		lecithinase	
γ-toxin			necrotizing, hemolytic		lipase	
δ-toxin			hemolytic			
ε-toxin			hemolytic			
ζ-toxin			hemolytic			
Cl. perfringens alpha α-toxin	53,000	zinc metalloenzyme	necrotizing, hemolytic	200 mouse LD$_{50}$/1 mg	lecithinase phospholipase C	
β-toxin						
γ-toxin						
δ-toxin						
ε-toxin						
η-toxin			necrotizing			
θ-toxin			hemolysin			
τ-toxin						
κ-toxin	80,000				collagenase	
λ-toxin					proteinase	
ν-toxin					DNase	
enterotoxin type C, A, D enterotoxin type D	35,000		diarrhoea vomiting			sporulation-spore coat protein
Cl. septicum α-toxin			hemolytic, lethal, necrotizing			
Cl. tetani tetanospasmin	140,000	H 87,000 L 48,000	neurotoxic	2×10^8 mouse MLD/mgN		plasmid
Cl. welchii α-toxin			cell necrosis hemolysis toxemia		phospholipase	

(1978). The lipid A moiety has been well established as responsible for the toxicity of these bacterial components.

A more descriptive term should be sought to replace 'endotoxin' which would point up the differences in biological and pharmacological action between pure protein toxins and these cell membrane components. Bonventre (1970) has suggested 'endobacterial poison'.

2. PURIFICATION

The complex problems of producing and purifying protein toxins have been reviewed many times in the past. The history of much of the early work has been covered by Pappenheimer (1948), Pillemer and Robbins (1949), van Heyningen (1954), Oakley (1954). More recently Alouf and Raynaud (1970) reviewed high resolution methods developed in the 1960's, namely, gel permeation, ion exchange chromatography, and electrophoretic methods. Wadström (1978) reviewed more modern toxin purification techniques of the 1970's, such as affinity chromatography and immunosorbent methods, isoelectric focusing, and isotachophoresis.

The purification of certain proteins from crude mixtures has become possible only recently with the development of novel methods of separation by immunoadherence, charge differences, etc. The 'purity' of toxin preparations can now be evaluated by SDS polyacrylamide electrophoresis and isoelectric focusing in polyacrylamide gel. Two dimensional immunoelectrophoresis methods, i.e., crossed immunoelectrophoresis, crossed immunoelectrofocusing, crossed disc immunoelectrophoresis, can be used to study the micro-heterogeneity of purified proteins.

These new techniques have created a need for a term such as 'isotoxin'. The extracellular toxins of *Staphylococcus aureus* are prime examples. Isoelectric focusing studies have revealed multiple forms of the α, γ, δ, hemolytic toxins (Bernheimer and Schwartz, 1963; Taylor and Bernheimer, 1974; Kreger *et al.*, 1971). The staphylococcal enterotoxins A, B, C_1, C_2 have 3–8 forms each (Bergdoll, 1972); while 2 or more epidermolytic toxins are recognized (Wiley and Rogolsky, 1977; Johnson *et al.*, 1979).

The existence of multiple molecular forms, as shown by isoelectric focusing, indicates the need for further investigations into the physical, chemical, and biological properties of these alternative forms of individual toxins. Such findings also indicate that careful scrutiny is required for possible post-synthetic modifications of toxins in culture fluids or during purification procedures yielding multiple molecular forms. Reports of such toxin modifications include deamination of staphylococcal enterotoxin B (Metzger *et al.*, 1975), and protease modification of both botulinum toxin (Duncan, 1975), and *E. coli* heat labile enterotoxin (Dorner, 1975).

Thus the problems of purity assessment remain and can only be defined in a negative manner, i.e., when no impurities can be detected by the best currently available methods. Ideally, a 'pure' protein would be shown to consist of a single molecular species with a unique amino acid sequence.

To date, several toxins have been completely or almost completely sequenced either by chemical analysis of the protein itself or from the nucleotide sequence of the coding gene(s): diphtheria toxin (Kaczorek *et al*, 1983; Ratti *et al*, 1983), staphylococcal enterotoxin B (Huang and Bergdoll, 1970a, b, c), staphylococcal delta toxin (Fitton *et al*, 1980), cholera and *E. coli* heat labile enterotoxins (Spicer *et al*, 1981) and the *E. coli* heat-stable enterotoxins STIa, b and STII (So and McCarthy, 1980; Moseley *et al*, 1983a; Moseley *et al*, 1983b; Lazure *et al*, 1983; Lee *et al*, 1983).

3. MEASUREMENT OF TOXICITY

The level of lethality of a toxin usually is indicated by the LD_{50} dose, which is the median dose that kills 50 per cent of the animals inoculated within a stated period of time. The LD_{50} is most readily computed by the method of Reed and Muench (1938).

While it is possible to measure the level of toxicity of those bacterial toxins that have been purified, it is not possible to make meaningful comparison of different toxins since there are differences in animals, such as species, breed, sex, age and weight, as well as inoculation route. In addition, the toxin preparation may have different modes of action on different tissues. The lethal amounts of various bacterial toxins as well as some plant and animal proteins have been tabulated by Gill (1982).

Bacterial toxins may be assayed by measuring one or more of the following properties: (1) biological potency; (2) enzymatic activity; and (3) antibody reactivity.

3.1. BIOLOGICAL POTENCY

Measurement of biological potency generally entails the determination of an LD_{50} in a susceptible animal species. However, one can also determine the least dose which produces a cytotoxic effect in a tissue culture system, hemolyzes a certain proportion of red cells, produces a certain size area of erythema or necrosis in animal skin, etc. Such assays have the advantage of measuring the amount of toxin that is biologically active. Often bacterial toxins can be detected and quantitated by using a number of *in vivo* and *in vitro* assay methods which may vary in sensitivity. For example, *E. coli* heat-labile enterotoxin (LT) causes fluid accumulation in the rabbit ligated ileal loop and also causes mouse Yl adrenal cells and Chinese hamster ovary tissue culture lines to undergo a morphological change and increased secretion of their respective hormones. The tissue culture techniques are approximately 100 times more sensitive than the rabbit loop reaction for detecting *E. coli* LT. However, morphological changes in tissue culture cells should only be interpreted as a *possible* indication of an LT-like enterotoxin; such findings should be confirmed in all instances by demonstration of a specific biochemical alteration (adenylate cyclase stimulation or increased steroidogenesis) or by correlation with an assay system involving the target organ (i.e. intestinal cells). Similarly, caution should be taken in the interpretation of positive results with other bacterial toxins. When possible confirmation should be made by employing a target organ assay system.

3.2. ENZYME ACTIVITY

With well-characterized and purified toxins of known enzyme action, determinations of toxin activity by measuring enzyme activity would be a reliable method. However, studies with crude or only partially purified culture filtrates could be misleading because enzymatic activities and toxicity can be easily attributed to one substance when in reality more bacterial components are present. Bacteria produce a wide variety of extracellular proteins (approximately 23 by *Staphylococcus aureus*, Wadström, 1978), and enzyme activity *per se*, does not constitute toxicity. Degradative enzymes are produced by pathogenic bacteria, yet few of these substances have been shown to be directly responsible for pathogenic properties; therefore, these enzymes should be categorized as potential auxiliary virulence factors, rather than as toxins.

3.3. ANTIGENIC REACTIVITY

Since toxins usually are large molecular weight proteins, they are highly antigenic. Immunological methods can be utilized to detect and quantitate small amounts of toxins, as well as recognize different classes of bacterial toxins. Two techniques currently in use are radioimmunoassay (RIA) and the enzyme linked immunosorbent assay (ELISA). The only disadvantage to immunologic methods is that although they are highly specific, they do not necessarily measure biologically active toxin.

4. TOXIGENICITY

The ability of a particular organism to produce toxin is influenced by a variety of factors, including the strain of organism, culture medium, and physiologic conditions of culture.

Great variation in the capacity to produce toxin can be found among different toxigenic strains of the same organism, even when grown under similar conditions. On repeated subculture, toxigenic strains may lose their ability to produce toxin. For this reason it is important to freeze-dry fresh isolates of toxigenic strains.

Investigators have often reported that the intestinal passage of hypotoxinogenic mutants of *V. cholerae* in animals and humans could result in enrichment of phenotypic revertants capable of producing more toxin *in vitro*. Recently Mekalanos (1983) has shown duplication and amplification of toxin genes in El Tor variants of *V. cholerae* selected by intestinal passage in rabbits. These hypertoxinogenic variants have large tandem duplications of the cholera toxin genes. The selective pressures operative in the gut which mediate enrichment for derivatives with tandem repeats remain unclear.

In certain cases, i.e, diphtheria, streptococcal, erythrogenic, *E. coli* shiga-like cytotoxin, and botulinum toxins, toxigenicity is dependent on the presence of a lysogenic bacteriophage infection of the organism (Tables 1, 2 and 4). Toxin production in other organisms i.e., staphylococcal exfoliative toxin B and α-toxin, *E. coli* LT and ST enterotoxins, tetanus toxin, anthrax virulence components, and a lepidopteran toxin, is controlled by plasmids (Tables 1–4). Study of the association between toxin production and extrachromosomal DNA species has led to a better understanding of the causes of strain variation in toxin production as well as the molecular nature of toxins. Genetic manipulation of structural genes for toxins on plasmids allowed for amplification of toxin production. The enterotoxin LT gene has been cloned and the toxin synthesized by a mini-cell *in vitro* protein synthesizing system (Dallas and Falkow, 1979). DNA probes derived from the cloned LT genes, *elt*A and *elt*B, hybridize to the cholera toxin genes (Moseley and Falkow, 1980). Molecular characterization of the cholera toxin genes (*ctx*) (Pearson and Mekalanos, 1982) has confirmed that the two subunit genes *ctxA* and *ctxB* are organized into a single transcriptional unit. Although the LT gene is encoded by a wide variety of plasmids, the cholera toxin operon is on the *V. cholerae* chromosome. Southern blot analysis indicates that *V. cholerae* of the classical biotypes may have multiple copies of the toxin operon while strains of the El Tor biotype usually have a single copy (Moseley and Falkow, 1980; Kaper *et al*, 1981).

Although the heat-labile enterotoxins of *E. coli* are homogeneous with regard to their molecular weight and mode of action, the heat-stable enterotoxins exhibit considerable heterogeneity. The two main types STI (STa) and STII (STb) differ from each other in mode of action and response in animal enterotoxin assays. STI stimulates guanylate cyclase in intestinal cells, and produces water secretion in the intestine of infant mice and piglets. Two heterologous DNA sequences (STIa, STIb) have been shown to encode for products of similar if not identical biological activities (Moseley *et al*, 1983a and Moseley *et al*, 1983b).

The second type STII produces water secretion in piglets, but not in infant mice, and its mode of action is unclear. Like the STIa,b genes, the nucleotide sequence of the STII gene has been determined (Picken *et al*, 1983; Lee *et al*, 1983). The size and overall structure of STII are similar to those of STI, but the amino acid composition of the two ST enterotoxins are completely different. Lazure *et al*, 1983 has shown a common 6-residue sequence (Cys-Cys-Asn-Pro-Ala-Cys) which the STI toxins share in common with conotoxins isolated from the venom of marine snails *Conus geographus* and *Conus vagus*.

The use of appropriate culture medium for toxin production cannot be over-emphasized. As van Heyningen noted (1970), the culture medium that promotes good growth of a particular toxigenic organism may not necessarily facilitate optimal toxin production. Generally, factors such as pH, organic and inorganic constituents, and the gas phase must be monitored in order to develop the best culture conditions. A thorough description of the effects of these factors on production of various toxins is given by van Heyningen in his review (1970).

Although a 'rich' complex medium often gives high toxin yields, this generality was not fulfilled when a defined medium was used for production of *E. coli* ST enterotoxin by Alderete and Robertson (1977) and Staples *et al*. (1980). The Staples group used a minimal medium that resulted in enterotoxin elaboration 6–10 fold greater than that produced in complex medium. A further 10–20 fold increase was achieved with constant bubbling of oxygen into the culture medium.

Another ploy to increase toxin yield involves incubation of cells with a surface-active antibiotic. *E. coli* heat-labile (LT) enterotoxin was found to be released from cells following treatment with polymyxin B (Evans *et al.*, 1974).

Toxin production can also be potentiated or adversely affected by production of a proteolytic enzyme by the toxigenic organism. With a toxin-destroying protease, the toxin yield depends on the relative timing of synthesis of toxin and enzyme and the length of time the two are together in the culture medium. Examples of proteolytic enzyme enhancement of toxin activity are also known: *Clostridium botulinum* type A toxin (Boroff and DasGupta, 1971) and *E. coli* LT toxin (Rappaport *et al.*, 1976).

5. MOLECULAR STRUCTURE

Microbial toxins that have been characterized can be placed in two classes: simple and complex. A simple toxin is synthesized as a single, homogeneous protein molecule which exhibits full biological activity. It can exist as a monomer, dimer or larger aggregate of identical subunits, all of which possess equal toxicity. Staphylococcal α-toxin is an example of a simple toxin which also exists in a polymeric form.

A second type of simple toxin is one which is synthesized as an inactive or partially inactive precursor, termed a protoxin or 'prototoxin' by Bonventre (1970). The nontoxicity or decreased toxicity exhibited by prototoxins can be explained in a number of ways, all of which involve blockade of the active site of the molecule. For example, changes in specific activity may be due to polymerization, or altered tertiary structural conformation, requiring activation by depolymerization, or proteolytic treatment. An example of a simple toxin which undergoes proteolytic activation is botulinum toxin, type A. Some degree of activation probably occurs under natural conditions since *Cl. botulinum* produces pro- teolytic enzymes during its late growth phase which enhance toxic activity of the culture (Boroff and Das Gupta, 1971). Like the toxins of proteolytic botulinum cultures, tetanus toxin is synthesized as a single polypeptide chain and is nicked into a dichain molecule enzymatically once the toxin becomes extracellular (Table 4). A discussion of the similarities of these toxins has been published (Sugiyama, 1980).

A complex toxin requires two or more distinct components which must be bound to each other by covalent binding or hydrogen binding for toxicity to be expressed *in vivo*. Four complex toxins which have been extensively studied have been shown to consist of an 'active' subunit 'A' and a 'binding' subunit 'B'. These toxins first attach to eukaryotic cell receptors followed by cell entry of the active subunit leading to an intracellular metabolic change. The complex toxins detailed in Tables 1 and 2 include diphtheria toxin and *Pseudomonas aeruginosa* exotoxin A, both of which cause inhibition of protein synthesis by ADP ribosylation of elongation factor 2.

Cholera toxin and *E. coli* heat labile (LT) enterotoxin are remarkably similar complex toxins involving binding components (B subunits) which react with GM-1 ganglioside and active fragments 'A' which activate the adenylate cyclase of the intoxicated cell.

Recently, attention has focused on the possibility that soluble adenylate cyclases secreted by pathogenic bacteria could play a role in virulence. The bacterial cyclases differ from the eukaryotic enzymes in that they are more active, soluble, heat stable and are not regulated by guanine nucleotides (Van Heyningen, 1982).

Leppla (1982) showed that EF (edema factor) toxin of *Bacillus anthracis* is a highly active cyclase *in vitro* in the presence of a CHO cell lysate (Table 1). In whole cells EF required the presence of PA (protective antigen) for activity; the latter presumably functions in some way to aid entry of EF into the cells. EF is the first example of a bacterial adenylate cyclase that enters mammalian cells and is activated by a mammalian protein. Since none of the three proteins produced by *B. anthracis* has much biological effect by itself, combinations of PA with EF produce skin edema, and PA with LF are lethal. The relevance of the effects of this adenylate cyclase to the disease anthrax is still unclear.

Bordetella pertussis, responsible for whooping cough, also produces an adenylate cyclase that is like the *B. anthracis* cyclase in that it is heat-stable and activated by calmodulin (Greenlee *et al*, 1982). Along with many other antigens, *B. pertussis* also secretes the islet-activating protein "pertussis toxin" which is not a cyclase but like cholera toxin works by activating the cyclase of the intoxicated cell. Like cholera and diphtheria toxins, it also catalyses the transfer of ADP-ribose from NAD + to a receptor protein (Katada and Ui, 1982). Thus *B. pertussis* secretes both a cyclase and a protein which can activate a mammalian cyclase. The recognition of bacterial proteins which have such similar properties to mammalian cyclases (and which can be activated by the mammalian protein calmodulin) and other proteins which can stimulate mammalian cyclases should stimulate studies into the function of increases in cyclic AMP used by invading bacteria in the establishment of a disease state.

6. NOMENCLATURE

At present, one of the main problems in toxin nomenclature is the lack of a uniform set of guidelines for use of symbolic notations to identify toxins, isotoxins, and their component parts. As a result, investigators continue to use arbitrarily capital and Greek letters, Arabic and Roman numerals, and various other symbols in their reports. Whatever notation system is finally employed, a few specific rules should be followed. These were previously outlined by Bonventre (1970) in his review, but bear repeating. A toxin nomenclature symbol should be used:

(1) only when two or more independently acting toxins are produced by the same organism.

(2) only for toxic bacterial substances, i.e., proteins which injure animals or cell culture preparations. Other substances not directly toxic should be termed 'virulence factors'.

(3) when coupled with the specific generic and species name of the organism for example, *C. perfringens*, *C. septicum*, and *C. novyi* all produce different α-toxins.

(4) until such time as the biochemical properties of the toxin are revealed. Then the name of the toxin should be changed to reflect the mode of action, thus, *S. aureus*-β toxin should be described as *S. aureus* sphingomyelinase C.

Greek letters have been used for identification of products associated with *Staphylococcus aureus* and clostridia of the gas gangrene group (Tables 3 and 4). Unfortunately, Greek letters also have been assigned to some bacterial products which should not be classified legitimately as toxins.

The capital letter system of nomenclature has been employed to signify staphylococcal enterotoxins (Table 1). These toxins are immunologically distinct proteins of similar molecular size (27,800–34,100) and presumably have the same active site and mechanism of action *in vivo*. The neurotoxins of *C. botulinum* also are identified by capital letters, and they are immunologically distinct toxins (Table 4).

The toxin nomenclature system can only become more confusing if both Greek and capital letters are employed by toxicologists to indicate subunit components of toxins. A universal symbolic notation must be sought in order to describe clearly multi-component toxins. Bonventre (1970) has proposed the term MT as the symbol for a multi-component toxin. Each individual component could then be designated as MT 1, MT 2, etc. This system has not been accepted in the toxin literature. For the four multi-component toxins best described to date, capital letters have been used to signify the 'Active' component(s) (A) and the 'binding' component(s) (B). A subscript number is added to indicate the production of more than one Active or Binding component (Tables 1 and 2).

If this nomenclature is adopted universally, it would establish a uniform and consistent system. Whatever the symbol chosen to indicate a toxin initially, a descriptive toxin terminology should be established as soon as possible. Eventually, the name of the toxin should reflect its mode of action.

REFERENCES

ALDERETE, J. F. and ROBERTSON, D. C. (1977) Nutrition and enterotoxin synthesis by enterotoxigenic strains of *Escherichia coli*: defined medium for production of heat-stable enterotoxin. *Infect. Immun.* **15**: 781–788.

ALOUF, J. E. and RAYNAUD, M. (1970) Isolation and purification of bacterial toxic proteins. In *Microbial Toxins*, Vol. 1, pp. 119–182, AJL, S. J., KADIS, S. and MONTIE C. (Eds). Academic Press, New York.

BERGDOLL, M. S. (1972) The enterotoxins. In *The Staphylococci*, pp. 301–331, COHEN J. O. (Ed.). John Wiley, New York.

BERNHEIMER, A. W. and SCHWARTZ, L. L. (1963) Isolation and composition of staphylococcal alpha toxin. *J. Gen. Microbiol.* **30**: 445–468.

BOIVIN, I. and MESROBEANU, L. (1935) Recherches sur les antigènes somatiques et sur les endotoxines des bactéries. *Revue d'Immunologie* **1**: 553–569.

BONVENTRE, P. F. (1970) The nomenclature of microbial toxins: problems and recommendations. In *Microbial Toxins*, Vol. 1, pp. 29–66, AJL, S. J., KADIS, S. and MONTIE, T. C. (Eds). Academic Press, New York.

BOROFF, D. A. and DASGUPTA, B. R. (1971) Botulinum toxin. In *Microbial Toxins*, Vol. IIA, pp. 1–68, KADIS, S., MONTIE, T. C. and AJL, S. J. (Eds). Academic Press. New York.

DALLAS, W. S. and FALKOW, S. (1979) The molecular nature of heat-labile enterotoxin (LT) of *Escherichia coli*. *Nature* **277**: 406–407.

DORNER, F. (1975) *Escherichia coli* enterotoxin: purification and partial characterization. In *Microbiology—1975*, pp. 242–251, SCHLESSINGER, D. (Ed.). American Society for Microbiology, Washington, D. C.

DUNCAN, D. L. (1975) Role of clostridial toxins in pathogenesis. In *Microbiology—1975*, pp. 283–291, SCHLESSINGER, D. (Ed.). American Society of Microbiology, Washington, D. C.

EVANS, D. J. JR., EVANS, D. G. and GORBACH, S. L. (1974) Polymyxin-B-induced release of low-molecular weight, heat labile enterotoxin from *Escherichia coli*. *Infect. Immun.* **10**: 1010–1017.

FITTON, J. E., DELL, A. and SHAW, W. V. (1980) The amino acid sequence of the delta haemolysin of *Staphylococcus aureus*. *FEBS Lett* **115**: 209–212.

GILL, D. M. (1982) Bacterial toxins: a table of lethal amounts. *Microbiol. Rev.* **46**: 86–94.

GILL, D. M., PAPPENHEIMER, A. M. JR., BROWN, R. and KURNICK, J. T. (1969) Studies on the mode of action of diphtheria toxin VII. Toxin-stimulated hydrolysis of nicotinamide adenine dinucleotide in mammalian cell extracts. *J. Exp. Med.* **129**: 1–21.

GREENLEE, D. V., ANDREASEN, T. J. and STORM, D. R. (1982) Calcium-independent stimulation of *Bordetella pertussis* adenylate cyclase. *Biochem.* **21**: 2759–2764.

HONJO, T., NISHIZUKA, Y. and HAYAISHI, O. (1969) Adenosine diphosphoribosylation of aminoacyl transferase II by diphtheria toxin. *Cold Spring Harbor Symp. Quant. Biol.* **34**: 603–610.

HONJO, T., NISHIZUKA, Y., KATO, I. and HAYAISHI, O. (1971) Adenosine diphosphate ribosylation of aminoacyl transferase II and inhibition of protein synthesis by diphtheria toxin. *J. Biol. Chem.* **246**: 4251–4260.

HUANG, I. -Y. and BERGDOLL, M. S. (1970a) The primary structure of staphylococcal enterotoxin B. *J. Biol. Chem.* **245**: 3493–3510.

HUANG, I. -Y. and BERGDOLL, M. S. (1970b) The primary structure of staphylococcal enterotoxin B. II Isolation, composition, and sequence of chymotryptic peptides. *J. Biol. Chem.* **245**: 3511–3517.

HUANG, I. -Y. and BERGDOLL, M. S. (1970c) The primary structure of staphylococcal enterotoxin B. III The cyanogen bromide peptides of reduced aminoethylated enterotoxin B, and the complete amino acid sequence. *J. Biol. Chem.* **245**: 3518–3525.

JOHNSON, A. D., SPERO, L., CADES, J. S. and DE CICCO, B. T. (1979) Purification and characterization of different types of exfoliative toxin from *Staphylococcus aureus*. *Infect. Immun.* **24**: 679–684.

KABIR, S., ROSENSTREICH, D. L. and MERGENHAGEN, S. E. (1978) Bacterial endotoxins and cell membranes. In *Bacterial Toxins and Cell Membranes*, pp. 59–87, JELJASZEWICZ, J. and WADSTRÖM, T. (Eds). Academic Press Inc., London.

KACZOREK, M., DELPEYROUX, F., CHENCINER, N., STREECK, R. E., MURPHY, J. R., BOQUET, P. and TIOLLAIS, P. (1983) Nucleotide sequence and expression of the diphtheria tox 228 gene in *Escherichia coli*. *Science* **221**: 855–858.

KAPER, J. B., MOSELEY, S. L. and FALKOW, S. (1981) Molecular characterization of environmental and nontoxinogenic strains of *Vibrio cholerae*. *Infect. Immun.* **32**: 661–667.

KATADA, T. and UI, M. (1982) Direct modification of the membrane-adenylate cyclase system by islet-activating protein due to ADP-ribosylation of a membrane protein. *Proc. Natl. Acad. Sci. U.S.A.* **79**: 3129–3133.

KREGER, A. S., KIM, K. -S., ZABORETZKY, F. and BERNHEIMER, A. W. (1971) Purification and properties of staphylococcal delta hemolysin. *Infect. Immun.* **3**: 449–465.

LAZURE, C., SEIDAH, N. G., CHRETIEN, M., LALLIER, R. and ST. PIERRE, S. (1983) Primary structure determination of *Escherichia coli* heat-stable enterotoxin of porcine origin. *Can. J. Biochem. Cell. Biol.* **61**: 287–292.

LEE, C. H., MOSELEY, S. L., MOON, H. W., WHIPP, S. C., GYLES, C. L. and SO, M. (1983) Characterization of the gene encoding heat-stable toxin II and preliminary molecular epidemiological studies of enterotoxigenic *Escherichia coli* heat-stable toxin II producers. *Infect. Immun.* **42**: 264–268.

LEPPLA, S. H. (1982) Anthrax toxin edema factor: a bacterial adenylate cyclase that increases cyclic AMP concentrations in eukaryotic cells. *Proc. Natl. Acad. Sci. U.S.A.* **79**: 3162–3166.

LOEFFLER, F. (1884) Untersuchungen über die Bedeutung der Mikroorganismen für die Entstehung der Diphtherie beim Menschen, bei der Taube und beim Kalbe. *Mitt. Reichsgesundheitsant* **2**: 421–499.

MEKALANOS, J. J. (1983) Duplication and amplification of toxin genes in *Vibrio cholerae*. *Cell* **35**: 253–263.

METZGER, J. F., JOHNSON, A. D. and SPERO, L. (1975). Intrinsic and chemically produced microheterogeneity of *Staphylococcus aureus* enterotoxin type C. *Infect. Immun.* **12**: 93–97.

MOSELEY, S. L. and FALKOW, S. (1980) Nucleotide sequence homology between the heat-labile enterotoxin gene of *Escherichia coli* and *Vibrio cholerae* DNA. *J. Bacteriol.* **144**: 444–446.

MOSELEY, S. L., HARDY, J. W., HUQ, M. I., ECHEVERRIA, P. and FALKOW, S. (1983a) Isolation and nucleotide sequence determination of a gene encoding a heat-stable enterotoxin of *Escherichia coli*. *Infect. Immun.* **39**: 1167–1174.

MOSELEY, S. L., SAMADPOUR-MOTALEBI, M. and FALKOW, S. (1983b) Plasmid association and nucleotide sequence relationships of two genes encoding heat-stable enterotoxin production in *Escherichia coli* H-10407. *J. Bacteriol.* **156**: 441–443.

OAKLEY, C. L. (1954) Bacterial toxins. Demonstration of antigenic components in bacterial filtrates. *A. Rev. Microbiol.* **8**: 411–428.

PAPPENHEIMER, A. M. JR. (1948) Proteins of pathogenic bacteria. *Adv. Protein Chem.* **4**: 123–151.

PEARSON, G. D. N. and MEKALANOS, J. J. (1982) Molecular cloning of *Vibrio cholerae* enterotoxin genes in *Escherichia coli* K12. *Proc. Natl. Acad. Sci. U.S.A.* **79**: 2976–2980.

PICKEN, R. N., MAZAITIS, A. J., MAAS, W. K., REY, M. and HEYNEKER, H. (1983) Nucleotide sequences of the gene for heat-stable enterotoxin II of *Escherichia coli. Infect. Immun.* **42**: 269–275.

PILLEMER, L. and ROBBINS, K. C. (1949) Chemistry of toxins. *A. Rev. Microbiol.* **3**: 265–288.

RAPPAPORT, R. S., SAGIN, J. F., PIERZCHALA, W. A., BONDE, G., RUBIN, B. A. and TINT, H. (1976) Reactivation of heat-labile *Escherichia coli* enterotoxin by trypsin. *J. Infect. Dis.* **133**: S41–S54.

RATTI, G., RAPPUOLI, R. and GIANNINI, G. (1983) The complete nucleotide sequence of the gene coding for diphtheria toxin in the corynephage omega (tox[+]) genome. *Nucleic Acids Research* **11**: 6589–6595.

REED, L. J. and MUENCH, H. (1938) A simple method of estimating fifty per cent endpoints. *Am. J. Hyg.* **27**: 493–497.

ROUX, E. and YERSIN, A. (1888) Contribution à l'étude de la diphtérie. *Ann. Inst. Pasteur* (Paris) **2**: 629–661.

SO, M. and McCARTHY, B. J. (1980) Nucleotide sequence of the bacterial transposon Tn1681 encoding a heat-stable (ST) toxin and its identification in enterotoxigenic *Escherichia coli* strains. *Proc. Natl. Acad. Sci. U.S.A.* **77**: 4011–4015.

SPICER, E. K., KAVANAUGH, W. M., DALLAS, W. S., FALKOW, S., KONIGSBERG, W. H. and SCHAFER, D. E. (1981) Sequence homologies between A subunits of *Escherichia coli* and *Vibrio cholerae* enterotoxins. *Proc. Natl. Acad. Sci. U.S.A.* **78**: 50–54.

STAPLES, S. J., ASHER, S. E. and GIANNELLA, R. A. (1980) Purification and characterization of heat-stable enterotoxin produced by a strain of *E. coli* pathogenic for man. *Biol. Chem.* **255**: 4716–4721.

SUGIYAMA, H. (1980) *Clostridium botulinum* neurotoxin. *Microbiol. Rev.* **44**: 419–448.

TAYLOR, A. G. and BERNHEIMER, A. W. (1974) Further characterization of staphylococcal gamma-hemolysin. *Infect. Immun.* **10**: 54–59.

VAN ERMENGEN, E. (1897) De l'étiologie du botulisme. *Compt. Rend. Soc. Biol.* **49**: 155.

VAN HEYNINGEN, W. E. (1954) Toxic proteins. In *The Proteins*, Vol. II, pp. 345–387, NEURATH, H. and BAILEY K. (Eds). Academic Press. New York.

VAN HEYNINGEN, W. E. (1970) General characteristics. In *Microbiol. Toxins*, Vol. 1, pp. 1–28, AJL, S. J., KADIS, S. and MONTIE, T. C. (Eds). Academic Press, New York.

VAN HEYNINGEN, S. (1982) Bacterial toxins and cyclic AMP. *Nature* **299**: 782.

VON BEHRING, E. and KITASATO, S. (1890) Ueber das Zustandekommen der Diphtherie-Immunität und der Tetanus-Immunität bei Thieren. *Deut. Med. Wochschr.* **16**: 1113–1114

WADSTRÖM, T. (1978) Advances in the purification of some bacterial protein toxins. In *Bacterial Toxins and Cell Membranes*, pp. 9–57, JELJASZEWICZ, J. and WADSTRÖM, T. (Eds). Academic Press, New York.

WILEY, B. V. and ROGOLSKY, M. (1977) Molecular and serological differentiation of staphylococcal exfoliative toxin synthesized under chromosomal and plasmid control. *Infect. Immun.* **18**: 487–494.

CHAPTER 3

GENETIC ASPECTS OF TOXIGENESIS IN BACTERIA

WERNER K. MAAS

New York University School of Medicine, New York, NY 10016

ABSTRACT

The application of recently developed methods of *molecular genetics* has made important contributions to our understanding of toxinogenesis. Examples of toxins studied by such genetic methods are reviewed. The following genetic aspects of toxin production are considered: 1. *Structure* of genes controlling toxins, including nucleotide sequences of these genes. 2. *Expression* of these genes, including transcription, translation and post-translational processing. 3. *Location* (chromosomal, plasmid, phage) and *movement* of the genes. Detailed genetic information is available for only a few toxins and for most toxins genetic investigations are projects for the future. Genetic studies are important not only for the understanding of the basic biology of toxin production, but also for practical applications, such as the *development of vaccines* and *gene probes* for diagnostic purposes.

1. INTRODUCTION

Bacterial toxins are substances that cause damage to host cells and that are often implicated in pathogenesis. Most of them are proteins and some of them have a demonstrable enzymatic activity. Toxin production belongs to the general category of genetic traits that are concerned with interactions of the bacteria with their host. Causing damage may at first glance appear to be harmful to the bacteria, since it weakens or kills the host, but presumably the harmful effects are offset by other advantages, for example, in the case of enteric pathogens, dispersal to other susceptible hosts. In general, the usefulness of toxin production to the bacteria is attested by the fact that many bacterial species produce one or more toxins. In the course of history, some toxigenic species have become less prominent and others have become more prevalent. These changes reflect the emergence of new bacterial populations in response to changes in the environment. Examples are the present lower frequency of *Vibrio cholerae* infections and the rise in toxic shock syndrome-producing staphylococci. From past history, it seems that toxigenic pathogens are a constant feature of our environment. The study of the genetics of toxin production is therefore an area of inquiry that is instrumental for our understanding of infectious disease.

Genetic studies dealing with toxin production can be considered under 3 headings: 1. *Structure* of the genes controlling toxin production. 2. *Gene expression* and its control. This involves the transfer of information from DNA to other macromolecules, such as messenger RNA and proteins. 3. *Location* and *movement* of genes within cells and between cells. Gene expression gives information about the mechanism of toxin biosynthesis; one often uses mutants affecting toxin production to study gene expression and its regulation. The study of location and movement of genes is important chiefly for epidemiology and the evolution and spreading of toxin-producing strains.

Studies on the genetics of bacterial toxins are for the most part of recent origin. During most of its 40-year history, bacterial genetics has dealt largely with basic cellular processes, first, the elucidation of metabolic pathways and their controls and later the analysis of gene replication and recombination and the formation and function of macromolecular structures, such as ribosomes and membranes. The study of extrachromosomal elements, plasmids and phages, has been a significant part in these developments. As our knowledge of the genetic machinery of the cell expanded, it became easier to manipulate genes and to isolate mutants and this culminated in the sophisticated cloning and sequencing procedures used in the present-day recombinant DNA technology. Genetic methods are now used in the study of almost all cellular activities.

One reason for the late arrival of genetic studies of toxins is the difficulty of isolating mutants in the absence of direct selection procedures. With the refinement of mutagenesis procedures, involving site specific mutagenesis, and the application of restriction enzyme technology, it is now much easier to isolate mutants affecting toxin production than it was 20 years ago. In addition, many bacterial toxins are produced by organisms for which genetic analysis has become available only recently. Examples can be found among gram-positive bacteria, such as staphylococci and clostridia.

The aim of this chapter is to review mainly recent studies on the genetics of toxins, which are the outcome of the application of the methods of molecular genetics. There has been a great deal of activity in this field and one reason for this is the frequent occurrence of toxin genes in plasmids. With the current interest in plasmid biology, these genes have received much attention.

We shall first consider toxins produced by gram-negative bacteria and then toxins produced by gram-positive bacteria. In each case we shall discuss the above-mentioned aspects, structure of the genes, gene expression, and location and movement of the genes. The toxins to be considered, together with some of their salient features, are listed in Table 1.

2. TOXINS PRODUCED BY GRAM-NEGATIVE BACTERIA

2.1. ENTEROTOXINS OF *ESCHERICHIA COLI*

The enterotoxins of *E. coli* have been thoroughly investigated genetically. These toxins bring about fluid secretion in the intestine and play an important role in the pathogenesis of diarrhoea. Two kinds of toxin have been described, heat labile toxin (LT) and heat stable toxin (ST). LT is similar to cholera toxin (CT) in its function and chemical structure. Like CT, it consists of 2 subunits, A and B, with 5 copies of B surrounding 1 copy of A (Gill *et al.*, 1981). The molecular weight is about 85,000, similar to that of CT, with A contributing about 25,000 and each of the B subunits about 11,800. Further details of the structure and mode of action are described in Chapter 5. LT toxins isolated from different strains have the same

TABLE 1.   *Genes Controlling Toxin Production*

Genes controlling	Type and location of gene	Producing organism
heat labile enterotoxin (LT)	structural—plasmid regulatory—chromosome	*E. coli*
heat stable enterotoxin (ST)	structural—plasmid regulatory(?)—chromosome	*E. coli*
cholera toxin (CT)	structural—chromosome regulatory—chromosome	*V. cholerae*
exotoxin A	structural—chromosome regulatory—chromosome	*P. aeruginosa*
diphtheria toxin (DT)	structural—phage regulatory—phage, chromosome	*C. diphtheriae*
exfoliative toxin (ET)	structural (?)—plasmid structural (?)—chromosome	*S. aureus*
enterotoxin B	structural (?)—chromosome	*S. aureus*
toxic shock syndrome exotoxin (TSSE)	structural (?)—chromosome	*S. aureus*
tetanus toxin	structural (?)—plasmid	*C. tetani*
botulinum toxin	structural or regulatory?—phage	*C. botulinum*
α-toxin	structural or regulatory?—phage	*C. novyi*

mode of action, but antigenic differences have been observed (Honda *et al.*, 1981; Holmes *et al.*, 1983; Geary *et al.*, 1982). ST is a smaller protein than LT, consisting of a single polypeptide with a molecular weight of about 5,000. Properties of ST are described in Chapter 6. ST toxins isolated from different strains are heterogeneous. Two types exist, ST I (or STa) and ST II (or STb), that can be distinguished from each other in regard to their mode of action (Greenberg *et al.*, 1981) and behavior in animal assays (Gyles, 1979).

The genes for LT and ST are generally located in plasmids, called Ent plasmids. Exceptional cases of location of a gene for LT in the chromosome (Green *et al.*, 1983) and in a bacteriophage (Takeda and Murphy, 1978) have been described. Some Ent plasmids carry genes for LT, others for ST and others for both. The plasmids range in size from 20 to 150 kilobases (kb), but most of them are in the 80–100 kb range. Many of them are transmissible by conjugation. For most Ent plasmids, toxin production is the only recognizable trait besides conjugal transfer ability, but some chimeric Ent plasmids have been described that carry additional genes for drug resistance (Gyles *et al.*, 1977; McConnell *et al.*, 1979; Silva *et al.*, 1983) and for the production of colonization factor antigens (Smith *et al.*, 1979; Reis *et al.*, 1980b; Penaranda *et al.*, 1983).

In this connection it should be noted that the production of a colonization factor antigen (CFA) is essential for virulence. These antigens are proteinaceous surface appendages that promote the adherence of the bacteria to the epithelial cells of the small intestine. They are host-species specific. Well known examples are K88 for porcine strains, K99 for bovine strains and CFA/I and CFA/II for human strains. The genes for CFA/I and CFA/II have been found in chimeric Ent plasmids, whereas the genes for K88 and K99 are present in separate plasmids. The genetics of colonization factor antigens is discussed in 2 recent reviews (Elwell and Shipley, 1980; Gaastra and De Graaf, 1982).

The structures of several LT and ST genes have been studied by cloning short DNA segments containing an LT or ST gene and determining their nucleotide sequences. The first determination for LT was carried out with the plasmid P307, originally present in a porcine strain. This plasmid is very similar to the chimeric Ent plasmid pCG86, except that the latter contains additional genes for drug resistance (Mazaitis *et al.*, 1981). An 8.1 kb *Bam* HI fragment was cloned and found to contain genes for LT and ST II (Dallas *et al.*, 1979; Mazaitis *et al.*, 1981). On further subcloning, 2 genes for LT, corresponding to the A and B subunits, were localized within a 1.8 kb segment. The 2 genes are adjacent to each other, with a single promoter preceding the gene for the A subunit (Dallas *et al.*, 1979). The 2 genes therefore constitute a unit of transcription. The nucleotide sequences of both genes have been determined (Dallas and Falkow, 1980; Spicer *et al.*, 1981; Spicer and Noble, 1982) and the corresponding amino acid sequences have been deduced. Each of the deduced amino acid sequences contains a segment at the amino terminal end that has a composition typical of a signal peptide. These signal peptides, consisting largely of hydrophobic amino acids, are required for the transport of the toxin molecules across the inner membrane. They are not present in the mature LT molecules. A feature of interest of the LT genes is a 2 base-pair overlap between the end of the A gene and the beginning of the B gene (Spicer and Noble, 1982). As might be expected from the similarities between LT and CT in regard to mode of action and size and arrangements of subunits, there is considerable homology between the amino acid sequences for both the A (Spicer *et al.*, 1981) and the B (Dallas and Falkow, 1980) subunits.

Recently the nucleotide sequences of the A and B genes, located in a plasmid of a human strain, were determined. In a preliminary report, some divergence from the corresponding genes in plasmid P307 is noted (Yamamoto *et al.*, 1982).

For ST, nucleotide sequences for 2 ST I genes and 2 ST II genes have been determined. The source of one of the ST I genes was a plasmid from a bovine strain (So and McCarthy, 1980), of the other, a plasmid from a human strain (Moseley *et al.*, 1983). The 2 genes are of similar size with about 210 base pairs, and both code for a signal peptide. However, there is 31 % divergence in the base composition of the sequences. The STII genes, whose sequences were determined, were derived from plasmids P307 (Lee *et al.*, 1983) and pCG86 (Picken *et al.*, 1986). In this case, the sequences for the toxins are identical and there is only one base-pair difference in the promoter region. Again, in each gene there is a sequence corresponding to a signal peptide. Although the size of the STII genes is very similar to the size of the STI genes, the base compositions are completely different. This is in agreement with the difference in mode of action between STI and STII.

Gene expression of the LT and ST genes, as for other secreted proteins, is a complicated process. For LT it involves transcription and translation of the A and B genes, passage of the precursor molecules through the inner cell membrane and assembly of the subunits, presumably at the outer cell membrane (Wensink et al., 1978; Gankema et al., 1980; Yamamoto and Yokota, 1982). Further stages in the processing of LT molecules are the release from the outer membrane and proteolytic cleavage of the A subunit to generate the enzymatically active A1 moiety.

Information about gene expression of LT has been obtained indirectly from considerations of the structure of the A and B genes. Thus because of the single promoter, there is presumably a single messenger RNA for both genes. Translation and passage through the inner membrane probably occur separately for the 2 genes, since there is a signal peptide for each gene. Information about gene expression can also be gained from the study of mutants affecting LT synthesis. We have developed a method for the enrichment of such mutants and have isolated a variety of them, including temperature-sensitive ones (Silva et al., 1978). Recently, 20 mutants were characterized immunologically and enzymatically and they were found to fall into 5 classes in terms of defects in the A and B subunits (Hirschfeld, 1983). Complementation tests employing a cloned fragment containing only the A gene (Dallas et al., 1979) showed that most mutants defective in A (but not in B) could be complemented by the cloned A fragment to produce active LT. With mutants producing only A or only B, it was shown that the product of the gene, like complete LT, accumulated in the cell envelope (Hirschfeld, 1983). These results with mutants support the notion that translation and processing of the products of the A and B genes occur separately and that assembly occurs either in the periplasmic space or in the outer membrane. Studies on the formation of the B subunit in minicells also support this notion (Palva et al., 1981).

Mutants were also found to be useful for the study of the regulation of gene expression of the LT genes. Nitrosoguanidine-induced mutants that produce increased amounts of LT (Htx mutants) have been isolated in a pCG86 carrying strain (Bramucci et al., 1981). Such mutants can be scored for hemolytic zones surrounding the colonies on blood agar plates, following exposure of the plates to antibody against LT and complement (Bramucci and Holmes, 1978). In some mutants total LT production was increased, but in others there was only an increased release of LT into the medium. In all these mutants the mutation had occurred in the chromosome. We have also isolated Htx mutants in a pCG86-carrying strain, following transposon insertion either into the chromosome or into the plasmid (Maas et al., 1981). The transposons used were Tn3 and Tn5. The chromosomal Htx insertion mutants may be in the same genes as the mutants isolated by Bramucci and Holmes. Since the transposons contain a selective marker gene (ampicillin resistance for Tn3, kanamycin resistance for Tn5), this will facilitate the mapping of the genes affecting LT synthesis. The plasmid insertion Htx mutants were obtained mainly with Tn3. We have mapped the insertion sites in 17 such mutants and have found them to be in the same region of the plasmid, in a gene involved in the regulation of plasmid copy number (Picken et al., 1983b). Increased LT production in these mutants is presumably due to an increase in the number of LT genes. We found in these mutants a 4 to 8 fold increase in plasmid copy number and a corresponding 4 to 8 fold increase in LT production. It is interesting that, with an increase of LT formation as a result of increased gene dosage, a large fraction of the toxin (about 50 %) is excreted.

Studies on the expression of ST genes have been hampered by the difficulty of carrying out assays for these toxins. The 4 ST genes which have been sequenced code for signal peptides. Most of the ST produced by the cell appears to be excreted. These 2 findings indicate that, as with LT, gene expression involves further steps beyond the transcription and translation of the genes. Passage through the inner membrane presumably requires the presence of signal peptides, as with other excreted proteins, and they are cleaved off subsequently. How ST gets through the outer membrane is not known. There may be a special mechanism for secretion, since very few proteins of *E. coli* are secreted into the culture medium. That such a mechanism exists is suggested by the finding of chromosomal mutants unable to produce secreted STII (Silva *et al.*, 1978). There may also be further proteolytic cleavage, beyond the removal of the signal peptides. That this is the case is indicated by the finding that the excreted STI contains 18 amino acids, whereas the nucleotide sequence of the mature toxin codes for about 50 amino acids (Chan and Giannella, 1981).

In regard to regulation of gene expression, it has been shown that the production of STI is controlled by catabolite repression (Alderete and Robertson, 1977). This mechanism is mediated by cyclic AMP and it has been shown that in mutants unable to synthesize cyclic AMP, STI is not produced, unless cyclic AMP is supplied. Mutants blocked in cyclic AMP binding protein are unable to produce STI (Martinez–Cadena *et al.*, 1981). It may be that cyclic AMP and its binding protein act directly on the promoter of the STI gene. It is also possible that the effect is an indirect one, via a system that is required for STI processing or secretion.

It should be noted that cell-free synthesis of STI has been achieved, using a cloned STI gene as a template (Lathe *et al.*, 1980). This system offers further possibilities for studying gene expression and its regulation. Cell-free synthesis for LT has also been achieved with P307 LT DNA as template (Dorner *et al.*, 1979). This system was strongly stimulated by cyclic AMP, but no such stimulation could be demonstrated *in vivo* in adenylcyclase deficient mutants (Hirschfeld, 1983).

Movement of enterotoxin genes has been shown to occur between cells and between different genetic elements within the same cell. Conjugal transfer of pCG86, which has selectable marker genes, has been demonstrated not only to other *E. coli* strains, but also to other genera, such as *Shigella*, *Klebsiella*, *Citrobacter*, *Salmonella* and *Vibrio* (Neill *et al.*, 1983a; Neill *et al.*, 1983b). It is, therefore, surprising that most enterotoxigenic isolates from clinical material have been found to belong to relatively few serotypes of *E. coli* (Reis *et al.*, 1980a; McConnell *et al.*, 1980; Echeverria *et al.*, 1982). Why there is this preference of Ent plasmids for certain serotypes is not understood. It may be related to the stability of these plasmids in different host strains. Whatever the underlying cause may be, the association of toxigenicity with only a few serotypes is of practical importance in the diagnosis of enteric infections.

Intracellular transposition from one genetic element to another has been demonstrated for an STI gene located in a plasmid of bovine origin (So *et al.*, 1979). It was shown that the DNA region containing the STI gene is flanked by inverted repeat DNA segments, suggestive of a transposon, and that the inverted DNA segments are practically identical with the known insertion element IS1 (So *et al.*, 1979). This STI gene is thus part of a transposon and was named Tn 1681. In the plasmid pCG86, the gene for STII, but not the LT gene complex, was also found to be located in a DNA segment flanked by inverted repeats (Mazaitis *et al.*, 1981). So far, transposition for this ST gene has not been demonstrated. The inverted repeat segments and the length of the segments between the repeats are different in pCG86 from those described above for the STI plasmid.

2.2. CHOLERA TOXIN

Cholera toxin (CT), as mentioned before, is very similar to LT in structure and mode of action. Studies on the chemistry of CT have been facilitated by the availability of a strain of *V. cholerae*, 569B, that excretes large amounts of CT. The protein is available in pure form and the amino acid sequences of the B subunit (Lai, 1977; Kurosky *et al.*, 1977) and part of the A subunit (Kurosky *et al.*, 1976; Klapper *et al.*, 1976; Lai *et al.*, 1979; Duffy *et al.*, 1981) have been determined. These amino acid sequences were used for the comparison with the amino acid sequences of LT deduced from the nucleotide sequences (Dallas and Falkow, 1980; Spicer *et al.*, 1981).

The structural genes for the A and B subunits have been cloned in *E. coli* in the vector pBR322 (Pearson and Mekalanos, 1982). The 2 genes are near each other in the cloned fragment, but it is not yet known, if they are adjacent, as they are for LT. There are similarities in the pattern of restriction enzyme sites between the LT genes and the CT genes. So far, the CT genes have not been sequenced.

The expression of the CT genes in *V. cholerae* strain 569B is quite different from that of the LT genes in *E. coli*, in that much larger amounts of toxin are produced and are excreted. However, the expression of the CT genes in the cloned fragment of strain 569B in *E. coli* is very much like that of LT (Pearson and Mekalanos, 1982). The total amount of CT produced is greatly reduced and the toxin remains largely cell-associated. Conversely, when plasmid pCG86 was introduced into strain 569B, the LT produced was largely excreted (Neill *et al.*, 1983b). It is clear from these results that host genes play an important role in the expression of the toxin genes, at least in the latter stages. Another host effect was observed at the stage of proteolytic cleavage of the A subunit to A1 and A2, which seems to be reduced in *E. coli* as compared to *V. cholerae* (Pearson and Mekalanos, 1982). This defect in proteolytic processing might be related to the decrease in CT excretion.

The earlier stages of gene expression are not well understood. It was shown that translation of the toxin genes occurs on free polysomes, but not on membrane-bound polysomes (Nichols *et al.*, 1980). A 52,000 molecular weight precursor of the toxin was found to be produced in the cytoplasm, which reacts with anti-A antibodies, but not with anti-B antibodies. A second precursor was found with a molecular weight of 45,000, which reacts with both antibodies. The nature of these precursors and the further steps leading to the mature toxin remain to be elucidated. From the little we know, the steps in the formation of CT appear to be different from those in the formation of LT.

Regulation of gene expression has been studied with the aid of regulatory mutants. Some time ago, mutants were isolated that prevent toxin production (Finkelstein *et al.*, 1974) and they were mapped in the chromosome near a gene for histidine biosynthesis (Vasil *et al.*, 1975). At first it was thought that these mutations were in the structural gene for the toxin, but later it turned out that they were in a regulatory gene, since the mutant strains produced small amounts of normal toxin (Holmes *et al.*, 1978). In addition to these hypoproducing mutants, hyperproducing mutants have been isolated (Mekalanos and Murphy, 1980). These were mapped in the chromosome near genes for streptomycin resistance and rifampicin resistance. From these mutants, secondary hypoproducing mutants were isolated that mapped in the same region and were possibly intragenic suppressor mutations in the same gene. It was suggested that this regulatory gene near the streptomycin resistance gene codes for a negative control element, such as a repressor (Mekalanos and Murphy, 1980). From these studies it is apparent that there are at least 2 chromosomal genes that are functioning in the regulation of CT production.

The structural genes for CT have been shown to be located in the chromosome. This was first done by using radiolabelled probes of LT DNA and hybridizing them by Southern blotting with restriction enzyme fragments of chromosomal DNA (Moseley and Falkow, 1980). It was found that strain 569B contains 2 sets of structural genes. More recently, it was shown that certain lysogenic phages that behave like phage Mu in being able to insert in different chromosomal sites, can bring about insertional inactivation and deletion of the structural genes for CT in the chromosome of an El Tor strain (Mekalanos *et al.*, 1982). Deletions were demonstrated by absence of hybridization with radiolabeled LT probes. The strains with deletions for CT grew normally in culture media and in intestinal loops of rabbits. Thus the toxin genes do not appear to be important for growth and metabolism of the cell. The DNA segments containing the structural genes for CT that were cloned in *E. coli* were obtained from digests of chromosomal DNA (Pearson and Mekalanos, 1982). Further evidence for chromosomal location of the structural genes has been obtained by mapping alleles that determine antigenic differences in CT in different strains (Saunders *et al.*, 1982). It is curious that the structural genes for CT and LT that are so similar in function, and probably in structure, should be located in different genetic elements in their respective hosts.

2.3. Exotoxin A of *Pseudomonas aeruginosa*

This toxin, like LT and CT, has ADP-ribosylating enzymatic activity. Its mode of action is very similar to that of diphtheria toxin, inhibition of protein synthesis by ADP-ribosylation of elongation factor EF2. However, its antigenic specificity and amino acid composition are different from those of diphtheria toxin (Iglewski and Kabat, 1975; Leppla, 1976).

The structural gene for exotoxin A has recently been mapped in the chromosome of *P. aeruginosa* strain PAO (Hanne *et al.*, 1983). This was done by testing for linkage to known chromosomal genes in mating experiments. The recipient strain used in these matings was a mutant that produces antigenically active, but biologically and enzymatically inactive toxin (Cryz *et al.*, 1980). A segment of the *Pseudomonas* chromosome has been cloned in *E. coli* and was shown to produce toxin (Gill, R., Kagan, J. and Falkow, S., personal communication). So far the gene for exotoxin A has not been sequenced.

In regard to gene expression, 2 mutants have been isolated and mapped in strain PAO, which produce reduced amounts of toxin (Gray and Vasil, 1981). The mutations are near each other, but not in the vicinity of the structural gene. The 2 genes appear to be involved in the regulation of toxin synthesis. One of the mutants is pleiotropic and affects the secretion of several proteins. This gene may have a function in the secretory mechanism for releasing the toxin. The other mutant is defective only in toxin production and the step in toxin production affected by it is not known. It should be noted that the production of exotoxin A, like that of diphtheria toxin, is controlled by the level of iron in the culture medium (Bjorn *et al.*, 1978). Mutants have been isolated in which the inhibition of toxin production is no longer inhibited by iron (Sokol *et al.*, 1982). Two kinds of mutants were distinguished. The first kind had lowered iron transport and affected the production of other substances, whose formation is controlled by iron. The second kind affected only toxin production. The mutation in this case was in a regulatory gene specific for the toxin.

3. TOXINS PRODUCED BY GRAM-POSITIVE BACTERIA

3.1. Diphtheria Toxin

In this group of toxins, by far the best studied example is diphtheria toxin (DT). This toxin is a single polypeptide of molecular weight 62,000, with 2 domains, one with ADP-ribosylating activity, the other involved in binding to host cell receptors. Mutants affecting the structure of the toxin, especially chain-terminating nonsense mutants, have been instrumental in elucidating relationships between the structure of the toxin and functions of different regions of the molecule (for review, see Collier, 1975; Pappenheimer, 1977; Murphy, 1976).

The structural gene for DT is located in a temperate phage (Uchida *et al.*, 1971). Phage-mediated toxin synthesis was reported in 1951 (Freeman, 1951) and since then genetic studies on the toxin have gone hand in hand with studies on the phage. Although several phages have been shown to carry the gene for DT (*tox*) (Holmes and Barksdale, 1970), most studies have been done with phage *β*, which in some ways resembles phage *λ* of *E. coli*. Phage *β* has been well characterized in regard to its biological properties, such as host range, immune specificity and plaque morphology (for review, see Singer, 1976). Genetic analysis and map construction were at first carried out by classical methods, involving crosses with mutants and the scoring of recombinants, then more recently by the methods of molecular genetics, utilizing cloning of restriction enzyme fragments. With the classical methods, maps of the vegetative phage (Singer, 1976) and the integrated prophage (Laird and Groman, 1976a) were constructed and it was shown that the prophage map is a circular permutation of the vegetative map, as it is in the case of phage *λ*. The *tox* gene was found to be located near the chromosomal insertion site (attachment site) and this led to the suggestion that the *tox* gene was originally located in the chromosome and was incorporated into the phage genome following abnormal excision during phage induction, similar to the formation of specialized transducing particles of phage λ. The orientation of the *tox* gene has been determined both in the vegetative map (Holmes, 1976) and in the prophage map (Laird and Groman, 1976b). For this purpose, crosses with mutants in the *tox* gene and in flanking genes were carried out.

Physical mapping of β-phage DNA with restriction enzymes and by electron microscope heteroduplex analysis have confirmed and extended the findings obtained by conventional genetic analysis (Buck and Groman, 1981a; Costa *et al.*, 1981). The attachment site was located in the phage. It was shown that the β-phage, like phage λ, has cohesive ends, through which linear phage DNA is circularized prior to integration. Another phage, γ, which is very closely related to phage β, but does not confer toxigenicity, was analyzed in the same way as phage β. There were only slight differences between the 2 phages, one being the insertion of a 1.1 kb fragment into the *tox* gene, which is presumably responsible for the Tox⁻ phenotype of the γ-phage (Buck and Groman, 1981a, 1981b, 1981c; Michel *et al.*, 1982). The detailed restriction enzyme analysis has made it possible to clone a portion of the *tox* gene in *E. coli* (Leong *et al.*, 1983). This cloned fragment expresses the ADP-ribosylating activity of the *tox* gene.

In regard to gene expression, mutants have been isolated that produce no detectable toxin or immunologically cross-reaching material (CRM). They map near the N-terminal end of the *tox* gene and it is possible that these mutations are in the control region of the gene (Holmes, 1976). With the presently available cloning and sequencing methodology, further studies of these mutants may throw light on the transcription of the *tox* gene and its control. Translation of the *tox* gene has been shown to occur on membrane-bound polysomes and not on free polysomes (Smith *et al.*, 1980). Initially, a 68,000 molecular weight precursor form of the toxin is produced, which is converted to active toxin during or after passage through the cell membrane (Smith, 1980). Presumably, the precursor contains a signal peptide at the N-terminal end of the toxin, which is cleaved off to form the mature toxin with a molecular weight of 62,000.

Regulation of gene expression is of special interest since it has been known for a long time that toxin synthesis is inhibited by the iron present in the usual culture media. On the basis of the properties of iron-insensitive phage mutants it was postulated that iron acts as a co-repressor, in conjunction with a repressor protein (Murphy *et al.*, 1976). Such a mutant has been mapped (Welkos and Holmes, 1981b) and again the mutation was found to be near the N-terminal end of the *tox* gene. The expression of the mutation is *cis*-dominant (Welkos and Holmes, 1981a). This mutation appears, therefore, to be in a control element of the *tox* gene, such as an operator or attenuator site.

Besides the phage mutants, chromosomal mutants have been isolated that produce high levels of toxin in the presence of iron (Kanei *et al.*, 1977). These and other similar mutants appear to be defective in the transport of iron into the cell (Cryz *et al.*, 1983). Of great interest would be the isolation of mutants in the postulated repressor protein, which, according to studies on *in vitro* toxin synthesis (Murphy *et al.*, 1974) should be the product of a chromosomal gene, but such mutants have not yet been described for DT. As mentioned above, for Pseudomonas exotoxin A, one class of mutants is possibly of this type.

Movement of the gene for DT between strains of Corynebacteria has not been studied extensively, presumably because of the difficulties in carrying out genetic experiments with these organisms.

3.2. STAPHYLOCOCCAL TOXINS

Although many staphylococcal toxins have been described, only a few have been studied genetically. The genetic studies that have been carried out have concentrated on the location and movement of toxin gene and little is known about gene structure and gene expression. Here we shall discuss the genetics of 3 toxins, exfoliative toxin (ET), enterotoxin B and toxic shock syndrome exotoxin (TSSE).

ET is implicated in a condition known as scalded skin syndrome. There are at least 2 serologically distinct types of ET with molecular weights between 20,000 and 40,000 (for review, see Rogolsky, 1979). Genetic determinants have been found in both the chromosome (Rosenblum and Tyrone, 1976) and in plasmids (Rogolsky *et al.*, 1974).

Restriction enzyme analysis of a number of plasmids carrying the gene for ET has been carried out and they were found to have similar patterns of restriction fragments (Warren, 1980). A restriction map of one of these plasmids has been constructed (Warren, 1981). It appears that in different strains of *S. aureus*, the same type of plasmid, called ET plasmid, determines the production of the toxin. The gene for the chromosomally determined ET has not been mapped.

Genetic studies on enterotoxin B production have been carried out for about 12 years and have led to the realization that this genetic system is complicated and difficult to unravel. For some time it was believed that toxin production is mediated by a 1.3 kb plasmid, but extensive studies of this plasmid, including nucleotide sequencing, led to the conclusion that it is not involved in toxin production (Khan and Novick, 1982). The gene for the toxin appears to be located in the chromosome (Shafer and Iandolo, 1979). There seems to be, however, an association of the toxin gene with the plasmid in gene transfer experiments. To explain these findings Khan and Novick have proposed that the toxin gene is part of a 'hitchhiking transposon,' by analogy with a transposon for the transfer of erythromycin resistance and spectinomycin resistance (Phillips and Novick, 1979).

Toxic shock syndrome, due to infection by *S. aureus*, has attracted much attention during recent years. The toxin associated with this disease was identified and purified by 2 groups and was named enterotoxin F by one (Bergdoll *et al.*, 1981) and pyrogenic exotoxin C by the other (Schlievert *et al.*, 1981). It is now called toxic shock syndrome exotoxin (TSSE) (Kreiswirth *et al.*, 1982). In a recent report, the suggestion was made that the gene for this toxin is located in a temperate phage (Schutzer *et al.*, 1983). This suggestion was based on circumstantial evidence involving an association between TSSE production and lysogeny. More incisive experiments, involving the expression of cloned fragments of chromosomal DNA in *E. coli* and in *S. aureus* have demonstrated clearly that there is a chromosomal gene for TSSE (Kreiswirth *et al.*, 1983). No evidence could be found for lysogenic conversion with temperate phages produced by induction of TSSE producing strains.

3.3. CLOSTRIDIAL TOXINS

Genetic studies on clostridial toxins, like those with staphylococcal toxins, have been largely concerned with location and movement of toxin genes.

Evidence has been obtained that a gene for tetanus toxin is located in a plasmid (Laird *et al.*, 1980). This evidence is based on the observation that curing of toxigenic strains of *C. tetani* of a large (about 90 kb) plasmid leads to loss of toxin production by these strains.

In *Clostridium botulinum* there are 8 types of neurotoxin, based on antigenic differences. For 2 of these types, C, and D, dependence of toxin production on a lysogenic phage has been demonstrated (Inoue and Iida, 1971). Lysogenic strains, when cured of their phages, become nontoxigenic and reinfection with the phage restores toxigenicity (Eklund *et al.*, 1972). This conversion is phage specific: a cured, nontoxigenic type C strain, when infected by a phage from type D toxigenic strain, becomes toxigenic for type D toxin, and vice versa (Eklund and Poysky, 1974). These converting phages are not stably integrated into the host's genome, as the phage can be lost following growth of the strain in the presence of antiserum against the phage (Eklund *et al.*, 1971). This condition is known as pseudolysogeny (Barksdale and Arden, 1974).

It is not known if the gene carried on the phage is the structural gene for the toxin or a regulatory gene that turns on toxin production. So far no phage mutants have been reported that result in altered toxin production. Thus, beyond the demonstrated control of toxin production by phages, very little is known about the genetics of botulinum toxin production. For a full account of these toxins, and the role of phages in toxin production, the reader is referred to 2 review articles (Sugiyama, 1980; DasGupta and Sugiyama, 1977).

In a bacterium related to *Clostridium botulinum*, *Clostridium novyi*, toxin production has also shown to be controlled by a phage. *Clostridium novyi* type A, which is frequently involved in gas gangrene, and *Clostridium novyi* type B, which can cause necrotic hepatitis in sheep and other animals, produce a toxin called α-toxin. Here also, strains cured of their phages become nontoxigenic and reinfection with a phage obtained from the same type restores toxigenicity (Eklund *et al.*, 1976). Moreover, when *Clostridium botulinum* type C, cured of its prophage is infected with phage NA1 derived from *Clostridium novyi* type A, it is converted to a *Clostridium novyi* type A strain and produces α-toxin (Eklund *et al.*, 1974). These findings have broad implications for the role played by phage conversion in the creation of pathogenic species of bacteria.

4. CONCLUSIONS

From the examples discussed in the preceding pages it is evident that genetic studies have made considerable inroads into the elucidation of the machinery of bacterial toxin production, but only for a few toxins. For these much has been learned about the structure of the genes controlling toxin synthesis, about the location—plasmid, phage or chromosomal—of these genes and about the steps occurring between gene transcription and the release of mature toxin molecules from the cell. Mutants affecting toxin production have been very useful in the analysis of these aspects of toxin production. Another use of mutants has been in the study of structure 1-activity relationships of toxin molecules. This aspect, which deals with mutants as tools to investigate the mode of action of toxins rather than with basic genetic processes, has not been discussed in this chapter.

The methods that are employed in current genetic studies include those of classical genetic analysis, involving crosses and subsequent characterizations of the different types of offspring and those of molecular genetics, such as electron microscope heteroduplex analysis, cloning of restriction enzyme fragments, hybridization with gene probes and sequencing of genes. The methods of molecular genetics have made it easier to carry out genetic investigations with organisms for which classical methods of genetic analysis have not been fully developed.

As stated above, the number of toxins that have been studied by genetic means is small in comparison with the total number of known bacterial toxins. Exploration of most toxins by genetic methods is therefore largely a task for the future. From what we have seen, it is clear that this will lead to a fuller understanding of the production of bacterial toxins than is available at present.

There are some questions of biological interest, to which genetic studies might provide answers. The evolution of toxins is shrouded in mystery at present. How did these molecules, which in many instances resemble mammalian hormones and which seem to be specifically designed to interact with mammalian cells, arise? It is hoped that with genetic methods it will be possible to discover the sources of the DNA that evolved into toxin genes and the nature of the cellular proteins that are the precursor molecules of toxins. Another question is how the production of toxins is controlled. What are the environmental signals that regulate the rate at which toxins are produced? For biosynthetic and catabolic pathways we have a good understanding of this kind of regulation, but for toxins, we know little about control mechanisms and genetic studies in this area may give clues about the way in which control of toxin production is achieved.

In addition to providing answers to basic biological questions, genetic studies are useful for attacking practical problems. For example, the development of vaccines is aided by the availability of mutants and gene fragments that carry genetic determinants for antigenicity. This applies to the *in vitro* production of specific proteins used for vaccination and to the construction of live vaccine strains. Another practical use of genetic methods is in the construction of gene probes for diagnostic bacteriology. Some toxins, such as ST, are difficult to assay biologically or serologically and in such cases the availability of specific gene probes is advantageous for clinical diagnosis as well as for epidemiological studies.

ACKNOWLEDGEMENT

The author is the holder of Public Health Service Research Career Award GM-15129 from the National Institute of General Medical Science.

REFERENCES

ALDERETE, J. F. and ROBERTSON, D. C. (1977) Repression of heat-stable enterotoxin synthesis in enterotoxigenic *Escherichia coli*. *Infect. Immun.* **17**: 629–633.

BACHA, P., MURPHY, J. R. and MOYNIHAN, M. (1980) Toxicity of diphtheria toxin-related proteins produced by suppression of nonsense mutations. *J. Biol. Chem.* **255**: 10658–10662.

BARKSDALE, L. and ARDEN, S. B. (1974) Persisting bacteriophage infections, lysogeny, and phage conversions. *Ann. Rev. Microbiol.* **28**: 265–299.

BERGDOLL, M. S., CROSS, B. A., REISER, R. F., ROBBINS, R. N. and DAVIS, J. P. (1981) A new staphylococcal enterotoxin, enterotoxin F, associated with toxic-shock-syndrome *Staphylococcus aureus* isolates. *Lancet* **1**: 1017–1021.

BJORN, M. J., IGLEWSKI, B. H., IVES, S. K., SADOFF, J. C. and VASIL, M. L. (1978) Effect of iron on yields of exotoxin A in cultures of *Pseudomonas aeruginosa* PA-103. *Infect. Immun.* **19**: 785–791.

BOQUET, P. and PAPPENHEIMER, A. M., JR. (1978) Interaction of diphtheria toxin with mammalian cell membranes. *J. Biol. Chem.* **251**: 5770–5778.

BRAMUCCI, M. G. and HOLMES, R. K. (1978) Radial passive immune hemolysis assay for detection of heat-labile enterotoxin produced by individual colonies of *Escherichia coli* or *Vibrio cholerae*. *J. Clin. Microbiol.* **8**: 252–255.

BRAMUCCI, M., TWIDDY, E. M., BAINE, W. B. and HOLMES, R. K. (1981) Isolation and characterization of hypertoxinogenic (htx) mutants of *Escherichia coli* KL320 (pCG86) *Infect. Immun.* **32**: 1034–1044.

BUCK, G. A. and GROMAN, N. B. (1981a) Physical mapping of β-converting and γ-nonconverting coryne-bacteriophage genomes. *J. Bact.* **148**: 131–142.

BUCK, G. A. and GROMAN, N. B. (1981b) Genetic elements novel for *Corynebacterium diphtheriae*: specialized transducing elements and transposons. *J. Bact.* **148**: 143–152.

BUCK, G. A. and GROMAN, N. B. (1981c) Identification of deoxyribonucleic acid restriction fragments of β-converting corynebacteriophages that carry the gene for diphtheria toxin. *J. Bact.* **148**: 153–162.

CHAN, S. K. and GIANNELLA, R. A. (1981) Amino acid sequence of heat-stable enterotoxin produced by *Escherichia coli* pathogenic for man. *J. Biol. Chem.* **256**: 7744–7746.

COLLIER, R. J. (1975) Diphtheria toxin: mode of action and structure. *Bact. Rev.* **39**: 54–85.

COSTA, J. J., MICHEL, J. L., RAPPUOLI, R. and MURPHY, J. R. (1981) Restriction map of corynebacteriophages β_c and β_{vir} and physical localization of the diphtheria *tox* operon. *J. Bact.* **148**: 124–130.

CRYZ, S. J. JR., FRIEDMAN, R. L. and IGLEWSKI, B. H. (1980) Isolation and characterization of a *Pseudomonas aeruginosa* mutant producing a nontoxic, immunologically crossreactive toxin A protein. *Proc. Natn. Acad. Sci. USA* **77**: 7199–7203.

CRYZ, S. J. JR. and HOLMES, R. K. (1979) Defective transport of ferric iron in mutants of *Corynebacterium diphtheriae* C7(B) that produce diphtheria toxin under high-iron conditions. *Abstr. Ann. Meeting Am. Soc. Microbiol.* p. 16.

CRYZ, S. J., RUSSELL, L. M. and HOLMES, R. K. (1983) Regulation of toxinogenesis in *Corynebacterium diphtheriae*: mutations in the bacterial genome that alter the effects of iron on toxin production. *J. Bact.* **154**: 245–252.

DALLAS, W. S., GILL, D. M. and FALKOW, S. (1979) Cistrons encoding *Escherichia coli* heat-labile toxin. *J. Bact.* **139**: 850–858.

DALLAS, W. S. and FALKOW, S. (1980) Amino acid sequence homology between cholera toxin and the *Escherichia coli* heat-labile toxin. *Nature* **288**: 499–501.

DASGUPTA, B. R. and SUGIYAMA, H. (1977) Biochemistry and pharmacology of botulinum and tetanus neurotoxins. In: *Perspectives in Toxinology* p. 87–119, BERNHEIMER, A. W. (ed) John Wiley and Sons, New York.

DORNER, F., HUGHES, C., NAHLER, G. and HÖGENAUER, G. (1979) *Escherichia coli* heat-labile enterotoxin: DNA-directed *in vitro* synthesis and structure. *Proc. Natn. Acad. Sci. U.S.A.* **76**: 4832–4836.

DUFFY, L. K., PETERSON, J. W. and KUROSKY, A. (1981) Covalent structure of the γ chain of the A subunit of cholera toxin. *J. Biol. Chem.* **256**: 12252–12256.

ECHEVERRIA, P., ORSKOV, F., ORSKOV, I. and PLIANBANGCHANG, D. (1982) Serotypes of enterotoxigenic *Escherichia coli* in Thailand and the Philippines. *Infect. Immun.* **36**: 851–856.

EKLUND, M. W., POYSKY, F. T., REED, S. M. and SMITH, C. A. (1971) Bacteriophage and the toxigenicity of *Clostridium botulinum* type C. *Science* **172**: 480–482.

EKLUND, M. W., POYSKY, F. T. and REED, S. M. (1972) Bacteriophage and the toxigenicity of *Clostridium botulinum* type D. *Nature New Biology* **235**: 16–17.

EKLUND, M. W. and POYSKY, F. T. (1974) Interconversion of type C and D strains of *Clostridium botulinum* by specific bacteriophages. *Appl. Microbiol.* **27**: 251–258.

EKLUND, M. W., POYSKY, F. T., MEYERS, J. A. and PELROY, G. A. (1974) Interspecies conversion of *Clostridium botulinum* type C to *Clostridium novyi* type A by bacteriophage. *Science* **186**: 456–458.

EKLUND, M. W., POYSKY, F. T., PETERSON, M. E. and MEYERS, J. A. (1976) Relationship of bacteriophages to alpha toxin production in *Clostridium novyi* types A and B. *Infect. Immun.* **14**: 793–803.

ELWELL, L. P. and SHIPLEY, P. L. (1980) Plasmid-mediated factors associated with virulence of bacteria to animals. *Ann. Rev. Microbiol.* **34**: 465–496.

FINKELSTEIN, R. A., VASIL, M. L. and HOLMES, R. K. (1974) Studies on toxinogenesis in *Vibrio cholerae*. I. Isolation of mutants with altered toxinogenicity. *J. Infect. Dis.* **129**: 117–123.

FREEMAN, V. J. (1951) Studies on the virulence of bacteriophage-infected *Corynebacterium diphtheriae*. *J. Bact.* **61**: 675–688.

GAASTRA, W. and DE GRAAF, F. K. (1982) Host-specific fimbrial adhesins of noninvasive enterotoxigenic *Escherichia coli* strains. *Microbiol. Rev.* **46**: 129–161.

GANKEMA, H., WENSINK, J., GUINEE, P. A. M., JANSEN, W. H. and WITHOLD, B. (1980) Some characteristics of the outer membrane material released by growing enterotoxigenic *Escherichia coli*. *Infect. Immun.* **29**: 704–713.

GEARY, S. J., MARCHLEWICZ, B. A. and FINKELSTEIN, R. A. (1982) Comparison of heat-labile enterotoxin from porcine and human strains of *Escherichia coli*. *Infect. Immun.* **36:** 215–220.

GILL, D. M., CLEMENTS, J. D., ROBERTSON, D. C. and FINKELSTEIN, R. A. (1981) Subunit number and arrangement in *Escherichia coli* heat-labile enterotoxin. *Infect. Immun.* **33:** 677–682.

GRAY, G. L. and VASIL, M. L. (1981) Isolation and genetic characterization of toxin-deficient mutants of *Pseudomonas aeruginosa* PAO. *J. Bact.* **147:** 275–281.

GREEN, B. A., NEILL, R. J., RUYECHAN, W. T. and HOLMES, R. K. (1983) Evidence that a new enterotoxin of *Escherichia coli* which activates adenylate cyclase in eucaryotic target cells is not plasmid-mediated. *Infect. Immun.* **41:** 383–390.

GREENBERG, R. N., CHANG, B., SAUCER, K., MURAD, F. and GUERRANT, R. L. (1981) Effects of a third type of *Escherichia coli* enterotoxin on cyclic nucleotide metabolism. *Clinical Research* **29:** 385A.

GYLES, C. L., PALCHAUDHURI, S. and MAAS, W. K. (1977) Naturally occurring plasmid carrying genes for enterotoxin production and drug resistance. *Science* **198:** 198–199.

GYLES, C. L. (1979) Limitations of the infant mouse test for *Escherichia coli* heat stable enterotoxin. *Can. J. Comp. Med.* **43:** 371–379.

HANNE, L. F., HOWE, T. R. and IGLEWSKI, B. H. (1983) Locus of the *Pseudomonas aeruginosa* toxin A gene. *J. Bact.* **154:** 383–386.

HIRSCHFELD, S. (1983) Biosynthesis and regulation of heat-labile enterotoxin from *Escherichia coli*. Ph.D. Thesis, New York University, New York, N.Y.

HOLMES, R. K. and BARKSDALE, L. (1970) Comparative studies with *tox*⁺ and *tox*⁻ corynebacteriophages. *J. Virol.* **5:** 783–794.

HOLMES, R. K. (1976) Characterization and genetic mapping of nontoxinogenic (*tox*) mutants of coryne-bacteriophage Beta. *J. Virol.* **19:** 195–207.

HOLMES, R. K., BAINE, W. B. and VASIL, M. L. (1978) Quantitative measurements of cholera enterotoxin in cultures of toxigenic wild-type and nontoxigenic mutant strains of *Vibrio cholerae* by using a sensitive and specific reversed passive hemagglutination assay for cholera enterotoxin. *Infect. Immun.* **19:** 101–106.

HOLMES, R. K., TWIDDY, E. M. and NEILL, R. J. (1985) Recent advances in the study of heat-labile enterotoxins of *Escherichia coli*. In Y. TAKEDA (Ed.) *Bacterial Diarrhoeal Disease: An International Symposium*. Marcel Dekker, Inc. New York, N.Y.

HONDA, T. and FINKELSTEIN, R. A. (1979) Selection and characteristics of a *Vibrio cholerae* mutant lacking the A (ADP-ribosylating) portion of the cholera enterotoxin. *Proc. Natn. Acad. Sci. U.S.A.* **76:** 2052–2056.

HONDA, T., TSUJI, T., TAKEDA, Y. and MIWATANI, T. (1981). Immunological non identity of heat-labile enterotoxins from human and porcine enterotoxigenic *Escherichia coli*. *Infect. Immun.* **34:** 337–340.

IGLEWSKI, B. H. and KABAT, D. (1975) NAD-dependent inhibition of protein synthesis by *Pseudomonas aeruginosa* toxin. *Proc. Natn. Acad. Sci. U.S.A.* **72:** 2284–2288.

INOUE, K. and IIDA, H. (1971) Phage-conversion of toxigenicity in *Clostridium botulinum* types C and D. *Jap. J. Med. Sci. Biol.* **24:** 53–56.

KANEI, C., UCHIDA, T. and YONEDA, M. (1977) Isolation from *Corynebacterium diphtheriae* C7 (β) of bacterial mutants that produce toxin in medium with excess iron. *Infect. Immun.* **18:** 203–209.

KHAN, S. A. and NOVICK, R. P. (1982) Structural analysis of plasmid pSN2 in *Staphylococcus aureus*: No involvement in enterotoxin B production. *J. Bact.* **149:** 642–649.

KLAPPER, D. G., FINKELSTEIN, R. A. and CAPRA, I. D. (1976) Subunit structure and N-terminal amino acid sequence of the three chains of cholera enterotoxin. *Immunochemistry* **13:** 605–611.

KREISWIRTH, B. N., NOVICK, R. P., SCHLIEVERT, P. M. and BERGDOLL, M. S. (1982) Genetic studies on staphylococcal strains from patients with toxic shock syndrome. *Ann. Intern. Med.* **96** Pt. 2: 974–977.

KREISWIRTH, B. N., LÖFDAHL, S., BETELY, J., O'REILLY, M., SCHLIEVERT, P. M., BERGDOLL, M. S. and NOVICK, R. P. (1983) Cloning and characterization of the toxic shock syndrome exotoxin gene from *Staphylococcus aureus*: no prophage involvement. *Nature* **305:** 709–712.

KUROSKY, A., MARKEL, D. E., TOUCHSTONE, B. and PETERSON, J. W. (1976) Chemical characterization of the structure of cholera toxin and its natural toxoid. *J. Infect. Dis.* **133:** 514–522.

KUROSKY, A., MARKEL, D. E. and PETERSON, J. W. (1977) Covalent structure of the γ chain of cholera enterotoxin. *J. Biol. Chem.* **252:** 7257–7264.

LAI, C. Y. (1977) Determination of the primary structure of cholera toxin B subunit. *J. Biol. Chem.* **252:** 7249–7256.

LAI, C. Y., CANCEDDA, F. and CHANG, D. (1979) Primary structure of cholera toxin subunit A, isolation, partial sequences and alignment of the BrCN fragments *FEBS Biochem. Lett.* **100:** 85–89.

LAIRD, W. and GROMAN, N. (1976a) Prophage map of converting corynebacteriophage Beta. *J. Virol.* **19:** 208–219.

LAIRD, W. and GROMAN, N. (1976b) Orientation of the *tox* gene in the prophage of corynebacteriophage Beta. *J. Virol.* **19:** 228–231.

LAIRD et al. (1980) (p. 25).

LATHE, R., HIRTH, P., DEWILDE, M., HARFORD, N. and LECOCQ, J. (1980) Cell-free synthesis of enterotoxin of *E. coli* from a cloned gene. *Nature* **284:** 473–474.

LEE, C. H., MOSELEY, S. L., MOON, H. W., GYLES, C. L. and SO, M. (1983) Characterization of the gene encoding STII toxin and preliminary molecular epidemiologic studies of ETEC STII producers. *Infect. Immun.* **42:** 264–268.

LEONG, D., COLEMAN, K. D. and MURPHY, J. R. (1983) Cloned fragment A of diphtheria toxin is expressed and secreted into the periplasmic space of *Escherichia coli* K12. *Science* **220:** 515–517.

LEPPLA, S. H. (1976) Large-scale purification and characterization of the exotoxin of *Pseudomonas aeruginosa*. *Infect. Immun.* **14:** 1077–1086.

MAAS, W. R., MAAS, R. and MAZAITIS, A. J. (1981) Enterotoxin genes: mapping and regulation studies. In: *Microbiology-1981*, SCHLESINGER, D. (ed) American Society of Microbiology, Washington, D.C. p. 133–136.

MARTINEZ-CADENA, M. G., GUZMAN-VERDUZCO, L. M., STIEGLITZ, H. and KUPERSZTOCH-PORTNOY, Y. M. (1981) Catabolite repression of *Escherichia coli* heat-stable enterotoxin activity. *J. Bact.* **145:** 722–728.

MAZAITIS, A. J., MAAS, R. and MAAS, W. K. (1981) Structure of a naturally occurring plasmid with genes for enterotoxin production and drug resistance. *J. Bact.* **145:** 97–105.

MCCONNELL, M. M., WILLSHAW, G. A., SMITH, H. R., SCOTLAND, S. M. and ROWE, B. (1979) Transposition of ampicillin resistance to an enterotoxin plasmid in an *Escherichia coli* strain of human origin. *J. Bact.* **139**: 346–355.

McCONNELL, M. M., SMITH, H. R., WILLSHAW, G. A., SCOTLAND, S. M. and ROWE, B. (1980) Plasmids coding for heat-labile enterotoxin production isolated from *Escherichia coli* 078: comparison of properties. *J. Bact.* **143**: 158–167.

MEKALANOS, J. J., MOSELEY, L. S., MURPHY, J. R. and FALKOW, S. (1982) Isolation of enterotoxin structural gene deletion mutations in *Vibrio cholerae* induced by two mutagenic vibriophages. *Proc. Natn. Acad. Sci. USA* **79**: 151–155.

MEKALANOS, J. J. and MURPHY, J. R. (1980) Regulation of cholera toxin production in *Vibrio cholerae*: genetic analysis of phenotypic instability in hypertoxinogenic mutants. *J. Bact.* **141**: 570–576.

MICHEL, J. L., RAPPUOLI, R., MURPHY, J. R. and PAPPENHEIMER, A. M. JR. (1982) Restriction endonuclease map of the nontoxigenic corynephage γc and its relationship to the toxigenic corynephage βc *J. Virol.* **42**: 510–518.

MOSELEY, S. L. and FALKOW, S. (1980) Nucleotide sequence homology between the heat-labile enterotoxin gene of *Escherichia coli* and *Vibrio cholerae* deoxyribonucleic acid. *J. Bact.* **144**: 444–446.

MOSELEY, S. L., HARDY, J. W., HING, M. I., ECHEVERRIA, P. and FALKOW, S. (1983) Isolation and nucleotide sequence determination of a gene encoding a heat-stable enterotoxin of *Escherichia coli. Infect. Immun.* **39**: 1167–1174.

MURPHY, J. R., PAPPENHEIMER, A. M., JR. and DE BORMS, S. T. (1974) Synthesis of diphtheria *tox* gene products in *Escherichia coli* extracts. *Proc. Natn. Acad. Sci. U.S.A.* **71**: 11–15.

MURPHY, J. R. (1976) Structure activity relationship of diphtheria toxin. In: *Mechanisms in Bacterial Toxinology* p. 31–51, BERNHEIMER, A. W. (ed) John Wiley and Sons, New York.

MURPHY, J. R., SKIVER, J. and McBRIDE, G. (1976) Isolation and partial characterization of a corynebacteriophage β, *tox* operator constitutive-like mutant lysogen of *Corynebacterium diphtheriae. J. Virol.* **18**: 235–244.

NEILL, R. J., TWIDDY, E. M. and HOLMES, R. K. (1983a) Synthesis of plasmid-coded heat-labile enterotoxin in wild type and hypertoxigenic strains of *Escherichia coli* and in other genera of the Enterobacteriaceae. *Infect. Immun.* **41**: 1056–1061.

NEILL, R. J., IVINS, B. E. and HOLMES, R. K. (1983b) Synthesis and secretion of the plasmid-coded heat-labile enterotoxin of *Escherichia coli* in *Vibrio cholerae. Science* **221**: 289–291.

NICHOLS, J., MURPHY, J. R., ROBB, M., ESCHEVERRIA, P. and CRAIG, J. P. (1979) Isolation and characterization of *Vibrio cholerae* mutants which produce defective cholera toxin p. 192–199, Proceedings of the 14th Joint Conference, U.S.–Japan Cooperative Medical Science Program, Cholera Panel, TAKEYA, K. and ZINNAKA, Y. (eds).

NICHOLS, J. C., TAI, P. C. and MURPHY, J. R. (1980) Cholera toxin is synthesized in precursor form on free polysomes in *Vibrio cholerae* 569B. *J. Bact.* **144**: 518–523.

PALVA, E. T., HIRST, T. R., HARDY, S. J. S., HOLMGREN, J. and RANDALL, L. (1981) Synthesis of a precursor to the B subunit of heat-labile enterotoxin in *Escherichia coli. J. Bact.* **146**: 325–330.

PAPPENHEIMER, A. M., JR. (1977) Diphtheria toxin. *Ann. Rev. Biochem.* **46**: 69–94.

PEARSON, G. D. N. and MEKALANOS, J. J. (1982) Molecular cloning of *Vibrio cholerae* enterotoxin genes in *Escherichia coli* K12. *Proc. Natn. Acad. Sci. U.S.A.* **79**: 2976–2980.

PENARANDA, M. E., EVANS, D. G., MURRAY, B. E. and EVANS, D. J. (1983) ST:LT:CFA/II plasmids in enterotoxigenic *Escherichia coli* belonging to serogroups 06, 08, 080, 085 and 0139. *J. Bact.* **154**: 980–983.

PHILLIPS, S. and NOVICK, R. D. (1979) Tn554-a site-specific repressor-controlled transposon in *Staphylococcus aureus. Nature* **278**: 476–478.

PICKEN, R. N., MAZAITIS, A. J., MAAS, W. K., REY, M. and HEYNEKER, H. (1983a) Nucleotide sequence of the gene for the heat-stable enterotoxin II of *Escherichia coli. Infect. Immun.* **42**: 269–275.

PICKEN, R., MAZAITIS, A. J., MAAS, R. and MAAS, W. K. (1986) Increased production of heat-labile enterotoxin as a result of Tn3 insertion into a chimeric R/Enf plasmid. In Y. TAKEDA (Ed.) *Bacterial Diarrhoeal Disease: An International Symposium.* Marcel Dekker, Inc. New York, N.Y.

REIS, M. H. L., MATOS, D. P., DE CASTRO, A. F. P., TOLEDO, M. R. F. and TRABULSI, L. R. (1980a) Relationship among enterotoxigenic phenotypes, serotypes, and sources of strains in enterotoxigenic *Escherichia coli. Infect. Immun.* **28**: 24–27.

REIS, M. H. L., ALFONSO, H. T., TRABULSI, L. R., MAZAITIS, A. J., MAAS, R. and MAAS, W. K. (1980b) Transfer of a CFA/I plasmid promoted by a conjugative plasmid in a strain of *Escherichia coli* of serotype 0128:H12. *Infect. Immun.* **29**: 140–143.

ROGOLSKY, M. (1979) Nonenteric toxins of *Staphylococcus aureus. Microbiol. Rev.* **43**: 320–360.

ROGOLSKY, M., WARREN, R., WILEY, B. B., NAKAMURA, H. T. and GLASGOW, L. A. (1974) Nature of the genetic determinant controlling exfoliative toxin production in *Staphylococcus aureus. J. Bact.* **117**: 157–165.

ROSENBLUM, E. D. and TYRONE, S. (1976) Chromosomal determinants for exfoliative toxin production in two strains of staphylococci. *Infect. Immun.* **14**: 1259–1260.

SAUNDERS, D. W., SCHANBACHER, K. J. and BRAMUCCI, M. G. (1982) Mapping of a gene in *Vibrio cholerae* that determines the antigenic structure of cholera toxin. *Infect. Immun.* **38**: 1109–1116.

SCHLIEVERT, P. M., SHANDS, K. N., DAN, B. B., SCHMID, G. P. and NISHIMURA, R. D. (1981) Identification and characterization of an exotoxin from *Staphylococcus aureus* associated with toxic shock syndrome. *J. Infect. Dis.* **143**: 509–516.

SCHUTZER, S. E., FISCHETTI, V. A. and ZABRISKIE, J. B. (1983) Toxic shock syndrome and lysogeny in *Staphylococcus aureus. Science* **220**: 316–318.

SHAFER, W. M. and IANDOLO, J. J. (1979) Genetics of staphylococcal enterotoxin B in methicillin-resistant isolates of *Staphylococcus aureus. Infect. Immun.* **25**: 902–911.

SILVA, M. L. M., MAAS, W. K. and GYLES, C. L. (1978) Isolation characterization of enterotoxin-deficient mutants of *Escherichia coli. Proc. Natn. Acad. Sci. U.S.A.* **75**: 1384–1388.

SILVA, M. L. M., SCALETSKY, I. C. A., REIS, M. H. L., ALFONSO, H. T. and TRABULSI, L. R. (1983) Plasmid coding for drug resistance and production of heat-labile and heat-stable toxins harbored by an *Escherichia coli* strain of human origin. *Infect. Immun.* **39**: 970–973.

SINGER, R. A. (1976) Lysogeny and toxinogeny in *Corynebacterium diphtheriae.* In: *Mechanisms in Bacterial*

Toxinology p. 1–30, BERNHEIMER, A. W. (ed). John Wiley and Sons, New York.

SMITH, H. R., CRAVIATO, A., WILLSHAW, G. A., MCCONNELL, M. M., SCOTLAND, S. M., GROSS, R. J. and ROWE, B. (1979) A plasmid coding for the production of colonization factor antigen I and heat-stable enterotoxin in strains of *Escherichia coli* of serogroup 078. *FEMS Microbiol. Lett.* **6**: 255–260.

SMITH, W. P., TAI, P. C., MURPHY, J. R. and DAVIS, B. D. (1980) Precursor in cotranslational secretion of diphtheria toxin. *J. Bact.* **141**: 1894–189 .

SMITH, W. P. (1980) Cotranslational secretion of diphtheria toxin and alkaline phosphatase *in vitro*: involvement of membrane protein(s). *J. Bact.* **141**: 1142–1147.

SO, M., BOYER, H. W., BETLACH, M. and FALKOW, S. (1976) Molecular cloning of an *Escherichia coli* plasmid determinant that encodes for the production of heat-stable enterotoxin. *J. Bact.* **128**: 463–472.

SO, M., DALLAS, W. S. and FALKOW, S. (1978) Characterization of an *Escherichia coli* plasmid encoding for synthesis of heat-labile toxin; molecular cloning of the toxin determinant. *Infect. Immun.* **21**: 405–411.

SO, M., HEFFRON, F. and MCCARTHY, B. S. (1979) The *E. coli* gene encoding heat-stable toxin is a bacterial transposon flanked by inverted repeats of IS1. *Nature* **277**: 453–455.

SO, M. and MCCARTHY, B. J. (1980) Nucleotide sequence of the bacterial transposon Tn1681 encoding a heat-stable (ST) toxin and its identification in enterotoxigenic *E. coli* strains. *Proc. Natl. Acad. Sci. U.S.A.* **77**: 4011–4015.

SOKOL, P. A., COX, C. D. and IGLEWSKI, B. H. (1982) *Pseudomonas aeruginosa* mutants altered in their sensitivity to the effect of iron on toxin A or elastase yields. *J. Bact.* **151**: 783–787.

SPICER, E. K., KAVANAUGH, W. M., DALLAS, W. S., FALKOW, S., KONIGSBERG, W. H. and SCHAFER, D. E. (1981) Sequence homologies between A subunits of *E. coli* and *V. cholerae* enterotoxins. *Proc. Natn. Acad. Sci. U.S.A.* **78**: 50–54.

SPICER, E. K. and NOBLE, J. A. (1982) *Escherichia coli* heat-labile enterotoxin. Nucleotide sequence of the A subunit gene. *J. Biol. Chem.* **257**: 5716–5721.

SUGIYAMA, H. (1980) *Clostridium botulinum* neurotoxin. *Microbiol. Rev.* **44**: 419–448.

TAKEDA, Y. and MURPHY, J. R. (1978) Bacteriophage conversion of heat-labile enterotoxin in *Escherichia coli*. *J. Bact.* **133**: 172–177.

UCHIDA, T., GILL, D. M. and PAPPENHEIMER, A. M. JR. (1971) Mutation in the structural gene for diphtheria toxin carried by temperate phage. *Nature New Biology* **233**: 8–11.

VASIL, M. L., HOLMES, R. K. and FINKELSTEIN, R. A. (1975) Conjugal transfer of a chromosomal gene determining production of enterotoxin in *Vibrio cholerae*. *Science* **187**: 849–850.

WARREN, R., ROGOLSKY, M., WILEY, B. B. and GLASGOW, L. A. (1975) Isolation of extrachromosomal DNA for exfoliative toxin from phage group 2 *Staphylococcus aureus*. *J. Bact.* **122**: 99–105.

WARREN, R. L. (1980) Exfoliative toxin plasmids of bacteriophage group 2 *Staphylococcus aureus*: sequence homology. *Infect. Immun.* **30**: 601–606.

WARREN, R. L. (1981) Restriction endonuclease map of phage group 2 *Staphylococcus aureus* exfoliative toxin plasmid. *Infect. Immun.* **33**: 7–10.

WELKOS, S. L. and HOLMES, R. K. (1981a) Regulation of toxinogenesis in *Corynebacterium diphtheriae*. I. Mutations in phage that alter the effects of iron on toxin production. *J. Virol.* **37**: 936–945.

WELKOS, S. L. and HOLMES, R. K. (1981b) Regulation of toxinogenesis in *Corynebacterium diphtheriae*. II. Genetic mapping of a *tox* regulatory mutation in phage. *J. Virol.* **37**: 946–954.

WENSINK, J., GANKENA, H., JANSEN, W. H., GUINEE, P. A. M. and WITHOTT, B. (1978) Isolation of the membranes of an enterotoxigenic strain of *Escherichia coli* and distribution of enterotoxin activity in different subcellular fractions. *Biochim. biophys. Acta.* **514**: 128–136.

YAMAMOTO, T., YOKOTA, T. and KUWAHARA, S. (1982) Nucleotide sequence of the LT operon originating in human enterotoxigenic *E. coli*. In Proceedings of the 18th Joint Conference on Cholera. Kurashiki, Japan.

YAMAMOTO, T. and YOKOTA, T. (1982) Release of heat-labile enterotoxin subunits by *Escherichia coli*. *J. Bact.* **150**: 1482–1484.

CHAPTER 4

AN OVERVIEW OF TOXIN-RECEPTOR INTERACTIONS

Harry Le Vine and Pedro Cuatrecasas

The Wellcome Research Laboratories, 3030 *Cornwallis Road, Research Triangle Park, North Carolina* 27709, *U.S.A.*

ABSTRACT

This article summarizes current knowledge of bacterial and other toxin receptors on eukaryotic cells and the process of internalization allowing expression of their toxicity. The apparent subversion of physiological pathways of uptake of cell surface molecules efficiently delivers the toxic activity to its site of action. The study of strategies adopted by organisms evolving such potent toxins allows the use of toxins as tools to probe cellular processes, perhaps leading to clinical exploitation in the control of disease.

1. INTRODUCTION

Since several recent reviews dealing with the physical and chemical properties of the major bacterial toxins are available, this article will present a summary of the current level of understanding of the mode of action of a number of toxins, focusing on the toxin−receptor interaction and other early events in the intoxication process at the cell surface. The number of toxins about which sufficient information about ligand−receptor interactions has been accumulated for a meaningful review is fairly small as this aspect has been passed over in favor of studying the cell function(s) altered by the toxin. The emphasis of this article will be to describe the current knowledge of toxin receptors, and to draw analogies with toxins from other kingdoms in an attempt to underline a common strategy in the 'choice' of receptor molecules on the cell surface. Finally, the use of some of these toxins as natural affinity labels to study membrane signal transducing mechanisms and other membrane-associated regulatory events will be considered.

Ligand−receptor interactions are probed by a variety of techniques tailored to be suitable for the particular range of affinities and receptor numbers encountered with each system. Complications in the methodology or its interpretation depend upon the nature of the receptor and its environment. Extensive studies of hormone−receptor binding on whole mammalian cells or fractions derived from the plasma membrane have allowed investigators to characterize the initial binding event, its specificity and cofactor requirements as well as to generate models for the transmission of a signal across the membrane. Whole cell studies have shown that the problem is considerably more complex with the presence of 'spare' sites and a multiplicity of internalization routes some of which may allow a biological response and others which may not. A similar situation obtains for bacterial toxins where internalization by some mechanism has been unambiguously shown to be required for toxin action. For certain bacterial toxins there is the additional complication of each toxin ligand being capable of interacting with multiple receptor sites, i.e. cholera toxin or *E. coli* heat-labile enterotoxin, with G_{M1} yielding an essentially irreversible complex. Nevertheless, binding sites can be quantitated with some accuracy providing the binding experiment is performed with the appropriate controls for internalization and irreversible association.

Because of the lack of purified toxin labeled to a high enough specific radioactivity in some toxin binding studies workers are forced to measure binding indirectly by competition with potential mono- or oligosaccharide ligands and assessing residual toxic activity. Additional difficulties encountered with whole cells and metabolism have confused earlier work. These problems will be identified and the experimental results on the receptor–ligand interaction evaluated when the individual toxins are discussed. A treatment of binding techniques for hormones and toxins and the interpretation of results may be found in Cuatrecasas and Hollenberg (1976).

The word 'toxin' in this review will be used to refer only to polypeptides or protein-aceous material that when bound to, or internalized by a cell, cause irreversible alteration of some component of the cell and its physiology. In this context it might be instructional to consider a toxin as an irreversible polypeptide hormone with an analogous receptor moiety and internalization mechanism. This possible analogy will be considered in the latter part of this review.

Bacterial protein toxins may be classified into two general categories, cytolytic and cytotoxic. The first category consists of a variety of toxins whose function is the destruction of the permeability barrier of the target cells, usually leading to lysis and cell death. Specific receptors for these toxins may not be required, or if they are demonstrable, very little definite work has been published on their characterization. Most simply require the presence of any of the common phospholipids or cholesterol to function. Although this class of toxins is outside the scope of this review because of the lack of information on receptors, they will be discussed briefly since they represent examples of water-soluble molecules that are converted, mostly by processes that are not clearly understood, into lipophilic molecules that will penetrate and perturb a bilayer. This class of toxins could represent an evolutionary stage in the development of a toxic molecule that would efficiently penetrate cells to modify an intracellular target. A similar cytotoxic system has evolved in the higher vertebrate as the complement system (with extensive control mechanisms) to aid in the removal of foreign cells and molecules from the host.

2. CYTOLYTIC TOXINS

J. E. Alouf (1977) points out in a recent review that a great number of cytolytic activities have been reported to be secreted by bacteria. A small fraction of these have been purified to homogeneity so that the assignment of toxic activity to a molecular entity could be made. Of these defined cytolytic toxins, an even smaller proportion have had their molecular mechanisms of action elucidated. Representative examples will be discussed in the following sections.

2.1. SURFACTANTS

The simplest form of membrane modification is a detergent-like solubilization. Surfactin is a heptapeptide with an N-glutamyl-3-hydroxy-13-methyltetradecanoic acid in amide linkage produced by *Bacillus subtilis* (Bernheimer and Avigad, 1970). This material will produce a concentration-dependent leakage of cell components and lysis. Streptolysin S, a polypeptide of 12,000 m.w., functions cytolytically as a surfactant when complexed with polyribonuc-leotides, serum albumin, and certain detergents (Ginsberg, 1970). Staphylococcal δ-toxin is also reported to act as a detergent in cytolysis.

2.2. THIOL-ACTIVATED TOXINS

Another class of cytolytic toxins is distinguished by their ability to polymerize to ring forms circumscribing structures of $\sim$ 50 nm diameter in erythrocyte membranes. These are the thiol-activated toxins represented here by Streptolysin O and *Clostridium perfringens* θ-toxin (McDonel, 1980). They are immunologically similar and share the cholesterol molecule as a receptor (Bernheimer, 1974). Liposomes and cells containing cholesterol in their membranes are rendered permeable by these toxins while cholesterol deficient bilayers are not attacked. It is still questionable whether or not these ring structures are actual holes in the membrane. The size of molecules released from cells or liposomes is inconsistent with the large ring structures being freely permeable.

2.2.1. *Streptolysin O*

The binding of Streptolysin O, a 68,000 m.w. or 130,000 m.w. (dimer) polypeptide is rapid, temperature independent, and irreversible during the prelytic period. Binding is inhibited by exposure of the toxin to p-chloromercuribenzoate, oxidative conditions, or to cholesterol. Antibody raised to Streptolysin O not previously allowed to proceed through the lytic phase will inhibit binding and subsequent lysis although it is unable to prevent lysis if the toxin is bound to the membrane before the antibody is added.

The lytic phase of Streptolysin O action is, in contrast, toxin concentration- and temperature-dependent and is sensitive to formaldehyde and photo inactivation. The bound but unprocessed toxin is not affected by these agents. Added cholesterol has no effect on the lytic form of the toxin. An antibody prepared against the lytic form of the toxin (before binding to membranes) will inhibit binding or if added subsequent to binding, the lytic event. Antibody raised to the bound form of the toxin will not inhibit lysis. Monospecific antibodies obtained by the monoclonal antibody technique were used in these studies to obtain the required specificity.

The ring structures observed are probably polymers of the toxin molecule. Further work is needed to clearly define the molecular events of ring formation and the role of cholesterol as the membrane receptor.

2.3. Non-Thiol Requiring Toxins

Other cytolytic toxins are less well characterized as to their mode of action. The best studied example of a non-enzymatic cytolytic toxin not related to the thiol-requiring toxins is the staphylococcal leukocidin.

2.3.1. *Staphylococcal Leukocidin*

The cytotoxic action of leukocidin is cell type specific, attacking only leukocytes (Woodin, 1970). Presumably a specific membrane molecule or process found only in leukocytes accounts for this specificity. Cytolytic action requires the synergistic function of two proteins, F (32,000 m.w.) and S (38,000 m.w.). The F protein binds to the bilayer, possibly providing the specificity of the interaction with leukocytes. A conformational change induced in F by the phospholipids of the bilayer allows S to adsorb to F. The S protein then interacts with a specific lipid, triphosphoinositide, altering the conformation of δ and forming a channel which is primarily cation selective. S, probably with the triphosphoinositide still bound, is released in an inactive form into the external solution and F returns to its original bound state ready to begin another cycle with a fresh molecule of S. It is not known whether the removal of the triphosphoinositide is in itself responsible for the cation permeability or whether it is removed from the annulus of a particular membrane protein such as the Na^+, K^+-ATPase (Freer and Arbuthnott, 1983).

2.3.2. *Staphylococcal α-Toxin*

Another cytolytic toxin, non-SH dependent, and nonenzymatic is the staphylococcal α-toxin (Freer and Arbuthnott, 1983). Erythrocytes from sensitive species, i.e. rabbit, possess 5000 high affinity, protease-sensitive binding sites for α-toxin (Cassidy and Harshman, 1976). Originally, α-toxin was observed to form large ring-like structures with sensitive erythrocytes. Recent work has shown that these ring structures are found only on cells treated with sufficient toxin to occupy 10^3 or 10^4 times the number of high affinity sites available and equivalent to 10^4 to 10^5 times the LD_{50} value. The rings are therefore probably artifactual structures. Staphylococcal α-toxin will also act on pure liposome structures to destroy their osmotic barrier (Weissman *et al.*, 1966), but this may not be physiologically relevant as osmotically effective concentrations are 10^3-times the LD_{50} value for cells.

There is some recent evidence using ^{125}I-labeled α-toxin that following the initial binding event, the toxin, which is normally 3S (28,000 m.w.), associates in a multivalent fashion with a ganglioside-like or ganglioside-containing membrane macromolecule (Kato and Naiki, 1976) forming a monomer—receptor complex with apparent m.w. of 1.6×10^5. An N-acetylneuraminic acid—galactose—N-acetylglucosamine structure is required for the binding of toxin. Ganglioside derivatives devoid of the terminal N-acetylneuraminic acid or substituted with N-glycolylneuraminic acid will not inactivate or precipitate α-toxin.

Differential proteolytic digestion of intact erythrocytes with pronase or trypsin suggests that the glycoprotein Band 3 is a receptor for α-toxin. Band 3 isolated from red cells of sensitive (rabbit) but not resistant (human) species is capable of binding and preventing toxicity of the toxin in solution. Concanavalin A on whole cells or in solution will similarly bind to Band 3 and block binding of toxin in a parallel fashion (Maharaj and Fackrell, 1980). The abundance of this major transmembrane protein as well as its role in anion transport make it an attractive choice for a toxin receptor as well as a site of action at physiologic toxin concentration.

The monomeric toxin-receptor units associate to form 12S hexamers of apparent m.w. 1.1×10^6 which then either (1) form dodecamers of toxin molecules and their associated receptors or (2) each toxin molecule in the hexamer binds an additional receptor molecule to form a 12S conglomerate, $\sim 1.5 \times 10^5$ m.w. From the estimated m.w. of the monomeric α-toxin of 28,000, the toxin receptor would be around 130,000 m.w. based on SDS gel electrophoresis (Cassidy and Harshman, 1979). Binding of a toxin molecule to multiple receptors could account for the observed decrease in remaining binding sites when cells are pretreated with a subsaturating amount of toxin. Internalization of binding sites is not a problem with erythrocytes.

Photoaffinity labeling of the toxin from within the bilayer by an amphipathic probe implies the penetration of the toxin into the hydrophobic region of the red cell membrane. By contrast, the clostridial θ-toxin (Section 2.2) which apparently interacts with cholesterol and does not intercalate into the membrane is not labeled by the same procedure (Thelestam *et al.*, 1983).

These findings are in line with the observational dissection of cell damage by α-toxin into a sequential series of events: (1) a relatively rapid but time and α-toxin concentration-independent binding of free α-toxin; (2) a less rapid time- and α-toxin concentration-dependent phase of generation of foci of damage to the cell membrane leading to K^+ release, and (3) osmotic effects on the cell. In neural tissue, the effects of α-toxin may be mediated by the demyelination of nerve sheaths as well as by action of the toxin on the nerve membrane (Harshman, 1979).

The role of the receptor molecule in the pathogenesis of the toxic condition may reflect its role in cellular physiology. There are few of these molecules available for α-toxin binding. Their small number may indicate a strictly regulated role in physiology or a limited accessibility for binding. Work in the field is now concentrating on the characterization and elucidation of the normal function of the receptor molecule. Relevant information such as the possible role, if any, of glycosyl residues either protein- or lipid-bound in analogy to other membrane-bound bacterial toxins should be soon forthcoming.

Numerous toxins have been described as cytotoxic or lytic whose mechanisms of action remain to be elucidated or do not seem to follow established routes. Of these, relatively few have been investigated in terms of receptor interactions.

2.3.3. *Clostridium perfringens* Δ-Toxin

In addition to the multitude of toxic activities produced by *Clostridia* spp., variously described as lethal or necrotizing, including numerous enzymatic activities, several distinct toxins have been purified and a receptor-mediated process implicated in their biological action. Of these, the Δ-toxin is the best characterized.

Clostridial Δ-toxin is a basic, single polypeptide, MW 42,000, with a restricted species specificity. Following rapid binding to cell surface receptors a slower, temperature-dependent irreversible ionic permeability change occurs, similar to that reported for staphylococcal α-toxin. Bound toxin is extremely resistant to dissociation except by chaotropic agents but is not released by nonionic detergents, suggesting a firm but not a purely hydrophobic interaction with the membrane. This conclusion has also been supported by experiments with photoreactive probes within the lipid bilayer (Thelestam *et al.*, 1983). Binding to erythrocytes correlates well, although not perfectly, with susceptibility of the cells to lysis. Sheep erythrocytes bind 7,000 toxin molecules to a single type of site per cell with an apparent affinity of 4.4×10^{-8} M. Gangliosides interfere with the binding and toxicity with an efficacy; $GM_1 < G_{D1a} < G_{M2}$. Other lipids were inactive. Enzymatic treatment of the membranes provide further insight into the receptor moiety. Cleavage of sialic acid from membrane G_{M2} decreases binding of toxin while sialic acid removal from glycoproteins was without effect. Yet pronase treatment but not trypsin digestion degrades all binding suggesting participation of a protein component in binding. Cell types other than erythrocytes from resistant species are not necessarily resistant to Δ-toxin suggesting that masking of receptor may be important in toxin sensitivity.

2.4. ENZYMATIC TOXINS

A large group of cytolytic toxins involve various enzymatic activities directed against either the lipids or proteinaceous components of the membrane. The phospholipases appear to exert their toxic activity by releasing local high concentrations of polar lipid headgroups and diglyceride which act as membrane destabilizing agents or detergents to disrupt the permeability barrier of the membrane. These enzymes work on both pure and biomembrane-incorporated lipid. Of the phospholipase C type of enzymes, the staphylococcal β-toxin (Bernheimer, 1974, Freer and Arbuthnott, 1983) (sphingomyelin-specific), the *Clostridium perfringens* α-toxins (Smyth and Arbuthnott, 1974, McDonel, 1980) (phosphatidylcholine- and sphingomyelin-specific), and the *Acinetobacter calcoaceticus* toxin (Lehman, 1972) have been characterized. A phospholipase D-related cytotoxic activity has been purified from *Corynebacterium ovis* (Soucek *et al.*, 1971). A phospholipase activity alone, however, does not imply cytotoxicity. *Bacillus cereus* produces a non-toxic and non-lytic phospholipase C (Wadström *et al.*, 1974, Turnbull, 1981). Special characteristics of the phospholipase molecule including the ability to partially penetrate the bilayer or to interact with membrane components other than lipids may be important in the cytolytic action of the toxins.

In general, the molecular mechanisms of the cytolytic action of these toxins have moved from vague explanations to the present level of understanding primarily because of the recent availability of homogeneous toxin preparations and advances in biochemical technology that have allowed quantitation of various events. More detailed mechanisms should be available in the future as the study of cytolytic toxins moves more from the microbiological realm into that of biochemistry.

3. CYTOTOXIC TOXINS

A second general category of bacterial toxins can be loosely defined as cytotoxic. In contrast to the cytolytic toxins which seem to destroy the permeability barrier of the plasma membrane, the cytotoxic toxins cause specific lesions in processes distinct from the permeability barrier. Their effects may be on molecules associated with the plasma membrane or upon cytoplasmic components. Given the toxins whose mechanism is sufficiently well understood at present, it appears, perhaps spuriously, that toxins that penetrate into the cytosol to act upon cytosolic structures are usually lethal to the cell. By comparison, cytotoxins which act on membrane components seem to select for processes that are not essential for cell viability. The organism, on the other hand, may suffer dire consequences due to interference with a specialized function of a particular group of cells or tissue, i.e. intestinal mucosa (cholera or *E. coli* enterotoxins) or neurons (botulinum and tetanus toxins). While the end result of the two types of cytotoxic toxins are similar, organism demise, there is an apparent dichotomy in the types of functions altered. This difference may have its origin in the development of membranes in cells as a repository for modulatory functions along with certain critical transport functions.

One group of cytotoxins, as classified by its target system, has been studied in detail over the last decade. This is the group of exotoxins that use intracellular NAD^+ to inactivate the protein synthetic machinery of the cell. The protein synthesizing mechanism of the cell is a favorite target, for both plants and bacteria produce toxins that attack the same functional mechanism, albeit different components. The following section will consider the similarities and differences of these ribosome-modifying toxins.

3.1. *CORYNEBACTERIUM DIPHTHERIAE* EXOTOXIN

Diphtheria toxin is elaborated only by strains of *C. diphtheriae* which are either lysogenic for or vegetatively infected by particular bacteriophage growing in the presence of a critical concentration of iron. It is clear that the phage DNA carries the structural gene for the toxin, as a cell-free system of *Escherichia coli* will synthesize the toxin when corynephage β DNA is added (Murphy *et al.*, 1974). The question of the evolution of the toxin from a parent phage protein of unknown function is an interesting but unresolved issue.

3.1.1. *Properties of the Toxin*

Diphtheria toxin is synthesized as a single polypeptide chain of around 60,000 to 63,000 m.w. containing two intrachain disulfide bridges but no free -SH groups (Collier and Kandel, 1971; Gill and Dinius, 1971). This holotoxin is toxic to animal cells as is its limited proteolytic cleavage product whose two large fragments A (24,000 m.w.) and B (39,000 m.w.) are still held together by the disulfide linkages. Much of the toxin found in the bacterial culture filtrate is this 'nicked' form, which may represent the biologically active form since cells also appear to have the capacity to nick the toxin at these trypsin-sensitive sites.

The action of the toxin is to cause the cessation of protein synthesis by the covalent attachment of adenosine diphosphoribose from a donor NAD^+ molecule through the $1''$ position of the second ribose to a modified histidine residue (Bodley *et al.*, 1979) of elongation factor-2 (EF-2) of eukaryotic organisms. Bacterial (EF-G) and mitochondrial EF-2 are not substrates for the toxin (Johnson *et al.*, 1968; Richter and Lipmann, 1970). The ADP-ribosyltransferase activity resides solely in the A fragment of the toxin. This enzymatic activity has the rather unusual property of being unaltered by heating at 100°C. Unnicked whole toxin does not ADP-ribosylate EF-2 and does not have NAD^+-hydrolase activity. Upon reduction of the intrachain disulfide links the nicked toxin molecule separates into two physically and functionally distinct polypeptide chains. The 24,000 m.w. A fragment bearing the ADP-ribosyltransferase activity is non-toxic to whole cells although it retains full inhibitory activity with respect to protein synthesis in cell-free systems. The 39,000 m.w. B fragment is devoid of any enzymatic activities and is non-toxic in both whole cell and cell-free systems. This polypeptide appears to have a role in the fixation of the holotoxin to specific receptors on the plasma membrane. Binding of this fragment to membrane receptors and the role of the receptors in the entry of the toxic A fragment into the cytosolic compartment and in species resistance to diphtheria toxin will be discussed in a later section of this review.

3.1.2. *Intracellular Intoxication Process*

Following exposure of cells to diphtheria toxin, inhibition of protein synthesis begins after an absolute lag phase of from 15 min to 3 hr at saturating toxin concentration, depending upon the target cell type (Moehring *et al.*, 1967). The transfer of amino acids from preformed aminoacyl-tRNA is strongly inhibited while the synthesis of the aminoacyl-tRNA's is unhindered (Kato and Pappenheimer, 1960). The GTP-dependent events of aminoacyl-tRNA attachment to the ribosome complex (EF-1) and the translocation of the mRNA (EF-2) are differentially effected with EF-2 receiving a covalent modification shutting down protein synthesis. The covalent modification event is not influenced by physiological concentrations of GTP or GDP and does not require the presence of divalent cations although it is inhibited by increasing ionic strength (Collier and Kandel, 1971; Traugh and Collier, 1971). The ADP-ribosylated EF-2 binds GTP normally (Montanaro *et al.*, 1971) and binds to ribosomes (Bermek, 1972). There is some kinetic evidence for the ADP-ribose modification blocking EF-2 interaction with the mRNA and thus the translocation-dependent hydrolysis of GTP (Traugh and Collier, 1971). EF-2 bound to a ribosomal complex is protected from derivatization by diphtheria toxin, a fact which may partially explain the initial lag phase in whole cells by the inaccessibility of EF-2 to toxin actions as 75% of EF-2 is bound to ribosomes in liver (Gill *et al.*, 1969).

The ADP-ribosylation of EF-2 is considered to be the primary toxic event in the cell. No early effects on the permeability of the plasma membrane were noted either on K^+ uptake (Kato and Pappenheimer, 1960), retention of ^{32}P-labeled compounds in ^{32}P-labeled cells (Strauss, 1960), or on the transport rate or amount of amino acid uptake (Pappenheimer and Brown, 1968). This is in marked contrast to those toxins considered to be cytolytic whose major consequence is disruption of the plasma membrane permeability barrier. The relevance of ADP-ribosylation of EF-2 to the cessation of protein synthesis and cell death has been established as follows: (1) EF-2 factor activity in the cytosol of whole cells treated with diphtheria toxin drops during the lag phase before the inhibition of protein synthesis; (2) EF-2 activity may be regenerated in a diphtheria toxin and nicotinamide-dependent fashion from extracts of intoxicated cells, and finally, (3) specific mutants (structural gene or corynephage β) have been isolated that show that ADP-ribosyltransferase activity is obligatory for toxicity in cell-free systems.

3.1.3. *Binding and Penetration of Toxin*

The relatively thorough understanding of the mechanism of inhibition of protein synthesis by toxin-mediated chemical modification of EF-2 is in decided contrast to the rather sketchy information concerning the process of transportation of the A fragment from the cell surface to the interior of the cell. During the last several years, this aspect of the intoxication process has received considerable attention resulting in the definition of some of the steps of the binding recognition and penetration phenomena.

Diphtheria toxin, nicked or unnicked, will bind to the plasma membrane of a variety of cells either sensitive or resistant to the protein synthesis inhibition activity of the toxin. The key observation is that on some types of cells (HeLa) the total binding is comprised of a relatively small number ($\sim 4,200$ per cell) of 'specific' binding sites with a $K_d \sim 10^{-8}$ M and a much larger number (nine-fold or more) of nonspecific sites (Boquet and Pappenheimer, 1976). The specificity of the sites is defined as the ability of diphtheria toxin to enter the cell through these sites and to effectively inhibit protein synthesis. Material bound at specific and non-specific sites suffer different fates and are not equally effective at inhibiting protein synthesis.

The B fragment of the toxin (39,000 m.w.) has been identified with the binding function. This was accomplished by the study of the toxicity of point mutant toxins altered in the C terminal portion of the B fragment and finally by the use of stable isolated B fragment (Burgoyne *et al.*, 1976). CRM45, an immunologically cross-reacting structural mutant of diphtheria toxin that harbors a point mutation within the terminal 17,000 m.w. portion of the B fragment thereby destroying specific binding, retains an unmodified A fragment possessing ADP-ribosyltransferase activity. This mutant is relatively non-toxic to whole cells but is fully active against cell-free systems. A hydrophobic component of the cell membrane-toxin interaction has been retained in the CRM45 mutant in that the mutant toxin will bind to Triton X-100 detergent micelles. This binding activity is destroyed by heating at 100°C for 10 min leaving the ADP-ribosyltransferase activity and therefore the toxicity to cell-free systems unaltered. Another mutant of the toxin, CRM197, contains a point mutation in the A fragment of the toxin destroying the ADP-ribosyltransferase activity without affecting the binding characteristics of the toxin. This mutant will block specific binding of holodiphtheria toxin and is used in whole cell experiments to block specific entry of the wild type toxin and therefore its toxicity. CRM197 is non-toxic for both whole cells and cell-free systems. Using either the mutants or a large excess of unlabeled wild type diphtheria toxin, Boquet and Pappenheimer (1976) were able to differentiate two steps in diphtheria toxin processing at the level of the plasma membrane and to discriminate between specific uptake and endocytotic or pinocytotic uptake and their effects on protein synthesis. A similar division has also been made by Dorland *et al.* (1979) involving binding and degradation linked with toxicity.

The first event is the rapid and reversible binding of the C-terminal portion of the B fragment to a small number of saturable sites on sensitive cells. Specific binding sites in this case are defined as these sites blocked by the addition of a low but saturating concentration of CRM197 and the resulting resistance to wild type diphtheria toxin added subsequently. Binding of toxin to these sites will occur at low temperatures while internalization and intoxication will not occur at low temperatures. HeLa cells possess ~ 4200 specific sites per cell, $K_d \sim 10^{-8}$ M, while mouse L929 cells, which are resistant to diphtheria toxin action, have no detectable specific binding sites. Cell-free preparations of L929 cells are, however, fully susceptible to diphtheria toxin. This is supportive evidence for the role of specific receptors in the intoxication process.

A second event is the slow and irreversible association of the B fragment with the receptor blocking the entry of additional toxin through that specific site. The conversion into an irreversibly associated form of the B fragment followed by protein synthesis inhibition does not occur if the cells are exposed to toxin below 15–20°C. Raising the cells to a permissive temperature will allow the bound toxin molecules to proceed through the irreversible binding stage to intoxicate the cells. Ammonium salts and other primary amines also prevent the second phase of toxin processing even at 37°C (Saelinger *et al.*, 1976) as does monensin, a H^+ ionophore which dissipates the pH gradient across endocytic vesicles which normally would allow the toxin to penetrate the bilayer to the cytosol (Marnell *et al.*, 1982).

Pinocytosis is unaffected in HEp-2 cells at the concentrations of ammonium chloride required to observe the effect on diphtheria toxin uptake. The site of action of the ammonium chloride is such that the toxin remains on the surface of the cell in a more slowly dissociating form and in a state susceptible to antidiphtheria toxin antibody (Ivins *et al.*, 1975) but not to trypsin. This could be in addition to the known inhibition of lysosome fusion and hydrolase activity by ammonium salts. Diphtheria toxin in the first stage of binding (bound at 4°C) is susceptible both to trypsin and antibody, and is dissociable by dilution or by pronase-inositol hexaphosphate treatment (Dorland *et al.*, 1979). These effects of primary amines on the internalization of the toxin are dependent on the presence of the ammonium salts, as intoxication resumes following their removal. The effects are not at the level of the toxin molecule as fragment A toxicity in cell-free systems is not modified by ammonium chloride. Other monovalent or divalent metal cations have no effect on intoxication. Penetration of diphtheria toxin is facilitated by lowering the pH of the extracellular medium, the effect of which is to cause the conformational change that would have occurred in the acidified endocytic vesicle inducing penetration of the plasma membrane (Sandvig and Olsnes, 1980.)

Non-specific internalization of diphtheria toxin presents a considerable background which confounded early investigations of diphtheria toxin binding and subsequent processing. HeLa cells, for example, will internalize 1.2% of the total cell volume per hour at 30°C as determined with several different markers. Toxin internalized via this alternate route, i.e. not through the specific receptors, does not disturb protein synthesis and therefore is not relevant to the intoxication event (Boquet, 1977; Boquet and Pappenheimer, 1976). Cells that are actively phagocytic magnify the difference between the non-specific uptake of diphtheria toxin and the specific relevant toxin binding. In macrophages, uptake of diphtheria toxin is increased 10-fold over that observed in HEp-2 cells.

Apparently, in this system receptor-bound toxin is phagocytosed along with the toxin internalized by pinocytosis. Diphtheria toxin is not maintained on the surface of the macrophage in an antitoxin antibody-sensitive state by ammonium ions, and the ammonium ions do not protect against intoxication unless present up to the moment of the protein synthetic rate measurement suggesting a lysosomal fusion-activation event for toxicity. Specific receptors capable of binding relatively small amounts of internalized diphtheria toxin in a toxic form are also expressed in phagocytic cells. Diphtheria toxin covalently immobilized on small beads is phagocytosed maintaining the external surface of the former plasma membrane to the lumen of the vesicle. Whatever mechanisms operating at the plasma membrane to transport diphtheria toxin to the cytosol appear to operate also on these vesicles. Sensitive phagocytic cells may be intoxicated by the specific receptor-bound toxin (Bonventre et al., 1975) while the resistant cells defective in the ability to translocate toxin internalize the toxin but are unaffected by it. Preexposure of macrophages and HEp-2 cells to the general metabolic inhibitors KCN and NaF prevent intoxication of cells and retain the bound diphtheria toxin in a form accessible to antibody, however, these compounds are such broad-spectrum poisons that a detailed interpretation is not possible. Maintenance of receptor sites on the cell surface requires constant expenditure of cellular energy (Middlebrook, 1981).

Several laboratories have used cell types that contain a much larger number of specific diphtheria toxin binding sites than HeLa cells for studies of uptake. Middlebrook and Dorland (1977) screened 22 cultured mammalian cell lines and found that Vero cells (a kidney line) were highly sensitive and that these and other cell lines were sensitive to the toxin in proportion to the number of measurable receptors. Resistant lines displayed virtually nondetectable amounts of specific diphtheria toxin binding. Vero cells contain 1.6×10^5 specific binding sites per cell with an average affinity of 9×10^8 M^{-1}, consistent with the affinity found for HeLa cells (Boquet and Pappenheimer, 1976) which contain only 4200 diphtheria toxin-specific binding sites per cell. High pH and the presence of adenine nucleotides reduced the binding of toxin to Vero cells in parallel with effects on cytotoxicity which argues for the biological relevance of the measured binding sites. Chang and Neville (1978) have applied standard binding techniques to the binding of diphtheria toxin to mammary gland and liver membrane preparations. This is an intrinsically more favorable system for the study of binding sites since internalization is not a problem here. They found that while Middlebrook et al. (1978) demonstrated one type of binding site for ^{125}I-diphtheria toxin in their cells, liver membranes gave non-linear Scatchard plots but a similar range of binding constants, 5×10^{-8} M to 1.8×10^{-7} M, and number of binding sites, 3.4–16 pmoles mg^{-1} protein ($1-3 \times 10^5$ sites per liver cell). Diphtheria toxin binding in membrane preparations was competitively inhibited by triphosphate nucleotides and requires the presence of Mg^{2+}, while unrelated peptides do not compete with the binding. Association and dissociation rates of the toxin with the binding site are high at 4°C. In comparing sensitive to resistant species, i.e. rabbit or guinea pig rat or mouse, Chang and Neville (1978) find no significant differences in specific diphtheria toxin binding site number in membranes between the species and only a slight decrease in the association and dissociation rates of toxin binding in the resistant species. They conclude that differences between resistant and sensitive cells are manifested beyond the binding step in the transport step since cell-free preparations from sensitive and resistant cells are equally sensitive to the A fragment of the toxin. In order to bring these findings into line with the observations of others (Boquet and Pappenheimer, 1976; Middlebrook and Dorland, 1977; Middlebrook et al., 1978) that receptor numbers correlate with sensitivity, one must postulate that either different species vary in the type of lesion responsible for resistance, i.e. binding or transport, or that 'cryptic' receptors are exposed in membranes that are unavailable in resistant whole cells. In this light it may be of interest that diphtheria toxin resistance is often accompanied by an increased resistance to certain RNA viruses where the virus is adsorbed normally but is not uncoated or transported into the cytosol (Moehring and Moehring, 1972). One determinant for whole cell sensitivity to diphtheria toxin has been localized on human chromosome 5 using mouse–human hybrid cells (resistant-sensitive) (Creagan et al., 1975). The cell-free extracts of the parental and the somatic hybrids are equally sensitive to A fragment intoxication. The parental and hybrid cells also have equivalent endocytotic activities. These cells have yet to be characterized with respect to their diphtheria toxin binding activity.

3.1.4. *Role of Toxin Fragments*

The requirement of the diphtheria toxin B fragment for the introduction of the toxic A fragment into the cytosol of cells and for the expression of toxicity has been examined by the synthesis of a variety of chimeric molecules all bearing the diphtheria toxin A fragment attached to the binding subunit of another protein, lectin, or hormone. For reviews on chimeric toxins see Olsnes and Pihl (1982) or Thorpe and Ross (1982) for toxin-antibody complexes. The association of these hybrids with cells was dependent on the specificity of the conjugated binding subunit. Holodiphtheria toxin randomly coupled to anti-SV40 antigen immunoglobulins by glutaraldehyde was only two-fold more selective than free diphtheria toxin against SV40 transformed tumor cells (Moolten *et al.*, 1975), but an anti-human lymphocytic globulin conjugate using chlorambucil as the crosslinking agent was 1000-fold more active against human lymphoblastoid CLA4 cells than unconjugated diphtheria toxin (Thorpe *et al.*, 1978). One possible explanation for this increased efficacy is that the membrane-bound (via the I_gG Fe receptor) antigen-antibody interaction increased the local concentration of diphtheria toxin to a level at which it could more efficiently bind to specific receptors. Since these cells lines are also phagocytic, the immune complex itself could induce phagocytic internalization of receptor-bound toxin which is also active. A series of lectins were also investigated.

Diphtheria toxin A fragment has been linked to the F_{ab} of I_gG raised against L1210 cell total surface antigens and has been shown to be selectively cytotoxic to this normally resistant cell line (Masuho *et al.*, 1979). Uchida *et al.* (1978) linked the A fragment of diphtheria toxin to the monovalent binding subunit of *Wisteria floribunda* lectin which binds to N-acetyl-D-glucosamine residues, via a cleavable —S—S—cross-linking agent. When this conjugate was applied to mouse L cells which are resistant to the action of diphtheria toxin, it was found to be 30-fold more toxic to the cells than the unconjugated diphtheria toxin. The monovalent lectin binding subunit alone has no effect on the cell viability and when mixed with the holotoxin did not synergise toxin action. An analogous experiment using Concanavalin A–A fragment produced comparable results (Gilliland *et al.*, 1978). Experiments with a diphtheria A fragment–ricin conjugate have shown that lactose which blocks ricin-mediated uptake of toxic activity prevents diphtheria toxin ADP-ribosylation of EF-2 while ammonium chloride which blocks diphtheria toxin uptake but not ricin uptake is ineffective. These workers conclude that the binding specificity controls the uptake mechanism (Youle and Neville, 1979). Similar conclusions were obtained using ricin A-diphtheria B which expressed toxicity through the diphtheria intoxication pathway. The corresponding diphtheria A-ricin B was inactive in whole cell studies (Sundan *et al.*, 1982).

The efficacy of receptor-mediated uptake in promoting inhibiton of protein synthesis by A fragment has been investigated by the construction of chimeric hybrids between A fragment and various other molecules targeted to specific receptors for uptake. A hybrid toxin formed from the β (binding) subunit of human placental lactogen coupled via—S—S—linkage(s) to the A fragment of diphtheria toxin showed the expected binding activity and cell-free enzymatic activity of the parent molecules (Chang *et al.*, 1977). When tested against mammary gland explants this conjugate proved to be inactive at inhibiting protein synthesis in this tissue, implying that the lactogenic receptor is unable to mediate the entry of the A fragment of diphtheria toxin into the cytosol in such a way as to express toxicity. This suggests that the mechanism of diphtheria toxin transport across the cell membrane is not related to the transport of lactogenic hormones and that the transported material is presented to the cell interior in a different form, i.e. a pinocytotic uptake mechanism for prolactin would not allow expression of diphtheria toxin internalized by this route. Alternatively, the processing route of the lactogenic hormones may inactivate the toxin by, for example, exposure to lysosomal proteases. Both of these aspects require further investigation. Diphtheria A-asialoorosomucoid conjugates were only toxic in the presence of inhibitors of asialoglycoprotein degradation; colchicine > chloroquine > NH_4Cl > leupeptin > cytochalasin B. Two separate pathways for entry were distinguished with these inhibitors (Chang and Kullberg, 1982). Other workers found in the same cultured hepatocyte system that the diphtheria A-asialofetuin conjugate was toxic through the same receptor system in the absence of inhibitors of degradation (Cawley *et al.*, 1981). Diphtheria A-epidermal growth factor (EGF) which enters through a similar pathway was nontoxic to 3T3 cells while ricin A-EGF retained full toxicity (Cawley *et al.*, 1980). Enzymatically active A fragment of diphtheria toxin that had been conjugated via a cystamine linkage to insulin showed toxic specificity only to insulin responsive cultured 3T3 cells (Miskimins and Shimizu, 1979). A fragment targeted to membrane receptors for lysosomal hydrolases by coupling monophosphopentamannose to the enzymatic unit via reductive amination was inactive although ADP-ribosyltransferase activity and membrane binding characteristics were normal (Youle *et al.*, 1979). The ricin–monophosphopentamannose analog, on the other hand, was toxic and demonstrated the appropriate sensitivity.

HJV (Sendai virus) envelopes and CRM45 (Uchida *et al.*, 1977), or liposomes with incorporated HJV spike protein and A fragment of diphtheria toxin (Uchida et al., 1979) have also been used to overcome the permeability barrier of resistant L cells to the toxin. The fusegenic properties of the HJV spike proteins cause the fusion of the cell membrane and the lipid bilayer enclosing or bearing the diphtheria toxin moiety allowing penetration of the active A fragments of the diphtheria toxin to the cytosol and subsequent inhibition of protein synthesis. These types of experiments utilize the unique property of the fusion system to bypass the normal entrance pathway. Thus, special processing of the toxin at the cell surface is not obligatory for toxicity. Unfortunately in the studies considered here the amount and efficiency of toxin incorporation into the cells were not determined.

The B fragment of diphtheria toxin is not simply a passive binding appendage of the A fragment. Once bound to the membrane, it is able to promote the penetration of vaccinia virus-specific toxic protein into HeLa cells (Burgoyne *et al.*, 1976). B fragment dissociated with guanidine-HCl and thiols and separated from A fragment was recombined with the viral protein and the dissociating agents removed by dialysis. The resultant conjugate was active on HeLa cells while the viral protein alone was inactive unless the cells were first made permeable by hypertonic salt treatment.

Other evidence that the B fragment of diphtheria toxin plays more than a passive role in toxin penetration has been obtained with artificial membrane systems. A fragment is water soluble and does not associate with liposomes. B fragment and CRM45 contain hydrophobic sites and are incorporated oriented to the outside of the liposome when incubated with preformed bilayer structures (Boquet, 1979). CRM45 will irreversibly form assymetric voltage-dependent ion permeability channels in planar bilayers which are open when the *cis*-side (side of incorporation) is positive and closed when it is negative (Kagan and Finkelstein, 1979). Uncharged molecules such as glucose do not pass out of liposomes containing incorporated CRM45 (Boquet, 1979). The bound protein spans the bilayer as judged by its destruction by pronase added to the *trans*-side of the bilayer. The implications for this perturbation of the bilayer are that the ion channel should be closed under physiological conditions (outside of cell negative) but that the B fragment has the potential of becoming incorporated into the bilayer. The underlying assumption here is that the CRM45 will insert in a manner similar to the wild type toxin and that incorporation into a protein-containing biological membrane maintains the same assymetry. CRM45 may not be an acceptable analog of diphtheria toxin because the C-terminal receptor binding region has been deleted and thus the interaction of the toxin with the bilayer may be different than for a fragment containing only the hydrophobic interaction region, such as CRM45. The channel-forming properties of the binding subunit of diphtheria toxin are interesting and suggestive. However, studies using mutants in the A fragment such as CRM197 which retain an unmodified binding polypeptide, would be more conclusive.

Although the high affinity, low capacity biologically relevant receptor for diphtheria toxin appears to be a glycoprotein, the toxin must also interact with the bilayer. Model systems with liposomes (Iglewski *et al.*, 1979), indicate that the polar phosphate head group portion of the phospholipid is also important in the binding event and that the fatty acyl chain length and possibly a requirement for more fluid regions of the membrane will modulate this binding. Various phosphate salts, including nucleotide triphosphates, will prevent binding to normally receptive liposomes as they will also interfere with binding of the toxin to cells or membranes (Chang and Neville, 1978; Middlebrook *et al.*, 1978). These interactions are probably secondary to the primary interaction with the binding glycoprotein or glycolipid. Further studies including the incorporation of the glycoprotein receptor into liposomes will be needed to determine the relative importance of the bilayer and the receptor molecules.

3.1.5. *Receptor Moiety*

A number of lines of evidence have implicated glycolipids and/or glycoproteins in the binding and fixation of diphtheria toxin to the cell surface. Competitive inhibition of intoxication of Chinese hamster V79 cells by diphtheria toxin was observed when Concanavalin A, succinylated Concanavalin A (monomeric) or wheat germ agglutinin, but not *Proteus vulgaris* agglutinin or *abrus* agglutinin were preincubated with the cells before the diphtheria toxin was added (Draper *et al.*, 1978a). Washing the lectin-treated cells failed to relieve the inhibition. The effects of the inhibitory lectins were reversed by the addition of α-methylmannopyranoside to the Concanavalin A-treated cells and N-acetyl-glucosamine to the wheat germ agglutinin-treated cells. The inability of the relevant monosaccharides (Draper *et al.*, 1978a) or various glycolipids (Pappenheimer, 1977) to inhibit diphtheria toxin action suggested that a specific oligosaccharide structure was necessary for the inhibition. Competition studies with a variety of mannose- and N-acetylglucosamine-containing polymers revealed that the ovalbumin glycopeptide and the *Salmonella cholera suis* 5210 polysaccharide were effective. This evidence plus the observation that mannosidase treatment of the ovalbumin glycopeptide destroyed its effectiveness (Draper *et al.*, 1978b), suggest that N-acetylglucosamine as a terminal residue and that the critical mannose(s) are internal. This combination of specificities explains the inability in some studies of the neuraminidase, lysozyme, and hyaluronidase treatments of cells to alter diphtheria toxin sensitivity (Duncan and Groman, 1969). Specific neuraminidases from different sources, however, were able to increase sensitivity of human FL cells to diphtheria toxin as well as to ricin (Mekada *et al.*, 1979).

The observation that an oligosaccharide moiety was involved in at least the expression of diphtheria toxin binding if not actually in the receptor itself allowed the isolation of a putative diphtheria toxin receptor from guinea pig lymph node cells by affinity chromatography of detergent-solubilized extracts on lentil lectin-Sepharose (Proia *et al.*, 1979). Purification was achieved by binding diphtheria toxin to the ^{125}I-labeled glycoprotein fraction that had been eluted from the lectin column with α-methylmannopyranoside, and immunoprecipitating the diphtheria toxin-associated component with antitoxin antibody. The only ^{125}I-labeled band in the dissociated immunoprecipitate appeared to be heavily glycosylated as judged by its aberrant behavior on SDS-polyacrylamide gel electrophoresis; 168,000 m.w. in 5% acrylamide, 145,000 m.w. in 7.5% acrylamide and greater than 250,000 m.w. in agarose/2.5% acrylamide. The observation that the immunoprecipitated band comprised only 0.1 to 0.2% of the ^{125}I-labeled cell surface membrane components and only a small fraction of the labeled components eluting from the lectin column is consistent with a small number of receptors per cell. The immunoprecipitation of ^{125}I-labeled material required the presence of a functional B fragment as either diphtheria toxoid or A fragment alone gave no labeled precipitation with antitoxin although both forms of the toxin will precipitate with the antibody. Holotoxin and CRM197, a mutant diphtheria toxin with a nonfunctional A fragment, but an intact B fragment precipitate the same ^{125}I-labeled component. A toxin with an unrelated receptor, cholera enterotoxin, reported to bind to glycolipid and possibly glycoprotein did not precipitate ^{125}I-labeled material when incubated with the lentil lectin column eluate and then reacted with anti-cholera toxin antibody.

Receptor binding of diphtheria toxin is modulated by polyanions, specifically poly-phosphates which interact with a polycationic P-site located on the carboxyterminal 8,000 m.w. CNBr peptide of the 40,000 m.w. B fragment. This region is present within the 17,000 m.w. portion of the B fragment deleted in the CRM45 molecule which predictably fails to bind polyanions or to cell surface receptors. This site is occupied *in vivo* by a slowly dissociating dinucleotide ligand, ApUp (Barbieri *et al.*, 1981), interfering with cytotoxicity and with binding to the solubilized glycoprotein receptor (Proia *et al.*, 1981). Dissection of the solubilized glycoprotein receptor from hamster thymocytes with papain yields two immunoprecipitable glycoproteins that can be isolated by lentil-Sepharose affinity chromatography and then immunoprecipitated, one of 88,000 m.w. and the other of 74,000 m.w. by SDS-PAGE and that bind diphtheria toxin in a polyphosphate-resistant fashion (Eidels *et al.*, 1982). These glycopeptides, which represent two different modes of cleavage of the receptor molecule are postulated to contain an X' site distinct from the P' (polyanion) site on the receptor, secondary to the polyanion-sensitive site in the cell membrane. Other evidence from studies with Fab fragment antibodies to portions of CRM45 also suggest a site other than the P site on the toxin involved in cell binding (Boquet and Deflot, 1981). The non-toxic CRM197 toxin which has a point mutation in A fragment enzymatic activity and a B fragment that binds to cell surface receptors but does not respond to polyanions, may be binding to the X' site but not to the P' site due to an altered conformational state. The X' site may also represent an interaction important in a subsequent entry step. Further experiments directed at this question both with additional toxin mutants and in further characterization of the previously described mutants in terms of the new data on binding sites is needed.

A diphtheria toxin-resistant mouse L cell line was found not to contain the ^{125}I-labeled glycoprotein diphtheria toxin binding site when the mouse cells were treated in the same manner as the guinea pig lymph node cells. Unfortunately, the question of whether the location of the biochemical lesion of the diphtheria toxin resistance in these mouse cells is in the binding site or in a transport mechanism remains unresolved since there are outstanding questions regarding the availability of all of the potential and biologically pertinent diphtheria toxin binding sites to the lactoperoxidase-catalyzed radioiodination reaction, the percentage of the potential binding sites solubilized retained on, and eluted from the lectin column. Despite these caveats, the isolation of a specific membrane glycoprotein component which may have biological relevance since it is not present in resistant cells which are reported to have low numbers of specific receptors (Boquet and Pappenheimer, 1976; Middlebrook and Dorland, 1977; Middlebrook *et al.*, 1978) is a significant advance in the study of the diphtheria toxin receptor moiety.

The possibility of the involvement of a glycoprotein in the binding of diphtheria toxin may be significant with regard to the species of glycoproteins and glycolipids exposed on the cell surface and their modulation by various stimuli which effect hormonal sensitivity or cell differentiation and in general reflect the metabolic state of the cell (Fishman and Brady, 1976; Spiegel *et al.*, 1979). The toxin receptor is most probably a normal cell membrane component 'selected' by the toxin on the basis of its widespread presence and relative indispensability to cellular function. A number of polypeptide hormone receptors appear to exhibit some overlap in binding specificity with some toxins, namely thyroid stimulating hormone (TSH) with tetanus toxin, cholera toxin, and interferon (Ledley *et al.*, 1977; Lee *et al.*, 1979). Moehring *et al.* (1971) report that interferon protects cells against the toxicity of diphtheria toxin, possibly at the cell entry stage. TSH and cholera toxin, whose binding and action depend on glycoprotein/glycolipid interaction are also effected by interferon treatment (Kohn, *et al.*, 1976; Kohn, 1978). However, there is some evidence based on the differential effects of cholera toxin action on the anticellular and antiviral activities of interferon to suggest that cholera toxin does not act directly on the binding site for interferon (Fuse and Kuwata, 1979). These types of cross-reactivities will be discussed later in an overview of possible toxin receptor normal physiology.

3.2. *Pseudomonas aeruginosa* Exotoxin A

The exotoxin produced by most cytotoxic *P. aeruginosa* strains is a material similar in many ways to diphtheria toxin. Compared to the diphtheria toxin prototype, very little detailed work has been done on the pseudomonas toxin, especially in terms of the requirements for the intoxication of whole cells. Most of the published work is with the inhibition of protein synthesis in cell-free systems. Therefore, the discussion of this toxin will be notably brief, concentrating as have most of the studies, on the similarities and differences between diphtheria toxin and pseudomonas toxin.

3.2.1. Properties of the Toxin and the Intracellular Intoxication Process

Pseudomonas toxin inhibits eukaryotic polypeptide chain elongation by using intracellular NAD^+ to ADP-ribosylate EF-2 at a site similar to that modified by diphtheria toxin (Iglewski and Kabat, 1975). In fact, fragment A of diphtheria toxin will remove, in a nicotinamide-dependent fashion, ADP-ribose incorporated into EF-2 by pseudomonas toxin, reversing the inactivation of EF-2 (Chang and Collier, 1977) and vice versa (Collier, 1977). Despite these similarities, there are a number of differences in the structure of the toxins and their detailed mechanism of action even at the level of present knowledge. Significant regions of sequence homology is apparently not present at least as reflected in secondary or tertiary structure based on the lack of crossreactivity of either toxin, or fragments derived therefrom, with antisera raised against the other holotoxin (Leppla, 1976). While diphtheria toxin enzymatic activity is thermostable, pseudomonas toxin ADP-ribosylating activity is destroyed at 50°C. The pseudomonas toxin is a slightly larger, 66,000–77,000 m.w. single polypeptide chain containing four intrachain —S—S— bridges but no free —SH groups (Leppla, 1976). Reduction of the toxin followed by alkylation of the —SH groups generated destroys toxic activity against whole cells but increases enzymatic activity (if denaturing agents are included in the chemical modification step) and toxicity in the cell-free protein synthesis system. It has not proven possible to generate enzymatically active fragments from pseudomonas toxin with trypsin or other standard proteases. The pseudomonas holotoxin molecule is enzymatically active in contrast to diphtheria toxin which requires proteolytic cleavage and reduction to generate enzymatic activity. Activation of pseudomonas toxin may be accomplished by treatment with denaturing and reducing agents alone, a process unaccompanied by detectable proteolytic action.

A 26,000 m.w. proteolytic fragment of pseudomonas toxin, apparently generated by a specific endogenous Pseudomonas protease, is present in partially purified toxin preparations. This fragment is enzymatically active in a cell-free system but is non-toxic to whole cells (Chang and Collier, 1977). A 45,000 m.w. b-fragment has been tentatively identified as the portion removed from the intact pseudomonas toxin to form the 26,000 m.w. enzymatically active fragment. This b-fragment has been postulated to be analogous to the B or binding fragment of diphtheria toxin (Vasil et al., 1977).

3.2.2. Binding and Penetration of the Toxin

As was found for diphtheria toxin, an absolute lag phase is observed before inhibition of protein synthesis by pseudomonas toxin begins (Iglewski and Kabat, 1975). Although pseudomonas toxin is taken up by the cells at a linear rate, washing Vero cells after up to three hours of exposure to various concentrations of the toxin reverses the toxic effect (Pavlovskis and Gordon, 1972). However, as subsequent work showed, the Vero cell line was a poor choice for this type of experiment due to its relative insensitivity to pseudomonas toxin. The locus of the Vero cell resistance has not been identified. A striking difference between diphtheria toxin and pseudomonas toxin and one with clear implications as to the receptor sites for the toxins since lysates of all cell types are equally sensitive, are the different ranges of sensitivity of cell lines to the two toxins. While diphtheria toxin shows a marked species dependence of activity on whole cells: monkey > hamster > human > rat ~ mouse (increasing resistance), pseudomonas toxin demonstrates no interspecies differences while cell lines or clones within the same species can differ greatly in their sensitivity. For example, the tissue culture LD_{50} in ng/ml for L-929 mouse cells for pseudomonas toxin is 0.21 compared to > 1000 for diphtheria toxin. Whole Vero cells show the opposite relationship, pseudomonas toxin = 15 and diphtheria toxin = 0.01. These results (Middlebrook and Dorland, 1977) and others (Moehring and Moehring, 1977) clearly imply different receptors for the two toxins. A series of somatic hybridization experiments with diphtheria toxin-resistant mutants have shown that diphtheria toxin will not penetrate these resistant cells but pseudomonas toxin will, again supporting the concept of different receptors and not just a toxin transport defect (Draper *et al.*, 1979). Unfortunately, the battery of mutants used to characterize the binding and processing of diphtheria toxin is not presently available for pseudomonas toxin nor are the various structural mutants (CRM's) in both the binding and enzymatic portions of the toxin molecule. As a result, detailed information on the number of receptors, their affinity, and an explanation for the varied sensitivity of cell lines has not been forthcoming. Differential sensitivity to neuraminidases from different sources of binding sites on human FL cells for diphtheria toxin and pseudomonas toxin suggest separate receptors (Mekada *et al.*, 1979).

The mechanism of uptake of pseudomonas toxin, specific and non-specific, has been intensively studied only recently and the results are somewhat contradictory. Middlebrook and Dorland (1977) found that ammonium salts did *not* inhibit intoxication of whole cells by pseudomonas toxin when it was present throughout the incubation time up to the estimation of protein synthesis. In contrast, diphtheria toxin intoxication of whole cells *is* prevented by the presence of ammonium salts and other primary amines at the stage of irreversible binding prior to internalization.

On the other hand, using LM mouse fibroblasts, Fitzgerald *et al.* (1980) found that a variety of amines blocked internalization and intoxication. Their electron microscopic studies showed that the toxin concentrated in coated pits and was internalized via a 'receptosome' pathway. Internalization was shown to require extracellular Ca^{+2} (Fitzgerald *et al.*, 1982) as has been found for diphtheria toxin and the plant toxins as discussed (Sandvig and Olsnes, 1982b.) Studies with epidermal growth factor (EGF) and adenovirus, both of which are known to enter via the coated pit-receptosome pathway show that both agents are present in the same receptosome vesicles. Adenovirus, which escapes into the cytosol by disrupting receptosome structure, was shown to enhance the efficacy of EGF-pseudomonas toxin conjugates and toxin-collidal gold conjugates by a receptosome-disruptive process (Fitzgerald *et al.*, 1983). These studies conclusively show that at least for this cell type receptor-mediated endocytosis is the mechanism by which pseudomonas toxin is delivered to the cytosol. The apparent conflict of experimental results may indicate that different pathways of endocytosis may prevail in different cell types. Another possibility is that a secondary mechanism may take over if one system is blocked, a caveat in studies using perturbants.

In summary, while diphtheria toxin and pseudomonas toxin share a common mechanism in the modification of EF-2, they differ in immunological reactivity, receptor specificity, cell and species sensitivity, and perhaps in the processing of the toxin into an active form.

3.3. *PSEUDOMONAS AERUGINOSA* EXOENZYME S

Another example of an exotoxin catalyzing an NAD^+-dependent inhibition of protein synthesis is *Pseudomonas aeruginosa* exoenzyme S isolated from the culture filtrate of a strain of *P. aeruginosa* that does not produce pseudomonas exotoxin A (Iglewski *et al.*, 1978). Several properties of the exoenzyme S distinguish this protein from exotoxin A; its relative heat stability, the lack of effect of antiexotoxin A antibody on the ADP-ribosyl-transferase activity of exoenzyme S, the lack of a stimulatory effect on the enzymatic activity in lysates when the toxin was treated with denaturing agents in the presence or absence of reducing conditions, and the transfer of a single ADP-ribose moiety not to EF-2 or a number of other proteins including lysozyme (a substrate of several viral ADP-ribosyltransferases) but apparently to EF-1 and a different group of other proteins. This toxin is not simply a variant of exotoxin A since some strains of *P. aeruginosa* produce both exotoxin A and exoenzyme S.

Extracts from a polyoma virus-transformed BHK-21 cell line that is insensitive to both diphtheria toxin and Pseudomonas toxin A are not ADP-ribosylated by the latter two toxins but can be efficiently modified by exoenzyme S (Sokol *et al.*, 1981).

Further work is needed on the purification and characterization of the toxin as well as its effects on whole cells before more than the general comparisons made in this section can be concluded.

3.4. NON-NAD$^+$-DEPENDENT INHIBITION OF PROTEIN SYNTHESIS: ABRIN, RICIN, VISCUMIN AND MODECCIN

A second subgroup of toxins that inhibit protein synthesis but through a non-NAD$^+$-dependent mechanism are the toxic plant proteins abrin (found in the seeds of *Abrus precatorius*), ricin (found in the seeds of *Ricinus communis*), modeccin (from the root of *Adenia digitata*) and viscumin (from leaves of *Viscum album* L. [mistletoe]).

These toxins which are found in nature together with their related lectins which are toxic in their own right, are separate molecular species from the lectins and have a different mode of intoxication. Although they are not bacterial products, these toxins accomplish a similar task, inhibiting protein synthesis in animal cells. They also appear to approach intoxication in a fashion analogous to those bacterial toxins already described by binding to cell surface receptors followed by internalization of an active component of the toxin, and finally inhibition of protein synthesis at the ribosomal level. A systematic study of the internalization mechanism has been initiated including the accumulation of appropriate cell mutants with variable sensitivities among these toxins as well as a differential sensitivity to diphtheria toxin. For this reason they are being discussed here along with the bacterial toxins which they resemble in a number of ways. A summary of the salient features of these plant toxins is presented in Table 1. Diphtheria toxin and shigella cytotoxin are included here for reference purposes.

3.4.1. *Properties of the Toxins*

The physical properties of the four plant toxins, although they are immunologically distinct molecules (Olsnes *et al.*, 1974), are quite similar. They are composed of two polypeptide chains (Table 1) joined by disulfide bridges required for toxic activity on whole cells, and are heat-labile. As with the prototype diphtheria toxin, the polypeptide chains may be separated by treatment with thiols but without prior proteolysis. Abrin and ricin hybrids and the converse hybrids containing the respective catalytic and binding chains may be formed by treating a mixture of the toxins or thiol-treated, separated chains with thiols and removing the reducing agents. The resulting hybrid molecules are active on whole cells (Olsnes *et al.*, 1974). Once again, the A-chains exhibit the enzymatic activity which may be expressed as the inhibition of protein synthesis in any convenient cell-free system. The B-chain appears to function in binding the holotoxin to the cell surface and is non-toxic by itself

TABLE 1. *Relative Ability to Inhibit Intoxication by 50% (HeLa)[c]*

Toxin	A-Chain[a] m. w.	B-Chain[a] m. w.	D-Galactose	T-Antigen[d]	Fetuin[d]	LD$_{50}$ pg/ml (HeLa)[c]	No. of Binding Sites (HeLa)[c] per cell
Abrin	30,000	35,000	1.3	11	550	250	10[7]
Ricin	32,000	34,000	1.0	11	33	50	10[7]
Modeccin	28,000	38,000	2.3	1.0	1.0	1.25	10[5]
Diphtheria	24,000[b]	39,000[b]	—	—	—	100[e]	10[3e]
Viscumin	29,000[f]	34,000[f]	1.0	—	—	6,000[f]	>10[8f]
Shigella	30,500[g]	5,000[g]	—	—	—	0.5[g]	10[6g]

(a) Data from Olsnes and Pihl (1977)
(b) Data from Collier (1977)
(c) Data from Olsnes *et al.* (1976)
(d) Pretreated with neuraminidase and normalized to molar galactose content (Olsnes *et al.* 1978)
(e) Data from Boquet and Pappenheimer (1976)
(f) Data from Stirpe *et al.* (1982)
(g) Data from Olsnes *et al.* (1981)

against either whole cells or in cell-free systems. Like the diphtheria toxin B fragment, the B-chain of abrin and ricin is unstable when free in solution and will precipitate unless denaturing solute or ligand is added. The relative specificities of the binding portions of the different toxins will be discussed in a later section.

3.4.2. *Intracellular Intoxication Process*

The site of action of abrin, ricin, viscumin, and modeccin is found on the 60S subunit of eukaryotic ribosomes. The A-chains of these toxins act on the 60S subunit to enzymatically release an 8S complex of 5S RNA and a single ribosomal protein (Grummt *et al.*, 1974; Benson *et al.*, 1975) inhibiting a GTPase activity found on the released complex. The net effect of this modification is a decrease in the affinity of the ribosome binding site for EF-2, (which may be overcome with excess EF-2), thereby decreasing the rate of polypeptide chain elongation. The presence of bound EF-2 protects the 60S ribosome from abrin and ricin action while sensitizing it to modeccin indicating a dichotomy of sites attacked by abrin and ricin, and modeccin. Guanyl nucleotides protect the ribosome against the first three toxins while their effect on viscumin is unknown. Since these toxins catalyze an irreversible modification of the ribosome, it is not possible to decide whether abrin and ricin attack the same site and conditions have not yet been found to separate their specificities on the ribosome.

This particular mode of inhibition of protein synthesis is apparently a conserved mechanism for toxicity. A series of protein toxins from other plants, distinct from their lectins, include *Phytolacca americana* peptide (pokeweed) or Croton II from *Croton tiglium*, α-sarcin from the fungus *Aspergillus giganteus* (Endo *et al.*, 1983) and others. A single phosphodiester linkage is cleaved in the 3' terminal region of the 28S RNA of the 60S ribosomal subunit effecting EF-1 mediated binding of aminoacyl-tRNA to ribosomes coupled to GTP hydrolysis by blocking EF-2-dependent translocation of the acceptor site aminoacyl t-RNA to the donor site (Gessner and Irvin, 1980). Although equipotent in lysates, these small (1.2×10^4 m.w.) basic polypeptides lack the receptor binding subunits observed for abrin, ricin, modeccin, and viscumin and therefore are considerably less toxic to whole cells. Illustrating this point, gelonin (from *Gelonium multiflorum*), another single chain toxin lacking a binding moiety demonstrated toxicity to whole cells when linked through a disulfide budge to Concanavalin A (Stirpe *et al.*, 1980).

3.4.3. *Binding and Penetration of the Toxin*

The series of events involved in the action of these plant toxins on cells is superficially similar to that of diphtheria toxin. Several observations suggest caution in the wholesale application of this paradigm. Ammonium salts do not protect sensitive cell lines against the toxic effects of abrin or ricin (not done with modeccin) (Olsnes and Pihl, 1977; Gahmberg and Hakomori, 1975). Ammonium chloride and chloroquine apparently block the entry of modeccin into cells but actually sensitize the cells to abrin and ricin (Sandvig *et al.*, 1979). Since primary amine treatment is reported to prevent endocytosis but not pinocytosis, a pinocytotic uptake mechanism may be able to deliver active phytotoxin to the cytosolic compartment. Calcium is required for uptake of the phytotoxins (Sandvig and Olsnes, 1982a). Contrary to the findings for diphtheria toxin, the toxicity of the phytotoxins is maximal at neutral pH or higher (Sandvig and Olsnes, 1982b).

Active diphtheria toxin is apparently *not* transported by this mechanism. Modeccin may be more like diphtheria toxin than abrin or ricin in this respect. Whether pinocytotic uptake is the physiological mechanism or an artifactual bypass in endocytosis-blocked cells remains to be determined. It should be noted here that these studies utilizing uptake inhibitors indirectly imply that toxin prevented from inhibiting protein synthesis is not readily dissociable from the surface and is not being internalized. An alternative interpretation is rather that these agents which prevent lysosomal processing are blocking the production of an active cytosolic toxin entity. Most studies to date have not addressed this question.

Internalization of the plant toxins is required for the inhibition of protein synthesis. Reticulocytes, which do not internalize surface-bound material, bind abrin and ricin, but their protein synthesis is unaffected. Diphtheria toxin also does not affect protein synthesis in intact reticulocytes (Refsnes et al., 1974).

Toxin binding to the cell surface saturates within ten minutes at 4°C. Lactose, a receptor analog, added during the binding step or within fifteen minutes of subsequently raising the temperature to 37°C will prevent intoxication. Uptake of toxin occurs only when the temperature is raised to 37°C, causing removal of toxin binding sites but not concanavalin A binding sites (Oliver et al., 1974). Ricin labeled with ferritin for visualization by electron microscopy shows clustering and uptake of bound toxin. Colchicine or vinblastin block the removal of toxin receptor sites from the cell surface along with prevention of intoxication implying a role for microtubules in ricin internalization (Refsnes et al., 1974). Toxin-bound mannose residues appear to be required for conformation and in the endocytic process but not for binding of the toxin to cells (Simeral et al., 1980). A ricin-resistant mutant has been isolated that binds ricin but does not cluster the occupied binding sites (Nicolson et al., 1976). Unfortunately, there is no information about other functions of this mutant that are known to be mediated by microtubular action. Not all cell surface binding events result in the transport of phytotoxin molecules and probably not all forms of transported toxin are capable of inhibiting protein synthesis. This suggests that a subpopulation of specific toxin binding sites is responsible for biologically relevant transport of the toxins, a finding similar to that for diphtheria toxin.

3.4.4. Role of Toxin Fragments

The role of the B-chain in determining the specificity of the toxin action has been examined with hybrid forms of the toxin in a manner similar to that used for diphtheria toxin (Olsnes and Pihl, 1982; Thorpe and Ross, 1982). Protein synthesis in mouse macrophages is inhibited by ricin A-chain·B-chain·AntiB-chain I_gG complexes but not by AntiA·I_gG·ricin A·B complexes which have no A-chain enzymatic activity (Refsnes and Munthe–Kaas, 1976). The toxicity of the first complex is abolished by the addition of soluble I_gG-antiI_gG complexes and is therefore F_c receptor mediated. The efficiency of ricin-antibody complexes is impaired compared to the free toxin, but the effect of blockage of the F_c receptor indicates that the phagocytosed enzymatically active material still will undergo internalization into the cytosolic compartment in a significant quantity. These results are similar to some of the earlier work of this type with diphtheria toxin. A more convincing demonstration of the role of the B-chain of ricin was presented by Oeltmann and Heath (1979) who chemically crosslinked the binding subunit of human chorionic gonadotropin (hCG) via a —S—S— linkage to the A-chain of ricin. Using either isolated rat Leydig cells or a R2C Leydig tumor cell line capable of binding hCG and mouse L cells which do not bind gonadotropin, the hybrid toxin inhibited protein synthesis only in the Leydig cells. This toxicity was blocked by the addition of hCG to the Leydig cells. Both cell types were susceptible to intact ricin: Thus, it is apparent that the B-chain is an important determinant in the specificity of toxin action towards different cell types and that the difference in the specificities of abrin, ricin, and modeccin probably resides in the B-chain of the toxins.

3.4.5. Receptor Moiety

The binding site specificity for abrin and ricin are quite similar but not identical involving D-galactose residues in both cases with each toxin molecule possessing one binding site for monomeric β-D-galactopyranoside, $K_a \sim 10^4$ M^{-1} at 20°C (van Wauwe et al., 1973). D-mannose, L-fucose, and N-acetyl-D-glucosamine are inactive as inhibitors of binding. Binding to carbohydrate also induces a conformational change in the toxin molecule which is temperature dependent. This change could be related to an early step in the irreversible association of toxin with the membrane. Comparing the low affinity of the toxins for the monomeric sugar to the high affinity for their membrane receptor, $\sim 10^8$ M^{-1} (HeLa), it is likely that the true receptor molecule contains D-galactose incorporated into a sequence of carbohydrate residues. Terminal galactose residues are apparently required. Sialic acid-blocked chains are inactive as a competitor of receptors unless the sialylated sequences are first treated with neuraminidase. This enzymatic treatment of HeLa cells can increase the number of abrin binding sites 2.3-fold and the number of modeccin binding sites ten-fold (Olsnes et al., 1978; Refsnes et al., 1977). Gangliosides have also been found to bind abrin and ricin when incorporated into liposomes, $K_a \sim 10^6$ M^{-1} at $4°$ (Surolin et al., 1975). Although Olsnes et al. (1978) found that added gangliosides did not prevent any of the three toxins from binding to HeLa cells, they did not specify whether the toxins were preincubated with the gangliosides or whether the cells were preincubated, then exposed to the toxins. In the latter case, the amphipathic ganglioside molecules could insert into the bilayer and act as receptors themselves (see later section on cholera toxin and GM_1), whereas the former type of experiment should prevent binding of toxin to the cells if gangliosides compete for the binding sites.

The possibility of a glycoprotein receptor containing oligosaccharide units attached by various linkages was addressed in two ways. Simple inhibition of binding was assessed (Olsnes et al., 1978) by adding several desialylated serum glycoproteins to HeLa cells (Table 1); T-antigen (O, NN blood group antigen), fetuin, α_1-acid glycoprotein, and mucin. After normalization to molar galactose content, the data showed all of these proteins to be more effective than free galactose. In addition, it was clear from the relative abilities to prevent binding of the toxins that abrin, ricin, and modeccin have different carbohydrate specificities for binding. This implies that there are different receptor molecules for each of the toxins although they may have some structural similarities.

Support for the notion of separate receptor molecules for each of the toxins is available from the study of mutants resistant to the action of one or more of the toxins. CHO cells (Gottlieb et al., 1974), BHK cells (Meager et al., 1975), and HeLa cell variants have been isolated by selective growth in toxin-containing media or by ultraviolet irradiation followed by growth in a selective medium. Mutants deficient in receptor number due either to the lack of the proper glycosyl transferase or to excess sialic acid incorporation as well as mutants in the internalization process were obtained by these procedures. Some of the mutants were sensitive to a particular toxin with few or minimal effects on the sensitivity to the other toxins. One HeLa cell line, R^R III (Olsnes et al., 1978), was initially resistant to 5,000 times as much of all three plant toxins as well as to diphtheria toxin than the wild type cells. Neuraminidase treatment of these cells regenerated the original sensitivities to diphtheria toxin and modeccin. The enzyme treated cells retained a resistance to 10–15 times more abrin and ricin than the wild type cells, although the number of binding sites for abrin and ricin returned to the wild type level. This observation again argues for the presence of more than one type of receptor with the same carbohydrate moiety, one (or more) which will allow biologically relevant internalization of the toxins and another type of nonspecific binding site. The regulation of expression of these sites is distinguishable on the basis of the experiments involving mutagenesis and selection.

Glycoproteins have been implicated in the receptor moiety for the abrin, ricin, and modeccin phytotoxins by several groups (Olsnes et al., 1976; Nicolson et al., 1976). Lactoperoxidase-catalyzed iodination of cell surface reactive tyrosine residues or in vivo (tissue culture) labeling with radioactive sugars of BW 5147 murine lymphoma cells and mutant cells possessing 30–50 % of the BW 5147 parent cell high affinity ricin binding sites revealed the conversion of a labeled 80,000 m.w. polypeptide into a 70,000 m.w. polypeptide and a diminution in the amount of a 35,000 m.w. polypeptide (m.w. by SDS— gel electrophoresis) in the mutant cells (Robbins et al., 1977). The 80,000 m.w. and 70,000 m.w. polypeptides both bind to ricin-Sepharose when solubilized from the cells with the nonionic detergent Nonidet P40. Finally, an antibody preparation made against the total membrane protein complement of the parent cell line will precipitate both the parental 80,000 m.w. polypeptide and the mutant cell 70,000 m.w. polypeptide (Nicolson and Poste, 1978; Robbins et al., 1977). The fact that the same pattern of proteins are generated both by the endogenous labeling of glycoproteins with radioactive sugar residues and by the membrane surface-accessible iodination lends credence to the idea of the structural difference of the mutant residing in the apparent change in molecular weight of the ricin binding proteins. An alternative explanation for the apparent change in molecular weight might be a change in the glycosylation of the glycoproteins which often migrate anomalously upon SDS— gel electrophoresis. In erythrocytes the Band III group of glycoproteins, m.w. 100,000, will bind abrin and ricin (Hyman *et al.*, 1974). These proteins, which include anion and glucose transport systems, also correspond to the intramembranous particles (Triche *et al.*, 1975). Glycophorin, one of the constituents of the intramembranous particles, is sialylated and does not bind abrin and ricin. Unfortunately, merely binding the toxins is not sufficient evidence for the identification of a biologically relevant receptor molecule. The receptor function of these proteins remains as a postulate.

For the four phytotoxins discussed, abrin, ricin, viscumin, and modeccin, it is possible that a relatively nonspecific mechanism for competent uptake may be operating (but not for diphtheria toxin) where any membrane associated molecule that appears to possess the appropriate carbohydrate residues would be a receptor. Only a certain percentage of these receptors would be associated with internalization machinery at any particular time. This view could be supported by the observation that ricin A-β-chain hCG is effective on cells with the appropriate receptor while diphtheria toxin A fragment-β-chain hCG is nontoxic in cells that should respond and contain gonadotropin receptor. Equally likely, however, for the phytotoxins is that the Band III complex with its associated transport functions is a true receptor and its normal transport duties facilitate the entry of the A-chain of the bound toxin molecules. A precedent for this can be found with the colicin E2, E3 system where the vitamin B_{12} transport protein is the receptor moiety for these bacteriocidal molecules as well as for several phages (Holland, 1977). These toxins take advantage of the properties of a transport protein to penetrate the complicated Gram-negative cell surface. Some specific process of this type may be operating in the abrin—ricin—modeccin system since endocytosis cannot account for the insensitivity of abrin and ricin intoxication to ammonium salts (Sandvig *et al.*, 1979). Although pinocytosis has not been ruled out, other mechanisms such as phagocytosis may serve as a default for it. This contrast with the diphtheria toxin and possibly the modeccin situation where ammonium salts prevent entry into the cells and subsequent intoxication, leading one to believe that endocytosis is important for these two toxins. Whether these differences are real or apparent will have to be decided by future experiments on the details of early events after the binding of toxin molecules to the membrane and their subsequent fate.

3.5. *SHIGELLA SHIGAE* CYTOTOXIN

Shigella shigae strains produce at least three distinguishable toxic activities, a neurotoxin, an enterotoxin, and a cytotoxin. Of these, the latter has been characterized most completely.

3.5.1. *Properties of the Toxin*

The native toxin, m.w. 68,000, is composed of a 30,500 m.w. disulfide cross-linked chain and six to seven B chains of approximately 5,000 m.w. (Olsnes *et al.*, 1981). A_1 fragment, a 27,000 m.w. proteolytic derivative of the A chain, is capable of enzymatically irreversibly inactivating the 60S component of 80S ribosomes in cell lysates but is non-toxic to whole cells. Unlike other toxins, the isolated B chain fails to bind to cells or block toxicity of holotoxin; however, the same phenomenon of binding subunit inactivation after dissociation of protein subunits is also observed for the glycoprotein hormones.

3.5.2. *Intracellular Intoxication Process*

The lethal activity of the toxin derives from its ability to inhibit protein synthesis. Unlike the plant toxins abrin and ricin which can modify isolated 60S ribosomal subunits, Shigella cytotoxin requires the assembled 80S ribosomal, much like colicin E_3 which modifies the 30S bacterial ribosomal subunit only when it is coupled with the 50S subunit (Holland, 1977). The function inhibited is the elongation of the polypeptide chain but not the ability to form a peptide bond, while an effect on chain initiation has not yet been ruled out.

3.5.3. *Binding and Penetration of the Toxin*

Development of cytotoxic effects in susceptible cell lines shows a characteristic dose-dependent lag phase during the early part of which the toxin is susceptible to added antibody, followed by irreversible fixation of toxin (Keusch *et al.*, 1972). This sequestration and development of toxicity is impeded by low temperature and various metabolic inhibitors, suggestive of an active process for uptake. Inhibitors of microfilament and microtubule function and corticosteroids also blunt toxin action. Ammonium chloride and chloroquine, which appear to interfere with lysosomal and endocytic vesicle function similarly inhibit (Keusch *et al.*, 1982). Putative transglutaminase inhibitors are less effective. Given what is known about cellular uptake of other toxins, there seems to be ample evidence for involvement of receptor-mediated (see next section) endocytosis in the uptake of Shigella cytotoxin. HeLa S3 cells (sensitive) contain up to 1.3×10^6 sites per cell while an insensitive clone possessed only 2.5×10^5 sites per cell. Both receptor affinities were in the range of 10^{-10} M. On the other hand, resistant cell lines including some other human carcinoma cell lines or non-epithelial cells from a variety of human and animal tissue showed no detectable binding (Eiklid and Olsnes, 1980).

3.5.4. *Receptor Moiety*

The initial event in toxin fixation by cells is binding to a surface receptor containing oligomeric N-acetyl-D-glucosamine. Susceptibility to proteolytic enzymes or lysozyme but not neuraminidase, galactose oxidase, or β-galactosidase suggested a glycoprotein moiety. Competitive inhibition studies with soluble mono- or oligo-saccharide ligands showed that only oligomeric lysozyme substrates of (N-acetyl-glucosamine)3–4 were effective inhibitors of cytotoxin toxicity. Finally, several lectins with different monosaccharide specificities; phytohemagutanin (N-acetyl-galactosamine) or concanavalin A (α-methylmannoside) were ineffective while wheat germ agglutinin (N-acetyl-glucosamine) inhibited toxic action (Keusch and Jacewicz, 1977). This chitotriose-like receptor concept has been utilized in affinity purification of the toxin (Keusch *et al.*, 1977).

4. BACTERIAL TOXINS AFFECTING THE NERVOUS SYSTEM

This section will deal with two bacterial toxins which have their loci of action in the nervous system. Although the particular part of the nervous system attacked is not the same, these differences may be more apparent than real in term of the molecular mechanism of action at the nerve terminal for the tetanus and botulinum toxins. Both toxins have presynaptic target sites and result in the blockade of Ca^{2+}-dependent neurotransmitter release (Bigalke *et al.*, 1978). The route of introduction of the toxic substances, the different types of nerves involved, and the physical pathways of the neural network may govern the characteristic expression of tetanus or botulism. The following section will attempt to emphasize the homology of the mechanisms of the toxic actions of these two proteins.

4.1. CLOSTRIDIUM TETANI TOXIN

4.1.1. *Properties of the Toxin*

Tetanus toxin is a single polypeptide chain of m.w. 150,000 (Mangalo *et al.*, 1968) containing six free—SH groups and two disulfide linkages (Bizzini *et al.*, 1970) produced by some *Clostridium tetani* strains and released upon cell autolysis and in the presence of O_2

(Vinet and Fredette, 1970). Although initially secreted as a single polypeptide chain, clostridial proteases of the culture medium or *in vitro* treatment with papain nick the polypeptide into fragments which upon reduction and SDS gel electrophoresis under denaturing conditions give a light 50,000 m.w., α-chain, and a heavier 100,000 m.w. β-chain (Bizzini, 1978). Gangliosides, specifically GD_{1b} and G_{T1}, were determined to fix and detoxify the tetanus toxin (van Heyningen, 1961). Subsequently, a subfragment of 47,000 m.w. derived via protease digestion from the β-chain was found to be the portion of the toxin responsible for the interaction with ganglioside (Bizzini, 1978; van Heyningen, 1976). By analogy with other bacterial toxins, and the lack of toxicity of the β-chain alone, the α-chain was proposed as the toxic component (van Heyningen, 1976). Unfortunately, as an assay for the biochemical target of the toxic action in broken cells has yet to be developed, this hypothesis has not been tested directly.

4.1.2. *Intracellular Intoxication Process*

Tetanus toxin is transported intra-axonally along motor neurons from the muscle injection site (the usual route of exposure) up to its site of action in the central nervous system. The toxin is taken up by the motor nerve endings and migrates along the corresponding nerve trunk via the ventral roots and fibers within the spinal cord. This retrograde transport of toxin is unique to this molecule as will be discussed in a later section. Movement within the nerve fibers is rapid, reaching velocities approaching 5 mm per hr (Habermann, 1970). Although toxin carried by this route can reach the brain stem, free toxin in the blood stream does not cross the blood-brain barrier (Stöckel *et al.*, 1975). The toxin is not found among the glial elements or in the extracellular space surrounding the nerve fibers but is concentrated along the nerve fiber route. Only a small proportion of the toxin injected into a muscle, 1 %, is taken up and transported, with the remainder either fixed at the site of injection or excreted (Habermann, 1970). Blood levels are extremely low. Subsequent to its transport into the central nervous system, the toxin passes trans-synaptically to the nerve terminals of the spinal neurons impinging on the dendrites of the peripheral motor neuron. This is the point at which the toxin blocks the release of the inhibitory neurotransmitter glycine. This blockade destroys inhibitory input to the motor neurons causing hyperactivity of these neurons with tetanic muscle contraction as a result. A number of events, while effectively described, are not defined on a molecular level. The toxin's primary effect *in vivo* is on inhibitory neurons, specifically on the glycine but not gamma aminobutyric acid (GABA) synapses (Osborne and Bradford, 1973). Secretion of glycine is interfered with presynaptically, causing accumulation of flattened vesicles (inhibitory vesicles) in the presynaptic terminals and a decrease in chloride and potassium permeability causing a depolarization of the terminal). These effects are distinct from processes on the postsynaptic membrane. Sensitivity to glycine is unaffected by tetanus intoxication (Curtis and deGroat, 1968) whereas strychnine, a classical glycine receptor antagonist (Young and Snyder, 1974) blocks function, mimicking tetanus symptomology. The focus of the toxin lesion appears to lie in the chemically mediated synaptic transmission mechanism. Acetylcholine-mediated synaptic transmission is similarly disturbed by tetanus toxin presynaptically (local muscle tetanus). Acetylcholine is metabolized and taken up by toxin-treated synapses normally, but none is released although sensitivity to externally applied acetylcholine remains (Bigalke *et al.*, 1978). thus, the effect of the toxin may be on the events leading to the fusion of synaptic vesicles and release of their contents at specific sites in the presynaptic membrane, an event common to both inhibitory and excitatory terminals. A general membrane effect rendering the neurons incapable of nerve impulse transmission is ruled out by the observation that toxin-blocked synapses respond normally to direct (electrical) stimulation (Kryzhanovsky *et al.*, 1974 as referenced in Bizzini, 1977).

Kryzhanovsky *et al.* (1974) as referenced in Bizzini 1977 have presented evidence for tetanus toxin binding to and altering some of the properties of an 'actomyosin-like' protein localized specifically in the synaptic membrane (Puszkin and Berl, 1972; Bizzini, 1979). This contractile protein displays Ca^{2+}, Mg^{2+}-ATPase activity and has been postulated to respond to the passive influx of calcium during nervous impulse transmission by contraction with concomitant release of neurotransmitter from vesicles. This contractability and ATPase activity are inhibited by bound tetanus toxin, and the effect of the toxin may be partially overcome by high concentrations of ATP. In lieu of further analysis this observation would suggest that the affinity of the actomyosin for ATP is lowered. Although the actomyosin-like protein may represent the toxin target, much more work needs to be done to clarify this. Tetanus toxin appears to alter the synaptosomal membrane potential (Ramos *et al.*, 1979), an observation which is consistent with the actomyosin-like ATPase protein target.

4.1.3. *Binding and Penetration of the Toxin*

The binding of tetanus toxin to specific gangliosides is well established (van Heyningen, 1961; van Heyningen, 1976; Helting *et al.*, 1977; van Heyningen, 1959). N-acetyl-neuraminic acid (sialic acid) residues are important in the interaction, fixation requiring the presence of at least two sialic acid residues one of which is coupled to lactose via a neuraminidase-sensitive bond (van Heyningen and Miller, 1961). The predominant gangliosides of nervous tissue are those possessing toxin binding activity, with G_{D1b} and G_{T1} being the most potent (van Heyningen, 1961). In addition, ganglioside-bound tetanus toxin is taken up by cells (Bizzini *et al.*, 1977; Yavin *et al.*, 1981). Neuronal cells from all parts of the nervous system will bind tetanus toxin (Mirsky *et al.*, 1978) implying that specificity of action is regulated at some step subsequent to binding. In contrast to cholera toxin, bound tetanus toxin does not protect the sialic acid residues from digestion by neuraminidase. Treatment with this enzyme will release bound tetanus toxin from the membrane.

Binding of the toxin via the β-chain has been shown to be required for expression of toxin activity as the separate chains are not toxic to whole cells (Bizzini, 1978). As demonstrated for diphtheria toxin (previous section), portions of the toxin subserve different functions (Morris *et al.*, 1980). A hydrophobic domain on the 50,000 m.w. terminal polypeptide of the heavy chain (β) will cause ion channel formation in synthetic lipid vesicles at low pH (Boquet and Duflot, 1982). Thus, penetration of the toxin may be enhanced in the acidified environment of endocytic vesicles as has been suggested for diphtheria toxin (Donovan *et al.*, 1981, 1982) and the asialoglycoprotein receptor (Blumenthal *et al.*, 1980).

Antitoxin antibodies interact with the toxin molecule affecting toxicity and binding to gangliosides in a complex fashion depending upon the relative concentrations of toxin, antitoxin, ganglioside, and cerebrosides (Bondartchuk *et al.*, 1971; and Kryzhanovski *et al.*, 1970 as referenced in Bizzini, 1977; Helting *et al.*, 1977).

Tetanus toxin and thyrotropin share a similar affinity for G_{D1b} and G_{T1} and affect each others' binding to thyroid plasma membranes (Ledley *et al.*, 1977). This interaction appears to be at the level of the ganglioside component of the thyrotropin receptor complex. Tetanus toxin will bind to liposomes with the specific gangliosides incorporated but not to liposomes containing only the glycoprotein component of the thyrotropin receptor (Lee *et al.*, 1979). This 'naked' receptor in liposomes will bind thyrotropin normally. Some crossreaction of thyrotropin and tetanus toxin is implied *in vivo* with the observation that mice injected subcutaneously (some therefore reaching the bloodstream) with one minimum lethal dose of the toxin respond with an increased release of radioiodine from the prelabeled thyroid (Curtis *et al.*, 1973). This may be an example of an effect of clustering, or co-clustering, on the receptor moieties triggering a response similar to the mimicking of the insulin response of adipocytes by multivalent anti-insulin receptor antibodies (Jacobs *et al.*, 1978).

Zimmerman and Piffaretti (1977) have studied the initial events associated with tetanus toxin binding to mouse neuroblastoma cells. These cells were chosen to represent the nervous system on the basis of their capability to elaborate neurotransmitters, generate action potentials in response to electrical stimulation *in vitro*, and to produce neuronal processes (differentiate) upon serum deprivation. Two classes of receptors were distinguished based on the ability to bind toxin molecules, to cause the cells to internalize these molecules, and to respond by withdrawing neuronal processes and becoming detached from the substratum.

The loss of adhesiveness was determined not be related to cell death. Binding and internalization of the toxin molecule as detected by assay with ^{125}I-tetanus toxin and with fluorescently tagged antitetanus toxin antibodies (after intoxication) are not sufficient for toxic expression. Patching of bound toxin molecules on the cell surface is prevented by the addition of toxin-anti-toxin complex which may destroy multivalent interactions between a toxin molecule and several ganglioside molecules as is the case for cholera toxin. When the cells are treated with neuraminidase or β-galactosidase, binding to sites which are internalized but that do not cause process retraction in differentiating cells is no longer detectable. The toxin sites modified by these treatments probably correspond to material destined for destruction in lysosomal vesicles. Stimulation of pinocytosis by polyanions increases the uptake of ineffectually bound toxin without an increase in the response or sensitivity of the cells. Ammonium chloride treatment prevented clustering and uptake of toxin in cells incubated under growth conditions with serum while preventing detectable binding, uptake, or biological effect on differentiated cells in serum-free medium. These results suggest that the biologically relevant receptor is relatively resistant to digestion with neuraminidase and β-galactosidase and that uptake of the toxin molecule by a mechanism other than routine pinocytosis is required for biological expression. The diffuse binding patterns observed upon enzyme treatment and the interpretation derived therefrom are, of course, subject to the limited sensitivity of fluorescence microscopy. Reduction of the number of binding sites to a few thousand or even a few tens of thousands if diffusely distributed would not be detectable by their fluorescence although that number of binding sites would be perfectly within the range of the number of specific binding sites found on HeLa cells for diphtheria toxin. Nevertheless, this work has addressed the question of specific vs. non-specific sites and serves as an important statement of progress in this area.

Ultrastructural studies (Montesano *et al.*, 1981) indicate that at least in a liver cell system, tetanus toxin is not taken up through a coated pit-mediated process. However, this is a non-neural tissue and may lack part of the transport system. Chloroquine, which is proportioned to block part of the cellular internalization process including lysosomal processing, is ineffective against tetanus blockage of neuromuscular transmission in intact tissue, while it does interfere with diphtheria toxin in the same preparation which is believed to follow such a route (Simpson, 1982).

In line with the effects of neuraminidase, it is not unexpected that tetanus toxin coinjected with neuraminidase is taken up and transported effectively with its normal toxic effects (Habermann and Erdmann, 1978).

4.1.4. *Retrograde Axonal Transport and Selective Retrograde Trans-synaptic Transfer*

A variety of molecules are known to be more or less specifically taken up at nerve endings and transported within a given neuron. These include such diverse materials as cholera toxin, wheat germ agglutinin (Stöckel *et al.*, 1977; Schwab *et al.*, 1979), ricin, phytohemagglutinin (Schwab *et al.*, 1979; Dumas *et al.*, 1979a,b) antibodies raised against adrenergic neuron dopamine β-hydroxylase (Fillenz *et al.*, 1976), and nerve growth factor (NGF) (Dumas *et al.*, 1979b). Uptake and transport of these toxins and lectins follow a pattern common to all peripheral and central neurons. NGF, on the other hand, is specifically taken up and transported only by peripheral adrenergic and sensory neurons (Stöckel *et al.*, 1975). Antibodies to the dopamine β-hydroxylase are taken up exclusively by adrenergic neurons (Fillenz *et al.*, 1976). Tetanus toxin is taken up by all peripheral and central neurons (Stöckel *et al.*, 1977; Schwab *et al.*, 1977), although classically by motor neurons, and is transported via smooth vesicles and smooth endoplasmic reticulum-like tubules and cisternae. This mode of transport is indistinguishable from that of all of the previously mentioned materials as well as horseradish peroxidase, ferritin, and colloidal thorium oxide. The apparent fate of these vesicles containing these materials is to fuse with lysosomes (Bunge, 1977; Weldon, 1975). However, in the case of tetanus toxin, a sizeable proportion of toxin-containing vesicles or cisternae fuse with the membrane in the synaptic terminal releasing their contents which are then bound to the presynaptic terminal membrane (Schwab *et al.*, 1979). This trans-synaptic transfer appears to be the point at which the toxin specificity is manifested. The signal distinguishing toxin-containing vesicles from those containing other materials is not known but may be part of the toxin molecule itself (Grob et al., 1980; Bizzini et al., 1981), perhaps a portion of the molecule spanning the bilayer or it may be a function of the putative receptor for the toxin molecule. Transfer of the entire toxin molecule is achieved, measured radiochemically, immunologically, and by subsequent repeat bioassay (Habermann et al., 1977). However, only a small percentage of the molecules are transported across the synapse and these may be altered in some subtle way undetectable in the average. The transfer may also occur through a chain of two neurons (Dumas et al., 1979a). The neural ascent of toxin molecules and toxic action is blocked by agents or treatments that interfere with axoplasmic flow, i.e. nerve ligation and colchicine treatment, indicating that some molecular component must be transported to the dendritic region.

The possibility that tetanus toxin may be taking advantage of pathways normally used in the anterograde and retrograde exchange of specific signals between neurons, or neurons and their target organs is an intriguing one. It may be possible to use tetanus toxin as a probe of this trophic signal transfer as well as some of the processes involved in the release of neurotransmitters (Schwab, 1980).

4.2. CLOSTRIDIUM BOTULINUM TOXIN TYPE A

Clostridium botulinum produces a variety of neurotoxins (types A through F) which differ in size, antigenicity, and heat stability. The Type A toxin is the most toxic and the most heavily investigated of this group (Simpson, 1977) and thus will be the focus of this next section. What is known about its mechanism of action suggests that the tetanus and botulinum toxins share at least a similar strategy in the disruption of nervous impulse transmission (Bigalke et al., 1978).

4.2.1. Properties of the Toxin

Botulinum type A toxin has been purified and shown to be a single component of m.w. 150,000 (Boroff and DasGupta, 1971, Simpson, 1981) which may be cleaved into two smaller fragments of m.w. 97,000 and 53,000 by treatment with thiols (DasGupta and Sugiyama, 1972). Whether or not these fragments represent a single polypeptide chain which was subsequently cleaved to yield fragments held together by disulfide bond(s) releasable by reduction is unknown. The reduced fragments are inactive against whole cells as were the cytotoxic toxins discussed in previous sections. Much of the structural chemistry of botulinum toxin is unresolved since the neurotoxic properties are extremely labile. Workers have concentrated on the pharmacology of toxin action and on its use as a tool to study the cholinergic synapse.

4.2.2. Binding and Intoxication Process

The physiological site of action of botulinum toxin was early discovered to be nerve endings in the peripheral nervous system rather than in the brain (Dickson and Shevky, 1923a; Dickson and Shevky, 1923b; Edmunds and Long, 1923; Schubel, 1923). Three major sites of action were defined; 1) nerve endings of preganglionic fibers from the parasympathetic and sympathetic autonomic nervous system, 2) nerve endings of postganglionic fibers of the parasympathetic nervous system, and 3) nerve endings of motor fibers that innervate striated muscle. Despite this knowledge, the molecular locus of the toxin action has not been fixed with certainty. A postsynaptic target has been eliminated from consideration by the fact that the acetylcholinesterase is not inhibited by toxin treatment, and that the responsiveness of a synapse to exogenous acetylcholine is undiminished (Guyton and MacDonald, 1947). Likewise, presynaptic effects on the metabolism of acetylcholine, such as the uptake of choline by the nerve terminal and resynthesis into acetylcholine can be explained by consideration of a feedback mechanism involving unreleased acetylcholine

(Gundersen and Howard, 1978). The current belief is that botulinum toxin acts by preventing the release of acetylcholine from the cholinergic nerve terminals, first demonstrated by Burgen *et al.* (1949). However, the mechanism by which this is accomplished is not clear at this time.

Toxin-induced paralysis of the neuromuscular junction can be divided into two stages (Simpson, 1974). The first stage involves the binding of the toxin which displays a weak temperature dependence and is poorly reversible but blockable by the presence of antitoxic antibody. The binding event is not facilitated by transmitter release (nerve stimulation), a characteristic of botulinum intoxication (Hughes and Whaler, 1962). The second stage involves the highly temperature dependent processing of the toxin into an irreversibly bound form (or environment) that is unaffected by antitoxin antibody, and is dependent upon nervous stimulation.

The presence of chloroquine inhibits the internalization process, maintaining the toxin in an antitoxin-sensitive site and preventing expression of toxicity (Simpson, 1982). Direct binding studies subsequently have excluded a direct effect on toxin binding (Williams *et al.*, 1983).

The requirement for nervous stimulation for toxicity expression has been shown to be coupled with membrane changes associated with release of acetylcholine rather than changes associated with the nerve action potential (Simpson, 1971; Simpson, 1973). Botulinum toxin paralysis does not effect sodium flux, the resting membrane potential, the propagation of the action potential, or the transmembrane flux of calcium (Simpson, 1978). Although the toxin can block neurotransmitter release triggered by intracellular calcium, this may be overcome by extremely high (10–20 mM) extracellular calcium in the presence of the calcium ionophore A23187 (Wonnacott *et al.*, 1978). It is possible that the toxin could, directly or indirectly, inhibit the loading of acetylcholine into synaptic vesicles (Boroff *et al.*, 1974), since there appears to be preferential release of 'old' acetylcholine before newly resynthesized material (Gundersen and Howard, 1978). Experiments with black widow toxin and batrachotoxin showed that separate pools of vesicles containing acetylcholine either do not exist or are in relatively rapid equilibrium. The spider venom-induced release is not blocked by botulinum toxin, and it exhausts batrachotoxin (sodium channel)-releaseable acetylcholine. Botulinum toxin, on the other hand, blocks batrachotoxin-induced release (Simpson, 1978). Hanig and Lamanna (1979) proposed a model in which botulinum toxin physically blocks efflux of acetylcholine by attaching stoichiometrically to the finite number of active sites on the end plate for efflux of acetylcholine-containing vesicles. This binding event is postulated to occur at the moment of vesicle fusion with the presynaptic membrane which exposes a receptor-site. This model is based upon the agreement of the number of toxin molecules reaching the implate after a minimum lethal dose, the number of vesicles released per impulse, and the number of active release sites on the synaptic membrane. While based primarily upon theoretical calculations, the model has predictive potential and should help in designing future investigations.

Other experiments suggest a more indirect interference with transmitter release (Gundersen *et al.*, 1981).

4.2.3. *Receptor Moiety*

The binding site for botulinum toxin has been demonstrated to be at least related to certain gangliosides. Particular gangliosides have been shown to neutralize botulinum toxin toxicity (Simpson and Rapport, 1971a,b) ($G_{T1} > G_{D1a} > G_{D1b} > G_{M1} > G_{M2} >$ asialoG_{M1} > asialoG_{M2}). While this sequence resembles that for tetanus toxin and thyrotropin it is not identical, with the isomeric G_{D1a} being more effective than G_{D1b} in preventing binding and toxicity.

Recently, a preparation of the toxin labeled to high specific radioactivity (1 mole ^{125}I per mole) retaining up to 85 % of its original biological activity has been obtained (Williams *et al.*, 1983). These workers were able to demonstrate a high affinity (0.6 nM), low capacity (60 fmol/mg) probably proteinaceous binding site on rat cerebrocortical synaptosomes that could be abolished by protease treatment or by heating. A large number of low affinity sites were also detected, Kd > 25 nM, but these were not affected by the heat or protease treatment. Neuramidinase treatment reduced binding to both types of sites over 70% suggesting that sialic acid is involved in the binding moiety. The involvement of gangliosides in the lower affinity binding (that studied by previous workers) is quite probable although the high affinity binding is unaltered by preincubation of synaptosomes with gangliosides. High affinity binding activity resides in the 97,000 m.w. subunit of the toxin and is specific in that the related Type B botulinum toxin or a number of other presynaptic neurotoxins do not compete for high affinity binding sites although at high concentrations tetanus toxin has some effect. This technological advance should speed the inquiry into the identity of the receptor moiety and the molecular mechanism of intoxication.

A glycoprotein could be intimately involved in neurotransmitter secretion process. Botulinum and tetanus toxins could be used to investigate this and any possible homology between excitatory and inhibitory neuro-transmitter secretory processes. Bigalke *et al.* (1978) have stressed the similarities in modes of action of the botulinum and tetanus toxins and propose that routes of exposure (botulinum-blood stream), (tetanus-injection) may play a major role in their selectivity. A major difference between tetanus toxin and botulinum toxin is that the tetanus toxin is transported specifically through a chain of two or more neurons to a site of action while the botulinum toxin is apparently confined to the cholinergic synapse.

Another level of specificity must exist within the toxin molecule itself, to produce this restriction since the same receptor, be it ganglioside or glycoprotein, would bind both toxins. It would be interesting and informative if hybrid nicked tetanus and botulinum toxins ($\alpha_B\beta_T$, $\alpha_T\beta_B$) could be generated as was done for diphtheria toxin, abrin, and ricin and their specificity of toxic activity determined to decide the relative functions of the α and β units. Presumably, the β subunit would be responsible for the binding specificity and perhaps the trans-synaptic specificity as well, although this is merely conjecture at this point. Also, development of procedures to study interactions on the cytosolic side of the dendritic processes of the motor neurons would allow the determination whether the transported toxin was promoting its own "secretion" into the proximal synaptic region, or whether it was taking advantage of some pre-existing pathway in the terminal. Other questions are: Is the retrograde axonal transport of toxin and processing required for toxicity at the inhibitory nerve ending? What is the nature of the interaction of the toxin with the inhibitory terminal? Are gangliosides involved at this point? What is the fate of the previously bound ganglioside? All of these questions require an answer before we will understand the true similarities and differences between the tetanus and botulinum toxins.

5. ENTEROTOXINS

Another group of toxins are elaborated by several enteric bacteria. These enterotoxins characteristically produce a hypersecretion of fluid from the intestinal mucosa by a mechanism independent of cytolytic events. The efflux of water is passive following the active secretion of chloride ions into the intestinal lumen (Field *et al.*, 1969). Early work had shown that the enteric application of 3'-5'-cyclic AMP (cAMP) to the luminal surface generated a similar sequence of events (Field *et al.*, 1968a; Field *et al.*, 1968b). In general, these toxins are considered to exert their effects by perturbations of the cylic nucleotide system at the level of the cyclizing enzyme. As such, the enterotoxins have become a valuable diagnostic tool in the study of the rule of cyclic nucleotides in cellular processes. The following sections will deal with cholera toxin, and the *Escherichia coli* heat-labile and heat-stable toxins. The *Shigella* and *Salmonella* exotoxins which are discussed in other reviews in this volume have insufficient data published on receptors for consideration here.

5.1. *VIBRIO CHOLERAE* ENTEROTOXIN

Vibrio cholerae produces a heat-labile exotoxin, choleragen, that is capable of inducing the massive water fluxes and diarrhoea characteristic of clinical cholera. This toxin has been the prototype for the study of enterotoxins in general and a great deal of work has been done on its association with cells and the mechanism of action on its target, the adenylate cyclase enzyme found in the luminal plasma membrane of intestinal cells and in the plasma membrane of virtually all other cell types (Bennett and Cuatrecasas, 1977).

5.1.1. *Properties of the Toxin*

Compared to the other toxins discussed in earlier sections of this review choleragen is a complicated multisubunit molecule of m.w. 84,000 (LoSpalluto and Finkelstein, 1972). Functionally it may be divided into a binding domain (B subunits) and a catalytic or active domain (A subunit). The binding domain is composed of 5 to 6 identical monomers m.w. 8,000–10,000 which self-associate in a ring structure. The ring associates with the A subunit (Gill, 1976a) to form a molecular assembly which is toxic to whole cells (Cuatrecasas *et al.*, 1973). The B subunit assembly, choleragenoid (m.w. 56,000) is non-toxic by itself and will associate with cell surfaces blocking a subsequent binding of choleragen. This multisubunit binding component allows for multivalent binding to receptors in the cell membrane. The significance of this possibility will be discussed in a later section. The A subunit of choleragen is a hydrophobic protein of m.w. 36,000 which is itself a dimer linked by an S—S linkage. The A_1 polypeptide (26,000 m.w.) possesses the toxic activity of the choleragen molecule. The function of the A_2 fragment (m.w. 8,000–10,000) is not known with certainty, although it may serve to inactivate the ADP-ribosyltransferase activity of the A_1 polypeptide until the A subunit is exposed to the reducing conditions of the target cell cytosol. The A subunit is toxic by itself to whole cells albeit with extremely poor efficiency (Sahyoun and Cuatrecasas, 1975). Thus, the role of the B subunit seems to be to bind to receptors and to localize the attached A subunit of the toxin at the surface of the cell membrane.

5.1.2. *Intoxication Process*

The A subunit of purified choleragen was shown to possess an NAD^+ hydrolase (Moss *et al.*, 1976c) and ADP-ribosyltransferase activities (Moss and Vaughan, 1977b). The expression of these activities required reducing conditions and therefore presumably the separation of the A_1 and A_2 polypeptides. Earlier studies had demonstrated that NAD^+ was required in broken cell systems for the expression of toxin activity, the activation of the adenylate cyclase enzyme, and that the A subunit (A_1 under the conditions applied) and not the B subunit contained the toxic activity (Gill, 1975; Gill and King, 1975; van Heyningen and King, 1975; Gill, 1976b; Martin *et al.*, 1977; Johnson and Bourne, 1977). The use of $[\alpha\text{-}^{32}P]$ NAD^+ of high specific radioactivity leads to the identification of a 43,000 m.w. membrane bound polypeptide as the acceptor for covalently bound ADP-ribose in pigeon erythrocyte membranes (Gill and Meren, 1978; Cassel and Pfeuffer, 1978) and a 45,000 m.w. polypeptide and a doublet of polypeptides at 52,000–53,000 m.w. in S49 lymphoma cells (Johnson *et al.*, 1978a). A series of elegant affinity isolation and reconstitution (Cassel and Pfeuffer, 1978) and transfer experiments with mutant S49 cells defective in various components of the hormonally-sensitive adenylate cyclase system (Gill and Meren, 1978; Johnson *et al.*, 1978a; Johnson *et al.*, 1978b) suggest that the ADP-ribosylated proteins are probably involved in altering the adenylate cyclase response. These same proteins are also ADP-ribosylated in whole cells (Hebdon *et al.*, 1980). The ADP-ribosylated component(s) are probably GTP-binding protein(s) (Pfeuffer, 1977; Pfeuffer, 1979) involved in the hormonal activation of the enzyme (Cassel and Selinger, 1977; Cassel *et al.*, 1979).

The state of knowledge concerning the molecular mechanism of cholera toxin activation of adenylate cyclase is intermediate between that of the protein synthesis modifiers diphtheria toxin, pseudomonas toxin, abrin, ricin, and modeccin, whose precise targets are known, soluble and characterized, and that of the tetanus, and botulinum toxins whose targets are largely unknown in molecular terms. Part of the problem with the cholera system has been the small number of adenylate cyclase molecules per cell (probably a few hundred to a few thousand copies), the fact that most of the components involved are membrane-bound and hydrophobic, and the inability to purify (to date) any of the components for characterization. However, the molecular mechanism is presently under intense study from which new understanding should develop.

5.1.3. *Binding and Penetration of the Toxin*

^{125}I-Choleragen binds rapidly, irreversibly and with saturation kinetics to rat liver plasma and microsomal membranes within 15 min at 4°C, and within 5 min at 25°C with levels of toxin < 10^{-10} M (Cuatrecasas, 1973a,b,c). Unlabeled choleragenoid and choleragen when preincubated with the membranes will specifically prevent this binding with an apparent K_i of 10^{-10} M. Similar results obtain for a variety of cells and tissues, see Bennett and Cuatrecasas (1977) for examples and references. The true binding affinity is difficult to determine because in analogy to diphtheria toxin, a portion of the membrane-bound choleragen is permanently attached to the membrane (Cuatrecasas, 1973b) and is inaccessible to exogenously applied anticholeragen antibody (Gill, 1976b). This is, however, not due to the classical internalization process which leads to degradation of surface adsorbed molecules in lysosomes. Classical internalization of cholera toxin has not, in general, been observed and is apparently not required for toxin action since intoxication occurs with erythrocytes (Bennett and Cuatrecasas, 1975a) which are not capable of endocytosis. Neural elements which appear to transport adsorbed materials intra-axonally in a retrograde fashion will take up and transport choleragen (Stöckel et al., 1977; Schwab et al., 1979) but this material is apparently not biologically active in the neuron.

The binding site for choleragen on the cell surface has been determined to be a carbohydrate portion of a specific ganglioside, G_{M1}, by a variety of observations of neutralization (van Heyningen et al., 1971; Pierce, 1973), competitive binding and antagonist activity (Cuatrecasas, 1973b; King and van Heyningen, 1973), and increase in binding and biological effects by incorporation of exogenous G_{M1} or its enzymatic generation in cell membranes (Cuatrecasas, 1973e; Holmgren et al., 1973; King and van Heyningen, 1973; Holmgren et al., 1975; Hollenberg et al., 1974; O'Keefe and Cuatrecasas, 1977; Moss et al., 1976a,b). The lipid moiety also plays a role in the intoxication process since replacing the fatty acyl group with an acetyl group increases the efficacy of the toxin in cells (Fishman et al., 1980). Although a number of experiments have indicated that the binding of choleragen to some membranes involves the sphingolipid G_{M1}, the involvement of a glycoprotein in the process remains to be excluded concretely, especially in the light of recent studies showing the possible role of gangliosides and a glycoprotein with the binding of TSH and its subsequent biological action. The possible involvement of proteins in the binding and processing of cholera toxin will be discussed in more detail in the subsequent section explicitly concerned with choleragen receptors.

After binding to the cell surface, cholera toxin undergoes a time- and temperature-dependent change in accessibility on the membrane surface, including a reduction in multivalent potential of the binding and apparent separation of the A subunit from the B subunit (Sahyoun and Cuatrecasas, 1975) and the redistribution of receptor and choleragen ligands in the plane of the membrane (Craig and Cuatrecasas, 1975; Sedlacek et al., 1976; Schlessinger et al., 1977). The multivalent attachment of the toxin appears to be an important step in the interaction of choleragen with the cell and the sequence of events leading to adenylate cyclase activation (Bennett et al., 1976; Brady and Fishman, 1979). The A subunit (A_1—S—S—A_2) becomes associated with the bilayer and available for labeling by photochemical glycolipid probes whose reactive group is restricted to the center of the bilayer (Wisnieski and Bramhall, 1979; Wisnieski et al., 1979). The adenylate cyclase-stimulating activity becomes inaccessible to externally applied antibody to choleragen (which is capable of crossreacting with the separated A subunit) with the same time course including a lag phase (Gill and King, 1975). During this period of redistribution there is no activation of adenylate cyclase or ADP-ribosylation. The length of the lag period is dependent upon the concentration of bound toxin and the temperature but cannot be decreased below 20–30 min (Bennett and Cuatrecasas, 1975b; Gill and King, 1975). The lag phase is not due to slow conversion of toxin into an active soluble form and release or secretion of active cellular metabolites (Cuatrecasas, 1973b). Events occurring at this time do so in the presence of inhibitors of RNA synthesis and protein synthesis and disrupters of microtubule and microfilament function (Bennett and Cuatrecasas, 1975b). The choleragen-mediated ADP-ribosylation of the 43,000 m.w. membrane component in pigeon erythro-cytes or a 45,000 m.w. component and doublet of polypeptides around 52,000–53,000 m.w. in $3T3L_1$ fibroblasts also displays a similar lag phase (Hebdon et al., 1980). Addition of a second dose of choleragen to partially activated cells does not affect the length of the lag period (Bennett and Cuatrecasas, 1975b) indicating that the rate-limiting process is not processing of a cell component or inhibitor but the rearrangement of the choleragen A subunit into a form, still membrane bound, that possesses ADP-ribosyltransferase activity and has access to specific cell membrane component substrate(s).

The lag phase may be abolished in favor of a linear time course for adenylate cyclase activation by either using high concentrations of A subunit on whole or broken cells (Sahyoun and Cuatrecasas, 1975) or by abolishing the membrane barrier and adding NAD^+ to the lysate with low concentrations of choleragen (Gill, 1975). The lysate also contains a small 13,000 m.w. (LeVine and Cuatrecasas, 1981) or 20,000 m.w. (Enomoto and Gill, 1979) macromolecular cytosolic factor that is required for both toxin-specific ADP-ribosylation and adenylate cyclase activation. The initial step of binding to ganglioside is circumvented with broken cells as conditions that allow activation of adenylate cyclase promote the dissociation of the toxin molecule and choleragenoid has no effect on the activation process. Thus, the lag phase appears to be a processing of the multisubunit toxin into a dissociated form where the A subunit is capable of ADP ribosyltransferase activity. The ADP-ribosylated membrane component has been shown not to have adenylate cyclase activity (Cassel and Pfeuffer, 1978). Although the mechanism of adenylate cyclase activation by this component is unknown, the ADP-ribosylated polypeptide is believed to be a GTP-binding protein or GTPase important in the regulation of adenylate cyclase activity by hormones. This is consistent with the effects of choleragen on the kinetics of the adenylate cyclase and its response to hormones and nucleotides (Bennett and Cuatrecasas, 1975a; Bennett and Cuatrecasas, 1975b; Gill and King, 1975; Beckman et al., 1974; Bennett et al., 1975a,b). The intoxicated enzyme is stably activated by GTP and its apparent activity is lowered by sodium fluoride, whereas the unmodified form of the enzyme is only slightly stimulated by this nucleotide and is greatly stimulated by NaF.

5.1.4. Receptor Moiety

As was found for diphtheria toxin, there appear to be a variable number of receptors for choleragen on cells. Far fewer choleragen molecules are needed to maximally stimulate the adenylate cyclase than there are binding sites available on the cell surface for a variety of cell types; K_{app} for activation $\sim$1,000–3,000 sites per cell in toad erythrocytes (Bennett and Cuatrecasas, 1975b) cultured melanocytes (O'Keefe and Cuatrecasas, 1974) and fibroblasts (Hollenberg et al., 1974) while the K_{app} for binding was between 20,000 and 50,000 sites per cell. Use of the competive antagonist choleragenoid suggest(s) that these excess binding sites represent equivalent receptors (Bennett et al., 1975b) as was concluded for diphtheria toxin (Habermann and Erdmann, 1978). The function of these extra receptors is not known. While the monosialoganglioside G_{M1} has been shown to bind choleragen with high affinity and to promote binding to and activation of adenylate cyclase when incorporated into membranes deficient in that ganglioside (Hollenberg et al., 1974; Moss et al., 1976a; O'Keefe and Cuatrecasas, 1977) only a small number of these receptors are needed for adenylate cyclase activation. This large discrepancy may be accounted for by the intervention of some other membrane component(s) that may guide the toxin molecule through a normal physiological pathway to the internal surface of the plasma membrane bilayer where the adenylate cyclase and the guanyl nucleotide-dependent regulatory protein reside (Farfel et al., 1979). This pathway may be bypassed as in the situation with broken cells where the ganglioside-specific receptors are not functional. The mechanistic problem remains to explain the transfer of the

A subunit of cholera toxin across the bilayer without endocytosis or related processes and without affecting the barrier properties of the plasma membrane.

Ganglioside causes a change in the circular dichroism spectrum of choleragen upon binding of the oligosaccharide chain to the B subunit(s) (Fishman et al., 1978). This change might facilitate interaction of the A subunit of the toxin with the lipid bilayer and other membrane components. The activation of adenylate cyclase by toxin adsorbed to the external surface of the cell requires the integrity of the cell membrane. Choleragen adsorbed to the surface of intact cells is not capable of activating adenylate cyclase once the cell is broken even when the cytosolic macromolecule, ATP, NAD^+, and reducing agents are supplied. The adsorbed toxin remains bound to the membranes and cytosol from activated cells has no effect on adenylate cyclase activity. Activation of adenylate cyclase occurs in broken cells only when free toxin is added to the lysate and this activation is unaffected by the addition of either ganglioside or choleragenoid. Choleragen remaining bound to whole cells after washing is still capable of activating adenylate cyclase.

The possibility that the A subunit of cholera toxin is associating with membrane macromolecules has been presented in the form of comigration of ^{125}I-choleragen (80% of the label in the A subunit), and adenylate cyclase activity in a nonionic detergent-solubilized preparation corresponding to about 1,000 choleragen molecules per adipocyte only when activation was allowed to take place before solubilization (Bennett et al., 1975b). Adenylate cyclase activity is precipitable by antibody to cholera toxin anti-A subunit only after activation of the adenylate cyclase has taken place (Sahyoun and Cuatrecasas, 1975). Once formed, the macromolecular complex containing choleragen is dissociated only with difficulty and only under specific conditions which are indicative, but not proof, of an association with cytoskeletal elements (Sahyoun et al., 1981). Table 2 shows the conditions required for elution of ^{125}I-labeled cholera toxin bound to pigeon erythrocyte membranes. Under optimal conditions nonionic detergents at low ionic strength at 37°C release only 1/3 of the bound toxin. The solubilized toxin migrates as a complex in the void volume of an Ultrogel 34 gel filtration column (m.w. > 350,000). SDS-polyacrylamide gel electrophoresis reveals that all of the radioactive label co-migrates with authentic ^{125}I-labeled A_1 subunit. Association of choleragen with the cytoskeleton has been demonstrated in studies of patching and capping (Craig and Cuatrecasas, 1975; Schlessinger et al., 1977; Sedlacek et al., 1976) with fluorescently labeled cholera toxin. Whether this sequestration of membrane-bound toxin, is a specific event in the sequence leading to toxin-dependent activation of adenylate cyclase or a mechanistically unimportant artifact related only to the multivalent nature of the toxin-ganglioside interaction is unknown.

The ganglioside-toxin complex within the membrane is capable of perturbing the structure of the bilayer sufficiently to allow previously impermeant molecules to traverse the barrier.

TABLE 2. *Differential Solubilization of ^{125}I-Cholera Toxin Bound to Pigeon Erythrocyte Membranes*

	Treatment* HEPES A	(^{125}I cpm solubilized $\times 10^{-3}$)
(A)	2% Lubrol PX (w/v) in HEPES A	28
(B)	2% Triton X-100 (w/v) in HEPES A	33
(C)	2% Nonidet P40 (w/v) in HEPES A	40
(D)	0.1 mM EDTA, pH 7.6	61
(E)	0.1 mM EDTA, pH 7.6 + 0.2%	
	Triton X-100 (w/v)	520
	(B) after (D)	12
	(D) after (B)	42
	(E) after (B)	580

* Aliquots of membranes containing 1.4×10^6 cpm bound ^{125}I-cholera toxin were treated as described for 30 min at 37°C and then centrifuged at $40,000 \times g_{max}$ at 4°C for 10 min. Composition of HEPES A buffer detailed in Gill (1975).

Binding of choleragen to G_{M1} incorporated into artificial vesicles protects the galactose residues from oxidation by galactose oxidase (Fishman et al., 1977). If the vesicles are preloaded with glucose, either choleragen (Moss et al., 1976b) or choleragenoid (Moss et al., 1977a) engender the release of the trapped marker. The release is specific for G_{M1} as other gangliosides do not substitute. Similarly, planar black lipid membranes of glycerol-monooleate preformed with G_{M1} incorporated reacted to the addition of choleragen by the development of randomly opening and closing ion conducting channels (Tosteson and Tosteson, 1978). The channels show no selectivity for sodium over potassium but the permeability to monovalent cations is twice as great as for chloride. No channels are formed in response to cholera toxin if either no gangliosides are added to the membranes, G_{M2} is incorporated into the bilayer instead of G_{M1}, or the toxin is premixed with G_{M1} before adding the mixture to a G_{M1}-containing or an undoped membrane. The concentration of choleragen needed for $\frac{1}{2}$ of the maximum conductance change response is 1.2×10^{-10} M, over a 10-fold range of G_{M1}: glycerolmonooleate ratios. This is also the biologically effective concentration range.

As with the analogous observations made for a diphtheria toxin mutant, the significance of these ionic changes in terms of the physiological mechanisms in whole cells is not known. If binding subunits alone are sufficient to trigger the membrane conductivity changes, unless those changes are in concert with other events initiated by the holotoxin, such changes while possibly playing a role in penetration are probably not important in the final mechanism of toxic action since binding domains of diphtheria toxin and cholera toxin do not exert toxic effects. A role in the processing of the holotoxin molecule such as a local change in membrane fluidity, cytoskeletal organization, protease or enzymatic activities, such that the active domain can exert its effects, cannot be supported or refuted at this point.

This possibility of the participation of other membrane components such as proteins in cholera toxin receptor function has been tested in several ways. There is precedence for such an interaction in the thyroid stimulating hormone (TSH) system. This possibility is made more appealing by the sequence homologies found between the A and α, and the B and β subunit of choleragen and TSH (Kohn, 1978). The TSH receptor is reported to be composed of a glycoprotein and a glycolipid portion, both of which are required for a hormonal response to be generated.

The concept of gangliosides initially binding hormones (and toxins) which then would associate with membrane macromolecules prompted Reidler et al. (1978) to use the fluorescence photobleaching-recovery technique with a G_{M1} substituted with fluorescein in place of the sphingosine moiety to label 3T3 mouse fibroblast and artificial lipid vesicles. They found that although the ganglioside in the membranes had restricted lateral mobility, ($D = 5.5 \times 10^{-9}$ cm^2 sec^{-1}) compared with lipid molecules ($D \sim 10^{-10}$ cm^2 sec^{-1}), it was twenty-five-fold more mobile than membrane proteins ($D = 1.5 \times 10^{-7}$ cm^2 sec^{-1}). This mobility was independent of the cell type or the presence of various metabolic poisons or cytoskeletal perturbing drugs. The addition of cholera toxin led to the immobilization of about 50% of the labeled G_{M1} in the membranes or artificial lipid bilayers and a 2-fold reduction of the diffusion coefficient of the remaining labeled G_{M1}. Their interpretation of these results, given the altered structure of the G_{M1} used, indicate that free labeled G_{M1} does not exhibit long-lived interactions with slowly moving or stationary membrane structures in cell membranes. The immobilization of G_{M1} after choleragen binding may be of importance in the later responses of the cells. Bound choleragen will patch and cap (Craig and Cuatrecasas, 1975; Sedlacek et al., 1976) and these movements are affected by anti-microtubule agents. Galactocerebroside has been detected immunologically in colchicine-sensitive cytoskeletal structures resembling tubulin in cultured cells (Sakakibara et al., 1981). Somehow the G_{M1} molecules (or the toxin molecules) become associated with the cytoskeleton (Sahyoun et al., 1981; Streuli et al., 1981; Hagmann and Fishman, 1982). Perhaps the 'freezing' of the glycolipids promotes their association with cytoskeletal elements. The generalization of these results to the small fraction of the total binding of choleragen required for intoxication may not be warranted, especially in view of non-quantitative recovery of fluorescence in which the signal due to the 1% or so 'relevant' sites might be neglected. It is clear from these results, however, that free added ganglioside is largely mobile within the plane of the bilayer. Ganglioside added to deficient cells restores a choleragen response, thereby suggesting that if ganglioside by itself is not the receptor that added ganglioside will function along with whatever other components are the true receptor moiety to produce intoxication.

The isolation of a membrane macromolecule associated with bound choleragen has been attempted by several groups following the solubilization of membranes containing bound toxin with nonionic detergents (to minimize the disaggregation of protein-protein complexes) using anticholeragen antibodies. While this approach was successful for diphtheria toxin and lactoperoxidase surface-iodinated proteins (Proia et al., 1979), no specifically immunoprecipitable material could be detected in similar experiments with cholera toxin. However, Bennett et al. (1975b) were able to immunoprecipitate adenylate cyclase activity with anticholeragen antibody only from toxin-treated adipocytes. Thus, evidence for membrane macromolecule participation in the receptor function is available, but it is not patently convincing. Isolation and reconstitution of such a membrane macromolecule as was done for the thyrotropin receptor (Kohn, 1978) will be required to study its role in the intoxication process and its link, if any, with glycoprotein portion of the thyrotropin receptor.

5.2. ESCHERICHIA COLI HEAT-STABLE ENTEROTOXIN

Strains of *Escherichia coli* infected with a toxigenic plasmid secrete two toxins that are capable of inducing massive efflux of water in the small intestine (Sack, 1975, Richards and Douglas, 1978). One type designated ST for its resistance to boiling has attracted relatively little experimental attention probably because of the tedious *in vivo* assay method. This toxin seems unrelated to choleragen. The short section devoted to this toxin will serve to illustrate the paucity of information available about this molecule and will perhaps stimulate more work on the subject. A recent review may be found in Greenberg and Guerrant (1981).

The heat-labile toxin (LT) is in many ways similar to choleragen and will be considered briefly in that regard. Investigators of the mechanism of action of LT have benefited greatly by the previous work done on choleragen with which it shares many properties.

The heat-stable enterotoxin (ST) elaborated by some strains of *E. coli* is a small molecular weight molecule with m.w. between 1,000 and 10,000 (Bywater, 1972; Jacks and Wu, 1974; Alderete and Robertson, 1978; Takeda et al., 1979). Physiological effects of the toxin, namely a rapid and transient efflux of water with no lag period from the intestinal epithelium (Evans et al., 1973) are best demonstrated with the suckling mouse assay (Giannella, 1976) within 1–3 hr of exposure to the toxin. Field et al. (1979) suggest that ST may be specifically inhibiting Na^+-coupled Cl^- absorption across the ileal brush border while cAMP will affect both this process as well as Cl^- secretion. In contrast to choleragen and LT, ST and its effects may be readily washed away (Nalin and Richardson, 1973). There is presently very little information available on the binding properties of ST other than some evidence that it does not bind to ganglioside (Pierce, 1973). The mechanism of action of ST is equally poorly understood. There is recent evidence for a rapid elevation of cGMP levels and guanylate cyclase activity (Field et al., 1978) in rabbit intestine unaccompanied by an increase in cAMP levels (Hughes et al., 1978). Classically, 8-bromo-cGMP mimics this rapid onset of fluid secretion. The molecular mechanism of ST action remains at this level of understanding.

Structural work on this small molecule has advanced rapidly. Both the nucleotide (So and McCarthy, 1980) and the amino acid (Takao et al., 1983) sequences have been determined for both the porcine and human strains. The m.w. from mass spectral analysis is 1970 daltons.

5.3. ESCHERICHIA COLI HEAT-LABILE ENTEROTOXIN

5.3.1. *Properties of the Toxin*

E. coli LT in contrast to ST has received a great deal of attention mostly due to the similarities between choleragen and LT in mode of action. Despite the effort invested, LT has not been purified to homogeneity in sufficient quantity to allow chemical characterization. Multiple forms of LT have confused the issue, being reported varying in m.w. from 20,000 to several million (Evans *et al.*, 1974; Dorner *et al.*, 1976; Finkelstein *et al.*, 1976; Robertson *et al.*, 1979). This apparent heterogeneity may arise from cellular processing stages or to differences in the plasmid-carried structural gene. Recent studies involving cloning of the LT structural gene and translation of the chimeric plasmid product in *E. coli* minicells have established the structure of LT as being made up of a 25,500 m.w. protein possessing adenylate cyclase stimulating activity and NADase activity, and a 11,500 m.w. protein, both of which react with anticholeragen antisera (Dallas and Falkow, 1979; Dallas *et al.*, 1979). LT crossreacts immunologically primarily with antisera directed against choleragen B subunit (Evans *et al.*, 1974; Gill *et al.*, 1976; Gyles, 1974; Klipstein and Engert, 1977). This observation has been cited as an indication of homology at least between the binding subunits (or domains) of the two toxins. Cholera toxin and LT activate adenylate cyclase and both toxins potentiate the effect of hormones on adenylate cyclase activity. Like choleragen, LT requires NAD^+ for the activation of adenylate cyclase in disrupted cell systems (Gill *et al.*, 1976) and possesses NAD^+-glycohydrolase and ADP-ribosyl transferase activity (Moss and Richardson, 1978). The stereospecificity of the ADP-ribosyl transfer to arginine is the α-anomeric configuration (Moss *et al.*, 1979a) as for choleragen (Oppenheimer, 1978). Identity of the product or of the labeling site have yet to be demonstrated. The kinetics of activation of adenylate cyclase are also similar, including a lag phase (Kantor *et al.*, 1974; Zenser and Metzger, 1974) although there is some evidence that LT-induced adenylate cyclase stimulation is more readily reversed than with choleragen-treated cells (Finkelstein *et al.*, 1976, Zenser and Metzger, 1974).

5.3.2. *Binding and Penetration of the Toxin*

In addition to sharing immunological determinants with the B (binding) subunit of choleragen, LT appears to also bind to the ganglioside G_{M1} either in solution or in membranes with some degree of specificity (Pierce, 1973; Zenser and Metzger, 1974; Holmgren, 1973; Cole *et al.*, 1977; Nalin and McLaughlin, 1978; Moss *et al.*, 1979b). This interaction may not be as avid for LT as the amounts of G_{M1} needed to neutralize activity are somewhat larger than for choleragen, although the relative order and magnitude of the differences are the same (Kantor *et al.*, 1974; Zenser and Metzger, 1974). However, the LT used in these studies was not purified to homogeneity so it is difficult to make quantitative comparisons between the two toxins. Some of the LT activity, unlike choleragen, is removable by washing, also indicating a less avid interaction (Finkelstein *et al.*, 1976; Zenser and Metzger, 1974). This may stem from a difference in the number of binding subunits for toxin molecules which would alter the multivalent binding characteristics. Two sites for binding of *E. coli* LT have been delineated in the intestinal mucosa; the glycocalix, and the plasma membrane of the microvilli. Crude intestinal mucosa components will block fixation of LT at the plasma membrane level, but not in the glycocalix (Cole *et al.*, 1977). The glycocalix sites are also not blocked by added choleragenoid. Thus, there may be some differences in specificity of the binding reaction of choleragen and LT at the level of the intestinal mucosa, but interaction with cell membranes appear to involve similar specificities for gangliosides. Moss *et al.* (1979b) have shown that a line of fibroblasts previously non-responsive to choleragen because of the absence of G_{M1} in the cell membrane become responsive to both choleragen and LT when G_{M1}, and exclusively G_{M1}, is added exogenously and allowed to incorporate before exposure of the cell to the toxin. Again, as for choleragen, the difficulty of ruling out ganglioside-protein or ganglioside-glycoprotein interactions in the physiological receptor due to the small number of molecules involved in the biological reaction prevents a more complete description of the receptor-membrane event at this time.

5.4. *Bordetella pertussis* Toxin (islet activating protein)

Another toxin effecting the adenylate cyclase system at the level between receptor and catalytic unit is the *Bordetella pertussis* islet-activating protein (IAP). This multisubunit protein of m.w. 117,000 (Tamura *et al.*, 1982) potentiates secretory responses (Yajima *et al.*, 1978 and references therein) and abolish receptor-mediated decreases in cellular cAMP content (Katada and Ui, 1981; Katada *et al.*, 1982). This was traced to the loss of the inhibitory function of a guanine nucleotide regulatory component of the adenylate cyclase system distinct from that modified by choleragen (Katada and Ui, 1982; Burns *et al.*, 1983; Murayama *et al.*, 1983). Further biochemical evidence showed that one of the six non-identical subunits of IAP (28,000 m.w.) was capable of ADP-ribosylating a membrane component, m.w. 41,000, that was correlated with the loss of responsiveness of adenylate cyclase to inhibitory hormones (Katada and Ui, 1982; Murayama and Ui, 1983.) While the toxin is a glycoprotein, little is known about the receptor moiety, as most of the work has focused on the biochemical target of the toxin.

The purified target of IAP is comprised of two subunits of 41,000 and 35,000 m.w. with the 41,000 m.w. subunit containing a binding site for GTP. Hydrodynamic characterization suggests that the IAP substrate undergoes alterations in the presence of ligand changing from 82,000 M_r to 51,000 M_r. Work is presently in progress to determine homology between the IAP substrate and other known GTP binding proteins. Current speculation is that the catalytic activity of adenylate cyclase is reciprocally modulated by a homologous pair of nucleotide-binding regulatory proteins. Although such a possibility had been postulated previously, clear proof required the clear distinction of the proteins provided by the pertussis toxin.

6. TOXIN RECEPTORS—THEIR RELATIONSHIP TO NORMAL MODES OF HORMONE AND GROWTH FACTOR ACTION

Far from being irrelevant, generalized poisons, bacterial and other exotoxins exploit a variety of mechanisms to effect cell surface components or to penetrate that barrier to interfere with some particular internal process of the cell. From the accumulating information, it appears that a number of the more complex toxins, i.e. those that do not act simply by nonspecific destruction of the cell membrane permeability barrier, subvert a variety of mechanisms that the cell normally utilizes to obtain information about its environment and to communicate with other cells. Some toxins such as tetanus toxin and botulinum toxin appear to interfere with a presynaptic neurosecretory membrane component whose function is directly affected at the membrane surface. Other toxins exploit uptake processes and perhaps pathways to arrive at the internal cellular compartment and from there to attack various cytosolic processes. The subunit structure and sequence homologies between the β (binding) subunits of TSH, LH, hCG, FSH and the α ('active') subunits of the same hormones and the corresponding subunits of choleragen may be significant in this regard (Kohn, 1978). Such a stratagem of attacking an evolutionarily conserved process would provide substantial protection against changes resulting in resistance of the cell to the bacterial toxin.

Hormonal signal transduction and control of cell sensitivity to hormones may be envisioned as occurring by a variety of mechanisms. Model hormone systems exist for some of these mechanisms although they are far from being proven. A number of the non-peptide hormones seem to act at the cell surface and do not appear to be taken up into the cytosolic compartment although signal transduction through the membrane occurs, i.e. ion transport or adenylate cyclase activation. For these substances (catecholamines and other neurotransmitter or neuromodulatory materials, prostaglandins and a variety of other factors too numerous to mention here), internalization does not appear to be important for function. Desensitization phenomena involving loss of response to a hormone occur primarily at the coupling level between receptor and function, however that is accomplished, followed on a longer time scale by a decrease in receptor number (Harden *et al.*, 1979). The opiate peptides also exert their action at the level of the cell membrane without requiring internalization. For many hormones, though, a requirement or lack thereof, for receptor and/or hormone internalization has not been vigorously investigated.

Several systems that appear to require some form of internalization of hormone receptor have been documented and these bear directly on the mode of action of some of the bacterial toxins. Uptake in the present discussion is limited to specific and biologically relevant uptake, i.e. leads to action on a target, and does not address generalized uptake into vesicles destined for lysosomal destruction. This nonspecific uptake is a process which often overshadows specific uptake by several hundred-fold. Some mechanism, as yet not elucidated, controls the difference. The uptake of lipoproteins into cells after binding to specific receptor sites and movement to specialized areas of the cell membrane occurs at these 'coated pits' (Goldstein *et al.*, 1979). Subsequent degradation of the protein portion of the molecule but recycling of the receptor moiety to the cell surface and deesterification and usage of cholesterol has been described. The existence of pathways for directing components of endocytosed vesicles to different sites implies that bacterial toxins may be able to take advantage of these targeting pathways to avoid destruction in lysosomes (Steinman *et al.*, 1983). Similar processing of epidermal growth factor (EGF) has been detected although direct proof is not yet available, particularly since the target of the EGF function is not known in molecular terms. Insulin may be another candidate for this processing, although direct evidence for biological relevance of internalization is sketchy and the pleiotrophic responses to this hormone confuse the issue still further.

Diphtheria toxin, Pseudomonas exotoxin A, abrin, ricin, modeccin, and tetanus toxin all appear to undergo some form of receptor-mediated endocytosis to penetrate the membrane. They somehow avoid destruction in lysosomes, escape from the vesicles and proceed to their intracellular targets. Tetanus toxin improves upon this by directing its own internalization, retrograde axonal transport and secretion for reuptake into the second of a chain of two neurons, whereas other endocytosed materials including some of the aforementioned toxins are not. The normal cell component analog of this is the uptake of nerve growth factor whose action is in maintaining the differentiated state of neurons. Thus, tetanus toxin may be taking advantage of this normal hormonal (growth factor) pathway to reach its target in the central nervous system.

The toxin receptors and their apparent resemblance or partial identity to some hormone receptors, in particular for the glycoprotein hormones, have provided some clues as to hormone receptor function. The binding characteristics of hormones such as glucagon, insulin, prolactin and ACTH are not modulated by gangliosides. Gangliosides seem to be involved in the binding of many of the toxins discussed in this review as well as the glycoprotein hormones, thyroid stimulating hormone (TSH) and interferon (Lee *et al.*, 1977a; Lee *et al.*, 1979; Kohn *et al.*, 1976). Cell lines (Meldolesi *et al.*, 1976) and disease states (Lee *et al.*, 1977b) lacking the specific gangliosides fail to respond to TSH although protein glycosylation could also play a role. It was subsequently found that there was also a glycoprotein embedded in the membrane that was responsible for TSH binding (Tate *et al.*, 1975) but that the ganglioside was probably responsible for the signal transduction (Winand and Kohn, 1975) although the mechanism for this is unclear. It is possible that the oligosaccharide portion of the glycoprotein is similar to that of the G_{D1b} or G_{T1} (Tonegawa and Hakomori, 1977) which would present a superficial explanation. However, both ganglioside and the glycoprotein are required for a response to hormone binding. Phospholipids may play a modulatory role (Aloj *et al.*, 1979) with phosphatidylinositol controlling binding of hormone as well as being associated with ionic fluxes (Michell, 1979). It has also been observed that the insulin receptor and the EGF receptor are glycoproteins (Maturo and Hollenberg, 1978; Nexø *et al.*, 1979) and that insulin receptor affinity for insulin is modulated by associated glycoprotein (Maturo and Hollenberg, 1978).

In view of these observations, it is possible that the action of some toxins may also depend upon the presence of a membrane glycoprotein as a part of the receptor. Diphtheria toxin is the only clear demonstration of such a glycoprotein receptor (Proia *et al.*, 1979), and it is present in only small amounts compared to the total number of membrane binding sites for the toxin. The lack of certain gangliosides due to metabolic deficiencies has produced examples of resistant cells for most of the nonlytic toxins described in this review. The resistance could also be due to a concomitant lack of oligosaccharide chains on the glycoprotein or the need for a ganglioside-coupling reaction as for TSH.

Many of the toxins discussed in this review will through the study of the mechanism by which they interact with and penetrate the cell membrane allow investigators to deduce some of the subtle processes of transmembrane signal transmission between hormone receptors and effectors within the cell. Useful mutant cell lines are now being developed that appear to be defective in various portions of the endocytic pathway (Robbins *et al.*, 1983). Medicine has expended much effort to free mankind from the death and suffering caused by the toxins elaborated by pathogenic organisms. It is now time to use these same poisons to understand more about life.

REFERENCES

ALDERETE, J. F. and ROBERTSON, D. C. (1978) Purification and chemical characterization of the heat-stable enterotoxin produced by porcine strains of the enterotoxigenic *Escherichia coli*. *Infect. Immun.* **19**: 1021–1030.

ALOJ, S. M., LEE, G., GROLLMAN, E. F., BEGUINOT, F., CONSIGLIO, E. and KOHN, L. D. (1979) Role of phospholipids in the structure and function of the thyrotropin receptor. *J. Biol. Chem.* **254**: 9040–9049.

ALOUF, J. E. (1977) Cell membranes and cytolytic bacterial toxins. In: *Receptors and Recognition* Series B Volume 1 pp. 219–270. CUATRECASAS, P. (Ed). Chapman and Hall, London.

BARBIERI, J. T., CARROLL, S. F., COLLIER, R. J. and McCLOSKEY, J. A. (1981) An endogenous dinucleotide bound to diphtheria toxin. Adenylyl-(3′, 5′)-uridine-3′-monophosphate *J. Biol. Chem.* **256**: 12247–12251.

BECKMAN, B., FLORES, J., WITKUM, P. A. and SHARP, G. W. G. (1974) Studies on the mode of action of cholera toxin. Effects on the solubilized adenylate cyclase. *J. Clin. Invest.* **53**: 1202–1205.

BENNETT, V., CRAIG, S., HOLLENBERG, M. D., O'KEEFE, E., SAHYOUN, N and CUATRECASAS, P. (1976) Structure and function of cholera toxin and hormone receptors. *J. Supramol. Struct.* **4**: 99–120.

BENNETT, V. and CUATRECASAS, P. (1977) Cholera toxin: membrane gangliosides and activation of adenylate cyclase. In: *Receptors and Recognition* Series B Volume 1 pp. 3–66, CUATRECASAS, P. (Ed). Chapman and Hall, London.

BENNETT, V. and CUATRECASAS, P. (1975a) Mechanism of action of *Vibrio cholerae* enterotoxin. Effects on adenylate cyclase of toad and rat erythrocyte plasma membranes. *J. Membrane Biol.* **22**: 1–28.

BENNETT, V and CUATRECASAS, P. (1975b) Mechanism of activation of adenylate cyclase by *Vibrio cholerae* enterotoxin. *J. Membrane Biol.* **22**: 29–52.

BENNETT, V., MONG, L. and CUATRECASAS, P. (1975a) Mechanism of activation of adenylate cyclase by *Vibrio cholerae* enterotoxin. Relations to the mode of activation by hormones. *J. Membrane Biol.* **24**: 107–129.

BENNETT, V., O'KEEFE, E., CUATRECASAS, P. (1975b) Mechanism of action of cholera toxin and the mobile receptor theory of hormone receptor-adenylate cyclase interaction. *Proc. Natl. Acad. Sci. U.S.A.* **72**: 33–37.

BENSON, S., OLSNES, S., PIHL, A., SKORVE, J. and ABRAHAM, A. K. (1975) On the mechanism of protein-synthesis inhibition by abrin and ricin. Inhibition of the GTP-hydrolysis site on the 60-S ribosomal subunit. *Eur. J. Biochem.* **59**: 573–580.

BERMEK, E. (1972) Formation of a complex involving ADP-ribosylated human translocation factor, guanosine nucleotide and ribosomes. *FEBS Lett.* **23**: 95–99.

BERNHEIMER, A. W. (1974) Interactions between membranes and cytolytic bacterial toxins. *Biochim. Biophys. Acta* **344**: 27–50.

BERNHEIMER, A. W. and AVIGAD, L. S. (1970) Nature and properties of a cytolytic agent produced by *Bacillus subtilis*. *J. Gen. microbiol.* **61**: 361–369.

BIGALKE, H., DIMPFEL, W. and HABERMAN, E. (1978) Suppression of ^{3}H-acetylcholine release from primary nerve cell cultures by tetanus and botulinum A toxin. *Naunyn-Schmiedeberg's Arch. Pharmak.* **303**: 133–138.

BIZZINI, B. (1979) Tetanus toxin, *Microbiol. Rev.* **43**: 224–240.

BIZZINI, B. (1978) Chemical studies on a pharmacologically active polypeptide fragment isolated from tetanus toxin. *Toxicon* **15**: 141.

BIZZINI, B. (1977) Tetanus toxin structure as a basis for elucidating its immunological and neuropharmacological activities. In: *Receptors and Recognition* Series B Volume 1 pp. 177–218. CUATRECASAS, P. (Ed). Chapman and Hall, London.

BIZZINI, B., BLASS, J., TURPIN, A. and RAYNAUD, M. (1970) Chemical characterization of tetanus toxin and toxoid. Amino acid composition, number of SH and S-S groups and N-terminal amino acid. *Eur. J. Biochem.* **17**: 100–105.

BIZZINI, B., GROB, P. and AKERT, K. (1981) Papain-derived fragment IIc of tetanus toxin: its binding to isolated synaptic membranes and retrograde axonal transport. *Brain Res.* **210**: 291–299.

BIZZINI, B., STÖCKEL, K. and SCHWAB, M. (1977) An antigenic polypeptide fragment isolated from tetanus toxin: Chemical characterization, binding to gangliosides and retrograde axonal transport in various neuron systems. *J. Neurochem.* **28**: 529–542.

BLUMENTHAL, R., KLAUSNER, R. D. and WEINSTEIN, J. N. (1980) Voltage-dependent translocation of the asialoglycoprotein receptor across lipid membranes. *Nature, Lond.* **288**: 333–338.

BODLEY, J. W., VANNESS, B. G., BROWN, B. A. and HOWARD, J. B. (1979) The site in elongation factor 2 of ADP-ribosylation by diphtheria toxin. *Fed. Proc.* **38**: 618.

BOKOCH, G. M., KATADA, T., NORTHUP, J. K., HEWLETT, E. L. and GILMAN, A. G. (1983) Identification of the predominant substrate for ADP-ribosylation by islet-activating protein. *J. Biol. Chem.* **258**: 2072–2075.

BONVENTRE, P. F., SAELINGER, C. B., IVINS, B., WOSCINSKI, C and AMORINI, M. (1975) Interaction of cultured mammalian cells with [^{125}I]diphtheria toxin *Infect. Immun.* **11**: 675–684.

BOQUET, P. (1979) Interaction of diphtheria toxin fragments a, b and protein crm 45 with liposomes. *Eur. J. Biochem.* **100:** 483–489.

BOQUET, P. (1977) Transport of diphtheria toxin fragment a across mammalian cell membranes. *Biochem. Biophys. Res. Commun.* **75:** 696–702.

BOQUET, P. and DUFLOT, E. (1982) Tetanus toxin fragment forms channels in lipid vesicles at low pH. *Proc. Natl. Acad. Sci. USA* **79:** 7614–7618.

BOQUET, P. and DUFLOT, E. (1981) Studies on the role of a nucleotide-phosphate-binding site of diphtheria toxin in the binding of toxin to Vero cells or liposomes. *Eur. J. Biochem.* **121:** 93–98.

BOQUET, P., PAPPENHEIMER, JR., A. M. (1976) Interaction of diphtheria toxin with mammalian cell membranes. *J. Biol. Chem.* **251:** 5770–5778.

BOROFF, D. A. and DASGUPTA, B. R. (1971) Botulinum toxin. In: *Microbial Toxins* Vol. 2A pp. 1–68, AJL, S. J. (Ed). Academic Press, New York and London.

BOROFF, D. A., DELCASTILLO, J., EVOY, W. H. and STEINHARDT, R. A. (1974) Observations on the action of type a botulinum toxin on frog neuromuscular junctions. *J. Physiol., Lond.* **240:** 227–253.

BRADY, R. O. and FISHMAN, P. H. (1979) Biotransducers of membrane-mediated information. *Adv. Enzymol.* **50:** 303–323.

BUNGE, M. B. (1977) Initial endocytosis of peroxidase or ferritin by growth cones of cultured nerve cells. *J. Neurocytol.* **6:** 407–439.

BURGEN, A. S. V., DICKENS, F. and ZATMAN, L. J. (1949) The action of botulinum toxin on the neuromuscular junction. *J. Physiol., London.* **109:** 10–24.

BURGOYNE, R. D., WOLSTENHOLME, J. and STEPHEN, J. (1976) The preparation of stable, biologically active b fragment of diphtheria toxin. *Biochem. Biophys. Res. Commun.* **71:** 920–925.

BURNS, D. L., HEWLETT, E. L., MOSS, J. and VAUGHAN, M. (1983) Pertussis toxin inhibits enkephalin stimulation of GTPase of NG108-15 cells. *J. Biol. Chem.* **258:** 1435–1438.

BYWATER, R. J. (1972) Dialysis and ultrafiltration of a heat-stable enterotoxin from *Escherichia coli. J. Med. Microbiol.* **5:** 337–343.

CASSEL, D., ECKSTEIN, F., LOWE, M. and SELINGER, Z. (1979) Determination of the turn-off reaction for the hormone-activated adenylate cyclase. *J. Biol. Chem.* **254:** 9835–9838.

CASSEL, D. and PFEUFFER, T. (1978) Mechanism of cholera toxin action: covalent modification of the guanyl nucleotide-binding protein of the adenylate cyclase system. *Proc. Natl. Acad. Sci. U.S.A.* **75:** 2669–2673.

CASSEL, D. and SELINGER, Z. (1977) Mechanism of adenylate cyclase activation by cholera toxin: inhibition of GTP hydrolysis at the regulatory site. *Proc. Natl. Acad. Sci. U.S.A.* **74:** 3307–3311.

CASSIDY, P. and HARSHMAN, S. (1979) Characterization of detergent-solubilized iodine-125-labeled staphylococcal α-toxin bound to rabbit erythrocytes and mouse diaphragm muscle. *Biochemistry* **18:** 232–236.

CASSIDY, P. and HARSHMAN, S. (1976) Studies on the binding of staphylococcal ^{125}I-labeled α-toxin to rabbit erythrocytes. *Biochemistry* **15:** 2348–2355.

CAWLEY, D. B., HERSCHMAN, H. R., GILLILAND, D. G. and COLLIER, R. J. (1980) Epidermal growth factor—toxin A chain conjugates: EGF-ricin A is a potent toxin while EGF-diphtheria fragment A is non-toxic. *Cell* **22:** 563–570.

CAWLEY, D. B., SIMPSON, D. L. and HERSCHMAN, H. R. (1981) Asialoglycoprotein receptor mediates the toxic effects of an asialofetuin-diphtheria toxin fragment A conjugate on cultured rat hepatocytes. *Proc. Natl. Acad. Sci. USA* **78:** 3383–3387.

CHANG, D. W. and COLLIER, R. J. (1977) Enzymatically active peptide from the adenosine diphosphate-ribosylating toxin of *Pseudomonas aeruginosa. Infect. Immun.* **16:** 832–841.

CHANG, T.-M., DAZORD, A. and NEVILLE, JR., D. M. (1977) Artificial hybrid protein containing a toxic protein fragment and a cell membrane receptor-binding moiety in a disulfide conjugate. *J. Biol. Chem.* **252:** 1515–1522.

CHANG, T.-M. and KULLBERG, D. W. (1982) Studies of the mechanism of cell intoxication by diphtheria toxin fragment A-asialoorosomucoid hybrid toxins. Evidence for utilization of an alternative receptor-mediated transport pathway. *J. Biol. Chem.* **257:** 12563–12572.

CHANG, T.-M. and NEVILLE, JR., D. M. (1978) Demonstration of diphtheria toxin receptors on surface membranes from both toxin-sensitive and toxin-resistant species. *J. Biol. Chem.* **253:** 6866–6871.

COLE, H. D., STALEY, T. E. and WHIPP, S. C. (1977) Reduction of reactivity of *Escherichia coli* enterotoxins by intestinal mucosal components. *Infect. Immun.* **16:** 374–381.

COLLIER, R. J. (1977) Inhibition of protein synthesis by exotoxins from *Corynebacterium diphtheriae* and *Pseudomonas aeruginosa.* In: *Receptors and Recognition* Series B Volume 1 pp. 67–98, CUATRECASAS, P. (Ed). Chapman and Hall, London.

COLLIER, R. J. and KANDEL, J. (1971) Structure and activity of diphtheria toxin. I. Thiol-dependent dissociation of a fraction of toxin into enzymatically active and inactive fragments. *J. Biol. Chem.* **246:** 1496–1503.

CRAIG, S. and CUATRECASAS, P. (1975) Mobility of cholera toxin receptors on rat lymphocyte membranes. *Proc. Natl. Acad. Sci. U.S.A.* **72:** 3844–3848.

CREAGAN, R. P., CHEN, S. and RUDDLE, F. H. (1975) Genetic analysis of the cell surface: association of human chromosome 5 with sensitivity to diphtheria toxin in mouse–human somatic cell hybrids. *Proc. Natl. Acad. Sci.* **72:** 2237–2241.

CUATRECASAS, P. and HOLLENBERG, M. D. (1976) Membrane receptors and hormone action. *Adv. Protein Chem.* **30:** 251–451.

CUATRECASAS, P. (1973a) Cholera toxin-fat cell interaction and the mechanism of activation of the lipolytic response. *Biochemistry* **12:** 3567–3577.

CUATRECASAS, P. (1973b) *Vibrio cholerae* choleragenoid. Mechanism of inhibition of cholera toxin action. *Biochemistry* **12:** 3577–3581.

CUATRECASAS, P. (1973c) Interaction of *Vibrio cholerae* enterotoxin with cell membranes. *Biochemistry* **12:** 3547–3558.

CUATRECASAS, P. (1973d) Interaction of wheat germ agglutinin and concanavalin a with isolated fat cells. *Biochemistry* **12:** 1312–1322.

CUATRECASAS, P. (1973e) Gangliosides and membrane receptors for cholera toxin. *Biochemistry* **12**: 3558–3566.

CUATRECASAS, P., PARIKH, I. and HOLLENBERG, M. D. (1973) Affinity chromatography and structural analysis of *Vibrio cholerae* enterotoxin-ganglioside agarose and the biological effects of ganglioside-containing soluble polymers. *Biochemistry* **12**: 4253–4264.

CURTIS, D. R. and DEGROAT, W. C. (1968) Tetanus toxin and spinal inhibition. *Brain Res., Osaka* **10**: 208–212.

CURTIS, D. R., FELIX, D., GAME, C. J. A. and MCCULLOCH, R. M. (1973) Tetanus toxin and the synaptic release of GABA. *Brain Res., Osaka* **51**: 358–362.

DALLAS, W. S. and FALKOW, S. (1979) The molecular nature of the heat-labile enterotoxin (LT) of *Escherichia coli*. *Nature, Lond.* **277**: 406–407.

DALLAS, W. S., GILL, D. M. and FALKOW, S. (1979) Cistrons encoding *Escherichia coli* heat-labile toxin. *J. Bact.* **139**: 850–858.

DASGUPTA, B. R. and SUGIYAMA, H. (1972) A common subunit structure in *Clostridium botulinum* type a, b and e toxins. *Biochem. Biophys. Res. Commun.* **48**: 108–112.

DICKSON, E. C. and SHEVKY, R. (1923a) Botulism, studies on the manner in which the toxin of *Clostridium botulinum* acts upon the body. I. The effect upon the autonomic nervous system. *J. Exp. Med.* **37**: 711–731.

DICKSON, E. C. and SHEVKY, R. (1923b) Botulism, studies on the manner in which the toxin of *Clostridium botulinum* acts upon the body. II. The effect on the voluntary nervous system. *J. Exp. Med.* **38**: 327–346.

DONOVAN, J. J., SIMON, M. I., DRAPER, R. K. and MONTAL, M. (1981) Diphtheria toxin forms transmembrane channels in planar lipid bilayers. *Proc. Natl. Acad. Sci. U.S.A.* **78**: 172–176.

DONOVAN, J. J., SIMON, M. I. and MONTAL, M. (1982) Insertion of diphtheria toxin into and across membranes: role of phosphoinositide asymmetry. *Nature, Lond.* **298**: 669–672.

DORLAND, R. B., MIDDLEBROOK. J. L. and LEPPLA, S. H. (1979) Receptor-mediated internalization and degradation of diphtheria toxin by monkey kidney cells. *J. Biol. Chem.* **254**: 11337–11342.

DORNER, F., JAKSCHE, H. and STÖCKEL, W. (1976) *Escherichia coli* enterotoxin: purification, partial characterization, and immunological observations. *J. Infect. Dis.* **133** (suppl) S142–S156.

DRAPER, R. K., CHIN, D., EUREY–OWENS, D., SCHEFFLER, I. E. and SIMON, M. I. (1979) Biochemical and genetic characterization of three hamster cell mutants resistant to diphtheria toxin. *J. Cell. Biol.* **83**: 116–125.

DRAPER, R. K., CHIN, D. and SIMON, M. I. (1978a) Diphtheria toxin has the properties of a lectin. *Proc. Natl. Acad. Sci. U.S.A.* **75**: 261–265.

DRAPER, R. K., CHIN, D., STUBBS, L. and SIMON, M. I. (1978b) Studies of the diphtheria toxin receptor on Chinese hamster cells. *J. Supramol. Struct.* **9**: 47–55.

DUMAS, M., SCHWAB, M. E., BAUMANN, R. and THOENEN, H. (1979a) Retrograde transport of tetanus toxin through a chain of two neurons. *Brain Res. Osaka* **165**: 354–357.

DUMAS, M., SCHWAB, M. E. and THOENEN, H. (1979b) Retrograde axonal transport of specific macromolecules as a tool for characterizing nerve terminal membranes. *J. Neurobiol.* **10**: 179–197.

DUNCAN, J. L. and GROMAN, N. B. (1969) Activity of diphtheria toxin. II. Early events in the intoxication of HeLa cells. *J. Bact.* **98**: 963–969.

EDMUNDS, C. W. and LONG, P. H. (1923) Contribution to the pathologic physiology of botulism. *J. Am. Med. Assoc.* **81**: 542–547.

EIDELS, L., ROSS, L. L. and HART, D. A. (1982) Diphtheria toxin-receptor interaction: A polyphosphate-insensitive diphtheria toxin-binding domain. *Biochem. Biophys. Res. Commun.* **109**: 493–499.

EIKLID, K. and OLSNES, S. (1980) Interaction of *Shigella shigae* cytotoxin with receptors on sensitive and insensitive cells. *J. Recept. Res.* **1**: 199–213.

ENDO, Y., HUBER, P. W. and WOOL, I. G. (1983) The ribonuclease activity of the cytotoxin α-sarcin. *J. Biol. Chem.* **258**: 2662–2667.

ENOMOTO, K. and GILL, D. M. (1979) Requirement for guanosine triphosphate in the activation of adenylate cyclase by cholera toxin. *J. Supramol. Struct.* **10**: 51–60.

EVANS, D. J., JR., EVANS, D. G. and GORBACH, S. L. (1974) Polymyxin B-induced release of low molecular weight, heat-labile enterotoxin from *Escherichia coli*. *Infect. Immum.* **10**: 1010–1017.

EVANS, D. G., EVANS, D. J. JR. and PIERCE, N. F. (1973) Differences in the response of rabbit small intestine to heat-labile and heat-stable enterotoxins of *Escherichia coli*. *Infect. Immum.* **7**: 873–880.

FARFEL, Z., KASLOW, H. R. and BOURNE, H. R. (1979) A regulatory component of adenylate cyclase is located on the inner surface of human erythrocyte membranes. *Biochem. Biophys. Res. Commun.* **90**: 1237–1241.

FERNANDEZ-PUENTES, C. and VAZQUEZ, D. (1977) Effects of some proteins that inactivate the eukaryotic ribosome. *FEBS Lett.* **78**: 143–146.

FIELD, M., FROMM, D., WALLACE, C. K. and GREENOUGH, W. B. III (1969) Stimulation of active chloride secretion in small intestine by cholera exotoxin. *J. Clin. Invest.* **48**: 24a.

FIELD, M., GRAF, JR. L. H., GUANDALINI, S., LAIRD, W. J., RAS, M. and SMITH, P. L. (1979) Mechanism of action of heat-stable *Escherichia coli* enterotoxin. In: *Symposium on Cholera*, Karatsu, Japan 1978. pp. 227–235, TAKEYA, K. and ZINNAKA, Y. (Eds). U.S.-Japan Cooperative Medical Science Program.

FIELD, M., GRAF, JR., L. H., LAIRD, W. J. and SMITH, P. L. (1978) Heat-stable enterotoxin of *Escherichia coli*: in vitro effects on guanylate cyclase activity, cyclic GMP concentration, and ion transport in small intestine. *Proc. Natl. Acad. Sci. U.S.A.* **75**: 2800–2804.

FIELD, M., PLOTKIN, G. R. and SILEN, W. (1968a) Effects of vasopressin, theophylline, and cyclic adenosine monophosphate on short-circuit current across isolated rabbit ileal mucosa. *Nature, Lond.* **217**: 469–471.

FIELD, M., PLOTKIN, G. R. and SILEN, W. (1968b) Cyclic AMP-induced secretion of chloride by rabbit ileum in vitro. *Gastroenterology* **54**: 1233.

FILLENZ, M., GAGNON, C., STÖCKEL, K. and THOENEN, H. (1976) Selective uptake and retrograde axonal transport of dopamine β-hydroxylase antibodies in peripheral adrenergic neurons. *Brain Res. Osaka* **114**: 293–303.

FINKELSTEIN, R. A., LARUE, M. K. JOHNSTON, D. W., VASIL, M. C., CHO, G. J. and JONES, J. R. (1976) Isolation and properties of heat-labile enterotoxin(s) from enterotoxigenic *Escherichia coli*. *J. Infect. Dis.* **133** (Suppl) S120–S137.

FISHMAN, P. H. and BRADY, R. O. (1976) Biosynthesis and function of gangliosides. *Science* **194**: 906–915.

FISHMAN, P. H., Moss, J. and OSBORNE, JR. J. C. (1978) Interaction of choleragen with the oligosaccharide of ganglioside GM_1: evidence for multiple oligosaccharide binding sites. *Biochemistry* **17**: 711–716.

FISHMAN, P. H., Moss, J., RICHARDS, R. L., BRADY, R. O. and ALVING, C. R. (1977) Liposomes as model membranes for ligand- receptor interactions: studies with choleragen and glycolipids. *Biochemistry* **16**: 2562–2567.

FISHMAN, P. H., PACUSZKA, T., HOM, B. and Moss, J. (1980) Modification of ganglioside G_{M1}. Effect of lipid moiety on choleragen action. *J. Biol. Chem.* **255**: 7657–7664.

FITZGERALD, D., MORRIS, R. E. and SAELINGER, C. B. (1982) Essential role of calcium in cellular internalization of Pseudomonas toxin. *Infect. Immun.* **35**: 715–720.

FITZGERALD, D., MORRIS, R. E. and SAELINGER, C. B. (1980) Receptor-mediated internalization of Pseudomonas toxin by mouse fibroblasts. *Cell* **21**: 867–873.

FITZGERALD, D., PADMANABHAN, R., PASTAN, I. and WILLINGHAM, M. C. (1983) Adenovirus-induced release of epidermal growth factor and Pseudomonas toxin into the cytosol of KB cells during receptor-mediated endocytosis. *Cell* **32**: 607–617.

FREER, J. H. and ARBUTHNOTT, J. P. (1983) Toxins of *Staphylococcus aureus*. *Pharmac. Ther.* **19**: 55–106.

FUSE, A. and KUWATA, T. (1979) Effect of cholera toxin on the antiviral and anticellular activities of human leukocyte interferon. *Infect. Immun.* **26**: 235–239.

GAHMBERG, C. G. and HAKOMORI, S.-I. (1975) Surface carbohydrates of hamster fibroblasts. II. Interaction of hamster NIL cell surface with *Ricinus communis* lectin and concanavalin a as revealed by surface galactosyl label. *J. Biol. Chem.* **250**: 2447–2451.

GESSNER, S. L. and IRVIN, J. D. (1980) Inhibition of elongation factor 2-dependent translocation by the pokeweed antiviral protein and ricin. *J. Biol. Chem.* **255**: 3251–3253.

GIANNELLA, R. A. (1976) Suckling mouse model for detection of heat-stable *Escherichia coli* enterotoxin: characteristics of the model. *Infect. Immun.* **14**: 95–99.

GILL, D. M. (1976a) The arrangement of subunits in cholera toxin. *Biochemistry* **15**: 1242–1248.

GILL, D. M. (1976b) Multiple roles of erythrocyte supernatant in the activation of adenylate cyclase by *Vibrio cholerae* toxin *in vitro*. *J. Infect. Dis.* **133** (Suppl.) S555–S563.

GILL, D. M. (1975) Involvement of NAD in the action of cholera toxin *in vitro*. *Proc. Natl. Acad. Sci. U.S.A.* **72**: 2064–2068.

GILL, D. M. and DINIUS, L. L. (1971) Observations on the structure of diphtheria toxin. *J. Biol. Chem.* **246**: 1485–1491.

GILL, D. M., EVANS, JR., D. J. and EVANS, D. G. (1976) Mechanism of activation of adenylate cyclase *in vitro* by polymyxin-released, heat-labile enterotoxin of *Escherichia coli*. *J. Infect. Dis.* **133** (Suppl.) S103–S107.

GILL, D. M. and KING, C. A. (1975) The mechanism of action of cholera toxin in pigeon erythrocyte lysates. *J. Biol. Chem.* **250**: 6424–6432.

GILL, D. M. and MEREN, R. (1978) ADP-ribosylation of membrane proteins catalyzed by cholera toxin: basis of the activation of adenylate cyclase. *Proc. Natl. Acad. Sci. U.S.A.* **75**: 3050–3054.

GILL, D. M., PAPPENHEIMER, JR., A. M., BROWN, R. and KURNICK, J. J. (1969) Studies on the mode of action of diphtheria toxin. VII. Toxin-stimulated hydrolysis of nicotinamide adenine dinucleotide in mammalian cell extracts. *J. Exp. Med.* **129**: 1–21.

GILLILAND, D. G., COLLIER, R. J., MOEHRING, J. M. and MOEHRING, T. J. (1978) Chimeric toxins: toxic disulfide-linked conjugate of concanavalin a with fragment a from diphtheria toxin. *Proc. Natl. Acad. Sci. U.S.A.* **75**: 5319–5323.

GINSBERG, I. (1970) Streptolysins. In: *Microbial Toxins* Volume 3 pp. 99–171. MONTIE, T. C., KADIS, S. and AJL, S. J. (Eds). Academic Press, New York and London.

GOLDSTEIN, J. L., ANDERSON, R. G. W. and BROWN, M. S. (1979) Coated pits, coated vesicles, and receptor-mediated endocytosis. *Nature, Lond.* **279**: 679–685.

GOTTLIEB, C., SKINNER, S. A. M. and KORNFELD, S. (1974) Isolation of a clone of Chinese hamster ovary cells deficient in plant lectin-binding sites, *Proc. Natl. Acad. Sci. U.S.A.* **71**: 1078–1082.

GREENBERG, R. N. and GUERRANT, R. L. (1981) *E. coli* heat-stable enterotoxin. *Pharmac. Ther.* **13**: 507–531.

GROB, P., AKERT, K., GLICKSMAN, M. A. and BIZZINI, B. (1980) Studies on the retrograde neuronal transport of various tetanus toxin fragments. *Experientia* **36**: 746.

GRUMMT, F., GRUMMT, I. and ERDMANN, V. A. (1974) ATPase and GTPase activities isolated from rat liver ribosomes. *Eur. J. Biochem.* **43**: 343–348.

GUNDERSEN, JR., C. B. and HOWARD, B. D. (1978) The effects of botulinum toxin on acetylcholine metabolism in mouse brain slices and synaptosomes. *J. Neurochem.* **31**: 1005–1013.

GUNDERSEN, C. B., KATZ, B. and MILEDI, R. (1981) The reduction of endplate responses by Botulinum toxin. *Proc. R. Soc. Lond.* B **213**: 489–493.

GUYTON, A. C. and MACDONALD, M. A. (1947) Physiology of botulinum toxin. *Archs. Neurol. Psychiat.* **57**: 578–592.

GYLES, G. L. (1974) Relationship among heat-labile enterotoxins of *Escherichia coli* and *Vibrio cholerae*. *J. Infect. Dis.* **129**: 277–283.

HABERMANN, E. (1970) Pharmakokinetische Besonderheiten des Tetanustoxins und ihre Beziehungen zur Pathogenese des lokalen bzw. generalisierten Tetanus. *Naunyn-Schmiedeberg's Arch. Pharmak.* **267**: 1–19.

HABERMANN, E. and ERDMANN, G. (1978) Pharmacokinetic and histoautoradiographic evidence for the intraaxonal movement of toxin in the pathogenesis of tetanus. *Toxicon* **16**: 611–623.

HABERMANN, E., WELLHÖNER, H. H. and RAKER, K. O. (1977) Metabolic fate of ^{125}I-tetanus toxin in the spinal cord of rats and cats with early local tetanus. *Naunyn-Schmiedeberg's Arch. Pharmak.* **299**: 187–196.

HAGMANN, J. and FISHMAN, P. H. (1982) Detergent extraction of cholera toxin and gangliosides from cultured cells and isolated membranes. *Biochim. Biophys. Acta* **720**: 181–187.

HANIG, J. P. and LAMANNA, C. (1979) Toxicity of botulinum toxin: a stoichiometric model for the locus of its extraordinary potency and persistence at the neuromuscular junction. *J. Theor. Biol.* **77**: 107–113.

HARDEN, T. K., SU, Y.-F. and PERKINS, J. P. (1979) Catecholamine-induced desensitization involves an uncoupling of β-adrenergic receptors and adenylate cyclase. *J. Cyc. Nucleotide Res.* **5**: 99–106.

HARSHMAN, S. (1979) Action of staphylococcal α-toxin on membranes: some recent advances. *Molec. and Cell. Biochem.* **23**: 143–152.

HEBDON, G. M., LeVINE, H., III, SAHYOUN, N. E., SCHMITGES, C. J. and CUATRECASAS, P. (1980) Demonstration of choleragen-dependent ADP-ribosylation in whole cells and correlation with the activation of adenylate cyclase. *Life Sci.* **26**: 1385–1396.

HELTING, T. B., ZWISLER, O. and WIEGANDT, H. (1977) Structure of tetanus toxin. II. Toxin binding to ganglioside, *J. Biol. Chem.* **252**: 194–198.

HOLLAND, I. B. (1977) Colicin E$_3$ and related bacteriocins: penetration of the bacterial surface and mechanism of ribosome inactivation. In: *Receptors and Recognition* Series B Volume 1 pp. 100–127, CUATRECASAS, P. (Ed). Chapman and Hall, London.

HOLLENBERG, M. D., FISHMAN, P. H., BENNETT, V. and CUATRECASAS, P. (1974) Cholera toxin and cell growth: role of membrane gangliosides. *Proc. Natl. Acad. Sci. U.S.A.* **71**: 4224–4228.

HOLMGREN, J. (1973) Comparison of the tissue receptors for *Vibrio cholerae* and *Escherichia coli* enterotoxins by means of gangliosides and natural cholera toxoid. *Infect. Immun.* **8**: 851–859.

HOLMGREN, J., LÖNNROTH, I., MANSSON, J.-E. and SVENNERHOLM, L. (1975) Interaction of cholera toxin and membrane G$_{M1}$ ganglioside of small intestine. *Proc. Natl. Acad. Sci. U.S.A.* **72**: 2520–2524.

HOLMGREN, J., LÖNNROTH, I. and SVENNERHOLM, L. (1973) Tissue receptor for cholera exotoxin: postulated structure from studies with G$_{M1}$ ganglioside and related glycolipids. *Infect. Immun.* **8**: 208–214.

HUGHES, J. M., MURAD, F., CHANG, B. and GUERRANT, R. L. (1978) Role of cyclic GMP in the action of heat-stable enterotoxin of *Escherichia coli*. *Nature, Lond.* **271**: 755–756.

HUGHES, R. and WHALER, B. C. (1962) Influence of nerve-ending activity and of drugs on the rate of paralysis of rat diaphragm preparations by *Clostridium botulinum* type a toxin. *J. Physiol. Lond.* **160**: 221–233.

HYMAN, R., LACORBIERE, M., STAVAREK, S., NICOLSON, G. (1974) Derivation of lymphoma variants with reduced sensitivity to plant lectins. *J. Natl. Cancer Inst.* **52**: 963–969.

IGLEWSKI, B. H., ALVING, C. R., URBAN, K. A., MOSS, J. and SADOFF, J. C. (1979) Binding of diphtheria toxin to phospholipids in liposomes. *Fed. Proc.* **38**: 824.

IGLEWSKI, B. H. and KABAT, D. (1975) NAD-dependent inhibition of protein synthesis by *Pseudomonas aeruginosa* toxin. *Proc. Natl. Acad. Sci. U.S.A.* **72**: 2284–2288.

IGLEWSKI, B. H., SADOFF, J., BJORN, M. J. and MAXWELL, E. S. (1978) *Pseudomonas aeruginosa* exoenzyme S. Adenosine diphosphoribosyltransferase distinct from toxin A. *Proc. Natl. Acad. Sci. U.S.A.* **75**: 3211–3215.

IVINS, B., SAELINGER, C. B., BONVENTRE, P. F. and WOSCINSKI, C. (1975) Chemical modulation of diphtheria toxin action on cultured mammalian cells. *Infect. Immun.* **11**: 665–674.

JACKS, T. M. and WU, B. J. (1974) Biochemical properties of *Escherichia coli* low-molecular weight heat-stable enterotoxin. *Infect. Immun.* **9**: 342–347.

JACOBS, S., CHANG, K.-J. and CUATRECASAS, P. (1978) Antibodies to purified insulin receptor have insulin-like activity. *Science* **200**: 1283–1284.

JOHNSON, G. L. and BOURNE, H. R. (1977) Influence of cholera toxin on the regulation of adenylate cyclase by GTP. *Biochem. Biophys. Res. Commun.* **78**: 792–798.

JOHNSON, G. L., KASLOW, H. R. and BOURNE, H. R. (1978a) Genetic evidence that cholera toxin substrates are regulatory components of adenylate cyclase. *J. Biol. Chem.* **253**: 7120–7123.

JOHNSON, G. L., KASLOW, H. R. and BOURNE, H. R. (1978b) Reconstitution of cholera toxin-activated adenylate cyclase. *Proc. Natl. Acid. Sci. U.S.A.* **75**: 3113–3117.

JOHNSON, W. R., KUCHLER, R. J. and SOLOTOROVSKY, M. (1968) Site in cell-free protein synthesis sensitive to diphtheria toxin. *J. Bact.* **96**: 1089–1098.

JOLIVET-REYNAUD, C. and ALOUF, J. E. (1983) Binding of *Clostridium perfringens* ^{125}I-labeled Δ-toxin to erythrocytes. *J. Biol. Chem.* **258**: 1871–1877.

KAGAN, B. L. and FINKELSTEIN, A. F. (1979) Channels formed in planar bilayer membranes by mutant diphtheria toxin. *Biophys. J.* **25**: A181.

KANTOR, H. S., TAO, P. and GORBACH, S. L. (1974) Stimulation of intestinal adenyl cyclase by *Escherichia coli* enterotoxin: comparison of strains from an infant and an adult with diarrhoea *J. Infect. Dis.* **129**: 1–9.

KATADA, T., AMANO, T. and UI, M. (1982) Modulation by islet-activating protein of adenylate cyclase activity in C-6 glioma cells. *J. Biol. Chem.* **257**: 3739–3746.

KATADA, T. and UI, M. (1982) Direct modification of the membrane adenylate cyclase system by islet-activating protein due to ADP-ribosylation of a membrane protein. *Proc. Natl. Acad. Sci. U.S.A.* **79**: 3129–3133.

KATADA, T. and UI, M. (1981) Islet-activating protein. A modifier of receptor-mediated regulation of rat islet adenylate cyclase. *J. Biol. Chem.* **256**: 8310–8317.

KATO, I. and NAIKI, M. (1976) Ganglioside and rabbit erythrocyte membrane receptor for staphylococcal alpha-toxin. *Infect. Immun.* **13**: 289–291.

KATO, I. and PAPPENHEIMER, JR., A. M. (1960) An early effect of diphtheria toxin on the metabolism of mammalian cells growing in culture. *J. Exp. Med.* **112**: 329–349.

KEUSCH, G. T., DONOHUE-ROLFE, A. and JACEWICZ, M. (1982) *Shigella* toxin(s): description and role in diarrhoea and dysentery. *Pharmac. Ther.* **15**: 403–438.

KEUSCH, G. T. and JACEWICZ, M. (1977) Pathogenesis of shigella diarrhoea. VII. Evidence for a cell membrane toxin receptor involving β1→4 linked N-acetyl-D-glucosamine oligomers. *J. Exp. Med.* **146**: 535–546.

KEUSCH, G. T., JACEWICZ, M. and HIRSCHMAN, Z. (1972) Quantitative microassay in cell culture for enterotoxin of *Shigella dysenteriae* 1. *J. Infect. Dis.* **125**: 539–541.

KEUSCH, G. T., PARIKH, I. and JACEWICZ, M. (1977) Affinity chromatography purification of *Shigella* toxin (ST) on a Sepharose-chitin column. *Clin. Res.* **25**: 490A.

KING, C. A. and VAN HEYNINGEN, W. E. (1973) Deactivation of cholera toxin by a sialidase-resistant monosialo-ganglioside. *J. Infect. Dis.* **127**: 639–647.

KLIPSTEIN, F. A. and ENGERT, R. F. (1977) Immunological interrelationships between cholera toxin and the heat-labile and heat-stable enterotoxins of coliform bacteria. *Infect. Immun.* **18**: 110–117.

KOHN, L. D. (1978) Relationships in the structure and function of receptors for glycoprotein hormones, bacterial toxins, and interferon. In: *Receptors and Recognition* Series A Volume 5 pp. 135–212, CUATRECASAS, P. and GREAVES, M. F. (Eds). Chapman and Hall, London.

KOHN, L. D., FRIEDMAN, R. M., HOLMES, J. M. and LEE, G. (1976) Use of thyrotropin and cholera toxin to probe the mechanism by which interferon initiates its antiviral activity. *Proc. Natl. Acad. Sci. U.S.A.* **73**: 3695–3699.

LEDLEY, F. D., LEE, G., KOHN, L. D., HABIG, W. H. and HARDEGREE, M. C. (1977) Tetanus toxin interactions with thyroid plasma membranes: implications for structure and function of tetanus toxin receptors and potential pathophysiological significance. *J. Biol. Chem.* **252**: 4049–4055.

LEE, G., ALOJ, S. M. and KOHN, L. D. (1977a) The structures and function of glycoprotein hormone receptors: ganglioside interactions with lutenizing hormone. *Biochem. Biophys. Res. Commun.* **77**: 434–441.

LEE, G., GROLLMAN, E. F., ALOJ, S. M., KOHN, L. D. and WINAND, R. J. (1977b) Abnormal adenylate cyclase activity and altered membrane gangliosides in thyroid cells from patients with Graves' disease. *Biochem. Biophys. Res. Commun.* **77**: 139–146.

LEE, G., GROLLMAN, E. F., DYER, S., BEGUINOT, I., KOHN, L. D., HABIG, W. H. and HARDEGREE, M. C. (1979) Tetanus toxin and thyrotropin interactions with rat brain membrane preparations. *J. Biol. Chem.* **254**: 3826–3832.

LEHMAN, V. (1972) Properties of purified phospholipase c from *Acinetobacter calcoaceticus*. *Acta Path. Microbiol. Scand.* **80B**: 827–834.

LEPPLA, S. H. (1976) Large scale purification and characterization of the exotoxin of *Pseudomonas aeruginosa*. *Infect. Immun.* **14**: 1077–1086.

LE VINE, III, H. and CUATRECASAS, P. (1981) Activation of pigeon erythrocyte adenylate cyclase by cholera toxin: Partial purification of an essential macromolecular factor from horse erythrocyte cytosol. *Biochim. Biophys. Acta* **672**: 248–261.

LOSPALLUTO, J. J. and FINKELSTEIN, R. A. (1972) Chemical and physical properties of cholera exo-enterotoxin (choleragen) and its spontaneously formed toxoid (choleragenoid). *Biochim. Biophys. Acta* **257**: 158–166.

MAHARAJ, I. and FACKRELL, H. B. (1980) Rabbit erythrocyte band 3: a receptor for staphylococcal alpha toxin. *Can. J. Microbiol.* **26**: 524–531.

MANGALO, R. B., BIZZINI, B., TURPIN, A. and RAYNARD, M. (1968) The molecular weight of tetanus toxin. *Biochim. Biophys. Acta* **168**: 583–584.

MARNELL, M. H., STOOKEY, M. and DRAPER, R. K. (1982) Monensin blocks the transport of diphtheria toxin to the cell cytoplasm. *J. Cell Biol.* **93**: 57–62.

MARTIN, B. R., HOUSLAY, M. D. and KENNEDY, E. L. (1977) Cholera toxin requires oxidized NAD to activate adenylate cyclase in purified rat liver plasma membranes. *Biochem. J.* **161**: 639–642.

MASUHO, Y., HARA, T. and NOGUCHI, T. (1979) Preparation of a hybrid of fragment Fab of antibody and fragment a of diphtheria toxin and its cytotoxicity. *Biochem. Biophys. Res. Commun.* **90**: 320–326.

MATURO, J. M. III and HOLLENBERG, M. D. (1978) Insulin receptor: interaction with non-receptor glycoprotein from liver cell membranes. *Proc. Natl. Acad. Sci. U.S.A.* **75**: 3070–3074.

MCDONEL, J. L. (1980) *Clostridium perfringens* toxins (Type A, B, C, D, E). *Pharmac. Ther.* **10**: 617–655.

MEAGER, A., UNGKITCHANUKIT, A., NAIRN, R. and HUGHES, R. C. (1975) Ricin resistance in baby hamster kidney cells. *Nature, Lond.* **257**: 137–139.

MEKADA, E., UCHIDA, T. and OKADA, Y. (1979) Modification of the cell surface with neuraminidase increases the sensitivities of cells to diphtheria toxin and pseudomonas toxin: *Exptl. Cell Res.* **123**: 137–146.

MELDOLESI, M. F., FISHMAN, P. H., ALOJ, S. M., KOHN, L. D. and BRADY, R. O. (1976) Relationship of ganglioside to the structure and function of thyrotropin receptors: their absence on plasma membranes of a thyroid tumor defective in thyrotropin receptor activity. *Proc. Natl. Acad. Sci. U.S.A.* **73**: 4060–4064.

MICHELL, R. H. (1979) Inositol phospholipids in membrane function. *Trends Biochem. Sci.* **4**: 128–131.

MIDDLEBROOK, J. L. (1981) Effect of energy inhibitors on cell surface diphtheria toxin receptor numbers. *J. Biol. Chem.* **256**: 7898–7904.

MIDDLEBROOK, J. L. and DORLAND, R. B. (1977) Response of cultured mammalian cells to the exotoxins of *Pseudomonas aeruginosa* and *Corynebacterium diphtheriae*: differential cytotoxicity. *Can. J. Microbiol.* **23**: 183–189.

MIDDLEBROOK, J. L., DORLAND, R. B. and LEPPLA, S. H. (1978) Association of diphtheria toxin with Vero cells. Demonstration of a receptor. *J. Biol. Chem.* **253**: 7325–7330.

MIRSKY, R., WENDON, L. M. B., BLACK, P., STOLKIN, C. and BRAY, D. (1978) Tetanus toxin: a cell surface marker for neurones in culture. *Brain Res. Osaka* **114**: 251–259.

MISKIMINS, W. K. and SHIMIZU, N. (1979) Synthesis of a cytotoxic insulin cross-linked to diphtheria toxin fragment a capable of recognizing insulin receptors. *Biochem. Biophys. Res. Commun.* **91**: 143–151.

MOEHRING, T. J. and MOEHRING, J. M. (1977) Selection and characterization of cells resistant to diphtheria toxin and pseudomonas exotoxin a: presumption translational mutants. *Cell* **11**: 447–454.

MOEHRING, T. J. and MOEHRING, J. M. (1972) Response of cultured mammalian cells to diphtheria toxin. V. Concurrent resistance to ribonucleic acid viruses in diphtheria toxin-resistant KB cell strains. *Infect. Immun.* **6**: 493–500.

MOEHRING, T. J., MOEHRING, J. M., KUCHLER, R. J. and SOLOTOROVSKY, M. (1967) The response of cultured mammalian cells to diphtheria toxin. I. Amino acid transport, accumulation and incorporation in normal and intoxicated sensitive cells. *J. Exp. Med.* **126**: 407–422.

MOEHRING, T. J., MOEHRING, J. M. and STINEBRING, W. R. (1971) Response of interferon-treated cells to diphtheria toxin. *Infect. Immun.* **4**: 747–752.

MONTANARO, L., SPERTI, S. and MATTIOLI, A. (1971) Interaction of ADP-ribosylated aminoacyltransferase II with GTP and with ribosomes. *Biochim. Biophys. Acta* **238**: 493–497.

MONTESANO, R., ROTH, J., ROBERT, A. and ORCI, L. (1981) Ultrastructural visualization of binding and internalization of cholera and tetanus toxin. *C. R. Séances Acad. Sci.* [III] **293**: 563–566.

MOOLTEN, F. L., CAPPARELL, N. J., ZAJDEL, S. H. and COOPERBAND, S. R. (1975) Antitumor effects of antibody-diphtheria toxin conjugates. II. Immunotherapy with conjugates directed against tumor antigens induced by simian virus 40. *J. Natl. Cancer Inst.* **55**: 473–477.

MORRIS, N. P., CONSIGLIO, E., KOHN, L. D., HABIG, W. H., HARDEGREE, M. C. and HELTING, T. B. (1980) Interaction of fragments B and C of tetanus toxin with neural and thyroid membranes and with gangliosides. *J. Biol. Chem.* **255**: 6071–6076.

MOSS, J., FISHMAN, P. H., MANGANELLO, V. C., VAUGHAN, M. and BRADY, R. O. (1976a) Functional incorporation of ganglioside into intact cells: induction of choleragen responsiveness. *Proc. Natl. Acad. Sci. U.S.A.* **73**: 1034–1037.

MOSS, J., FISHMAN, P. H., RICHARDS, R. L., ALVING, C. R., VAUGHAN, M. and BRADY, R. O. (1976b) Choleragen-mediated release of trapped glucose from liposomes containing ganglioside G_{M1}. *Proc. Natl. Acad. Sci. U.S.A.* **73**: 3480–3482.

MOSS, J., GARRISON, S., OPPENHEIMER, N. J. and RICHARDSON, S. H. (1979a) NAD-dependent ADP-ribosylation of arginine and proteins by *Escherichia coli* heat-labile enterotoxin. *J. Biol. Chem.* **254**: 6270–6272.

MOSS, J., GARRISON, S., FISHMAN, P. H. and RICHARDSON, S. H. (1979b) Gangliosides sensitize unresponsive fibroblasts to *Escherichia coli* heat-labile enterotoxin. *J. Clin. Invest.* **64**: 381–384.

MOSS, J., MANGANIELLO, V. C. and VAUGHAN, M. (1976c) Hydrolysis of nicotinamide adenine dinucleotide by choleragen and its protomer: possible role in the activation of adenylate cyclase. *Proc. Natl. Acad. Sci. U.S.A.* **73**: 4424–4427.

MOSS, J., RICHARDS, R. L., ALVING, C. R. and FISHMAN, P. H. (1977a) Effect of the a and b protomers of choleragen on release of trapped glucose from liposomes containing or lacking ganglioside G_{M1}. *J. Biol. Chem.* **252**: 797–798.

MOSS, J. and RICHARDSON, S. H. (1978) Activation of adenylate cyclase by heat-labile *Escherichia coli* enterotoxin. Evidence for ADP-ribosyl-transferase activity similar to that of choleragen. *J. Clin. Invest.* **62**: 281–285.

MOSS, J. and VAUGHAN, M. (1977b) Mechanism of action of choleragen. Evidence for ADP-ribosyltransferase activity with arginine as acceptor. *J. Biol. Chem.* **252**: 2455–2457.

MURAYAMA, T., KATADA, T. and UI, M. (1983) Guanine nucleotide activation and inhibition of adenylate cyclase as modified by islet-activating protein, pertussis toxin, in mouse 3T3 fibroblasts. *Arch. Biochem. Biophys.* **221**: 381–390.

MURAYAMA, T. and UI, M. (1983) Loss of the inhibitory function of the guanine nucleotide regulatory component of adenylate cyclase due to its ADP-ribosylation by islet-activating protein, pertussis toxin, in adipocyte membranes. *J. Biol. Chem.* **258**: 3319–3326.

MURPHY, J. R., PAPPENHEIMER, JR., A. M. and DEBORMS, S. T. (1974) Synthesis of diphtheria *tox*-gene products in *Escherichia coli* extracts. *Proc. Natl. Acad. Sci. U.S.A.* **71**: 11–15.

NALIN, D. R. and MCLAUGHLIN, J. C. (1978) Effects of choleragenoid and glucose on the response of dog intenstine to *Escherichia coli* enterotoxins. *J. Med. Microbiol.* **11**: 177–186.

NALIN, D. R. and RICHARDSON, S. H. (1973) Diarrhoea resembling cholera induced by *Escherichia coli* culture filtrate. *Lancet* 677–678.

NEXØ, E., HOCK, R. A. and HOLLENBERG, M. D. (1979) Lectin-agarose immobilization, a new method for detecting soluble membrane receptor. *J. Biol. Chem.* **254**: 8740–8743.

NICOLSON, G. C. and POSTE, G. (1978) Mechanism of resistance to recin toxin in selected mouse lymphoma cell lines. *J. Supramol. Struct.* **8**: 235–245.

NICOLSON, G. L., ROBBINS, J. C. and HYMAN, R. J. (1976) Cell surface receptors and their dynamics on toxin-treated malignant cells. *J. Supramol. Struct.* **4**: 15–26.

OELTMANN, T. N. and HEATH, E. C. (1979) A hybrid protein containing the toxic subunit of ricin and the cell-specific subunit of human chorionic gonadotropin. *J. Biol. Chem.* **254**: 1028–1032.

O'KEEFE, E. and CUATRECASAS, P. (1977) Persistence of exogenous, inserted ganglioside G_{M1} on the cell surface of cultured cells. *Life Sci.* **21**: 1649–1654.

O'KEEFE, E. and CUATRECASAS, P. (1974) Cholera toxin mimics melanocyte stimulating hormone in inducing differentiation in melanoma cells. *Proc. Natl. Acad. Sci. U.S.A.* **71**: 2500–2504.

OLIVER, J. M., UKENA, T. E. and BERLIN, R. D. (1974) Effects of phagocytosis and colchicine on the distribution of lectin-binding sites on cell surfaces. *Proc. Natl. Acad. Sci. U.S.A.* **71**: 394–398.

OLSNES, S., PAPPENHEIMER, JR., A. M. and MEREN, R. (1974) Lectins from *Abrus precatorius* and *Ricinus communis*. II. Hybrid toxins and their interaction with chain-specific antibodies. *J. Immun.* **113**: 842–847.

OLSNES, S. and PIHL, A. (1982) Chimeric toxins. *Pharmac. Ther.* **15**: 355–381.

OLSNES, S. and PIHL, A. (1977) Abrin, ricin and their associated agglutinins. In: *Receptors and Recognition* Series B Volume 1 pp.129–173, CUATRECASAS, P. (Ed). Chapman and Hall, London.

OLSNES, S., REISBIG, R. and EIKLID, K. (1981) Subunit structure of *Shigella* cytotoxin. *J. Biol. Chem.* **256**: 8732–8738.

OLSNES, S. and SANDVIG, G. (1983) Entry of toxic proteins into cells. In: *Receptors and Recognition* Series B, Vol. 15. pp. 187–231, CUATRECASAS, P. (Ed.) Chapman and Hall, London.

OLSNES, S., SANDVIG, K., EIKLID, K. and PIHL, A. (1978) Properties and action mechanism of the toxic lectin modeccin: interaction with cell lines resistant to modeccin, abrin, and ricin. *J. Supramol. Struct.* **9**: 15–25.

OLSNES, S., SANDVIG, K., REFSNES, K. and PIHL, A. (1976) Rates of different steps involved in the inhibition of protein synthesis by the toxic lectins abrin and ricin. *J. Biol. Chem.* **251**: 3985–3992.

OPPENHEIMER, N. J. (1978) Structural determination and stereospecificity of the choleragen-catalyzed reaction of NAD^+ with guanidines. *J. Biol. Chem.* **253**: 4907–4910.

OSBORNE, R. H. and BRADFORD, H. F. (1973) Tetanus toxin inhibits amino acid release from nerve endings *in vitro*. *Nature New Biol.* **244**: 157–158.

PAPPENHEIMER, JR. A. M. (1977) Diphtheria toxin. *Ann. Rev. Biochem.* **46**: 69–94.

PAPPENHEIMER, JR., A. M. and BROWN, R. (1968) Studies on the mode of action of diphtheria toxin. VI. Site of the action of toxin in living cells. *J. Exp. Med.* **127**: 1073–1086.

PAVLOVSKIS, O. R. and GORDON, F. B. (1972) Pseudomonas a exotoxin: effect on cell cultures. *J. Infect. Dis.* **125**: 631–636.

PFEUFFER, T. (1979) Guanine nucleotide-controlled interactions between components of adenylate cyclase. *FEBS Lett.* **101**: 85–89.

PFEUFFER, T. (1977) GTP-binding proteins in membranes and the control of adenylate cyclase activity: *J. Biol. Chem.* **252**: 7224–7234.

PIERCE, N. F. (1973) Differential inhibitory effects of cholera toxoids and ganglioside on the enterotoxins of *Vibrio cholerae* and *Escherichia coli*. *J. Exp. Med.* **137**: 1009–1023.

PROIA, R. L., EIDELS, L. and HART, D. A. (1981) Diphtheria toxin: receptor interaction. Characterization of the receptor interaction with the nucleotide-free toxin, the nucleotide-bound toxin, and the B-fragment of the toxin. *J. Biol. Chem.* **256**: 4991–4997.

PROIA, R. L., HART, D. A., HOLMES, R. K., HOLMES, R. V. and EIDELS, L. (1979) Immunoprecipitation and partial characterization of diphtheria toxin-binding glycoproteins from surface of guinea pig cells. *Proc. Natl. Acad. Sci. U.S.A.* **76**: 685–689.

PUSZKIN, S. and BERL, S. (1972) Actomyosin-like protein from brain: separation and characterization of the actin-like component. *Biochim. Biophys. Acta* **256**: 695–709.

RAMOS, S., GROLLMAN, E. F., LAZO, P. S., DYER, S. A., HABIG, W. H., HARDEGREE, M. C., KABACK, H. R. and KOHN, L. D. (1979) Effect of tetanus toxin on the accumulation of the permeant lipophilic cation tetraphenylphosphonium by guinea pig brain synaptosomes. *Proc. Natl. Acad. Sci. U.S.A.* **76**: 4783–4787.

REFSNES, K., HAYLETT, T., SANDVIG, K. and OLSNES, S. (1977) Modeccin—a plant toxin inhibiting protein synthesis. *Biochem. Biophys. Res. Commun.* **79**: 1176–1183.

REFSNES, K. and MUNTHE-KAAS, A. C. (1976) Introduction of b-chain-inactivated ricin into mouse macrophages and rat Kupffer cells via their membrane F_c receptors. *J. Exp. Med.* **143**: 1464–1474.

REFSNES, K., OLSNES, S. and PIHL, A. (1974) On the toxic proteins abrin and ricin. Studies of their binding to and entry into Ehrlich ascites cells. *J. Biol. Chem.* **249**: 3557–3562.

REIDLER, J., EDRIDGE, C., SCHLESSINGER, Y., ELSON, E. and WIEGANDT, H. (1978) Lateral mobility of a fluorescent ganglioside G_{M1} analog in cell membranes. *J. Supramol. Struct.* **9** (Suppl. 2): 124.

REISBIG, R., OLSNES, S. and EIKLID, K. (1981) The cytotoxic activity of *Shigella* toxin. Evidence for catalytic inactivation of the 60S ribosomal subunit. *J. Biol. Chem.* **256**: 8739–8744.

RICHARDS, K. L. and DOUGLAS, S. D. (1978) Pathophysiological effects of *Vibrio cholerae* and enterotoxigenic *Escherichia coli* and their exotoxins on eucaryotic cells. *Microbiol. Rev.* **42**: 592–613.

RICHTER, D. and LIPMANN, F. (1970) Separation of mitochondrial and cytoplasmic peptide chain elongation factors from yeast. *Biochemistry* **9**: 5065–5070.

ROBBINS, A. R., PENG, S. S. and MARSHALL, J. L. (1983) Mutant Chinese hamster ovary cells pleiotrophically defective in receptor-mediated endocytosis. *J. Cell Biol.* **96**: 1064–1071.

ROBBINS, J. C., STALLINGS, V. and NICOLSON, G. C. (1977) Cell-surface changes in a *Ricinus communis*, toxin (ricin) resistant variant of a murine lymphoma *J. Natl. Cancer Inst.* **58**: 1027–1033.

ROBERTSON, D. C., KUNKEL, S. L. and GILLIGAN, P. H. (1979) Purification and characterization of heat-labile enterotoxin produced by ent+ *Escherichia coli*: application of hydrophobic chromatography and use of defined media. In: *Symposium on Cholera*, Karatsu, Japan 1978, pp. 250–265. TAKEYA, K. and ZINNAKA, Y. (Eds). U.S. Japan Cooperative Medical Science Program.

SACK, R. B. (1975) Human diarrhoeal disease caused by enterotoxigenic *Escherichia coli*. *Ann. Rev. Microbiol.* **29**: 333–353.

SAELINGER, C. B., BONVENTRE, P. F., IVINS, B. and STRAUS, D. (1976) Uptake of diphtheria toxin and its fragment a moiety by mammalian cells in culture. *Infect. Immun.* **14**: 742–751.

SAHYOUN, N. E. and CUATRECASAS, P. (1975) Mechanism of activation of adenylate cyclase by cholera toxin. *Proc. Natl. Acad. Sci. U.S.A.* **72**: 3438–3442.

SAHYOUN, N., SHATILA, T., LE VINE III, H. and CUATRECASAS, P. (1981) Cytoskeletal association of the cholera toxin receptor in rat erythrocytes. *Biochem. Biophys. Res. Commun.* **102**: 1216–1222.

SAKAKIBARA, K., MOMOI, T., UCHIDA, T. and NAGAI, Y. (1981) Evidence for association of glycosphingolipid with a colchicine-sensitive microtubule-like cytoskeletal structure of cultured cells. *Nature, Lond.* **293**: 76–79.

SANDVIG, K. and OLSNES, S. (1982a) Entry of the toxic proteins abrin, modeccin, ricin and diphtheria toxin into cells. I. Requirement for calcium. *J. Biol. Chem.* **257**: 7495–7503.

SANDVIG, K. and OLSNES, S. (1982b) Entry of the toxic proteins abrin, modeccin, ricin, and diphtheria toxin into cells. II. Effect of pH, metabolic inhibitors and ionophores, and evidence for toxin penetration from endocytotic vesicles. *J. Biol. Chem.* **257**: 7504–7513.

SANDVIG, K. and OLSNES, S. (1980) Diphtheria toxin entry into cells is facilitated by low pH. *J. Cell Biol.* **87**: 828–832.

SANDVIG, K. OLSNES, S. and PIHL, A. (1979) Inhibitory effect of ammonium chloride and chloroquine on the entry of the toxic lectin modeccin into cells. *Biochem. Biophys. Res. Commun.* **90**: 648–655.

SCHLESSINGER, J., BARAK, L. S., HAMMES, G. G., YAMADA, K. M., PASTAN, I., WEBB, W. W. and ELSON, E. L. (1977) Mobility and distribution of a cell surface glycoprotein and its interaction with other membrane components. *Proc. Natl. Acad. Sci. U.S.A.* **74**: 2909–2913.

SCHUBEL, K. (1923) On botulinal toxin. *Arch. Exp. Path. Pharmak.* **96**: 193–259.

SCHWAB, M. E. (1980) Axonal transport from the nerve ending to the nerve cell body: a pathway for trophic signals and neurotoxins. *Bull. Schweiz. Akad. Med. Wiss.* **36**: 7–19.

SCHWAB, M. E., AGID, Y., GLOWINSKI, J. and THOENEN, H. (1977) Retrograde axonal transport of ^{125}I-tetanus toxin as a tool for tracing fiber connections in the central nervous system; connections of the rostral part of the rat neostriatum. *Brain Res. Osaka* **126**: 211–224.

SCHWAB, M. E., SUDA, K. and THOENEN, H. (1979) Selective retrograde transsynaptic transfer of a protein, tetanus toxin, subsequent to its retrograde axonal transport. *J. Cell Biol.* **82**: 798–810.

SEDLACEK, H. H., STÄRK, J., SEILER, F. R., ZIEGLER, W. and WIEGANDT, H. (1976). Cholera toxin-induced redistribution of sialoglycolipid receptor at the lymphocyte membrane. *FEBS Lett.* **61**: 272–276.

SIMERAL, L. S., KAPMEYER, W., MACCONNELL, W. P. and KAPLAN, N. O. (1980) On the role of the covalent carbohydrate in the action of ricin. *J. Biol. Chem.* **255**: 11098–11101.

SIMPSON, L. L. (1982) The interaction between aminoquinolines and presynaptically acting neurotoxins. *J. Pharmac. Exp. Ther.* **222:** 43–48.

SIMPSON, L. L. (1981) The origin, structure, and pharmacological activity of botulinum toxin. *Pharmac. Rev.* **33:** 155–188.

SIMPSON, L. L. (1978) Pharmacological studies on the subcellular site of action of botulinum toxin type a. *J. Pharmac. Exp. Ther.* **206:** 661–669.

SIMPSON, L. L. (1977) Presynaptic actions of botulinum toxic and β-bungarotoxin. In: *Receptors and Recognition* Series B Volume 1 pp. 273–295. CUATRECASAS, P. (Ed)., Chapman and Hall, London.

SIMPSON, L. L. (1974) Studies on the binding of botulinum toxin type a to the rat phrenic nerve-hemidiaphragm preparation. *Neuropharmac.* **13:** 689–691.

SIMPSON, L. L. (1973) Interaction between divalent cations and botulinum toxin type a in the paralysis of the rat phrenic nerve-hemidiaphragm preparation. *Neuropharmac.* **12:** 165–176.

SIMPSON, L. L. (1971) Ionic requirements for the neuromuscular blocking action of botulinum toxin: implications with regard to synaptic transmission. *Neuropharmac.* **10:** 673–684.

SIMPSON, L. L. and RAPPORT, M. M. (1971a) Ganglioside inactivation of botulinum toxin. *J. Neurochem.* **18:** 1341–1343.

SIMPSON, L. L. and RAPPORT, M. M. (1971b) The binding of botulinum toxin to membrane lipids: sphingolipids, steroids and fatty acids. *J. Neurochem.* **18:** 1751–1759.

SMYTH, C. and ARBUTHNOTT, J. P. (1974) Properties of *Clostridium perfringens* (*welchii*) type A λ-toxin (phospholipase c) purified by electrofocusing. *J. Med. Microbiol.* **7:** 41–66.

SO, M. and McCARTHY, B. J. (1980) Nucleotide sequence of the bacterial transposon Tn 1681 encoding a heat-stable (ST) toxin and its identification in enterotoxigenic *Escherichia coli* strains. *Proc. Natl. Acad. Sci. U.S.A.* **77:** 4011–4015.

SOKOL, P. A., IGLEWSKI, B. H., HAGER, T. A., SADOFF, J. C., CROSS, A. S., McMANUS, A., FARBER, B. F. and IGLEWSKI, W. J. (1981) Production of exoenzyme S by clinical isolates of *Pseudomonas aeruginosa. Infect. Immun.* **34:** 147–153.

SOUCEK, A., MICHALEX, C. and SOUCKOVA, A. (1971) Identification and characterization of a new enzyme of the group 'phospholipase d' isolated from *Corynebacterium ovis. Biochim. Biophys. Acta* **227:** 116–128.

SPIEGEL, S., RAVID, A. and WILCHEK, M. (1979) Involvement of gangliosides in lymphocyte stimulation. *Proc. Natl. Acad. Sci. U.S.A.* **76:** 5277–5281.

STEINMAN, R. M., MELLMAN, I. S., MULLER, W. A. and COHN, Z. A. (1983) Endocytosis and the recycling of plasma membrane. *J. Cell. Biol.* **96:** 1–27.

STIRPE, F., SANDVIG, K., OLSNES, S. and PIHL, A. (1982) Action of viscumin, a toxic lectin from mistletoe, on cells in cultures. *J. Biol. Chem.* **257:** 13271–13277.

STIRPE, F., OLSNES, S. and PIHL, A. (1980) Gelonin, a new inhibitor of protein synthesis, nontoxic to intact cells. Isolation, characterization and preparation of complexes with concanavalin A. *J. Biol. Chem.* **255:** 6947–6953.

STÖCKEL, K., SCHWAB, M. E. and THOENEN, H. (1977) Role of gangliosides in the uptake and retrograde axonal transport of cholera and tetanus toxin as compared to nerve growth factor and wheat germ agglutinin. *Brain Res. Osaka* **132:** 273–285.

STÖCKEL, K., SCHWAB, M. and THOENEN, H. (1975) Comparison between the retrograde axonal transport of nerve growth factor and tetanus toxin in motor sensory and adrenergic neurons. *Brain Res. Osaka* **99:** 1–16.

STRAUSS, N. (1960) The effect of diphtheria toxin on the metabolism of HeLa cells. I. Effect on nucleic acid metabolism. *J. Exp. Med.* **12:** 351–359.

STREULI, C. H., PATEL, B. and CRITCHLEY, D. R. (1981) The cholera toxin receptor ganglioside GM remains associated with triton X-100 cytoskeletons of BALB/c-3T3 cells. *Exp. Cell. Res.* **136:** 247–254.

SUNDAN, A., OLSNES, S., SANDVIG, K. and PIHL, A. (1982) Preparation and properties of chimeric toxins prepared from the constituent polypeptides of diphtheria toxin and ricin. Evidence for entry of ricin A chain via the diphtheria toxin pathway. *J. Biol. Chem.* **257:** 9733–9739.

SUROLIN, A., BACHHAWAT, B. K. and PODDLER, S. K. (1975) Interaction between lectin from *Ricinus communis* and liposomes containing ganglioside. *Nature, Lond.* **257:** 802–804.

TAKAO, T., HITOUJI, T., AIMOTO, S., SHIMONISHI, Y., HARA, S., TAKEDA, T., TAKEDA, Y. and MIWATANI, T. (1983) Amino acid sequence of a heat-stable enterotoxin isolated from enterotoxigenic *Escherichia coli* strain 18D *FEBS Lett.* **152:** 1–5.

TAKEDA, Y., TAKEDA, T., YANO, T. and MIWATANI, T. (1979) Purification and some properties of heat-stable enterotoxin of *Escherichia coli*. In: *Symposium on Cholera*. Karatsu, Japan 1978, pp. 236–249. TAKEYA, K. and ZINNAKA, Y. (Eds)., U.S.—Japan Cooperative Medical Science Program.

TAMURA, M., NOGIMORI, K., MURAI, S., YAJIMA, M., ITO, K., KATADA, T., UI, M. and ISHII, S. (1982) Subunit structure of islet-activating protein, pertussis toxin, in conformity with the A–B model. *Biochemistry* **21:** 5516–5522.

TATE, R. L., HOLMES, J. M., KOHN, L. D. and WINAND, R. J. (1975) Characteristics of a solubilized thyrotropin receptor from bovine thyroid plasma membrane. *J. Biol. Chem.* **250:** 6527–6533.

THELESTAM, M., JOLIVET–REYNAUD, C. and ALOUF, J. E. (1983) Photolabeling of staphylococcal α-toxin from within rabbit erythrocyte membranes. *Biochem. Biophys. Res. Commun.* **111:** 444–449.

THORPE, P. E. and ROSS, W. C. J. (1982) The preparation and cytotoxic properties of antibody-toxin conjugates. *Immunological Rev.* **62:** 119–158.

THORPE, P. E., ROSS, W. C. J., CUMBER, A. J., HINSON, C. A., EDWARDS, D. C. and DAVIES, A. J. S. (1978) Toxicity of diphtheria toxin for lymphoblastoid cells is increased by conjugation to antilymphocytic globulin. *Nature, Lond.* **271:** 752–755.

TONEGAWA, Y. and HAKOMORI, S. (1977) Ganglioprotein and globoprotein: the glycoprotein reacting with antiganglioside and antigloboside antibodies and the ganglioprotein change associated with transformation. *Biochem. Biophys. Res. Comm.* **76:** 9–17.

TOSTESON, M. T. and TOSTESON, D. C. (1978) Bilayers containing gangliosides develop channels when exposed to cholera toxin. *Nature, Lond.* **275:** 142–144.

TRAUGH, J. A. and COLLIER, R. J. (1971) Interaction of transferase II with polynucleotides and inhibition of the interaction by guanosine nucleotides. *Biochemistry* **10**: 2357–2366.

TRICHE, T. J., TILLACK, T. W. and KORNFELD, S. (1975) Localization of the binding sites for the *Ricinus communis, Agaricus hisporus* and wheat germ lectins on human erythrocyte membranes. *Biochim. Biophys. Acta* **394**: 540–549.

TURNBULL, P. C. B. (1981) *Bacillus cereus* toxins. *Pharmac. Ther.* **13**: 453–505.

UCHIDA, T., KIM, J., YAMAIZUMI, M., MIYAKE, Y. and OKADA, Y. (1979) Reconstitution of lipid vesicles associated with HVJ (sendaj virus) spikes. Purification and some properties of vesicles containing nontoxic fragment a of diphtheria toxin. *J. Cell Biol.* **80**: 10–20.

UCHIDA, T., YAMAIZUMI, M., MEKADA, E., OKADA, Y., TSUDA, M., KUROKAWA, T. and SUGINO, Y. (1978) Reconstitution of hybrid toxin from fragment a of diphtheria toxin and a subunit of *Wistaria floribunda* lectin. *J. Biol. Chem.* **253**: 6307–6310.

UCHIDA, T., YAMAIZUM, M. and OKADA, Y. (1977) Reassembled HVJ (sendai virus) envelopes containing non-toxic mutant proteins of diphtheria toxin show toxicity to mouse L cell. *Nature, Lond.* **266**: 839–840.

VAN HEYNINGEN, S. (1980) Tetanus toxin. *Pharmacol. Ther.* **11**: 147–157.

VAN HEYNINGEN, S. (1976) Binding of ganglioside by the chains of tetanus toxin. *FEBS Lett.* **68**: 5–7.

VAN HEYNINGEN, W. E. (1961) The fixation of tetanus toxicity by ganglioside. *J. Gen. Microbiol.* **24**: 107–119.

VAN HEYNINGEN, S. and KING, C. A. (1975) Subunit a from cholera toxin is an activator of adenylate cyclase in pigeon erythrocytes. *Biochem. J.* **146**: 269–271.

VAN HEYNINGEN, W. E. (1959) Chemical assay of the tetanus toxin receptor in nervous tissue. *J. Gen. Microbiol.* **20**: 301–309.

VAN HEYNINGEN, W. E., CARPENTER, W. B., PIERCE, N. F. and GREENOUGH, W. B. III (1971) Deactivation of cholera toxin by ganglioside. *J. Infect. Dis.* **124**: 415–418.

VAN HEYNINGEN, W. E. and MILLER, P. A. (1961) The fixation of tetanus toxin by ganglioside. *J. Gen. Microbiol.* **24**: 107–119.

VAN WAUWE, J. P., LOONTIENS, F. G. and DE BRUYNE, C. K. (1973) The interaction of *Ricinus communis* hemagglutinin with polysaccharides and low molecular weight carbohydrates. *Biochim. Biophys. Acta* **313**: 99–105.

VASIL, M. L., KABAT, D. and IGLEWSKI, B. H. (1977) Structure-activity relationships of an exotoxin of *Pseudomonas aeruginosa. Infect. Immun.* **16**: 353–361.

VINET, G. and FREDETTE, V. (1970) Influence du mode de culture dans la toxinogénèse de *Plectridium tetani. Can. J. Microbiol.* **16**: 135–136.

WADSTRÖM, T., THELESTAM, M. and MÖLLBY, R. (1974) Biological properties of extracellular proteins from staphylococcus. *Ann. NY. Acad. Sci.* **236**: 343–361.

WEISSMAN, G., SESSA, G. and BERNHEIMER, A. W. (1966) Staphylococcal alpha-toxin: effects on artificial lipid spherules. *Science* **154**: 772–774.

WELDON, P. R. (1975) Pinocytotic uptake and intracellular distribution of colloidal thorium dioxide by cultured sensory neurities. *J. Neurocytol.* **4**: 341–356.

WILLIAMS, R. S., TSE, C.-K., DOLLY, J. O., HAMBLETON, P. and MELLING, J. (1983) Radio-iodination of botulinum neurotoxin type A with retention of biological activity and its binding to brain synaptosomes. *Eur. J. Biochem.* **131**: 437–445.

WINAND, R. J. and KOHN, L. D. (1975) Thyrotropin effects on thyroid cells in culture: effects of trypsin on the thyrotropin receptor and on thyrotropin-mediated cyclic 3′:5′-AMP changes. *J. Biol. Chem.* **250**: 6534–6540.

WISNIESKI, B. J. and BRAMHALL, J. S. (1979) Labeling of the active subunit of cholera toxin from within the membrane bilayer. *Biochem. Biophys. Res. Commun.* **87**: 308–313.

WISNIESKI, B. J. SHIFLETT, M. A., MEKALANOS, J. and BRAMHALL, J. S. (1979) Analysis of transmembrane dynamics of cholera toxin using photoreactive probes. *J. Supramol. Struct.* **10**: 191–197.

WONNACOTT, S., MARCHBANKS, R. M. and FIOL, C. (1978) Ca^{2+} uptake by synaptosomes and its effect on the inhibition of acetylcholine release by botulinum toxin. *J. Neurochem.* **30**: 1127–1134.

WOODIN, A. M. (1970) Staphylococcal leukocidin. In: Microbial. Toxins Volume 3. pp. 327–355. MONTIE, T. C., KADIS, S. and AJL, S. J. (Eds). Academic Press, New York.

YAJIMA, M., HOSODA, K., KANBAYASHI, Y., NAKAMURA, T., NOGIMORI, K., MIZUSHIMA, Y., NAKASE, Y. and UI, M. (1978) Islets-activating protein (IAP) in *Bordetella pertussis* that potentiates insulin secretory responses of rats. *J. Biochem., Tokoyo,* **83**: 295–303.

YAVIN, E., YAVIN, Z., HABIG, W. H., HARDEGREE, M. C. and KOHN L. D. (1981) Tetanus toxin association with developing neuronal cell cultures. Kinetic parameters and evidence for ganglioside-mediated internalization. *J. Biol. Chem.* **256**: 7014–7022.

YOULE, R. J., MURRAY, G. J. and NEVILLE, JR., D. M. (1979) Ricin linked to monophosphopentamannose binds to fibroblast lysosomal hydrolase receptors, resulting in a cell type-specific toxin. *Proc. Natl. Acad. Sci. U.S.A.* **76**: 5559–5562.

YOULE, R. J. and NEVILLE, JR. D. M. (1979) Receptor-mediated transport of the hybrid protein ricin-diphtheria toxin fragment a with subsequent ADP-ribosylation of intracellular elongation factor II. *J. Biol. Chem.* **254**: 11089–11096.

YOUNG, A. B. and SNYDER, S. H. (1974) Strychnine binding associated with glycine receptors of the central nervous system. *Proc. Natl. Acad. Sci. U.S.A.* **70**: 2832–2836.

ZENSER, T. V. and METZGER, J. F. (1974) Comparison of the action of *Escherichia coli* enterotoxin on the thymocyte adenylate cyclase-cyclic adenosine monophosphate system to that of cholera toxin and prostaglandin E_1. *Infect. Immun.* **10**: 503–509.

ZIMMERMAN, J. M. and PIFFARETTI, J.-C. (1977) Interaction of tetanus toxin and toxoid with cultured neuroblastoma cells. *Naunyn-Schmiedeberg's Arch. Pharmak.* **296**: 271–277.

CHAPTER 5

E. COLI HEAT-LABILE ENTEROTOXIN

Donald C. Robertson,* James L. McDonel† and Friedrich Dorner††

*Dept. of Microbiology, University of Kansas, 735 Haworth Hall, Lawrence, Kansas 66045, U.S.A., †Route 7, Box 94B, Roanoke, VA 24018, U.S.A. and ‡IMMUNO AG, Industriestrasse 72, A-1220 Vienna, Austria

1. INTRODUCTION

Enterotoxigenic *Escherichia coli* (ETEC) can cause diarrheal disease by several mechanisms including the production of either one or two different protein enterotoxins, called LT (heat-labile toxin) and ST (heat-stable toxin). The structure, chemical characteristics, genetic control, mode of action, clinical presentation and ecological distribution of these two toxins are in many ways diversely different. The following sections describe in detail those two toxins, their differences and similarities, and their apparent role in diarrheal disease.

2. BACKGROUND

Perhaps the major cause during the 19th century of infant mortality in most countries, where such records were kept, was 'summer diarrhea'. It generally affected infants during the first month, if not the first week, of life, and caused rapid dehydration and demise. In 1885, Professor Escherich of Vienna, Austria, isolated from several infants with summer diarrhea an organism which he called *Bacterium coli*. Subsequently, this organism was shown to be a constituent of the normal bowel flora (Escherich, 1887). Moro, working in Escherich's clinic, published in 1905 the important observation that the source of *B. coli* was food and breast milk, and that the type of the organism, as determined by laboratory culture, changed when an infant became sick. Massini, working in Ehrlich's department in Frankfurt, Germany, showed in 1907 that, when injected intraintestinally into rabbits, *B. coli* strains from diarrheal patients caused diarrhea in all the rabbits while only 4 of 10 rabbits injected with *B. coli* from healthy patients developed diarrhea.

Similar observations were made by veterinarians studying the diarrhea of calves. Adam, working in Heidelberg, Germany, published a study in 1923 that classified the pathogenic *B. coli* responsible for dyspepsia and intestinal intoxication on the basis of sugar fermentation patterns. This group also published a serological classification of strains isolated from children with enteritis.

As early as 1925 Smith and Orcutt postulated that diarrhea, or 'scours', of calves is associated with the probable "absorption of toxins produced and set free during multiplication" of *B. coli*. However, disagreement with this idea was also prevalent at that time (Jones and Little, 1931a,b; Jones *et al.*, 1932).

Other sporadic reports appeared during the next 15 years but the etiological role of the *coli* group of bacteria was never clearly established until the late 1940s. The realization in 1944 of a comprehensive serological classification scheme by Kauffmann and the availability of reference antisera allowed the development of adequate epidemiological data to associate this organism, by then called *Escherichia coli* by some (Wallick and Stuart, 1943), with diarrhea.

The serological typing system was used during the 1950s to show that the strains which normally live in the intestine, known as commensals, differed from those responsible for hospital outbreaks of diarrhea (Ewing, 1962).

E. coli can cause diarrhea by at least three different pathogenic mechanisms (Rowe, 1979): destruction of the intestinal epithelial cells' brush border, invasion, and toxin production. These mechanisms are used to classify pathogenic *E. coli* into three major groups: enteropathogenic *E. coli* (EPEC), enteroinvasive *E. coli* (EIEC), and enterotoxigenic *E. coli* (ETEC). The EPEC are represented by those serotypes initially described during the 1940s and 1950s which are associated with diarrhea in infants. The EIEC were first described in 1967 by Sakazaki *et al.* The ETEC were the most recently characterized and currently are the best understood.

The etiological relationship between *E. coli* and diarrhea was most firmly demonstrated by a series of animal experiments during the 1960s. In 1967 Gyles and Barnum developed a pig model to show that *E. coli* strains isolated from humans, calves and pigs are all effective in reproducing the disease. For the first time since Smith and Orcutt (1925) it was again proposed, in 1966, that *E. coli* causes diarrhea in the rabbit model through the mechanism of a toxin (Taylor and Bettelheim, 1966). The following year Smith and Halls (1967a,b) using strains isolated from pigs and calves, showed that *E. coli* could produce an enterotoxin. They went on to show (Smith and Halls, 1968) that the gene coding for the enterotoxin was on a transmissible factor and in 1969 Gyles and Barnum described an *E. coli* strain from pigs that produced a heat-labile (activity destroyed by heating at o0°C for 30 min) factor which, quite interestingly, displayed antigenic cross-reactivity to cholera toxin.

A second form of the enterotoxin, a heat-stable (retained most of its activity after 30 min at 100°C, but was inactivated after 30 min at 121°C) form was described by Smith and Gyles in 1970. The accepted nomenclature today for the two enterotoxin types is LT (heat-labile) and ST (heat-stable) toxin.

In 1971 Sack *et al.* and Gorbach *et al.* isolated enterotoxin-producing strains from humans with cholera-like diarrhea. Later, heat-labile-toxin producing strains were shown to be responsible for traveler's diarrhea, a syndrome with many eponyms (Gorbach *et al.*, 1975; Merson *et al.*, 1976). Subsequently, many investigators have confirmed the antigenic re atedness of heat-labile forms of *E. coli* enterotoxin and cholera toxin (Smith and Sack, 1973; Gyles, 1974a,b; Clements and Finkelstein, 1978a,b). It is now known that clinical isolates of *E. coli* may make one or both types of toxin.

3. EPIDEMIOLOGY AND CLINICAL PRESENTATION

Infectious diarrheas are the third leading cause of morbidity and mortality in the world and the major cause of infant mortality in developing countries (Lee and Kean, 1978; Holmgren, 1981). There are an estimated one billion cases per year in children under five years of age and an estimated five million deaths. These account for one-third to one-half of all infant mortality. Furthermore, incidence rates as high as 50% have been reported for traveler's diarrhea suffered by millions throughout the world each year (Steffen *et al.*, 1983). Although there are varied etiologies, approximately 50% of diarrhea is due to enterotoxins (Holmgren, 1981). A large proportion of identified clinical isolates in many series of cases is *E. coli* (Guerrant *et al.*, 1975; Sack, 1975, 1980; Pickering *et al.*, 1978). Epidemiological studies by Merson *et al.* (1979a) and Orskov *et al.* (1976) showed that strains, isolated from many parts of the world, which produce *E. coli* enterotoxin belong to relatively few serogroups, and that these differ from the known EPEC serogroups. This led to the speculation by Orskov that these were clones of a small number of strains that had spread throughout the world. Similar results were obtained by Reis *et al.* (1980a).

The importance of *E. coli* enterotoxin in the production of diarrhea has been emphasized (Plotkin *et al.*, 1979) in studies involving infants and children (Otnaess and Halvorsen, 1981; Gorbach and Khurana, 1972; Guerrant *et al.*, 1975, 1976; Toledo *et al.*, 1983; Evans *et al.*, 1977b; Klipstein *et al.*, 1978; Pickering *et al.*, 1978; Sack *et al.*, 1975a; Wadström *et al.*, 1976), soldiers (DuPont *et al.*, 1971), adults in general (Evans *et al.*, 1977a; Sack, 1975; Sack *et al.*, 1977b; Shore *et al.*, 1974), and patients with 'non-vibrio cholera' (Sack *et al.*, 1971). Presence of LT in disease is most frequently reported in countries with relatively poor hygienic conditions, but antibodies against it have been found in many adult Americans as well (Donta *et al.*, 1974b) which suggests that ETEC may be widespread throughout the world. Indeed, the ability to produce LT is distributed throughout a wide range of serotypes, both inside and outside the classical enteropathogenic serotypes of *E. coli* (EPEC) (Otnaess and Halvorsen, 1981).

A more severe diarrhea is produced by strains that produce ST as well as LT. Most strains identified in hospitals and treatment centers have been found to be LT^+/ST^+ and belong most commonly to O serogroups 6, 8, 12, 20, 25, 62, 63, 78, 115, 128, 148, 153 and 159 (Black *et al.*, 1981b; Echeverria *et al.*, 1982; Merson *et al.*, 1979a,b, 1980a; Orskov *et al.*, 1976; Orskov and Orskov, 1977; Reis *et al.*, 1980a). In non-hospitalized persons, including infants and travelers in underdeveloped countries, LT^+/ST^- strains, while important, have been found to be less prevalent than LT^-/ST^+ strains in causing diarrhea (Black *et al.*, 1981a, 1982; Guerrant *et al.*, 1980c; Merson *et al.*, 1976; Sack *et al.*, 1978). In these studies, 20–30% of isolates were found to be LT^+/ST^- and 30–40% were LT^+/ST^+. Nearly 50% were devoid of LT (LT^-/ST^+). Strains producing only LT or ST represent a much wider array of O serotypes than those which express both toxin types. Ericsson *et al.* (1983) have reported that ETEC associated with humans generally produces both toxins (LT^+/ST^+).

Some correlations, in both human and pig strains of *E. coli* have been noted between enterotoxin production and the presence of various adhesins (Gaastra and de Graaf, 1982). LT production has been associated only with the presence of K88, CFA/I and CFA/II antigens either alone or in combination with ST production.

Disease due to enterotoxigenic *E. coli* results from specific attachment to the gut wall and elaboration of toxins, and is characterized by non-invasive, highly secretory diarrhea. Traveler's diarrhea, a common manifestation of ETEC-induced diarrhea, involving LT alone or LT and ST, has been attributed in some studies to about 37% of cases (Sack *et al.*, 1977a; Guerrant *et al.*, 1980b). Its typical presentation has been described (DuPont, 1981) as beginning within 10 days of arriving in the endemic area with the average illness consisting of 13 unformed stools over a 5-day period. Other symptoms were described as abdominal cramps 92%, nausea 55%, anal irritation 36%, a sense of urgency 27%, fever 20%, and vomiting 20%. The symptoms of this disease are likely, however, to vary from region to region depending upon the distribution of LT, ST, and LT/ST producing strains. Age of persons, and normal living environment are also important in the clinical presentation of ETEC disease.

4. PATHOGENESIS AND PATHOPHYSIOLOGY OF ENTEROTOXIGENIC *ESCHERICHIA COLI* (ETEC) DISEASE

The association of *Escherichia coli* with diarrheal disease has been appreciated since the 1940s. Enteropathogenic *E. coli* (EPEC) were first identified as the causative agent of infantile diarrhea (Neter, 1976; Rowe, 1979; Sack, 1980). Such strains belong to a restricted group of O serotypes (Goldschmidt and DuPont, 1976; Gurwith *et al.*, 1977; Wadström, 1978; Sack, 1980) and their mode of pathogenesis is essentially unknown but recent evidence suggests that an enterotoxin is involved (Klipstein *et al.*, 1978; Ryder *et al.*, 1979; Scheftel *et al.*, 1980; Scotland *et al.*, 1980). Enteroinvasive *E. coli* (EIEC) invade mucosal epithelial cells leading to inflammation and necrosis similar to that observed in shigellosis (Formal *et al.*, 1978; O'Brien *et al.*, 1979). In addition to the two mechanisms of pathogenesis just noted, enterotoxigenic *E. coli* (ETEC) were first recognized in veterinary medicine when they were isolated from neonatal calves and piglets suffering from acute diarrheal disease otherwise known as colibacillosis (Smith and Halls, 1967a,b; Kohler, 1968; Gyles and Barnum, 1969; Stevens *et al.*, 1972). ETEC have since been implicated in sporadic outbreaks and epidemics of diarrheal disease in both human infants and adults throughout the world (Sack, 1975, 1980; Gyles, 1978; Merson *et al.*, 1978; Polotsky *et al.*, 1977; Robertson, 1978).

The pathogenesis of ETEC summarized in Fig. 1 is mediated by at least two virulence factors: (1) pili (fimbriae) which enable the bacilli to specifically adhere to mucosal epithelial cells; and (2) production of two kinds of enterotoxins: a heat-stable enterotoxin

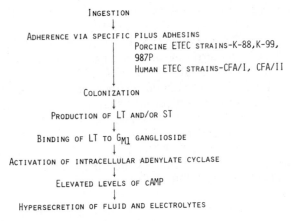

IMPORTANCE OF HEAT LABILE ENTEROTOXIN(LT)
IN PATHOGENESIS OF ETEC

INGESTION
↓
ADHERENCE VIA SPECIFIC PILUS ADHESINS
      PORCINE ETEC STRAINS-K-88,K-99,
      987P
      HUMAN ETEC STRAINS-CFA/I, CFA/II
↓
COLONIZATION
↓
PRODUCTION OF LT AND/OR ST
↓
BINDING OF LT TO G_{M1} GANGLIOSIDE
↓
ACTIVATION OF INTRACELLULAR ADENYLATE CYCLASE
↓
ELEVATED LEVELS OF cAMP
↓
HYPERSECRETION OF FLUID AND ELECTROLYTES

FIG. 1.

(ST) and a heat-labile enterotoxin (LT). Without surface pili, the bacteria cannot overcome intestinal motility and other host factors and ultimately colonize the small intestine (Freter, 1978; Moon et al., 1979; Gianella, 1981). Genes for both enterotoxins and pilus antigens, referred to as adhesins (Jones, 1977), are present on plasmids (Smith and Linggood, 1971b,c). Strains containing either the K-88 plasmid and/or the enterotoxin (ENT) plasmid were constructed using a K-12 E. coli strain cured of all plasmids (Smith and Linggood, 1971b). The strain containing the ENT plasmid did not colonize the small intestine and was avirulent while the strain containing the K-88 plasmid, but lacking the ENT plasmid, colonized the small intestine and caused a mild diarrhea. In contrast to strains carrying either the K-88 or ENT plasmids, the strain carrying both plasmids colonized the small intestine and caused severe diarrhea with a high incidence of mortality. The surface pili of ETEC protrude from the bacterial cell surface, bind to specific receptors on the surface of epithelial cells (Kearns and Gibbons, 1979; Faris et al., 1980), and are composed of protein which can be visualized by electron microscopy (Stirms et al., 1967; Moon et al., 1977, 1979). Three different chemical and antigenic types of pili (K-88, K-99, 987P) have been identified on porcine and bovine ETEC strains (Moon et al., 1980) and human ETEC strains possess at least two well characterized antigenic types, CFA/I and CFA/II (Evans et al., 1975; Evans and Evans, 1978). Other antigenic types may be found in association with animal strains of ETEC similar to observations recently made with human strains (Deneke et al., 1979; Thorne et al., 1979).

Pili determine species specificity of ETEC, that is, human strains do not cause disease in piglets and animal strains do not cause disease in humans. Pilus antigens may also be responsible for the age-dependent disease observed in piglets (Moon et al., 1980). Bacteria with K-99 and 987P pilus antigens are usually associated with diarrheal disease in piglets less than two weeks of age. Although not absolute, most of these strains produce heat-stable enterotoxin. The K-88 pilus antigen, common for porcine ETEC strains throughout the world, is often produced along with LT. The presence of plasmid-coded surface pili on porcine and human ETEC correlates with increased hydrophobicity as measured by hydrophobic interaction chromatography (Smyth et al., 1978; Wadström et al., 1978b; Faris et al., 1981). Hydrophobic interactions may provide the driving force necessary to overcome the net negative charge on bacterial and intestinal cell surfaces prior to adherence and colonization. The evidence for pili being important in the pathogenesis of ETEC can be summarized as follows: (1) loss of genetic information which codes for a specific pilus antigen leads to decreased virulence; and (2) anti-pilus antibodies block pilus function and protect animals against challenge by homologous strains (Isaacson et al.,

1978). It has been suggested that a trivalent vaccine against the three major porcine pilus types (K-88, K-99, and 987P) should protect piglets against diarrheal disease (Moon *et al.*, 1980). Immunization with LT and/or immunogenic forms of ST in combination with pilus antigens will likely provide the most effective form of protection (Smith and Linggood, 1971a; Pierce, 1977; Levine *et al.*, 1979b). Several reviews are available on the structure and function of pili (adhesins) in diarrheal disease (Freter, 1978; Duguid and Old, 1980; Moon *et al.*, 1979; Moon, 1980).

The somatic, or O, antigen of enteric bacilli most likely contributes to pathogenesis through increased resistance to phagocytosis, and resistance to complement-mediated killing by specific or cross-reacting (natural) antibodies. As noted previously, EPEC belong to a restricted group of O serotypes (Goldschmidt and DuPont, 1976; Gurwith *et al.*, 1977; Wadström, 1978; Sack, 1980), thus, information on the number and distribution of O serogroups associated with ETEC may assist identification and characterization. Although not widely accepted over the past 10 years, recent evidence suggests that serotyping may be clinically useful since a limited number of serotypes have been identified with diarrheal disease of piglets, calves and humans (Orskov and Orskov, 1979; Sack, 1980). Even though over 10,000 O:K:H serotypes are possible, approximately 12 are responsible for most disease in piglets throughout the world and 8 serotypes have been found associated with ETEC disease in calves. Of 109 strains isolated from humans in Bangladesh (Merson *et al.*, 1979a), 86% of LT/ST strains belonged to four O serotypes (O6, O8, O78 and O115) and 81% belonged to one of six O:K:H groups. Thirty four strains which produced ST were distributed over 15 serogroups. Reis *et al.* (1980b) made similar observations on strains isolated in Brazil. Certain combinations of O and H antigens almost assure that the strain will be enterotoxigenic (Sack, 1980). For example, O78:H11, O78:H12 and O6:H16 serotypes are usually enterotoxigenic whereas serogroups with other H antigens are not enterotoxigenic. Further, there can be a correlation between serotype and enterotoxin type (Merson *et al.*, 1979a; Orskov and Orskov, 1977). For example, serotype O6:H16 usually produces LT and ST whereas serotype O128:H almost always produces ST (Reis *et al.*, 1979). Another study on ETEC isolated from Ethiopian children (Bäck *et al.*, 1980) showed that: (1) like in previous studies, only a few O antigens account for most isolates, with O6, O8 and O78 serogroups being the most frequently identified; (2) enterotoxigenicity (LT) can be associated with a variety of O serogroups including the classical enteropathogenic O111; (3) *E. coli* with O antigens other than O6, O8 and O78 as well as non-*E. coli* rapidly lose the ability to produce enterotoxins; and (4) O78 strains possess CFA/I whereas O6 and O8 strains are associated with CFA/II. Eleven of the serotypes found throughout the world have been detected in ETEC isolated in the United States (DeBoy *et al.*, 1980). Enterotoxigenicty occurs more often in strains possessing a specific H antigen in conjunction with a specific O antigen. Also, ETEC which produce LT and ST belong to a smaller number of serotypes than those which produce ST or LT alone. Distinctive patterns of loss of enterotoxin production have been correlated with serotype (Evans *et al.*, 1977a). These observations probably can be explained by plasmid incompatibilities (McConnell *et al.*, 1980). Despite the fact that enteropathogenic serogroups usually do not produce LT and/or ST, enterotoxin production has been noted in serogroups O44, O14 and O128 (Scotland *et al.*, 1981). Most of these isolates were from tropical or developing countries. A low molecular weight form of LT was detected in culture supernatants of serogroup O55 (Ketyi *et al.*, 1979). It appears that serotyping is indeed useful in identification and characterization of ETEC, and once a genetic basis is established, it should be possible to explain the association of certain combinations of serotypes, pilus antigens and enterotoxins.

The pathogenesis of ETEC is closely intertwined with the production of LT and ST enterotoxins (Gyles and Barnum, 1969; Gyles, 1971; Kohler, 1971; Smith and Gyles, 1970b). LT has been shown to be immunologically related to cholera toxin (Gyles, 1974a,b; Clements and Finkelstein, 1978a,b; Holmgren and Svennerholm, 1979) and possesses a similar subunit structure and mechanism of action (Holmgren and Lönnroth, 1975; Gill, 1976; Gill *et al.*, 1981). The B monomeric units of *E. coli* LT and cholera toxin differ by a limited number of amino acid residues (Dallas and Falkow, 1980; Moseley and Falkow, 1980; Yamamoto and Yokota, 1983). The A subunit of LT which carries out ADP-ribosylation of a GTP binding protein with concomitant activation of adenylate cyclase (Gill and Richardson, 1980) shares some regions of homology with the analogous subunit of cholera toxin (Spicer et al., 1981; Yamamoto et al., 1984). The chemistry and subunit structure of cholera toxin have been the subject of several reviews (Finkelstein, 1973; Bennett and Cuatrecasas, 1976; Fishman, 1980; Lai, 1980).

The heat-stable toxin (ST) is a low-molecular-weight methanol-soluble polypeptide of 18–19 amino acid residues (Staples et al., 1980; Aimoto et al., 1982; Lallier et al., 1982; Rönnberg et al., 1983; Saeed et al., 1983; Dreyfus et al., 1983) which induces a secretory response in the small bowel through activation of guanylate cyclase (Field et al., 1978; Guerrant et al., 1980a). At least two kinds of STs have been identified, one with biological activity in suckling mice and piglets (ST_A) and another with biological activity only in piglets (ST_B) (Burgess et al., 1978). The chemical properties of ST_A produced by porcine, bovine and human ETEC strains include unique heat stability, stability to acid but not alkaline pH, high content of half-cystines, and absence of several amino acids commonly found in proteins (Alderete and Robertson, 1978; Kapitany et al., 1979; Takeda et al., 1979a,b; Madsen and Knopp, 1980; Staples et al., 1980; Dreyfus et al., 1983). Recently it was shown that ST_As produced by ETEC of different host origins exhibit immunological homogeneity (Frantz and Robertson, 1981; Giannella et al., 1981). Despite the observation that bovine strains of ETEC always produce ST (Sivasamy and Gyles, 1976), LT serum antibodies have been detected (Whipp and Donta, 1976; Dobrescu, 1979), and in vivo production of LT and ST has been demonstrated (Donta et al., 1974c).

It is likely that LT binds to a G_{M1} ganglioside receptor on small intestinal epithelial cells. (Donta and Viner, 1975; Donta, 1976; Moss et al., 1981) yet it was not explained until recently why preincubation of ligated rabbit ileal loops with choleragenoid (B subunits of cholera toxin) does not inhibit binding and the secretory response due to E. coli LT, and further, why cholera toxin is more efficiently bound and deactivated by gangliosides than LT (Pierce, 1973). A glycoprotein receptor for LT with no affinity for cholera toxin has been detected on surfaces of rabbit intestinal epithelial cells (Holmgren et al., 1982); thus, cholera toxin binds selectively to G_{M1} ganglioside, whereas LT binds to both G_{M1} ganglioside and a glycoprotein receptor. LT has been shown to stimulate adenylate cyclase in rabbit ileal mucosa (Evans et al., 1972; Kantor et al., 1974a; Kantor, 1975), isolated fat cells (Hewlett et al., 1974), thymocytes (Zenser and Metzger, 1974), canine jejunum (Guerrant et al., 1973), liver (Tait et al., 1980), cat heart myocardial preparations (Dorner and Mayer, 1975) and pigeon erythrocytes (Gill et al., 1976; Gill and Richardson, 1980). Increased levels of cyclic AMP have been demonstrated in Y-1 adrenal cells (Donta and Smith, 1974), Chinese hamster ovary (CHO) cells (Guerrant et al., 1974; Guerrant and Brunton, 1977) and Vero cells (Stavric et al., 1978).

The secretory response of rabbits and piglets to LT is virtually the same as the response to cholera toxin (Moon et al., 1971; Sherr et al., 1973; Hamilton et al., 1978b). Moon et al. (1971) have compared the effects of LT and cholera toxin on rabbit and swine small intestine. Histological changes in loops treated with the two enterotoxins were almost identical. The only change noted was the loss of goblet cell mucus and slight inflammatory lesions in some loops which was likely due to hydrostatic pressure since the lesions were more noticeable at 16 hr than at 8 hr. Villus adsorptive cells and other epithelial cells were normal in controls and toxin-treated loops. Compared with serum, rabbit ileal and pig jejunal loop fluids were low in protein, Mg^{2+} and Ca^{2+} and high in K^+, Na^+ and HCO_3^-.

Absorption of sugars and amino acids is not impaired in patients with severe watery diarrhea due to ETEC or V. cholerae and, in fact, oral rehydration with glucose and electrolytes is a recommended course of treatment (Greenough, 1978). Severity of ETEC-mediated disease can range from mild to a cholera-like condition (Finkelstein et al., 1976b). Thus, dehydration and metabolic acidosis may develop if the fluid loss is not reversed. More extensive reviews on the pathophysiology of E. coli LT compared with cholera toxin are available (Banwell and Sherr, 1973; Field, 1974; Kimberg, 1974; Moon, 1978; Richards and Douglas, 1978; Sack, 1978; Whipp, 1978; Field, 1979a,b).

5. ASSAYS FOR *E. COLI* LT

5.1. WHOLE ANIMALS

5.1.1. Ligated Loops

Ligated small intestinal loops of rabbits and piglets were extensively used in early studies on pathogenesis of ETEC (Smith and Halls, 1967a,b; Moon and Whipp, 1971; Smith and Gyles, 1970b; Lariviere *et al.*, 1972; Evans *et al.*, 1973b; Enweani *et al.*, 1975a,b; Hamilton *et al.*, 1978a,b,c). Despite its expense and being rather time consuming, the assay can be used to study the effects on both secretion and absorption, in rabbit ileal loops and pig jejunal loops, induced by enterotoxins and other pharmacological agents. Pig jejunum and rabbit ileum were used because these areas were found to be the most sensitive to enterotoxins (Moon and Whipp, 1971). Other advantages of the assay are that either live bacterial suspensions or enterotoxin preparations at various stages of purity can be assayed. Also, neutralization by specific antibodies can be measured. Fluid produced in response to either cholera toxin or *E. coli* LT is similar with respect to electrolyte and protein composition (Moon *et al.*, 1971; Sherr *et al.*, 1973; Hamilton *et al.*, 1978b). In general, preparations are tested in duplicate in a random sequence and in different animals. False–positive and false–negative reactions are common; therefore, multiple controls must be run. Samples injected into loops should be similar in osmolarity and electrolyte composition. Accumulation of fluid in rabbit ileal loops in response to *E. coli* LT reaches a maximum at about 18 hr with a ratio of volume (ml) to length (cm) of about 2–2.5. Whipp *et al.* (1981) improved quantitative aspects of the assay by using an inert volume marker, (^{14}C) polyethylene glycol (PEG), to measure fluid movement which reflects changes in absorption and/or secretion. Myers *et al.* (1975) found that as many as 150 isolates could be assayed in one calf with little problem caused by false–positive reactions.

5.1.2. Infant Rabbits

Although used as an assay for *E. coli* LT (Smith, 1972; Burgess *et al.*, 1979), the infant rabbit assay does not appear to offer an advantage over the loop assay unless the objective is to observe colonization followed by a diarrheagenic response. The assay can be performed with either broth suspensions or partially purified enterotoxin preparations. The sample to be assayed is introduced into the stomach by force feeding with a plastic tube or by direct injection following a surgical incision. The entire gastrointestinal tract is removed after the animal is sacrificed. The data is expressed as a ratio of gut weight to body weight. Infant rabbits exhibit a reproducible increase in intestinal fluid content in response to LT which is maximal at 5 hr following oral administration. They remain responsive to LT until 14 days of age. After this time, gastric pH apparently causes inactivation of LT.

5.1.3. Rat Perfusion

Perfusion of the rat jejunum provides a sensitive assay for both *E. coli* enterotoxins (Klipstein *et al.*, 1976, 1979). The assay has been shown to be reproducible, sensitive, and exhibits a dose-dependent response. A single jejunal segment of an anesthetized rat is perfused with one of the following solutions, an isosmolar balanced electrolyte solution, an electrolyte solution containing enterotoxin, or an electrolyte solution plus enterotoxin incubated with antitoxin. After a period of time to reach a steady rate, fractions are collected at timed intervals to measure net transport of water. The assay has been extensively used to monitor the secretory response of immunized animals compared with normal controls (Klipstein and Engert, 1977, 1978, 1979, 1980, 1981a,b; Klipstein *et al.*, 1980b). More important, the perfusion assay can detect toxins produced by enteric bacilli which induce secretion but are not positive in conventional enterotoxin assays. Following termination of the experiment, mucosal cells can be removed by scraping and assayed for various enzymatic activities and cyclic nucleotide content.

5.1.4. Canine Models

Dogs have been used to a limited extent for assay of LT and studies on pathogenesis of ETEC. Chronic Thiry–Vella loops are the most satisfactory for studying the secretory effect of multiple jejunal challenges (Guerrant et al., 1973; Sack et al., 1976). Disease has not been observed after orogastric challenge. The assay can be used to detect and quantitate a local immune response to LT, and the secretory response to ST can be distinguished from that due to LT.

5.1.5. Skin Permeability Assay

The skin permeability assay developed by Craig for determination of the biological activity of cholera toxin (Craig, 1971) can also be used to detect LT and its neutralization by specific antibodies (Evans et al., 1973b). Hair must be clipped, or removed with depilatory cream, followed by injection of 0.1 ml of sample per injection site. Each rabbit can receive 40–50 injections. After 18 hr, the animals receive an intravenous injection of 2% Evans blue dye in phosphate buffered saline. The areas of bluing or induration are measured in millimeters two hours later. Based on the results of Craig, varying amounts of LT should be mixed with antitoxin to generate a broad sigmoidal response instead of a steep dose response with unacceptable reproducibility. Either cholera antitoxin or E. coli LT antitoxin can be used for neutralization. Several concentrations of toxin and appropriate controls should be run to avoid misinterpretation due to a 'blanching factor' (Finkelstein et al., 1976a). A significant advantage of the assay is that it permits rapid screening of large numbers of samples. On the other hand, the assay is difficult, somewhat complicated, and requires considerable experience. Ketyi et al. (1978) have compared the sensitivity of the rabbit skin permeability test with Chinese hamster ovary (CHO) cells and rabbit ileal loop assays. The skin permeability assay has proven to be the most sensitive and useful of the three for screening clinical isolates for the presence of ETEC.

5.2. TISSUE CULTURE ASSAYS

5.2.1. Y-1 Adrenal Cells

Various tissue culture assays have simplified detection and quantitation of enterotoxins produced by enteric pathogens, especially *Vibrio cholerae* and ETEC. Mouse adrenal tumor (Y-1) cells in tissue culture respond to picogram amounts of cholera toxin (Donta et al., 1973) and E. coli (LT) (Donta et al., 1974a; Kwan and Wishnow, 1974) with a pronounced morphological change ('rounding response') and increased production of Δ^4-3-ketosteroids. The amount of rounding by LT can be estimated as a semi-quantitative assay, or steroids can be extracted and quantitated by fluorometry. The assay is somewhat limited by the fact that steroid production by cells declines after 8–10 passages, causing a significant decrease in sensitivity. Cells become granular and less suitable for rounding assays after 15–20 passages. Culture supernatants of ETEC are positive at dilutions from 1:4 up to 1:10.

A cytotoxin produced by some strains of ETEC can hinder detection of enterotoxin activity or give a false-positive reaction (Konowalchuk et al., 1978; O'Brien and LaVeck, 1983). The original assay has been modified to detect and measure the extent of neutralization by antibodies (Donta et al., 1974b; Donta and Smith, 1974; Wachsmuth et al., 1977), and to permit rapid screening of a large number of clinical specimens (Sack and Sack, 1975; Gurwith, 1977).

5.2.2. Chinese Hamster Ovary Cells

Chinese hamster ovary (CHO) cells respond to both E. coli LT and cholera toxin with morphological changes and increased intracellular levels of cAMP (Guerrant et al., 1974;

Guerrant and Brunton, 1977). The CHO cell assay has been recently modified by growing cells in monolayers followed by addition of enterotoxin (Nozawa *et al.*, 1978). Cells not incubated with LT or cholera toxin are released upon subsequent incubation whereas those treated with toxin contain more attached cells and fewer floating cells. Floating cells can be enumerated using a Coulter counter which alleviates the tedium of counting elongated cells stained with dilute Giemsa stain. The sensitivities of the Y-1 adrenal cells and CHO cells are similar. It is a matter of personal choice whether one wishes to estimate the degree of rounding, determine steroid content of culture media, or count the number of elongated cells within a population of 100–400 cells. Both Y-1 and CHO cells have been extensively used in clinical studies on ETEC-mediated diarrhea (Sack *et al.*, 1975a,b, 1977b; Morris *et al.*, 1976; Donta *et al.*, 1977; Echeverria *et al.*, 1978; Merson *et al.*, 1980b).

5.2.3. Vero Cells

Vero (African Green Monkey kidney) cells respond with morphological changes when treated with LT (Spiers *et al.*, 1977; Stavric *et al.*, 1978). Vero cells can be cultured quickly in quantity, and stock cultures require no maintenance for up to three weeks which results in considerable savings in time and labor. Vero cells tend to be sensitive to cytotoxins present in some crude enterotoxin preparations. The dose response of Vero cells treated with LT is comparable to Y-1 and CHO cells.

5.2.4. Henle Intestinal Cells

Human embryonic intestinal cells in monolayer cultures treated with *E. coli* LT exhibit increased adenylate cyclase activity (Kantor *et al.*, 1974b). Use of this intestinal cell line, compared with non-intestinal cells described above, appears to offer little advantage in the study of enterotoxin structure and function. The assay requires determination of either cAMP or adenylate cyclase activity. The cells may be useful to study receptors involved in binding of *E. coli* enterotoxins.

5.3. ENZYMATIC ASSAYS

5.3.1. Pigeon Erythrocyte Lysate Assay

Lysates of pigeon erythrocytes can be used for the assay of *E. coli* LT in culture supernatants (Gilligan and Robertson, 1979). The assay requires only the A or A_1 fragment of the toxin and can be used to screen large numbers of samples and correlates well with other bioassays which require the binding component in addition to an enzymatically active peptide. The A fragment reacts directly with a GTP-binding protein associated with adenylate cyclase (Gill *et al.*, 1976; Gill and Richardson, 1980). Activation of adenylate cyclase occurs with transfer of adenosine diphosphate ribose (ADPR) to the GTP-binding protein. The assay consists of three steps: (1) activation of adenylate cyclase by LT; (2) timed accumulation of cyclic AMP before the reaction mixture is stopped with dilute acid; and (3) determination of cyclic AMP by either a protein binding assay or radio-immunoassay. Despite the fact that LT remains associated primarily with the cell envelope of ETEC (Gankema *et al.*, 1980), the PEL assay is maximally stimulated with 20–40 μl of ETEC culture supernatant. Dilutions are routinely carried out in the presence of dilute sodium dodecylsulfate (SDS) which increases the amount of stimulation of adenylate cyclase by the A subunit. The assay can be used for quantitation of LT in culture supernatants and studies on the mechanism of the toxin.

5.3.2. Cat Heart Myocardial Assay

Another broken cell assay which responds to LT employs myocardial fractions from in heart (Dorner and Mayer, 1975). The assay can be used like the PEL assay to *ly, the* preparations at various stages of purity and antitoxin titers in sera. P mechanism of stimulation of adenylate cyclase is similar to that in other systems, i.e. ADP-ribosylation of a GTP-binding protein involved in regulation of adenylate cyclase.

5.3.3. NAD-Glycohydrolase and ADP-Ribosyltransferase Activities

Enzymatic activities intrinsic to the A subunit of LT can be measured by following the release of (carbonyl-^{14}C) nicotinamide from (carbonyl-^{14}C) NAD in the presence and absence of arginine or arginine methyl ester which acts as a receptor (Moss and Richardson, 1978; Moss et al., 1979b, 1981). The release of nicotinamide is dependent upon the presence of both dithiothreitol and arginine or arginine methyl ester. ^{14}C-Nicotinamide can be resolved from other reaction components by thin layer chromatography or use of ion exchange resins. The utility of the assay is limited by the expense of radioactive NAD. A less expensive assay for the enzymatic activity of E. coli LT and cholera toxin has been described by Mekalanos et al. (1979) which employs ^{125}I-N-guanyltyramine (^{125}I-GT) as an ADP-ribose acceptor in a reaction mixture containing thiol-treated cholera toxin and excess unlabeled NAD. ADP-ribosyl-^{125}I-GT can be readily quantitated by ion exchange fractionation to remove unreacted ^{125}I-GT. The radioactive substrate exhibits a high affinity for the ADP-ribosyltransferase reaction in contrast to other protein receptors which contain variable amounts of arginine. The use of ^{125}I-N-guanyltyramine as an ADP-ribose acceptor is a simpler system than using membranes which require unknown soluble factors for activation of adenylate cyclase (Moss and Vaughan, 1977; Enomoto and Gill, 1980).

5.4. Immunological Assays

5.4.1. Solid Phase Radioimmunoassays and ELISA

Solid phase radioimmunoassays (RIA) and enzyme linked immunoadsorbent assays (ELISA) have been developed based upon the antigenic cross-reactivity of cholera toxin and E. coli LT (Greenberg et al., 1977, 1979; Yolken et al., 1977; Ceska et al., 1978; Ketyi and Pacsa, 1980).

In the solid phase RIA, LT antigen is incubated in antibody-coated wells of microtiter plates followed by reaction with ^{125}I-anti-cholera toxin. The ELISA assay involves coating wells of microtiter plates with rabbit anti-cholera toxin, addition of samples containing LT, reaction with guinea pig anti-cholera toxin, use of anti-guinea pig IgG immunoglobulin conjugated to alkaline phosphatase, and incubation with substrate solution to measure the amount of bound alkaline phosphatase. The solid phase RIA can be modified to detect specific antibodies to E. coli LT (Greenberg et al., 1979). The sensitivity of both assays is comparable to the Y-1 adrenal assay. Another quantitative method has been devised based on specific binding of LT to polystyrene-adsorbed G_{M1} ganglioside, incubation with an appropriate dilution of rabbit anti-LT, and reaction with anti-rabbit IgG conjugated with alkaline phosphatase (Svennerholm and Holmgren, 1978). The G_{M1} ELISA is sensitive, reproducible, and yields results almost identical to the Y-1 adrenal cell assay. A micro-scale modification for large-scale screening of clinical specimens from patients with diarrhea has been described (Sack et al., 1980). The G_{M1}-ELISA assay compares favorably with Y-1 adrenal cells and is slightly more sensitive for identification of strains of ETEC producing LT (Bäck et al., 1979). The original G_{M1}-ELISA has been modified with the objectives of decreased performance time, increased simplicity, and ability to be read with the naked eye (Svennerholm and Wiklund, 1983; Beutin et al., 1984). Results from the G_{M1}-ELISA assay usually compare favorably with the Biken test (Sen et al., 1984).

Comparison of the G_{M1}-ELISA assay with the Y-1 adrenal cell assay, counter immunoelectrophoresis, and the Biken test revealed that the G_{M1}-ELISA is more sensitive as po~ of the other assays and can be used to detect LT in stool supernatants as well with the ~e supernatants (Morgan et al., 1983). In contrast to other studies, results ~oprecipitation test were somewhat disappointing.

Ristaino *et al.* (1983) attempted to improve the sensitivity of the G_{M1}-ELISA with anti-cholera toxin as the detecting reagent. The net optical density was increased using (1) a Casamino acids medium supplemented with glucose; (2) lincomycin; and (3) polymyxin B to release LT from bacterial pellets. The *E. coli* strains to be tested were grown directly in G_{M1}-coated wells of microtiter plates which saved assay time, materials, and reagents. The direct assay can be performed in about one-half of the time required for the Biken test and can use cholera antiserum which is commercially available. Optimal results are obtained with the G_{M1}-ELISA and other serological tests when homologous antisera against porcine and human heat-labile enterotoxins are used to identify porcine and human strains of ETEC, respectively (Gustafsson and Möllby, 1982).

5.4.2. Passive Immune Hemolysis

Sheep erythrocytes sensitized with partially purified LT incubated in the presence of anti-LT or anti-cholera toxin have been used in a passive immune hemolysis assay for detection and quantitation of LT (Evans and Evans, 1977a,b; Evans *et al.*, 1977b; Serafim *et al.*, 1979, 1981; DeCastro *et al.*, 1980; Tsukamoto *et al.*, 1980). Strains isolated from numerous sources (humans, swine, food and water) have been examined using both the Y-1 adrenal cell assay and passive immune hemolysis using antiserum produced against a crude LT preparation produced by human ETEC strain H-10407 (Serafim *et al.*, 1979). Strains isolated from pigs, sausage and water were not detected with antiserum raised against strain H-10407 which suggests that LTs from human and porcine strains of ETEC are not immunologically identical. Cholera antitoxin and anti-choleragenoid both were more effective than antisera raised against partially purified LT in detecting LT-producing strains.

5.4.3. Staphylococcal Agglutination Technique

The staphylococcal coagglutination technique has been applied to detection of LT in culture supernatants (Brill *et al.*, 1979; Rönnberg and Wadström, 1983; Honda *et al.*, 1983). Cholera antitoxin or anti-LT serum is absorbed with protein A-bearing staphylococci. The sensitized staphylococci agglutinate when mixed with LT antigen. The assay is performed in capillary tubes and requires cholera antitoxin which is readily available. Test results using the assay agree with CHO cell and passive immune hemolysis assays. Specialized equipment is not required which makes the test applicable to diagnosis of ETEC disease in developing countries.

5.4.4. Biken Test

The method combines principles of the Elek test and Oucherlony double gel diffusion test (Honda *et al.*, 1981a). Four isolates of *E. coli* to be tested are applied to a Biken agar plate followed by incubation for 48 hr. Filter paper disks containing polymyxin B are placed near each of the four areas of growth. After 5 hr mcubation at 37°C, anti-LT serum is placed in a well cut in the center of the four strains. If any of the isolates produce LT, precipitin lines form in about 24 hr. Pieces of agar near the colonies can be removed, extracted with buffer, and the gel supernatant assayed for ST by the suckling mouse assay. A total of 2,129 strains of *E. coli* isolated from patients with diarrhea were tested for LT production by the Biken test and CHO cell assay (Honda *et al.*, 1982). A total of 578 strains were positive in both assays, 22 strains were positive by one of the two assays, and 1,629 strains were negative with both assays.

5.4.5. Latex Particle Agglutination Test

A simple, rapid and economical test for *E. coli* LT, which can be applie~~ic~~ media, isolated from primary cultures of stool specimens on common enteri~~ ~~

has been developed (Finkelstein *et al.*, 1983). Latex particles sensitized with anti-LT serum are mixed with polymyxin B extracts of emulsified colonies. After 3 min incubation, the mixture is observed for agglutination using transmitted oblique illumination. Several factors are important for optimal results with the assay: (1) high quality specific antiserum; (2) the quality and source of latex preparation; (3) use of polymyxin B to release intracellular and periplasmic LT; and (4) careful titration of the antibody preparation. The assay will detect LT produced by porcine *E. coli* isolates using antiserum raised against either human or porcine LTs (Finkelstein *et al.*, 1983). An automated latex agglutination method for detection of cholera toxin and *E. coli* LT has also been described (Ito *et al.*, 1983).

5.5. Detection of Individual Colonies Producing LT

A novel DNA colony hybridization technique has been developed for detection of ETEC (Mosley *et al.*, 1980). The method is based on detection of genes that code for LT and ST instead of the enterotoxins themselves. Clinical isolates of ETEC, stools, or rectal swabs are spotted directly on nitrocellulose filters overlaid on MacConkey's agar plates. Radioactive DNA probes are prepared by *in vitro* labeling of restriction endonuclease fragments of genes which encode for LT or ST. After growth of the bacteria, colonies are lysed and DNA denaturation *in situ* carried out on the nitrocellulose filter. The filter is then incubated with radiolabeled DNA fragments under conditions which favor hybridization of homologous DNA sequences. Hybridization is detected by radioautography. The assay detects all LT-producing strains but does not detect all ST-producing strains which suggests that ST genes are more chemically heterogeneous than LT genes. The Y-1 assay has also been used to detect LT-producing colonies on membrane filters (Calderon and Levin, 1981). The assay can quantitate ETEC producing LT in fecal specimens and environmental samples where large volumes must be filtered.

Several techniques recently have been described for detection of hypertoxinogenic or hypotoxinogenic mutant colonies following mutagenesis (Silva *et al.*, 1978). The passive immune hemolysis assay has been modified to detect halos in agar layers of sheep red blood cells mixed with bacteria and covered with a soft agar overlay of complement and specific antibody (Bramucci and Holmes, 1978). LT binds to gangliosides on RBC cell surfaces and fixes antibody prior to lysis by complement. The ganglioside filter assay described by Mekalanos *et al.* (1978a) should be readily applicable to selection of LT mutants. Alternatively, polyvinyl plastic discs can be coated with specific antibody (anti-LT or anti-cholera toxin) and applied to plates with bacterial colonies (Broome and Gilbert, 1978; Shah *et al.*, 1982). The immobilized antigen can be detected with radioiodinated antibody. The G_{M1}-ELISA assay can be modified to screen individual colonies and thus avoid use of radioactive reagents (Czerkinsky and Svennerholm, 1983).

6. PURIFICATION AND CHARACTERIZATION OF LT

Despite the fact that the enterotoxins of *Vibrio cholerae* and ETEC share similar roles in pathogenesis, techniques successful in purification of cholera toxin are, for the most part, not applicable to purification of *E. coli* LT. Molecular weights ranging from 23,000 to approximately 1,000,000 have been reported for *E. coli* LT (Jacks *et al.*, 1973; Lariviere *et al.*, 1973; Evans *et al.*, 1974; Mitchell *et al.*, 1974; Söderlind *et al.*, 1974; Dorner, 1975; Möllby *et al.*, 1975; Schenkein *et al.*, 1976; Wadström *et al.*, 1977; Konowalchuk *et al.*, 1978; Lallier and Lariviere, 1978). Thus, in the early and mid-1970s investigators were faced with a bewildering array of molecular weights which until recently could not be explained. In addition to the heterogeneous molecular weights, most reports described the purification of only minute amounts of LT, and further, antiserum prepared against LT anal laboratory showed lack of reactivity, or only partial cross-reactivity by Ouchterlony found the Schenkein *et al.*, 1976). The situation was made even more confusing when it was weights and produced by one strain grown in different media has different molecular genic specificities (Finkelstein *et al.*, 1976a).

More recent data show that LT is a hydrophobic protein which remains associated with the cell envelope (inner and outer membranes) and, depending on the strain, is released in high molecular weight vesicles (Wensink *et al.*, 1978; Gankema *et al.*, 1980) or as a small amount of free LT protein. LT was finally purified through use of alternative approaches such as use of hydrophobic interaction chromatography to resolve LT from membrane components (Robertson *et al.*, 1978; Kunkel and Robertson, 1979), use of immunological assays to better quantitate amounts of LT in various fractions (Clements and Finkelstein, 1979; Clements *et al.*, 1980), and purification of LT from hypertoxinogenic mutants (Holmes *et al.*, 1979).

6.1. NUTRITION AND RELEASE OF LT

6.1.1. Nutritional Factors

When Robertson and coworkers began their work on LT, it appeared that a chemically defined medium would be advantageous for at least three reasons: (1) the amount of ultraviolet absorbing substances contributed by peptones in complex media would be eliminated, or at least decreased; (2) if media were standardized between laboratories, the likelihood of isolating similar preparations would be increased; and (3) factors affecting release and processing of extracellular toxin might be more easily identified and studied. They observed that amino acids, carbon sources, pH, oxygen tension, divalent cations, growth temperature and protease activity all affect the amount of LT in culture supernatants of ETEC (Gilligan and Robertson, 1979; Kunkel and Robertson, 1979).

Methionine and lysine were the most stimulatory amino acids when added to a basal salts medium containing morpholinopropane sulfonate (MOPS) and 0.5% D-glucose. Either aspartic acid or glutamic acid in the presence of methionine and lysine further increased levels of LT produced by porcine and human strains of ETEC, respectively. The data in Table 1 show that levels of LT produced in the defined media were approximately four-fold higher in a complex Casamino acids-yeast extract medium and at least three-fold higher than M-9 minimal salts media containing 0.5% D-glucose. There is no correlation between growth (OD_{620}) and the amount of LT present in culture supernatants. The reason for the higher levels of LT in the defined media compared with Casamino acids-yeast extract medium is that several amino acids are inhibitory to LT synthesis. In particular, branched-chain amino acids (leucine, isoleucine and valine) were often inhibitory, as was histidine for some strains. The importance of glucose in the growth medium is shown in Experiments No. 4 and 5 of Table 1. In the presence of amino acids found to be optimal for synthesis of ST (Alderete and Robertson, 1979) and those which stimulate LT synthesis, LT is not detected until addition of 0.5% glucose. Higher levels of glucose decrease the pH and yield lower amounts of extracellular LT. Other carbon sources which exhibit a high degree of catabolite repression support synthesis of LT, but less than with D-glucose. There are no vitamin or unusual growth factor requirements, and Fe^{3+} is not required although it slightly stimulates LT synthesis by porcine strains grown in the

TABLE 1. *Effects of Nutritional Conditions on Synthesis of LT by ETEC Strain 1362**

Expt	OD_{620}†	Medium	cAMP (pmol)‡
1	3.4	Salts	86
2	3.2	+ Met + Lys + Asp§	240
3	3.3	+ ST amino acids (no glucose)‖	20
4	3.5	As 3 + Met + Lys + Asp	22
5	4.8	As 4 + 0.5% glucose	190
6	4.3	Casamino acids-yeast extract	66

*Gilligan and Robertson (1979).
†OD_{620}, optical density at 620 nm.
‡Equivalent of 2 μl of culture supernatant used in PEL assay.
§Methionine, lysine, aspartic acid; 200 μg/ml.
‖Alderete and Robertson (1977).

Table 2. *LT Antigen Produced in different Growth Media by ETEC Strain 286C$_2$*

Medium	OD$_{620}$	pH	Concentration of LT μg/ml*
Defined†	3.8	6.8	4.60
Brain–heart infusion	6.7	8.25	1.16
Casamino acids-yeast extract	4.8	8.45	0.17
Syncase‡	3.8	7.95	0.78
Trypticase soy broth	5.7	8.25	0.13

*Determined as LT antigen by solid-phase RIA. All preparations were concentrated 10-fold by PM-10 ultrafiltration before assay.
†Gilligan and Robertson (1979).
‡Finkelstein *et al.* (1966).

presence of the three amino acids and D-glucose. The stimulation appears to be on the overall physiology of the bacteria and not directly on LT synthesis.

Amounts of LT produced in several complex media and the defined medium containing three amino acids have been measured using a solid-phase RIA (Table 2). Antiserum raised against purified 286C$_2$ LT was used to coat polystyrene tubes. Minimal amounts of LT were produced during growth in Trypticase-soy broth, Casamino acids-yeast extract and Syncase medium (Finkelstein *et al.*, 1966), as compared with the defined medium. Growth in Brain–heart infusion (BHI) broth resulted in about four-fold less LT antigen than in the defined medium. The amount of LT measured in the defined medium was about two-fold less than is normally detected due to losses during ultrafiltration. All culture supernatants were concentrated 10-fold by Amicon PM-10 ultrafiltration. A Tryptone-yeast extract medium coupled with vigorous aeration (Landwall and Möllby, 1978) yielded the most extracellular LT in fermentor cultures compared with a glucose–salts medium (Mitchell *et al.*, 1974). BHI has been shown to be optimal with shake flask cultures (Wadström *et al.*, 1978a).

Addition of mitomycin C to growth media will also increase the amount of LT in culture supernatants (Isaacson and Moon, 1975; Yoh *et al.*, 1983) due to cell lysis caused by induction of temperate bacteriophage (Gemski *et al.*, 1978; Takeda and Murphy, 1978). While this seems to be a convenient method of increasing the yield of extracellular LT, not all strains of ETEC are susceptible to mitomycin C induced lysis. Only about one-half of the porcine and human strains used in Robertson's laboratory for nutritional studies lyse upon incubation with the antibiotic. LT purified from ETEC strain H-10407 treated with mitomycin C exhibits a molecular weight of about 30,000 which may correspond to the A subunit of LT (Takeda *et al.*, 1979a). Thus, the molecular nature of LT released by mitomycin-treated cells is unclear.

Lincomycin, an inhibitor of protein synthesis, significantly increases amounts of LT antigen which reacts with anti-cholera toxin (Levner *et al.*, 1977). Amino acids present in the defined media may increase intracellular pools and ultimately increase the synthesis of LT similar to the proposed mechanism of action of lincomycin which has been shown to increase the synthetic rate and periplasmic pool of cholera toxin within *Vibrio cholerae* 569B (Levner *et al.*, 1980).

6.1.2. Release of Cell Associated LT

The pH of the defined medium decreases during growth from 7.5 to 6.8 even when highly buffered. Therefore, it is necessary to adjust the pH of culture supernatants of stationary-phase cells grown in the defined medium to approximately 8 in order to effect complete release of LT. The pH effect observed for release of cell-associated LT by ETEC is similar to that observed in studies on release of cholera toxin by *Vibrio cholerae* 569B (Callahan and Richardson, 1973), except that the critical pH for release of LT is about a 0.5 unit lower. The basis of the pH effect and its role in the release of LT are unknown at the present time. Callahan and Richardson (1973) suggested that ionic interactions are important in the release of cholera toxin by *Vibrio cholerae*. Alternatively, pH adjustment may be necessary to permit a protease to effect release of LT from the outer membrane. The effect of pH on the amount of LT in culture supernatants has also been observed by Mundell *et al.* (1976).

Extracellular LT rapidly appears in culture supernatants following pH adjustment and reaches maximum levels in 20–30 min. The release of LT occurs in the absence of cell lysis and LT synthesis parallels growth if the pH is maintained above 7.5. Incubation with protease inhibitors prior to pH adjustment decreases levels of extracellular LT. Likewise, pre-incubation with trypsin enhances toxin release.

Temperature also exerts a dramatic influence on the processing and/or release of LT (Kunkel and Robertson, 1979). Cell-associated LT is not released by pH adjustment when bacteria are grown at 21°C, but, polymyxin-B treatment of bacteria releases a toxin species of 30,000 daltons with biological activity in the pigeon erythrocyte lysate (PEL) assay. As the growth temperature is increased to 37°C, polymyxin-B treatment releases two additional species of LT which are active in either the PEL assay or exhibit both PEL and Y-1 adrenal tumor cell activity. Polymyxin-B extracts of ETEC in early log phase grown at 37°C exhibit only PEL activity whereas extracts from cells in late-log and early-stationary phase exhibit biological activity in both assay systems. No LT is released by pH adjustment of early log phase cells but LT released in later phases of growth is active in both assay systems. Gel electrophoresis of polymyxin-B extracts and elution of toxin activity from gel slices indicates the presence of at least three molecular species active in either the PEL (22,000 and 30,000 daltons) or Y-1 adrenal tumor cell assay (72,000 daltons), depending on the growth temperature. These data suggest that a subunit of LT with PEL activity analogous to the A subunit of cholera toxin is synthesized at low growth temperatures and early log phase when cells are grown at 37°C. Later in the growth cycle, the binding component is synthesized and associates with the A subunit already inserted into the outer membrane. The 30,000 dalton species with PEL activity, but no Y-1 activity, may be a precursor form of the A subunit which has not been processed by a protease.

The high molecular weight species of *E. coli* LT encountered by many investigators and in Robertson's laboratory can now be explained by recent observations (Wensink *et al.*, 1978; Gankema *et al.*, 1980). These workers have shown that non-pathogenic *E. coli* and ETEC normally release vesicles containing LT during growth as well as other outer membrane components. The medium vesicles account for 3–5% of the total protein. A second fraction released by growing cells consists mostly of lipopolysaccharide with a very low protein content. The LT content of medium vesicles is 3–4 times that of the outer membrane based on protein content, and likely arises by release from sites of outer membrane synthesis. More recently, Middeldorp and Witholt (1981) studied the binding of inner membrane and outer membranes, periplasmic vesicles, and medium vesicles, and whole cells to isolated porcine brush border membranes. Preparations enriched in K-88 antigen selectively bind to porcine brush borders. It was suggested that local patches of outer membrane 'bud out' and, once the bacteria bind to epithelial cells in the small intestine, outer membrane fragments (medium vesicles) containing K-88 and LT may function as carriers which efficiently deliver the enterotoxin to its site of action.

Amounts of LT associated with membrane fractions and the cytoplasm of two strains of ETEC are shown in Table 3. The bacteria were disrupted using a French press and centrifuged at $30,000 \times g$ to pellet the cell envelope (inner and outer membranes). The cell envelope was resuspended in 0.12 M Tris (pH 8.5) and incubated at 37°C for 60 min with gentle shaking to release cell associated toxin.

Strain 286C$_2$ releases about 20% of its total LT whereas strain 263 releases 10–20-fold less extracellular toxin. Strain 286C$_2$ is a human ETEC strain (Morris *et al.*, 1976) and strain 263 is a porcine isolate. Decreased levels of toxin in culture supernatants of strain 263 correlate with decreased amounts associated with the inner and outer membranes and increased amounts of LT in the cytoplasmic fraction. Some of the problems associated with purification of LT are brought out by these data. Strain 286C$_2$ produces at least 10-fold less extracellular material than does *V. cholerae* 569$_B$ (Mekalanos *et al.*, 1978b).

TABLE 3. *Distribution of Cell Associated and Extracellular LT in Cell Fractions of ETEC**

Strain	Fraction	Toxin production (μg/ml)†
263	Culture supernatant (pH adjusted)	0.06–0.11
	Cell-associated‡	
	Cytoplasm	3.8
	Cell envelope (inner + outer membrane)	0.5
286C$_2$	Culture supernatant (pH adjusted)	1.1
	Cell-associated‡	
	Cytoplasm	2.9
	Cell envelope (inner + outer membrane)	1.7
V. cholerae 598B	Culture supernatant	10§

*Robertson (unpublished data).
†Determined as LT antigen by solid-phase RIA.
‡Volume of each fraction adjusted to be the same as culture supernatant.
§Mekalanos *et al.* (1978b).

Purification of 263 LT from culture supernatants requires large amounts of cells. Methods need to be developed to isolate enterotoxin species associated with the periplasmic space, inner and outer membranes and the cytoplasmic fraction. It appears that strain 286C$_2$ releases more toxin rather than being a hypertoxinogenic (htx) producer. Bramucci *et al.* (1981) have recently described isolation and characterization of htx mutants of ETEC produced by mutagenesis with *N*-methyl-*N*-nitro-nitrosoguanidine. Four phenotypically distinct classes with respect to the amounts of cell-associated and extracellular LT have been isolated. Type 1 and 2 htx mutants produce increased amounts of cell-associated LT, with slight to moderate increases in extracellular LT, whereas Type 3 and Type 4 htx mutants produce normal or decreased amounts of cell-associated LT and moderate to markedly increased levels of extracellular LT. Thus, it is possible to isolate mutants that produce more LT with only small changes in the levels of extracellular toxin, produce the same amount of LT but release more, or produce and release more LT.

6.2. APPROACHES TO PURIFICATION

A comparison of the three schemes which have yielded homogeneous LT are summarized in Fig. 2. The results of Robertson and coworkers with pH-adjusted cells suggest

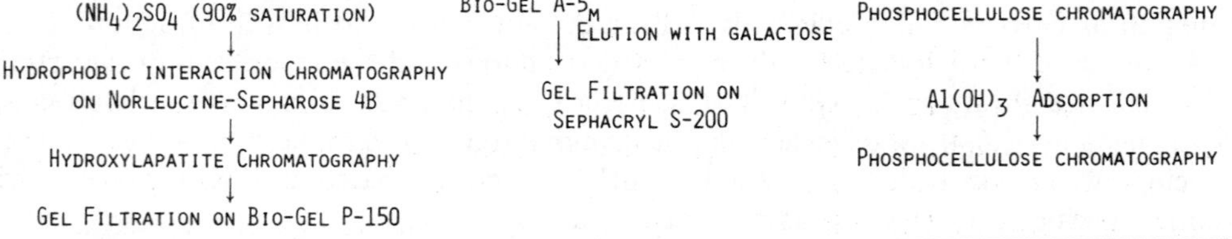

PURIFICATION SCHEME FOR E. COLI LTs

ETEC STRAIN

286C$_2$[A]	P307[B]	KL320 (pCG86-T65)[C]
pH EXTRACT[D]	CFS[E], WCL[3] OR NaCl EXTRACT[G]	WCL
↓	↓	↓
ULTRAFILTRATION WITH PM-10 DIAFLO MEMBRANES	$(NH_4)_2SO_4$ (60% SATURATION)	$(NH_4)_2SO_4$ (40–70% SATURATION)
↓	↓	↓
$(NH_4)_2SO_4$ (90% SATURATION)	BIO-GEL A-5$_M$	PHOSPHOCELLULOSE CHROMATOGRAPHY
↓	↓ ELUTION WITH GALACTOSE	
HYDROPHOBIC INTERACTION CHROMATOGRAPHY ON NORLEUCINE-SEPHAROSE 4B	GEL FILTRATION ON SEPHACRYL S-200	Al(OH)$_3$ ADSORPTION
↓		↓
HYDROXYLAPATITE CHROMATOGRAPHY		PHOSPHOCELLULOSE CHROMATOGRAPHY
↓		
GEL FILTRATION ON BIO-GEL P-150		

(A) ROBERTSON, ET AL. (1978), KUNKEL AND ROBERTSON (1979).
(B) CLEMENTS AND FINKELSTEIN (1979).
(C) HOLMES, ET AL. (1979).
(D) pH EXTRACT-CELL ASSOCIATED LT RELEASED BY ADJUSTMENT OF CELLS FROM pH 6.8 TO 8.0.
(E) CFS-CELL FREE SUPERNATANT.
(F) WCL-WHOLE CELL LYSATE.
(G) NaCl EXTRACT-PERIPLASMIC FRACTION.

FIG. 2.

that it might facilitate purification to wash cells at low pH, thereby removing loosely associated LPS and other membrane components, and then resuspend cells at pH 8 to release cell-associated LT. The release of outer membrane components occurs in Tris buffer and is enhanced by EDTA. Addition of EDTA does not increase the amount of extracellular LT and various cations have no effect on the amount of LT released by pH adjustment. Maximum amounts of LT with minimal cell lysis are obtained with hypotonic 0.12 M Tris buffer (pH 8.5). It is interesting that two of the three purification schemes employ hydrophobic interaction chromatography (HIC). The adsorption to BIO-GEL A-5m with subsequent elution by galactose probably represents a modified form of HIC. In Robertson's laboratory HIC was considered to be a useful purification step for *E. coli* LT because: (1) LT was one of the most hydrophobic proteins in pH extracts of four different ETEC strains; (2) LT might be resolved from other hydrophobic outer membrane components, especially lipopolysaccharide which readily associates with LT; (3) chromatography on DEAE BIO-GEL A and other anion-exchange resins yielded three peaks of LT activity, three active in the PEL assay and only one active against Y-1 adrenal cells; and (4) the amount of LT activity in pH extracts from most porcine strains of ETEC which bound to anion-exchange resins was much less than the amount of toxin activity which passed through the column. Following concentration and $(NH_4)_2SO_4$ fractionation, partially purified LT preparations were applied to a HIC column of norleucine covalently coupled to Sepharose 4B. Elution was accomplished using a linear decreasing ammonium sulfate gradient combined with an increasing ethylene glycol gradient. Addition of ethylene glycol was necessary to minimize spreading of LT activity. Hydroxylapatite chromatography of fractions containing LT from the hydrophobic column yield an essentially pure preparation. In the final purification step, BIO-GEL P-150 was used since gel filtration of partially purified LT on agarose resins (e.g. Bio-Rad A-5m and Ultragel AcA(44)) leads to aggregation and low recoveries of LT activity.

Clements and Finkelstein (1979) observed that LT adsorbs to column supports containing agarose and can be eluted in almost pure form with D-galactose. Since galactose is a component of G_{MI} ganglioside, it is not surprising that LT interacts with the agarose backbone. Adsorption is likely due to hydrophobic forces, and D-galactose causes a conformational change which decreases the association of the agarose with hydrophobic regions of LT. The purification scheme of Holmes *et al.* (1979) couples phosphocellulose chromatography used for purification of cholera toxin and its subunits (Mekalanos *et al.*, 1978b) with $Al(OH)_3$ adsorption chromatography. The yield of LT obtained from the $Al(OH)_3$ step is low but this apparently is necessary to obtain homogeneous material from the second phosphocellulose chromatography step. Affinity chromatography using an anti-cholera toxin immunoglobulin-Sepharose column has also been used to purify LT. A protein of 50,000 daltons, presumably the B subunit of LT, has been isolated by Dafni *et al.* (1978), while Wolk *et al.* (1980) have isolated both A and B subunits. The yield of LT antigen is about 50% but the skin permeability and PEL assays indicate that only partial reassociation of the subunits occurs during dialysis to remove guanidine hydrochloride.

6.3. Chemical and Biological Properties of *E. coli* LT

The chemical properties of all three LT preparations are remarkably similar (Table 4). The molecular weight of $286C_2$ LT has been determined to be 73,000 by gel electrophoresis and 64,000–66,000 by sedimentation equilibrium, while P307 LT exhibits a molecular weight of 93,000 as determined by sedimentation equilibrium. Purified $286C_2$ LT retains biological activity over a range of storage conditions, and at alkaline pHs, but rapidly loses enterotoxin activity below pH 6.0. Purified preparations are heat-labile as measured by the Y-1 adrenal cell assay but heating at 65°C does not destroy biological activity associated with the A subunit measured by the PEL assay. Neither $286C_2$ LT or P307 LT are contaminated with lipopolysaccharide or contained carbohydrate. The amino acid composition of two purified LTs is presented in Table 5 with cholera toxin included for comparison. The amino acid compositions of the two LTs are quite different and both are

TABLE 4. *Chemical Properties of* E. coli *LTs*

	ETEC strain			
Characteristic	286C$_2$*	P307†	KL320 (pCG86-T65)‡	Cholera toxin§
Molecular weight	74,000	92,000	—	84,000
Subunit composition	AB$_5$‖	AB$_5$‖	—	AB$_5$
Subunit molecular units				
B oligomer	42–46,000	60–70,000	58,000	59,000
B monomer	11,500	11,500	11,500	11,000
A subunit	28,200	28,000	30,000	29,000
A$_1$ fragment	24,000	21,000	21,000	23–24,000
A$_2$ fragment	5,100	7,000	7,000	6–7,000
pI	7.55¶	8.0		6.87
Terminal residues				
A subunit				
Amino	Asparagine	Asparagine**	—	Asparagine
Carboxyl	—	Glycine††	—	Tyrosine
B subunit				
Amino	Threonine	Alanine**	—	Threonine
Carboxyl	—	Asparagine††	—	Asparagine
Biological activity				
Y-1 adrenal cells‡‡	50	20	—	50§§
ADP-ribosyl transferase‖‖				
− Trypsin	78	—	—	144
+ Trypsin	248	—	—	134

*Kunkel and Robertson (1979); Robertson *et al.* (1979).
†Clements and Finkelstein (1979); Clements *et al.* (1980).
‡Holmes *et al.* (1979).
§Gill (1977); Lai (1980).
‖Gill *et al.* (1981).
¶Kunkel and Robertson (unpublished data).
**Dallas and Falkow (1980).
††Spicer and Noble (1982).
‡‡picograms/ml of toxin which give a 50% rounding response.
§§Donta *et al.* (1973).
‖‖nmol min^{-1} mg^{-1} of (carbonyl-^{14}C) nicotinamide released, Moss *et al.* (1981).

TABLE 5. *Amino Acid Composition of* E. coli *LTs*

	Concentration (g/100 g of amino acids) ETEC strain		
Amino acid	286C$_2$*	P307†	Cholera toxin‡
Aspartic acid	9.20	11.62	11.2
Threonine	6.19	10.39	7.8
Serine	4.4	9.94	6.6
Glutamic acid	12.33	11.70	10.8
Proline	1.82	3.68	4.3
Glycine	2.44	6.44	5.8
Alanine	3.5	5.74§	9.9
Half-cystine	5.41	—	1.6
Valine	5.56	3.84	4.3
Methionine	5.48	3.74	3.2
Isoleucine	8.80	9.97	7.4
Leucine	6.41	5.84	5.9
Tyrosine	8.37	4.17	4.3
Phenylalanine	4.44	2.25	3.1
Histidine	3.54	1.19	2.3
Lysine	7.09	6.82	6.9
Arginine	5.33	3.79	4.5
Tryptophan	ND‖	ND‖	—

*Kunkel and Robertson (1979).
†Clements and Finkelstein (1979).
‡Finkelstein (1973).
§Value represents alanine + half-cystine content.
‖Not determined.

unique compared with cholera toxin. Hydrophobic residues (valine, isoleucine and leucine) of 286C$_2$ constitute about 20% of total amino acids expressed on a weight basis and may explain the hydrophobic properties of the protein and interaction with norleucine-Sepharose 4B. The two purified *E. coli* LTs and cholera toxin have different isoelectric points as might be predicted from their amino acid compositions.

LT purified from strain 286C$_2$ (Robertson *et al.*, 1978; Kunkel and Robertson, 1979) is cell-associated enterotoxin released by pH adjustment of cells whereas Clements and Finkelstein (1979) have isolated extracellular LT, periplasmic and cytoplasmic forms of toxin. Preparations described by Holmes *et al.* (1979) likely represented a mixture of all three forms of LT since the starting material consisted of sonicated cell lysates. The biological activities of the three forms described by Clements and Finkelstein (1979) were markedly different, with varying degrees of activation by trypsin. For example, the extracellular form was only slightly activated by treatment with trypsin compared with the periplasmic and cytoplasmic forms which were activated 500-fold, and about 200-fold, respectively. The toxin produced by strain 286C$_2$ was activated three–four-fold by treatment with trypsin (Moss *et al.*, 1981). Purified 286C$_2$ LT exhibited biological activity compared to that of cholera toxin in bioassays specific for the two enterotoxins (Y-1 adrenal tumor cells, Chinese hamster ovary cells, pigeon erythrocyte lysates and skin permeability test).

Like cholera toxin, the receptor for *E. coli* LT appears to be G$_{M1}$ ganglioside based on the following evidence: (1) the toxin binds to rat glioma cells that have incorporated G$_{M1}$ ganglioside but not to cells that have been preincubated with gangliosides G$_{M2}$, G$_{D1a}$ or G$_{D1b}$; (2) the tryptophanyl fluorescence spectra of LT and LT-B are 'blue shifted' in the presence of the oligosaccharide moiety of G$_{M1}$, whereas neuramin lactose and the oligosaccharide moiety of G$_{D1a}$ have no effect; (3) the concentrations of G$_{M1}$ oligosaccharide necessary to 'blue shift' the tryptophanyl fluorescence spectrum of LT are similar to those effective for cholera toxin.

The receptors on Y-1 adrenal cells for *E. coli* LT and cholera toxin have been characterized (Donta *et al.*, 1982). Only one class of receptors is detected for each toxin with a K_a of $1.5–2.0 \times 10^9$ M^{-1}. About three-fold fewer receptors for cholera toxin need to be occupied prior to induction of a morphological change, whereas there is a strong correlation between the amount of LT bound and the subsequent biological response. The data suggest that there are 'spare receptors' present on Y-1 adrenal cells for cholera toxin but not for LT. Each toxin competitively inhibits binding by both enterotoxins. However, two-fold more LT is needed to inhibit 50% of the binding of cholera toxin compared with the amount of cholera toxin required to inhibit 50% of the binding of LT, or the same amount of inhibition by either homologous unlabeled enterotoxin. In contrast to binding of LT-B, LT-A does not affect binding of ^{125}I-LT but inhibits the binding of ^{125}I-CT by 20–30%, which is similar to results obtained with the A subunit of cholera toxin. These data suggest that LT-A and CT-A exist in different conformation states which may explain the differences in biological activities of the two toxins against different tissue culture cell lines.

The requirements for expression of ADP-ribosyltransferase activity of *E. coli* LT have been examined (Moss and Richardson, 1978; Moss *et al.*, 1981). Incubation of 286C$_2$ LT with trypsin increases the ADP-ribosyltransferase activity over 200%. The specific enzyme activity of trypsin-treated LT is similar to that of cholera toxin which does not increase with trypsin treatment. The A subunit of 286C$_2$ LT is only partially nicked by a protease while the A fragment of cholera toxin is completely nicked but remains linked by a disulfide bridge. Trypsin enhances the enzymatic activity of LT-A but is not absolutely essential for enzymatic activity. However, a reducing agent such as dithiothreitol is necessary for maximal expression of catalytic activity.

6.4. EVIDENCE FOR AB SUBUNIT STRUCTURE

In the presence of 0.1% SDS (pH 7.0) LT dissociates into two species which migrate with mobilities similar to those of the A subunit and B protomer of cholera toxin (Fig.

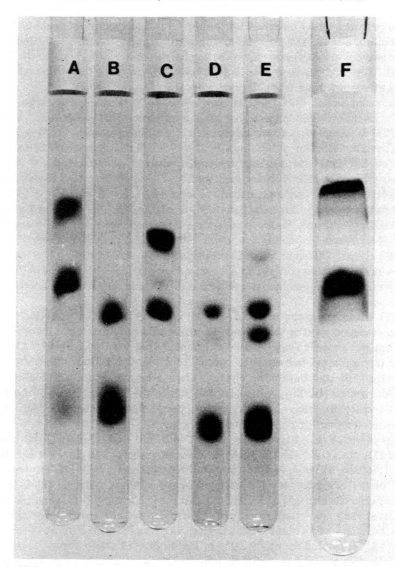

Fig. 3. SDS and acid-urea gel electrophoresis of cholera toxin and LT. Gels: A, non-reduced cholera toxin; B, heated and reduced cholera toxin; C, non-reduced 286C$_2$ LT; D, heated 286C$_2$ LT; E, heated and reduced 286C$_2$ LT; F, acid-urea gel of non-reduced LT.

3). Heating reduces the size of the larger LT component and causes it to migrate in the region of heated and reduced B protomer of cholera toxin but does not affect the faster migrating band. Heating and reduction partially dissociate the LT component which migrates just ahead of the A subunit of cholera toxin. The two components of LT also can be resolved by acid urea gel electrophoresis. LT purified from a porcine strain of ETEC (strain 263) has a similar subunit structure (Kunkel and Robertson, 1979).

As shown in Table 4, the molecular weight of the B oligomers of the three LTs ranges from 42,000 to 70,000, yet the monomeric molecular weights measured by SDS-gel electrophoresis following heating and reduction with reducing agents are almost identical. Recent data by Gill *et al.* (1981) demonstrate that the B oligomers of 286C$_2$ LT and P307 LT possess different conformations. The faster form of 286C$_2$ LT, with a migration corresponding to 42,000–46,000 daltons, can be converted to a diffuse, slower band, which migrates to a position between 60,000 and 70,000 daltons, by incubating it at 50°C or at 37°C with 0.2 M galactose.

Even though 286C$_2$ LT is released by pH adjustment of washed cells, it is unique compared with cholera toxin since only a small percentage of the A subunit appears to be nicked and can be subsequently reduced by dithiothreitol. The low molecular weight fragment of reduced LT-A, like the A2 fragment of cholera toxin, cannot be readily stained using Coomassie blue following SDS gel electrophoresis. Both the 28,200 and 24,000 dalton species catalyze the NAD-dependent activation of adenylate cyclase and are active against Y-1 adrenal cells at concentrations 100-fold higher than LT holotoxin. The subunits of *E. coli* LT can be purified on a preparative scale by acid urea gel filtration in the presence of 6 M urea, 0.1 M glycine (pH 3.5).

The subunit structure of *E. coli* LT has been established using bifunctional cross-linking reagents (Gill *et al.*, 1981; Kunkel and Robertson, unpublished data) similar to the approach used in studies on the subunit structure of cholera toxin (Gill, 1976). Incubation of the B oligomer of either LT or cholera toxin with dimethylpimelimidate (DMP) generates five bands which migrate with similar mobilities on SDS gels. Higher concentrations of cross-linking agents form species of 6B to 10B. All possible cross-linked forms of A5B have been identified when LT holotoxin is reacted with DMP. However, the A3B, A4B and A5B forms of LT are more difficult to visualize than the corresponding forms of cholera toxin. The cross-linked forms of the B oligomers are readily apparent in each holotoxin preparation.

The subunit structure of *E. coli* LT has been confirmed by Dallas and Falkow (1979) and by Dorner *et al.* (1979). The LT gene has been cloned (So *et al.*, 1978), linked to plasmid PBR322 and minicells used to express the cloned LT gene products (Dallas *et al.*, 1979). The labeled minicell proteins have been immunoprecipitated with anti-cholera toxin. SDS gel electrophoresis of the protein products revealed two protein bands at 25,500 and 11,500 daltons. The larger subunit stimulates adenylate cyclase analogous to the A subunit of cholera toxin. The lower molecular weight species migrated with the mobility of the B monomer of cholera toxin. Dorner (1979) has used the purified P307 plasmid and studied the synthesis of LT in a cell-free protein synthesizing system. He found that the synthesis of LT is stimulated 10-fold by cyclic AMP, and spermidine (a polyamine) lowered the optimal concentration of magnesium from 17 mM to 4 mM. Analysis of immunoprecipitated products by SDS polyacrylamide gel electrophoresis reveals two bands with adenylate cyclase stimulating activity at 26,000 and 23,000 daltons and a species at 11,500 daltons with the mobility of the B monomeric subunit of cholera toxin.

The amino acid composition of the A and B subunits of 286C$_2$ LT, P307 LT, and cholera toxin are presented in Table 6. Comparison of the amino acid composition of the B subunit of both LTs and the B subunit of cholera toxin reveals striking similarities. Only six amino acids of 286C$_2$ LT-B differ significantly from the amino acid composition of the B monomer of cholera toxin. The amino acid composition of the A subunit of LT appears to be quite different compared with the analogous subunit of cholera toxin, which explains the differences in amino acid composition between 286C$_2$ LT and cholera toxin noted in Table 5. The binding component of the toxin appears to have been more conserved through evolution, whereas the enzymatically active component has been altered. The nucleotide sequences of the subunit B genes of human (h) and porcine (p) LTs have been determined (Dallas and Falkow, 1980; Yamamoto *et al.*, 1982; Yamamoto and Yokota, 1983). Hydrophobic leader sequences were detected on both LT-B genes. Eighty of the 102 amino acid residues of LTp-B and CT-B toxins are identical, and of the 22 amino acid residues that are different, a single base change accounts for 20 of the changes. The existence of a leader sequence associated with secretion of LTp-B has been verified (Palva *et al.*, 1981). The homologies between LTh and LTp, between LTh-B and CT-B, and between LTp and CT-B were 96, 81 and 79%, respectively. As might be expected, LTh-B appears more closely related to CT-B than does LTp-B.

The nucleotide sequences of the A subunits of LTp and LTh have also been determined (Spicer and Noble, 1982; Yamamoto *et al.*, 1984). The LTp-A subunit comprises 254 amino acids, whereas LTh-A consists of 258 amino acids. Comparison of the two subunit A genes reveals several large identical sequences with insertions or deletions of nucleotides in the LTp-A gene which resulted in non-homologous amino acid sequences or deletion of four amino acid residues. Extensive homology exists between the pre-subunit A

TABLE 6. *Amino Acid Composition of* E. coli *LT Subunits**

Amino acid	LT-A			LT-B		
	286C₂†	P307‡	CT-A§	286C₂†	P307‡	CT-B§
Aspartic acid	33	21	35	10	9	10
Threonine	11	11	11	10	11	9
Serine	22	15	20	9	6	5
Glutamic acid	32	8	35	14	11	11
Proline	7	17	19	3	3	3
Glycine	26	29	28	4	3	3
Alanine	16	21‖	19	6	5‖	10
Cystine	2	—	2	2	—	2
Valine	12	11	13	4	3	3
Methionine	5	14	4	4	4	3
Isoleucine	12	17	15	11	10	7
Leucine	16	22	21	5	5	6
Tyrosine	18	22	19.	4	4	3
Phenylalanine	6	6	8–9	2	2	2
Histidine	4	9	12–13	1	2	7
Lysine	13	4	11	9	9	3
Arginine	19	24	17	4	5	2
Tryptophan	ND	ND	—	ND	ND	—
	254	254	291–293	102	92	90

*Data expressed as best whole numbers of residues.
†Kunkel and Robertson (unpublished data).
‡Clements *et al.* (1980).
‖Klapper *et al.* (1976).
§Alanines + half-cystine.

sequences of LTp, LTh and cholera toxin. No sequences were present in LTh-A which were not present in CT-A; however, unique sequences were present in LTp-A, which makes the two genes readily distinguishable. Nucleotide sequence homology between LTp-A and LTh-A ranged from 92.9 to 98.5% in different regions of the polypeptide chains (Honda *et al.*, 1981b). Comparison with LTh-A and LTp-A with CT-A showed ranges of homology from 70.4 to 93.5% and 71.9 to 93.5%, respectively. As noted with the B subunit genes, the A subunit of LTh is more closely related to CT-A than is the A subunit gene of LTp.

6.5. IMMUNOLOGICAL RELATIONSHIPS

The immunological cross-reactivity between *E. coli* LT and cholera toxin has been documented by several investigators (Gyles, 1974a,b; Clements and Finkelstein, 1978a,b; Holmgren and Svennerholm, 1979). To further characterize the nature of the antigenic determinants of *E. coli* LT an cholera toxin, high titered antiserum was raised in rabbits against LTs purified from strains 286C₂, and 263, a human and porcine strain of ETEC, respectively (Gilligan and Robertson, unpublished data). Sera from rabbits immunized with 100 μg of 286C₂ LT contained high levels of anti-LT activity, measured as neutralizing antibody, prior to incubation with Y-1 adrenal cells. Neutralizing activity reached peak values at five weeks and remained at maximum titers for up to 15 weeks. When antisera against 286C₂ LT was incubated with pH extracts from several strains of ENT⁺ *E. coli*, the extent of neutralization was variable. In general, LTs produced by heterologous ETEC strains were less efficiently neutralized than 286C₂ LT by antiserum against 286C₂ LT, and LTs produced by human strains were neutralized better than LTs from porcine strains. In contrast to the data obtained with anti-286C₂ antisera, anti-263 LT neutralized pH-extracts of porcine and human strains of ETEC with equal efficiency. Similar results have been noted with solid-phase RIAs. That is to say, pH-extracts of human and porcine ETEC did not compete with ¹²⁵I-286C₂ LT for binding to anti-286C₂ LT, but competition was observed using ¹²⁵I-263 LT and homologous anti-263 LT. Experiments are in progress to distinguish between three possible explanations for these data: (1) there are differences in the affinities of the two kinds of antibodies for each enterotoxin; (2) the differences in neutralization and binding reflect a difference in hydrophobicity of the two toxins; and (3) the antigenic determinants of the B subunits of the two toxins are different.

Despite the differences in neutralization of pH extracts of ETEC, anti-286C$_2$ LT immunoglobulin strongly neutralized cholera toxin (Gilligan *et al.*, 1983). Data from neutralization assays with 286C$_2$ LT, cholera toxin and their antisera showed that LT was more effectively neutralized by homologous anti-LT than CT (3.7-fold). Anti-CT was only slightly more effective in neutralization of homologous CT compared with LT (1.9-fold). Antisera raised against choleragenoid exhibited higher neutralization against CT than LT (5.8-fold), however, the amount of CT neutralized by anti-choleragenoid was about four-fold less than anti-CT. Based on these data, it appears that anti-CT serum contained neutralizing antibodies reactive with a shared determinant formed by interaction of the A and B subunits; whereas anti-LT and anti-choleragenoid sera did not. The contribution of antibodies to the unique determinants of each enterotoxin to neutralization activity may be greater than anticipated. These data do not agree with previous results (Holmgren *et al.*, 1973; Smith and Sack, 1973; Gyles, 1974a; Klipstein and Engert, 1977) in which it was shown that anti-cholera toxin neutralized LT and cholera toxin, but anti-LT neutralized cholera toxin at a level which is 10–30% that of homologous antigen. It should be noted that most early LT preparations used for raising antisera were not highly purified. Ouchterlony analysis has shown that 286C$_2$ LT and cholera toxin have at least one antigenic determinant in common, and each has at least one unique antigenic determinant. The nature of the antigenic determinants shared and unique to *E. coli* LT and cholera toxin were further characterized using solid-phase RIA's and antisera to each toxin (Gilligan *et al.*, 1983). The data in Fig. 4 show that both LT and CT competed only with homologus radioiodinated toxin for binding to each homologous antibody. However, when radio-iodinated enterotoxins were incubated with heterologous antibody in the presence of either LT or CT, both enterotoxins competed equally well.

Structural and antigenic differences have been observed in the B subunits of LTs produced by human and porcine strains of ETEC (Honda *et al.*, 1981c; Tsuji *et al.*, 1982; Geary *et al.*, 1982; Clements *et al.*, 1982). Immunodiffusion analysis showed the presence

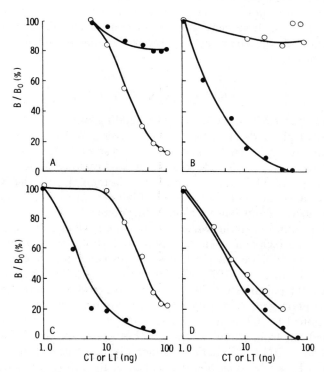

Fig. 4. Homologous and heterologous interactions between anti-286C$_2$ LT, anti-cholera toxin, and each purified enterotoxin: (○——○), 286C$_2$ LT; (●——●), cholera toxin. (A) anti-286C$_2$ LT, ^{125}I-286C$_2$ LT. (B) anti-cholera toxin, ^{125}I-cholera toxin. (C) anti-286C$_2$ LT, ^{125}I-cholera toxin. (D) anti-cholera toxin, ^{125}I-286C$_2$ LT.

of unique and shared antigenic determinants. The molecular weights of LTp-B differed by about 1,000, with LTp-B migrating faster than LTh-B.

Since each subunit consists of 103 amino acid residues, substitution of a limited number of residues leads to pronounced conformational differences. Extensive antigenic analysis of LTp, LTh and CT have been carried out using polyclonal antisera (Honda et al., 1981; Takeda et al., 1983; Marchlewicz and Finkelstein, 1983). These studies have shown that: (1) each enterotoxin has unique antigenic determinants; (2) at least one antigenic determinant is common to all three enterotoxins; (3) LTh and CT share an antigenic determinant not present on LTp; and (4) LTh and LTp share an antigenic determinant not present on CT.

It should be a simple matter to isolate specific antibodies directed against the shared determinant of LT and CT, as well as the unique antigenic determinants present on each enterotoxin (Lindholm et al., 1983; Belisle et al., 1984). Finkelstein et al. (1983) have recently reported the use of monoclonal antibodies against various forms of LT to study the roles of individual amino acids in determining the specific epitopes of the cholera/coli family of enterotoxins. As is to be expected, monoclonal antibodies directed against domains shared by the various toxin moieties of different origins recognize their respective counterparts.

Single amino acid substitutions have been made in porcine LT B subunit such that the amino acid residues at positions 102, 46, 13 and 4 are those of human LT B subunit. Many monoclonal antibodies against genetically engineered hybrid human LT B subunit oligomers do not recognize porcine LT antigens but do recognize the hybrid molecules with particular amino acid substitutions. Apparently, amino acid 46, the *ala* residue shared by CT and human LT, but not porcine LT, is especially important. Other monoclonals have been found to be specific for human LT, or to recognize combinations such as human and porcine LT but not CT, or, human LT and CT but not porcine LT. In some cases CT from different strains of *V. cholerae* (Marchlewicz and Finkelstein, 1983) could be distinguished. And, some monoclonals have recognized only the A subunit, in one instance reacting with human and porcine LT A subunit, but not the CT A subunit.

Observations such as these may hopefully lead to the development of antigens biologically engineered, or, chemically synthesized antigens which could prove to be completely cross-protective.

7. GENETIC CONTROL OF LT

Plasmids, designated ENT, contain the genes coding for both LT and ST. There are three groups of ENT plasmids based on their size (averaged, 100 kilobases; range, 30–150 kilobases), incompatibility reactions, and ability to restrict *E. coli* K-12 phages (Gyles et al., 1974; Willshaw et al., 1980). Hybridization studies have shown DNA homology, between these groups, of 40–70%, and up to 40% homology with the R plasmids which code for drug-resistance factors (So et al., 1975; Gyles et al., 1977; McConnell et al., 1980; Willshaw et al., 1980). Many plasmids, including many ENT plasmids, are capable of conjugal transfer to other bacteria, which requires the synthesis of adhesive factors (pili) for attachment to the recipient bacteria (Smith and Halls, 1968; Smith and Linggood, 1971b; Skerman et al., 1972). Some ENT plasmids also code for adhesions for attachment to epithelial cells (Smith et al., 1979; McConnell et al., 1981). There is evidence which suggests that the ENT plasmids may be hybrids of plasmids carrying the toxin genes and plasmids which contain genes for drug resistance, conjugal transfer, or adhesions. So et al. (1978) have cloned an LT gene from a porcine strain, and Yamamoto and Yokota (1980) have cloned one from a human strain. In both cases the structural information for LT is contained in a DNA fragment of under two kilobases. The gene consists of a promoter followed by a ribosome binding sequence, the information for the A peptide, a second ribosome binding sequence, and the information for the B peptide. Both the A and the B peptide-coding regions have information coding for an amino terminal peptide not found in the native molecule. Each also has a region characteristic of a signal sequence.

In the case of the B subunit this has been directly demonstrated by Palva *et al.* (1981) and Hirst *et al.* (1983), who have shown that a precursor exists with a 3,000 dalton segment that is cleaved from the amino terminus to form the mature molecule. There is 79% homology between the predicted amino acid sequence from the porcine strain B gene and the B chain of cholera toxin (Dallas and Falkow, 1980). The LT gene from the human strain differs from that of the porcine strain in that it is found in a large DNA sequence flanked by inverted repeats that contain both the ST and LT genes. The ST gene within the large sequence is flanked by inverted repeats (Yamamoto and Yokota, 1981). They also differ in that there is the presence, in the human strain gene, of an intervening sequence between the A and B peptide-coding regions. The differences in gene structure among ENT plasmids coding for LT can explain the observation that, while producing similar biological effects, the immunologic cross-reactivity with each other and with cholera toxin varies among LT molecules isolated from different sources.

8. IMMUNE RESPONSE

Nearly 80% of persons with ETEC infections demonstrate a serum (IgM) and intestinal secretory (IgG) antibody response against the homologous O antigen, with peak titers usually occurring 8–10 days after onset of infection (Deetz *et al.*, 1979; Levine *et al.*, 1977, 1979b, 1982, 1984). In contrast to ST, which appears not to induce neutralizing or binding antibodies during ETEC infection, LT causes a significant rise in antibodies in most persons who develop diarrhea due to an LT-producing strain of *E. coli* (Evans *et al.*, 1978; Greenberg *et al.*, 1979; Levine *et al.*, 1979b, 1982, 1984). When human volunteers were fed LT-producing *E. coli*, 77% of those who developed diarrhea demonstrated a rise in serum IgG neutralizing antibodies against LT (Levine *et al.*, 1983b). Similar experimental infections have been reported to cause rises as well in intestinal fluid levels of SIgA antibody against LT (Levine *et al.*, 1982, 1984).

9. VACCINES

Because of the importance of both adherence of ETEC to the gut and toxin production in this disease, the most effective vaccines against ETEC diarrhea will likely combine anti-adhesion as well as anti-toxic immunity (Svennerholm and Ahren, 1982). Also, because the obvious site of challenge by ETEC and its toxin(s) is the intestine, intestinal mucosal (secretory IgA) antibodies are certain to be the target for stimulation by antigens or attenuated strains for immunization. The toxoid portion of such a vaccine would have to stimulate anti-LT and ST antibodies which are capable of neutralizing each toxin. As with cholera toxin, *E. coli* LT, when heated under controlled conditions, becomes a polymerized, non-toxic protein antigen ('procoligenoid') similar to procholeragenoid. The vaccine could include a combination of linked molecules such as ST linked to LT, procoligenoid, colonizing factors (pili), or even procholeragenoid. However, whatever combinations are used, such isolated antigens generally are not good or lasting stimulators of the secretory immune response. Until better adjuvant systems are developed, simple oral administration of isolated antigens does not seem to offer great promise.

Perhaps more promising for vaccine development is the application of attenuated strains of *E. coli* which produce antigens which will give rise to protective immunity (Levine, 1983b; Levine *et al.*, 1984). An attenuated strain would be capable of colonizing the gut after only one oral administration. During colonization the organism would produce a steady supply of the immunizing antigens which would eventually result in significant secretory mucosal immunity. The hope for development of such an *E. coli* strain seems to lie in the realm of genetic engineering. Indeed, the genes encoding porcine and human LT or their subunits have already been successfully cloned (Clements *et al.*, 1983; Dallas, 1983; Dallas and Falkow, 1979; Dallas *et al.*, 1979; Yamamoto *et al.*, 1981). Ideally, a strain would be constructed which simultaneously produces the critical adhesion factors, the B subunit of LT and even an inactive form of ST. However, success has not yet been reported in cloning just the genes for the important colonization factors. In one case, isolation of the genes for CFA/I has not been successful to the exclusion of apparently closely-associated ST genes as well (McConnell *et al.*, 1981; Reis *et al.*, 1980a; Willshaw *et al.*, 1983).

An *E. coli* strain has been reported (Levine, 1983b; Levine *et al.*, 1984) which previously was LT$^+$/ST$^+$ CFA$^+$, but spontaneously lost the LT and ST traits. Most adult volunteers fed this organism in experimental studies developed a serological response, though 2 of 19 volunteers also developed mild diarrhea. A similar result has been observed in man and piglets after oral inoculation with enterotoxin-negative, adhesive strains of *E. coli* (Smith and Linggood, 1971b) and *Vibrio cholerae* (Levine *et al.*, 1983a). These mutant strains which are toxin-negative, adhesion-positive could serve as excellent recipients for plasmid vectors coding for protective antigens such as LT B subunit and CFA/I. An initial bout of mild diarrhea may prove to be the price to be paid for immunization against the more severe forms of this disease.

The potential for application of toxoids or non-toxic subunits of toxins to develop immunity to *E. coli* diarrhea has been demonstrated in several animal models. Piglets can be protected from ETEC diarrhea if they are suckled on sows immunized parenterally with porcine LT (Dobrescu and Huygelen, 1976; Dorner *et al.*, 1980). However, common toxoiding agents such as glutaraldehyde and formalin, while working to alter toxicity, are not likely to be useful because these agents have not produced good immunogens with the closely related cholera toxin (Curlin *et al.*, 1975; Levine *et al.*, 1979a).

The porcine LT B subunit and LT holotoxin have been used (Klipstein and Engert, 1981a) to immunize rats orally, parentally, or in combination. Both agents demonstrated induction of protection against challenge with toxigenic strains or purified toxin, with holotoxin being the most efficacious of the two. Hopefully, this work can be expanded to human LT now that the LT genes have been successfully cloned into a high-copy vector (Yamamoto *et al.*, 1981).

Procholeragenoid, which has nearly 100% of the immunogenicity, but only 1% of the toxicity of cholera toxin (Finkelstein *et al.*, 1971; Germanier *et al.*, 1976), has been shown to protect piglets, which suckled on sows immunized with procholeragenoid, against ETEC infection (Fürer *et al.*, 1982). If large quantities of human LT can be produced with the aid of gene cloning methodologies, heat possibly could be used to produce an LT 'procoligenoid' with the same useful properties observed with procholeragenoid.

Cross-linking of ST to LT (Klipstein *et al.*, 1982) has produced a toxoid with less than 0.15% of the biological activity of native ST or LT. Rats immunized with this cross-linked material developed protection against intestinal loop challenge with the toxins or strains producing the toxins.

Studies have also been done with cross-linked synthetic ST (Klipstein *et al.*, 1983c) and porcine LT B subunit (Klipstein *et al.*, 1983a,b,d). This toxoid, while stimulating neutralizing antibodies and a significant rise in mucosal IgA antibodies, apparently is devoid of undesirable biological activity. The rats immunized with this toxoid, when challenged with human or porcine strains (LT$^+$ or ST$^+$) or pure toxin (LT or ST), experienced up to 80% less secretory response than controls (Klipstein *et al.*, 1983a). A similar protective effect was noted in rabbits and rats which were immunized orally with three doses of this toxoid (Klipstein *et al.*, 1983d).

REFERENCES

Adam, A. (1923) Über die Biologie der Dyspepsie coli und ihre Beziehung zur Pathogenese der Dyspepsie und Intoxication. *J.b. Kinderheilk. Berlin 1923* 3. F. **LI**: 295–314.

Aimoto, S., Takao, T., Shimonishi, Y., Hara, S., Takeda, T., Takeda, Y. and Miwatani, T. (1982) Amino acid sequence of a heat-stable enterotoxin produced by human enterotoxigenic *Escherichia-coli*. *Eur. J. Biochem.* **129**: 257–263.

Alderete, J. F. and Robertson, D. C. (1977) Nutrition and enterotoxin synthesis by enterotoxigenic strains of *Escherichia coli:* defined medium for production of heat-stable enterotoxin. *Infect. Immun.* **15**: 781–788.

Alderete, J. F. and Robertson, D. C. (1978) Purification and chemical characterization of the heat-stable enterotoxin produced by porcine strains of enterotoxigenic *Escherichia coli*. *Infect. Immun.* **19**: 1021–1030.

BÄCK, E., MÖLLBY, R., KAIJSER, G., STINTZING, G., WADSTRÖM, T. and HABTE, D. (1980) Enterotoxigenic *Escherichia coli* and other Gram-negative bacteria and infantile diarrhea: and surface antigens, hemagglutinins, colonization factor antigen, and loss of enterotoxigenicity. *J. infect. Dis.* **142**: 318–327.

BÄCK, E., SVENNERHOLM, A. M., HOLMGREN, J. and MÖLLBY, R. (1979) Evaluation of a ganglioside immunoassay for detection of *Escherichia coli* heat-labile enterotoxin. *J. clin. Microbiol.* **10**: 791–795.

BANWELL, J. G. and SHERR, H. (1973) Effect of bacterial enterotoxins on the gastrointestinal tract. *Gastroenterology* **65**: 467–497.

BELISLE, B. W., TWIDDY, E. M. and HOLMES, R. K. (1984) Characterization of monoclonal antibodies to heat-labile enterotoxin encoded by a plasmid from a clinical isolate of *Escherichia-coli*. *Infect. Immun.* **43**: 1027–1032.

BENNET, V. and CUATRECASAS, P. (1976) Cholera toxin: membrane gangliosides and activation of adenylate cyclase. In: *Receptors and Recognition*, Series B, Vol. 1, pp. 3–66, CUATRECASAS, P. (ed.) Chapman and Hall, London.

BEUTIN, L., BODE, L., RICHTER, T., PELTRE, G. and STEPHAN, R. (1984) Rapid visual detection of *Escherichia coli* and *Vibrio cholerae* heat-labile enterotoxins by nitrocellulose enzyme-linked immunosorbent assay. *J. clin. Microbiol.* **19**: 371–375.

BLACK, R. E., BROWN, K. H., BECKER, S., ALIM ABDUL, A. R. M. and HUQ, I. (1982) Longitudinal studies of infectious diseases and physical growth of children in rural Bangladesh. II. Incidence of diarrhea and association with known pathogens. *Am. J. Epidemiol.* **115**: 315–324.

BLACK, R. E., MERSON, M. H., HUQ, I., ALIM, A. R. M. A. and YUNUS, M. (1981a) Incidence and severity of rota-virus and *Escherichia coli* diarrhoea in rural Bangladesh. *Lancet* **i**: 141–143.

BLACK, R. E., MERSON, M. H., ROWE, B., TAYLOR, P., ABDUL ALIM, A. R. M. A., GROSS, R. J. and SACK, D. A. (1981b) Enterotoxigenic *Escherichia coli* diarrhoea: acquired immunity and transmission in an endemic area. *Bull. Wld Hlth Org.* **59**: 263–268.

BRAMUCCI, M. G. and HOLMES, R. K. (1978) Radial passive immune hemolysis assay for detection of heat-labile enterotoxin produced by individual colonies of *Escherichia coli* or *Vibrio cholerae*. *J. clin. Microbiol.* **8**: 252–255.

BRAMUCCI, M. G., TWIDDY, E. M., BAINE, W. B. and HOLMES, R. K. (1981) Isolation and characterization of hypertoxigenic mutants of *Escherichia coli* KL320 (pCG86). *Infect. Immun.* **32**: 1034–1044.

BRILL, B. M., WASILAUSKAS, B. L. and RICHARDSON, S. H. (1979) Adaptation of the staphylococcal-coagglutination technique for detection of heat-labile enterotoxin of *Escherichia coli*. *J. clin. Microbiol.* **9**: 49–55.

BROOM, S. and GILBERT, W. (1978) Immunological screening method to detect specific translation products. *Proc. natn. Acad. Sci. U.S.A.* **75**: 2746–2749.

BURGESS, M. N., BYWATER, R. J., COWLEY, C. M., MULLAN, N. A. and NEWSOME, P. M. (1978) Biological evaluation of a methanol-soluble, heat-stable *Escherichia coli* enterotoxin in infant mice, pigs, rabbits, and calves. *Infect. Immun.* **21**: 526–531.

BURGESS, M. N., COWLEY, C. M., MELLING, J., MULLAN, N. A. and NEWSOME, P. M. (1979) Assay of the heat-labile enterotoxin of *Escherichia coli* in infant rabbits. *J. med. Microbiol.* **12**: 291–302.

CALDERON, R. L. and LEVIN, M. A. (1981) Quantitative method for enumeration of enterotoxigenic *Escherichia coli*. *J. clin. Microbiol.* **13**: 130–134.

CALLAHAN, L. T., III and RICHARDSON, S. H. (1973) Biochemistry of *Vibrio cholerae* virulence. III. Nutritional requirements for toxin production and the effects of pH on toxin elaboration in chemically defined media. *Infect. Immun.* **7**: 567–572.

CASKA, M., GROSSMÜLLER, F. and EFFENBERGER, F. (1978) Solid-phase radioimmunoassay method for determination of *Escherichia coli* enterotoxin. *Infect. Immun.* **19**: 347–352.

CLEMENTS, J. D. and FINKELSTEIN, R. A. (1978a) Immunological cross-reactivity between a heat-labile enterotoxin(s) of *Escherichia coli* and subunits of *Vibrio cholerae* enterotoxin. *Infect. Immun.* **21**: 1036–1039.

CLEMENTS, J. D. and FINKELSTEIN, R. A. (1978b) Demonstration of shared and unique immunological determinants in enterotoxins from *Vibrio cholerae* and *Escherichia coli* cultures. *Infect. Immun.* **22**: 709–713.

CLEMENTS, J. D. and FINKELSTEIN, R. A. (1979) Isolation and characterization of homogeneous heat-labile enterotoxins with high specific activity from *Escherichia coli* cultures. *Infect. Immun.* **24**: 760–769.

CLEMENTS, J. D., FLINT, D. C., ENGERT, R. F. and KLIPSTEIN, F. A. (1983) Cloning and molecular characterization of the B subunit of *Escherichia coli* heat-labile enterotoxin. *Infect. Immun.* **40**: 653–658.

CLEMENTS, J. D., FLINT, D. C. and KLIPSTEIN, F. A. (1982) Immunological and physicochemical characterization of heat-labile enterotoxins isolated from two strains of *Escherichia coli*. *Infect. Immun.* **38**: 806–809.

CLEMENTS, J. D., YANCEY, R. J. and FINKELSTEIN, R. A. (1980) Properties of homogeneous heat-labile enterotoxin from *Escherichia coli*. *Infect. Immun.* **29**: 91–97.

CRAIG, J. P. (1971) Cholera toxins. In: *Microbial Toxins*, Vol. 2A, pp. 189–254, MONTIE, T. C., KADIS, S. and AJL, S. J. (eds) Academic Press, New York.

CURLIN, G., LEVINE, R., AZIZ, K. M. A., MINZANUR RAHMAN, A. C. M. and VERWAY, W. F. (1975) Field trial of cholera toxoid. In: *Proceedings of the 11th Joint Conference on Cholera, U.S. Japan Cooperative Medical Science Program*, pp. 314–329, New Orleans.

CZERKINSKY, C. C. and SVENNERHOLM, A.-M. (1983) Ganglioside G_{M1} enzyme-linked immunospot assay for simple identification of heat-labile enterotoxin-producing *Escherichia coli*. *J. clin. Microbiol.* **17**: 965–969.

DAFNI, Z., SACK, R. B. and CRAIG, J. P. (1978) Purification of heat-labile enterotoxin from four *Escherichia coli* strains by affinity immunoadsorbent: evidence for similar subunit structure. *Infect. Immun.* **22**: 852–860.

DALLAS, W. S. (1983) Conformity between heat-labile toxin genes from human and porcine enterotoxigenic *Escherichia coli*. *Infect. Immun.* **40**: 647–652.

DALLAS, W. S. and FALKOW, S. (1979) The molecular nature of heat-labile enterotoxin (LT) of *Escherichia coli*. *Nature* **277**: 406–407.

DALLAS, W. S. and FALKOW, S. (1980) Amino acid sequence homology between cholera toxin and *Escherichia coli* heat-labile toxin. *Nature* **288**: 499–501.

DALLAS, W. S., GILL, D. M. and FALKOW, S. (1979) Cistrons encoding *Escherichia coli* heat-labile toxin. *J. Bact.* **139**: 850–858.

DEBOY, J. M., II, WACHSMITH, I., KAYE, and DAVIS, B. R. (1980) Serotypes of enterotoxigenic *Escherichia coli* isolated in the United States. *Infect. Immun.* **29**: 361–368.

DECASTRO, A. F. P., SERAFIM, M. B., FOMES, J. A. and GATTI, M. S. V. (1980) Improvements in the passive immuno hemolysis test for assaying enterotoxigenic *Escherichia coli*. *J. clin. Microbiol.* **12**: 714–717.

DEETZ, T. R., EVANS, D. J., JR., EVANS, D. G. and DUPONT, H. L. (1979) Serologic responses to somatic O and colonization-factor antigens of enterotoxigenic *Escherichia coli* in travelers. *J. infect. Dis* **140**: 114–118.

DENEKE, C. F., THORNE, G. M. and GORBACH, S. L. (1979) Attachment pili from enterotoxigenic *Escherichia coli* pathogenic for humans. *Infect. Immun.* **26**: 362–368.

DOBRESCU, L. (1979) Heat-labile enterotoxin antibodies in calves. *Res. vet. Sci.* **27**: 133–134.

DOBRESCU, L. and HUYGELEN, C. (1976) Protection of piglets against neonatal *E. coli.* enteritis by immunization of the sow with vaccine containing heat-labile enterotoxin (LT). *Zentbl. Vet Med.* **23**: 79–88.

DONTA, S. T. (1976) Interactions of choleragenoid and Gm_1 ganglioside with enterotoxins of *Vibrio cholera* and *Escherichia coli* in cultured adrenal cells. *J. infect. Dis.* **133**: S115–S119.

DONTA, S. T. and SMITH, D. M. (1974) Stimulation of steroidogenesis in tissue culture by enterotoxigenic *Escherichia coli* and its neutralization by specific antiserum. *Infect. Immun.* **9**: 500–505.

DONTA, S. T. and VINER, J. P. (1975) Inhibition of the steroidogenic effects of cholera and heat-labile *Escherichia coli* enterotoxins by Gm_1 ganglioside: Evidence for a similar receptor site for the two toxins. *Infect. Immun.* **11**: 982–985.

DONTA, S. T., KING, M. and SLOPER, K. (1973) Induction of steroidogenesis in tissue culture by cholera enterotoxin. *Nature* **243**: 246–247.

DONTA, S. T., MOON, H. W. and WHIPP, S. C. (1974a) Detection of heat-labile *Escherichia coli* enterotoxin with the use of adrenal cells in tissue culture. *Science* **183**: 334–336.

DONTA, S. T., MOON, H. W., WHIPP, S. C. and SKARTVEDT, S. M. (1974c) *In vivo* production and inactivation of *Escherichia coli* enterotoxin. *Gastroenterology* **67**: 983–990.

DONTA, S. T., POINDEXTER, N. J. and GINSBERG, B. H. (1982) Comparison of the binding of cholera and *E. coli* enterotoxins to Y_1 adrenal cells. *Biochemistry* **21**: 660–664.

DONTA, S. T., SACK, D. A., WALLACE, R. B., DUPONT, H. L. and SACK, R. B. (1974b) Tissue culture assay of antibodies to heat-labile *Escherichia coli* enterotoxins. *New Engl. J. Med.* **291**: 117–121.

DONTA, S. T., WALLACE, R. B., WHIPP, S. C. and OLARTE, J. (1977) Enterotoxigenic *Escherichia coli* and diarrheal disease in Mexican children. *J. infect. Dis.* **135**: 482–485.

DORNER, F. (1975) *Escherichia coli* enterotoxin-purification and partial characterization. *J. biol. Chem.* **250**: 8712–8719.

DORNER, F. and MAYER, P. (1975) *Escherichia coli* enterotoxin: Stimulation of adenylate cyclase in broken-cell preparations. *Infect. Immun.* **11**: 429–435.

DORNER, F., HUGHES, C., NAHLER, G. and HÖGENAUER, G. (1979) *Escherichia coli* heat-labile enterotoxin: DNA-directed synthesis and structure. *Proc. natn. Acad. Sci. U.S.A.* **76**: 4832–4836.

DORNER, F., MAYER, P. and LESKOVA, R. (1980) Immunity to *Escherichia* in piglets: the role of colostral antibodies directed against heat-labile enterotoxin in experimental neonatal diarrhea. *Zentbl. VetMed.* **27**: 207–221.

DREYFUS, L. A., FRANTS, J. C. and ROBERTSON, D. C. (1983) Chemical properties of heat-stable enterotoxins produced by enterotoxigenic *Escherichia coli* of different host origins. *Infect. Immun.* **42**: 539–548.

DUGUID, J. P. and OLD, D. C. (1980) Adhesive properties of enterobacteriaceae. In: *Bacterial Adherence, Receptors and Recognition*, Series B, Vol. 6, pp. 185–218, BEACHEY, E. (ed.) Chapman and Hall, London.

DUPONT, H. L. (1981) Traveller's Diarrhoea. *Clin. Res. Rev.* **1**: 225–234.

DUPONT, H. L., FORMAL, S. B., HORNICK, R. B., SNYDER, M. J., LIBONATI, J. P., SHEAHAN, D. G., LABREC, E. H. and KALAS, J. P. (1971) Pathogenesis of *Escherichia coli* diarrhea. *New Engl. J. Med.* **285**: 1.

ECHEVERRIA, P., ORSKOV, F., ORSKOV, I. and PLIANBANGCHANG, D. (1982) Serotypes of enterotoxigenic *Escherichia coli* in Thailand and the Philippines. *Infect. Immun.* **36**: 851–856.

ECHEVERRIA, P., VERHEART, L., ULYANCO, C. V. and SANTIAGO, L. T. (1978) Detection of heat-labile enterotoxin-like activity in stools of patients with cholera and *Escherichia coli* diarrhea. *Infect. Immun.* **19**: 343–344.

ENOMOTO, K. and GILL, D. M. (1980) Cholera toxin activation of adenylate cyclase. Role of nucleoside triphosphates and a macromolecular factor in the ADP-ribosylation of the GTP-dependent regulatory component. *J. biol. Chem.* **255**: 1252–1258.

ENWEANI, C. C., GYLES, C. L. and BARNUM, D. A. (1975a) The effect of antisera on porcine enteropathogenic *Escherichia coli* in ligated segments of pig intestine. *Can J. comp. Med.* **39**: 46–53.

ENWEANI, C. C., GYLES, C. L. and BARNUM, D. A. (1975b) Antibacterial activity of antisera against homologous and heterologous *Escherichia coli* of porcine origin. *Can. J. comp. Med.* **39**: 54–60.

ERICSSON, D. D., DUPONT, H. L., SULLIVAN, P., GALINDO, E., EVANS, D. G. and EVANS, D. J. (1983) Bicozamycin, a poorly absorbable antibiotic effectively treats traveler's diarrhea. *Ann. intern. Med.* **98**: 20–25.

ESCHERICH, T. (1885) Die Darmbakterien des Neugeborenen und Säuglings. *Fortschr. Med., Berlin 1885* **III**: 231–236.

ESCHERICH, T. (1887) Über Darmbakterien im Allgemeinen und diejenigen der Säuglinge im Besonderen, sowie die Beziehung der letzteren zur Äthiologie der Darmerkrankungen. *Zentlbl. Bakt. Parasitkde Jena 1887* **I**: 705–713.

EVANS, D. J., JR. and EVANS, D. G. (1977a) Direct serological assay for the heat-labile enterotoxin of *Escherichia coli*, using passive immune hemolysis. *Infect. Immun.* **16**: 604–609.

EVANS, D. J., JR. and EVANS, D. G. (1977b) Inhibition of immune hemolysis: Serological assay for the heat-labile enterotoxin of *Escherichia coli*. *J. clin. Microbiol.* **5**: 100–105.

EVANS, D. G. and EVANS, D. J., JR. (1978) New surface-associated heat-labile colonization factor antigen (CFA/II) produced by enterotoxigenic *Escherichia coli* of Serogroups O6 and O8. *Infect. Immun.* **21**: 638–647.

EVANS, D. J., JR., CHEN, L. C., CURLIN, G. T. and EVANS, D. G. (1972) Stimulation of adenyl cyclase by *Escherichia coli* enterotoxin. *Nature* **236**: 137–138.

EVANS, D. J., JR., EVANS, D. G., DUPONT, H. L., ORSKOV, F. and ORSKOV, I. (1977a) Patterns of loss of enterotoxigenicity by *Escherichia coli* isolated from adults with diarrhea: Suggestive evidence for an interrelationship with serotype. *Infect. Immun.* **17**: 105–111.

EVANS, D. G., EVANS, D. J. and GORBACH, S. L. (1973a) Identification of enterotoxigenic *Escherichia coli* and serum antitoxin activity by the vascular permeability factor assay. *Infect. Immun.* **8**: 731–735.

EVANS, D. J., JR., EVANS, D. G. and GORBACH, S. L. (1974) Polymyxin B-induced release of low-molecular-weight heat-labile enterotoxin from *Escherichia coli*. *Infect. Immun.* **10**: 1010–1017.

EVANS, D. G., EVANS D. J., JR. and PIERCE, N. F. (1973b) Differences in the response of rabbit small intestine to heat-labile and heat-stable enterotoxins of *Escherichia coli*. *Infect. Immun.* **7**: 873–880.

EVANS, D. G., OLARTE, J., DUPONT, H. L., EVANS, D. J., GALINDO, E., PORTNOY, B. L. and CONKLIN, R. H. (1977b) Enteropathogens associated with pediatric diarrhea in Mexico City. *J. Pediat.* **91**: 65–68.

EVANS, D. J., JR., RUIZ-PALACIOS, G., EVANS, D. G., DUPONT, H. L., PICKERING, L. K. and OLARTE, J. (1977c) Humoral immune response to the heat-labile enterotoxin of *Escherichia coli* in naturally acquired diarrhea and antitoxin determination by passive immune hemolysis. *Infect. Immun.* **16**: 781–788.

EVANS, D. G., SATTERWHITE, T. K., EVANS, D. J., JR. and DUPONT, H. L. (1978) Differences in serological responses and excretion patterns of volunteers challenged with enterotoxigenic *Escherichia coli* with and without the colonization factor antigen. *Infect. Immun.* **19**: 883–888.

EVANS, D. G., SILVER, R. P., EVANS, D. J., JR., CHASE, D. G. and GORBACH, S. L. (1975) Plasmid-controlled colonization factor associated with virulence in *Escherichia coli* enterotoxigenic for humans. *Infect. Immun.* **12**: 656–667.

EWING, W. H. (1962) Sources of *E. coli* cultures that belonged to O A6 groups associated with infantile diarrheal disease. *J. infect. Dis.* **110**: 114–120.

FARIS, A., LINDAHL, M. and WADSTRÖM, T. (1981) GM$_2$-like glycoconjugate as possible erythrocyte receptor for the CFA/I and K-99 hemagglutinatinins of enterotoxigenic *Escherichia coli*. *FEMS Micro. Lett.* **7**: 265–269.

FIELD, M. (1974) Intestinal secretion. *Gastroenterology.* **66**: 1063–1084.

FIELD, M. (1979a) Mechanisms of action of cholera and *Escherichia coli* enterotoxins. *Am. J. clin. Nutr.* **32**: 189–196.

FIELD, M. (1979b) Intracellular mediators of secretion in the small intestine. In: *Mechanisms of Intestinal Secretion*, pp. 83–91, BINDER, H. J. (ed.) Alan R. Liss, New York.

FIELD, M., GRAF, L. H., LAIRD, W. J. and SMITH, P. L. (1978) Heat-stable enterotoxin of *Escherichia coli: In vitro* guanylate cyclase activity, cyclic GMP concentration, and ion transport in small intestine. *Proc. natn. Acad. Sci. U.S.A.* **75**: 2800–2804.

FINKELSTEIN, R. A. (1973) Cholera. *Crit. Rev. Microbiol.* **2**: 553–623.

FINKELSTEIN, R. A. and YANG, Z. (1983) Rapid test for identification of heat-labile enterotoxin-producing *Escherichia coli* colonies. *J. clin. Microbiol.* **18**: 23–28.

FINKELSTEIN, R. A., ATTHASAMPUNNA, P., CHULASAMAYA, M. and CHARUNMETHEE, P. (1966) Pathogenesis of experimental cholera: biological activities of purified procholeragen A. *J. Immun.* **96**: 440–449.

FINKELSTEIN, R. A., BURKS, M., RIEKE, L., MCDONALD, R., BROWNE, S. and DALLAS, W. S. (1983) Structural and immunological (including monoclonal antibody) analyses of the cholera-related enterotoxin family. In: Proceedings of the 19th Joint Conference on Cholera, U.S.–Japan Cooperative Medical Science Program. *Advances in Research on Cholera and Related Diarrheas.* KTK Scientific Publishers, Tokyo.

FINKELSTEIN, R. A., FUJITA, K. and LOSPALLUTO, J. J. (1971) Procholeragenoid: an aggregated intermediated in the formation of choleragenoid. *J. Immun.* **107**: 1043–1051.

FINKELSTEIN, R. A., LARUE, M. K., JOHNSTON, D. W., VASIL, M. L., CHO, G. J. and JONES, J. R. (1976a) Isolation and properties of heat-labile enterotoxin(s) from enterotoxigenic *Escherichia coli*. *J. infect. Dis.* **133**: S120–S137.

FINKELSTEIN, R. A., VASIL, M. L., JONES, J. R., ANDERSON, R. A. and BARNARD, T. (1976b) Clinical cholera caused by enterotoxigenic coli. *J. clin. Microbiol.* **3**: 382–384.

FINKELSTEIN, R. A., YANG, Z., MOSELEY, S. L. and MOON, H. W. (1983) Rapid Latex particle agglutination test for *Escherichia coli* strains of porcine origin producing heat-labile enterotoxin. *J. clin. Microbiol.* **18**: 1417–1418.

FISHMAN, P. H. (1980) Mechanism of action of cholera toxin: Events on the cell surface. In: *Secretory Diarrhea*, pp. 85–106, FIELD, M., FORDTRAN, J. S. and SCHULTZ, S. G. (ed.) Am. Physiol. Soc., Bethesda, Maryland. Williams & Wilkens, Baltimore, Maryland.

FORMAL, S. B., O'BRIEN, A., GEMSKI, P. and DOCTOR, B. P. (1978) Invasive *Escherichia coli*. *J. Am. vet. med. Ass.* **173**: 596–598.

FRANTZ, J. C. and ROBERTSON, D. C. (1981) Immunological properties of *Escherichia coli* heat-stable enterotoxins: Development of a radioimmunoassay specific for heat-stable enterotoxins with suckling mouse activity. *Infect. Immun.* **33**: 193–198.

FRETER, R. (1978) Association of enterotoxigenic bacteria with the mucosa of the small intestine: Mechanisms and pathogenic implications. In: *Cholera and Related Diarrheas*, pp. 155–170, OUCHTERLONY, O. and HOLMGREN, J. (eds) S. Karger, Basel.

FÜRER, E., CRYZ, S. J., JR., DORNER, F., NICOLE, J., WANNER, M. and GERMANIER, R. (1982) Protection against colibacillosis in neonatal piglets by immunization of dams with procholeragenoid. *Infect. Immun.* **35**: 887–894.

GAASTRA, W. and DE GRAAF, F. (1982) Host-specific fimbrial adhesions of noninvasive enterotoxigenic *Escherichia coli* strains. *Microb. Rev.* **46**: 129–161.

GANKEMA, H., WENSINK, J., GUINEE, P. A. M., JANSSEN, W. H. and WITHOLT, B. (1980) Some characteristics of the outer membrane released by growing enterotoxigenic *Escherichia coli*. *Infect. Immun.* **29**: 704–713.

GEARY, S. J., MARCHLEWICZ, B. A. and FINKELSTEIN, R. A. (1982) Comparison of heat-labile enterotoxins from porcine and human strains of *Escherichia coli*. *Infect. Immun.* **36**: 215–220.

GEMSKI, P., O'BRIEN, A. D. and WOHLHIETER, J. A. (1978) Cellular release of heat-labile enterotoxin of *Escherichia coli* by bacteriophage induction. *Infect. Immun.* **19**: 1076–1082.

GERMANIER, R., FÜRER, E., VARALLYAY, S. and INDERBITZIN, T. M. (1976) Preparation of a purified antigenic cholera toxoid. *Infect. Immun.* **13**: 1692–1698.

GIANELLA, R. A. (1981) Pathogenesis of acute bacterial diarrheal disorders. *Ann. Rev. Med.* **32**: 341–357.

GIANELLA, R. A., DRAKE, K. W. and LUTTRELL, M. (1981) Development of a radioimmunoassay for *Escherichia coli* heat-stable enterotoxin: Comparison with the suckling mouse assay. *Infect. Immun.* **33**: 186–192.

GILL, D. M. (1976) The arrangement of subunits in cholera toxin. *Biochemistry (ACS)* **15**: 1242–1248.

GILL, D. M. (1977) Mechanism of action of cholera toxin. In: *Advances in Cyclic Nucleotide Research*, Vol. 8, pp. 85–118. Raven Press, New York.

GILL, D. M. and RICHARDSON, S. H. (1980) Adenosine diphosphate-ribosylation of adenylate cyclase catalyzed by heat-labile enterotoxin of *Escherichia coli:* comparison with cholera toxin. *J. infect. Dis.* **141**: 64–70.

GILL, D. M., CLEMENTS, J. D., ROBERTSON, D. C. and FINKELSTEIN, R. A. (1981) Subunit number and arrangement in the heat-labile enterotoxin of *Escherichia coli. Infect. Immun.* **33**: 677–682.

GILL, D. M., EVANS, D. J., JR. and EVANS, D. G. (1976) Mechanism of activation of adenylate cyclase *in vitro* by polymyxin-released, heat-labile enterotoxin of *Escherichia coli. J. infect. Dis.* **133**: S103–S107.

GILLIGAN, P. H. and ROBERTSON, D. C. (1979) Nutritional requirements for synthesis of heat-labile enterotoxin by enterotoxigenic strains of *Escherichia coli. Infect. Immun.* **23**: 99–107.

GILLIGAN, P. H., BROWN, J. C. and ROBERTSON, D. C. (1983) Immunological relationships between cholera toxin and *Escherichia coli* heat-labile enterotoxin. *Infect. Immun.* **42**: 683–691.

GOLDSCHMIDT, M. C. and DUPONT, H. L. (1976) Enteropathogenic *Escherichia coli:* lack of correlation of serotype with pathogenicity. *J. infect. Dis.* **133**: 153–156.

GORBACH, S. L. and KHURANA, C. M. (1972) Toxigenic *Escherichia coli:* A cause of infantile diarrhea in Chicago. *New Engl. J. Med.* **287**: 791.

GORBACH, S. L., BANWELL, I. G., CHATTERJEE, B. D., JACOBS, B. and SACK, R. B. (1971) Acute undifferentiated human diarrhea in the tropics. I. Alterations in intestinal microflora. *J. clin. Invest.* **50**: 881–889.

GORBACH, S. L., KEAN, B. H., EVANS, D. G., EVANS, D. J., JR. and BESSUDO, D. (1975) Travelers' diarrhea and toxigenic *Escherichia coli. New Engl. J. Med.* **292**: 933–936.

GREENBERG, H. B., LEVINE, M. M., MERSON, M. H., SACK, R. B., SACK, D. A., VALDEVUSO, J. R., NALIN, D. R., HOOVER, D., CHANOCK, R. M. and KAPIKIAN, A. Z. (1979) Solid-phase microtiter radioimmunoassay blocking test for detection of antibodies to *Escherichia coli* heat-labile enterotoxin. *J. clin. Microbiol.* **9**: 60–64.

GREENBERG, H. B., SACK, D. A., RODRIGUEZ, W., SACK, R. B., WYATT, R. G., KALICA, A. R., HORSWOOD, R. L., CHANOCK, R. M. and KAPIKIAN, A. Z. (1977) Microtiter solid-phase radioimmunoassay for detection of *Escherichia coli* heat-labile enterotoxin. *Infect. Immun.* **17**: 541–545.

GREENOUGH, W. B., III (1978) Principles and prospects in the treatment of cholera and related dehydrating diarrheas. In: *Cholera and Related Diarrheas 1978*, pp. 211–218, OUCHTERLONY, O. and HOLMGREN, J. (eds) 43rd Nobel Symp., S. Karger, Basel 1980.

GUERRANT, R. L. and BRUNTON, L. L. (1977) Characterization of the Chinese hamster ovary cell assay for the enterotoxins of *Vibrio holerae* and *Escherichia coli* and for antitoxin: Differential inhibition by gangliosides, specific antisera, and toxoid. *J. infect. Dis.* **135**: 720–728.

GUERRANT, R. L., BRUNTON, L. L., SCHNAITMAN, T. C., RUBHUN, L. I. and GILMAN, A. G. (1974) Cyclic adenosine monophosphate and alteration of Chinese hamster ovary cell morphology: a rapid, sensitive *in vitro* assay for the enterotoxins of *Vibrio cholerae* and *Escherichia coli. Infect. Immun.* **10**: 320–327.

GUERRANT, R. L., DICKENS, M. D., WENZEL, R. P. and KAPIKIAN, A. Z. (1976) Toxigenic bacterial diarrhea: Nursery outbreak involving multiple bacterial strains. *J. Pediat.* **89**: 885–891.

GUERRANT, R. L., GANGULY, U., CASPER, A. G., MOORE, E. J., PIERCE, N. F. and CARPENTER, C. C. (1973) Effect of *Escherichia coli* on fluid transport across canine small bowel. Mechanism and time-course with enterotoxin and whole bacterial cells. *J. clin. Invest.* **52**: 1707–1714.

GUERRANT, R. L., HUGHES, J. M., CHANG, B., ROBERTSON, D. C. and MURAD, F. (1980a) Activation of intestinal cyclase by heat-stable enterotoxin of *Escherichia coli:* studies of tissue specificity, potential receptors and intermediates. *J. infect. Dis.* **142**: 220–228.

GUERRANT, R. L., MOORE, R. A., KIRSCHENFELD, P. M. and SANDE, M. A. (1975) Role of toxigenic and invasive bacteria in acute diarrhea of childhood. *New Engl. J. Med.* **293**: 567–573.

GUERRANT, R. L., ROUSE, J. D. and HUGHES, J. M. (1980b) Turista among the Yale Glee Club in Latin America: Studies of enterotoxigenic bacteria, *E. coli* serotypes and rotaviruses. *Am. J. trop. Med. Hyg.* **29**: 895–900.

GUERRANT, R. L., ROWE, J. D., HUGHES, J. M. and ROWE, B. (1980c) Turista among members of the Yale Glee Club in Latin America. *Am. J. trop. Med. Hyg.* **29**: 895–900.

GURWITH, M. J. (1977) Rapid Screening method of enterotoxigenic *Escherichia coli. J. clin. Microbiol.* **6**: 314–316.

GURWITH, M. J., WISEMAN, D. A. and CHOW, P. (1977) Clinical and laboratory assessment of the pathogenicity of serotyped enteropathogenic *Escherichia coli. J. infect. Dis.* **135**: 736–743.

GUSTAFSSON, B. and MÖLLBY, R. (1982) G_{M1} ganglioside enzyme-linked immunosorbent assay for detection of heat-labile enterotoxin produced by human and porcine *Escherichia coli* strains. *J. clin. Microbiol.* **15**: 298–301.

GYLES, C. L. (1971) Heat-labile and heat-stable forms of the enterotoxin from *E. coli* strains enteropathogenic for pigs. *Ann. N.Y. Acad. Sci.* **176**: 314–316.

GYLES, C. L. (1974a) Relationships among heat-labile enterotoxins of *Escherichia coli* and *Vibrio cholerae. J. infect. Dis.* **129**: 277–283.

GYLES, C. L. (1974b) Immunological study of the heat-labile enterotoxins of *Escherichia coli* and *Vibrio cholerae. Infect. Immun.* **9**: 564–570.

GYLES, C. L. (1978) Comments on detection and importance of enteropathogenic *Escherichia coli* in diarrheal disease of human beings. *J. Am. vet. med. Assoc.* **173**: 598–600.

GYLES, C. L. and BARNUM, D. A. (1967) *Escherichia coli* in ligated segments of pig intestine. *J. Path. Bact.* **94**: 189–194.

GYLES, C. L. and BARNUM, D. A. (1969) A heat-labile enterotoxin from strains of *Escherichia coli* entero-pathogenic for pigs. *J. infect. Dis.* **120**: 419–426.

GYLES, C. L., PALCHANDHURI, S. and MAAS, W. K. (1977) Naturally occurring plasmid carrying genes for enterotoxin production and drug resistance. *Science* **198**: 198–199.

HOLMGREN, J. and SVENNERHOLM, A.-M. (1979) Immunological cross-reactivity between *Escherichia coli* heat-labile enterotoxin and cholera toxin A and B subunits. *Curr. Microbiol.* **2**: 55–58.

HOLMGREN, J., FREDMAN, P., LINDBLAD, M., SVENNERHOLM, A.-M. and SVENNERHOLM, L. (1982) Rabbit intestinal glycoprotein receptor for *Escherichia coli* heat-labile enterotoxin lacking affinity for cholera toxin. *Infect. Immun.* **38**: 424–433.

HOLMGREN, J., SÖDERLIND, O. and WADSTRÖM, T. (1973) Cross-reactivity between heat-labile enterotoxins *Vibrio cholerae* and *Escherichia coli* in neutralization tests in rabbit ileum and skin. *Acta path. microbiol. scand. Sect. B* **81**: 757–762.

HONDA, T., ARITA, M., TAKEDA, Y. and MIWATANI, T. (1982) Further evaluation of the Biken test (modified ELEK test) for detection of enterotoxigenic *Escherichia coli* producing heat-labile enterotoxin and application of the test sampling of heat-stable enterotoxin. *J. clin. Microbiol.* **16**: 60–62.

HONDA, T., SAMAKOSES, R., SORNCHAI, C., TAKEDA, T. and MIWATANI, T. (1983) Detection by a staphylococcal coagglutination test of heat-labile enterotoxin-producing enterotoxigenic *Escherichia-coli.* *J. clin. Microbiol.* **17**: 592–595.

HONDA, T., TAGA, S., TAKEDA, Y. and MIWATANI, T. (1981a) Modified elek test for detection of heat-labile enterotoxin of enterotoxigenic *Escherichia coli.* *J. clin. Microbiol.* **13**: 1–5.

HONDA, T., TAKEDA, Y. and MIWATANI, T. (1981b) Isolation of special antibodies which react only with homologous enterotoxins from *Vibrio cholerae* and enterotoxigenic *Escherichia coli.* *Infect. Immun.* **34**: 333–336.

HONDA, T., TSUJI, T., TAKEDA, Y. and MIWATANI, T. (1981c) Immunological nonidentity of heat-labile enterotoxins from human and porcine enterotoxigenic *Escherichia coli.* *Infect. Immun.* **34**: 337–340.

ISAACSON, R. E. and MOON, H. W. (1975) Induction of heat-labile enterotoxin synthesis in enterotoxigenic *Escherichia coli* by mitomycin C. *Infect. Immun.* **12**: 1271–1275.

ISAACSON, R. E., FUSCO, P. A., BRINTON, C. C. and MOON, H. W. (1978) *In vitro* adhesion of *Escherichia coli* to porcine small intestinal epithelial cells: pili as adhesive factors. *Infect. Immun.* **21**: 392–397.

ITO, T., KUWAHARA, S. and YOKOTA, T. (1983) Automatic and manual latex agglutination tests for measurement of cholera toxin and heat-labile enterotoxin of *Escherichia coli.* *J. clin. Microbiol.* **17**: 7–12.

JACKS, T. M., WU, B. J., BREAEMER, A. C. and BIDLACK, D. E. (1973) Properties of the enterotoxic component in *Escherichia coli* enteropathogenic for swine. *Infect. Immun.* **7**: 178–189.

JONES, F. S. and LITTLE, R. B. (1931a) Etiology of infectious diarrhea (winter scours) in cattle. *JEM* **53**: 835–843.

JONES, F. S. and LITTLE, R. B. (1931b) Vibrionic enteritis in calves. *JEM* **53**: 845–851.

JONES, F. S., ORCUTT, M. and LITTLE, R. B. (1932) Atypical (slow) lactose fermenting *B. coli.* *J. Bact.* **23**: 267–279.

JONES, G. W. (1977) The attachment of bacteria to the surfaces of animal cells, microbial interactions. pp. 139–176, REISSIG, G. W. (ed.) Chapman & Hall, London.

KANTOR, H. S. (1975) Enterotoxins of *Escherichia coli* and *Vibrio cholera*: Tools for the molecular biologist. *J. infect. Dis.* **131**: S22–S32.

KANTOR, H. S., TAO, P. and GORBACH, S. L. (1974a) Stimulation of intestinal adenyl cyclase by *Escherichia coli* enterotoxin: Comparison of strains from an infant and an adult with diarrhea. *J. infect. Dis.* **129**: 1–9.

KANTOR, H. S., TAO, P. and WISDOM, C. (1974b) Action of *Escherichia coli* enterotoxin: Adenylate cyclase behavior of intestinal epithelial cells in culture. *Infect. Immun.* **9**: 1003–1010.

KAPITANY, R. A., SCOOT, A., FORSYTH, G. W., MCKENZIE, S. L. and WORTHINGTON, R. W. (1979) Evidence for two heat-stable enterotoxins produced by enterotoxigenic *Escherichia coli.* *Infect. Immun.* **24**: 965–966.

KAUFFMANN, F. (1944) Zur Serologie der Coli-Gruppe. *Acta path. microbiol. scand.* **21**: 20.

KEARNS, M. J. and GIBBONS, R. A. (1979) The possible nature of the pig intestinal receptor for the K-88 antigen of *Escherichia coli.* *FEMS Micro. Lett.* **6**: 165–168.

KETYI, I. and PACSA, A. S. (1980) Estimation of *Vibrio cholerae* and *Escherichia coli* heat-labile enterotoxin by enzyme linked immunosorbent assay (ELISA). *Acta Microbiol.* **27**: 89–97.

KETYI, I., CZIROK, E., VERTENYI, A., MALOVICS, I. and PACSA, S. (1978) Comparison of *Escherichia coli* enterotoxin tests. *Acta microbiol. hung.* **25**: 23–36.

KETYI, I., EMODY, L., PACSA, S., VERTENYI, A. and KONTROHR, T. (1979) An altered heat-labile enterotoxin (LT′) produced by *Escherichia coli* serogroup O55 strain. *Acta Microbiol.* **26**: 255–262.

KIMBERG, D. V. (1974) Cyclic nucleotides and their role in gastrointestinal secretion. *Gastroenterology* **67**: 1023–1064.

KLAPPER, D. G., FINKELSTEIN, R. A. and CAPRA, M. D. (1976) Subunit structure and *N*-terminal amino acid sequence of the three chains of cholera enterotoxin. *Immunochemistry* **13**: 605–611.

KLIPSTEIN, F. A. and ENGERT, R. F. (1977) Immunological interrelationships between cholera toxin and the heat-labile and heat-stable enterotoxins of coliform bacteria. *Infect. Immun.* **18**: 110–117.

KLIPSTEIN, F. A. and ENGERT, R. F. (1978) Immunological relationship of different preparations of coliform enterotoxins. *Infect. Immun.* **21**: 771–778.

KLIPSTEIN, F. A. and ENGERT, R. F. (1979) Protective effect of active immunization with purified *Escherichia coli* heat-labile enterotoxin in rats. *Infect. Immun.* **23**: 592–599.

KLIPSTEIN, F. A. and ENGERT, R. F. (1980) Influence of route of administration on immediate and extended protection in rats immunized with *Escherichia coli* heat-labile enterotoxin. *Infect. Immun.* **27**: 81–86.

KLIPSTEIN, F. A. and ENGERT, R. F. (1981a) Protective effect of immunization of rats with holotoxin or B subunit of *Escherichia coli* heat-labile enterotoxin. *Infect. Immun.* **31**: 144–150.

KLIPSTEIN, F. A. and ENGERT, R. F. (1981b) Respective contributions to protection of primary and booster immunization with *Escherichia coli* heat-labile enterotoxin in rats. *Infect. Immun.* **31**: 252–260.

KLIPSTEIN, F. A., ENGERT, R. F. and CLEMENTS, J. D. (1982) Development of a vaccine of cross-linked ST-LT that protects against *Escherichia coli* heat-labile and heat-stable enterotoxins. *Infect. Immun.* **37**: 550–557.

KLIPSTEIN, F. A., ENGERT, R. F., CLEMENTS, J. D. and HOUGHTEN, R. A. (1983a) Protection against human and porcine enterotoxigenic strains of *Escherichia coli* in rats immunized with a cross-linked toxoid vaccine. *Infect. Immun.* **40**: 924–929.

KLIPSTEIN, F. A., ENGERT, R. F., CLEMENTS, J. D. and HOUGHTEN, R. A. (1983b) Vaccine for enterotoxigenic *Escherichia coli* based on synthetic heat-stable toxin cross-linked to the B subunit of heat-labile toxin. *J. infect. Dis.* **147**: 318–326.

KLIPSTEIN, F. A., ENGERT, R. F. and HOUGHTEN, R. A. (1983c) Properties of synthetically produced *Escherichia coli* heat-stable enterotoxin. *Infect. Immun.* **39**: 117–121.

KLIPSTEIN, F. A., ENGERT, R. F. and HOUGHTEN, R. A. (1983d) Protection in rabbits immunized with a vaccine of *Escherichia coli* heat-stable toxin cross-linked to the heat-labile toxin B subunit. *Infect. Immun.* **40**: 888–893.

KLIPSTEIN, F. A., ENGERT, R. F. and SHORT, H. D. (1980) Immunological cross-reactivity of heat-labile enterotoxins produced by enterotoxigenic and enteropathogenic strains of *Escherichia coli*. *Immunology* **41**: 115–121.

KLIPSTEIN, F. A., GUERRANT, R. L., WELLS, J. G., SHORT, H. B. and ENGERT, R. F. (1979) Comparison of assay in coliform enterotoxins by conventional techniques versus *in vivo* intestinal perfusion. *Infect. Immun.* **25**: 146–152.

KLIPSTEIN, F. A., LEE, C. and ENGERT, R. F. (1976) Assay of *Escherichia coli* enterotoxins by *in vivo* perfusion in the rat jejunum. *Infect. Immun.* **14**: 1004–1010.

KLIPSTEIN, F. A., ROWE, B., ENGERT, R. F., SHORT, H. B. and GROSS, R. J. (1978) Enterotoxigenicity of enteropathogenic serotypes of *Escherichia coli* isolated from infants with epidemic diarrhea. *Infect. Immun.* **21**: 171–178.

KOHLER, E. M. (1968) Enterotoxic activity of filtrates of *Escherichia coli* in young pigs. *Am. J. vet. Res.* **29**: 2263–2274.

KOHLER, E. M. (1971) Observations on enterotoxins produced by enteropathogenic *Escherichia coli*. *Ann. N. Y. Acad. Sci.* **176**: 212–219.

KONOWALCHUK, J., DICKIE, N., STAVRIC, S. and SPEIRS, J. I. (1978) Comparative studies of five heat-labile toxic products of *Escherichia coli*. *Infect. Immun.* **22**: 644–648.

KUNKEL, S. L. and ROBERTSON, D. C. (1979) Purification and chemical characterization of the heat-labile enterotoxin produced by enterotoxigenic *Escherichia coli*. *Infect. Immun.* **25**: 586–596.

KWAN, C. N. and WISHNOW, R. M. (1974) *Escherichia coli* enterotoxin induced steroidogenesis in cultured adrenal tumor cells. *Infect. Immun.* **10**: 146–151.

LAI, C. Y. (1980) The chemistry and biology of cholera toxin. In: *CRC Critical Reviews in Biochemistry* **9**: 171–206.

LALLIER, R. and LARIVIERE, S. (1978) Effect of different treatments on activity of heat-labile enterotoxin of *Escherichia coli* F11 (P155). *Can. J. comp. Med.* **42**: 214–218.

LALLIER, R., BERNARD, F., GENDREAU, M., LAZURE, C., SEIDAH, N. G., CHRETIEN, M. and ST-PIERRE, S. A. (1982) Isolation and purification of *Escherichia coli* heat-stable enterotoxin of porcine origin. *Anal. Biochem.* **127**: 267–275.

LANDWALL, P. and MÖLLBY, R. (1978) Production of *Escherichia coli* heat-labile enterotoxin in fermenter dialysis culture. *J. appl. Bact.* **44**: 141–149.

LARIVIERE, S., GYLES, C. L. and BARNUM, D. A. (1972) A comparative study of the rabbit and pig gut loop systems for the assay of *Escherichia coli* enterotoxin. *Can. J. comp. Med.* **36**: 319–328.

LARIVIERE, S., GYLES, C. L. and BARNUM, D. A. (1973) Preliminary characterization of the heat-labile enterotoxin of *Escherichia coli*. *J. infect. Dis.* **128**: 312–320.

LEE, J. A. and KEAN, B. H. (Chairman and Convener) (1978) International conference on the diarrhea of traveler—new directions in research: A summary. *J. infect. Dis.* **137**: 355–368.

LEVINE, M. M. (1983) Traveler's diarrhoea: prospects for successful immunoprophylaxis. *Scand. J. Gastroenterol.* **84** (Suppl. 18): 121–134.

LEVINE, M. M., BLACK, R. E., BRINTON, C. C., JR., CLEMENTS, M. L., FUSCO, P., HUGHES, T. P., O'DONNELL, S., ROBINS-BROWNE, R., WOOD, S. and YOUNG, C. (1982a) Reactogenicity, immunogenicity, and efficacy studies of *Escherichia coli* type 1 somatic pili parental vaccine in man. *Scand. J. infect. Dis.* **33** (Suppl.): 83–95.

LEVINE, M. M., BLACK, R. E., CLEMENTS, M. L., YOUNG, C. R., BRINTON, C. C., JR., FUSCO, P., WOOD, S., BOEDEKER, E., CHENEY, C., SCHADL, P. and COLLINS, H. (1984) Prevention of enterotoxigenic *Escherichia coli* diarrheal infection in man by vaccines that stimulate anti-adhesion (anti-pili) immunity. In: *Attachment of organisms to the gut mucosa*, Vol. II, Chapt. 23, pp. 223–244, BOEDEKER, E. C. (ed.) CRC Press, Boca Raton, Florida.

LEVINE, M. M., BLACK, R. E., CLEMENTS, M. L., YOUNG, C. R., LANATA, C., SEARS, S., HONDA, T. and FINKELSTEIN, R. (1983a) Texas Star-SR: Attenuated *Vibrio cholerae* oral vaccine candidate. *Dev. Biol. Stand.* **53**: 59–65.

LEVINE, M. M., CAPLAN, E. S., WATERMAN, D., CASH, R., HORNICK, R. B. and SNYDER, M. J. (1977) Diarrhea caused by *Escherichia coli* that produce only heat-stable enterotoxin. *Infect. Immun.* **17**: 78–82.

LEVINE, M. M., KAPER, J. B., BLACK, R. E. and CLEMENTS, M. L. (1983b) New knowledge on pathogenesis of bacterial enteric infections as applied to vaccine development. *Microbiol. Rev.* **47**: 510–550.

LEVINE, M. M., NALIN, D. R., CRAIG, J. P., HOOVER, D., BERGQUIST, E. J., WATERMAN, D., HOLLEY, H. P., HORNICK, R. B., PIERCE, N. P. and LIBONATI, J. P. (1979a) Immunity to cholera in man: relative role of antibacterial versus antitoxic immunity. *Trans. R. Soc. trop. Med. Hyg.* **73**: 3–9.

LEVINE, M. M., NALIN, D. R,, HOOVER, D. L., BERGQUIST, E. J., HORNICK, R. B. and YOUNG, C. R. (1979b) Immunity to enterotoxigenic *Escherichia coli*. *Infect. Immun.* **23**: 729–736.

LEVNER, M. H., URBANO, C. and RUBIN, B. A. (1980) Lincomycin increases synthetic rate and periplasmic pool size for cholera toxin. *J. Bact.* **143**: 441–447.

LEVNER, M. H., WIENER, F. P. and RUBIN, B. A. (1977) Induction of *Escherichia coli* and *Vibrio cholerae* enterotoxins by an inhibitor of protein synthesis. *Infect. Immun.* **15**: 132–137.

LINDHOLM, L., HOLMGREN, J., WIKSTROM, M., KARLSSON, U., ANDERSSON, K. and LYCKE, N. (1983) Monoclonal antibodies to cholera toxin with special reference to cross reactions with *Escherichia-coli* heat-labile enterotoxin. *Infect. Immun.* **40**: 570–576.

MADSEN, G. L. and KNOOP, F. C. (1980) Physicochemical properties of a heat-stable enterotoxin produced by *Escherichia coli* of human origin. *Infect. Immun.* **28**: 1051–1053.

MARCHLEWICZ, B. A. and FINKELSTEIN, R. A. (1983) Immunologic differences among the cholera/coli family of enterotoxins. *Diag. Microbiol. infect. Dis.* **1**: 129–138.

MASSINI, R. (1907) Über eine in biologischer Beziehung interessanten Kolistamm (Bact. coli mutabile); ein Beitrag zur Variation bei Bakterien. *Arch. Hyg.* **LI**: 250–292.

McCONNELL, M. M., SMITH, H. R., WILLSHAW, G. A., FIELD, A. M. and ROWE, B. (1981) Plasmids coding for colonization factor antigen I and heat-stable enterotoxin production isolated from enterotoxigenic *Escherichia coli*: comparison of their properties. *Infect. Immun.* **32**: 927–936.

McCONNELL, M. M., SMITH, H. R., WILLSHAW, G. A., SCOTLAND, S. M. and ROWE, B. (1980) Plasmids coding for heat-labile enterotoxin production isolated from *Escherichia coli* O78: comparison of properties. *J. Bact.* **143**: 158–167.

MEKALANOS, J. J., COLLIER, R. J. and ROMIG, W. R. (1978a) Affinity filters, a new approach to isolation of tox mutants of *Vibrio cholerae*. *Proc. natn. Acad. Sci. U.S.A.* **75**: 941–945.

MEKALANOS, J. J., COLLIER, R. J. and ROMIG, W. R. (1978b) Purification of cholera toxin and its subunits: new methods of preparation and the use of hypertoxinogenic mutants. *Infect. Immun.* **20**: 552–558.

MEKALANOS, J. J., COLLIER, R. J. and ROMIG, W. R. (1979) Enzymatic activity of cholera toxin. I. New method of assay and the mechanism of ADP-ribosyl transfer. *J. biol. Chem.* **254**: 5849–5854.

MERSON, J. H., MORRIS, G. K., SACK, D. A., WELLS, J. G., FEELEY, J. C., SACK, R. B., CREECH, W. B., KAPIKIAN, A. Z. and GANGAROSA, E. J. (1976) Traveler's diarrhea in Mexico: A prospective study of physicians and family members attending a congress. *New Engl. J. Med.* **294**: 1299–1305.

MERSON, J. H., MORRIS, G. K., SACK, D. A., WELLS, J. G., FEELEY, J. C., SACK, R. B, CREECH, W. B., KAPIKIAN, A. Z. and GANGAROSA, E. J. (1976) Travelers diarrhea in Mexico: A prospective study of physicians and family members attending a congress. *New Engl. J. Med.* **294**: 1299–1305.

MERSON, M. H., ORSKOV, F., ORSKOV, I., SACK, R. B., HUQ, I. and KOSTER, F. T. (1979a) Relationship between enterotoxin production and serotypes in enterotoxigenic *Escherichia coli*. *Infect. Immun.* **23**: 325–329.

MERSON, M. H., ROWE, B., BLACK, R. E, HUQ, I., GROSS, R. J. and EUSOF, A. (1980a) Use of antisera for identification of enterotoxigenic *Escherichia coli*. *Lancet* ii: 222–224.

MERSON, M. H., SACK, R. B. and KIBRIYA, A. K. M. G. (1979b) The use of colony pools for diagnosis of enterotoxigenic *Escherichia coli* diarrhoea. *J. clin. Microbiol.* **9**: 493–497.

MERSON, M. H., YOLKEN, R. H., SACK, R. B., FROEHLICH, J. L., GREENBERT, H. B., HUQ, I. and BLACK, R. W. (1980b) Detection of *Escherichia coli* enterotoxins in stools. *Infect. Immun.* **29**: 108–113.

MIDDELDORP, J. M. and WITHOLT, R. B. (1981) K88-mediated binding of *Escherichia coli* outer membrane fragments to porcine intestinal epithelial cell brush borders. *Infect. Immun.* **31**: 42–51.

MITCHELL, I. DE C., TAME, M. J. and KENWORTHY, R. J. (1974) Separation and purification of enterotoxins from a strain of *Escherichia coli* pathogenic for pigs. *J. med. Microbiol.* **7**: 439–450.

MÖLLBY, R., HJALMARSSON, S. G. and WADSTRÖM, T. (1975) Separation of *E. coli* heat-labile enterotoxin by preparative isotachophoresis. *FEBS Lett.* **56**: 30–33.

MOON, H. W. (1978) Mechanisms in pathogenesis of diarrhea—Review. *J. vet. med. Ass.* **172**: 443–448.

MOON, H. W. (1980) Luminal and mucosal factors of small intestine affecting pathogenic colonization. In: *Secretory Diarrhea*, pp. 127–139, FIELD, M., FORTRAN, J. S. and SCHULTZ, S. G. (ed.) Am. Physiol. Soc., Bethesda, Maryland. Williams & Wilkins, Baltimore, Maryland.

MOON, H. W. and WHIPP, S. C. (1971) Systems for testing the enteropathogenicity of *Escherichia coli*. *Ann. N.Y. Acad. Sci.* **176**: 197–211.

MOON, H. W., ISAACSON, R. E. and POHLENZ, J. (1979) Mechanisms of association of enteropathogenic *Escherichia coli* with intestinal epithelium. *Am. J. clin. Nutr.* **32**: 119–127.

MOON, H. W., KOHLER, E. M., SCHNEIDER, R. A. and WHIPP, S. C. (1980) Prevalence of pilus antigens, enterotoxin types and enteropathogenicity among K88-negative enterotoxigenic *Escherichia coli* from neonatal pigs. *Infect. Immun.* **27**: 222–230.

MOON, H. W., NAGY, B. and ISAACSON, R. E. (1977) Intestinal colonization and adhesion by enterotoxigenic *Escherichia coli*: Ultrastructural observations on adherence to ileal epithelium of the pig. *J. infect. Dis.* **136**: S124–S129.

MOON, H. W., WHIPP, S. C. and BAETZ, A. L. (1971) Comparative effects of enterotoxins from *Escherichia coli* and *Vibrio cholerae* on rabbit and swine small intestine. *Lab. Invest.* **25**: 133–140.

MORGAN, D. R., DuPONT, H. L., WOOD, L. V. and ERICSSON, C. D. (1983) Comparison of methods to detect *Escherichia coli* heat-labile enterotoxin in stool and cell-free culture supernatants. *J. clin. Microbiol.* **18**: 798–802.

MORO, E. (1905) Morphologische und biologische Untersuchungen über die Darmbakterien des Säuglings. *Jb. K. Berlin 1905* **XIX**: 500–502.

MORRIS, G. K., MERSON, M. H., SACK, D. A., WELLS, J., MARTIN, W. T., DeWITT, W. E., FEELEY, J. C., SACK, R. B. and BESSUDO, D. M. (1976) Laboratory investigation of diarrhea in travelers to Mexico: Evaluation of methods for detecting enterotoxigenic *Escherichia coli*. *J. clin. Microbiol.* **3**: 486–495.

MOSELEY, S. L. and FALKOW, S. (1980) Nucleotide sequence homology between the heat-labile enterotoxin gene of *Escherichia coli* and *Vibrio cholerae* deoxyribonucleic acid. *J. Bact.* **144**: 444–446.

MOSELEY, S. L., HUQ, I., ALIM, A. R. M. A., SO, M., SAMADPOUR-MOTALEBI, M. and FALKOW, S. (1980) Detection of enterotoxigenic *Escherichia coli* by DNA colony hybridization. *J. infect. Dis.* **142**: 892–898.

Moss, J. M. and Richardson, S. H. (1978) Activation of adenylate cyclase by heat-labile *Escherichia coli* enterotoxin. Evidence for ADP-ribosyl-transferase activity similar to that of choleragen. *J. clin. Invest.* **62**: 271–285.

Moss, J. and Vaughan, M. (1977) Choleragen activation of solubilized adenylate cyclase-requirement for GTP and protein activator for demonstration of enzymatic activity. *Proc. natn. Acad. Sci. U.S.A.* **74**: 4396–4400.

Moss, J. M., Garrison, S., Oppenheimer, N. J. and Richardson, S. H. (1979) NAD-dependent ADP-ribosylation of arginine and proteins by *Escherichia coli* heat-labile enterotoxin. *J. biol. Chem.* **254**: 6270–6272.

Moss, J. M., Osborne, J. C., Fishman, P. H., Nakaya, S. and Robertson, D. C. (1981) *Escherichia coli* heat-labile enterotoxin: Ganglioside specificity and ADP-ribosyltransferase activity. *J. biol. Chem.* **256**: 12861–12865.

Mundell, D. H., Anselmo, C. R. and Wishnow, R. M. (1976) Factor influencing heat-labile *Escherichia coli* enterotoxin activity. *Infect. Immun.* **14**: 383–388.

Myers, L. L., Newman, F. S., Warren, G. R., Catlin, J. E. and Anderson, C. L. (1975) Calf ligated intestinal segment test to detect enterotoxigenic *E. coli. Infect. Immun.* **11**: 588–591.

Neter, E. (1976) *Escherichia coli* as a pathogen. *J. pediat.* **89**: 166–168.

Nozawa, R. T., Yokota, T. and Kuwahara, S. (1978) Assay method for *Vibrio cholerae* and *Escherichia coli* enterotoxins by automated counting of floating Chinese hamster ovary cells in culture medium. *J. clin. Microbiol.* **7**: 479–485.

O'Brien, A. D. and LaVeck, G. D. (1983) Purification and characterization of a *Shigella dysenteriae* I-like toxin produced by *Escherichia coli. Infect. Immun.* **40**: 675–683.

O'Brien, A. D., Gentry, M. K., Thompson, M. R., Doctor B. P., Gemski, P. and Formal, S. G. (1979) Shigellosis and *Escherichia coli* diarrhea: relative importance of invasive and toxigenic mechanisms. *Am. J. clin. Nutr.* **32**: 229–233.

Orskov, F. and Orskov, I. (1979) Special *Escherichia coli* serotypes from enteropathies in domestic animals and man. In: Escherichia coli *Infections in Domestic Animals, Advances in Veterinary Medicine*, Vol. 29, pp. 7–14, Willinger, H. and Weber, A. (eds).

Orskov, F., Orskov, I., Evans, D. J., Jr., Sack, R. B., Sack, D. A. and Wadström, T. (1976) Special *Escherichia coli* serotypes among enterotoxigenic strains from diarrhoea in adults and children. *Med. Microbiol. Immun.* **162**: 73–80.

Orskov, I. and Orskov, F. (1977) Special O:K:H serotypes among enterotoxigenic *E. coli* strains from diarrhea in adults and children. Occurrence of the CH (colonization factor) antigen and hemagglutinating abilities. *Med. Microbiol. Immun.* **163**: 99–110.

Otnaess, A.-B. and Halvorsen, S. (1981) Identification of low levels of heat-labile enteroxin in *Escherichia coli* from children with diarrhoea. *Acta path. microbiol. scand. Sect. B* **89**: 173–177.

Palva, T. E., Hirst, T. R., Hardy, S. J. S., Holmgren, J. and Randall, L. (1981) Synthesis of a precursor to the B subunit of heat-labile enteroxin in *Escherichia coli. J. Bact.* **146**: 325–333.

Pickering, L. K., Evans, D. J., Munòz, O., DuPont, H. L., Coello-Ramirez, P., Vollet, J. J., Conklin, R. H., Olarte, J. and Kohl, S. (1978) Prospective study of enteropathogens in children with diarrhea in Houston and Mexico. *J. Pediat.* **93**: 383–388.

Pierce, N. F. (1973) Differential inhibitory effects of cholera toxoids and ganglioside on the enterotoxins of *Vibrio cholera* and *Escherichia coli. J. exp. Med.* **137**: 1009–1023.

Pierce, N. F. (1977) Protection against challenge with *Escherichia coli* heat-labile enterotoxin by immunization of rats with cholera toxin/toxoid. *Infect. Immun.* **18**: 338–341.

Plotkin, G. R., Kluge, R. M. and Waldman, R. H. (1979) Gastroenteritis: etiology, pathophysiology and clinical manifestations. *Medicine* **58**: 95–114.

Polotsky, Y. E., Dragunskaya, E. M., Seliverstava, V. G., Avdeeva, V. G., Chakhutinskaya, M. G., Ketyi, I., Vertenyi, A., Ralovich, B., Emody, L., Malovics, I., Safonova, N. V., Snigierevskaya, E. S. and Karyagina, E. I. (1977) Pathogenic effect of enterotoxigenic *Escherichia coli* and *Escherichia coli* causing infantial diarrhoea. *Acta microbiol. hung.* **24**: 221–236.

Reis, M. H. L., Affonso, M. H. T., Tabulsi, L. R., Oh, A. J., Maas, R. and Maas, W. K. (1980a) Transfer of a CFA/I-ST plasmid promoted by a conjugative plasmid in a strain of *Escherichia coli* of serotype O128ac:H12. *Infect. Immun.* **29**: 140–143.

Reis, M. H. L., DeCastro, A. F. P., Toledo, M. R. F. and Trabulski, L. R. (1979) Production of heat-stable enterotoxin by the O128 serogroup of *E. coli. Infect. Immun.* **24**: 289–290.

Reis, M. H. L., Matos, D. P., DeCastro, A. F. P., Toledo, M. R. F. and Trabulsi, L. R. (1980b) Relationship among enterotoxigenic phenotypes, serotypes and sources of strains in enterotoxigenic *Escherichia coli. Infect. Immun.* **28**: 24–27.

Richards, K. L. and Douglas, S. D. (1978) Pathophysiological effects of *Vibrio cholerae* and enterotoxigenic *Escherichia coli* and their exotoxins on eucaryotic cells. *Microbiol. Rev.* **42**: 592–613.

Ristaino, P. A., Levine, M. M. and Young, C. R. (1983) Improved G_{M1}-enzyme-linked immunosorbent assay for detection of *Escherichia coli* heat-labile enterotoxin. *J. clin. Microbiol.* **18**: 808–815.

Robertson, D. C. (1978) Chemistry and biology of the heat-stable *Escherichia coli* enterotoxin. In: *Cholera and Related Diarrheas*, pp. 115–126, Ouchterlony, O. and Holmgren, J. (eds) S. Karger, Basel.

Robertson, D. C., Kunkel, S. L. and Gilligan, P. H. (1978) Purification and characterization of heat-labile enterotoxin produced by ENT$^+$ *Escherichia coli:* Application of hydrophobic chromatography and use of defined media. In: *Proceedings of the 14th Joint Conference, U.S.–Japan Cooperative Medical Science Program*, pp. 250–265, Takeya, K. and Zinnaka, Y. (eds) Fuji Printing, Tokyo.

Robertson, D. C., Kunkel, S. L. and Gilligan, P. H. (1979) Structure and function of *E. coli* heat-labile enterotoxin. In: *Proceedings of the 15th Joint Conference, U.S.–Japan Cooperative Medical Science Program*, pp. 389–400. National Institutes of Health (Publication No. 80-2003), Bethesda.

Rönnberg, B. and Wadström, T. (1983) Rapid detection by a co-agglutination test of heat-labile enterotoxin in cell lysates from blood agar-grown *Escherichia coli. J. clin. Microbiol.* **17**: 1021–1025.

RÖNNBERG, B., WADSTRÖM, T. and JORNVALL, H. (1983) Structure of heat-stable enterotoxin produced by a human strain of *Escherichia coli:* differences from the toxin of another human strain suggest the presence of compensated amino acid exchanges. *FEBS Lett.* **155**: 183–185.

ROWE, B. (1979) The role of *Escherichia coli* in gastroenteritis. *Clin. Gastroenterol.* **8**: 625–644.

RYDER, R. W., KASLOW, R. A. and WELLS, J. G. (1979) Evidence for enterotoxin production by a classic enteropathogenic serotype of *Escherichia coli. J. infect. Dis.* **140**: 626–628.

SACK, D. A. and SACK, R. B. (1975) Test for enterotoxigenic *Escherichia coli* using Y-1 adrenal cells in miniculture. *Infect. Immun.* **11**: 334–336.

SACK, D. A., HUDA, S., NEOGI, P. K. B., DANIEL, R. R. and SPIRA, W. M. (1980) Microtiter ganglioside enzyme-linked immunosorbent assay for *Vibrio* and *Escherichia coli* heat-labile enterotoxins and antitoxin. *J. clin. Microbiol.* **11**: 35–40.

SACK, D. A., KAMINSKY, D. C., SACK, R. B., ITOTIA, J. N., ARTHUR, R. R., KAPIKIAN, A. Z., ORSKOV, F. and ORSKOV, I. (1978) Prophylactic doxycycline for travelers' diarrhea. *New Engl. J. Med.* **298**: 758–763.

SACK, D. A., KAMINSKY, D. C., SACK, R. B., WAMOLA, I. A., ORSKOV, I., SLACK, R. C. B., ARTHUR, R. R. and KAPIKIAN, A. Z. (1977a) Enterotoxigenic *Escherichia coli* diarrhea of travelers: A prospective study of American Peace Corps volunteers. *John Hopkins Med. J.* **141**: 63–70.

SACK, D. A., MCLAUGHLIN, J. C., SACK, R. B., ORSKOV, F. and ORSKOV, I. (1977b) Enterotoxigenic *Escherichia coli* isolated from patients in a hospital in Dacca. *J. infect. Dis.* **135**: 275–280.

SACK, D. A., MEHLMAN, I. J., ORSKOV, F. and ORSKOV, I. (1977c) Enterotoxigenic *Escherichia coli* isolated from food. *J. infect. Dis.* **135**: 313–317.

SACK, R. B. (1975) Human diarrheal disease caused by enterotoxigenic *Escherichia coli. Ann. Rev. Microbiol.* **29**: 333–353.

SACK, R. B. (1980) Enterotoxigenic *Escherichia coli.* Identification and characterization. *J. infect. Dis.* **142**: 279–286.

SACK, R. B., GORBACH, S. L., BANWELL, J. G., JACOBS, B., CHATTERJEE, B. D. and MITRA, R. C. (1971) Enterotoxigenic *Escherichia coli* isolated from patients with severe cholera-like disease. *J. infect. Dis.* **123**: 378–385.

SACK, R. B., HIRSCHHORN, N., BROWNLEE, I., CASH, R. A., WOODWARD, W. A. and SACK, D. A. (1975a) Enterotoxigenic *Escherichia coli*-associated diarrheal diseases in Apache children. *New Engl. J. Med.* **292**: 1041–1045.

SACK, R. B., HIRSCHHORN, N., WOODWARD, W. E., SACK, D. A. and CASH, R. A. (1975b) Antibodies to heat-labile *Escherichia coli* enterotoxin in Apaches in White River, Arizona. *Infect. Immun.* **12**: 1475–1477.

SACK, R. B., JOHNSON, J., PIERCE, N. F., KEREN, D. F. and YARDLEY, J. H. (1976) Challenge of dogs with live enterotoxigenic *Escherichia coli* and effects of repeated challenge on fluid secretion in jejunal Thiry-Vella loops. *J. infect. Dis.* **134**: 15–24.

SAEED, A. M. K., SRIRANGANATHAN, N., COSAND, W. and BURGER, D. (1983) Purification and characterization of heat-stable enterotoxin from bovine enterotoxigenic *Escherichia coli Infect. Immun.* **40**: 701–707.

SAKAZAKI, R., TAMURA, K. and SAITO, M. (1967) Enteropathogenic *Escherichia coli.* associated with diarrhea in children and adults. *Jap. J. med. Sci. Biol.* **20**: 387–399.

SCHEFTEL, J. M., MARTIN, C., BOBER, C. and MONTEIL, H. (1980) Isolation of an enterotoxigenic factor elaborated by human enteropathogenic *Escherichia coli. FEMS Microbiol. Lett.* **9**: 125–130.

SCHENKEIN, I., GREEN, R. F., SANTOS, D. S. and MAAS, W. K. (1976) Partial purification and characterization of a heat-labile enterotoxin of *Escherichia coli. Infect. Immun.* **13**: 1710–1720.

SCOTLAND, S. M., DAY, N. P., CRAVIOTO, A., THOMAS, L. V. and ROWE, B. (1981) Production of heat-labile or heat-stable enterotoxins by strains of *Escherichia coli* belonging to serogroups O44, O114, and O128. *Infect. Immun.* **31**: 500–503.

SCOTLAND, S. M., DAY, N. P. and ROWE, B. (1980) Production of a cytotoxin affecting Vero cells by strains of *Escherichia coli* belonging to traditional enteropathogenic serogroups. *FEMS Microbiol. Lett.* **7**: 15–17.

SEN, D., SAHA, M. R. and PAL, S. C. (1984) Evaluation of three simple and rapid immunological tests for detection of heat-labile enterotoxin of enterotoxigenic *Escherichia coli. J. clin. Microbiol.* **19**: 194–196.

SERAFIM, M. B., DECASTRO, A. F. P., LEMOS DOS REIS, M. H. and TRABULSI, L. R. (1979) Passive immune hemolysis for detection of heat-labile enterotoxin produced by *Escherichia coli* isolated from different sources. *Infect. Immun.* **24**: 606–610.

SERAFIM, M. B., DECASTRO, A. F. P., LEONARDO, M. B. and MONTEIRO, A. R. (1981) Single radial immune hemolysis test for detection of *Escherichia coli* thermolabile enterotoxin. *J. clin. Microbiol.* **14**: 473–478.

SHAH, D. B., KAUFFMAN, P. E., BOUTIN, B. K. and JOHNSON, C. H. (1982) Detection of heat-labile-enterotoxin-producing colonies of *Escherichia coli* and *Vibrio cholerae* by solid-phase sandwich radioimmunoassays. *J. clin. Microbiol.* **16**: 504–508.

SHERR, H. P., BANWELL, J. G., ROTHFIELD, A. and HENDRIX, T. R. (1973) Pathophysiological response of rabbit jejunum to *Escherichia coli* enterotoxin. *Gastroenterology* **65**: 895–902.

SHORE, E. G., DEAN, A. G., HOLIK, K. J. and DAVIS, B. R. (1974) Enterotoxin-producing *Escherichia coli* and diarrheal disease in adult travelers: A prospective study. *J. infect. Dis.* **129**: 577–582.

SILVA, M. L. M., MAAS, W. K. and GYLES, C. L. (1978) Isolation and characterization of enterotoxin-deficient mutants of *Escherichia coli. Proc. natn. Acad. Sci. U.S.A.* **75**: 1384–1388.

SIVASWAMY, G. and GYLES, C. L. (1976) Prevalence of enterotoxigenic *Escherichia coli* in the feces of calves with diarrhea. *Can. J. comp. Med.* **40**: 241–246.

SKERMAN, F. J., FORMAL, S. B. and FALKOW, S. (1972) Plasmid-associated enterotoxin production in a strain of *Escherichia coli* isolated from humans. *Infect. Immun.* **5**: 622–624.

SMITH, H. R., CRAVIOTO, A., WILLSHAW, G. A., MCCONNELL, M. M., SCOTLAND, S. M., GROSS, R. J. and ROWE, B. (1979) A plasmid coding for the production of colonization factor antigen I and heat-stable enterotoxin in strains of *Escherichia coli* of serogroup O78. *FEMS Microbiol. Lett.* **6**: 255–260.

SMITH, H. W. (1972) The production of diarrhoea in baby rabbits by the oral administration of cell-free preparations of enteropathogenic *Escherichia coli* and *Vibrio cholerae:* The effect of antisera. *J. Med. Microbiol.* **5**: 299–303.

Smith, H. W. and Gyles, C. L. (1970a) The relationship between two apparently different enterotoxins produced by enteropathogenic strains of *Escherichia coli*. *J. Med. Microbiol.* **3**: 387–401.

Smith, H. W. and Gyles, C. L. (1970b) The effect of cell-free fluids prepared from cultures of human and animal enteropathogenic strains of *Escherichia coli* on ligated intestinal segments of rabbits and pigs. *J. Med. Microbiol.* **3**: 403–409.

Smith, H. W. and Halls, S. (1967a) Observations by the ligated intestinal segment and oral inoculation methods on *Escherichia coli* infections in pigs, calves, lambs and rabbits. *J. Path. Bact.* **93**: 499–529.

Smith, H. W. and Halls, S. (1967b) Studies on *Escherichia coli* enterotoxin. *J. Path. Bact.* **93**: 531–543.

Smith, H. W. and Halls, S. (1968) The transmissible nature of the genetic factor in *Escherichia coli* that controls enterotoxin production. *J. gen. Microbiol.* **52**: 319–334.

Smith, H. W. and Linggood, M. A. (1971a) The transmissible nature of enterotoxin production in a human enteropathogenic strain of *Escherichia coli*. *J. Med. Microbiol.* **4**: 301–305.

Smith, H. W. and Linggood, M. A. (1971b) Observation on the pathogenic properties of the K-88, Hly and Ent plasmids of *Escherichia coli* with particular reference to porcine diarrhoea. *J. Med. Microbiol.* **4**: 467–485.

Smith, N. M. and Sack, R. B. (1973) Immunologic cross-reactions of enterotoxins from *Escherichia coli* and *Vibrio cholerae*. *J. infect. Dis.* **127**: 164–170.

Smith, T. and Orcutt, M. L. (1925) Bacteriology of intestinal tract of young calves with special reference to early diarrhea ("scours"). *JEM 1925* **41**: 89–106.

Smith, C. J., Jonnsson, P., Olsson, E., Söderlind, O., Rosengren, J., Hjerten, S. and Wadström, T. (1978) Differences in hydrophobic surface characteristics of porcine enteropathogenic *Escherichia coli* with or without K-88 antigen as revealed by hydrophobic interaction chromatography. *Infect. Immun.* **22**: 462–472.

So, M., Crosa, I. H. and Falkow, S. (1975) Polynucleotide sequence relationship among Ent plasmids and the relationship between Ent plasmids and other plasmids. *J. Bact.* **121**: 234–238.

So, M., Dallas, W. S. and Falkow, S. (1978) Characterization of an *Escherichia coli* plasmid encoding for synthesis of heat-labile toxin: molecular cloning of the toxin determinant. *Infect. Immun.* **21**: 405–411.

Söderlind, O., Möllby, R. and Wadström, T. (1974) Purification and some properties of a heat-labile enterotoxin from *Escherichia coli*. *Zentbl. Bakt. Parasitkde Abt. 1 Orig. Reihe A* **229**: 190–204.

Speirs, J. I., Stavric, S. and Konowalchuk, J. (1977) Assay of *Escherichia coli* heat-labile enterotoxin with Vero cells. *Infect. Immun.* **16**: 617–622.

Spicer, E. K. and Noble, J. A. (1982) *Escherichia coli* heat-labile enterotoxin: Nucleotide sequence of the A subunit gene. *J. biol. Chem.* **257**: 5716–5721.

Spicer, E. K., Kavanaugh, W. M., Dallas, W. S., Falkow, S., Konigsberg and Schafer, D. E. (1981) Sequence homologies between A subunits of *Escherichia coli* and *Vibrio cholerae* enterotoxins. *Proc. natn. Acad. Sci. U.S.A.* **78**: 50–54.

Staples, S. J., Asher, S. E. and Gaianella, R. A. (1980) Purification and characterization of heat-stable enterotoxin produced by a strain of *E. coli* pathogenic for man. *J. biol. Chem.* **255**: 4716–4721.

Stavric, S., Speirs, J. I., Konowalchuk, J. and Jeffrey, D. (1978) Stimulation of cyclic AMP secretion in Vero cells by enterotoxins of *Escherichia coli* and *Vibrio cholerae*. *Infect. Immun.* **21**: 514.

Steffen, R., van der Linde, F., Gyr, K. and Schär, M. (1983) Epidemiology of diarrhea in travelers. *JAMA* **249**: 1176–1180.

Stevens, J. B., Gyles, C. L. and Barnum, D. A. (1972) Production of diarrhea in pigs in response to *Escherichia coli* enterotoxin. *Am. J. vet. Res.* **33**: 2511–2526.

Stirm, S., Orskov, F., Orskov, I. and Birch-Anderson, A. (1967) Episome-carried surface antigen K-88 of *Escherichia coli*, III. Morphology. *J. Bact.* **93**: 740–748.

Svennerholm, A.-M. and Ahren, C. (1982) Immune protection against enterotoxigenic *E. coli:* search for synergy between antibodies to enterotoxin and somatic antigens. *Acta. path. microbiol. immun. scand. Sect. C* **90**: 1–6.

Svennerholm, A.-M. and Holmgren, J. (1978) Identification of *Escherichia coli* heat-labile enterotoxin by means of a ganglioside immunosorbent assay (Gm_1-ELISA) procedure. *Curr. Microbiol.* **1**: 19–23.

Svennerholm, A.-M. and Wiklund, G. (1983) Rapid G_{MI}-enzyme linked immunosorbent assay with visual reading for identification of *Escherichia coli* heat-labile enterotoxin. *J. clin. Microbiol.* **17**: 596–600.

Tait, R. M., Booth, B. R. and Lambert, P. A. (1980) ADP-ribosylation of a rat liver membrane protein catalyzed by heat-labile enterotoxin from *E. coli*. *Biochem. biophys. Res. Commun.* **96**: 1024–1031.

Takeda, Y. and Murphy, J. R. (1978) Bacteriophage conversion of heat-labile enterotoxin in *Escherichia coli*. *J. Bact.* **133**: 172–177.

Takeda, T., Honda, T., Sima, H., Tsuji, T. and Miwatani, T. (1983) Analysis of antigenic determinants in cholera enterotoxin and heat-labile enterotoxins from human and porcine enterotoxigenic *Escherichia coli*. *Infect. Immun.* **41**: 50–53.

Takeda, Y., Taga, S. and Miwatani, T. (1979a) Purification of heat-labile enterotoxin of *Escherichia coli*. *FEMS Microbiol. Lett.* **5**: 181–186.

Takeda, Y., Takeda, T., Yano, T., Yamamoto, K. and Miwatani, T. (1979b) Purification and partial characterization of heat-stable enterotoxin of enterotoxigenic *Escherichia coli*. *Infect. Immun.* **25**: 978–985.

Taylor, I. and Bettelheim, K. A. (1966) The action of chloroform-killed enteropathogenic *Escherichia coli* on ligated rabbit-gut segments. *J. gen. Microbiol.* **42**: 309–313.

Thorne, G. M., Deneke, C. F. and Gorbach, S. L. (1979) Hemagglutination and adhesiveness of toxigenic *Escherichia coli* isolated from humans. *Infect. Immun.* **23**: 690–699.

Toledo, M. R. F., Alvariza, M. C. B., Murahovschi, J., Ramos, S. R. T. S. and Trabulsi, L. R. (1983) Enteropathogenic *Escherichia coli* serotypes and endemic diarrhea in infants. *Infect. Immun.* **39**: 586–589.

Tsuji, T., Taga, S., Honda, T., Takeda, Y. and Miwatani, T. (1982) Molecular heterogeneity of heat-labile enterotoxins from human and porcine enterotoxigenic *Escherichia coli*. *Infect. Immun.* **38**: 444–448.

TSUKAMOTO, T., KINOSHITA, Y., TAGA, S., TAKEDA, Y. and MIWATANI, T. (1980) Value of passive immune hemolysis for detection of heat-labile enterotoxin produced by enterotoxigenic *Escherichia coli*. *J. clin. Microbiol.* **12**: 768–771.

WACHSMUTH, I. K., WELLS, J. G. and RYDER, R. W. (1977) *Escherichia coli* heat-labile enterotoxin: Comparison of antitoxin assays and serum antitoxin levels. *Infect. Immun.* **18**: 348–351.

WADSTRÖM, T. (1978) Relative importance of enterotoxigenic and invasive enteropathogenic bacteria in infantile diarrhea. *Zenbl. Bakt. Parasitkde. Abt. 1 Orig. Reihe A* **242**: 53–63.

WADSTRÖM, T., AUST-KETTIS, A., HABTE, D., HOLMGREN, J., MEEUWISSE, MÖLLBY, R. and SODERLIND, O. (1976) Enterotoxin-producing bacteria and parasites in stools of Ethiopian children with diarrhoeal disease. *Archs Dis. Childh.* **51**: 865–870.

WADSTRÖM, T., MÖLLBY, R. and SÖDERLIND, O. (1977) Heat-labile enterotoxins of *Escherichia coli*. *Toxicon* **15**: 511–519.

WADSTRÖM, T., MÖLLBY, R. and SÖDERLIND, O. (1978a) Production of heat-labile *Escherichia coli* enterotoxin. *FEMS Microbiol. Lett.* **3**: 61–64.

WADSTRÖM, T., SMYTH, C. J., FARIS, A., JONSSON, P. and FREER, J. J. (1978b) Hydrophobic adsorptive and hemagglutinating properties of enterotoxigenic *Escherichia coli* with different colonizing factors: K-88, K-99, and colonization factor antigens and adherence factor. In: *Second International Symposium on Neonatal Diarrhea*, pp. 29–55, October 3–5, 1978, University of Saskatchewan, Canada.

WALLICK, H. and STUART, C. A. (1943) Antigenic relationships of *E. coli* isolated from one individual. *J. Bact.* **45**: 121–126.

WENSINK, J., GANKEMA, H., JANSEN, W. H., GUINEE, P. A. M. and WITHOLT, B. (1978) Isolation of the membranes of an enterotoxigenic strain of *Escherichia coli* and distribution of enterotoxin activity in different subcellular fractions. *Biochem. biophys. Acta* **514**: 128–136.

WHIPP, S. C. (1978) Physiology of diarrhea-small intestines. *J. Am. vet. med. Ass.* **173**: 662–666.

WHIPP, S. C. and DONTA, S. T. (1976) Serum antibody to *Escherichia coli* heat-labile enterotoxin in cattle and swine. *Am. J. vet. Res.* **37**: 905–906.

WHIPP, S. C., MOON, H. W. and ARGENZIO, R. A. (1981) Comparison of enterotoxic activity of heat-stable enterotoxins from Class 1 and Class 2 *Escherichia coli* of swine origin. *Infect. Immun.* **31**: 245–251.

WILLSHAW, G. A., BARCKLAY, E. A., SMITH, H. R., MCCONNELL, M. M. and ROWE, B. (1980) Molecular comparison of plasmid encoding heat-labile enterotoxin isolated from *Escherichia coli* strains of human origin. *J. Bact.* **143**: 168–175.

WILLSHAW, G. A., SMITH, H. R. and ROWE, B. (1983) Cloning of regions encoding colonization factor antigen 1 and heat-stable enterotoxin in *Escherichia coli*. *FEMS Microbiol. Lett.* **16**: 101–106.

WOLK, M., SVENNERHOLM, A.-M. and HOLMGREN, J. (1980) Isolation of *Escherichia coli* heat-labile enterotoxin by affinity chromatography: characterization of subunits. *Curr. Microbiol.* **3**: 339–344.

YAMAMOTO, T. and YOKOTA, T. (1980) Cloning of deoxyribonucleic acid regions encoding a heat-labile and heat-stable enterotoxin originating from an enterotoxigenic *Escherichia coli* strain of human origin. *J. Bact.* **143**: 652–660.

YAMAMOTO, T. and YOKOTA, T. (1981) *Escherichia coli* heat-labile enterotoxin genes are flanked by repeated deoxyribonucleic acid sequences. *J. Bact.* **145**: 850–860.

YAMAMOTO, T. and YOKOTA, T. (1983) Sequence of heat-labile enterotoxin of *Escherichia coli* pathogenic for humans. *J. Bact.* **155**: 728–733.

YAMAMOTO, T., TAMURA, T.-A. and YOKOTA, T. (1984) Primary structure of heat-labile enterotoxin produced by *Escherichia coli* pathogenic for humans. *J. biol. Chem.* **259**: 5037–5044.

YAMAMOTO, T., TAMURA, T.-A., RYOJI, M., KAJI, A., YOKOTA, T. and TAKANO, T. (1982) Sequence analysis of the heat-labile enterotoxin subunit B gene originating in human enterotoxigenic *Escherichia coli*. *J. Bact.* **152**: 506–509.

YAMAMOTO, T., YOKOTA, T. and KAJI, A. (1981) Molecular organization of heat-labile enterotoxin genes originating in *Escherichia coli* of human origin and construction of heat-labile toxoid-producing strains. *J. Bact.* **148**: 983–987.

YOH, M., YAMAMOTO, K., HONDA, T., TAKEDA, Y. and MIWATANI, T. (1983) Effects of lincomycin and tetracycline on production and properties of enterotoxins of enterotoxigenic *Escherichia-coli*. *Infect. Immun.* **42**: 778–782.

YOLKEN, R. H., GREENBERG, H. B., MERSON, M. H., SACK, R. B. and KAPIKIAN, A. Z. (1977) Enzyme-linked immunosorbent assay for detection of *Escherichia coli* heat-labile enterotoxin. *J. clin. Microbiol.* **6**: 439–444.

ZENSER, T. V. and METZGER, J. F. (1974) Comparison of the action of *Escherichia coli* enterotoxin on the thymocyte adenylate cyclase-cyclic adenosine monophosphate system to that of cholera toxin and prostaglandin E. *Infect. Immun.* **10**: 503–509.

CHAPTER 6

E. COLI HEAT-STABLE ENTEROTOXIN

Richard N. Greenberg* and Richard L. Guerrant**

*Department of Internal Medicine, St. Louis University School of Medicine,
1325 S. Grand Blvd. St. Louis, Missouri 63104, U.S.A.

and

**Divisions of Geographic Medicine and Infectious Diseases, Department of Medicine,
Box No. 485 Medical Center, University of Virginia,
Charlottesville, Virginia 22908, U.S.A.

ABSTRACT

E. coli that produce a heat stable enterotoxin are increasingly recognized as one of the commonest causes of the devastating morbidity (including malnutrition) and mortality associated with diarrhea throughout the tropical developing world. As a classic example of the remarkably versatile ways that E. coli can cause diarrhea, ST-producing E. coli also provide a model of the pathogenesis of intralumenal infections: the microbial pathogen first adheres to a host surface, and then produces a toxin that alters normal host physiology to cause disease. In addition to its major role as a human pathogen, ST-producing E. coli has a massive economic impact as a veterinary pathogen (especially among calves and piglets).

Numerous recent advances in the recognition and assay of ST-producing E. coli, in the purification and characterization of different STs, and in the understanding of the transposable ST gene code and the pathogenesis and promising areas of control of ST-induced disease are reviewed. ST-producing E. coli constitute a major cause of diarrhea among childhood and adult residents in the tropics, as well as among foreign travelers to these areas.

Improved understanding of the nature of the initial colonization steps by enterotoxigenic E. coli and of the secretory effects of ST via newly recognized pathways that involve intestinal guanylate cyclase activation and cyclic GMP formation continues to open new basic concepts in the biochemistry of microbe: host cell interactions and in secretory physiology. Such advances in unravelling the pathogenesis of ST-producing E. coli diarrhea hold great promise for opening new avenues of potential pharmacologic or immunologic control of this widespread, life-threatening infection.

1. BACKGROUND

The ability of *Escherichia coli*, the predominant aerobic component of normal enteric bacterial flora, to cause diarrheal disease, was first suggested in the late 1800s and early 1900s by several veterinary workers studying calf scours (Nocard and Leclainche, 1898; Joest, 1903; Titze and Weichel, 1908; Jensen, 1913; Smith, T. and Orcutt, 1925). In 1933, Goldschmidt, R. demonstrated by slide agglutination that certain *E. coli* were associated with an institutional outbreak of infantile diarrhea, findings that were confirmed by Dulaney and Michelson (1935). In 1945, Bray identified serologically homogeneous *E. coli* from over 90% of cases of summer diarrhea in England. Several other serotypes of *E. coli* were subsequently associated with infant diarrhea over the ensuing decade (Kauffmann, F., 1947; Giles and Sangster, 1948; Kauffmann, F. and DuPont, 1950; Ewing, 1956). The emphasis was then slowly shifted by several medical and veterinary workers to enterotoxins produced by previously recognized and new strains of *E. coli*. De and his colleagues (De *et al.*, 1956), working in Calcutta, showed that whole broth cultures of several *E. coli* isolates, including three enteropathogenic *E. coli* serotypes, from patients with diarrhea resulted in a fluid secretory response in the rabbit upper small bowel. This response did not occur with a majority of strains isolated from controls, when large bowel loops were used, or when the pH was not maintained in a mildly alkaline range (pH = 8.4). Trabulsi (1964) also demonstrated enterotoxin production by recognized and previously unrecognized serotypes of *E. coli* from children with diarrhea in São Paulo, which he contrasted with non-enterotoxigenic *E. coli* from healthy controls. Taylor *et al.* (1961; Taylor and Bettelheim, 1966) demonstrated that viable organisms were not required to produce this secretory response and showed that enterotoxigenicity correlated poorly with the classically recognized serotypes. Meanwhile, several veterinary workers demonstrated additional enterotoxigenic *E. coli* strains associated with animal diarrhea (Moon *et al.*, 1966a, b, 1970; Smith, H. W. and Halls, 1967a; Kohler, 1968; Truszczynski and Pilaszek, 1969; Gyles and Barnum, 1969).

Other workers demonstrated an association of enterotoxigenic *E. coli* with 'acute undifferentiated diarrhea' in adult patients from Bengal. These organisms were usually not of the classically recognized enteropathogenic serotypes and were present only during acute illness. The enterotoxic material from culture filtrates of these organisms caused net upper small bowel secretion and appeared to be heat-labile, non-dialyzable and precipitable in 40% ammonium sulphate (Gorbach *et al.*, 1971; Banwell *et al.*, 1971; Sack, R. B. *et al.*, 1971).

Analogous to the usually short-lived human diarrheal illness associated with enterotoxigenic *E. coli* (Formal *et al.*, 1971), several workers noted a shorter time course with the secretory response to material prepared from enterotoxigenic *E. coli* culture filtrates (Pierce and Wallace, 1972; Pierce, 1973; Guerrant *et al.*, 1973). Further clarification of the enterotoxic material produced by *E. coli* suggested that at least two types of enterotoxins were produced: one, a heat-labile enterotoxin (LT) that has subsequently been demonstrated to be much like choleratoxin, and the other, a heat-stable enterotoxin (ST) (Smith, H. W. and Gyles, 1970a; Kohler, 1971; Moon and Whipp, 1971). Both enterotoxins were found to be plasmid-encoded traits which appear to be separable from the equally important plasmid-encoded adherence traits for pathogenesis (Smith, H. W. and Halls, 1968; Smith, H. W. and Linggood, 1971; Skerman *et al.*, 1972). The secretory responses to ST appeared immediate and reversible, while choleratoxin and LT effects followed a lag period and were relatively irreversible, perhaps pending renewal of the epithelium (Guerrant *et al.*, 1972; Evans, D. G. *et al.*, 1973; Nalin *et al.*, 1974).

Early work on the pathogenesis of enterotoxigenic *E. coli* diarrhea in animal models not only suggested that some *E. coli* enterotoxins had a shorter time course than choleratoxin, it also suggested that secretory responses to *E. coli* toxin or to whole, viable, toxigenic *E. coli* were often associated with activation of adenylate cyclase in intestinal mucosa that paralleled the fluid secretory responses (Pierce and Wallace, 1972; Evans, D. J. *et al.*, 1972; Guerrant *et al.*, 1973; Kantor *et al.*, 1974). Subsequent studies have clarified that only LT is associated with the longer time course and adenylate cyclase activation characteristic of choleratoxin responses in many cell systems. In contrast, early studies with ST failed to demonstrate an ST effect on non-intestinal assay systems (Mashiter *et al.*, 1973; Guerrant *et al.*, 1974; Donta *et al.*, 1974). ST required a different assay model, the suckling mouse assay (Dean, A. G. *et al.*, 1972; Giannella, 1976), and did not have antigenic cross-reactivity with LT or choleratoxin (Gyles, 1974). ST was subsequently shown to result in elevated intracellular cyclic GMP rather than cyclic AMP concentrations (Hughes *et al.*, 1978a; Field *et al.*, 1978), and the apparent early adenylate cyclase activation was likely due to the formation of some cyclic AMP *in vitro* by ST-activation guanylate cyclase (Guerrant *et al.*, 1973; Mittal and Murad, 1977a). ST could be inactivated by extremes of heat (Giannella, 1976; Alderete and Robertson, 1978; Guerrant *et al.*, 1980a) or pH (Kohler, 1968; Mullan *et al.*, 1978; Guerrant *et al.*, 1980a), by treatment with reducing agents or after performic acid oxidation (Staples *et al.*, 1980; Dreyfus *et al.*, 1980).

The existence of several different types of ST was first suggested by variations in the degree of heat-stability of different ST preparations (Whipp *et al.*, 1975; Burgess *et al.*, 1978). As the purification of ST has progressed, differences in amino acid content, methanol solubility and animal species specificity of different preparations from different sources further substantiate the existence of several distinct types of ST (Jacks and Wu, 1974; Whipp *et al.*, 1975; Mullan *et al.*, 1978; Burgess *et al.*, 1978; Alderete and Robertson, 1978; Kapitany *et al.*, 1979, Gyles, 1979; Moon *et al.*, 1980; Olsson and Söderlind, 1980; Whipp *et al.*, 1981; Kashiwazaki *et al.*, 1981a and 1981b). Additionally, molecular genetic studies utilizing DNA hybridization suggest that different plasmids are responsible for synthesis of ST_b that is positive in pigs but inactive in infant mice, and ST_a that is active both in pigs and infant mice (So and

McCarthy, 1980). Frantz and Robertson (1981) and Giannella *et al.* (1981) each have reported that their ST_a antibody does not bind to ST_b. Unlike ST_a, ST_b does not effect increases in intestinal intracellular cyclic GMP nor does it activate adenylate cyclase (Kennedy *et al.*, 1984; Guerrant *et al.*, 1985).

2. EPIDEMIOLOGY AND CLINICAL PRESENTATION

Although recognized as a cause of colibacillosis in several infant animal species (piglets, calves, lambs and rabbits) (Smith, H. W. and Halls, 1967b; Smith, H. W. and Gyles, 1970b; Gyles, 1971; Gyles *et al.*, 1971; Pesti and Semjen, 1973; Sivaswamy and Gyles, 1976; Larivière and Lallier, 1976; Acosta−Martinez *et al.*, 1980), ST-producing *E. coli* were first associated with human disease in studies of travelers' diarrhea. Shore *et al.* (1974) reported the isolation of enterotoxigenic *E. coli* (by suckling mouse test) from four of eleven travelers who had been to Latin America or Africa. *E. coli* which produce only ST were also associated with 5 of 51 (9.8 %) cases of acute diarrheal illness among gastroenterologists at a convention in Mexico over a 16-day period in October 1974 (Sack, D. A. *et al.*, 1975; Merson *et al.*, 1976; Morris, G. K. *et al.*, 1976). Three of these cases had no other pathogens found. Illnesses lasted 5−21 days, with up to 10 watery, non-bloody diarrheal episodes per day. Two had nausea, malaise and fever; one each had cramping and vomiting. In three other studies of traveler's diarrhea, both LT and ST were examined. These involved 39 American Peace Corps volunteers in Kenya (Sack, D. A. *et al.*, 1977a), 34 members of the Yale Glee Club, which toured 12 Latin American cities in the spring of 1975 (Guerrant *et al.*, 1980b) and 35 American Peace Corps volunteers in rural Thailand (Echeverria *et al.*, 1981). To summarize 114 cases from these 4 studies, 8 % were associated with *E. coli* that produced only ST, 18 % were associated with *E. coli* that produced ST + LT, and 22 % were associated with *E. coli* that are produced only LT (Table 1). Enterotoxigenic *E. coli* were found in 17 of 50 (34 %) of stool cultures taken from American student population in Mexico ill with diarrhea (7 were ST and LT, 7 were ST only and 3 were LT only); these students were participating in a subsalicylate bismuth drug trial to prevent or reduce travelers' diarrhea (DuPont *et al.*, 1980b). Ryder *et al.* (1981) reported that enterotoxigenic *E. coli* was not a frequent cause of travelers' diarrhea in Panamanian tourists visiting Mexico.

Diarrhea among travelers to tropical areas usually has its onset 5−15 days after arrival, and is typically manifested by malaise, anorexia, abdominal cramps and often explosive, non-inflammatory diarrhea. Nausea and vomiting occur in up to 25 % of cases, and approximately one-third may have a low grade fever. The duration is usually 1−5 days, but a number of cases may continue longer than one week.

The most definitive evidence for the type of illness caused by ST is from volunteer studies done by Levine *et al.* (1977) who found that 10^8-10^{10} organisms resulted in a 60−80 % attack rate of mild to moderate diarrheal illness. Illnesses were characterized much as described above for tropical travelers' diarrhea. The infecting organism (a non-typable *E. coli* that produced only ST and had been isolated from a patient who acquired Turista in

TABLE 1. *Association of Enterotoxigenic E. coli with Travelers' Diarrhea**

Study population	Gastroenterologists	Peace corps volunteers	Yale glee club	Peace corps volunteers	total
Number of Cases:	51	27	16	20	
Attack Rate:	49% in 16 days	69% in 5 weeks	74% in 1 month	57% in 5 weeks	
% of Cases with:					
Toxigenic *E. coli*	41%	52%	56%	50%	48%
ST only	10%	2%	19%	0%	8%
ST + LT	16%	15%	12%	30%	18%
LT only	16%	33%	25%	20%	22%

* Data from Merson *et al.* (1976), Sack, D. A. *et al.* (1977a), Guerrant and Hughes (1979), Guerrant *et al.* (1980b), Echeverria *et al.* (1981).

Mexico) became the predominant coliform organism in the stools of patients given 10^8 or more organisms, 80 % of whom also developed an increase in serum somatic antibody titer to this organism. The incubation periods ranged from 14–53 hours; illnesses lasted 1–3 days. With higher inoculae, illnesses tended to be more severe, with greater fever and frequency and duration of diarrhea.

The association of ST-producing E. coli with infantile diarrhea has been made in several studies. Ryder et al. (1976a) reported that 18 of 25 (72 %) symptomatic infants in the special care nurseries of a large hospital in Texas had ST-producing E. coli 078:K80:H12. This isolation rate was significantly greater than that from 14 of 55 asymptomatic infants in these units. This organism was resistant to multiple antibiotics and attempts at management with colistin failed. In the same year, Gross et al. (1976) reported on outbreak of diarrhea in an infant nursery involving 25 babies. Diarrhea lasted 1–11 days (mean was 4 days), and five patients required intravenous fluids. Twenty-four ill infants had E. coli 0159 isolated from their stools, and four of ten of these isolates produced ST. In other studies, an epidemic E. coli strain was recovered that produced only ST from a series of outbreaks of infantile diarrhea in a Mexican hospital nursery (Evans, D. G. et al., 1977a), from several family outbreaks of diarrhea in New Zealand (Bettelheim and Reeve, 1982), and it is the commonest recognized cause of diarrhea in both hospital and community settings in north-eastern Brazil where attacks rates may excede 7 diarrheal illness per year in small children (McLean et al., 1981; Guerrant et al., 1983). The potential for spread of the genetic code for enterotoxins among multiple bacterial strains in the hospital nursery has been raised by studies showing plasmid (Skerman et al., 1972) or even bacteriophage (Takeda, Y. and Murphy, 1978) transfer of enterotoxigenicity and, further, by outbreaks of diarrhea associated with multiple, simultaneous, enterotoxigenic (LT) organisms in the special host setting of a newborn intensive care unit (Guerrant et al., 1976) and aboard ships (Wachsmuth et al., 1979).

Studies of patients with non-cholera diarrhea in Bangladesh substantiate the role of ST-producing E. coli as enteric pathogens in this setting. To summarize two of these studies in which stools were examined for pathogens from 113 patients with acute diarrhea, ST-producing E. coli were isolated from there patients, ST + LT-producing E. coli from 27 patients, and LT-producing E. coli from four patients. The older the age group (> 10 years), the more likely that the patient had enterotoxigenic E. coli as a cause for non-cholera diarrhea (Ryder et al., 1976b; Sack, D. A. et al., 1977b). From another study of over 500 inpatients with diarrhea, the authors suggest that four cases of dehydrating diarrhea requiring hospitalization per 10,000 persons occur each year with ST-producing E. coli and another seven cases per 10,000 persons per year occur with ST + LT-producing E. coli. They suggest that ST and ST + LT-producing E. coli may be among the commonest causes of diarrhea in the tropics (Nalin et al., 1975). In a fourth report, two epidemiologic surveys were conducted in rural Bangladesh, one examining hospitalized patients with diarrhea and the other examining families and the environment of hospitalized patients. The authors conclude that: (1) enterotoxigenic E. coli (ST, LT or both) were the most frequent enteric pathogens in adults and second commonest, after rotaviruses, among hospitalized children; (2) among children less than 2 years old, ST-associated illnesses were more severe than illnesses associated with ST + LT- or LT-producing E. coli alone; (3) relatively few serotypes appear to be enterotoxigenic; (4) while humans represent the major reservoir, animals such as cows or calves may also be reservoirs of enterotoxigenic E. coli; (5) the principle incriminated vectors for spread were food and water; and (6) antitoxic immunity to LT and increasing infection to case ratios increase with age, but antitoxic immunity is not necessarily protective (Black et al., 1979). Black et al. (1980, 1982a) have recently reported data again identifying the importance of ST- or LT and ST-producing E. coli as etiologic agents of diarrhea in rural Bangladesh (20 % of episodes). In rural Bangladesh E. coli diarrhea occurred most frequently in the hot, wet months from April to September. Their studies suggest that repeated episodes of diarrhea due to enterotoxigenic E. coli which occurred throughout childhood were most likely due to the consumption of contaminated foods during weaning (Black et al., 1982b).

Studies from Mexico City (Evans, D. G. *et al.*, 1977c), Manitoba, Canada (Brunton *et al.*, 1980), rural Zaire (De Mol *et al.*, 1983), Addis Ababa, Ethiopia (Stintzing *et al.*, 1982), São Paulo, Brazil (Reis *et al.*, 1982), Costa Rica (Mata *et al.*, 1983) and Calcutta, India (Sen *et al.*, 1983), each identify enterotoxigenic *E. coli* (including ST-producing strains) as a cause of out-patient and inpatient isolates diarrhea. ST-producing isolates were reported in cases of non-cholera diarrhea as follows: 3 % in Calcutta and in Manitoba, 5 % in São Paulo, 13 % in Costa Rica, and 15 % in Addis Ababa. In these reports, ST-producing strains were isolated significantly more from children with diarrhea than from normal children.

ST-producing *E. coli* are not significantly associated with diarrheal illnesses among infants and young children in southern Brazil. However, in two controlled studies, adults from this region and Navajo adults from southwestern United States had ST-producing *E. coli* significantly associated with non-inflammatory, summer diarrhea (Korzeniowski *et al.*, 1978; Hughes *et al.*, 1980). One uncontrolled study performed in Lagos, Nigeria also reported ST-producing *E. coli* were found primarily in adults with diarrhea (Agbonlahor and Odugbemi, 1982). These latter observations raised the possibility that adults may remain susceptible to the poorly immunogenic ST while, having developed some measure of antitoxic immunity to LT, they may carry LT-producing *E. coli* asymptomatically. LT-producing organisms frequently cause diarrhea in small children in these same areas. In contrast to the infrequency of ST in association with childhood diarrhea in southern Brazil and in southwestern United States, recent studies done in northeastern Brazil show that ST-producing *E. coli* are the commonest recognized pathogens found among infants and small children with dehydrating diarrheal illnesses seen at a Rehydration Center during the peak diarrhea season (McLean *et al.*, 1981). Furthermore, prospective community surveillance in this area of the northeast of Brazil has revealed that ST-producing *E. coli* are the commonest recognized pathogens, and that these illnesses are associated with weight loss and occur in the wet season when they are found in large numbers in the water supplies (Shields *et al.*, 1982, Guerrant *et al.*, 1983).

While most reports of sporadic, community-acquired diarrheal illnesses in the United States fail to implicate enterotoxigenic *E. coli* (Echeverria *et al.*, 1975; Hughes *et al.*, 1978b), several reports demonstrate their potential roles in disease in the United States or similar temperate settings. A large outbreak of watery diarrhea at Crater Lake National Park was traced to an *E. coli* 06:K15:H16 that produced ST + LT, which was isolated from park water that was contaminated with raw sewage (Rosenberg *et al.*, 1977). Kudoh *et al.* (1977) reported seven outbreaks of diarrheal illness in Japan due to ST-producing *E. coli*; two of these outbreaks had food as a vehicle for transmission, two had well water. The overall attack rate was 48 % (306/633) of people exposed. Echeverria *et al.* (1982) found as much as 9 % of water samples taken from homes in rural Thailand contained enterotoxigenic bacteria that produced either ST, LT, or both enterotoxins, and Shields *et al* (1982) found that 12 % of water samples taken from household water sources in northeastern Brazil had enterotoxigenic *E. coli* often in large numbers ($> 10^4$/100 ml). Eight percent of 240 *E. coli* isolates from food and animal sources in the United States have been reportedly enterotoxigenic (LT or ST), thus raising the potential threat of foodborne transmission of enterotoxigenic *E. coli* in the United States (Sack, R. B. *et al.*, 1977).

Unlike ST (i.e., ST_a), the epidemiology of ST_b is poorly understood. ST_b is thought to be important in swine scours but little evidence exists to implicate the toxin as a cause of diarrhea in humans. Lee *et al.* used a *Hin*f I fragment from a cloned ST_b plasmid as a DNA probe and examined human and animal isolates reported to be pathogenic diarrhea strains of *Escherichia coli*. They found nomology for 38 animal isolates but for only one human isolate from a patient who had contact with pigs.

3. ASSAY METHODS

Because of the transmissible nature of the genetic code for ST-production, there are no reliable serologic or biochemical markers for its presence. Methods for identifying ST-producing *E. coli* are further limited by the lack of selective culture media (such as those commonly used to isolate salmonella or shigella) and the necessity to pick a few random colonies of *E. coli* for *in vitro* enterotoxin testing. Finally, the intestinal tissue specificity of ST effects (in contrast to the widespread effects of LT or choleratoxin on many tissues) has been limiting on the development of new assay models. Currently, the standard assay for ST is the suckling mouse assay, developed by Dean, A. G. *et al.* (1972) and modified by Giannella (1976). When examined at 3 or 4 hours, the suckling mouse assay is specific for ST and not influenced by the heat-labile toxin, LT. The ratio of intestinal weight to remaining body weight is then determined separately or in groups of three to six mice each. Depending on the laboratory and mouse strain used (de Castro *et al.*, 1978), ratios greater than 0.083–0.09 are considered positive, and ratios between 0.07–0.09 are considered intermediate. Although the original assay was done with filtrates or supernatants from trypticase soy broth (TSB) cultures shaken overnight, Giannella reported slightly better results with Casamino Acids-yeast extract broth cultures incubated 16–24 hours in roller tubes. Suckling mice are inoculated with 0.1 ml of test culture supernatants, with 2% Pontamine sky blue (6BX) or 2% Evans blue dye (two drops per ml) as a marker. After 3–4 hours at 28°C, the mice are sacrificed by decapitation, chloroform or cervical dislocation; the intestinal tract (without the stomach) is dissected and, if the blue marker dye is seen in the gastrointestinal tract, promptly weighed.

Other modifications proposed for the suckling mouse assay are less frequently employed. Jacks and Wu (1974) describes inoculation of 0.05 ml test material orally, using a blunt 23 gauge hypodermic needle; Moon *et al.* (1978, 1979) inject 0.1 ml orally by stomach tube attached to a 23 gauge needle. They have noted that the characteristic sluggish intestinal transit time of suckling mice can be increased by raising the temperature to 37°C or by using older mice. They suggest using 8-day-old mice, incubated at 37°C, and examining for dye mixed with feces. These older mice held at 37°C had low gut-to-carcass ratios but responded to ST with diarrhea after 4 hours. Stavric and Jeffrey (1977) have reported good results with shortening of the incubation period to 90 minutes, with mice held at 22°C. This earlier response may relate to oral toxin administration or to use of more concentrated toxin. Likewise, a 10-fold, concentrated, semi-purified ST caused positive secretory responses in mice up to 15 days of age (Mullan *et al.*, 1978).

Testing of fresh clinical isolates should be done as promptly as possible. Loss of the plasmid-mediated ST production has been described when strains are stored in the laboratory (Evans, D. J. *et al.*, 1977). The appropriate number of randomly picked *E. coli* to test for ST (in three to six mice each) from each stool sample is difficult to determine. Some have picked two to four colonies of different colony types, others have picked five to ten colonies, regardless of number of colony types, for enterotoxin testing. Still others have suggested pooling multiple *E. coli* colonies isolated from a single individual (Byers and DuPont, 1979). Screening with pools of five isolates or a combination of pooling plus individual testing will detect over 96% of toxigenic *E. coli* found by testing multiple individual isolates (Merson *et al.*, 1979a). Pooling of isolates has occasionally lead to false negative results (Brunton *et al.*, 1980). Murray *et al.* (1981) reported that storage or cultivation of enterotoxigenic *E. coli* may result in a false negative suckling mouse assay and a false negative Y-1 adrenal cell assay for LT if any of the isolates produce colicin(s).

Considerable concern has arisen over the possible lack of sensitivity of the suckling mouse assay for ST (Whipp *et al.*, 1975; Olsson and Söderlind, 1980; Merson *et al.*, 1980a). A number of strains isolated from children with diarrhea produced LT and some secretory response after heating in 6 hour rabbit ileal loop studies, but no significant response in the suckling mouse assay (Guerrant *et al.*, 1975). Sivaswamy and Gyles (1976) found that the suckling mouse results with isolates from calf scours paralleled those in calf ligated loops. However, they also noted that 27 of 72 strains that were positive in 7-day-old piglet loops were inactive in suckling mouse and calf loops. Other investigators, using perfused canine jejunal loops (Nalin *et al.*, 1978), *in vivo* perfusion of rat small intestine (Klipstein *et al.*, 1978, 1979), and 3- to 8-week-old piglet loops (Burgess *et al.*, 1978; Gyles, 1979; Olsson and Söderlind, 1980), report similar limitations and relative insensitivity of the suckling mouse assay for ST from certain *E. coli* strains. Burgess *et al.* (1978) have proposed that *E. coli* may secrete two forms of ST: ST_a, which is partially heat-stable, methanol soluble and active in infant mice and neonatal piglets; and ST_b, which is highly heat-stable, methanol insoluble, and inactive in suckling mice but active in ligated intestinal segments of older piglets and rabbits. However, Gyles (1979) recently reported another pattern among *E. coli* recovered from diarrheal samples of humans, pigs, and calves. Culture supernatants from these strains were all positive in the ligated pig intestine, some of which were also positive in ligated rabbit segments and in suckling mice (certain porcine strains were negative in the latter two tests). Several other investigators have since confirmed that certain porcine strains produce a ST that is inactive in suckling mice and rabbits (Olsson and Söderlind, 1980; Kashiwazaki *et al.*, 1981a; Kennedy *et al.*, 1984); this ST has been called ST_b. Unlike some porcine isolates, bovine ST-producing *E. coli* appear to produce ST_a and be active in mice and in young piglets (Gyles, 1979).

In addition to the widely-used suckling mouse assay, several other animal intestinal segment assays have been employed over the last two decades for detection of *E. coli* enterotoxins. In general, they involve more cost and technician time than the biologic or immunoassays commonly used for LT, and can be divided into two types: (1) those that measure total fluid accumulation over a period of time; and (2) those that determine net ionic or total volume fluxes, usually over shorter intervals, using a perfusion technique with labeled ions or a non-absorbable volume marker. In the former category, the ligated adult rabbit ileal segment model is one of the oldest and best defined. Originally developed by De and Chatterje in 1953 for studies with *Vibrio cholerae*, the rabbit 'loop' model has been modified for the detection of ST and LT in *E. coli* broth cultures (De *et al.*, 1956; Pierce and Wallace, 1972). When examined at 6 hours rather than 18 hours, rabbit segment volume-to-length ratios reflect primarily the early onset effects of ST and not the delayed effects of LT or choleratoxin (Evans, D. G. *et al.*, 1973). Fasted, young, 1–2 kg albino rabbits are anaesthetized and multiple, 3–10 cm, ligated segments are prepared, beginning in the terminal ileum, after a saline flush. Volume-to-length ratios at 6 hours of greater than 0.4 ml/cm are considered positive. However, because of considerable animal-to-animal variation, both positive and negative controls in each animal, as well as testing of each specimen in three different rabbits, is essential (Kasai and Burrows, 1966; Sack, R. B. 1975).

Seven- to nine-day-old infant rabbits have also been used for detection of ST and LT. One milliliter of broth culture is inoculated into the small intestine, either directly or through a surgically implanted gastric tube; the animals are sacrificed at 6 hours, and the whole bowel is dissected to determine the fluid-to-whole bowel weight ratio (greater than 0.2 is considered positive) (Dutta and Habbu, 1955; Sack, R. B. 1975). Reports vary regarding the sensitivity of this assay (Gorbach and Khurana, 1972; Sack, R. B. 1975), which is not widely used.

Ligated jejunal segments in 7- to 12-week-old piglets has been employed in a number of studies of veterinary *E. coli* enterotoxins (Smith, H. W. and Halls, 1967a, b, Gyles and Barnum, 1967). Most studies suggest that pig loop assays are more sensitive for porcine isolates and less sensitive for human or calf isolates. While older, weaned pigs are preferred by some (Burgess *et al.*, 1978), others have reported better results with 3- to 5-week old piglets for testing porcine and human *E. coli* (Moon and Whipp, 1970; Larivière and Lallier, 1976; Gyles, 1979).

To study bovine isolates, ligated calf intestinal segments have been used (Smith, H. W. and Halls, 1967a, b; Moon and Whipp, 1971; Myers *et al.*, 1975; Sivaswamy and Gyles, 1976; Burgess *et al.*, 1978). Less frequently used animal intestinal loop preparations used for the study of enterotoxins include lambs (Smith, H. W. and Halls, 1967b), adult mice (Dobrescu and Huygelen, 1973) and hamsters (Frisk *et al.*, 1978).

For several years, intestinal perfusion studies have been done in canine and, more recently, rat isolated small bowel segments *in vivo* (Nalin *et al.*, 1974, 1978; Klipstein *et al.*, 1978, 1979). Because the perfusion model provides an opportunity to detect decreased absorption (even in the absence of net secretion), these studies may provide a more sensitive assay for enterotoxins or other agents that affect fluid secretion.

Based on Craig's original work with choleratoxin (1965), several investigators have utilized the effects of ST and LT on rabbit skin permeability as an assay. Twenty-four hours after an intracutaneous injection of toxin, a blue dye is given intravenously to demonstrate the areas of increased skin permeability (Moon and Whipp, 1971; Evans, D. J. *et al.*, 1973; Takeda, Y. *et al.*, 1979). Takeda, Y. *et al.* (1979) have suggested that ST may provide a qualitatively different type of skin permeability alteration.

While cell culture assays for ST have been limited by its tissue specificity, Farkas–Himsley and Jessop (1978) have reported inhibition of proliferation and ^{3}H-thymidine uptake by L60T mouse fibroblasts exposed to ST-containing culture filtrates. Antiserum against both semi-purified ST (Lathe *et al.*, 1980) and purified ST have been prepared and a radioimmunoassay has been described (Kauffman, P. E. 1981; Frantz and Robertson, 1981; Giannella *et al.*, 1981). These groups report that their radioimmunoassay was specific for ST_a, measuring human, porcine, and bovine ST_a equally well and did not cross-react with ST_b, LT, CT or various gastrointestinal peptides. Giannella *et al.* (1981) comments that intact disulfide bridges in the ST_a were necessary for immunoreactive activity. The radioimmunoassay can detect as little as 50 pg of ST; the suckling mouse assay requires about 0.4 to 2.6 ng of ST (Alderete and Robertson, 1978; Staples *et al.*, 1980).

Detection of enterotoxigenic *E. coli* by DNA colony hybridization has recently been developed and identifies the genes that encode the enterotoxins (Mosley *et al.*, 1980). Genes encoding LT and ST have been characterized (So *et al.*, 1979; Lathe *et al.*, 1980). Gene fragments prepared by restriction endonuclease treatment are radiolabled and used to probe for DNA homology with *E. coli*. The technique of DNA colony hybridization requires *E. coli* strains to grow on a nitrocellulose filter overlaid with media. Lysed colonizes are exposed to the probe, washed, and autoradiographed. DNA homology is revealed by exposure of film over areas of filter where DNA from the probe annealed to the DNA from test strain. Two ST gene probes, ST-P (of porcine origin) and ST-H (of human origin) have been necessary to identify all strains that are positive in the suckling mouse assay (So *et al.*, 1981; Moseley *et al.*, 1982; Echeverria *et al.*, 1982; Georges *et al.*, 1983; Moseley *et al.*, 1983). A gene probe for ST_b-producing *E. coli* is being evaluated (Lee, C. H. *et al.*, 1983).

Enzyme-linked immunosorbent assays (ELISA) with high sensitivity and specificity for ST_a have been recently reported. The competitive ELISAs differ primarily in the solid phase antigen (Klipstein *et al.*, 1984; Lockwood and Robertson, 1984; Thompson *et al.*, 1984; Rönnberg *et al.*, 1985).

4. PURIFICATION AND CHARACTERIZATION OF ST

In 1968, Kohler reported several characteristics of an ST preparation from supernatants of shaken syncase 18-hour broth cultures. His lyophilized material retained activity after acid treatment (pH = 1.0), but was alkali-labile (pH = 10.5), extractable in methanol and, to a lesser extent, in ethanol. It was not extractable in ether. ST was adsorbed onto acidic cation or basic anion exchange resins (Kohler, 1968). From its elution just after sucrose with 0.02 M NaCl on a Sephadex G-15 column, he concluded that its molecular weight was relatively small (Kohler, 1971). Utilizing dialysis, acetone fractionation and ultrafiltration, Bywater (1972) concluded that ST had a molecular weight between 1,000–10,000 daltons, Others have confirmed this size, and have shown that ST is resistant to trypsin or pronase (Jacks and Wu, 1974) and is precipitable by ammonium sulfate (Klipstein *et al.*, 1976). Additional purification was reported with the use of isoelectric focusing (Madsen and Knoop, 1980; Burgess *et al.*, 1980; Saeed *et al.*, 1984), hydrophobic polymeric adsorbent column chromatography (Amberlite XAD-2 and Octyl-Sepharose CL-4B) gel filtration on Sephadex LH-20 (Field *et al.*, 1978; Stavric *et al.*, 1981) and HPLC (Saeed and Greenberg, 1985). Alderete and Robertson (1978) defined a basic medium (less complex than casamino acids-yeast extract), optimal growth times and added preparative gel electrophoresis, ion exchange chromatography and methanol-chloroform extraction to their purification scheme. They concluded that it was important to shake the growth medium vigorously under aerobic conditions in a medium free of D-glucose, D-gluconate and L-arabinose (which repress ST production). Their purified material from porcine strain 431 appears to be a polypeptide of 47 residues with a molecular weight of 4,400 (by SDS gel electrophoresis and gel filtration) to 5,133 (by calculation). They identified six half-cysteine residues, suggesting the presence of disulfide bonds, very few hydrophobic amino acids and a single amino-terminal residue of glycine. Biological activity was not affected by proteases, nucleases, phospholipase C or several organic solvents, and it exhibited no hemolytic or lipase activity. Although it did not stain with conventional protein or carbohydrate stains, it had a strong absorption at 260 nm, was only weakly antigenic (even when coupled to albumin) and had an effective dose in mice of 0.85 ng (Alderete and Robertson, 1977a, b, 1978). Since this work, Olsson (1982) has described a minimal salts-amino acid medium with a low quantity of a carbohydrate source that appears to improve ST yields, and Pesti and Lukacs (1981) have described a Coomassie brilliant blue G-250 staining technique for gels that identifies ST (both suckling mouse positive (ST_a) and negative (ST_b). Olsvik and Kapperud (1982) have shown that ST_a enterotoxin is not produced in sterile milk at 22°C or 4°C.

Others report different findings with different strains of *E. coli*. Klipstein *et al.*, (1976) report that their 'ST' material was elaborated in stationary aerobic and anaerobic broth cultures, but not in agitated aerobic cultures. Tewari *et al* (1981a, b) have reported that their human strains of ST-producing *E. coli* produce a ST that has two active lipid components as identified by agarosegel-electrophoresis. Johnson *et al.* (1978, 1979) noted that up to 20 % of ST activity from six other strains of *E. coli* was present in the cell lysate, and that yield increased when pH was maintained around 8.5 and when a synthetic medium without amino acids was used. Takeda *et al.* (1979, 1983) purified ST from *E. coli* 53402 A-1, which gave a positive Folin phenol reaction and an absorption maximum at 275 nm. As noted above, Burgess *et al.* (1978) have reported considerable variation in methanol solubility of ST from different *E. coli* strains; some producing methanol-soluble ST, others producing methanol-insoluble ST, and still others producing both. Purified ST preparations have now been described with considerably different molecular weights (1,500–10,000), different amino acid compositions (Fig. 1), different biological activities and different degrees of heat stability (Kapitany *et al.*, 1979; Lallier *et al.*, 1980; Staples *et al.*, 1980; Lathe *et al.*, 1980; Chan and Giannella, 1981; Aimoto *et al.*, 1982; Lallier *et al.*, 1982, Takao *et al.*, 1983; Saeed *et al.*, 1983; Rönnberg *et al.*, 1983). However, it now appears that these enterotoxins share a great deal of molecular and biological similarities (Saeed *et al.*, 1984; Thompson and Giannella, 1985). Aimoto *et al* (1983) have synthesized a 14 amino acid ST analog that includes 6 half-cysteine and is 2 to 5 times more potent than native ST.

Several other strains of bacteria besides *E. coli* have been reportedly capable of producing a heat-stable enterotoxin. That of *Yersinia enterocolitica* appears to share the guanylate cyclase activating mechanism of action with *E. coli* ST (Boyce *et al.*, 1979; Rao *et al.*, 1979a; Velin *et al.*, 1980; Okamoto *et al.*, 1982). *Y. entercolitica* ST appears to be more active in infant mice at 25°C than at 37°C and is produced more often in Pai-Mors medium (Serafim *et al.*, 1983). Mosimable and Gyles (1982) raise the issue of differences between *E. coli* mouse active ST and *Y. entercolitica* ST; they report discrepancies between the two toxins in the ability to induce intestinal fluid secretion in ligated intestinal loop in pigs (1 to 5 weeks old). Other organisms that have reportedly produced a heat-stable enterotoxin include *Klebsiella pneumoniae* (Klipstein *et al.*, 1975; Klipstein and Engert, 1976a), *Enterobacter cloacae* (Klipstein and Engert, 1976b), *Aeromonas hydrophilia* and *sobria* (Boulanger *et al.*, 1977; Pitarangsi *et al.*, 1982; Burke *et al.*, 1982) and *Salmonella species* (Koupal and Deibel, 1975; Sandefur and Peterson, 1976). Although less well characterized, these ST share some of the biological activities and low molecular weight with *E. coli* ST. It is now clear that there are several heat-stable enterotoxins produced by different *E. coli*, as well as by other enteric bacteria.

5. GENETIC CONTROL OF ST

Both LT and ST are genetically coded by plasmids that have been shown, under laboratory conditions, to be transferable to other *E. coli* strains, and potentially trans-posable into other gene sequences such as bacteriophage or plasmids of other species of Enterobacteriaceae (Smith, H. W. and Halls, 1968; Smith, H. W. and Gyles, 1970a; Smith,

Source	Sequence	Reference
Human	Asn-Thr-Phe-Tyr-Cys-Cys-Glu-Leu-Cys-Cys-Asn-Pro-Ala-Cys-Ala-Gly-Cys-Try	Takao et al., 1983; Rönnberg et al., 1983
Human	Asn-Thr-Phe-Tyr-Cys-Cys-Glu-Leu-Cys-Cys-Asn-Pro-Ala-Cys-Ala-Gly-Cys-Tyr-	Chan and Giannella, 1981; Thompson and Giannella, 1985
Transposon Tn 1681[a]	Asn-Thr-Phe-Tyr-Cys-Cys-Glu-Leu-Cys-Cys-Asn-Pro-Ala-Cys-Ala-Gly-Cys-Tyr	So and McCarthy, 1980
Human	Asn-Ser-Ser-Asn-Tyr-Cys-Cys-Glu-Leu-Cys-Cys-Asn-Pro-Ala-Cys-Tyr-Gly-Cys-Try	Aimoto et al, 1982
Swine	Asn-Thr-Phe-Try-Cys-Cys-Gly-Leu-Cys-Cys-Asn-Pro-Ala-Cys-Ala-Gly-Cys-Tyr	Lallier et al., 1982
Synthesized	Cys-Cys-Glu-Leu-Cys-Cys-Asn-Pro-Ala-Cys-Tyr-Gly-Cys-Tyr	Aimoto et al., 1983
Bovine	Asn-Thr-Phe-Tyr-Cys-Cys-Glu-Leu-Cys-Cys-Asn-Pro-Ala-Cys-Ala-Gly-Cys-Tyr	Saeed et al., 1984

Fig 1. Amino Acid Sequences of Mouse Active Heat-Stable Enterotoxin from Various Sources

H. W. and Linggood, 1971; Skerman et al., 1972; Gyles et al., 1974; Takeda, T. et al., 1981). To date, enterotoxigenic organisms have not been distinguishable from nontoxigenic strains on morphologic or biochemical bases. From ST + LT-producing E. coli of human and animal origin, a homogeneous plasmid species of DNA has been described to be approximately 60 megadaltons with 50 % guanosine and cytosine. In contrast, the plasmids from porcine strains that produce only ST appear to be heterogeneous. These ENT plasmids range in size from 20 to 80 megadaltons, and appear relatively unrelated by DNA sequence studies to the ST + LT plasmids (Gyles et al., 1974). From different human isolates of E. coli, both ST only and ST + LT plasmids have been described (Wachsmuth et al., 1976). From an outbreak of infantile diarrhea in Scotland, an E. coli strain was isolated that produced only ST and contained an R-factor conferring resistance to multiple antibiotics. Furthermore, the co-transfer of antibiotic resistance and ST was clearly demonstrated (Gross et al., 1976). While early experiences showed that some ENT plasmids were incompatible with some antibiotic resistance plasmids, the concurrence of ENT with R-factors that encode for resistance to multiple antibiotics, and their co-transfer to recipient transconjugates, has been documented in many areas (Gross et al., 1976; Wachsmuth et al., 1976; Gyles et al., 1977; Echeverria et al., 1978; McConnell et al., 1979; Smith, H. R. et al., 1979). Of 176 enterotoxigenic E. coli isolated from children and adults in the Far East, 61 % (40 of 66) of ST- and ST + LT-producing isolates were resistant to one or more antibiotics. All eight strains tested exhibited co-transfer of the antimicrobial resistance and ST (Echeverria et al., 1978). Furthermore, the ST codon has been demonstrated to be transposable; hence, the potential for the widespread occurrence of enterotoxigenicity under the selective pressure of antibiotic usage is very real (Smith, H. R. et al., 1979; So et al., 1979; Franklin et al., 1981). Indeed, the in vivo transfer of an enterotoxin and antibiotic-resistance plasmid has been demonstrated in newly weaned piglets (Gyles et al., 1978). Additionally, Sekizaki et al. (1982) have shown that ENT plasmids conferring ST-production can coexist with conjugative R plasmids conferring antimicrobial resistance.

Another mode of transfer for the ST genes has been reported by Reis et al. (1980a). They have isolated E. coli serotype 0128ac:H12 found in Brazilian children with diarrhea which produces ST and colonization factor CFA/I and carries 2 plasmids (97 and 64 Kilobases). Analysis of plasmid content revealed that genes for ST and CFA/I are carried on a large not self-transmissible plasmid whereas the smaller plasmid is without recognizable products but is conjugative and promotes cotransfer of the larger plasmid. Yamamoto and Yokota (1983) have studied the human enterotoxigenic E. coli strain H10407 and have shown (1) the presence of two non-self transmissible plasmids which encode for ST_a production, (2) that the two ST's produced have quantitative differences when neutralized by single ST_a anti-serum and differences in ST_a production suggesting heterogeneous DNA differences in ST encoded areas in the plasmids and (3) that with restriction endonuclease mapping the two different ST fragments differ from that previously described in a bovine *E. coli* isolate (So and McCarthy, 1980; So *et al.*, 1981). Their data suggest that these ST genes are not on the same transposon as that of bovine ST-producing *E. coli*. However, cloning and characterization of the gene that encodes for ST from another human *E. coli* isolate (strain 153837-2) was partially homologous to the bovine cloned DNA (So and McCarthy, 1980). Hybridization studies with this probe showed that 83 % of *E. coli* isolated from humans with diarrhea in Bangladesh possessed genes highly homologous to the ST gene from strain 153837-2 and from the bovine isolate of So *et al.* (Moseley *et al.*, 1983). The above studies suggest that ST_a may be transmitted in several modes and that while DNA encoding for ST_a may be relatively homogeneous in a particular geographic area, overall there are important differences in both DNA content and transmission.

In 1980, Lathe and co-workers reported the cloning of the ST-coding region from a bovine *E. coli* isolate (B-11). They synthesized an ST protein with a molecular weight of 10,000 daltons and an active enterotoxin fragment of 7000 daltons. Cloning of DNA regions encoding heat-stable enterotoxin of human, bovine, porcine origin has been described. The cloning studies have revealed that ST DNA regions are flanked by inverted repeats, suggesting that the DNA encoding for ST is on a transposon (So *et al.*, 1979; Yamamoto and Yokota, 1980; So *et al.*, 1981). Current efforts are being directed toward utilizing DNA hybridization to probe for different STs (i.e. ST_a and ST_b), and toward cloning strains that produce larger amounts or more antigenic forms of ST.

Little is known about the secretory export mechanism of ST from the intracellular to extracellular space. ST activity is known to be 160 times greater in the extracellular space than in the intracellular space. Current data suggest that ST is initially formed as an inactive pretoxin in the cytoplasmic space and becomes active as it is exported from the periplasmic space through the outer membrane (Guzman–Verduzco *et al.*, 1983).

6. PATHOLOGY

Smith, H. W. and Jones, studying the pathologic findings of scours in piglets due to *E. coli* (1963), reported that the internal organs, including the alimentary tract, were normal macroscopically, and there was no evidence of inflammatory exudate, cellular infiltration, epithelial desquamation or excessive mucus secretion. In all piglets, large numbers of *E. coli* (greater than 10^4) were found in the proximal small bowel. In studies of acute undifferentiated diarrhea in human adults in Calcutta, 8 of 17 cases were associated with enterotoxigenic *E. coli* (Banwell *et al.*, 1971). During acute illness, the intestinal microflora was predominated by *E. coli* in the numbers that usually exceeded anaerobic and other aerobic flora by one to three logs. In seven of these eight cases, $10^3–10^8$ *E. coli* per ml were found in the small bowel, and five of the seven had only a single serotype of *E. coli* recovered. In convalescence, 7–10 days after acute illness, only three of eight patients had *E. coli* in the upper small bowel (all three of which were non-toxigenic; two of three had different serotypes) and in all eight cases, the number of fecal anaerobic bacteria had increased one to four logs. Histologic studies in these cases revealed an intact mucosal architecture without tissue penetration by *E. coli*. In additional animal studies, neither animal and human enterotoxigenic *E. coli*, nor their enterotoxins, caused inflammatory or other gross or histologic changes in animal intestinal tracts (Moon *et al.*, 1971; Guerrant *et al.*, 1973). Rectal biopsies from symptomatic, infected human volunteers showed intact mucosal surface and glandular epithelial with normal goblet cells (Banwell *et al.*, 1971; DuPont *et al.*, 1971).

In detailed studies of enterotoxigenic *E. coli* in piglets, enterotoxigenic *E. coli* had a greater tendency to be associated with small bowel epithelium than non-toxigenic strains. Organisms tended to be distributed along the entire villus, and did not penetrate the epithelial cells (Bertschinger *et al.*, 1972a). They further showed that enterotoxigenic *E. coli* did not adhere to the same degree in different litters or in older piglets, suggesting that host variability and age were important factors in determining the susceptibility of animals to colonization by enterotoxigenic *E. coli* and, hence to symptomatic colibacillosis (Bertschinger *et al.*, 1972b).

While enterotoxigenic *E. coli* characteristically colonized the small bowel at the epithelial brush border, they did not elicit a destructive inflammatory response and did not invade the mucosa (Moon *et al.*, 1980). Using mouse inactive pig active ST_b, our studies (Kennedy *et al.*, 1984) and those of Kashiwazaki *et al.* (1981b) show intact small bowel histology without an inflammatory response upon exposure to ST_b for up to 16 hours. There is no evidence for colonic involvement by enterotoxigenic *E. coli* in these animal studies.

7. PATHOGENESIS

7.1. Colonization

Usually within a few days of birth, non-pathogenic *E. coli* promptly become the predominant aerobic organism in the normal human colon (Rosebury, 1962; Mata and Urrutia, 1971). In order to cause disease, ST-producing *E. coli* must first colonize the upper small bowel, where the effect of its enterotoxin is most apparent. The mechanism for their selection in the intestinal tract is unknown. Some investigators have suggested that in particular instances involving weaning piglets damaged small intestine epithelium (due to recent or concurrent Rotavirus infection) may produce an environment which favors growth and selection of enterotoxigenic *E. coli* (Lecce *et al.*, 1982, 1983). Certain serotypes tend to predominate (Rosebury, 1962). In the case of enterotoxigenic *E. coli*, elegant early studies in piglets revealed that an antigenic protein fimbriate adherence factor (K88) was essential for their colonization and proliferation in the proximal small bowel, and to cause diarrhea (Orskov *et al.*, 1961; Stirm *et al.*, 1967a,b; Smith, H. W. and Linggood, 1971; Jones and Rutter, 1972). The binding of K88 antigen to brush borders may involve galactosyl residues (Sellwood, 1980) and does not appear to vary with the age of the swine (Runnels *et al.*, 1980). The genetic code for this K88 antigen was found to be plasmid-mediated and separable from enterotoxigenicity (Smith, H. W. and Halls, 1967b).

Evans, D. G. *et al.* (1975) extended these findings to humans. They demonstrated a heat-labile, fimbriate 'colonization factor' or an enterotoxigenic *E. coli* from a patient with cholera-like diarrhea. This strain caused diarrhea in infant rabbits when 10^5 organisms/ml were introduced; they multiplied in the bowel to greater than 9×10^7 colony-forming units/g of tissue. They further demonstrated passive protection in infant rabbits with specific anti-colonization factor serum (which did not agglutinate a procine *E. coli* with K88 antigen) (Evans, D. G. *et al.*, 1975, 1977a,b, 1978a,b). Human volunteer studies have shown that, as in the piglets, the presence of a colonization factor was necessary in order for an enterotoxigenic *E. coli* to cause disease (Evans, D. G. 1978a). Among enterotoxigenic *E. coli* from adults with Turista acquired in Mexico, 86% had the colonization factor antigen (CFA/I), while only 18% of strains from asymptomatic controls had toxigenic *E. coli* with CFA/I (Evans, D. G. *et al.*, 1978b). Others have reported the prevalence of CFA/I in association with only 7–17% of case isolates of enterotoxigenic *E. coli* (Levine and Rennels, 1978; Gross *et al.*, 1978; Bergman *et al.*, 1981). CFA/I-positive *E. coli* typically causes hemagglutination of human group A erythrocytes, which resist 1% mannose. Evans, D. G. and Evans, D. J. (1978) have more recently described an antigenically distinct CFA/II in association with other human enterotoxigenic *E. coli*. CFA/II causes mannose-resistant hemagglutination of bovine erythrocytes, but not human group A red cells (Smyth *et al.*, 1979). Recent reports suggest that CFA/I tends to be associated with *E. coli* in 0 serogroups 15, 25, 63, 78, 114, 126, 128, 153 and production of ST only; while CFA/II tends to occur among *E. coli* in 0 groups 6, 8, 80, 85, 115, 139 and is associated with production of ST and LT. Both the particular colonization factor and the associated enterotoxins appear to be encoded on the same plasmid but at different sites (Freer *et al.*, 1978; Evans, D. G. and Evans, D. J., 1979; DuPont *et al.*, 1979; Smith, H. R. *et al.*, 1979, 1982, 1983; Reis *et al.*, 1980a; Willshaw *et al.*, 1982; Cravioto *et al.*, 1982; Thomas and Rowe, 1982; Murray *et al.*, 1983; Peñaranda *et al.*, 1983). To date, non-enterotoxigenic *E. coli* have not been found to possess CFA/I or /II. Several laboratories have suggested that additional colonization factors may be found in human enterotoxigenic *E. coli* such as the putative E8775 colonization factor found in 5 % of Asian strains of ETEC, the PCF 8775 antigens CS4, CS5 and CS6, and type 1 somatic pili (Gross *et al.*, 1978, Guerrant and Bergman, 1979; Deneke *et al.*, 1979, 1981, 1983; Levine, 1981; Thomas and Rowe, 1982; Gaastra and De Graaf, 1982; Zilberberg *et al.*, 1983; Levine *et al.*, 1983; Thomas *et al.*, 1985).

From calves and sheep, other types of colonizing antigens, K99, and F41, have been described (Ørskov *et al.*, 1975; Morris *et al.*, 1982), and another, 987P, from porcine enterotoxigenic *E. coli* (Moon *et al.*, 1980). Several porcine strains have expressed multiple pilus antigens, *e.g.* K88 and 987P (Schneider and To, 1982). K99 antigen appears to be associated primarily with young piglets, suggesting (unlike with K88) older animals become resistant to K99-associated adhesion (Runnels *et al.*, 1980; Smyth *et al.*, 1981; Tzipori *et al.*, 1982). Additionally, there are some enterotoxigenic strains of *E. coli* that produce none of these antigens, suggesting that still other unidentified adherence fimbriae may be important in porcine strains (Moon *et al.*, 1980; Awad–Masalmeh *et al.*, 1982). Interestingly, Haddad and Gyles (1982a, b) have identified a possible role for the capsular material as an adherence factor in *E. coli* enterotoxigenic in calves.

7.2. ENTEROTOXIN EFFECTS

Following the early studies of intestinal flux alterations in acute cholera, Banwell and his colleagues (1971) described a net jejunal secretory process in four of seven patients from Calcutta with enterotoxigenic *E. coli*-associated diarrhea. The isotonic fluid had slightly higher bicarbonate concentrations in the ileum than in the jejunum, and resembled the composition of fluid in the same regions of the intestinal tracts of normal individuals. This fluid was also similar in many respects to that seen during acute cholera.

Alteration of intestinal fluxes by enterotoxins were further examined by several investigators in acute and chronic Thiry–Vella canine loops. Pierce and Wallace (1972) demonstrated that a crude LT + ST *E. coli* preparation produced the rapid onset of a secretory response within 90 minutes of perfusion which was rinsable; normal absorptive fluxes returned within 30 minutes after removal of the toxin. This effect is in contrast to that of choleratoxin, which achieves a peak response only after $2\frac{1}{2}$–3 hours and which is sustained for more than 24 hours after removal of the choleratoxin (Guerrant *et al.*, 1972; Evans, D. G. *et al.*, 1973; Nalin *et al.*, 1974). This secretory response to crude *E. coli* resulted in no alteration in jejunal mucosal permeability to serum proteins or in the active absorption of glucose and glucose-coupled sodium. Likewise, the small bowel mucosa retains its capacity to maintain concentration gradients of chloride and bicarbonate between plasma and lumenal fluid. However, the maximal jejunal secretory response to this crude *E. coli* toxin was four-fold less than that achieved with purified choleratoxin.

Further studies utilizing crude enterotoxic material containing LT + ST demonstrated that a net secretory response occurred during the initial 10-min interval of exposure, that this effect was immediately rinsable during the subsequent 10-minute interval, that this material appeared to be consumed during its action in the loops and that this secretory response was associated with apparent increased adenylate cyclase activity in the intestinal mucosa (Guerrant *et al.*, 1973). Although a more prolonged activation of adenylate cyclase by whole cultures of enterotoxigenic *E. coli* was seen, this early effect was likely, in retrospect, due to ST and activated guanylate cyclase (Hughes *et al.*, 1978a). Pierce (1973) further demonstrated that, using rat and rabbit intestinal segments, neither cholera toxoid (choleragenoid) nor ganglioside G_{M1} altered the ST-induced secretion. In studies done with a partially-purified ST. Bywater (1972) demonstrated that the net secretory response in rabbit jejunum was associated with increased bicarbonate secretion and decreased sodium absorption.

The different time courses of *E. coli* ST and LT were clarified by D. G. Evans *et al.* (1973), who demonstrated maximal secretory response to ST at 4–6 hours, while maximum fluid accumulation with LT occurred only after approximately 10 hours in rabbit ligated intestinal segments. The latter was more comparable to the choleratoxin response. The rapid onset of ST, its reversibility, its resistance to choleragenoid and the intact glucose-coupled sodium absorptive responses were further demonstrated by Nalin in canine loops (Nalin *et al.*, 1974; Nalin and McLaughlin, 1978). In other experiments with swine, the distal jejunum and the colon appeared to respond to ST with an increased unidirectional sodium secretory flux suggesting that enterotoxin effects may vary with species, small or large bowel location and differences in exposure time in the bowel (Hamilton *et al.*, 1977; Argenzio and Whipp, 1981).

In Ussing chamber studies with stripped rabbit ileal mucosa mounted between separate fluid reservoirs, Field *et al.* (1978) have further clarified ST effects on secretory mechanisms. There is a 1–4 mV serosa-positive electrical potential (PD) across the ileal mucosa under basal conditions. To measure ion fluxes, the PD is nullified by a short circuit current. The presence of a net ion flux across the short-circuited membrane indicates active ion transport. The net flux is determined as the difference between opposing unidirectional fluxes measured with radioisotopes. Normally, the ileum generates net absorptive fluxes of sodium and chloride and a net secretory flux of bicarbonate. While the effect of cyclic AMP, theophylline, choleratoxin or LT are both to inhibit active sodium absorption and to stimulate chloride secretion, ST and cyclic GMP analogues appear primarily to reduce sodium and chloride absorption. The effect of ST on PD and the short-circuit current required to neutralize this difference is rapid in onset and promptly reversed when toxin is removed from the bathing solutions. Furthermore, the effect is observed in rabbit jejunum, ileum and cecum, but not in duodenum or distal colon. Although an effect has been demonstrated with as little as 0.1 ng ml, the maximal effect on PD and on ion fluxes was about half that of theophylline, with which it was not additive (Brasitus *et al.*, 1976; Field *et al.*, 1978; Rao *et al.*, 1979b; Field, 1979a,b; Guandalini *et al.*, 1982).

Because of an apparent early effect of *E. coli* enterotoxin on tissue adenylate cyclase activity, ST effects on cyclic nucleotide were re-examined and found to increase intestinal cyclic GMP concentrations, but not cyclic AMP concentrations (Hughes *et al.*, 1978a). Furthermore, ST-induced intestinal fluid secretion in suckling mice was mimicked by 8-bromo cyclic GMP (Hughes *et al.*, 1978a) and ST was independently shown to activate guanylate cyclase (Field *et al.*, 1978). Other studies have shown *in vivo* intestinal tissue specificity for ST-activation of particulate guanylate cyclase (Hughes *et al.*, 1978c; Guerrant *et al.*, 1980a). Rao and co-workers (1979b) have demonstrated that the rabbit jejunum and ileum respond specifically to lumenal ST, while (except for some response to serosal ST in proximal colon) duodenum and distal colon are unresponsive to ST. *In vivo* studies have shown ST binding to human intestinal cells (Henle 407) and jejunal brush border preparations (Giannella and Luttrell, 1982; Thomas and Knoop, 1983). Giannella and Luttrell (1982) report that disruption of disulfide bridges of ST prevents binding. Recently ST has been shown to bind to rat basophilic leukemic cells, resulting in a dose-dependent secretion of histamine (Thomas and Knoop, 1983). Thus, ST effects are quite different from choleratoxin and LT, which are widespread activation of adenylate cyclase in multiple cell types and exhibit a characteristic lag in onset in intact cells (Sharp and Hynie, 1971; Guerrant *et al.*, 1972; Evans, D. J. *et al.*, 1972; Mashiter *et al.*, 1973; Evans, D. G. *et al.*, 1973; Guerrant *et al.*, 1974; Gill *et al.*, 1976; Gill, 1977). The effects of ST on guanylate cyclase and cyclic GMP concentrations has been confirmed in several other laboratories (Newsome *et al.*, 1978; Giannella and Drake, 1979).

The following observations implicate a direct role for cyclic GMP in the secretory process induced by ST: (1) ST effects on both cyclic GMP accumulation and secretory responses in rabbit, mouse and Ussing chamber studies demonstrate a comparable rapid onset, time course and dose response. (2) The 8-bromo analogue of cyclic GMP mimics the ST effect on secretion, including location of intestinal responses (suggesting that some intestinal regional specificity may relate to responsiveness to the cyclic GMP nucleotides rather than to the ST 'receptor' differences). (3) Agents which prevent ST activation of guanylate cyclase consistently prevent the secretory responses. This includes alkaline treatment of ST (pH > 10.5), butylated hydroxyanisole (BHA) scavenging of free radicals (Guerrant *et al.*, 1980a), chlorpromazine (Abbey and Knoop, 1979; Greenberg *et al.*, 1980a) and quinacrine

(Greenberg *et al.*, 1982b), all of which inhibit ST activation of guanylate cyclase as well as the secretory responses (Fig. 2). (4) Hydroxylamine, an agent that had been shown to activate guanylate cyclase, presumably by free radical formation (Kimura *et al.*, 1975), also appears to cause intestinal ion transport alterations similar to those seen with ST (Field, 1979a).

Also consistent with a role for cyclic GMP in intestinal secretion is the existence of a brush border protein kinase in intestinal tissue that is more sensitive to cyclic GMP than to cyclic AMP (De Jonge, 1976; Kimberg *et al.*, 1979; De Jonge, 1984). Most guanylate cyclase activity in the mammalian small bowel is measured in villous brush border preparations (Ishikawa *et al.*, 1969; Kimura and Murad, 1975; Quill and Weiser, 1975; De Jonge, 1975; Walling *et al.*, 1978). However, the complexity of the role of cyclic GMP in intestinal secretory processes is demonstrated by the stimulation of sodium chloride *absorption* and *inhibition* of bicarbonate secretion when intestinal cyclic GMP was increased in response to α-adrenergic agents, muscarinic cholinergic agents, insulin or cholecystokinin (Brasitus *et al.*, 1976). Experiments with isolated ileal epithelial cell suggest that the effect of some of these agents on cyclic GMP levels may occur at a site other than the enterocyte or that other pathways may be overriding cyclic nucleotide effects or that different intracellular compartments of cyclic nucleotides may play opposite roles (Sheerin and Field, 1977; Field, 1979b; Guandalini *et al.*, 1982). In one experiment using the Ussing chamber, the increment in mucosal cyclic GMP concentration necessary to alter steady-state Cl fluxes and I_{sc} was greater than the increment produced by epinephrine (Guandalini *et al.*, 1982).

Roles for free radicals and the prostaglandin synthesis pathways have been implicated in the mechanism of action of ST; ST is inhibited by the free radical scavenger, butylated hydroxyanisole (BHA), aspirin and indomethacin. Each agent blocks guanylate cyclase activation and intestinal fluid secretory responses by ST. These agents do not inhibit the secretory response seen with 8-bromo cyclic GMP (Madsen and Knoop, 1978; Guerrant *et*

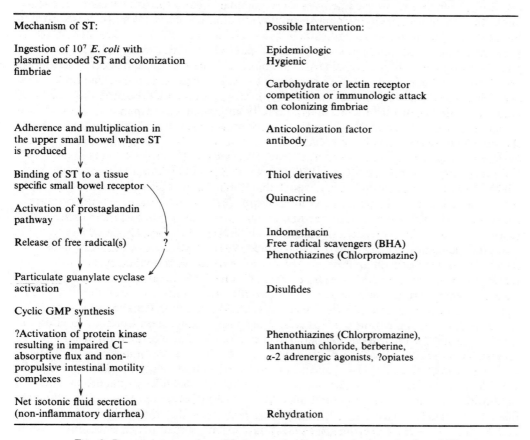

Mechanism of ST:	Possible Intervention:
Ingestion of 10^7 *E. coli* with plasmid encoded ST and colonization fimbriae	Epidemiologic Hygienic
	Carbohydrate or lectin receptor competition or immunologic attack on colonizing fimbriae
Adherence and multiplication in the upper small bowel where ST is produced	Anticolonization factor antibody
Binding of ST to a tissue specific small bowel receptor	Thiol derivatives
Activation of prostaglandin pathway	Quinacrine
Release of free radical(s) ?	Indomethacin Free radical scavengers (BHA) Phenothiazines (Chlorpromazine)
Particulate guanylate cyclase activation	Disulfides
Cyclic GMP synthesis	
?Activation of protein kinase resulting in impaired Cl⁻ absorptive flux and non-propulsive intestinal motility complexes	Phenothiazines (Chlorpromazine), lanthanum chloride, berberine, α-2 adrenergic agonists, ?opiates
Net isotonic fluid secretion (non-inflammatory diarrhea)	Rehydration

FIG. 2. Proposed steps and possible interventions in the mechanism of action of ST.

al., 1980a; Greenberg *et al.*, 1980a; Bruke and Gracey, 1980; Knoop and Abbey, 1981). The inhibitory effect of indomethacin can be overcome by increasing the dose of ST. Whether indomethacin is acting as a prostaglandin synthesis inhibitor is unclear; indeed, indomethacin at high concentration (0.1–1 mM) may act by a prostaglandin-independent mechanism (Smith, P. L. *et al.*, 1981). However, as indomethacin inhibits cyclo-oxygenase, which forms cyclic endoperoxides and free radicals from arachidonic acid (Nickander *et al.*, 1979), and as free radicals may activate guanylate cyclase (Mittal and Murad, 1977b), the indomethacin inhibition of ST may be by the prevention of free radical formation. Indomethacin has also been reported to reduce the secretory responses to choleratoxin (Jacoby and Marshall, 1972; Gots *et al.*, 1974; Wald *et al.*, 1977), *Shigella flexneri* (Gots *et al.*, 1974) and *Salmonella typhimurium* (Gots *et al.*, 1974; Giannella *et al.*, 1977). The mechanism for inhibition of choleratoxin-induced secretion may be related to inhibition of prostaglandin synthesis directly, as aspirin, steroids and phenylbutazone have also been shown to reduce choleratoxin-mediated secretion in rat and cat models (Jacoby and Marshall, 1972; Finck and Katz, 1972).

Divalent cations play important roles in the regulation of cyclic GMP responses to ST. While basal guanylate cyclase activity in intestinal tissues is substantially higher in the presence of 4 mM manganese, responses to ST are greater in the presence of the more physiologic 4 mM magnesium (Guerrant *et al.*, 1980a). A limiting role for calcium is suggested by effects of chlorpromazine, which binds to calmodulin (Wolff and Brostrom, 1979). Chlorpromazine reduces the effect of a submaximal but not maximal dose of ST on fluid secretion in suckling mice. In our studies chlorpromazine also reduces ST activation of guanylate cyclase; Robins–Browne and Levine (1981) did not find such reduction in ST-induced guanylate cyclase activity. However, chlorpromazine has consistently reduced the secretory response to 8-bromo cyclic GMP, suggesting that it interferes with the effects of ST, both prior to and after its activation of guanylate cyclase (Greenberg, *et al.*, 1980a). While the mechanism of chlorpromazine inhibition of ST effects is unknown, it is known to bind calmodulin, scavenge free radicals (Cohen and Heikkila, 1974), stabilize membranes or act as an antagonist to adrenergic agents, serotonin or histamine (Seeman, 1972; Goodman and Gilman, 1975). Chlorpromazine also inhibits adenylate cyclase activation by hormones and inhibits the intestinal secretory responses to choleratoxin, LT, prostaglandin E-1 and butyryl cyclic AMP (Holmgren *et al.*, 1978). One group has described the ability of chlorpromazine to disturb the normal continuity and contact between epethelial cells and basement membrane, possibly leading to interference of water transport and reduced intestinal fluid secretion (Olsvik *et al.*, 1981).

Other phenothiazine derivatives also reduce ST-induced fluid secretion and guanylate cyclase activation (Greenberg *et al.*, 1980b; Smith, P. L. and Field, 1980; Knoop and Abbey, 1981). Thomas and Knoop (1982) report that the calcium channel blockers diltiazem, nifedipine, and cromolyn sodium cause a significant decrease in ST-induced fluid secretion in suckling mice. They also have reported that diltiazem and lodoxamide tromethamine as well as quinacrine, and indomethacin significantly inhibit ST-induced histamine release from rat basophilic leukemia cells (Thomas and Knoop, 1983). Lanthanum chloride, a substance which acts as a calcium antagonist, also blocks ST-induced secretion. Lanthanum does not reduce ST-induced cyclic GMP levels and appears to block ST after activation of guanylate cyclase. Lanthanum potentiates the inhibitory effects of quinacrine and chlorpromazine (Greenberg *et al.*, 1982a). Another agent that has been shown to prevent enterotoxin-induced secretion is nicotinic acid. Having been shown to reverse choleratoxin effects in rabbit jejunum (Turjman *et al.*, 1978), it had been recently shown by Forsyth *et al.* (1979) to reverse ST-induced secretion in pig jejunum. Inhibition of secretion is seen with partially neutralized nicotinic acid (pH 4.5) and is not associated with a reduction in ST-induced cyclic GMP levels (Forsyth *et al.*, 1981b). While the mechanism of nicotinic acid inhibition of ST is unknown, it is felt to directly inhibit adenylate cyclase (Skidmore *et al.*, 1971), stimulate phosphodiesterase (Schwabe, 1971) and interfere with the NAD-requiring reactions (Turjman *et al.*, 1978). Forsyth *et al.* (1981a) have extended their observations on nicotinic acid to other weak acids including glutaric acid and para-aminobenzoic acid. Each appears to increase unidirectional absorption of sodium and block ST-induced fluid secretion in weaned pig intestinal loops. The beta-adrenergic antagonist propranolol also reduces ST-induced fluid secretion in suckling mice; the mechanism of inhibition of intestinal fluid secretion by propranolol is not clear but like chlorpromazine, propranolol is also active against choleratoxin (Donowitz *et al.*, 1979; Bertin, 1982).

We have reported that the anti-malarial compound quinacrine reduces ST-activation of guanylate cyclase and its stimulation of fluid secretion (Greenberg *et al.*, 1982b). Possibly by its inhibition of phospholipase A_2 (an enzyme that releases arachidonate from phospholipids and allows arachidonate to be a substrate for prostaglandin synthesis), the effects of quinacrine, like those of indomethacin, suggest a role for prostaglandin synthesis in ST activation of guanylate cyclase (Vargaftig and Dao Hai, 1972; Flower and Blackwell, 1976). Thomas and Knoop (1982) have also observed that quinacrine, as well as zomepirac, a cyclooxygenase inhibitor, cause a significant reduction in ST-induced fluid secretion in suckling mice.

Recently, we investigated thiol and disulfide compounds for inhibition of ST effects. Disulfide compounds (cystamine and cystine) and thiols (cysteamine, cysteine, and acetyl cysteine) reduced the ST-response in suckling mice as well as ST-activation of guanylate cyclase. Disulfide compounds had a non-specific inhibitory effect on guanylate cyclase activity. Neither group of agents inhibited 8-bromo cyclic GMP-induced intestinal fluid secretion. The study results suggested that the disulfides may be acting on cellular guanylate cyclase activity while the thiols might be inactivating ST by breaking its disulfide bridges or its receptor (Greenberg *et al.*, 1983).

An additional four other types of pharmacologic ST-inhibitors have recently been reported. Berberine, an isoquinoline alkaloid, and α-2 adrenergic agonists (e.g. clonidine and naphazoline) inhibit not only ST-effects and 8-bromo cyclic GMP-induced fluid secretion but also LT and choleratoxin-induced fluid secretion (Ahrens and Zhu, 1982b; Zhu and Ahrens, 1982; Sack, R. B. and Froehlich, 1982; Jacks *et al.*, 1983). The mechanism of action of each of these agents appears to be at a step distal to the production of degradation of cyclic AMP or cyclic GMP (Field and McColl, 1973; Tai *et al.*, 1981; Swabb *et al.*, 1981). Morphine, an opiate agonist, has been described to reduce the secretory response to ST in pig jejunum. The mechanism is not known but morphine has also been shown to inhibit intestinal fluid secretion by choleratoxin and PGE_1, (Lee and Coupar, 1980; Ahrens and Zhu, 1982b). Lastly, despite a report to the contrary (Guerrant *et al.*, 1980a), Ahrens and Zhu (1982a) show that atropine will effectively reduce net loss of water and electrolytes produced by ST in pig jejunum. They speculate that atropine might be blocking a cholinergic mediated secretory component of normal small bowel and its effect may be an indirect one.

Besides direct secretory actions, several studies have suggested that enterotoxins may act to cause diarrhea by altering small intestinal motility. In studies of the myoelectric activity in distal rabbit ileal loops, choleratoxin and LT were found to significantly prolong migrating action potential complex patterns (MAPC) (Mathias *et al.*, 1976; Burns *et al.*, 1978). ST, however, evoked a different pattern, one of a non-propulsive complex of repetitive bursts of myoelectric activity (RBAP) (Nogueira *et al.*, 1979). This latter effect may not be mediated through cyclic GMP as 8-bromo cyclic GMP does not alter motor activity when placed into the lumen of ligated ileal loops (Mathias *et al.*, 1982). By decreasing intralumenal flow, this effect to reduce gut motility could facilitate proliferation of the organism in the bowel lumen.

Overall, the pathogenesis of ST-producing *E. coli* diarrhea first appears to require a colonization factor that allows multiplication of the organism in the upper small bowel. There, as summarized in Fig. 2, ST is produced where its secretory effects appear to involve guanylate cyclase activation, impaired chloride absorption and alteration of motility by inducing non-propulsive complexes. Cyclic GMP appears to mediate these processes after the specific ST activation of particulate guanylate cyclase in intestinal mucosa. A number of pharmacologic inhibitors of ST suggest that ST may act through the prostaglandin synthesis pathway, may involve free radical activation of guanylate cyclase and may be regulated by intracellular calmodulin. However, recently Dreyfus *et al.* (1984) report that experiments with isolated rat intestinal epithelial cells and brush border membranes did not establish a role in the mechanism of action of ST for phospholipases A_2 and C_1 for calcium or calmodulin, for free radicals derived from oxygen, or for phospholipids. Alternatively, De Jonge (1984) and others speculate that ST may possibly interact directly with 'receptor' regions of a transmembrane guanylate cyclase. Their hypothesis is based on an analogy with the glycoprotein structure of particulate guanylate cyclase purified from sea urchin sperm flagellae (Garbers and Radany, 1981) and the sensitivity of the enzyme to thermotropic lipid transitions (Brasitus and Schachter, 1980).

Lastly, the mechanism of action for ST_b (mouse inactive, weaned pig active) is not yet known. Kennedy et al. (1984) and Guerrant et al., 1985 report that ST_b fails to activate adenylate cyclase or induce cyclic GMP formation in intestinal mucosal cells after 30 minutes and 6 hour incubations. They report that although ST_b has an early onset of action (by 30 minutes), it appears to have a mechanism of action different from the mouse active ST. Sears et al. (1982) also report that ST_b has a distinctly different profile of action than ST_a in Ussing chambers. Examining short circuit current (SCC) produced by stripped jejunal mucosa from 4- to 7-week-old pigs, ST_b induced a net increase in SCC and potential difference and decreased tissue resistance. ST_b and ST_a each caused immediate rises in the SCC but ST_b was maximal by 8 minutes whereas ST_a required 30 to 60 minutes for a maximal effect. ST_b-induced SCC declined gradually over several hours while ST_a-induced SCC persisted. Chlorpromazine appeared to inhibit the effects of both toxins.

8. SEROTYPES

Consistent with the transferable, plasmid-encoded nature of enterotoxigenicity, it is not limited to any specific serotype. Furthermore, many classically recognized 'enteropathogenic serotypes' (EPEC) do not produce typically recognizable ST or LT (Goldschmidt and DuPont, 1976; Gangarosa and Merson, 1977). However, there is a tendency for enterotoxigenic E. coli isolates from certain species to occur among a predominant group of serotypes. This group is different from the commonest E. coli serotypes comprising the normal flora, EPEC serotypes, or invasive E. coli serotypes. Many of the serotypes most frequently associated with enterotoxin production and human diarrhea are listed in Table 2. Predominant enterotoxigenic serotypes among porcine isolates include 0-groups 8, 9, 45, 64, 101, 116, 138, 141, 147, 149 and 157 (Smith, H. W. and Gyles, 1970a; Gyles et al., 1971; Larivière and Lallier, 1976; Moon et al., 1980; Olsson and Söderlind, 1980; Oliveira et al., 1981). The predominant serotypes among enterotoxigenic E. coli recovered from food specimens also tend to belong to these latter 0-groups (Sack, R. B. et al., 1977).

9. IMMUNITY TO ST-PRODUCING E. COLI

The limited quality of purified, small-molecular weight, poorly antigenic ST material has greatly hampered work on the immunology of ST. Numerous investigators have found both purified and crude ST preparations to be poorly antigenic, even when coupled to bovine serum albumin (Smith, H. W. and Gyles, 1970a; Sack, R. B. et al., 1976; Alderete and Robertson, 1977c, 1978; Klipstein and Engert, 1978a). Moon et al. (1983) recently evaluated purified ST_a coupled to bovine IgG as a vaccine. Gilts were vaccinated subcutaneously three times during pregnancy. Although gilts after vaccination had high titers of RIA antitoxin in serum and colostrum, the neutralization titers were much lower. Immunized gilts did not demonstrate protection to their pigs. As anti-ST antibody protection would be an avenue for possible vaccine development, work on chemical alterations of ST ·to enhance its immunogenicity and on possible roles of cell-mediated immunity are highly important. Klipstein et al. (1981a, b, 1983a, b, c) in a series of papers has described an ST-vaccine that is protective for rats. The vaccine is a synthetically produced ST coupled to a protein carrier and to B subunit of porcine heat-labile toxin. Immunization as a primary intraperitoneal injection and subsequent oral booster doses gave at least sixfold increases in mucosal IgA antitoxin titers and provided significant protection against heterologous serotypes of human

TABLE 2. *Serotypes of E. coli that Appear with Increased Frequency among ST + LT Enterotoxigenic Isolates in Humans*

Serotype	Reference
06:K15:H16	(Rosenberg *et al.*, 1977) (Merson *et al.*, 1979b)
08:K40:H9; 08:K25:H9; 08, 060:H9	(Evans, D. G. *et al.*, 1977b) (Merson *et al.*, 1979b)
011:H27	(Kudoh *et al.*, 1977)
015:H11; 015:H-	(Evans, D. G. *et al.*, 1977b) (DeBoy *et al.*, 1980a)
020:H-	(Evans, D. G. *et al.*, 1977b)
025:K7:H42; 025:K98:H-	(Evans, D. G. *et al.*, 1977b)
027:H7; 027:H20	(Sack, D. A. *et al.*, 1977a) (DeBoy *et al.*, 1980a)
063:K?:H-; 063:K-:H12	(Merson *et al.*, 1979b) (Reis *et al.*, 1980b)
078:H11; 078:K80:H12	(Ryder *et al.*, 1976a) (Smith, H. R. *et al.*, 1979)
080:H9	(Peñaranda *et al.*, 1983)
085:H7	(Peñaranda *et al.*, 1983)
0114:H21	(Scotland *et al.*, 1981)
0115:K-:H40; 0115:K-:(H51)	(Merson *et al.*, 1979b)
0126:H variable	(Bettleheim and Reeve, 1982) (Berry *et al.*, 1983)
0128:H7; 0128ac:H21; 0128ac:H12	(Merson *et al.*, 1979b) (Reis *et al.*, 1979)
0139:H28	(Reis *et al.*, 1980b)
0148:H28	(DeBoy *et al.*, 1980a)
0149:H10*	(Sack, R. B. 1978)
0159:H20	(Gross *et al.*, 1976) (Kudoh *et al.*, 1977)
0166:H27	(Gross *et al.*, 1985)
0167:H5; 0167:H4	(Gross *et al.*, 1983)

* Type of enterotoxin produced not identified.

Other references used for this table include the following: DuPont *et al* (1971); Ørskov *et al.* (1976, 1977); Morris *et al.* (1976); Sack, D. A. *et al.* (1977b); Rowe *et al.* (1977, 1978); Deetz *et al.* (1979); Ryder *et al.* (1979); Guerrant *et al.* (1980b); Merson *et al.* (1980b); Bäck *et al.* (1980); DeBoy *et al.* (1980b).

or porcine origin *E. coli* that made ST, LT or both toxins. This exciting work needs further testing in other animals and in man.

It is well recognized by veterinarians and farmers that certain sows and their litters are less prone to enteric colibacillosis than others, and that colostrum from sows immunized with certain strains of enterotoxigenic *E. coli* will have significantly higher indirect hemagglutination titers to the vaccine strain and will confer protection against whole bacterial challenges in animal loop studies (Barnum, 1971; Chidlow *et al.*, 1979; Logan and Meneely, 1981). Furthermore, antiserum prepared against strains that produce ST + LT were protective against whole bacterial challenges with strains that produced ST only. However, these antisera failed to neutralize the effect of cell-free ST preparations. Neither could the homologous immunity conferred by enterotoxigenic *E. coli* diarrhea be attributed to bactericidal or antisomatic (0 antigen) antibodies (Linggood and Ingram, 1978; Levine *et al.*, 1979). For these reasons, studies of protective immunity to ST-producing *E. coli* have focused primarily on antibody-mediated or other types of host resistance to colonization by ST-producing *E. coli*.

In animal studies, the fimbriate surface adhesive antigen, K88 is immunogenic in rabbits (Stirm *et al.*, 1967a), and appeared to be the primary antigen responsible for protection of calves born to dams vaccinated with enterotoxigenic *E. coli* (Wilson and Jutila, 1976). In one study, rabbits immunized with K88 antigen (intravenous injections of a culture of K12:K88 *E. coli*) was not protected (Molenda and Kozyrczak, 1983). However, several other vaccine studies have shown protection of young animals against diarrheal diseases when purified K88 or 987P suspensions or K99 extracts have been used in the active immunization of dams, cows and piglets (Morgan *et al.*, 1978; Nagy *et al.*, 1978; Nagy, 1980; Isaacson *et al.*, 1980; Moon, 1981; Acres *et al.*, 1982), and in the passive protection of lambs (Sojka *et al.*, 1978). The protected young were demonstrated to have fewer *E. coli* attached to their intestinal villous epithelium after challenge. In one study, the organism excreted by vaccinated (K88) pigs, although initially K88$^+$ quickly changed to K88$^-$. These results suggest a possible plasmid-curing upon vaccination (Porter and Linggood, 1983).

Antibody responses to colonization factor (CFA/I) have been documented in humans with naturally- and experimentally-acquired toxigenic *E. coli* (Satterwhite *et al.*, 1978; Deetz *et al.*, 1979). Boedeker *et al.* (1982) have reported a dose-related IgA response to purified CFA/II in rabbit intestinal loops. In addition to antibody-mediated protection, receptor competition may also be protective. Purified CFA/I retains an affinity for epithelial cells in rabbit small bowel and competitively blocks adherence of *E. coli* with CFA/I (Evans, D. G. *et al.*, 1979). Colonization factor antibodies may also affect bacterial expression of colonization factors. Antibody to CFA/I when present in the culture media appears to exert a switching-off effect on expression of the adherence antigen (Dean and Wansbrough–Jones, 1983). Finally, the nature of the mammalian cell receptors (possibly glycoproteins) for the lectin-like bacterial fimbriate adhesins is being defined genetically in animals (Sellwood *et al.*, 1975; Sellwood and Kearns, 1979), and explored in humans (Guerrant and Bergman, 1979). A multifaceted approach is therefore appropriate in the design of effective prevention and control of enterotoxigenic *E. coli* diarrhea, using immunologic (circulating and local), pharmacologic and receptor competition concepts.

10. MANAGEMENT AND PREVENTION

The mainstay of therapy of all diarrheal illnesses is adequate hydration. This can usually be accomplished with an oral glucose- or sucrose-electrolyte solution (Palmer *et al.*, 1977; McLean *et al.*, 1981). Glucose-coupled sodium absorption remains intact, despite choleratoxin, LT- or ST-induced secretion (Levinson and Schedl, 1968; Fordtran *et al.*, 1968; Sack, R. B. *et al.*, 1970; Klipstein and Engert, 1978b). The recommended oral therapy solution by The World Health Organization contains 3.5 g of sodium chloride, 2.5 g of sodium bicarbonate, 1.5 g of potassium chloride, and 20 g of glucose (or 40 g of sucrose) per liter of clean water. In order to simplify therapy, reduce cost, and provide nutrition, an oral rice powder electrolyte therapy (40 gm rice powder was substituted for sucrose and mixed with recommended electrolytes) has been studied and appears as efficient and safe as the World Health Organization recommended therapy (Molla *et al.*, 1982). Isotonic intravenous rehydration may become necessary if the patient is unable to tolerate the oral solution because of vomiting or lethargy.

Several studies in animals and in human volunteers suggest that antimicrobial agents will be effective treatment of ST-induced diarrhea. The mortality in calves due to colibacillosis with ST-producing *E. coli* has been reduced from 90 to 14%, weight loss reduced and diarrhea abbreviated to 1 day in calves treated with cephamycin C (Jacks *et al.*, 1980). In a double-blind study, diarrhea was induced in human volunteers with a ST + LT producing *E. coli* sensitive to the study antimicrobial agents. 111 volunteers responded to either trimethoprim alone or in combination with sulfamethoxazole with a 50% reduction in duration of diarrhea. Trimethoprim resistant *E. coli* were found in 5 of 10 trimethoprim volunteers after 48 hours of treatment and two of these volunteers developed a clinical relapse. No resistance of relapse was seen in the combination therapy group (Black *et al.*, 1982c). Similar findings have been noted by DuPont *et al.* (1982a); however, increasing emergence of combined, transferable sulfamethoxazole and trimethoprim resistance is alarming and may limit its usefulness (Murray *et al.*, 1982). Recently, bicozamycin, a poorly absorbed antimicrobial agent that interferes with cell wall synthesis in *E. coli*, has been shown to effectively treat Turista. The agent has several interesting characteristics including its lack of use for other diseases, poor absorption, and resistance not associated with resistance to other antimicrobial agents (Ericsson *et al.*, 1983; Hardford *et al.*, 1983). Whether antibiotics will be effective and without relapses if used on a large scale remains completely unknown.

Several antimicrobial agents have been demonstrated to be effective in preventing traveler's diarrhea over short periods. These include phthalylsulfathiazole (Kean *et al.*, 1962), streptotriad (streptomycin, sulfamethazine, sulfadiazine and sulfathiazole) (Turner, 1967), doxycycline (Sack, D. A. *et al.*, 1978; Sack, R. B. *et al.*, 1979; Freeman *et al.*, 1983), trimethoprim-sulfamethoxazole (DuPont *et al.*, 1980a, 1982b), trimethoprim alone (DuPont *et al.*, 1982b) and even iodochlorhydroxyquin (which may cause subacute myelo-optic atrophy) (Richards, 1970). However, several concerns raise serious questions about the advisability of widespread prophylactic use of antibiotics for this common problem. There is increasing information about the widespread frequency of antimicrobial resistance among enterotoxigenic *E. coli*, and the potential co-transfer of ST and antibiotic resistance (Echeverria *et al.*, 1978; Stieglitz *et al.*, 1980; Echeverria and Murphy, 1980; DeBoy *et al.*, 1980c; Panhotra and Agarwal, 1981; De Lopez *et al.*, 1982a, b; Wachsmuth *et al.*, 1983; Silva *et al.*, 1983). This information raises the concern about potential selection of enterotoxigenic organisms as well as questions about efficacy after extended use of an antimicrobial agent. In a study which reexamined the efficacy of prophylactic doxycycline (100/mg biweekly × 6 weeks), there was only marginal success in prevention of travelers' diarrhea (20 episodes among 24 individuals taking doxycycline versus 27 episodes among 22 individuals in the control group). These authors speculated that the failure of doxycycline to prevent Turista may have been due to a large number of doxycycline-resistant enterotoxigenic *E. coli* in the Honduras study area (Santosham *et al.*, 1980). Secondly, concern is raised by the potential for increasing the susceptibility to possibly more pathogens, such as shigella or salmonella, especially if normal flora and host resistant are eradicated (Rosenthal, 1969; Askerkoff and Bennett, 1969). Thirdly, the side-effects of these agents must be considered in the risk; benefit analysis. In particular, the currently popular doxycycline and trimethoprim-sulfamethoxazole regimens have a significant risk of severe photosensitivity reaction or skin rash, respectively. Therefore, at this time it seems appropriate to aim treatment primarily at reducing the risk of dehydration (i.e. appropriate fluids therapy), rather than at indiscriminate eradication of microorganisms.

Another approach to treatment of Turista due to enterotoxigenic *E. coli* has been to bind, absorb or otherwise inactivate the enterotoxin in the upper small bowel. Cholestyramine and other adsorbent resins have been examined in ligated porcine intestinal segments and have been given to suckling mice and neonatal piglets. Cholestyramine bound both LT and ST, and significantly reduced the secretory responses. However, it was not effective *in vivo* when milk was present in the intestinal tract (Mullan *et al.*, 1979). Bismuth subsalicylate (Pepto-Bismol) has also been reported to be effective in reducing enterotoxin-induced secretion in adult rabbit ileal segments if given before the toxins were bound to the intestinal mucosa (Ericsson *et al.*, 1977). In clinical studies, American students with Turista (due to toxigenic *E. coli* or shigella) experienced significant reduction in diarrheal stools and subjective relief after 30–60 ml bismuth subsalicylate every 30 minutes for 4 hours (eight doses) (DuPont *et al.*, 1977). Steinhoff *et al.* (1980) has also shown the agent to significantly reduce some symptoms of Norwalk viral gastroenteritis (but not the duration or quantity of diarrhea) in a human volunteer study. In other studies, bismuth subsalicylate was taken in an attempt to prevent travelers' diarrhea. In high doses (60 ml QID), which totaled over five liters per person during the 21 day trip, bismuth subsalicylate significantly reduced the occurrence of diarrheal illnesses and the acquisition of bacterial and viral pathogens among American students visiting Mexico (DuPont *et al.*, 1980b). While this large dose reduced enteric infections, the large amount of salicylate absorption is a particular concern in children (Pickering *et al.*, 1981) and one wonders if these doses actually reduced intake of the indigenous pathogenic flora. However, a small volunteer study using 300 mgm nougats of bismuth subsalicylate as prophylactic therapy has shown the effectiveness of a nougat form of bismuth subsalicylate in preventing enterotoxigenic *E. coli* diarrhea. Two 300 mgm nougats were taken 8 and 2 hours prior to challenge and at 2 and 4 hours after challenge and then QID for 3 days (Graham *et al.*, 1982).

Several potential avenues for pharmacological control of enterotoxin-induced secretion hold promise under pathophysiology above, one might predict that agents such as aspirin, indomethacin and chlorpromazine will reduce the secretory responses to ST or LT. While neither has been clinically tested specifically against ST-induced disease in humans, aspirin significantly decreased stool volume by 100 ml/day in Indonesian children hospitalized with acute gastroenteritis (Suharyono and Sunoto, 1980). Indomethacin (1.5 mg/kg q 8 h) has been shown to reduce the duration of non-specific watery diarrheal illnesses in Libyan children from 3.5–5 days to 1.5–2 days (Neumann, 1980). Chlorpromazine has been shown to reduce the duration and volume of diarrhea in piglets with ST + LT-producing *E. coli*

(Lönnroth *et al.*, 1979), and in humans with cholera (Rabbani *et al.*, 1979, 1982; Islam *et al.*, 1982). Anti-motility agents have demonstrated efficacy in reducing the amount of fluid loss. The pharmacologic effects of this family of agents warrant study for possible anti-secretory effects. Caution should be exercised to avoid use of antimotility agents in inflammatory enteritis, where they may worsen the illness.

Although no studies describe the ability of human or animal milk to inhibit ST-induced intestinal fluid secretion, human milk and colostrum has been shown to inhibit *E. coli* cell adhesion mediated by colonization factors as well as the binding of LT or choleratoxin to their receptors (Holmgren *et al.*, 1981). A non-immunoglobulin fraction of human milk will inhibit fluid secretion induced by LT or choleratoxin in rabbit ileal loops (Otnaess and Svennerholm, 1982). Lactoferrin (an unsaturated iron binding protein which inhibits the growth of *E. coli* and certain other microorganisms), lysozyme, nutrient carried proteins, bifidus factor, complement, as well as immunoglobulins and cellular components, are important constituents of breast milk. Breast feeding has been reported to reduce the incidence of diarrhea and dehydration in infants (Brock, 1980; Schmidt, 1983; Lodinova–Zadnikova and Tlaskalova–Hogenova, 1983; Guerrant *et al.*, 1983).

Finally, in an attempt to interfere with enterotoxin-producing *E. coli* (multiplication, toxin production or colonization) with organisms, *Saccharomyces boulardii*, *Lactobacillus acidophilus*, *Lactobacillus bulgaricus* and *Streptococcus faecalis* have been reported to reduce the enterotoxic effects of *E. coli* in test animals (Mitchell and Kenworthy, 1976; Underdahl *et al.*, 1982; Massot *et al.*, 1982). These findings require further examination. Some of these findings have not been reproduced by others (Turnbull *et al.*, 1978; Clements *et al.*, 1981).

11. HORIZONS FOR FUTURE CONSIDERATIONS

Diarrheal diseases rank highest as an obvious and fundamental influence on human welfare and an important deterrent to economic progress throughout the developing world (Lee and Kean, 1978). Snyder and Merson (1982) estimated over 4.6 million deaths/year due to diarrheal disease in Africa, Asia and Latin America. ST-producing *E. coli* (and possibly some other organisms) are widespread throughout the most populous areas of the world, where climates are warm and sanitation facilities are poor. In some areas where diarrheal diseases constitute the major cause of a 25% mortality in the first 5 years of life, ST-producing *E. coli* are the commonest identifiable enteric pathogens in children with diarrhea in this age group (McLean *et al.*, 1981; Guerrant *et al.*, 1983). Questions arise as to the presence of multiple enteric pathogens in these children and their chances for survival (Ljungstrom *et al.*, 1980). Likewise, ST-producing *E. coli* constitute a major problem for the animal food industry. Answers are needed to explain the occurrence of enterotoxigenic *E. coli* in young animals in connection with feed change, changing temperature, or travel (Shimizu and Terashima, 1982). For these reasons, a multifaceted, aggressive, investigative and field attack must be mounted to improve our understanding and control of ST- and other enterotoxin-induced diarrheas. A great deal of work is needed on the epidemiologic, immunologic and pharmacologic fronts to control this problem.

Epidemiologic studies have begun to demonstrate the widespread occurrence of ST-producing *E. coli* in association with travelers' diarrhea and childhood diarrhea in many areas, infantile diarrhea in newborn nurseries and among several domestic animals. However, this work has been hampered by the need for an improved, less expensive, more sensitive assay for ST than the *in vivo* animal models currently used. Perhaps hybrid DNA probes or ELISAs may be the answer. Likewise, a great deal needs to be learned about the now apparent differences in types of ST produced by organisms from different sources. Work is needed to define the molecular differences among STs, their immunologic and biologic differences, and whether all act through similar receptors and intracellular mechanisms to activate intestinal guanylate cyclase in different species. As ST-producing organisms have been isolated from food and water samples, it is clear that epidemiologic control of ST- associated diseases will require major efforts to improve the quality and quantity of available water and sanitation facilities. Improved understanding of animal and human species specificities will also aid in directing appropriate epidemiologic control measures.

On a global scale, the major deterrents to physiologic control are the complex difficulties of delivering safely-prepared oral glucose- or sucrose-electrolyte solutions. The critical goal of early treatment with appropriate, safe therapy solution is met with numerous obstacles when delivery to homes in remote areas (where it is needed the most) is attempted. Potential problems occur from the improper preparation of the potentially life-saving, oral therapy solution. Preparation and delivery of oral therapy solution must also be carefully incorporated into the existing social and cultural fabric in order to be accepted and successful at the important primary level.

With improved understanding of the mechanism of action of ST and the adherence ST-producing *E. coli* to intestinal mucosa, several very exciting avenues of *pharmacologic* attack are raised. While antimicrobial treatment or prophylaxis carries several potential drawbacks, much remains to be learned about potential means of pharmacologic reversal of ST-induced secretion and biochemical approaches toward 'elution' or prevention of bacterial attachment in the small bowel. With improved understanding of the chain of biochemical events preceding and following guanylate cyclase activation by ST come potential avenues of attack with single or multiple, possibly synergistic, blocking agents. Likewise, clarification of the possible lectin-like glycoprotein receptors involved in attachment of *E. coli* or their toxins in the upper small bowel will likely lead to new, safer, specifically-targeted 'receptor chemotherapy' (Keusch, 1979).

Finally, potential horizons for immunologic control of ST-induced disease include the avenues of vaccine development that provide either antitoxic, antiattachment or anti-bacterial immunity. Improved understanding of the potentially transmissible genetic codes for enterotoxigenicity or adherence traits will greatly aid our understanding of the variability of STs and colonizing antigens, their occurrence in nature, and potential differences in their receptors, mechanisms of action and immunogenicity. This type of multipronged attack holds the greatest promise for ultimate control of the widespread, often devastating problem of ST-induced diarrhea.

REFERENCES

ABBEY, D. M. and KNOOP, F. C. (1979) Effect of chlorpromazine on the secretory activity of *Escherichia coli* heat-stable enterotoxin. *Infect. Immun.* **26:** 1000–1003.

ACOSTA–MARTINEZ, F., GYLES, C. L. and BUTLER, D. G. (1980) *Escherichia coli* heat-stable enterotoxin in feces and intestines of calves with diarrhea. *Am. J. Vet. Res.* **41:** 1143–1149.

ACRES, S. D., FORMAN, A. J. and KAPITANY, R. A. (1982) Antigen-extinction profile in pregnant cows, using a K99-containing whole-cell bacterin to induce passive protection against enterotoxigenic colibacillosis of calves. *Am. J. Vet. Res.* **43:** 569–579.

AGBONLAHOR, D. E. and ODUGBEMI, T. O. (1982) Enteropathogenic, enterotoxigenic and enteroinvasive *Escherichia coli* isolated from acute gastroenteritis patients in Lagos, Nigeria. *Trans. R. Soc. Trop. Med. Hyg.* **76:** 265–267.

AHRENS, F. A. and ZHU, B. (1982a) Effects of indomethacin, acetozolamide, ethacrynate sodium, and atropine on intestinal secretion mediated by *Escherichia coli* heat-stable enterotoxin in pig jejunum. *Can. J. Physio. Pharmacol* **60:** 1281–1286.

AHRENS, F. A. and ZHU, B. L. (1982b) Effects of epinephrine, clonidine, L-phenylephrine, and morphine on intestinal secretion mediated by *Escherichia coli* heat-stable enterotoxin in pig jejunum. *Can. J. Physiol. Pharmacol* **60:** 1680–1685.

AIMOTO, S., TAKAO, T., SHIMONISHI, Y., HARA, S., TAKEDA, T., TAKEDA, Y. and MIWATANI, T. (1982) Amino-acid sequence of a heat-stable enterotoxin produced by human enterotoxigenic *Escherichia coli*. *Eur. J. Biochem.* **129:** 257–263.

AIMOTO, S., WATANOBE, H., IKEMURA, H., SHIMONISHI, Y., TAKEDA, T., TAKEDA, Y. and MIWATANI, T. (1983) Chemical synthesis of a highly potent and heat-stable analog of an enterotoxin produced by a human strain of enterotoxigenic *Escherichia coli*. *Biochem. Biophys. Commun.* **112:** 320–326.

ALDERETE, J. F. and ROBERTSON, D. C. (1977a) Repression of heat-stable enterotoxin synthesis in enterotoxigenic *Escherichia coli*. *Infect. Immun.* **17:** 629–633.

ALDERETE, J. F. and ROBERTSON, D. C. (1977b) Nutrition and enterotoxin synthesis by enterotoxigenic strains of *Escherichia coli*: Defined medium for production of heat-stable enterotoxin. *Infect. Immun.* **15:** 781–788.

ALDERETE, J. F. and ROBERTSON, D. C. (1977c) Purification and properties of ENT ⁺ *Escherichia coli* heat-stable enterotoxin. In: Proceedings of the Thirteenth Joint Conference of the United States–Japan Cooperative Medical Science Program Cholera Panel held in Washington, D. C. pp. 19–31.

ALDERETE, J. F. and ROBERTSON, D. C. (1978) Purification and chemical characterization of the heat-stable enterotoxin produced by porcine strains of enterotoxigenic *Escherichia coli. Infect. Immun.* **19**: 1021–1030.

ARGENZIO, R. A. and WHIPP, S. C. (1981) Effect of *Escherichia coli* heat-stable enterotoxin, cholera toxin and theophylline on ion transport in porcine colon. *J. Physiol.* **320**: 469–487.

ASKERKOFF, B. and BENNETT, J. V. (1969) Effect of antibiotic therapy in acute salmonellosis on the fecal excretion of salmonellae. *N. Engl. J. Med.* **281**: 636–640.

AWAD–MASALMEH, M., MOON, H. W., RUNNELS, P. L. and SCHNEIDER, R. A. (1982) Pilus production, hemagglutination, and adhesion by porcine strains of enterotoxigenic *Escherichia coli* lacking K88, K99, and 987P antigens. *Infect. Immun.* **35**: 305–313.

BÄCK, E., MÖLLBY, R., KAIJSER, B., STINTZING, G., WADSTRÖM, T. and HABTE, D. (1980) Enterotoxigenic *Escherichia coli* and other gram-negative bacteria of infantile diarrhea: surface antigens, hemagglutinins, colonization factor antigen, and loss of enterotoxigenicity. *J. Infect. Dis.* **142**: 318–326.

BANWELL, J. G., GORBACH, S. L., PIERCE, N. F., MITRA, R. and MONDAL, A. (1971) Acute undifferentiated human diarrhea in the tropics. II. Alterations in intestinal fluid and electrolyte movements. *J. Clin. Invest.* **50**: 890–900.

BARNUM, D. A. (1971) The control of neonatal colibacillosis of swine. *Ann. NY Acad. Sci.* **176**: 385–400.

BERGMAN, M. J., UPDIKE, W. S., WOOD, S. J., BROWN III, S. E. and GUERRANT, R. L. (1981) Attachment factors among enterotoxigenic *Escherichia coli* from patients with acute diarrhea from diverse geographic areas. *Infect. Immun.* **32**: 881–888.

BERRY, R. J., BETTELHEIM, K. A. and GRACEY, M. (1983) Studies on enterotoxigenic *Escherichia coli* isolated from persons without diarrhea in western Australia. *J. Hyg. Camb.* **90**: 99–106.

BERTIN, A. (1982) Effect of propranolol on the secretory activity of *Escherichia coli* heat-stable enterotoxin in the suckling mouse assay. *Zbl. Bakt. Hyg.* **251**: 522–528.

BERTSCHINGER, H. U., MOON, H. W. and WHIPP, S. C. (1972a) Association of *Escherichia coli* with the small intestinal epithelium. I. Comparison of enteropathogenic and non-enteropathogenic porcine strains in pigs. *Infect. Immun.* **5**: 595–605.

BERTSCHINGER, H. U., MOON, H. W. and WHIPP, S. C. (1972b) Association of *Escherichia* coli with the small intestinal epithelium. II. Variations in association index and the relationship between association index and enterosorption in pigs. *Infect. Immun.* **5**: 606–611.

BETTELHEIM, K. A. and REEVE, K. G. (1982) An outbreak of gastroenteritis due to enteropathogenic *Escherichia coli*, which are also enterotoxigenic. *N. Z. Med. J.* **95**: 215–216.

BLACK, R. E., MERSON, M. H., ROWE, B., TAYLOR, P. R., MIZANUR RAHMAN, A. S. M., HUQ, A., ALEEM, A. R. M. A., SACK, D. A. and CURLIN, G. T. (1979) Epidemiology of enterotoxigenic *Escherichia coli* in rural Bangladesh. In: Symposium on Cholera, TAKEYA, K. and ZINNAKA, Y. (Eds), held in Karatsu, 1978, Fuji Printing Company, Tokyo, Japan. p. 292–301.

BLACK, R. E., MERSON, M. H., RAHMAN, A. S. M. M., YUNUS, M., ALIM, A. R. M. A., HUQ, I., YOLKEN, R. H. and CURLIN, G. T. (1980) A two-year study of bacterial, viral, and parasitic agents associated with diarrhea in rural Bangladesh. *J. Infect. Dis.* **142**: 660–664.

BLACK, R. E., BROWN, K. H., BECKER, S., ALIM, A. R. M. A. and HUQ, I. (1982a) Longitudinal studies of infectious diseases and physical growth of children in rural Bangladesh. *Amer. J. Epidemiol.* **115**: 315–324.

BLACK, R. E., BROWN, K. H., BECKER, S., ALIM, A. R. M. A. and MERSON, M. H. (1982b) Contamination of weaning foods and transmission of enterotoxigenic *Escherichia coli* diarrhoea in children in rural Bangladesh. *Trans. R. Soc. Trop. Med. Hyg.* **76**: 259–264.

BLACK, R. E., LEVINE, M. M., CLEMENTS, M. L., CISNEROS, L. and DAYA, V. (1982c) Treatment of experimentally induced enterotoxigenic *Escherichia coli* diarrhea with trimethoprim, trimethoprim-sulfamethoxazole, or placebo. *Rev. Infect. Dis.* **4**: 540–545.

BOEDEKER, E. C., YOUNG, C. R., COLLINS, H. H., CHENEY, C. P. and LEVINE, M. M. (1982) Towards a vaccine for Traveler's diarrhea (TD): Mucosally administered *Escherichia coli* colonization factor antigens (CFAs) elicit a specific local immunoglobulin A response in isolated intestinal loops. *Gastroenterology* **82** (part 2): 1020.

BOULANGER, Y., LALLIER, R. and COUSINEAUU, G. (1977) Isolation of enterotoxigenic Aeromonas from fish. *Can. J. Microbiol.* **23**: 1161–1164.

BOYCE, J. M., EVANS, D. J. JR., EVANS, D. G. and DuPONT, H. L. (1979) Production of heat-stable, methanol-soluble enterotoxin by *Yersinia enterocolitica. Infect. Immun.* **25**: 532–537.

BRASITUS, T. A., FIELD, M. and KIMBERG, D. V. (1976) Intestinal mucosal cyclic GMP: Regulation and relation to ion transport. *Amer. J. Physiol.* **231**: 275–281.

BRASITUS, T. A. and SCHACHTER, D. (1980) Membrane lipids can modulate guanylate cyclase activity of rat intestinal microvillus membranes. *Biochim. Biophys. Acta.* **630**: 152–156.

BRAY, J. (1945) Isolation of antigenically homogeneous strains of *Bact. coli* neopolitanum from summer diarrhea of infants. *J. Path. Bact.* **57**: 239–247.

BROCK, J. H. (1980) Lactoferrin in human milk: its role in iron absorption and protection against enteric infection in the newborn infant. *Archives of Disease in Childhood* **55**: 417–421.

BRUNTON, J., HINDE, D., LANGSTON, C., GROSS, R., ROWE, B. and GURWITH, M. (1980) Enterotoxigenic *Escherichia coli* in Central Canada. *J. Clin. Microbiol.* **11**: 343–348.

BURGESS, M. N., BYWATER, R. J., COWLEY, C. M., MULLAN, N. A. and NEWSOME, P. M. (1978) Biological evaluation of a methanol-soluble, heat-stable *Escherichia coli* enterotoxin in infant mice, pigs, rabbits and calves. *Infect. Immun.* **21**: 526–531.

BURGESS, M. N., MULLAN, N. A., and NEWSOME, P. M. (1980) Heat-stable enterotoxins from *Escherichia coli* P. 16 *Infect. Immun.* **28**: 1038–1040.

BURKE, V. and GRACEY, M. (1980) Effects of salicylate on intestinal absorption: *in vitro* and *in vivo* studies with enterotoxigenic micro-organisms. *GUT* **21**: 683–688.

BURKE, V., ROBINSON, J., ATKINSON, H. M. and GRACEY, M. (1982) Biochemical characteristics of enterotoxigenic *Aeromonas* spp. *J. Clin. Microbiol.* **15**: 48–52.

BURNS, T. W., MATHIAS, J. R., CARLSON, G. M., MARTIN, J. L. and SHIELDS, R. P. (1978) Effect of toxigenic *Escherichia coli* on myoelectric activity of small intestine. *Amer. J. Physiol.* **235**: E311–E315.

BYERS, P. A. and DuPONT, H. L. (1979) Pooling method for screening large numbers of *Escherichia coli* for production of heat-stable enterotoxin and its application in field studies. *J. Clin. Microbiol.* **9**: 541–543.

BYWATER, R. J. (1972) Dialysis and ultrafiltration of a heat-stable enterotoxin from *Escherichia coli*. *J. Med. Microbiol.* **5**: 337–343.

CHAN, S.-K. and GIANNELLA, R. A. (1981) Amino acid sequence of heat-stable enterotoxin produced by *Escherichia coli* pathogenic for man. *J. Biol. Chem.* **256**: 7744–7746.

CHIDLOW, J. W., BLADES, J. A. and PORTER, P. (1979) Sow vaccination by combined oral and intramuscular antigen: a field study of maternal protection against neonatal *Escherichia coli* enteritis. *Veterinary Record* **105**: 437–440.

CLEMENTS, M. L., LEVINE, M. M., BLACK, R. E., ROBINS-BROWNE, R. M., CISNEROS, L. A., DRUSANO, G. L., LANATA, C. F. and SAAH, A. J. (1981) *Lactobacillus* prophylaxis for diarrhea due to enterotoxigenic *Escherichia coli*. *Antimicrob. Agents. Chemother.* **20**: 104–108.

COHEN, G. and HEIKKILA, R. E. (1974) The generation of hydrogen peroxide, superoxide radical and hydroxyl radical by 6-hydroxydopamine, dialuric acid and related cytotoxic agents. *J. Biol. Chem.* **249**: 2447–2452.

CRAIG, J. P. (1965) A permeability factor (toxin) found in cholera stools and culture filtrates and its neutralization by convalescent cholera sera. *Nature (London)* **207**: 614–616.

CRAVIOTO, A., SCOTLAND, S. M. and ROWE, B. (1982) Hemagglutination activity and colonization factor antigens I and II in enterotoxigenic and non-enterotoxigenic strains of *Escherichia coli* isolated from humans. *Infect. Immun.* **36**: 189–197.

DE, S. N., BHATTACHARYA, K. and SARKAR, J. K. (1956) A study of the pathogenicity of strains of *Bacterium coli* from acute and chronic enteritis. *J. Path. Bact.* **71**: 201–209.

DE, S. N. and CHATTERJE, D. N. (1953) An experimental study of the mechanism of action of *Vibrio cholerae* on the intestinal mucous membrane. *J. Path. Bact.* **66**: 559–562.

DEAN, A. G., CHING, Y., WILLIAMS, R. G. and HARDEN, L. B. (1972) Test for *Escherichia coli* enterotoxin using infant mice: Application in a study of diarrhea in children in Honolulu. *J. Infect. Dis.* **125**: 407–411.

DEAN, G. S. and WANSBROUGH-JONES, M. H. (1983) Loss of CFA/I expression by enteropathogenic *E. coli* following exposure to antibody. *Clin. Exp. Immunol.* **52**: 293–296.

DEBOY, J. M. II, WACHSMUTH, I. K. and DAVIS, B. R. (1980a) Serotypes of enterotoxigenic *Escherichia coli* isolated in the United States. *Infect. Immun.* **29**: 361–368.

DEBOY, J. M. II, WACHSMUTH, I. K. and DAVIS, B. R. (1980b) Hemolytic activity in enterotoxigenic and non-enterotoxigenic strains of *Escherichia coli*. *J. Clin. Microbiol.* **12**: 193–198.

DEBOY, J. M. II, WACHSMUTH, I. K. and DAVIS, B. R. (1980c) Antibiotic resistance in enterotoxigenic and non-enterotoxigenic *Escherichia coli*. *J. Clin. Microbiol.* **12**: 264–270.

DE CASTRO, A. F. P., SERAFIM, M. B., RANGEL, H. A. and GUERRANT, R. L. (1978) Swiss and inbred mice in the infant mouse test for the assay of *Escherichia coli* thermostable enterotoxin. *Infect. Immun.* **22**: 972–974.

DEETZ, T. R., EVANS, D. J. JR., EVANS, D. G. and DuPONT, H. L. (1979) Serologic responses to somatic 0 and colonization-factor antigens of enterotoxigenic *Escherichia coli* in travelers. *J. Infect. Dis.* **140**: 114–118.

DE JONGE, H. R. (1975). The localization of guanylate cyclase in rat small intestinal epithelium. *FEBS Lett.* **53**: 237–242.

DE JONGE, H. R. (1976) Cyclic nucleotide-dependent phosphorylation of intestinal epithelium proteins. *Nature* **262**: 590–593.

DE JONGE, H. R. (1984) The mechanism of action of *Escherichia coli* heat-stable toxin. *Biochem. Soc. Transact.* **12**: 180–184.

DE LOPEZ, A. G., KADIS, S. and SHOTTS, E. B. (1982a) Transfer of drug resistance and enterotoxin production in porcine *Escherichia coli* strains and relationship between K88 antigen and raffinose (Melitose) fermentation. *Am. J. Vet. Res.* **43**: 499–501.

DE LOPEZ, A. G., KADIS, S. and SHOTTS, E. B. (1982b) Enterotoxin production and resistance to antimicrobial agents in porcine and bovine *Escherichia coli* strains. *Am. J. Vet. Res.* **43**: 1286–1287.

DE MOL, P., HEMELHOF, W., BUTZLER, J. P., BRASSEUR, D., KALALA, T. and VIS, H. L. (1983) Enteropathogenic agents in children with diarrhea in rural Zaire. *Lancet* **1**: 516–518.

DENEKE, C. F., McGOWAN, K., THORNE, G. M. and GORBACH, S. L. (1983) Attachment of enterotoxigenic *Escherichia coli* to human intestinal cells. *Infect. Immun.* **39**: 1102–1106.

DENEKE, C. F., THORNE, G. M. and GORBACH, S. L. (1979) Attachment pili from enterotoxigenic *Escherichia coli* pathogenic for humans. *Infect. Immun.* **26**: 362–368.

DENEKE, C. F., THORNE, G. M. and GORBACH, S. L. (1981) Serotypes of attachment pili of enterotoxigenic *Escherichia coli* isolated from humans. *Infect. Immun.* **32**: 1254–1260.

DOBRESCU, L. and HUYGELEN, C. (1973) Susceptibility of the mouse intestine to heat-stable enterotoxin produced by enteropathogenic *Escherichia coli* of porcine origin. *Applied Microbiol.* **26**: 450–451.

DONOWITZ, M., CHARNEY, A. N. and HYNES, R. (1979) Propranolol prevention of cholera enterotoxin induced intestinal secretion in the rat. *Gastroenterology* **76**: 482–491.

DONTA, S. T., MOON, H. W. and WHIPP, S. C. (1974) Detection of heat-labile *Escherichia coli* enterotoxin with the use of adrenal cells in tissue culture. *Science* **183**: 334–335.

DREYFUS, L. A., FRANTZ, J. C. and ROBERTSON, D. C. (1980) Biochemical properties of *E. coli* heat-stable enterotoxins. Abstract of the annual meeting of the American Society for Microbiology, held in Miami, 1980, ⧣B115.

DREYFUS, L. A., JASO-FREIDMAN, A. L. and ROBERTSON, D. C. (1984) Characterization of the mechanism of action of *Escherichia coli* heat-stable enterotoxin. *Infect. Immun.* **44**: 493–501.

DULANEY, A. D. and MICHELSON, I. D. (1935) A study of *B. coli mutabile* from an outbreak of diarrhea in the newborn. *Am. J. Public Health* **25**: 1241–1251.

DuPONT, H. L., EVANS, D. G., EVANS, D. JR. and SATTERWHITE, T. K. (1979) Role of bacterial fimbriae in the pathogenesis of enterotoxigenic *Escherichia coli* diarrhea in man. In: *International Colloquium in Gastroenterology-Frontiers of Knowledge in the Diarrheal Diseases*, pp. 123–136. JANOWITZ, H. D. and SACHAR, D. B. (Eds), Projects in Health, Inc., Upper Montclair, New Jersey.

DuPONT, H. L., EVANS, D. G., RIOS, N., CABADA, F. J., EVANS, D. J. JR. and DuPONT, M. W. (1982b) Prevention of Travelers' diarrhea with trimethoprim-sulfamethoxazole. *Rev. Infect. Dis.* **4**: 533–539.

DuPONT, H. L., FORMAL, S. B., HORNICK, R. B., SNYDER, M. J., LIBONATI, J. P., SHEAHAN, D. G., LA BREC, E. H. and KALAS, J. P. (1971) Pathogenesis of *Escherichia coli* diarrhea. *N. Engl. J. Med.* **285**: 1–9.

DuPONT, H. L., GALINDO, E., EVANS, D. G., CABADA, F. J., SULLIVAN, P. and EVANS, D. J. JR. (1980a) Prevention of Travelers' diarrhea with trimethoprim-sulfamethoxazole and trimethoprim alone. *Gastroenterology* **84**: 75–80.

DuPONT, H. L., SULLIVAN, P., EVANS, D. G., PICKERING, L. K., EVANS, D. J. JR., VOLLET, J. J., ERICSSON, C. D., ACKERMAN, P. B. and TJOA, W. S. (1980b) Prevention of travelers' diarrhea (emporiatic enteritis) – prophylactic administration of subsalicylate bismuth. *J. Am. Med. Assoc.* **243**: 237–241.

DuPONT, H. L., SULLIVAN, P., PICKERING, L. K., HAYNES, G. and ACKERMAN, P. B. (1977) Symptomatic treatment of diarrhea with bismuth subsalicylate among students attending a Mexican university. *Gastroenterology* **73**: 715–718.

DuPONT, H. L., REVES, R. R., GALINDO, E., SULLIVAN, P. S., WOOD, L. V. and MENDIOLA, J. G. (1982a) Treatment of travelers' diarrhea with trimethoprim/sulfamethoxazole and with trimethoprim alone. *N. Engl. J. Med.* **307**: 841–844.

DUTTA, N. K. and HABBU, M. K. (1955) Experimental cholera in infant rabbits: A method for chemotherapeutic investigation. *Br. J. Pharmacol.* **10**: 153–159.

ECHEVERRIA, P., BLACKLOW, N. R. and SMITH, D. H. (1975) Role of heat-labile toxigenic *Escherichia coli* and reoviruslike agent in diarrhoea in Boston children. *Lancet* **ii**, 1113–1116.

ECHEVERRIA, P. and MURPHY, J. R. (1980) Enterotoxigenic *Escherichia coli* carrying plasmids for antibiotic resistance and enterotoxin production. *J. Infect. Dis.* **142**: 273–278.

ECHEVERRIA, P., ULYANGCO, C. V., HO, M. T., VERHAERT, L., KOMALARINI, S., ØRSKOV, F. and ØRSKOV, I. (1978) Antimicrobial resistance and enterotoxin production among isolates of *Escherichia coli* in the Far East. *Lancet* **ii**, 589–592.

ECHEVERRIA, P., BLACKLOW, N. R., SANFORD, L. B. and CUKOR, G. C. (1981) Travelers' diarrhea among American Pearce Corps volunteers in rural Thailand. *J. Infect. Dis.* **143**: 767–771.

ECHEVERRIA, P., SERIWATANA, J., CHITYOTHIN, O., CHAICUMPA, W. and TIRAPAT, C. (1982) Detection of enterotoxigenic *Escherichia coli* in water by hybridization with three enterotoxin gene probes. *J. Clin. Microbiol.* **16**: 1086–1090.

ERICSSON, C. D., DuPONT, H. L., SULLIVAN, P., GALINDO, E., EVANS, D. G. and EVANS, D. J. JR. (1983) Bicozamycin, a poorly absorbable antibiotic, effectively treats travelers' diarrhea. *Ann. Int. Med.* **98**: 20–25.

ERICSSON, D. C., EVANS, D. G., DuPONT, H. L., EVANS, D. J. JR. and PICKERING, L. K. (1977) Bismuth subsalicylate inhibits activity of crude toxins of *Escherichia coli* and *Vibrio cholerae. J. Infect. Dis.* **136**: 693–696.

EVANS, D. G. and EVANS, D. J. JR. (1978) New surface-associated heat-labile colonization factor antigen (CFA/II) produced by enterotoxigenic *Escherichia coli* of serogroup 06 and 08. *Infect. Immun.* **21**: 638–647.

EVANS, D. G. and EVANS, D. J. JR. (1979) Colonization factor antigens of enterotoxigenic *Escherichia coli*: Presnet status and future directions. In: *Symposium on Cholera*, TAKEYA, K. and ZINNAKA, Y. (Eds), held in Karatus, 1978. Fuji Printing Company, Tokyo, Japan. pp. 282–291.

EVANS. D. G., EVANS, D. J. JR., CLEGG, S. and PAULEY, J. A. (1979) Purification and characterization of the CFA/I antigen of enterotoxigenic *Escherichia coli. Infect. Immun.* **25**: 738–748.

EVANS, D. G., EVANS, D. J. JR., and DuPONT, H. L. (1977a) Virulence factors of enterotoxigenic *Escherichia coli. J. Infect. Dis.* (suppl.) **136**: S118–S123.

EVANS, D. G., EVANS, D. J. JR. and PIERCE, N. F. (1973) Differences in the response of rabbit small intestine to heat-labile and heat-stable enterotoxins of *Escherichia coli. Infect. Immun.* **7**: 873–880.

EVANS, D. G., EVANS, D. J. JR. and TJOA, W. (1977b) Hemagglutination of human group A erythrocytes by enterotoxigenic *Escherichia coli* isolated from adults with diarrhea: Correlation with colonization factor. *Infect. Immun.* **18**: 330–337.

EVANS, D. G., EVANS, D. J. JR., TJOA, W. S. and DuPONT, H. L. (1978b) Detection and characterization of colonization of enterotoxigenic *Escherichia coli* isolated from adults with diarrhea. *Infect. Immun.* **19**: 727–736.

EVANS, D. G., OLARTE, J., DuPONT, H. L., EVANS, D. J. JR., GALINDO, A., PORTNOY, B. L. and CONKLIN, R. H. (1977c) Enteropathogens associated with pediatric diarrhea in Mexico City. *J. Pediatr.* **91**: 65–68.

EVANS, D. G., SATTERWHITE, T. K., EVANS, D. J. JR. and DuPONT, H. L. (1978a) Differences in serological responses and excretion patterns of volunteers challenged with enterotoxigenic *Escherichia coli* with and without the colonization factor antigen. *Infect. Immun.* **19**: 883–888.

EVANS, D. G., SILVER, R. P., EVANS, D. J. JR., CHASE, D. G. and GORBACH, S. L. (1975) Plasmid-controlled colonization factor associated with virulence in *Escherichia coli* enterotoxigenic for humans. *Infect. Immun.* **12**: 656–667.

EVANS, D. J. JR., CHEN, L. C., CURLIN, G. T. and EVANS, D. G. (1972) Stimulation of adenyl cyclase by *Escherichia coli* enterotoxin. *Nature* (*New Biol*) **236**: 137–138.

EVANS, D. J. JR., EVANS, D. G., DuPONT, H. L., ØRSKOV, F. and ØRSKOV, I. (1977) Patterns of loss of enterotoxigenicity by *Escherichia coli* isolated from adults with diarrhea: Suggestive evidence for an interrelationship with serotype. *Infect. Immun.* **17**: 105–111.

EVANS, D. J. JR., EVANS, D. G. and GORBACH, S. L. (1973) Production of vascular permeability factor by enterotoxigenic *Escherichia coli* isolated from man. *Infect. Immun.* **8**: 725–730.

EWING, W. H. (1956) Enteropathogenic *Escherichia coli* serotypes. *Ann. NY Acad. Sci.* **66**: 61–70.

FARKAS–HIMSLEY, H. and JESSOP, J. (1978) Detection of heat-stable enterotoxin in cell culture. *Microbios. Letters* **7**: 39–48.

FIELD, M. (1979a) Modes of action of enterotoxins from *Vibrio cholrae* and *Escherichia coli. Rev. Infect. Dis.* **1**: 918–925.

FIELD, M. (1979b) Regulation of small bowel electrolyte transport by cyclic nucleotides and calcium. In: *International Colloquium in Gastroenterology–Frontiers of Knowledge in the Diarrheal Diseases*, pp. 27–35, JANOWITZ, H. D. and SACHAR, D. G. (Eds), Projects in Health, Inc., Upper Montclair, New Jersey.

FIELD, M., GRAF, L. H. JR., LAIRD, W. J. and SMITH, P. L. (1978) Heat-stable enterotoxin of *Escherichia coli*: In vitro effects on guanylate cyclase activity, cyclic GMP concentration, and ion transport in small intestine. *Proc. Natl. Acad. Sci. U.S.A.* **75**: 2800–2804.

FIELD, M. and McCOLL, I. (1973) Ion Transport in rabbit ileal mucosa III. Effects of catecholamines. *Am. J. Physiol.* **225**: 852–857.

FINCK, A. D. and KATZ, R. L. (1972) Prevention of cholera-induced intestinal secretion in the cat by aspirin. *Nature.* **238**: 273–275.

FLOWER, R. J. and BLACKWELL, G. J. (1976) The importance of phospholipase A_2 in prostaglandin biosynthesis. *Biochem. Pharm.* **25**: 285–291.

FORDTRAN, J. S., RECTOR, F. C. JR. and CARTER, N. W. (1968) The mechanism of sodium absorption in the human small intestine. *J. Clin. Invest.* **47**: 884–900.

FORMAL, S. B., DuPONT, H. L., HORNICK, R., SNYDER, M. J., LIBONATI, J. and LA BREC, E. H. (1971) Experimental models in the investigation of the virulence of dysentery bacilli and *Escherichia coli. Ann. NY Acad. Sci.* **176**: 190–196.

FORSYTH, G. W., KAPITANY, R. A. and HAMILTON, D. L. (1981a) Organic acid proton donors decrease intestinal secretion caused by enterotoxins. *Amer. J. Physiol.* **241**: G227–G234.

FORSYTH, G. W., KAPITANY, R. A. and SCOOT, A. (1981b) Nicotinic acid inhibits enterotoxin-induced jejunal secretion in the pig. *Can. J. Comp. Med.* **45**: 167–172.

FORSYTH, G. W., KAPITANY, R. A., SCOOT, A. and HAMILTON, D. L. (1979) Comparative effects of cholera toxin and *Escherichia coli* heat-stable enterotoxin in the pig. *Proceedings of the Fifteenth Joint Conference of the United States–Japan Cooperative Medical Science Program Cholera Panel*, held in Washington, D. C.

FRANKLIN, A., SÖDERLIND, O. and MOLLBY, R. (1981) Plasmids coating for enterotoxins, K88 antigen and colicins in porcine *Escherichia coli* strains of O-group 149. *Med. Microbiol. Immunol.* **170**: 63–72.

FRANTZ, J. C. and ROBERTSON, D. C. (1981) Immunological properties of *Escherichia coli* heat-stable enterotoxins: Development of a radioimmunoassay specific for heat-stable enterotoxins with suckling mouse activity. *Infect. Immun.* **33**: 193–198.

FREEMAN, L. D., HOOPER, D. R., LATHEN, D. F., NELSON, D. P., HARRISON, W. O. and ANDERSON, D. S. (1983) Brief prophylaxis with doxycycline for the prevention of travelers' diarrhea. *Gastroenterology* **84**: 276–280.

FREER, J. H., ELLIS, A., WADSTROM, T. and SMYTH, C. J. (1978) Occurrence of fimbriae among enterotoxigenic intestinal bacteria isolated from cases of human infantile diarrhea. *FEMS Microbiology Letter* **3**: 277–281.

FRISK, C. S., WAGNER, J. E. and OWENS, D. R. (1978) Enteropathogenicity of *Escherichia coli* isolated from hamsters (*Mesocricetus auratus*) with hamster enteritis. *Infect. Immun.* **20**: 319–320.

GAASTRA, W. and DE GRAAF, F. K. (1982) Host-specific fimbrial adhesins of non-invasive enterotoxigenic *Escherichia coli* strains. *Microbiological Reviews* **46**: 129–161.

GANGAROSA, E. J. and MERSON, M. H. (1977) Epidemiologic assessment of the relevance of the so-called enteropathogenic serogroups of *Escherichia coli* in diarrhea. *N. Engl. J. Med.* **296**: 1210–1213.

GARBERS, D. L. and RADANY, E. W. (1981) Characteristics of the soluble and particulate forms of guanylate cyclase. *Adv. Cyclic Nucleotide Res.* **14**: 241–254.

GEORGES, M. C., WACHSMUTH, I. K., BIRKNESS, K. A., MOSELEY, S. L. and GEORGES, A. J. (1983) Genetic probes for enterotoxigenic *Escherichia coli* isolated from childhood diarrhea in the Central African Republic. *J. Clin. Microbiol.* **18**: 199–202.

GIANNELLA, R. A. (1976) Suckling mouse model for detection of heat-stable *Escherichia coli* enterotoxin: Characteristics of the model. *Infect. Immun.* **14**: 95–99.

GIANNELLA, R. A. and DRAKE, K. W. (1979) Effect of purified *Escherichia coli* heat-stable enterotoxin on intestinal cyclic nucleotide metabolism and fluid secretion. *Infect. Immun.* **24**: 19–23.

GIANNELLA, R. A., DRAKE, K. W. and LUTTRELL, M. (1981) Development of a radio-immunoassay for *Escherichia coli* heat-stable enterotoxin: Comparison with the suckling mouse bioassay. *Infect. Immun.* **33**: 186–192.

GIANNELLA, R. A. and LUTTRELL, M. (1982) Binding of *E. coli* heat-stable enterotoxin to small intestinal brush border receptors. *Gastroenterology* **82**: 1065.

GIANNELLA, R. A., ROUT, W. R. and FORMAL, S. B. (1977) Effect of indomethacin on intestinal water transport in salmonella-infected rhesus monkeys. *Infect. Immun.* **17**: 136–139.

GILES, C. and SANGSTER, G. (1948) An outbreak of infantile gastroenteritis in Aberdeen. *J. Hyg.* **46**: 1–9.

GILL, D. M. (1977) Mechanism of action of cholera toxin. In: *Advances in Cyclic Nucleotide Research*, Volume **8**, pp. 85–118, GREENGARD, P. and ROBINSON, G. A. (Eds), Raven Press, New York.

GILL, D. M., EVANS, D. J. JR. and EVANS, D. G. (1976) Mechanism of activation of adenylate cyclase *in vitro* by polymixin-released, heat-labile enterotoxin of *Escherichia coli. J. Infect. Dis.* (suppl) **133**: S103–S107.

GOLDSCHMIDT, R. (1933) Untersuchungen zur Ätiology der Durchfalserkrankungen des Säuglings. *Jahrb. Kinderheilk.* **89**: 318–358.

GOLDSCHMIDT, M. C. and DuPONT, H. L. (1976) Enteropathogenic *Escherichia coli*: Lack of correlation of serotype with pathogenicity. *J. Infect. Dis.* **133**: 153–156.

GOODMAN, L. S. and GILMAN, A. (1975) *The Pharmacological Basis of Therapeutics*, Fifth Edition, MacMillan Company, New York, p. 152–200.

GORBACH, S. L., BANWELL, J. G., CHATTERJEE, B. D., JACOBS, B. and SACK, R. B. (1971) Acute undifferentiated human diarrhea in the tropics. I. Alterations in intestinal microflora. *J. Clin. Invest.* **50**: 881–889.

GORBACH, S. L. and KHURANA, C. M. (1972) Toxigenic *Escherichia coli*–A cause of infantile diarrhea in Chicago. *N. Engl. J. Med.* **287**: 791–795.

GOTS, R. E., FORMAL, S. B. and GIANNELLA, R. A. (1974) Indomethacin inhibition of *Salmonella typhimurium*,

Shigella flexneri, and cholera-mediated rabbit ileal secretion. *J. Infect. Dis.* **130:** 280–284.

GRAHAM, D. Y., ESTES, M. K. and SACKMAN, J. W. (1982) Rotavirus induces an osmatic diarrhea in miniature swine. *Gastroenterology* **82** (part 2): 1072.

GREENBERG, R. N., CHANG, B., MURAD, F. and GUERRANT, R. L. (1980b) Inhibition of *E. coli* heat-stable enterotoxin by phenothiazine derivatives and indomethacin. *Clin. Res.* **28:** 369A.

GREENBERG, R. N., DUNN, J. A. and GUERRANT, R. L. (1983) Reduction of the secretory response to *Escherichia coli* heat-stable enterotoxin by thiol and disulfide compounds. *Infect. Immun.* **41:** 174–180.

GREENBERG, R. N., GUERRANT, R. L., CHANG, B., ROBERTSON, D. C. and MURAD, F. (1982b) Inhibition of *Escherichia coli* heat-stable enterotoxin effects on intestinal guanylate cyclase and fluid secretion by quinacrine. *Biochem. Pharmac.* **31:** 2005–2009.

GREENBERG, R. N., MURAD, F., CHANG, B., ROBERTSON, D. C. and GUERRANT, R. L. (1980a) Inhibition of *Escherichia coli* heat-stable enterotoxin by indomethacin and chlorpromazine. *Infect. Immun.* **29:** 908–913.

GREENBERG, R. N., MURAD, F. and GUERRANT, R. L. (1982a) Lanthanum chloride inhibition of the secretory response to *Escherichia coli* heat-stable enterotoxin. *Infect. Immun.* **35:** 483–488.

GROSS, R. J., CRAVIOTO, A., SCOTLAND, S. M., CHEASTY, T. and ROWE, B. (1978) The occurrence of colonization factor (CF) in enterotoxigenic *Escherichia coli*. *FEMS Microbiology Letters* **3:** 231–233.

GROSS, R. J., ROWE, B., HENDERSON, A., BYATT, M. E. and MACAURIN, J. C. (1976) A new *Escherichia coli* O-group, 0159, associated with outbreaks of enteritis in infants. *Scand. J. Infect. Dis.* **8:** 195–198.

GROSS, R. J., THOMAS, L. V., CHEASTY, T., DAY, N. P., ROWE, B., TOLEDO, M. R. F. and TRABULSI, L. R. (1983) Enterotoxigenic and enteroinvasive *Escherichia coli* strains belonging to a new O-group, 0167. *J. Clin. Microbiol.* **17:** 521–523.

GROSS, R. J., THOMAS, L. V. and ROWE, B. (1985) Enterotoxigenic *Escherichia coli* strains belonging to a new serogroup, *Escherichia coli* 0166. *J. Clin. Microbiol.* **22:** 705–707.

GUANDALINI, S., RAO, M. C., SMITH, P. L. and FIELD, M. (1982) cGMP modulation of ileal ion transport: *in vitro* effects of *Escherichia coli* heat-stable enterotoxin. *Am. J. Physiol.* **243:** G36–G41.

GUERRANT, R. L., and BERGMAN, M. J. (1979) Attachment factors among enterotoxigenic *Escherichia coli*. In: *International Colloquium in Gastroenterology—Frontiers of Knowledge in the Diarrheal Diseases*, pp. 137–147, JANOWITZ, H. D. and SACHAR, D. B. (Eds), Projects in Health, Inc., Upper Montclair, New Jersey.

GUERRANT, R. L., BRUNTON, L. L., SCHNAITMAN, T. C., REBHUN, L. I. and GILMAN, A. G. (1974) Cyclic adenosine monophosphate and alteration of Chinese hamster ovary cell morphology: A rapid, sensitive *in vitro* assay for the enterotoxins of *Vibrio cholerae* and *Escherichia coli*. *Infect. Immun.* **10:** 320–327.

GUERRANT, R. L., CHEN, L. C. and SHARP, G. W. G. (1972) Intestinal adenyl-cyclase activity in canine cholera: Correlation with fluid accumulation. *J. Infect. Dis.* **125:** 377–381.

GUERRANT, R. L., DICKENS, M. D., WENZEL, R. P. and KAPIKIAN, A. Z. (1976) Toxigenic bacterial diarrhea: Nursery outbreak involving multiple bacterial strains. *J. Pediatr.* **89:** 885–891.

GUERRANT, R. L., GANGULY, U., CASPER, A. G. T., MOORE, E. J., PIERCE, N. F. and CARPENTER, C. C. J. (1973) Effect of *Escherichia coli* on fluid transport across canine small bowel: Mechanism and time course with enterotoxin and whole bacterial cells. *J. Clin. Invest.* **52:** 1707–1714.

GUERRANT, R. L., HOLMES, R. K., ROBERTSON, D. C. and GREENBERG, R. N. (1985) Roles of enterotoxins in the pathogenesis of *Escherichia coli* diarrhea, in *Microbiology—1985*, American Society for Microbiology, Washington, D. C.

GUERRANT, R. L. and HUGHES, J. M. (1979) Nausea, vomiting and non-inflammatory diarrhea. In: *Principles and Practice of Infectious Diseases*, Chapter 71, MANDELL, G. L., DOUGLAS, R. G., JR. and BENNETT, J. E. (Eds), John Wiley & Sons, New York.

GUERRANT, R. L., HUGHES, J. M., CHANG, B., ROBERTSON, D. C. and MURAD, R. (1980a) Activation of rat and rabbit intestinal guanylate cyclase by the heat-stable enterotoxin of *Escherichia coli*: Studies of tissue specificity, potential receptors and intermediates. *J. Infect. Dis.* **142:** 220–228.

GUERRANT, R. L., KIRCHHOFF, L. V., SHIELDS, D. S., NATIONS, M. K., LESLIE, J., DeSOUSA, M. A., ARAUJO, J. G., CORREIA, L. L., SAUER, K. T., McCLELLAND, K. E., TROWBRIDGE, F. L. and HUGHES, J. M. (1983) Prospective study of diarrheal illnesses in northeastern Brazil: Patterns of disease, nutritional impact, etiologies and risk factors. *J. Infect. Dis.* **48:** 986–997.

GUERRANT, R. L., MOORE, R. A., KIRSCHENFELD, P. M. and SANDE, M. A. (1975) Role of toxigenic and invasive bacteria in acute diarrhea of childhood. *N. Engl. J. Med.* **293:** 567–573.

GUERRANT, R. L., ROUSE, J. D. and HUGHES, J. M. (1980b) Turista among the Yale Glee Club in Latin America: Studies of enterotoxigenic bacteria, *E. coli* serotypes and rotaviruses. *Amer. J. Trop. Med. & Hyg.* **29:** 895–900.

GUZMÁN–VERDUZCO, L. M., FONSECA, R. and KUPERSZTOCH–PORTNOY. (1983) Thermo-activation of a periplasmic heat-stable enterotoxin of *Escherichia coli*. *J. Bacteriol.* **154:** 146–151.

GYLES, C. L. (1971) Discussion: Heat-labile and heat-stable forms of the enterotoxin from *E. coli* strains enteropathogenic for pigs. *Ann. NY Acad. Sci.* **176:** 314–322.

GYLES, C. L. (1974) Relationship among heat-labile enterotoxins of *Escherichia coli* and *Vibrio cholerae*. *J. Infect. Dis.* **129:** 277–283.

GYLES, C. L. (1979) Limitations of the infant mouse test for *Escherichia coli* heat-stable enterotoxin. *Can. J. Comp. Med.* **43:** 371–379.

GYLES, C. L. and BARNUM, D. A. (1967) *Escherichia coli* in ligated segments of pig intestine. *J. Path. Bact.* **94:** 189–194.

GYLES, C. L. and BARNUM, D. A. (1969) A heat-labile enterotoxin from strains of *Escherichia coli* enteropathogenic for pigs. *J. Infect. Dis.* **120:** 419–426.

GYLES, C. L., FALKOW, S. and ROLLINS, L. (1978) *In vivo* transfer of an *Escherichia coli* enterotoxin plasmid possessing genes for drug resistance. *Am. J. Vet. Res.* **39:** 1438–1441.

GYLES, C. L., PALCHAUDHURI, S. and MAAS, W. K. (1977) Naturally occurring plasmid carrying genes for enterotoxin production and drug resistance. *Science* **198:** 198–199.

GYLES, C., SO, M. and FALKOW, S. (1974) The enterotoxin plasmids of *Escherichia coli*. *J. Infect. Dis.* **130:** 40–49.

GYLES, C. L., STEVENS, J. B. and CRAVEN, J. A. (1971) A study of *Escherichia coli* strains isolated from pigs with gastro-intestinal disease. *Can. J. Comp. Med.* **35:** 258–266.

HADDAD, J. J. and GYLES, C. L. (1982a) The role of K antigens of enteropathogenic *Escherichia coli* in colonization of the small intestine of calves. *Can. J. Comp. Med.* **46:** 21–26.

HADDAD, J. J. and GYLES, C. L. (1982b) Scanning and transmission electron microscopic study of the small intestine of colostrum-fed calves infected with selected strains of *Escherichia coli*. *Am. J. Vet. Res.* **43:** 41–49.

HAMILTON, D. L., ROE, W. E. and NIELSEN, N. O. (1977) Effect of heat stable and heat labile *Escherichia coli* enterotoxins, cholera toxin and theophylline on undirectional sodium and chloride fluxes in the proximal and distal jejunum of weaning swine. *Can. J. Comp. Med.* **41:** 306–317.

HARFORD, P. S., MURRAY, B. E., DuPONT, H. L. and ERICSSON, C. D. (1983) Bacteriologic studies of the enteric flora of patients treated with Bicozamycin (CGP 3543/E) for acute nonparasitic diarrhea. *Antimicrob. Agents Chemother.* **23:** 630–633.

HOLMGREN, J., LANGE, S. and LÖNNROTH, I. (1978) Reversal of cyclic AMP-mediated intestinal secretion in mice by chlorpromazine. *Gastroenterology* **75:** 1103–1108.

HOLMGREN, J., SVENNERHOLM, A. -N. and AHRÉN, C. (1981) Nonimmunoglobulin fraction of human milk inhibits bacterial adhesion (hemagglutination) and enterotoxin binding of *Escherichia coli* and *Vibrio cholerae*. *Infect. Immun.* **33:** 136–141.

HUGHES, J. M., GWALTNEY, J. M. JR., HUGHES, D. H. and GUERRANT, R. L. (1978b) Acute gastrointestinal illness in Charlottesville: A prospective family study. *Clin. Res.* **26:** 28A.

HUGHES, J. M., MURAD, F., CHANG, B. and GUERRANT, R. L. (1978a) Role of cyclic GMP in the action of heat-stable enterotoxin of *Escherichia coli*. *Nature* **271:** 755–756.

HUGHES, J. M., MURAD, F. and GUERRANT, R. L. (1978c) Studies to elucidate the mechanism of action of heat-stable enterotoxin of *Escherichia coli*. *Clin. Res.* **26:**'524A.

HUGHES, J. M., ROUSE, J. D., BARADA, F. A. and GUERRANT, R. L. (1980) Etiology of summer diarrhea among the Navajo. *Am. J. Trop. Med. Hyg.* **29:** 613–619.

ISAACSON, R. E., DEAN, E. A., MORGAN, R. L. and MOON, H. W. (1980) Immunization of suckling pigs against enterotoxigenic *Escherichia coli* induced diarrheal disease by vaccinating dams with purified K99 or 987P pili: Antibody production in response to vaccination. *Infect. Immun.* **29:** 824–826.

ISHIKAWA, E., ISHIKAWA, S., DAVIS, J. W. and SUTHERLAND, E. W. (1969) Determination of guanosine 3',5'-monophosphate in tissues and of guanyl cyclase in rat intestine. *J. Biol. Chem.* **244:** 6371–6376.

ISLAM, M. R., SACK, D. A., HOLMGREN, J., BARDHAN, P. K. and RABBANI, G. H. (1982) Use of chlorpromazine in the treatment of cholera and other severe acute watery diarrheal diseases. *Gastroenterology* **82:** 1335–1340.

JACKS, T. M., LIKOFF, R. O., FRAZIER, E. A. and MILLER, B. M. (1983) Antidiarrheal properties of clonidine, berberine and chlorpromazine. *Abstracts of the annual meeting of American Society for Microbiology*, B134, held in New Orleans, Louisiana.

JACKS, T. M., SCHLEIN, K. D., JUDITH, F. R. and MILLER, B. M. (1980) Cephamycin C treatment of induced enterotoxigenic colibacillosis (scours) in calves and piglets. *Antimicrob. Agents. Chemother.* **18:** 397–402.

JACKS, T. M. and WU, B. J. (1974) Biochemical properties of *Escherichia coli* low molecular-weight, heat-stable enterotoxin. *Infect. Immun.* **9:** 342–347.

JACOBY, H. I. and MARSHALL, C. H. (1972) Antagonism of cholera enterotoxin by anti-inflammatory agents in the rat. *Nature* **235:** 163–164.

JENSEN, C. O. (1913) Handbuch der Pathogenen. *Microorganismen* **6:** 131–144.

JOEST, E. (1903) Untersuchungen über Kälberruhr. *Z. Tiermed.* **7:** 377–413.

JOHNSON, W. M., LIOR, H. and JOHNSON, K. G. (1978) Heat-stable enterotoxin from *Escherichia coli*: Factors involved in growth and toxin production. *Infect. Immun.* **20:** 352–359.

JOHNSON, K. G., McDONALD, I. J. and JOHNSON, W. M. (1979) Heat-stable enterotoxin production in chemostat cultures of *Escherichia coli*. In S. ACRES (Editor), *Proceedings of the Second International Symposium on Neonatal Diarrhea*, VIDO, October 3–5, 1978, Saskatoon, Sask, Canada. Stuart Brandle Publishing Service. pp. 75–91.

JONES, G. W. and RUTTER, J. M. (1972) Role of the K88 antigen in the pathogenesis of neonatal diarrhea caused by *Escherichia coli* in piglets. *Infect. Immun.* **6:** 918–927.

KANTOR, H. S., TAO, P. and GORBACH, S. L. (1974) Stimulation of intestinal adenyl cyclase by *Escherichia coli* enterotoxin: Comparison of strains from an infant and an adult with diarrhea. *J. Infect. Dis.* **129:** 1–9.

KAPITANY, R. A., FORSYTH, G. W., SCOOT, A., McKENZIE, S. F. and WORTHINGTON, R. W. (1979) Isolation and partial characterization of two different heat-stable enterotoxins produced by bovine and porcine strains of enterotoxigenic *Escherichia coli*. *Infect. Immun.* **26:** 173–177.

KASAI, G. J. and BURROWS, W. (1966) The titration of cholera toxin and antitoxin in the rabbit ileal loop. *J. Infect. Dis.* **116:** 606–614.

KASHIWAZAKI, M., AKAIKE, Y., MIYACHI, T., OGAWA, T., SUGAWARA, M. and ISAYAMA, Y. (1981a) Production of heat-stable enterotoxin component by *Escherichia coli* strains enteropathogenic for swine. *Natl. Inst. Anim. Health Q.* (Jpn.) **21:** 21–25.

KASHIWAZAKI, M., NAKAMURA, K., SUGIMOTO, C., ISAYAMA, Y. and AKAIKE, Y. (1981b) Diarrhea in piglets due to *Escherichia coli* that produce only porcine ileal loop-positive heat-stable enterotoxic component. *Natl. Inst. Anim. Health Q.* (Jpn.) **21:** 148–149.

KAUFFMANN, F. (1947) The serology of the coli group. *J. Immunol.* **57:** 71–100.

KAUFFMANN, F. and DUPONT, A. (1950) Escherichia strains from infantile epidemic gastro-enteritis. *Acta. Pathol. Microbiol. Scand.* **27:** 552–564.

KAUFFMAN, P. E. (1981) Production and evaluation of antibody to the heat-stable enterotoxin from a human strain of enterotoxigenic *Escherichia coli*. *Applied and Environmental Microbiol.* **42:** 611–614.

KEAN, B. H., SCHAFFNER, W., BRENNAN, R. W. and WATERS, S. R. (1962) The diarrhea of travelers. V. Prophylaxis with phthalysulfathiazole and neomycin sulphate. *J. Am. Med. Assoc.* **180:** 367–371.

KENNEDY, D. J., GREENBERG, R. N., DUNN, J. A., ABERNATHY, R., RYERSE, J. S. and GUERRANT, R. L. (1984) Effects of *Escherichia coli* heat-stable enterotoxin ST_b on intestines of mice, rats, rabbits and piglets. *Infect. Immun.* **46:** 639–643.

KEUSCH, G. T. (1979) Specific membrane receptors: Pathogenic and therapeutic implications in infectious diseases. *Rev. Infect. Dis.* **1:** 517–529.

KIMBERG, D. V., SHLATZ, L. J. and CATTIEU, K. A. (1979) Cyclic nucleotide-dependent phosphorylation of specific rat intestinal microvillus and basal-lateral membrane proteins by endogenous protein kinases. In: *International Colloquium in Gastroenterology – Frontiers of Knowledge in the Diarrheal Diseases*, pp. 63–80, JANOWITZ, H. D. and SACHAR, D. B. (Eds), Projects in Health, Inc., Upper Montclair, New Jersey.

KIMURA, H., MITTAL, C. K. and MURAD, F. (1975) Activation of guanylate cyclase from rat liver and other tissues by sodium azide. *J. Biol. Chem.* **250:** 8016–8022.

KIMURA, H. and MURAD, F. (1975) Subcellular localization of guanylate cyclase-Minierview. *Life Sciences* **17:** 837–843.

KLIPSTEIN, F. A. and ENGERT, R. F. (1976a) Purification and properties of *Klebsiella pneumoniae* heat-stable enterotoxin. *Infect. Immun.* **13:** 373–381.

KLIPSTEIN, F. A. and ENGERT, R. F. (1976b) Partial purification and properties of *Enterobacter cloacae* heat-stable enterotoxin. *Infect. Immun.* **13:** 1307–1314.

KLIPSTEIN, F. A. and ENGERT, R. F. (1978a) Immunological relationships of different preparations of coliform enterotoxins. *Infect. Immun.* **21:** 771–778.

KLIPSTEIN, F. A. and ENGERT, R. F. (1978b) Reversal of jejunal water secretion by glucose in rats exposed to coliform enterotoxins. *Gastroenterology* **75:** 255–262.

KLIPSTEIN, F. A., ENGERT, R. F. and CLEMENTS, J. D. (1981a) Immunization of rats with heat-labile entertoxin provides uniform protection against heterologous serotypes of enterotoxigenic *Escherichia coli. Infect. Immun.* **32:** 1100–1104.

KLIPSTEIN, F. A., ENGERT, R. F. and CLEMENTS, J. D. (1981b) Protection in rats immunized with *Escherichia coli* heat-stable enterotoxin. *Infect. Immun.* **34:** 637–639.

KLIPSTEIN, F. A., ENGERT, R. F., CLEMENTS, J. D. and HOUGHTEN, R. A. (1983a) Protection against human and porcine enterotoxigenic strains of *Escherichia coli* in rats immunized with a cross-linked toxoid vaccine. *Infect. Immun.* **40:** 924–929.

KLIPSTEIN, F. A., ENGERT, R. F., CLEMENTS, J. D. and HOUGHTEN, R. A. (1983b) Vaccine for enterotoxigenic Escherichia coli based on synthetic heat-stable toxin crossed-linked to the B subunit on heat-labile toxin. *J. Infect. Dis.* **147:** 318–326.

KLIPSTEIN, F. A., ENGERT, R. F. and HOUGHTEN, R. A. (1983c) Properties of a synthetically produced *Escherichia coli* heat-stable enterotoxin. *Infect. Immun.* **39:** 117–121.

KLIPSTEIN, F. A., ENGERT, R. F., HOUGHTEN, R. A. and ROWE, B. (1984) Enzyme-linked immunosorbent assay for *Escherichia coli* heat-stable enterotoxin. *J. Clin. Microbiol.* **19:** 798–803.

KLIPSTEIN, F. A., GUERRANT, R. L., WELLS, J. G., SHORT, H. B. and ENGERT, R. F. (1979) Comparison of assay of coliform enterotoxins by conventional techniques versus *in vivo* intestinal perfusion. *Infect. Immun.* **25:** 146–152.

KLIPSTEIN, F. A., HOROWITZ, I. R., ENGERT, R. F. and SCHENK, E. A. (1975) Effect of *Klebsiella pneumoniae* enterotoxin on intestinal transport in the rat. *J. Clin. Invest.* **56:** 799–807.

KLIPSTEIN, F. A., LEE, C. and ENGERT, R. F. (1976) Assay of *Escherichia coli* enterotoxins *in vivo* perfusion in the rat jejunum. *Infect. Immun.* **14:** 1004–1010.

KLIPSTEIN, F. A., ROWE, B., ENGERT, R. F., SHORT, H. B. and GROSS, R. J. (1978) Enterotoxigenicity of enteropathogenic serotypes of *Escherichia coli* from infants with epidemic diarrhea. *Infect. Immun.* **21:** 171–178.

KNOOP, F. C. and ABBEY, D. M. (1981) Effect of chemical and pharmacological agents on the secretory activity induced by *Escherichia coli* heat-stable enterotoxin. *Can. J. Microbiol.* **27:** 754–758.

KOHLER, E. M. (1968) Enterotoxic activity of filtrates of *Escherichia coli* in young pigs. *Am. J. Vet. Res.* **29:** 2263–2274.

KOHLER, E. M. (1971) Observations on enterotoxins produced by enteropathogenic *Escherichia coli. Ann. NY Acad. Sci.* **176:** 212–219.

KORZENIOWSKI, O. M., DANTAS, W. and GUERRANT, R. L. (1978) Role of ST-producing *E. coli* in sporadic adult diarrhea in Brazil. *Clin. Res.* **26:** 400A.

KOUPAL, L. R. and DEIBEL, R. H. (1975) Assay, characterization and localization of an enterotoxin produced by Salmonella. *Infect. Immun.* **11:** 14–22.

KUDOH, Y., HIROSHI, Z. -Y., MATSUSHITA, S., SAKAI, S. and MARUYAMA, T. (1977) Outbreaks of acute enteritis due to heat-stable enterotoxin-producing strains of *Escherichia coli. Microbiol. Immunol.* **21:** 175–178.

LALLIER, R., LARIVIÈRE, S. and ST–PIERRE, S. (1980) *Escherichia coli* heat-stable enterotoxin: Rapid method for purification and some characteristics of the toxin. *Infect. Immun.* **28:** 469–474.

LALLIER, R., BERNARD, F., GENDREAU, M., LAZURE, C., SEIDAH, N. G., CHRÉTIEN, M. and ST.–PIERRE, S. A. (1982) Isolation and purification of *Escherichia coli* heat-stable enterotoxin of porcine origin. *Analytical Biochem.* **127:** 267–275.

LARIVIÈRE, S. and LALLIER, R. (1976) *Escherichia coli* strains isolated from diarrheic piglets in the province of Quebec. *Can. J. Comp. Med.* **40:** 190–197.

LATHE, R., HIRTH, P., DE WILDE, M., HARFORD, N. and LECOCQ, J.-P. (1980) Cell-free synthesis of enterotoxin of *E. coli* from a cloned gene. *Nature* **284:** 473–474.

LECCE, J. G., BALSBAUGH, R. K., CLARE, D. A. and KING, M. W. (1982) Rotavirus and hemolytic enteropathogenic *Escherichia coli* in weaning diarrhea of pigs. *J. Clin. Microbiol.* **16:** 715–723.

LECCE, J. G., CLARE, D. A., BALSBAUGH, R. K. and COLLIER, D. N. (1983) Effect of dietary regimen of Rotavirus–*Escherichia coli* weaning diarrhea of piglets. *J. Clin. Microbiol.* **17:** 689–695.

LEE, C. H., MOSELEY, S. L., MOON, H. W., WHIPP, S. C., GYLES, C. L. and SO, M. (1983) Characterization of the gene encoding heat-stable toxin II and preliminary molecular epidemiology studies of enterotoxigenic *Escherichia coli* heat-stable toxin II producers. *Infect. Immun.* **42:** 264–268.

LEE, J. A. and KEAN, B. H. (Chairman and Convenor) (1978) International conference on the diarrhea of traveller – New directions in research: A summary. *J. Infect. Dis.* **137:** 355–368.

LEE, M. K. and COUPAR, I. M. (1980) Opiate receptor-mediated inhibition of rat jejunal fluid secretion. *Life Sciences* **27:** 2319–2325.

LEVINE, M. M. (1981) Adhesion of enterotoxigenic *Escherichia coli* in humans and animals in *Adhesion and Microorganism Pathogenicity*. Pitman Medical, Turnbridge Wells (Ciba Foundation Symposium 80) pp. 142–160.

LEVINE, M. M., CAPLAN, E. S., WATERMAN, D., CASH, R. A., HORNICK, R. B. and SNYDER, M. J. (1977) Diarrhea caused by *Escherichia coli* that produce only heat-stable enterotoxin. *Infect. Immun.* **17**: 78–82.

LEVINE, M. M., NALIN, D. R., HOOVER, D. L., BERGQUIST, E. J., HORNICK, R. B. and YOUNG, C. R. (1979) Immunity to enterotoxigenic *Escherichia coli. Infect. Immun.* **23**: 729–736.

LEVINE, M. M. and RENNELS, M. B. (1978) *E. coli* colonization factor antigen in diarrhea. *Lancet* **ii**: 534.

LEVINE, M. M., RISTAINO, P., SACK, R. B., KAPER, J. B., ØRSKOV, F. and ØRSKOV, I. (1983) Colonization factor antigens I and II and type 1 somatic pili in enterotoxigenic *Escherichia coli*: Relation to enterotoxin type. *Infect. Immun.* **39**: 889–897.

LEVINSON, R. A. and SCHEDL, H. P. (1968) Adsorption of sodium, chloride and water and simple sugars in rat small intestine. *Am. J. Physiol.* **215**: 49–55.

LINGGOOD, M. A. and INGRAM, P. L. (1978) The effect of oral immunization with heat-stable *Escherichia coli* antigens on the sensitivity of pigs to enterotoxins. *Research in Veterinary Science* **25**: 113–115.

LJUNGSTROM, I., HOLMGREN, J., HULDT, G., LANGE, S. and SVENNERHOLM, A. -M. (1980) Changes in intestinal fluid transport and immune responses to enterotoxins due to concomitant parasitic infection. *Infect. Immun.* **30**: 734–740.

LOCKWOOD, D. E. and ROBERTSON, D. C. (1984) Development of a competitive enzyme-linked immunosorbent assay (ELISA) for *Escherichia coli* heat-stable enterotoxin (ST$_a$). *J. Immunol. Methods* **75**: 295–307.

LODINOVÁ-ŽADNIKOVÁ, R. and TLASKALOVA-HOGENOVA. (1983) Role of breast-feeding for the nutrition and immunologic development of the infant in *Acute Diarrhea: Its Nutritional Consequences in Children*, edited by J. A. BELLANTI, Nestle, Vevey/Raven Press, New York, pp. 165–178.

LOGAN, E. F. and MENEELY, J. D. (1981) Effect of immunizing pregnant sows with different *Escherichia coli* vaccines on the antibody levels in the piglet sera. *Veterinary Record* **109**: 513–514.

LÖNNROTH, I., ANDRÉN, B., LANGE, S., MARTINSON, K. and HOLMGREN, J. (1979) Chlorpromazine reverses diarrhea in piglets caused by enterotoxigenic *Escherichia coli. Infect. Immun.* **24**: 900–905.

MADSEN, G. L. and KNOOP, F. C. (1978) Inhibition of the secretory activity of *Escherichia coli* heat-stable enterotoxin by indomethacin. *Infect. Immun.* **22**: 143–147.

MADSEN, G. L. and KNOOP, F. C. (1980) Physiological properties of a heat-stable enterotoxin produced by *Escherichia coli* of human origin. *Infect. Immun.* **28**: 1051–1053.

MASHITER, K., MASHITER, G. D., HAUGHER, R. L. and FIELD, J. B. (1973) Effects of cholera and *E. coli* enterotoxins on cyclic adenosine 3′: 5′ monophosphate levels and intermediary metabolism in the thyroid. *Endocrinology* **92**: 541–549.

MASSOT, J., DESCONCLOIS, M. and ASTOIN, J. (1982) Protection par *Saccharomyces boulardii* de la diarrhée à *Escherichia coli* du souriceau. *Ann. Pharmaceutiques françaises* **40**: 445–449.

MATA, L. J. and URRUTIA, J. J. (1971) Intestinal colonization of bread-fed children in a rural area of low socioeconomic level. *Ann. NY Acad. Sci.* **176**: 93–109.

MATA, L., SIMHON, A., PADILLA, R., GAMBOA, M. D. M., VARGAS, G., HERNÁNDEZ, F., MOHS, E. and LIZANO, C. (1983) Diarrhea associated with rotaviruses, enterotoxigenic *Escherichia coli*, *Campylobacter* and other agents in Costa Rican children, 1976–1981. *Amer. J. Trop. Med. Hyg.* **32**: 146–153.

MATHIAS, J. R., CARLSON, G. M., DI MARINO, A. J., BERTIGER, G., MORTON, H. E. and COHEN, S. (1976) Intestinal myoelectric activity in response to live *Vibrio cholerae* and cholera enterotoxin. *J. Clin. Invest.* **58**: 91–96.

MATHIAS, J. R., NOGUEIRA, J., MARTIN, J. L., CARLSON, G. M. and GIANNELLA, R. A. (1982) *Escherichia coli* heat-stable toxin: Its effect on motility of the small intestine. *Am. J. Physiol.* **242**: G360–G363.

McCONNELL, M. M., WILLSHAW, G. A., SMITH, H. R., SCOTLAND, S. M. and ROWE, B. (1979) Transposition of ampicillin resistance to an enterotoxin plasmid in an *Escherichia coli* strain of human origin. *J. Bacteriol.* **139**: 346–355.

McLEAN, M., BRENNAN, R., HUGHES, J. M., KORZENIOWSKI, O. M., AUXILIADORA DE SOUZA, M., AROUJO, J. G., BENEVIDES, T. and GUERRANT, R. L. (1981) Etiology and oral rehydration therapy of childhood diarrhea in northeastern Brazil. *Bull. Pan. Am. Health Org.* **15**: 318–326.

MERSON, M. H., BLACK, R. E., GROSS, R. J., ROWE, B., HUQ, I. and EUSOF, A. (1980b) Use of antisera for identification of enterotoxigenic *Escherichia coli. Lancet* **ii**: 222–224.

MERSON, M. H., MORRIS, G. K., SACK, D. A., WELLS, J. G., FEELEY, J. C., SACK, R. B., CREECH, W. B., KAPIKIAN, A. Z. and GANGAROSA, E. J. (1976) Travelers' diarrhea in Mexico: A prospective study of physicians and family members attending a congress. *N. Engl. J. Med.* **294**: 1299–1305.

MERSON, M. H., ØRSKOV, F., ØRSKOV, L., SACK, R. B., HUQ, I. and KOSTER, F. T. (1979b) Relationship between enterotoxin production and serotype in enterotoxigenic *Escherichia coli. Infect. Immun.* **23**: 325–329.

MERSON, M. H., SACK, R. B., KIBRIYA, A. K. M. G., AL-MAHMOOD, A., ADAMED, Q. S. and HUQ, I. (1979a) Use of colony pools for diagnosis of enterotoxigenic *Escherichia coli* diarrhea. *J. Clin. Microbiol.* **9**: 493–497.

MERSON, M. H., YOLKEN, R. H., SACK, R. B., FROEHLICH, J. L., GREENBERG, H. B., HUQ, I. and BLACK, R. W. (1980a) Detection of *Escherichia coli* enterotoxins in stools. *Infect. Immun.* **29**: 108–113.

MITCHELL, I. G. and KENWORTHY, R. (1976) Investigation on a metabolite from *Lactobacillus bulgaricus* which neutralizes the effect of enterotoxin from *Escherichia coli* pathogenic for pigs. *J. Applied Bacteriol.* **41**: 163–174.

MITTAL, C. K. and MURAD, F. (1977a) Formation of adenosine 3′: 5′-monophosphate by preparations of guanylate cyclase from rat liver and other tissues. *J. Biol. Chem.* **252**: 3136–3140.

MITTAL, C. K. and MURAD, F. (1977b) Properties and oxidative regulation of guanylate cyclase. *J. Cyclic Nucleotide Res.* **3**: 381–391.

MOLENDA, J. and KOZYRCZAK (1983) Influence of immunization with enteropathogenic and non-enteropathogenic *Escherichia coli* on the occurrence of loop dilation in rabbits. *Research in Veterinary Science* **34**: 1–4.

MOLLA, A. M., HOSSAIN, M., SARKER, S. A., MOLLA, A. and GREENOUGH, W. B. III (1982) Rice-powder electrolyte solution as oral therapy in diarrhea due to *Vibrio cholerae* and *Escherichia coli. Lancet* **i**: 1317–1319.

MOON, H. W. (1981) Protection against enteric colibacillosis in pigs suckling orally vaccinated dams: Evidence for pili as protective antigens. *Am. J. Vet. Res.* **42**: 173–177.

MOON, H. W., BAETZ, A. L. and GIANNELLA, R. A. (1983) Immunization of swine with heat-stable *Escherichia coli* enterotoxin coupled to a carrier protein does not protect suckling pigs against an *Escherichia coli* strain that produces heat-stable enterotoxin. *Infect. Immun.* **39**: 990–992.

MOON, H. W., FUNG, P. Y., ISSACSON, R. E. and BOOTH, G. D. (1979) Effects of age, ambient temperature and heat-stable *Escherichia coli* enterotoxin on intestinal transit in infant mice. *Infact. Immun.* **25**: 127–132.

MOON, H. W., FUNG, P. Y., WHIPP, S. C. and ISSACSON, R. E. (1978) Effects of age and ambient temperature on the response of infant mice to heat-stable enterotoxin of *Escherichia coli*: Assay modifications. *Infect. Immun.* **20**: 36–39.

MOON, H. W., KOHLER, E. M., SCHNEIDER, R. A. and WHIPP, S. C. (1980) Prevalence of pilus antigens, enterotoxin types, and enteropathogenicity among K88-negative enterotoxigenic *Escherichia coli* from neonatal pigs. *Infect. Immun.* **27**: 220–230.

MOON, H. W., SORENSEN, D. K. and SAUTTER, J. H. (1966a) *Escherichia coli* infection of the ligated intestinal loop of the newborn pig. *Amer. J. Vet. Res.* **27**: 1317–1325.

MOON, H. W., SORENSEN, D. K., SAUTTER, J. H. and HIGBEE, J. M. (1966b) Association of *Escherichia coli* with diarrheal disease of the newborn pig. *Amer. J. Vet. Res.* **27**: 1007–1011.

MOON, H. W. and WHIPP, S. C. (1970) Development of resistance with age by swine intestine to effects of enteropathogenic *Escherichia coli*. *J. Inf. Dis.* **122**: 220–223.

MOON, H. W. and WHIPP, S. C. (1971) Systems for testing the enteropathogenicity of *Escherichia coli*. *Ann. NY Acad. Sci.* **176**: 197–211.

MOON, H. W., WHIPP, S. C. and BAETZ, A. L. (1971) Comparative effects of enterotoxins from *Escherichia coli* and *Vibrio cholerae* on rabbit and swine intestine. *Lab. Invest.* **25**: 133–140.

MOON, H. W., WHIPP, S. C., ENGSTROM, G. W. and BAETZ, A. L. (1970) Response of the rabbit ileal loop to cell-free products of *Escherichia coli* enteropathogenic for swine. *J. Inf. Dis.* **121**: 182–187.

MORGAN, R. L., ISAACSON, R. E., MOON, H. W., BRINTON, C. C. and TO, C.-C. (1978) Immunization of suckling pigs against enterotoxigenic *Escherichia coli*-induced diarrheal disease by vaccinating dams with purified 987P or K99 pili: Protection correlated with pilus homology of vaccine and challenge. *Infect. Immun.* **22**: 771–777.

MORRIS, G. K., MERSON, M. H., SACK, D. A., WELLS, J. G., MARTIN, W. T., DEWITT, W. E., FEELEY, J. C., SACK, R. B. and BESSUDO, D. M. (1976) Laboratory investigation of diarrhea in travelers to Mexico: Evaluation of methods for detecting enterotoxigenic *Escherichia coli*. *J. Clin. Microbiol.* **3**: 486–495.

MORRIS, J. A., THORNS, C., SCOTT, A. C., SOJKA, W. J. and WELLS, G. A. (1982) Adhesion *in vitro* and *in vivo* associated with an adhesive antigen (F41) produced by a K99 mutant of the reference strain *Escherichia coli* B41. *Infect. Immun.* **36**: 1146–1153.

MOSELEY, S. L., HARDY, J. W., HUQ, M. I., ECHEVERRIA, P. and FALKOW, S. (1983) Isolation and nucleotide sequence determination of a gene encoding a heat-stable enterotoxin of *Escherichia coli*. *Infect. Immun.* **39**: 1167–1174.

MOSELEY, S. L., HUQ, M. I., ALIM, A. R.'M. A., SO, M., SAMADPOUR–MOTALEBI, M. and FALKOW, S. (1980) Detection of enterotoxigenic *Escherichia coli* by DNA colony hybridization. *J. Infect. Dis.* **142**: 892–898.

MOSELEY, S. L., ECHEVERRIA, P., SERIWATANA, J., TIRAPAT, C., CHAICUMPA, W., SAKULDAIPEARA, T. and FALKOW, S. (1982) Identification of enterotoxigenic *Escherichia coli* by colony hybridization using three enterotoxin gene probes. *J. Infect. Dis.* **145**: 863–869.

MOSIMABLE, F. and GYLES, C. L. (1982) The pathogenicity of *Yersinia entercolitica* strains isolated from various sources in four test systems. *Can. J. Comp. Med.* **46**: 70–75.

MULLAN, N. A., BURGESS, M. N., BYWATER, R. J. and NEWSOME, P. M. (1979) The ability of cholestyramine resin and other adsorbents to bind *Escherichia coli* enterotoxins. *J. Med. Microbiol.* **12**: 487–496.

MULLAN, N. A., BURGESS, M. N. and NEWSOME, P. M. (1978) Characterization of a partially purified, methanol soluble heat-stable *Escherichia coli* enterotoxin in infant mice. *Infect. Immun.* **19**: 779–784.

MURRAY, B. E., EVANS, D. J. JR., PEÑARANDA, M. E. and EVANS, D. G. (1983) CFA/I-ST plasmids: Comparison of enterotoxigenic *Escherichia coli* (ETEC) of serotype 025, 063, 078, and 0128 and mobilization from an R factor – containing epidemic ETEC isolate. *J. Bacteriol.* **153**: 566–570.

MURRAY, B. E., RENSIMEN, E. R. and DuPONT, H. L. (1982) Emergence of high level trimethoprim resistance in fecal *E. coli* during oral administration of trimethoprim or trimethoprim/sulfamethoxazole. *N. Engl. J. Med.* **306**: 130–135.

MURRAY, B. E., SERIWATANA, J. and ECHEVERRIA, P. (1981) Toxin detection after storage or cultivation of enterotoxigenic *Escherichia coli* with colicinogenic *Escherichia coli*: A possible mechanism for toxin-negative pools. *J. Clin. Microbiol.* **13**: 179–183.

MYERS, L. L., NEWMAN, F. S., WARREN, G. R., CATLIN, J. E. and ANDERSON, C. K. (1975) Calf ligated intestinal segment test to detect enterotoxigenic *Escherichia coli*. *Infect. Immun.* **11**: 588–591.

NAGY, B. (1980) Vaccination of cows with a K99 extract to protect newborn calves against experimental enterotoxic colibacillosis. *Infect. Immun.* **27**: 21–24.

NAGY, N., MOON., H. W., ISAACSON, R. E., TO, C.-C. and BRUNTON, C. C. (1978) Immunization of suckling pigs against enteric enterotoxigenic *Escherichia coli* infection by vaccinating dams with purified pili. *Infect. Immun.* **21**: 269–274.

NALIN, D. R., BHATTACHARJEE, A. K. and RICHARDSON, S. H. (1974) Cholera-like toxic effect of culture filtrates of *Escherichia coli*. *J. Infect. Dis.* **130**: 595–601.

NALIN, D. R., LEVINE, M. M., YOUNG, C. R., BERGQUIST, E. J. and McLAUGHLIN, J. C. (1978) Increased *Escherichia coli* enterotoxin detection after concentrating culture supernatants: Possible new enterotoxin detectable in dogs but not in infant mice. *J. Clin. Microbiol.* **8**: 700–703.

NALIN, D. R. and McLAUGHLIN, J. C. (1978) Effects of choleragenoid and glucose on the response of dog intestine to *Escherichia coli* enterotoxins. *J. Med. Microbiol.* **11**: 177–186.

NALIN, D. R., McLAUGHLIN, J. C., RAHAMAN, M., YUNUS, M. and CURLIN, G. (1975) Enterotoxigenic *Escherichia coli* and ideopathic diarrhea in Bangladesh. *Lancet* **ii**: 1116–1119.

NEUMANN, S. Z. (1980) Childhood diarrhea and its treatment with indomethacin in Libya. *Tropical Doctor* **10**: 24–28.

NEWSOME, P. M., BURGESS, M. N. and MULLAN, N. A. (1978) Effect of *Escherichia coli* heat-stable enterotoxin on cyclic GMP levels in mouse intestine. *Infect. Immun.* **22**: 290–291.

NICKANDER, R., MCMAHON, F. G. and RIDOLFO, A. S. (1979) Nonsteroidal anti-inflammatory agents. *Ann. Rev. Pharmacol. Toxicol.* **19**: 469–480.

NOCARD, E. and LECLAINCHE, E. (1898) Les maladies microbiennes des animaux, Second Edition, pp. 106–112, Masson, Paris, France.

NOGUEIRA, J., MARTIN, J. L., CARLSON, G. M., MATHIAS, J. R. and GIANNELLA, R. A. (1979) *Escherichia coli* heat-stable toxin—Its effect on the motility of the small intestine. *Clin. Res.* **27**: 742A.

OKAMOTO, K., INOUE, T., SHIMIZU, K., HARA, S. and MIYAMA, A. (1982) Further purification and characterization of heat-stable enterotoxin produced by *Yersinia entercolitica*. *Infect. Immun.* **35**: 958–964.

OLIVEIRA, M. S., DE CASTRO, A. F. P. and SARAFIN, M. B. (1981) Mannose-resistant haemagglutination and colonization factors among *Escherichia coli* strains isolated from pigs. *Veterinary Record* **109**: 275–278.

OLSSON, E. (1982) Cultural methods for the production of heat-stable enterotoxin by porcine strains of *Escherichia coli* and its detection by the infant mouse test. *Veterinary Microbiol.* **7**: 253–266.

OLSSON, E. and SÖDERLIND, O. (1980) Comparison of different assays for definition of heat-stable enterotoxigenicity of *Escherichia coli* porcine strains. *J. Clin. Microbiol.* **11**: 6–15.

OLSVIK, Ø., BERGAN, T. and ØYE, I. (1981) Shedding of intestinal epithelium induced by chlorpromazine as mechanism inhibiting enterotoxin diarrhea. *Current Microbiology* **6**: 263–268.

OLSVIK, Ø. and KAPPERUD, G. (1982) Enterotoxin production in milk at 22°C and 4°C by *Escherichia coli* and *Yersinia entercolitica*. *Appl. Environ. Microbiol.* **43**: 997–1000.

ØRSKOV, I., ØRSKOV, F., SOJKA, W. J. and LEACH, J. M. (1961) Simultaneous occurrence of *E. coli* and B and L antigens in strains from diseased swine. *Acta. Pathol. Microbiol. Scand. Sect. B.* **53**: 404–422.

ØRSKOV, F., ØRSKOV, I., EVANS, D. J., SACK, R. B., SACK, D. A. and WADSTROM, T. (1976) Special *Escherichia coli* serotypes among enterotoxigenic strains from diarrhea in adults and children. *Med. Microbiol. Immunol.* **162**: 73–80.

ØRSKOV, I., ØRSKOV, F., JANN, B. and JANN, K. (1977) Serology, chemistry and genetics of O and K antigens of *Escherichia coli*. *Bacteriol. Rev.* **41**: 667–710.

ØRSKOV, I., ØRSKOV, F., SMITH, H. W. and SOJKA, W. J. (1975) The establishment of K99, a thermolabile, transmissible, *Escherichia coli* K antigen, previously called "Kco," possessed by calf and lamb enterotoxigenic strains. *Acta. Pathol. Microbiol. Scand. Sect. B* **83**: 31–36.

OTNAESS, A.-B. and SVENNERHOLM, A.-M. (1982) Non-immunoglobulin fraction of human milk protects rabbits against enterotoxin-induced intestinal fluid secretion. *Infect. Immun.* **35**: 738–740.

PALMER, D. L., KOSTER, F. T., ISLAM, A. F. M. R., RAHMAN, A. S. M. M. and SACK, R. B. (1977) Comparison of sucrose and glucose in the oral electrolyte therapy of cholera and other severe diarrheas. *N. Engl. J. Med.* **297**: 1107–1110.

PANHOTRA, B. R. and AGARWAL, K. C. (1981) Plasmids carrying genes for enterotoxin production and drug resistance in *Escherichia coli* of human origin. *Indian J. Med. Res.* **74**: 652–655.

PEÑARANDA, M. E., EVANS, D. G., MURRAY, B. E. and EVANS, D. J. JR. (1983) ST:LT:CFA/II plasmid in enterotoxigenic *Escherichia coli* belonging to serogroups 06, 08, 080, 085, and 0139. *J. Bacteriol.* **154**: 980–983.

PESTI, L. and LUKÁCS, K. (1981) Staining technique for peptides of *Escherichia coli* heat-stable enterotoxin. *Infect. Immun.* **33**: 944–947.

PESTI, L. and SEMJEN, G. (1973) Studies on enteropathogenicity, loop dilating effect and enterotoxin producing capacity of *Escherichia coli* strains isolated from enteric disease of swine. *Acta. Vet. Hung.* **23**: 227–236.

PICKERING, L. K., FELDMAN, S., ERICSSON, C. D. and CLEARLY, T. G. (1981) Absorption of salicylate and bismuth from a bismuth subsalicylate-containing compound (Pepto-Bismol). *J. Pediatr.* **99**: 654–656.

PIERCE, N. F. (1973) Differential inhibitory effects of cholera toxoids and gangliosides on the enterotoxins of *Vibrio cholerae* and *Escherichia coli*. *J. Exp. Med.* **137**: 1009–1023.

PIERCE, N. F. and WALLACE, C. K. (1972) Stimulation of jejunal secretion by a crude *Escherichia coli* enterotoxin. *Gastroenterology* **63**: 439–448.

PITARANGSI, C., ECHEVERRIA, P., WHITMIRE, R., TIRAPAT, C., FORMAL, S., DAMMIN, G. J. and TINGTALAPONG, M. (1982) Enteropathogenicity of *Aeromonas hydrophilia* and *Plesiomonas shigelloides*: Prevalence among individuals with and without diarrhea in Thailand. *Infect. Immun.* **35**: 666–673.

PORTER, P. and LINGGOOD, M. A. (1983) Development of oral vaccines for preventing diarrhoea caused by enteropathogenic *Escherichia coli*. *Journal of Infection* **6**: 111–121.

QUILL, J. and WEISER, M. M. (1975) Adenylate and guanylate cyclase activities and cellular differentiation in the small intestine. *Gastroenterology* **69**: 470–478.

RABBANI, G. H., GREENOUGH, W. B. III, HOLMGREN, J. and KIRKWOOD, B. (1982) Controlled trial of chlorpromazine as antisecretory agent in patients with cholera hydrated intravenously. *Brit. Med. J.* **284**: 1361–1364.

RABBANI, G. H., HOLMGREN, J., GREENOUGH, W. B. III and LÖNNROTH, I. (1979) Chlorpromazine reduces fluid loss in cholera. *Lancet* **i**: 410–412.

RAO, M. C., GUANDALINI, S., LAIRD, W. J. and FIELD, M. (1979a) Effects of heat-stable enterotoxin of *Yersinia enterocolitica* on ion transport and cyclic guanosine 3′-5′-monophosphate metabolism in rabbit ileum. *Infect. Immun.* **26**: 875–878.

RAO, M. C., GUANDALINI, S., LAIRD, W. J., SMITH, P. L. and FIELD, M. (1979b) Heat-stable enterotoxins: Mechanisms of action. *Proceedings of the Fifteenth Joint Conference of the United States–Japan Cooperative Medical Science Program Cholera Panel*, held in Washington, D.C.

REIS, M. H. L., CASTRO, A. F. P., TOLEDO, M. R. F. and TRABULSI, L. R. (1979) Production of heat-stable enterotoxin by the 0128 serogoup of *Escherichia coli*. *Infect. Immun.* **24**: 289–290.

REIS, M. H. L., GUTH, B. E. C., GOMES, T. A. T., MURAHOVSCHI, J. and TRABULSI, L. R. (1982) Frequency of *Escherichia coli* strains producing heat-labile toxin or heat-stable toxin or both in children with and without diarrhea in São Paulo. *J. Clin. Microbiol.* **15**: 1062–1064.

REIS, M. H. L., MATOS, D. P., PESTANA DE CASTRO, A. F., TOLEDO, M. R. F. and TRABULSI, L. R. (1980b) Relationship among enterotoxigenic phenotypes, serotypes, and sources of strains of enterotoxigenic *Escherichia coli*. *Infect. Immun.* **28**: 24–27.

REIS, M. H. L., AFFONSO, M. H. T. A., TRABULSI, L. R., MAZAITIS, A. J., MASS, R. and MAAS, W. K. (1980a) Transfer of CFA/I-ST Plasmid promoted by a conjugative plasmid in a strain of *Escherichia coli* of serotype 0128ac:H12. *Infect. Immun.* **29:** 140–143.

RICHARDS, D. A. (1970) A controlled trial in travelers' diarrhea. *Practitioner* **204:** 822–824.

ROBINS–BROWNE, R. M. and LEVINE, M. M. (1981) Effect of chlorpromazine on intestinal secretion mediated by *Escherichia coli* heat-stable enterotoxin and 8-Br-cyclic GMP in infant mice. *Gastroenterology* **80:** 321–326.

RONNBERG, B., SODERLINO, O. and WADSTROM, T. (1985) Evaluation of a competitive enzyme-linked immunosorbent assay for porcine *Escherichia coli* heat-stable enterotoxin. *J. Clin. Microbiol.* **22:** 893–896.

RÖNNBERG, B., WASTRÖM, T. and JÖRNVALL, H. (1983) Structure of heat-stable enterotoxin produced by a human strain of *Escherichia coli*. *FEBS Letters* **155:** 183–186.

ROSEBURY, T. (1962) *Microorganism indigenous to man.* McGraw-Hill Book Co., Inc., New York.

ROSENBERG, M. L., KOPLAN, J. P., WACHSMUTH, I. K., WELLS, J. G., GANGAROSA, E. J., GUERRANT, R. L. and SACK, D. A. (1977) Epidemic diarrhea at Crater Lake from enterotoxigenic *Escherichia coli*: A large, waterborne outbreak. *Ann. Intern. Med.* **86:** 714–718.

ROSENTHAL, S. L. (1969) Exacerbation of *Salmonella enteritis* due to ampicillin. *N. Engl. J. Med.* **280:** 147–148.

ROWE, B., GROSS, R. J., SCOTLAND, S. M., WRIGHT, A. E., SHILLOM, G. N. and HUNTER, N. J. (1978) Outbreak of infantile enteritis caused by enterotoxigenic *Escherichia coli* 06:H16. *J. Clin. Pathol.* **31:** 217–219.

ROWE, B., SCOTLAND, S. M. and GROSS, R. J. (1977) Enterotoxigenic *Escherichia coli* causing infantile enteritis in Britain. *Lancet* **i:** 90–91.

RUNNELS, P. L., MOON, H. W. and SCHNEIDER, R. A. (1980) Development of resistance with host age to adhesion of K99⁺ *Escherichia coli* to isolated intestinal epithelial cells. *Infect. Immun.* **28:** 298–300.

RYDER, R. W., KASLOW, R. A. and WELLS, J. G. (1979) Evidence for enterotoxin production by a classic enteropathogenic serotype of *Escherichia coli*. *J. Infect. Dis.* **140:** 626–628.

RYDER, R. W., SACK, D. A., KAPIKIAN, A. Z., MCLAUGHLIN, J. C., CHAKRABORTY, J., MIZANUR RAHMAN, A. S. M., MERSON, M. H. and WELLS, J. G. (1970b) Enterotoxigenic *Escherichia coli* and reovirus-like agent in rural Bangladesh. *Lancet* **i:** 659–662.

RYDER, R. W., WACHSMUTH, I. K., BUXTON, A. E., EVANS, D. G., DuPONT, H. L., MASON, E. and BARRETT, F. F. (1976a) Infantile diarrhea produced by heat-stable enterotoxigenic *Escherichia coli*. *N. Engl. J. Med.* **295:** 849–853.

RYDER, R. W., OQUIST, C. A., GREENBERG, H., TAYLOR, D. N., ØRSKOV, F., ØRSKOV, I., KAPIKIAN, A. Z. and SACK, R. B. (1981) Travelers' diarrhea in Panaminian tourists in Mexico. *J. Infect. Dis.* **144:** 442–448.

SACK, D. A., KAMINSKY, D. C., SACK, R. B., ITOTIA, J. N., ARTHUR, R. R., KAPIKIAN, A. Z., ØRSKOV, F. and ØRSKOV, I. (1978) Prophylactic doxycycline for travelers' diarrhea: Results of a prospective double-blind study of Peace Corps volunteers in Kenya. *N. Engl. J. Med.* **298:** 758–763.

SACK, D. A., KAMINSKY, D. C., SACK, R. B., WAMOLA, I. A., ØRSKOV, F., ØRSKOV, I., SLACK, R. C. B., ARTHUR, R. R. and KAPIKIAN, A. Z. (1977a) Enterotoxigenic *Escherichia coli* diarrhea of travelers: A prospective study of American Peace Corps volunteers. *Johns Hopkins Med. J.* **141:** 63–70.

SACK, D. A., MCLAUGHLIN, J. C., SACK, R. B., ØRSKOV, F. and ØRSKOV, I. (1977b) Enterotoxigenic *Escherichia coli* isolated from patients at a hospital in Daca, *J. Infect. Dis.* **135:** 275–280.

SACK, D. A., MERSON, M. M., WELLS, J. C., SACK, R. B. and MORRIS, G. K. (1975) Diarrhoea associated with heat-stable enterotoxin-producing strains of *Escherichia coli*. *Lancet* **ii:** 239–244.

SACK, R. B. (1975) Human diarrheal diseases caused by enterotoxigenic *Escherichia coli*. *Ann. Rev. Microbiol.* **29:** 333–353.

SACK, R. B. (1978) The epidemiology of diarrhea due to enterotoxigenic *Escherichia coli*. *J. Infect. Dis.* **137:** 639–640.

SACK, R. B., CASSELLS, J., MITRA, R., MERRITT, D., BUTLER, T., THOMAS, J., JACOBS, B., CHAUDHURI, A. and MONDAL, A. (1970) The use of oral replacement solutions in the treatment of cholera and other severe diarrheal disorder. *Bull. World Health Org.* **43:** 351–360.

SACK, R. B. and FROEHLICH, J. L. (1982) Berberine inhibits intestinal secretory response of *Bibrio cholerae* and *Escherichia coli* enterotoxins. *Infect. Immun.* **35:** 471–475.

SACK, R. B., FROEHLICH, J. L., ZULICH, A. W., SIDI HIDI, D., KAPIKIAN, A. Z., ØRSKOV, F., ØRSKOV, I. and GREENBERG, H. B. (1979) Prophylactic doxycycline for travelers' diarrhea–Results of a prospective double-blind study of Peace Corps volunteers in Morocco. *Gastroenterology* **76:** 1368–1373.

SACK, R. B., GORBACH, S. L., BANWELL, J. G., JACOBS, B., CHATTERJEE, B. D. and MITRA, R. C. (1971) Enterotoxigenic *Escherichia coli* isolated from patients with severe cholera-like disease. *J. Infect. Dis.* **123:** 378–385.

SACK, R. B., HIRSCHHORN, N., BROWNLEE, I., CASH, R. A., WOODWARD, W. E. and SACK, D. A. (1975) Enterotoxigenic *Escherichia coli*-associated diarrheal disease in Apache children. *N. Engl. J. Med.* **292:** 1041–1045.

SACK, R. B., JOHNSON, J., PIERCE, N. F., KEREN, D. F., and YARDLEY, J. H. (1976) Challenge of dogs with live enterotoxigenic *Escherichia coli* and effects of repeated challenges on fluid secretion of jejunal thirty-vella loops. *J. Infect. Dis.* **134:** 15–24.

SACK, R. B., SACK, D. A., MEHLAM, I. J., ØRSKOV, F. and ØRSKOV, I. (1977) Enterotoxigenic *Escherichia coli* isolated from food. *J. Infect. Dis.* **135:** 313–317.

SAEED, A. M. K. and GREENBERG, R. N. (1985) Preparative purification of *Escherichia coli* heat-stable enterotoxin. *Anal. Biochem.* **151:** (in press).

SAEED, A. M. K., MAGNUSON, N. S., SRIRANGANATHAN, N., BURGER, D. and COSAND, W. (1984) Molecular homogeneity of heat-stable enterotoxins produced by bovine enterotoxigenic *Escherichia coli*. *Infect. Immun.* **45:** 242–247.

SAEED, A. M. K., SPIRANGANATHAN, N., COSAND, W. and BURGER, D. (1983) Purification and characterization of heat-stable enterotoxin from bovine enterotoxigenic *Escherichia coli*. *Infect. Immun.* **40:** 701–707.

SANDEFUR, P. D. and PETERSON, J. W. (1976) Isolation of skin permeability factors from culture filtrates of *Salmonella typhimurim*. *Infect. Immun.* **14:** 671–679.

SANTOSHAM, M., SACK, R. B., FROEHLICH, J. L., AURELIAN, L., GREENBERG, H. B., YOLKEN, R., KAPIKIAN, A. Z.,

JAVIER, C., MEDINA, C., ØRSKOV, F. and ØRSKOV, I. (1980) Biweekly prophylactic doxycycline for travelers' diarrhea. In: *Current Chemotherapy and Infectious Disease*, pp. 922–924, American Society for Microbiology, Washington, D. C.

SATTERWHITE, T. K., EVANS, D. G., DuPONT, H. L. and EVANS, D. J. JR. (1978) Role of *Escherichia coli* colonization factor antigen in acute diarrhea. *Lancet* ii: 181–184.

SCHMIDT, B. J. (1983) Role of breast-feeding in the nutritional status of infants: *Comments in Acute Diarrhea: Its Nutritional Consequences in Children*, edited by J. A. BELLANTI, Nestle, Vevey/Raven Press, New York, pp. 179–180.

SCHNEIDER, R. A. and TO, S. C. M. (1982) Enterotoxigenic *Escherichia coli* strains that express K88 and 987P pilus antigens. *Infect. Immun.* 36: 417–418.

SCHWABE, U. (1971) Effect of nicotinic acid 3'5'-AMP-phosphate-diesterase activity in adipose tissue. In: *Metabolic Effects of Nicotinic Acid and Its Derivatives*, pp. 367–371, GEY, K. F. and CARLSON, L. A. (Eds). Hans Huber Publishers, Bern, Switzerland.

SCOTLAND, S. M., DAY, N. P., CRAVIOTO, A., THOMAS, L. V. and ROWE, B. (1981) Production of heat-labile or heat-stable enterotoxins by strains of *Escherichia coli* belonging to serogroups 044, 0114, and 0128. *Infect. Immun.* 31: 500–503.

SEARS, C., HEWLETT, E. and GUERRANT, R. (1982) Effects of *E. coli* heat-stable enterotoxins on pig jejunum. *Clin. Res.* 30: 877A.

SEEMAN, P. (1972) The membrane actions of anaesthetics and tranquilizers. *Pharmacol. Rev.* 24: 583–653.

SEKIZAKI, T., TERAKADO, N., UEDA, H. and HASHIMOTO, K. (1982) Isolation and characterization of plasmids encoding heat-stable enterotoxin from *Escherichia coli* of cattle origin. *Jpn. J. Vet. Sci.* 44: 619–627.

SELLWOOD, R. (1980) The interaction of the K88 antigen with porcine intestinal epithelial cell brush borders. *Biochim. Biophys. Acta* 632: 326–335.

SELLWOOD, R., GIBBONS, R. A., JONES, G. W. and RUTTER, J. M. (1975) Adhesion of enteropathogenic *Escherichia coli* to pig intestinal brush borders: The existence of two pig phenotypes. *J. Med. Microbiol.* 8: 405–411.

SELLWOOD, R. and KEARNS, M. (1979) Inherited resistance to *Escherichia coli* diarrhea in pigs: The genetics and nature of intestinal receptor. In: *International Colloquium in Gastroenterology–Frontiers of Knowledge in the Diarrheal Diseases*, pp. 113–122, JANOWITZ, H. D. and SACHAR, D. B. (Eds), Projects in Health, Inc., Upper Montclair, New Jersey.

SEN, D., SAHA, M. R., NIYOGI, S. K., BALAKRISH NAIR, G., DE, S. P., DATTA, P., DATTA, D., PAL, S. C., BASE, R. and ROYCHOWDHURY, J. (1983) *Trans. R. Soc. Trop. Med. Hyg.* 77: 212–214.

SERAFIM, M. B., MONTEIRO, A. R. and DE CASTRO, A. F. P. (1983) Factors affecting detection of *Yersinia enterocolitica* heat-stable enterotoxin by the infant mouse test. *J. Clin. Microbiol.* 17: 799–803.

SHARP, G. W. G. and HYNIE, S. (1971) Stimulation of intestinal adenyl cyclase by cholera toxin. *Nature* 299: 266–269.

SHEERIN, J. E. and FIELD, M. (1977) Ileal mucosal cyclic AMP and CL secretion: Serosal vs mucosal addition of cholera toxin. *Amer. J. Physiol.* 232: E210–E215.

SHIELDS, D. S., KIRCHHOFF, L. V., SAUER, K. T., NATIONS, M. K., ARAUJO, J. G., DeSOUSA, M. A. and GUERRANT, R. L. (1982) Abstract 867, 1982 Interscience Conference on Antimicrobial Agents and Chemotherapy.

SHIMIZU, M. and TERASHIMA, T. (1982) Appearance of enterotoxigenic *Escherichia coli* in piglets with diarrhea in connection with feed changes. *Microbiol. Immunol.* 26: 467–477.

SHORE, E. F., DEAN, A. G., HOLIK, K. J. and DAVIS, B. R. (1974) Enterotoxin-producing *Escherichia coli* and diarrheal disease in adult travelers: A prospective study. *J. Infect. Dis.* 129: 577–582.

SILVA, M. L. M., SCALETSKY, I. C. A., REIS, M. H. L., AFFONSO, M. H. T. and TRABULSI, L. R. (1983) Plasmid coding for drug resistance and production of heat-labile and heat-stable toxins harbored by an *Escherichia coli* strain of human origin. *Infect. Immun.* 39: 970–973.

SIVASWAMY, G. and GYLES, C. L. (1976) The prevalence of enterotoxigenic *Escherichia coli* in the feces of calves with diarrhea. *Can. J. Comp. Med.* 40: 241–246.

SKERMAN, F. J., FORMAL, S. B. and FALKOW, S. (1972) Plasmid-associated enterotoxin production in a strain of *Escherichia coli* isolated from humans. *Infect. Immun.* 5: 622–624.

SKIDMORE, I. F., SCHÖNHOFFER, P. S. and KRITCHEVSKY, D. (1971) Effects of nicotinic acid and some of its homologues on lipolysis, adenyl cyclase, phosphodiesterase and cyclic AMP accumulation in isolated fat cells. *Pharmacology* 6: 330–338.

SMITH, H. R., SCOTLAND, S. M. and ROWE, B. (1983) Plasmids that code for production of colonization factor antigen II and enterotoxin production of strains of *Escherichia coli*. *Infect. Immun.* 40: 1236–1239.

SMITH, H. R., WILLSHAW, G. A. and ROWE, B. (1982) Mapping of a plasmid, coding for colonization factor antigen I and heat-stable enterotoxin production, isolated from an enterotoxigenic strain of *Escherichia coli*. *J. Bacteriol.* 149: 264–275.

SMITH, H. R., CRAVIOTO, A., WILLSHAW, G. A., McCONNELL, M. M. SCOTLAND, S. M. GROSS, R. J. and ROWE, B. (1979) A plasmid coding for the production factor antigen 1 and heat-stable enterotoxin in strains of *Escherichia coli* of serogroup 078. *FEMS Microbiology Letters* 6: 255–260.

SMITH, H. W. and GYLES, C. L. (1970a) The relationship between two apparently different enterotoxin produced by enteropathogenic strains of *Escherichia coli* of porcine origin. *J. Med. Microbiol.* 3: 387–402.

SMITH, H. W. and GYLES, C. L. (1970b) The effect of cell-free fluids prepared from cultures of human and animal enteropathogenic strains of *Escherichia coli* on ligated intestinal segments of rabbits and pigs. *J. Med. Microbiol.* 403–409.

SMITH, H. W. and HALLS, S. (1967a) Studies on *Escherichia coli* enterotoxin. *J. Path. Bact.* 93: 531–543.

SMITH, H. W. and HALLS, S. (1967b) Observations by ligated intestinal segment and oral inoculation methods on *Escherichia coli* infections in pigs, calves, lambs and rabbits. *J. Path. Bact.* 93: 499–529.

SMITH, H. W. and HALLS, S. (1968) The transmissible nature of the genetic factor in *Escherichia coli* that controls enterotoxin production. *J. Gen. Microbiol.* 52: 319–334.

SMITH, H. W. and JONES, J. E. T. (1963) Observations on the alimentary tract and its bacterial flora in healthy and diseased pigs. *J. Path. Bact.* 86: 387–412.

SMITH, H. W. and LINGGOOD, M. A. (1971) Observations on the pathogenic properties of the K88, HLY and ENT plasmids of *Escherichia coli* with particular reference to porcine diarrhea. *J. Med. Micro.* **4**: 467–485.

SMITH, P. L., BLUMBERG, J. B., STOFF, J. S. and FIELD, M. (1981) Antisecretory effects of indomethacin on rabbit ileal mucosa *in vitro*. *Gastroenterology* **80**: 356–365.

SMITH, P. L. and FIELD, M. (1980) *In vitro* antisecretory effects of trifluoperazine and other neuroleptics in rabbit and human small intestine. *Gastroenterology* **78**: 1545–1553.

SMITH, T. and ORCUTT, M. L. (1925) The bacteriology of the intestinal tract of young calves with special reference to the early diarrhea ("scours"). *J. Exp. Med.* **41**: 89–196.

SMYTH, C. J., KAUSER, B., BÄCK, E., FARIS, A., MÖLLBY, R., SÖDERLIND, O., STINTZING, G. and WADSTRÖM, T. (1979) Occurrence of adhesins causing mannose-resistant hemagglutination of bovine erythrocytes in enterotoxigenic *Escherichia coli*. *FEMS Microbiology Letters* **5**: 85–90.

SMYTH, C. J., OLSSON, E., MONCALVO, C., SÖDERLIND, O., ØRSKOV, F. and ØRSKOV, I. (1981) K99 antigen-positive enterotoxigenic *Escherichia coli* from piglets with diarrhea in Sweden. *J. Clin. Microbiol.* **13**: 252–257.

SNYDER, J. D. and MERSON, M. M. (1982) The magnitude of the global problem of acute diarrhoeal disease: A review of active surveillance data. *Bull. WHO* **60**: 605–613.

SO, M., HEFFRON, F. and MCCARTHY, B. (1979) The *E. coli* gene encoding heat-stable toxin is a bacterial transposon flanked by inverted repeats of ISI. *Nature* **277**: 453–456.

SO, M. and MCCARTHY, B. J. (1980) Nucleotide sequence of the bacterial transposon Tn1681 encoding a heat stable (ST) toxin and its identification in enterotoxigenic *E. coli* strains. *Proc. Natl. Acad. Sci. U.S.A.* **77**: 4011–4015.

SO, M., ATCHISON, S., FALKOW, S., MOSELEY, S. and MCCARTHY, B. J. (1981) A study of the dissemination of Tn 1681: A bacterial transposon encoding a heat-stable toxin among enterotoxigenic *Escherichia coli* isolates. *Cold Spring Harbor Symp. Quant. Biol.* **45**: 53–58.

SOJKA, W. J., WRAY, C. and MORRIS, J. A. (1978) Passive protection of lambs against experimental enteric colibacillosis by colostral transfer of antibodies from K99-vaccinated ewes. *J. Med. Microbiol.* **11**: 493–499.

STAPLES, D. J., ASHER, S. E. and GIANNELLA, R. A. (1980) Purification and characterization of heat-stable enterotoxin produced by a strain of *E. coli* pathogenic for man. *J. Biol. Chem.* **255**: 4716–4721.

STAVRIC, S., DICKIE, N., GLEESON, T. M. and AKHTAR, M. (1981) Application of hydrophobic interaction chromatography to purification of *Escherichia coli* heat-stable enterotoxin. *Toxicon.* **19**: 743–747.

STAVRIC, S. and JEFFREY, D. (1977) A modified bioassay for heat-stable *Escherichia coli* enterotoxin. *Can. J. Microbiol.* **23**: 331–336.

STEINHOFF, M. C., DOUGLAS, R. G. JR., GREENBERG, H. B. and CALLAHAN, D. R. (1980) Bismuth subsalicylate therapy of viral gastroenteritis. *Gastroenterology* **78**: 1495–1499.

STINTZING, G., MOLLBY, R. and HABTE, D. (1982) Enterotoxigenic *Escherichia coli* and other enteropathogens in paediatric diarrhoea in Addis Ababa. *Acta Paediatr. Scand.* **71**: 279–286.

STIEGLITZ, H., FONSECA, R., OLARTE, J. and KUPERSZTOCH-PORTNOY, Y. M. (1980) Linkage of heat-stable enterotoxin activity and ampicillin resistance in a plasmid isolated from an *Escherichia coli* strain of human origin. *Infect. Immun.* **30**: 617–620.

STIRM, S., ØRSKOV, F., ØRSKOV, I. and BIRCH–ANDERSON, A. (1967b) Episome-carried surface antigen K88 of *Escherichia coli*. III. Morphology. *J. Bacteriol.* **93**: 740–748.

STIRM, S., ØRSKOV, F., ØRSKOV, I. and MANSA, B. (1967a) Episome-carried surface antigen K88 of *Escherichia coli*. II. Isolation and chemical analysis. *J. Bacteriol.* **93**: 731–739.

SUHARYONO, V. B. and SUNOTO, M. G. (1980) Reduction by aspirin of intestinal fluid-loss in acute childhood gastroenteritis. *Lancet* i: 1329–1330.

SWABB, E. A., TAI, Y. -H. and JORDAN, L. (1981) Reversal of cholera toxin-induced secretion in rat ileum by luminal berberine. *Am. J. Physiol.* **241**: G248–G252.

TAI, Y. -H., FESER, J. F., MARNANE, W. G., and DESJEUX, J. -F. (1981) Antisecretory effects of berberine in rat ileum. *Am. J. Physiol.* **241**: G253–G258.

TAKAO, T., HITOUJI, T., AIMOTO, S., SHIMONISHI, Y., HARA, S., TAKEDA, T., TAKEDA, Y. and MIWATANI, T. (1983) Amino acid sequence of a heat-stable enterotoxin isolated from enterotoxigenic *Escherichia coli* strain 18D. *FEBS Letters.* **152**: 1–5.

TAKEDA, Y. and MURPHY, J. (1978) Bacteriophage conversion of heat-labile enterotoxin in *Escherichia coli*. *J. Bacteriol.* **133**: 172–177.

TAKEDA, T., TAKEDA, Y. and MIWATANI, T. (1983) Improved method for purification of heat-stable enterotoxin of *Escherichia coli*. *FEMS Microbiol. Lettrs.* **16**: 81–84.

TAKEDA, T., TAKEDA, Y., MIWATANI, T., GREGORY, P., MORITA, T. and MATSUSHIRO, A. (1981) Genetic labeling of an ENT plasmid that encodes heat-stable enterotoxin of enterotoxigenic *Escherichia coli* isolated from patients. *Biken Journal* **24**: 127–135.

TAKEDA, Y., TAKEDA, T., YANO, T., YAMMOTO, K. and MIWATANI, T. (1979) Purification and partial characterization of heat-stable enterotoxin of enterotoxigenic *Escherichia coli*. *Infect. Immun.* **25**: 978–985.

TAYLOR, J. and BETTELHEIM, K. A. (1966) The action of chloroform-killed suspensions of enteropathogenic *Escherichia coli* on ligated rabbit-gut segments. *J. Gen. Microbiol.* **42**: 309–313.

TAYLOR, J., WILKINS, M. P. and PAYNE, J. M. (1961) Relation of rabbit gut reaction to enteropathogenic *Escherichia coli*. *Br. J. Exp. Pathol.* **42**: 43–52.

TEWARI, L., AGARWAL, S. K. and KUMAR, A. (1981b) A study of heat-stable enterotoxins of enteropathogenic *E. coli*: Part II chemical nature of toxic fractions. *Indian J. Med. Sci.* **35**: 104–108.

TEWARI, L., AGARWAL, S. K., NATU, S. M. and KUMAR, A. (1981a) A study on heat-stable enterotoxins of enteropathogenic *E. coli*: Part I fractionation by agar gel electrophoresis. *Indian J. Med. Sci.* **35**: 99–103.

THOMAS, D. D. and KNOOP, F. C. (1982) The effect of calcium and prostaglandin inhibitors on the intestinal fluid response to heat-stable enterotoxin of *Escherichia coli*. *J. Infect. Dis.* **145**: 141–147.

THOMAS, D. D. and KNOOP, F. C. (1983) Effect of heat-stable enterotoxin of *Escherichia coli* on cultured mammalian cells. *J. Infect. Dis.* **147**: 450–459.

THOMAS, L. V., McCONNELL, M. M., ROWE, B. and FIELD, A. M. (1985) The possession of three coli surface antigens by enterotoxigenic *Escherichia coli* strains positive for the putative colonisation factor PCF 8775. *J. Gen. Microbiol.* **131**: 2319–2326.

THOMAS, L. V. and ROWE, B. (1982) The occurrence of colonisation factors (CFA/I, CFA/II and E 8775) in enterotoxigenic *Escherichia coli* from various countries in South East Asia. *Med. Microbiol. Immunol.* **171**: 85–90.

THOMPSON, M. R., BRANDWEIN, H., LABINE-RACKE, M. and GIANNELLA, R. A. (1984) Simple and reliable enzyme-linked immunosorbent assay with monoclonal antibodies for detection of *Escherichia coli* heat-stable enterotoxin. *J. Clin. Microbiol.* **20**: 59–64.

THOMPSON, M. R. and GIANNELLA, R. A. (1985) Revised amino acid sequence for a heat-stable enterotoxin produced by an *Escherichia coli* strain (18D) that is pathogenic for humans. *Infect. Immun.* **47**: 834–836.

TITZE, C. and WEICHEL, T. (1908) Die Ätiologie der Kälberruhr. Berlin, Tierartzl. *Wochschr.* **26**: 457–458.

TRABULSI, L. R. (1964) Revelaçaõ de colibacilos associados as diarreias infantis pelo metodo infecçaõ experimental de alca ligade do intestino do coelho. *Rev. Inst. Med. Trop. S. Paulo* **6**: 197–203.

TRUSZCZYNSKI, M. and PILASZEK, J. (1969) Effects of injection of enterotoxins, endotoxin or live culture of *Escherichia coli* into the small intestine of pigs. *Rev. Vet. Sci.* **10**: 469–476.

TURJMAN, N., GOTTERER, G. S. and HENDRIX, T. R. (1978) Prevention reversal of cholera enterotoxin effects in rabbit jejunum by nicotinic acid. *J. Clin. Invest.* **61**: 1155–1160.

TURNBULL, P. C. B., GERSON, P. J. and STANLEY, G. (1978) Inability of selected lactobacilli to inhibit the heat-labile or heat-stable enterotoxin effects of *Escherichia coli* B7A. *J. Applied Bacteriol.* **45**: 157–160.

TURNER, A. C. (1967) Travelers' diarrhea: A survey of symptoms, occurrence and possible prophylaxis. *Br. Med. J.* **4**: 653–654.

TZIPORI, S., CHANDLER, O., SMITH, M., MAKIN, T. and HALPIN, C. (1982) Experimental colibacillosis in gnotobiotic piglets exposed to 3 enterotoxigenic serotypes. *Australian Veterinary J.* **59**: 93–95.

UNDERDAHL, N. R., TORRES–MEDINA, A. and DOSTER, A. R. (1982) Effect of *Streptococcus faecium* C-68 in control of *Escherichia coli*-induced diarrhea in gnotobiotic pigs. *Am. J. Vet. Res.* **43**: 2227–2232.

VARGAFTIG, R. B. and DAO HAI, N. (1972) Selective inhibition by mepacrine of the release of 'rabbit aorta contracting substance' evoked by the administration of bradykinin. *J. Pharm. Pharmacol.* **24**: 159–161.

VELIN, D., EMÖDY, L., PÁCSA, S. and KONTROHR, T. (1980) Enterotoxin production of *Yersinia enterocolitica* strains. *Acta Microbiol. Acad. Sci. Hung.* **27**: 299–304.

WACHSMUTH, K., DEBOY, J., BIRKNESS, K., SACK, D. and WELLS, J. (1983) Genetic transfer of antimicrobial resistance and enterotoxigenicity among *Escherichia coli* strains. *Antimicrob. Agents. Chemother.* **23**: 278–283.

WACHSMUTH, K., WELLS, J., SHIPLEY, P. and RYDER, R. (1979) Heat labile enterotoxin production in isolates from a shipboard outbreak of human diarrheal illness. *Infect. Immun.* **24**: 793–797.

WACHSMUTH, I. K., FALKOW, S. and RYDER, R. W. (1976) Plasmid-mediated properties of a heat-stable enterotoxin-producing *Escherichia coli* associated with infantile diarrhea. *Infect. Immun.* **14**: 403–407.

WALD, A., GOTTERER, G. S., RAJENDRA, G. R., TURJMAN, N. A. and HENDRIX, T. R. (1977) Effect of indomethacin on cholera induced fluid movement, undirectional sodium fluxes, and intestinal cAMP. *Gastroenterology* **72**: 106–110.

WALLING, M. W., MIRCHEFF, A. K., VAN OS, C. H. and WRIGHT, E. M. (1978) Subcellular distribution of nucleotide cyclases in rat intestinal epithelium. *Amer. J. Physiol.* **235**: E539–E545.

WHIPP, S. C., MOON, H. W. and ARGENZIO, R. A. (1981) Comparison of enterotoxic activities of heat-stable enterotoxins from class 1 and class 2 *Escherichia coli* of swine origin. *Infect. Immun.* **31**: 245–251.

WHIPP, S. C., MOON, H. W. and LYON, N. C. (1975) Heat-stable *Escherichia coli* enterotoxin produced *in vivo*. *Infect. Immun.* **12**: 240–244.

WILLSHAW, G. A., SMITH, H. R., MCCONNEL, M. M., BARCLAY, E. A., KRNJULAC, J. and ROWE, B. (1982) Genetic and molecular studies of plasmids coding for colonization factor antigen I and heat-stable enterotoxin in several *Escherichia coli* serotypes. *Infect. Immun.* **37**: 858–868.

WILSON, R. A. and JUTILA, J. W. (1976) Experimental neonatal colibacillosis in cows: Serological studies. *Infect. Immun.* **13**: 92–99.

WOLFF, D. J. and BROSTROM, C. O. (1979) Properties and functions of the calcium-dependent regulator protein. *Adv. Cyclic Nucleotide Res.* **11**: 27–88.

YAMAMOTO, T. and YOKOTA, T. (1980) Cloning of deoxyribonucleic acid regions encoding a heat-labile and heat-stable enterotoxin originating from an enterotoxigenic *Escherichia coli* strain of human origin. *J. Bacteriol.* **143**: 652–660.

YAMAMOTO, T. and YOKOTO, T. (1983) Plasmids of enterotoxigenic *Escherichia coli* H10407: Evidence for two heat-stable enterotoxin genes and a conjugal transfer system. *J. Bacteriol.* **153**: 1352–1360.

ZHU, and AHRENS, F. A. (1982) Effect of berberine on intestinal secretion mediated by *Escherichia coli* heat-stable enterotoxin in jejunum of pigs. *Am. J. Vet. Res.* **43**: 1594–1598.

ZILBERBERG, A., LAHAV, M., PERI, R. and GOLDHAR, J. (1983) Adherence properties of enterotoxigenic *Escherichia coli* (ETEC) isolated in the Tel-Aviv area. *Zbl. Bakt. Hyg.* **254**: 234–243.

CHAPTER 7

ANTITOXIN IMMUNITY IN CHOLERA AND ENTEROTOXIGENIC *ESCHERICHIA COLI* (ETEC) DIARRHEA

D. R. Morgan, L. V. Wood, H. L. DuPont and T. K. Satterwhite

The University of Texas Medical School at Houston,
Program in Infectious Diseases and Clinical Microbiology
Houston, Texas 77030, U.S.A.

ABSTRACT

Diarrheal disease is a major cause of childhood morbidity worldwide and mortality in developing nations. *Vibrio cholerae*, predominantly a threat in the Near and Far East, and enterotoxigenic *Escherichia coli*, common in most if not all developing countries produce diarrhea largely through elaboration of one or more enterotoxins. Human and animal studies have shown that antitoxin, as well as antibacterial, responses are measurable after natural and experimentally induced disease. Gut level immunity is believed to be of most importance in both diseases. Toxin and toxoid preparations have been shown to be effective immunogens in animal studies. It is probable that adequate immunoprophylaxis may be achieved in man by stimulating local antitoxin immunity with oral administration of such vaccines.

1. INTRODUCTION

Few enteric diseases have been as well characterized as gastroenteritis caused by *Vibrio cholerae* and enterotoxigenic *Escherichia coli* (ETEC). The first step in establishment of either infection is the ability of the organisms to adhere to and colonize the epithelial cells of the small bowel. In the case of ETEC, the ability to colonize the gut is dependent on the presence of specific fimbriae, called colonization factor antigens (CFA). Once attached to the small bowel wall, the bacteria secrete one or more enterotoxins causing an influx of fluids into the lumen of the gut. Infection caused by both *V. cholerae* and ETEC is, therefore, characterized by non-invasive, highly secretory diarrhea.

Both diseases show remarkable geographic limitations. In addition, immunity does seem to occur among indigenous populations within endemic areas. Although local secretory IgA responses may be more important in protection against disease, levels of both serum antitoxin and antibacterial immunoglobulins increase with age in these regions. The serum antibodies may, therefore, only serve as markers of prior exposure to prevalent organisms.

Asiatic cholera, a sometimes rapidly fatal disease, can be easily controlled by fluid and electrolyte replacement. Appropriate antimicrobial therapy is also recommended to reduce fluid requirements and to decrease excretion of the infecting strain. The drug of choice is tetracycline (DuPont and Pickering, 1980). ETEC induced diarrhea is commonly seen among children in developing countries constituting the major cause of illness in many areas. Adult tourists traveling from industrialized nations into these developing nations also commonly experience ETEC infection. This illness can be prevented or shortened in duration by administration of antimicrobial agents, such as doxycycline (Sack *et al.*, 1978) or trimethoprim-sulfamethoxazole (DuPont *et al.*, 1982). Because of antigenic homogeneity of prevalent strains and because there exists a predictable population at risk for cholera and for ETEC infection, it is probable that these important and sometimes life-threatening forms of acute gastroenteritis will ultimately be adequately controlled by immunoprophylaxis.

2. PATHOGENESIS OF INFECTION

2.1. Cholera

Classic cholera is caused by an enterotoxin-producing strain of serogroup 01 *V. cholerae*, a water-borne pathogen. Following an incubation period of 1–4 days after ingestion, the enterotoxigenic organisms produce a secretory diarrhea characterized by the passage of large volume rice water stools. Cholera toxin, a homogeneous protein of molecular weight 84K, is made up of two types of subunits. The interior A subunit possesses adenylate cyclase activity which causes fluid secretion after a 10–60 minutes lag (Greenough *et al.*, 1970; McGonagle *et al.*, 1969). During experimental cholera, the net movement of sodium is inhibited and the direction of chloride flux is reversed (Field *et al.*, 1969). The six superficial B subunits are responsible for the binding of the toxin to monosialoganglioside (GMI) residues of gut epithelial cells (van Heyningen, 1973).

2.2. ETEC Diarrhea

ETEC strains cause disease in a variety of animals, with a high degree of species specificity. This is related to the capacity of the strains to adhere to specific receptors of the small bowel. Several colonization factor antigen (CFA) types, characterized by their mannose-resistant hemagglutination of specific red blood cells, have been defined (D. G. Evans *et al.*, 1977, 1979; Thomas *et al.*, 1982). In man, these intestinal adhesins are morphologically similar to, yet functionally distinct from, type 1 or common pili. Colonization factors of human and animal strains are strictly serotype and species specific (DuPont and Pickering, 1980).

In addition to diverse attachment factors, ETEC produce a homogeneous cholera-like heat-labile enterotoxin (LT) and/or smaller molecular weight heterogeneous heat-stable enterotoxins (ST). LT is functionally, structurally, and immunologically similar to cholera toxin. Several ST molecules have been reported (DuPont and Pickering, 1980). They are all small proteins, reportedly of 2–10 K molecular weight, which cause fluid secretion rapidly by the stimulation of guanylate cyclase activity. Both toxins are coded for by extrachromosomal plasmid DNA, which explains the instability of toxin production in strains upon laboratory transfer. ETEC associated with human diarrhea generally produce both toxins (Ericsson *et al.*, 1983), although LT-only and ST-only strains have been found and associated with illness (Wood *et al.*, 1983b; Wachsmuth *et al.*, 1976; Levine *et al.*, 1977). There is no known difference in the clinical disease produced by ETEC that elaborate either or both toxins. ETEC are characteristically food-borne pathogens (Ericsson *et al.*, 1980; Wood *et al.*, 1983a, b).

3. CHOLERA IMMUNITY

3.1. Immunity Following Infection

In cholera endemic areas, a dramatic fall in incidence of illness occurs with increasing age (DuPont and Pickering, 1980). Persons convalescing from clinical cholera show a low frequency of reinfection suggesting that natural illness leads to immunity. Similarly, volunteers experimentally infected with *V. cholerae* show immunity when rechallenged 1 year after recovery from primary infection (Cash *et al.*, 1974). Up to 50% of populations in cholera endemic areas have elevated antibacterial or antitoxin titers, compared to less than 10% of surveyed populations in non-cholera endemic areas (Felsenfeld and Dutta, 1972). Immunity has been demonstrated to correlate with serum vibriocidal antibody titer (Mosely, 1969), although serum antitoxin levels may remain elevated for a longer time after infection (Benenson *et al.*, 1968; Snyder *et al.*, 1981). In experimental animal models, a protective role for both antibacterial and antitoxin antibody has been demonstrated (Svennerholm and Holmegren, 1976; Peterson, 1979). Gut level immunity, perhaps most important, is stimulated in both natural human infection and experimental infection in animals.

3.2. Antitoxin Immunity

Immunization with whole cell and isolated somatic antigen vaccines confers only a transient type-specific resistance to infection (Mosely *et al.*, 1970). Following the isolation and characterization of cholera toxin (Finkelstein *et al.*, 1964), the concept of both local and systemic antitoxin immunity was actively pursued. In natural and experimental cholera, vibrios and cholera toxin do not penetrate beyond the mucosal epithelial cells. Therefore, there is currently an emphasis on oral immunization to stimulate and monitor gut level mucosal immunity.

In humans, antitoxin responses are seen in serum and breast milk following cholera infection (Craig, 1965; Majumdar *et al.*, 1981, Majumdar and Ghose, 1981). These antibodies are generally of the IgG and IgA classes (Majumdar *et al.*, 1981; Majumdar and Ghose, 1981). In adult volunteers with experimentally-induced cholera, significant rises in serum IgG antitoxin were noted in all cases (Levine *et al.*, 1981). In this study, it was also demonstrated that serum antitoxin levels in volunteers with subclinical infection fell more rapidly than the corresponding levels of those with clinical cholera.

3.3. Vaccine Preparations

Antitoxin immunity appears to be mediated by antibodies to the B subunit. This indicates that the protective antibodies to toxin probably act by preventing the binding of the B subunit of toxin to GM_1 receptors of the intestinal epithelium rather than by interaction with active A subunit. The B subunit of cholera toxin (choleragenoid) may be an effective oral immunizing agent as it shares with toxin the property of binding to GM_1 receptors on lymphocyte membranes (Cuatrecasas, 1973). Choleragenoid does not produce diarrhea since it doesn't act to stimulate adenylate cyclase. However, choleragenoid is less effective as a mucosal immunogen than intact toxin (Pierce, 1978). Oral B subunit protects mice against challenge of intestinal segments with *V. cholerae* (Fujita and Finkelstein, 1972). An excellent candidate for cholera vaccine may be a non-virulent mutant of *V. cholerae* which produces only B subunit of cholera toxin (Honda and Finkelstein, 1979).

Toxoids free of somatic antigen have been produced by glutaraldehyde treatment of purified cholera toxin (Rappaport *et al.*, 1974). Difficulties have been encountered, however, in toxoid preparation. The commonly used method of detoxification with formaldehyde does not yield stable toxoid and reversion to partial toxicity occurs (Northrup and Chisari, 1972). Although glutaraldehyde treatment renders the toxoid stable, the immunogenicity is significantly reduced by the detoxification procedure (Saletti and Ricci, 1974). Heating, followed by formaldehyde treatment, may yield a stable, immunogenic toxoid immunogenic preparation (Germanier *et al.*, 1977).

Toxoids have been tested experimentally as both oral and parenteral immunizing agents. Toxoid given intraluminally or subcutaneously to rats was shown to prime the mucosal immune system although somewhat less than cholera toxin (Pierce *et al.*, 1978). Both were effective boosters. Antitoxin-containing plasma cells in jejunal lamina propria of rats correlated with the amount of antitoxin recovered in jejunal washings. This in turn correlated with protection against cholera toxin challenge. Parenteral administration of purified glutaraldehyde-treated toxoid to volunteers evoked high titers of circulating antitoxin (Levine *et al.*, 1978). A glutaraldehyde preparation has been tested as a parentally administered vaccine in Bangladesh where cholera is endemic and only minimal short lived immunity was induced (Curlin *et al.*, 1976).

Oral immunization, with or without parenteral immunization, employing a toxoid preparation may lead to protective immunity. Dogs immunized daily with oral toxoid developed protective immunity against *V. cholerae* even though no increase in serum antitoxin could be detected (Pierce *et al.*, 1978). The jejunal antitoxin was predominantly IgA. Repeated local application of antigen was associated with a rapid brief amnestic antibody response indicating that the gut secretory immune system possessed immunologic memory. Since at least two immune mechanisms are made operative by combining oral and parenteral antigens, an ideal approach may be to deliver the preparation by subcutaneous priming and subsequent oral boosting. Multiple antigens may be employed. Derivatives of cholera toxin, including both A and B subunits, heat-aggregated toxin (procholeragenoid) and glutaraldehyde-treated procholeragenoid were protective when administered orally and parenterally to rabbits (Peterson, 1979).

4. ETEC IMMUNITY

4.1. Immunity Following Infection

There is evidence to support the theory that indigenous populations possess lowered susceptibility to ETEC due to natural immunization following frequent exposure. DuPont *et al.* (1976) demonstrated that ETEC illness was more common among students who had recently arrived in Mexico than among students from Mexico and Venezuela. Not only was diarrhea and ETEC infection less common, it was also milder when disease did occur. The titer of baseline serum antibodies against heat-labile enterotoxin was also higher in students from Latin America (D. J. Evans *et al.*, 1977). Brown *et al.* (1982) showed that diarrhea in U.S. students in Mexico was mainly due to ETEC during the first one to two weeks after arrival. The incidence of illness decreased to low levels after one month. This is indirect evidence of lowered susceptibility following repeated exposure to ETEC. D. J. Evans *et al.* (1977) were able to demonstrate a significant correlation between rise in antitoxin titer and diarrhea caused by LT-producing *E. coli*. These authors concluded that humoral antitoxin titers were a useful indicator of immune status related to ETEC diarrhea. Black *et al.* (1981) found that in Bangladesh the rate of ETEC infection decreased with age. These authors suggested that immunity to both ST/LT and ST-only ETEC does develop. However, they noted that the presence of substantial serum antitoxic antibody prior to infection was not protective against disease. They also pointed out that development of immunity to ST-only producing ETEC implies that mechanisms of immunity other than antitoxin antibody production must be important, since ST is only slightly immunogenic. Based on the decreased rate of infection with age observed in their study, Black *et al.* (1981) suggested that antibacterial or anticolonization mechanisms of immunity might also be important. In volunteer studies, Levine *et al.* (1979) demonstrated that prior ETEC disease conferred homologous immunity against subsequent challenge. The mechanism of this protection was not bactericidal serum anti-O antibodies. However, heterologous protection was not produced when LT was the only common antigen. Hence they concluded that serum antitoxin to LT following infection was not protective.

4.2. Antitoxin Immunity

LT's from different human and animal ETEC apparently are similar, if not identical. There is strong cross neutralization when antiserum made from one strain is tested against antisera from other strains (Gyles and Barnum, 1969; Sack and Froehlich, 1977). The differences in LTs from different sources have been shown to reside in the B subunit (Geary *et al.*, 1982). Immunological similarities between the heat-labile enterotoxins of *E. coli* and *V. cholerae* have also been demonstrated (Gyles, 1974; Clements and Finkelstein, 1978 a, b). Antisera against *V. cholerae* toxin will neutralize the homologous antigen as well as heterologous *E. coli* LT. The heterologous neutralization is 1/3 to 1/10 that of homologous reaction. Similarly anti *E. coli* LT will neutralize *E. coli* LT and, to a far lesser degree, cholera toxin.

By immunodiffusion and biological neutralizing studies, LT of *E. coli* has antigenic determinants in common with both A and B subunits of cholera toxin (Clements and Finkelstein, 1978 a,b). Knowledge of the similarity between the toxins and experimental evidence that antitoxin-induced immunity against *V. cholerae* is protective against experimental cholera have given hope that ETEC might be controlled immunoprophylactically.

In 1973, Sack reported that rabbits immunized with a culture filtrate of an enterotoxigenic strain of *E. coli* were protected against homologous enterotoxin challenge. The sera of these animals contained anti-enterotoxin activity. Klipstein and Engert (1979) demonstrated using rats that active immunization with purified LT resulted in significant protection against both pure LT and viable LT-producing organisms. They found no protection against ST-producing strains. Immunization by an intraperitoneal prime followed by peroral booster doses was shown to be the optimal method conferring protection in rats against LT (Klipstein and Engert, 1980). This study demonstrated that immunization with LT is similar to that with cholera toxin since peroral immunization provided maximal extended protection by stimulation of the local immune response. Klipstein *et al.* (1983) recently showed that LT could be administered in pH-dependent microspheres to give the same serum and mucosal antitoxin levels and degree of protection as when LT was given after previous administration of cimetidine.

4.3. Vaccine Preparations

Two approaches have been taken to preparation of vaccines against ETEC. The first approach is to immunize with the enterotoxins produced by ETEC and the second is to immunize with fimbrial preparations (CFA's), aiming to prevent attachment of the organisms to the small intestine.

The ability of LT to stimulate mucosal secretory IgA antitoxin is dependent on the antigenicity, route and dosage of LT (Klipstein *et al.*, 1982). These authors further suggested that duration of protection in perorally immunized animals was related to secretory IgA levels which could be achieved. Ahren and Svennerholm (1982) demonstrated that the combination of antiserum directed against CFA/I or CFA/II with anti-enterotoxin gave a synergistic protective effect in rabbits. Protection conferred by anti-CFA/I has been shown by other authors (Clegg, Evans and Evans, 1980). Rats immunized with semipurified ST conjugated to a protein carrier were protected against challenge with semipurified or purified ST and viable ST-only producing organisms (Klipstein, Engert and Clements, 1981). However, when purified ST, coupled to bovine immunoglobulin G was used to immunize pregnant swine, neutralizing titers of serum and colostrum were comparatively low. Newborns suckling immunized dams were not protected against ST-producing *E. coli*.

Klipstein, Engert and Clements (1982) developed a vaccine using cross-linked ST and LT and obtained good protection in rats against ST or LT or viable heterologous strains. This approach has been refined with the development of a vaccine composed of synthetic ST cross-linked with the B (nontoxic) subunit of LT.

A vaccine directed against the fimbriae which mediate adhesion to the intestinal wall is currently being actively pursued. Preliminary trials in rabbits show high antitoxin levels and adequate protection (F. J. dela Cabada, D. G. Evans and D. J. Evans, Jr., Role of colonization factor antigen in immuno protection against enterotoxigenic *Escherichia coli* (ETEC) diarrhea. Interscience Conference on Antimicrobial Agents and Chemotherapy, Abstract 772, 1981). The polivalent pilus vaccine has been shown to be free of endotoxin and safe for human use. Clinical trials are currently under way by our group.

REFERENCES

Ahren, C. M. and Svennerholm, A-M. L. (1982) Synergistic protective effect of antibodies against *Escherichia coli* enterotoxin and colonization factor antigens. *Infect. Immun.* **38**: 74–79.

Benenson, A. S., Saad, A., Mosely, W. H. and Ahmed, A. (1968) Serological studies in cholera 3. Serum toxin neutralization-rise in titer in response to infection with *Vibrio cholerae*, and the level in the 'normal' population of East Pakistan. *Bull. Wld. Hlth. Org.* **38**: 287–295.

Black, R. E., Merson, M. H., Rowe, B., Taylor, P. R., Abdul Alim, A-R. M., Gross, R. J. and Sack, D. A. (1981) Enterotoxigenic *Escherichia coli* diarrhoea: acquired immunity and transmission in an endemic area. *Bull. Wld. Hlth. Org.* **59**: 263–268.

Brown, M. R., DuPont, H. L. and Sullivan, P. S. (1982) Effect of duration of exposure on diarrhoea due to enterotoxigenic *Escherichia coli* in travelers from the United States to Mexico. *J. Infect. Dis.* **145**: 582.

Cash, R. A., Music, S. I., Libonati, J. P., Craig, J. P., Pierce, N. F. and Hornick, R. B. (1974) Response of man to infection with *Vibrio cholerae* II. Protection from illness afforded by previous disease and vaccine. *J. Infect. Dis.* **130**: 325–333.

CLEGG, S., EVANS, D. G. and EVANS, D. J., JR. (1980) Enzyme-linked immunosorbent assay for quantitating the humoral immune response to the colonization factor antigen of *Escherichia coli*. *Infect. Immun.* **27**: 525–531.

CLEMENTS, J. D. and FINKELSTEIN, R. A. (1978a) Demonstration of shared and unique immunological determinants in enterotoxins from *Vibrio cholerae* and *Escherichia coli*. *Infect. Immun.* **22**: 709–713.

CLEMENTS, J. D. and FINKELSTEIN, R. A. (1978b) Immunological cross-reactivity between a heat-labile enterotoxin(s) of *Escherichia coli* and subunits of *Vibrio cholerae* enterotoxin. *Infect. Immun.* **21**: 1036–1039.

CRAIG, J. M. P. (1965) A permeability factor (toxin) found in cholera stools and culture filtrates and its neutralization by convalescent cholera sera. *Nature* (London) **207**: 614–616.

CUATRECASAS, P. (1973) *Vibrio cholerae* choleragenoid. Mechanism of inhibition of toxin action. *Biochemistry* **12**: 3577–3581.

CURLIN, G., LEVINE, K. M., AZIZ, K. M. A., RAHMAN, A. S. M. and VERWAY, W. F. (1976) Field trial of cholera toxoid *In* Proceedings of the 11th Joint Conference of the U. S.—Japan Cooperative Medical Science Program Symposium on Cholera. New Orleans, 1975, pp. 314–329. National Institute of Allergy and Infectious Diseases. Bethesda, MD.

DUPONT, H. L., OLARTE, J., EVANS, D. G., PICKERING, L. K., GALINDO, E. and EVANS, D. J. (1976) Comparative susceptibility of Latin American and United States students to enteric pathogens. *New England J. Med.* **295**: 1520–1521.

DUPONT, H. L. and PICKERING, L. K. (1980) Infections of the gastrointestinal tract. Microbiology, pathophysiology and clinical features. Plenum, New York.

DUPONT, H. L., REVES, R. R., GALINDO, E., SULLIVAN, P. S., WOOD, L. V. and MENDIOLA, J. G. (1982) Treatment of travelers' diarrhea with trimethoprim/sulfamethoxazole and with trimethoprim alone. *N. Engl. J. Med.* **307**: 841–844.

ERICSSON, C. D., DUPONT, H. L., SULLIVAN, P., GALINDO, E., EVANS, D. G. and EVANS, D. J. (1983) Bicozamycin, a poorly absorbable antibiotic, effectively treats travelers' diarrhea. *Ann. Int. Med.* **98**: 20–25.

ERICSSON, C. D., PICKERING, L. K., SULLIVAN, P. and DUPONT, H. L. (1980) The role of location of food consumption in the prevention of travelers' diarrhea in Mexico. *Gastroenterology* **79**: 812–816.

EVANS, D. G., EVANS, D. J., JR. and TJOA, W. (1977) Hemagglutination of human group A erythrocytes by enterotoxigenic *Escherichia coli* isolated from adults with diarrhea: Correlation with colonization factor. *Infect. Immun.* **18**: 330–337.

EVANS, D. J., JR., EVANS, D. G. and DUPONT, H. L. (1979) Hemagglutination patterns of enterotoxigenic *Escherichia coli* determined with human, bovine, chicken, and guinea pig erythrocytes in the presence and absence of mannose. *Infect. Immun.* **23**: 336–346.

EVANS, D. J., JR., RUIZ-PALACIOS, G., EVANS, D. G., DUPONT, H. L., PICKERING, L. K. and OLARTE, J. (1977) Humoral immune response to the heat-labile enterotoxin of *Escherichia coli* in naturally acquired diarrhea and antitoxin determination by passive immune hemolysis. *Infect. Immun.* **16**: 781–788.

FELSENFELD, O. and DUTTA, N. K. (1972) A serologic survey of cholera-free and cholera-infected areas. *J. Trop. Med. Hyg.* **75**: 209–212.

FIELD, M., FROMM, D., WALLACE, D. K., and GREENOUGH, W. B., III. (1969) Stimulation of active chloride secretion in small intestine by cholera exotoxin. *J. Clin. Invest.* **48**: 24a.

FINKELSTIN, R. A., NORRIS, H. T. and DUTTA, N. K. (1964) Pathogenesis of experimental cholera in infant rabbits. I. Observations on the intraintestinal injection and experimental cholera produced with cell free products. *J. Infect. Dis.* **114**: 203–216.

FUJITA, K. and FINKELSTEIN, R. A. (1972) Antitoxin immunity in experimental cholera: comparison of immunity induced perorally and parenterally in mice. *J. Infect. Dis.* **125**: 647–655.

GEARY, S. J., MARCHLEWICZ, B. A. and FINKELSTEIN, R. A. (1982) Comparison of heat-labile enterotoxins from porcine and human strains of *Escherichia coli*. *Infect. Immun.* **36**: 215–220.

GERMANIER, R., FURER, E., VARALLYAY, S. and INDERBITZIN, T. M. (1977) Antigenicity of cholera toxoid in humans. *J. Infect. Dis.* **135**: 512–516.

GREENOUGH, W. B., III, PIERCE, N. F., and VAUGHN, M. (1970) Titration of cholera enterotoxin and antitoxin in isolated fat cells. *J. Infect. Dis.* (Suppl.) **121**: S111–S113.

GYLES, C. L. (1974) Immunological study of the heat-labile enterotoxins of *Escherichia coli* and *Vibrio cholerae*. *Infect. Immun.* **9**: 564–570.

GYLES, C. L. and BARNUM, D. A. (1969) A heat-labile enterotoxin from strains of *Escherichia coli* enteropathogenic for pigs. *J. Infect. Dis.* **120**: 419–426.

HONDA, T. and FINKELSTEIN, R. A. (1979) Selection and characteristics of a *Vibrio cholerae* mutant lacking the A (ADP-ribosylating) portion of the cholera enterotoxin. *Proc. Natl. Acad. Sci. U.S.A.* **76**: 2052–2056.

KLIPSTEIN, F. A. and ENGERT, R. F. (1979) Protective effect of active immunization with purified *Escherichia coli* heat-labile enterotoxin in rats. *Infect. Immun.* **23**: 592–599.

KLIPSTEIN, F. A. and ENGERT, R. F. (1980) Influence of route of administration on immediate and extended protection in rats immunized with *Escherichia coli* heat-labile enterotoxin. *Infect. Immun.* **27**: 81–86.

KLIPSTEIN, F. A., ENGERT, R. F. and CLEMENTS, J. D. (1981) Immunization of rats with heat-labile enterotoxin provides uniform protection against heterologous serotypes of enterotoxigenic *Escherichia coli*. *Infect. Immun.* **32**: 1100–1104.

KLIPSTEIN, F. A., ENGERT, R. F. and CLEMENTS, J. D. (1982) Arousal of mucosal secretory immunoglobulin A antitoxin in rats immunized with *Escherichia coli* heat-labile enterotoxin. *Infect. Immun.* **37**: 1086–1092.

KLIPSTEIN, F. A., ENGERT, R. F. and SHERMAN, W. T. (1983) Peroral immunization of rats with *Escherichia coli* heat-labile enterotoxin delivered by microspheres. *Infect. Immun.* **39**: 1000–1003.

LEVINE, M. M., CAPLAN, E. S., WATERMAN, D., CASH, R. A., HORNICK, R. B. and SNYDER, M. J. (1977) Diarrhea caused by *Escherichia coli* that produce only heat-stable enterotoxin delivered by microspheres. *Infect. Immun.* **17**: 78–82.

LEVINE, M. M., HUGHES, T. P., YOUNG, C. R., O'DONNEL, S., CRAIG, J. P., HOLLY, H. P. and BERGQUIST, (1978) Antigenicity of purified glutaraldehyde-treated cholera toxoid administered orally. *Infect. Immun.* **21**: 158–162.

LEVINE, M. M., NALIN, D. M., HOOVER, D. L., BERGQUIST, E. J., HORNICK, R. B. and YOUNG, C. R. (1979) Immunity to enterotoxigenic *Escherichia coli*. *Infect. Immun.* **32**: 1–8.

LEVINE, M. M., YOUNG, C. R., HUGHES, T. P., O'DONNELL, S., BLACK, R. E., CLEMENTS, M. L., ROBINS–BROWNE, R. and LIM, Y.-L. (1981) Duration of serum antitoxin response following *Vibrio cholerae* infection in North Americans: relevance for seroepidemiology. *Am. J. Epidemiol.* **114**: 348–354.

MAJUMDAR, A. S., DUTTA, P., DUTTA, D. and GHOSE, A. C. (1981) Antibacterial and antitoxin responses in the serum and milk of cholera patients. *Infect. Immun.* **32**: 1–8.

MAJUMDAR, A. S. and GHOSE, A. C. (1981) Evaluation of the biological properties of different classes of human antibodies in relation to cholera. *Infect. Immun.* **32**: 9–14.

McGONAGLE, T. J., SEREBRO, H. H., BER, F. L., BAYLESS, T. M. and HENDRIX, T. R. (1969) Time of onset of cholera toxin in dog and rabbit. *Gastroenterology* **57**: 5–8.

MOSLEY, W. H. (1969) The role of immunity in cholera. A review of epidemiological and serological studies. *Texas Rep. Biol. Med.* (Suppl.) **27**: 227–241.

MOSLEY, W. H., WOODWARD, W. E., AZIZ, K. M. A., MIZANUR RAHMAN, A. S. M., ALAUDDIN CHOWDHURY, A. K. M., AHMED, A. and FEELEY, J. C. (1970) The 1968–1969 cholera-vaccine field trial in rural East Pakistan. Effectiveness of monovalent Ogawa and Inaba vaccines and a purified Inaba antigen, with comparative results of serological and animal protection tests. *J. Infect. Dis.* **121**: (Suppl.): S1–S9.

NORTHRUP, R. S. and CHISARI, F. V. (1972) Response of monkeys to immunization with cholera toxoid, toxin and vaccine: reversion of cholera toxoid. *J. Infect. Dis.* **125**: 471–479.

PETERSON, J. W. (1979) Synergistic protection against experimental cholera by immunization with cholera toxoid and vaccine. *Infect. Immun.* **26**: 528–533.

PIERCE, N. F. (1978) The role of antigen form and function in the primary and secondary intestinal immune response to cholera toxin and toxoid in rats. *J. Exp. Med.* **148**: 195–206.

PIERCE, N. F., CRAY, W. C., JR. and SIRCAR, B. K. (1978) Induction of a mucosal antitoxin response and its role in immunity to experimental canine cholera. *Infect. Immun.* **21**: 185–193.

RAPPAPORT, R. S. BONDE, G., McCANN, T., RUBIN, B. A. and TINT, H. (1974) Development of a purified cholera toxoid II. Preparation of a stable, antigenic toxoid by reaction of toxin with glutaraldehyde. *Infect. Immun.* **9**: 304–317.

SACK, R. B. (1973) Immunization with *Escherichia coli* enterotoxin protects against homologous enterotoxin challenge. *Infect. Immun.* **8**: 641–644.

SACK, R. B. and FROEHLICH, J. L. (1977) Antigenic similarity of heat-labile enterotoxins from diverse strains of *Escherichia coli*. *J. Clin. Microbiol.* **5**: 570–572.

SACK, D. A., KAMINSKY, D. C., SACK, R. B., ITOTIA, J. N., ARTHUR, R. R., KAPIKIAN, A. Z., ØRSKOV, F. and ØRSKOV, I. (1978) Prophylactic doxycycline for travelers' diarrhea. Results of a prospective double-blind study of Peace Corps volunteers in Kenya. *N. Eng. J. Med.* **298**: 758–763.

SALETTI, M. and RICCI, A. (1974). Experiments with cholera toxin detoxified with glutaraldehyde. *Bull. Wld. Hlth. Org.* **51**: 633–639.

SNYDER, J. D., ALLEGRA, D. T., LEVINE, M. M., CRAIG, J. P., FEELEY, J. C., DeWITT, W. E. and BLAKE, P. A. (1981) Serologic studies of naturally acquired infection with *Vibrio cholerae* serogroup 01 in the United States. *J. Infect. Dis.* **143**: 182–187.

SVENNERHOLM, A. M. and HOLMGREN, J. (1976) Synergistic protective effect in rabbits of immunization with *Vibrio cholerae* lipopolysaccharide and toxin/toxoid. *Infect. Immun.* **13**: 735–740.

THOMAS, L. V., CRAVIOTO, A., SCOTLAND, S. M. and ROWE, B. (1982) New fimbrial antigenic type (E8775) that may represent a colonization factor in enterotoxigenic *Escherichia coli* in humans. *Infect. Immun.* **35**: 1119–1124.

VAN HEYNINGEN, S. (1973) Cholera toxin: Interaction of subunits with ganglioside GMI. *Science* **183**: 656–657.

WACHSMUTH, I. K., FALKOW, S. and RYDER, R. W. (1976) Plasmid mediated properties of a heat-stable enterotoxin producing *Escherichia coli* associated with infantile diarrhea. *Infect. Immun.* **14**: 403–407.

WOOD, L. V., FERGUSSON, L. E., HOGAN, P., THURMAN, D., MORGAN, D. R., DuPONT, H. L. and ERICSSON, C. D. (1983a) Incidence of bacterial enteropathogens in food from Mexico. *Appl. Environ. Microbiol.* **46**: 328–332.

WOOD, L. V., WOLFE, W. H., RUIZ–PALACIOS, G., FOSHEE, W. S., CORMAN, L. I., McCLESKEY, F., WRIGHT, J. A. and DuPONT, H. L. (1983b) An outbreak of gastroenteritis due to a heat-labile enterotoxin (LT) producing strain of *Escherichia coli*. *Infect. Immun.* **41**: 931–934.

CHAPTER 8

CHOLERA ENTEROTOXIN (CHOLERAGEN)

Richard A. Finkelstein* and Friedrich Dorner†

*Department of Microbiology, School of Medicine, University of Missouri-Columbia, Columbia, Missouri 65212, U.S.A. and †Research Center Orth. Immuno A.G. Uferstraße 15, A 2304 Orth/Donau, Austria

1. HISTORY

The many reports and observations that have led to the current state of knowledge of cholera toxin have been summarized extensively elsewhere (Pollitzer, 1959; Finkelstein, 1973, 1975, 1976, 1981; Barua and Burrows, 1974; Bennett and Cuatrecasas, 1977; Gill, 1978; Moss and Vaughan, 1979; Ouchterlony and Holmgren, 1980, 1981; Giannella, 1981; Gill, 1982; S. van Heyningen, 1982; Moss and Vaughan, 1982; van Heyningen and Seal, 1983). For this reason this review will be confined primarily to a general description as well as a summary of recent progress in cholera research.

Cholera toxin was 'discovered' nearly 75 years after Koch's prediction, in the late 19th century (see Pollitzer, 1959), that cholera is a toxin-mediated disease. Reasonable data to support this prediction first became available in 1959 when two Indian researchers, working independently of one another, showed that cell-free preparations from *Vibrio cholerae* caused relevant symptomatology in animal models which they had developed (De, 1959; Dutta *et al.*, 1959). One model was the adult rabbit ligated ileal loop (De and Chatterje, 1953) which responded to sterile culture filtrates of an unidentified Ogawa serotype strain of *V. cholerae* with luminal fluid accumulation which suggested 'enterotoxicity' (De, 1959). The other model (Dutta and Habbu, 1955) was the infant rabbit which, when fed multiple doses of sterile lysates of heavy suspensions of the 569B Inaba strain of *V. cholerae* (Dutta *et al.*, 1959), responded with fatal choleraic diarrhea.

By 1964 it had been demonstrated that enterotoxic activity could be produced routinely and optimally by growing strain 569B Inaba with vigorous aeration in synthetic culture medium (Finkelstein and Lankford, 1955) supplemented with casamino acids (Finkelstein *et al.*, 1964). The putative cholera enterotoxin, which was shown not to be the cholera endotoxin, was then named choleragen—now an accepted synonym (Stedman's Medical Dictionary, 1972; Dorland's Medical Dictionary, 1974) for cholera toxin (CT) or cholera enterotoxin.

In subsequent years, as an outgrowth of basic research on cholera and the resulting increased understanding of its pathophysiology, a simple, economical and effective treatment regimen for diarrheal disease has been developed—oral rehydration therapy (ORT) (World Health Organization, 1983). Regarded as potentially the most important medical advance of the century, ORT will save countless millions of lives in the decade of the 1980s alone. However, completely satisfactory methods of preventing the disease or of interrupting its progress, when it occurs, remain to be developed.

2. PURIFICATION

Purification of cholera toxin to homogeneity was accomplished by 1969 using a sequence of $(NH_4)_2SO_4$ precipitation, ion exchange chromatography, and Agarose and Sephadex gel filtration chromatography (Finkelstein and LoSpalluto, 1969). During these studies, another product was isolated which, at first, appeared to be immunologically identical to choleragen but differed in size and charge, and did not have the biologic activity (toxicity) of choleragen. Both this material, called choleragenoid, and choleragen were successfully crystallized in 1972 (Finkelstein and LoSpalluto, 1972; Sigler *et al.*, 1977). A high molecular weight, relatively nontoxic polymer called 'procholeragenoid' has also been described (Finkelstein *et al.*, 1971). This material, produced by heating purified choleragen under certain conditions, is important in that it has been shown to be better than other forms of the toxin in inducing intestinal immunity (Fujita and Finkelstein, 1972). It is now clear that there are at least two immunologically related, but not completely identical, forms of cholera toxin (Finkelstein *et al.*, 1974b, 1984; Vasil *et al.*, 1974; Marchlewicz and Finkelstein, 1983) as well as a growing family of enterotoxins which are functionally, structurally and immunologically related to cholera toxin. Of these, the best known example is the heat-labile enterotoxin (LT) produced by *Escherichia coli* (Robertson *et al.*, 1986).

3. STRUCTURE

Choleragen is composed of two distinct species of subunits, called A and B, which are held in association by strong noncovalent forces (see Fig. 1). When separated, neither species has significant biological activity in animal models or intact cell systems. However, activity and normal properties of the holotoxin are recovered upon reassociation of the subunits (Finkelstein *et al.*, 1974a). The holotoxin contains five identical, non-covalently linked B subunits (each consisting of 103 amino acid residues with a total formula weight of 11,604) and one A subunit. The A subunit (MW ~28,000) consists of an A_1 peptide (MW 21,000–22,000) and an A_2 peptide (MW ~6,000) which are joined by a disulfide bond. The five non-covalently associated B subunits are responsible for specific binding of the holotoxin to receptors on target cell membranes which contain the oligosaccharide of the G_{M1} ganglioside. This pentamer of B subunits (which is synonymous to choler- agenoid) is also the portion of the cholera toxin molecule which is the predominant immunogen. The amino acid sequence of the B subunit is given in Fig. 2 (Kurosky *et al.*, 1977a; Kurosky *et al.*, 1977b; Lai, 1977). The A subunit amino acid sequence, derived from the nucleotide sequence of the cloned toxin operon, has been published recently (Mekalanos *et al.*, 1983).

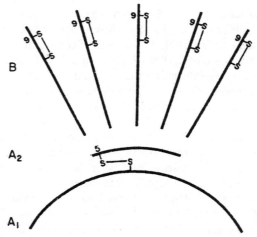

FIG. 1. Schematic representation of the molecular structure of the cholera enterotoxin (choleragen) (modified from Klapper *et al.*, *Immunochemistry* **13**: 605–611, 1976). The holotoxin is depicted as consisting of 5 identical noncovalently associated B subunits (MW ~ 11,500), which together constitute the choleragenoid or B-(binding) region (MW ~ 56,000) of the molecule, and a single A subunit (MW ~ 28,000) which consists of two fragments, A_1 (MW ~ 21,000) and A_2 (MW ~ 7,000), joined by a disulfide bond which is initiated at residue 5 from the amino terminus of the A_2 peptide. Of these, the A_1 peptide is responsible for the biological, i.e. enzymatic, activity of the enterotoxin, while the A_2 peptide is shown as providing the noncovalent link between the A and the B domains. Each B-subunit has an internal disulfide loop starting at position 9 and terminating at residue 86.

Thr Pro Gln Asn Ile⁵ Thr Asp Leu Cys Ala¹⁰ Glu Tyr His Asn Thr¹⁵ Gln Ile His Thr Leu²⁰

Asn Asn Lys Ile Phe²⁵ Ser Tyr Thr Glu Ser³⁰ Leu Ala Gly Lys Arg³⁵ Glu Met Ala Ile Ile⁴⁰

Thr Phe Lys Asn Gly⁴⁵ Ala Thr Phe Gln Val⁵⁰ Glu Val Pro Gly Ser⁵⁵ Gln His Ile Asp Ser⁶⁰

Gln Lys Lys Ala Ile⁶⁵ Glu Arg Met Lys Asn⁷⁰ Thr Leu Arg Ile Ala⁷⁵ Tyr Leu Thr Glu Ala⁸⁰

Lys Val Glu Lys Leu⁸⁵ Cys Val Trp Asn Asn⁹⁰ Lys Thr Pro His Ala⁹⁵ Ile Ala Ala Ile Ser¹⁰⁰

Met Ala Asn

FIG. 2. Amino acid sequence of the B subunit of cholera enterotoxin (CT). The sequence of CT-B is derived from A. Kurosky *et al.*, *J. Biol. Chem.* **252**: 7257–7264, 1977 and C.-Y. Lai, *Ibid*, pp. 7249–7256.

4. MODE OF ACTION

The A subunit is responsible for the biological activity of the molecule. It is an enzyme which is thought to be synthesized and secreted as a single protein (Gill and Rappaport, 1979), which is then nicked extracellularly by either trypsin-like enzymes (Mekalanos *et al.*, 1979) or possibly a specific *V. cholerae* protease (Finkelstein *et al.*, 1983) is homologous with, but not identical to, the analogous protein of the cholera-related heat-labile enterotoxin (LT) of *Escherichia coli* (Spicer and Noble, 1982; Spicer *et al.*, 1981). The A_1 portion of the holotoxin has been demonstrated, through studies with pigeon erythrocytes (Gill, 1982; Gill and King, 1975; Gill and Meren, 1978), to be the moiety responsible for the biological activity (see below) of cholera toxin. The function of the A_2 subunit appears to be confined to linking the A protomer to the B subunits. Reduction of nicked toxin in the presence of urea frees A_1 and results in an A_2–$B_{(5)}$ complex (Mekalanos *et al.*, 1979; Sattler *et al.*, 1975).

Cholera vibrios manage, through apparently complex mechanisms which may involve motility (Guentzel and Berry, 1975; Eubanks *et al.*, 1976; Yancey *et al.*, 1979; Attridge and Rowley, 1983), chemotactic activity (Freter *et al.*, 1981a; Freter *et al.*, 1981b), mucinase and possibly fibronectinase (Finkelstein *et al.*, 1983), and other possible factors (Hanne and Finkelstein, 1982), to evade the normally effective host defenses to colonize the surface small bowel without invading the tissue. During the resultant adhesion of the vibrios to gut epithelial cells (Nelson *et al.*, 1976), the cholera enterotoxin is assembled and secreted, binds to specific receptors on the epithelial cell membranes, is internalized, and finally exerts its biological activity. The net result is hypersecretion of Cl^-, CHO_3^- and water, which define the copious watery stools characteristic of cholera.

While most cholera toxin produced by *V. cholerae* is secreted (Holmes *et al.*, 1975), not much is known about the synthesis and assembly of the molecule by the bacterial cells. Interestingly, and in contrast to the situation in *E. coli*, when the *E. coli* enterotoxin plasmid is transferred into *V. cholerae*, the *E. coli* LT is also secreted by *V. cholerae* (Neill *et al.*, 1983). Thus *V. cholerae* is an unusual Gram-negative bacterium in terms of its ability to export proteins through the cell envelope. Also, in contrast to *E. coli* the genes which encode cholera toxin synthesis are located on the bacterial chromosome (Vasil *et al.*, 1975; Pearson and Mekalanos, 1982). Like the A subunits, the B subunits of the *E. coli* LTs are homologous with, but not identical to the B subunits of the cholera enterotoxin (Dallas and Falkow, 1980; Clements *et al.*, 1980; Geary *et al.*, 1982; Mekalanos *et al.*, 1983; Finkelstein *et al.*, 1984).

The genes are arranged in a single transcriptional unit with the A cistron (*ctx* A) preceding the B cistron (*ctx* B). *V. cholerae* strains of the classical biotype contain a non-tandem duplication of the *ctx* operon while most El Tor biotype strains have only a single copy (Mekalanos *et al.*, 1983). The molar ratio of synthesis of A and B subunits is unknown. The ratio of five B subunits for each A subunit in the holotoxin would suggest a different efficiency of expression of *ctx* A and *ctx* B. However, excess A subunits have been reported to be found in the bacterial cytosol (Gill and Rappaport, 1979; Ohtomo *et al.*, 1978). It is likely that both A and B subunits are generated through processing of larger precursor polypeptides (Fernandes *et al.*, 1979; Nichols *et al.*, 1980; Mekalanos *et al.*, 1983) containing hydrophobic, amino-terminal signal sequences.

However produced and secreted, once outside the vibrios, the cholera toxin must bind to specific receptors for activity to be expressed. The binding properties of choleragenoid (B region) are indistinguishable from those of holotoxin (Bennett and Cuatrecasas, 1977; LeVine and Cuatrecasas, 1981; van Heyningen and Seal, 1983), and, in fact, pretreatment of target cells with choleragenoid prevents further binding by holotoxin (Pierce, 1973). The cell receptors contain the G_{M1} ganglioside (GGnSLC) (Cuatrecasas, 1973; Holmgren *et al.*, 1973; van Heyningen and Seal, 1983). More precisely, it is the oligosaccharide portion of the ganglioside to which the toxin binds and a good correlation exists between G_{M1} content and binding ability of cells (Hollenberg *et al.*, 1974; Holmgren *et al.*, 1975; Moss *et al.*, 1976; Moss and Vaughan, 1979; LeVine and Cuatrecasas, 1981). Some evidence has implicated galactose-containing glycoproteins as possible receptors for cholera toxin (Morita *et al.*, 1980) but these do not appear to play a significant role (Critchley *et al.*, 1981; Critchley *et al.*, 1982). While cholera toxin normally has direct access in nature only to human intestinal epithelial cells, the ubiquity of G_{M1} ganglioside on the surface of other mammalian (and some other eucaryotic) cells has enabled the toxin to serve as an excellent experimental tool for studying cAMP-mediated reactions in a wide variety of cell systems (Finkelstein, 1973, 1976; Bennett and Cuatrecasas, 1977). Because of the nature of the biological activity of the toxin at least a portion of the molecule must penetrate the cytoplasmic membrane of the target cells (Gill, 1978, 1982; Moss and Vaughan, 1979). The oligomeric B subunits bind multivalently to G_{M1} which may facilitate entry of the A subunit (or A_1 peptide). Binding has been reported to result in increased glucose permeability, membrane conductance and channel formation in synthetic lipid bilayers (Moss *et al.*, 1977; Tosteson *et al.*, 1980). The A subunit is presumed to be available for entry through prior nicking (by either vibrio or host proteases) and separation from $A_2-B_{(5)}$ by reduction of the disulfide bond (Moss and Vaughan, 1979; Gill, 1982). Further observations which support the concept of binding followed by penetration and activity are: (a) the known binding activity, (b) the lag that exists between exposure of whole cells to intact cholera toxin and the resultant activity as contrasted to the immediate onset of activity in lysed cells which are exposed to the toxin and (c) the dependence of activity on internal host cell factors such as NAD and ATP (Gill, 1982). It has been suggested recently that the entire toxin molecule may enter the cell (Tsuru *et al.*, 1982; Fishman, 1982).

Cholera toxin was first shown to mimic the action of certain hormones by stimulating cAMP-mediated lipolysis in rat epididymal fat cells (Vaughan *et al.*, 1970; Greenough III *et al.*, 1970), and causing elevated levels of cAMP in intestinal epithelial cells from animals or humans exposed to cholera toxin (Schafer *et al.*, 1970; Sharp and Hynie, 1971; Chen *et al.*, 1971). Since these early studies it has been shown that every cell type examined which contains membrane G_{M1} responds to cholera toxin with an increase in adenylate cyclase activity (Finkelstein, 1973; Finkelstein, 1976; Bennett and Cuatrecasas, 1977). This elevation occurs via enzymatic transfer of ADP-ribose from NAD to a regulatory protein (RP) component of the cyclase complex as shown in the following equation:

$$NAD^+ + RP \overset{CT}{\rightleftharpoons} ADP\text{-ribosyl-RP} + nicotinamide + H^+$$

The regulatory protein, identified variously by the symbols 'N' (for the nucleotide binding), 'G' (binding of guanyl nucleotides) of 'G/F' (because cyclase activation is mediated by fluoride ions), has been reported to be a peptide of MW $\sim$42,000 (Gill, 1982). Activation of cyclase occurs when GTP is bound to the regulatory protein, while hydrolysis of the bound GTP results in the loss of cyclase activity. The formation of RP-GTP is increased by hormones, thereby activating adenylate cyclase, while ADP-ribosylation of RP reduces the hydrolysis to RP-GDP and thus locks the system in its 'on' mode (Gill, 1982).

Both NAD^+ hydrolase and ADP-ribosyltransferase activities are attributable to the A_1 subunit of choleragen. It has been found that arginine and other guanidino derivatives act as acceptors of ADP-ribose though the precise location of the RP has not yet been identified (Moss and Vaughan, 1979).

The events, after elevation of levels of cAMP, which lead to hypersecretion of Cl^- and HCO_3^- by intestinal crypt cells are undefined at this time. Further elucidation of these events could aid in the development of antisecretory drugs, such as chlorpromazine or by inhibiting or reversing some event in the cAMP-regulated subsequent cascade. These could be very useful for treatment of cholera and related secretory diarrheas (Holmgren, 1981).

It should be noted that other toxins have been shown to act via mechanisms similar to that of cholera toxin. Of these, most closely related are the *E. coli* heat-labile enterotoxins (LTs) which are very similar structurally, functionally and immunologically to cholera toxin. Diphtheria toxin and *Pseudomonas aeruginosa* exotoxin A, while synthesized as single peptide chains, are also activated by proteolytic nicking to form active A and binding B subunits and enzymatically transfer ADP-ribose from NAD to an acceptor protein (Thompson and Iglewski, 1982; Uchida, 1983). In these cases, the acceptor protein is elongation factor 2 (EF2) and their activity, unlike that of cholera toxin, results in cell death through inhibition of protein synthesis.

5. IMMUNITY

While parenterally adminstered, killed *V. cholerae* vaccines have been in use since the late 1800's, rigid scientifically controlled field studies of the efficacy of these vaccines were not carried out prior to the 1960's. The unfortunate conclusions from these studies (Joó, 1974; Finkelstein, 1975, 1981; Felley and Gangarosa, 1980) was that what little protection these whole cell (or vibrio lipopolysaccharide somatic antigen) vaccines afforded was also short lived. The most optimistic results were derived from studies in heavily endemic regions where the vaccines were likely serving merely as boosters of pre-existing, naturally acquired immunity. Most enlightened countries have now discontinued recommending or requiring the use of such 'conventional' cholera vaccines.

Large numbers of studies in animals have indicated that cholera antitoxin was protective and that various forms of cholera toxin antigens could serve as effective vaccines against experimental cholera (Finkelstein, 1975; Finkelstein, 1981). While the concept of antitoxic immunity in cholera is a reasonable one, especially in light of earlier successes with toxoid vaccines against diphtheria and tetanus, progress along these lines in humans has, thus far, been disappointing.

Complete detoxification of cholera toxin can be achieved by formaldehyde treatment but subsequent delayed reversion to toxicity has been enough of a problem to cause abandonment of large scale studies with such material in humans (Northrup and Chisari, 1972). A stably detoxified material can be produced by treating toxin with formalin in the presence of glycine, but, while it has been found to be antigenic, it has not been found to be immunogenic (that is, to prevent cholera disease) (Ohtomo, 1977; Noriki, 1977). A glutaraldehyde toxoid has been studied as well (Rappaport *et al.*, 1974) but was found to induce significant protection for only 24 weeks. After one year, protection was only in the range of 26% (Curlin *et al.*, 1976).

Cholera, the disease, is itself an immunizing process as indicated by both epidemiological evidence and by studies in volunteers. In heavily endemic areas, the highest incidence of disease is in children. The increase with age of a serum vibiocidal titer [primarily antibody against somatic lipopolysaccharide antigens (Finkelstein, 162)] is correlated with the decreasing incidence in older people (Mosley, 1969). And, volunteers who have convalesced from cholera, of either serotype, have been shown to be entirely resistant for at least three years to later challenge with heterologous or homologous serotype of biotype cholera vibrios (Levine *et al.*, 1981).

During the disease, the affected host is presented with all the products of the cholera vibrios (the enterotoxin, lipopolysaccharide, flagella, colonization factors, membrane proteins and other surface and extracellular factors) at the local level which should induce a maximal secretory IgA immune response. This information, coupled with the disappointing results of trials to induce immunity by the parenteral route, has led investigators to attempt to duplicate the effective immunity which results from the disease by peroral administration of various *V. cholerae* antigens.

Multiple doses of killed whole cell vibrios vaccines administered perorally have been shown (Freter and Gangarosa, 1963) to induce detectable intestinal and serum antibody titers. While a similar approach (Cash *et al.*, 1974) resulted in significant protection against subsequent homologous strain challenge in volunteers, the protection achieved was not equivalent to that provided by either parenterally administered vaccine or previous disease. However, these results should be kept in mind since they may indicate the feasibility (even if not necessarily the practicality) of oral immunization against cholera.

Choleragenoid, the nontoxic but immunologically dominant B region of cholera toxin first identified as a spontaneous by-product during toxin purification (Finkelstein and LoSpalluto, 1969; Finkelstein and LoSpalluto, 1970), can also be prepared from the holotoxin by mild acid treatment in urea (Finkelstein *et al.*, 1974a) or guanidine (Klapper *et al.*, 1976), by formic acid (Lai, 1980), or by cation exchange chromatography (Mekalanos *et al.*, 1978).

Since its discovery (Finkelstein and LoSpalluto, 1969), choleragenoid has been regarded as a promising candidate vaccine against cholera and it was soon found to induce immunity in rabbits (Finkelstein, 1970). However it was also reported to be an 'erratic' antigen in rats (Finkelstein and Hollingsworth, 1970). Nevertheless it has been shown to be immunogenic through parenteral or peroral administration in mice (Fujita and Finkelstein, 1972) and dogs (Pierce *et al.*, 1982, 1983), though it is generally less effective than crude culture filtrates, purified cholera toxin, or procholeragenoid (see also Holmgren, 1973). It is possible that the A subunit may be necessary for an adjuvant effect. The cholera holotoxin has been reported to be either an adjuvant or an immunosuppressant depending on the dose and time of administration (Finkelstein, 1981). Despite its relatively poor immunogenicity when separated from the A subunit, consideration has been given to using the B region of cholera toxin orally (Svennerholm *et al.*, 1983), and it has been noted that, in people in heavily endemic areas, peroral doses of 2.5 mg of choleragenoid induced a SIgA antibody response (Svennerholm *et al.*, 1983).

Although the mechanism is not clear, experimental evidence indicates that combination of enterotoxin antigen and lipopolysaccharide (LPS) somatic antigen (even from *E. coli*) may provide a synergistic protective effect (Svennerholm and Holmgren, 1976; Peterson, 1979a; Rappaport and Bonde, 1981) and a combination of such antigens, to be administered perorally, has been advocated (Svennerholm *et al.*, 1983). If such synergistic effects can be duplicated in humans, it should be recognized that such a vaccine could be quite expensive since, under present optimal conditions, nearly 250 ml of *V. cholerae* culture filtrate would be required to yield 2.5 mg of the purified antigen, and large doses of killed vibrios (or LPS) are also required.

Procholeragenoid (Finkelstein *et al.*, 1971) has been demonstrated to be a superior parenteral immunogen to other forms of cholera toxin antigen in mice and rabbits (Fujita and Finkelstein, 1972; Peterson, 1979a, b). Substantial immunity to enteric challenge with live vibrios can also be induced by peroral administration of procholeragenoid. When residual toxicity in procholeragenoid is reduced by formaldehyde it remains at least as effective as cholera toxin in inducing antitoxic antibodies (Germanier *et al.*, 1976) and it has been shown to protect swine against colibacillosis (Fürer *et al.*, 1983). Recently it has been proposed that procholeragenoid be combined with a whole cell oral vaccine (Pierce *et al.*, 1983) and trials with volunteers currently are under way using both whole cells and choleragenoid, as well as whole cells and procholeragenoid (M. M. Levine, personal communication).

Avirulent O group I *V. cholerae* strains isolated from the environment have been suggested and tested in animal models and humans as live vaccines (Mukerjee, 1963; Sanyal and Mukerjee, 1969; Cash *et al.*, 1974b; Levine *et al.*, 1982) but have proven ineffective in colonization or inducing immunity. A hypotoxigenic mutant strain (M-13; Finkelstein *et al.*, 1974b), which was found to be harmless in volunteers, did lead to substantial immunity against challenge with the virulent parent strain (Woodward *et al.*, 1976). However, potential of reversion to virulence limited further consideration of the use of that strain.

Another avirulent mutant, the Texas Star-SR (SR = streptomycin resistant) mutant strain which produces choleragenoid but not choleragen ($A^- B^+$ mutant) (Honda and Finkelstein, 1979), when administered intraintestinally into rabbits resulted in highly significant immunity against challenge by live virulent *V. cholerae* (Boesman-Finkelstein and Finkelstein, 1982). Highly significant protection against virulent challenge was also observed in human volunteer studies (Levine *et al.*, 1983). But, this vaccine strain, although apparently stably nontoxigenic, was observed to cause one or more (mild and non-inconveniencing) loose stools in 24% of the recipients regardless of the dose administered over the extreme range of 10^5 through 5×10^{10} live vibrios. The worst case of this side effect was in an individual who received the lowest dose of vaccine and who passed six stools, totaling less than 1500 ml, over a two day period. The latter observations may imply that the mere act of intestinal colonization can in itself elicit a diarrheal response in some people. It is conceivable that this side effect is the price that must be paid for an economical and effective vaccine against cholera.

Recent advances in recombinant DNA technology have enabled the construction of *V. cholerae* mutants with clear-cut deletions of the entire toxin, or of the A, gene (Kaper and Levine, 1981; Pearson and Mekalanos, 1982; Mekalanos *et al.*, 1983). Further work with these and other mutants which could be developed hopefully will enable an understanding the role of enterotoxin and of other antigens in inducing immunity to cholera and could result in an economical and effective vaccine with minimal and acceptable side effects. In this connection, it should be mentioned that the best protection yet obtained has been that provided by the living cholera vibrios growing *in vivo*. Recent evidence indicates that *in vivo*-grown *V. cholerae* express novel outer membrane proteins which could contribute to immunity (Sciortino and Finkelstein, 1983).

6. CONCLUSION

The intent of this article has been to summarize the recent research which continues to develop a more precise understanding of the cholera toxin molecule and its mode of action. The pathogenesis of cholera is today probably better understood than that of any other infectious disease. During the past decade and a half the toxin has been purified, its subunit structure defined, its cell membrane receptor identified, and its effect on cell function explained in considerable detail. In addition to illuminating the mechanism of the disease, cholera toxin research has provided important stimulation to studies dealing with other enterotoxin-mediated diseases. Concepts and methodologies elaborated for cholera toxin have proven to be very useful for research and other enterotoxins. Furthermore, by virtue of its specific ability to activate adenylate cyclase in all mammalian cells, cholera toxin has become an important experimental tool for studying the adenylate cyclase system in the wide variety of tissues which contain membrane G_{M1}.

Although more specific and immediate remedies or antidotes remain to be developed and applied, the understanding of the pathophysiology of cholera has led to an unexpected reward of incredible value—oral rehydration therapy—a practical treatment for diarrheal disease which will save millions of lives, particularly of children, annually.

Unfortunately, only rudimentary knowledge has yet been obtained of effective prevention of cholera, though current studies offer promise for the development of useful and practical methods for the prevention of cholera and related diarrheal disease.

Acknowledgement—Observations in the laboratory of one of the authors (R. A. Finkelstein) reported herein were supported in part by U.S. Public Health Service grants AI-16776 andAI-17312 from the (U.S.) National Institute of Allergy and Infectious Diseases.

REFERENCES

ATTRIDGE, S. R. and ROWLEY, D. (1983) The role of the flagellum in the adherence of *Vibrio cholerae*. *J. Infect. Dis.* **147**: 864–872.

BARUA, D. and BURROWS, W. (eds) (1974) *Cholera*. Saunders, W. B. Co.

BENNETT, V. and CUATRECASAS. P. (1977) Cholera Toxin: Membrane gangliosides and activation of adenylate cyclase. In: *The Specificity and Action of Animal, Bacterial and Plant Toxins* pp. 3–66, Chapman and Hall. London.

BOESMAN-FINKELSTEIN, M. and FINKELSTEIN, R. A. (1982) Protection in rabbits induced by the Texas Star-SR attenuated A⁻B⁺ mutant candidate live oral cholera vaccine. *Infect. Immunol.* **36**: 221–226.

CASH, R. A., MUSIC, S. I., LIBONATI, J. P., CRAIG, J. P., PIERCE, N. F. and HORNICK, R. B. (1974) Response of man to infection with *Vibrio cholerae*. II. Protection from illness afforded by previous disease and vaccine. *J. Infect. Dis.* **130**: 325–333.

CASH, R. A., MUSIC, S. I., LIBONATI, J. P., SCHWARTZ, A. R. and HORNICK, R. B. (1974b) Live oral cholera vaccine: Evaluation of the clinical effectiveness of two strains in humans. *Infect. Immunol.* **10**: 762–764.

CHEN, L. C., ROHDE, J. E. and SHARP, G. W. G. (1971) Intestinal adenyl-cyclase activity in human cholera. *Lancet* i: 939–941.

CLEMENTS. J. D., YANCEY, R. J. and FINKELSTEIN, R. A. (1980) Properties of homogeneous heat-labile enterotoxin(s) [LT(s)] with high specific activity from *Escherichia coli* cultures. *Infect. Immunol.* **24**: 760–769.

CRITCHLEY, D. R., MAGNANI, J. L. and FISHMAN, P. H. (1981) Interaction of cholera toxin with rat intestinal brush border membranes. Relative roles of gangliosides and galactoproteins as toxin receptors. *J. biol. Chem.* **256**: 8724–8731.

CRITCHLEY, D. R., STREULI, C. H., KELLIE, S., ANSELL, S. and PATEL, B. (1982) Characterization of the cholera toxin receptor on Balb/c 3T3 cells as a ganglioside similar to, or identical with, ganglioside G_{M1}. No evidence for galactoproteins with receptor activity. *Biochem. J.* **204**: 209–219.

CUATRECASAS, P. (1973) Gangliosides and membrane receptors for cholera toxin. *Biochemistry* **12**: 3558–3566.

CURLIN, G., LEVINE, R., AZIZ, K. M. A., RAHMAN, A. S. M. M. and VERWEY, W. F. (1976) Field trial of cholera toxoid. *Proceedings of the 11th Joint Conference on Cholera*, pp. 314–329. U.S.–Japan Cooperative Medical Science Program, New Orleans, 1975, National Institutes of Health.

DALLAS, W. S. and FALKOW, S. (1980) Amino acid sequence homology between cholera toxin and *Escherichia coli* heat-labile toxin. *Nature* **288**: 499–501.

DE, S. N. (1959) Enterotoxicity of bacteria-free culture filtrate of *Vibrio cholerae*. *Nature* **183**: 1533–1534.

DE, S. N. and CHATTERJE, D. N. (1953) An experimental study of the mechanism of action of *Vibrio cholerae* on the intestinal mucous membrane. *J. Path. Bacteriol.* **66**: 559–562.

DORLAND'S MEDICAL DICTIONARY (1974) 25th Edition, Saunders, W. B.

DUTTA, N. K. and HABBU. M. K. (1955) Experimental cholera in infant rabbits: A method for chemotherapeutic investigation. *Br. J. Pharmac. Chemother.* **10**: 153–159.

DUTTA, N. K., PANSE, M. W. and KULKARNI, P. R. (1959) Role of cholera toxin in experimental cholera. *J. Bacteriol.* **78**: 594–595.

EUBANKS, E. R., GUENTZEL, M. N. and BERRY, L. J. (1976) Virulence factors involved in the intraperitoneal infection of adult mice with *Vibrio cholerae*. *Infect. Immun.* **13**: 457–463.

FEELEY, J. C. and GANGAROSA, E. J. (1980) Field trial of cholera vaccine. In: *Cholera and Related Diarrheas*, pp. 204–210. OUCHTERLONY, O. and HOLMGREN, J. (eds) Karger, Basel.

FERNANDES, P. B., WELSH, K. M. and BAYER, M. E. (1979) Characterization of membrane-bound nicotinamide adenine dinucleotide glycohydrolase of *Vibrio cholerae*. *J. biol. Chem.* **254**: 9254–9261.

FINKELSTEIN, R. A. (1962) Vibriocidal antibody inhibition (VAI) analysis: a technique for the identification of the predominant vibriocidal antibodies in serum and for the recognition and identification of *Vibrio cholerae* antigens. *J. Immunol.* **89**: 264–271.

FINKELSTEIN, R. A. (1970) Antitoxic immunity in experimental cholera: observations with purified antigens and the ligated ileal loop model. *Infect. Immun.* **1**: 464–467.

FINKELSTEIN, R. A. (1973) Cholera. *CRC crit. Rev. Microbiol.* **2**: 553–623.

FINKELSTEIN, R. A. (1975) Immunology of cholera. *Curr. Top. Microbiol. Immunol.* **69**: 137–196.

FINKELSTEIN, R. A. (1976) Progress in the study of cholera and related enterotoxins. In: *Mechanisms in Bacterial Toxinology*, pp. 53–84, BERNHEIMER, A. (ed.) John Wiley and Sons, New York.

FINKELSTEIN, R. A. (1981) Immunology of *Vibrio cholerae*. In: *Comprehensive Immunology (series): Immunology of Human Infections*, pp. 291–315. NAHMIAS, A. J. and O'REILLY, R. J. (eds) Plenum Publishing Corp., New York.

FINKELSTEIN, R. A., BOESMAN-FINKELSTEIN, M. and HOLT, P. (1983) *Vibrio cholerae* hemagglutinin/lectin/protease hydrolyzes fibronectin and ovomucin: F. M. Burnet revisited. *Proc. natnl. Acad. Sci. U.S.A.* **80**: 1092–1095.

FINKELSTEIN, R. A., BOESMAN, M., NEOH, S. H., LARUE, M. K. and DELANEY, R. (1974a) Dissociation and recombination of the subunits of the cholera enterotoxin (choleragen). *J. Immunol.* **113**: 145–150.

FINKELSTEIN, R. A., BURKS, M. F., RIEKE, L. C., MCDONALD, R. J., BROWNE, S. K. and DALLAS, W. S. (1984) Application of monoclonal antibodies and genetically-engineered hybrid B-subunit proteins to the analysis of the cholera/coli enterotoxin family. *Dev. Biol. Stand.* in press.

FINKELSTEIN, R. A., FUJITA, K. and LoSPALLUTO, J. J. (1971) Procholeragenoid: An aggregated intermediate in the formation of choleragenoid. *J. Immunol.* **107**: 1043–1051.

FINKELSTEIN, R. A. and HOLLINGSWORTH, R. C. (1970) Antitoxic immunity in experimental cholera: observations with purified antigens and the rat foot edema model. *Infect. Immun.* **1**: 468–473.

FINKELSTEIN, R. A. and LANKFORD, C. E. (1955) Nutrient requirements of *Vibrio cholerae*. *Bacteriol. Proc.* **1955**: 49.

FINKELSTEIN, R. A. and LoSPALLUTO, J. J. (1969) Pathogenesis of experimental cholera: Preparation and isolation of choleragen and choleragenoid. *J. exp. Med.* **130**: 185–202.

FINKELSTEIN, R. A. and LoSPALLUTO, J. J. (1970) Production of highly purified choleragen and choleragenoid. *J. Infect. Dis.* **121** (Suppl.): S63–S72.

FINKELSTEIN, R. A. and LoSPALLUTO, J. J. (1972) Crystalline cholera toxin and toxoid. *Science* **175**: 529–530.

FINKELSTEIN, R. A., NORRIS, H. T. and DUTTA, N. K. (1964) Pathogenesis of experimental cholera in infant rabbits. I. Observations on the intraintestinal infection and experimental cholera produced with cellfree products. *J. Infect. Dis.* **114**: 203–226.

FINKELSTEIN, R. A., VASIL, M. L. and HOLMES, R. K. (1974b) Studies on toxinogenesis in *Vibrio cholerae*. I. Isolation of mutants with altered toxinogenicity. *J. Infect. Dis.* **129**: 117–123.

FISHMAN, P. H. (1982) Internalization and degradation of cholera toxin by cultured cells: relationship to toxin action. *J. cell. Biol.* **93**: 860–865.

FRETER, R., ALLWEISS, B., O'BRIEN, P. C. M., HALSTEAD, S. A. and MACSAI, M. S. (1981a) Role of chemotaxis in the association of motile bacteria with intestinal mucosa: In vitro studies. *Infect. Immun.* **34**: 241–249.

FRETER, R. and GANGAROSA, E. J. (1963) Oral immunization and production of coproantibody in human volunteers. *J. Immunol.* **91**: 724–729.

FRETER, R., O'BRIEN, P. C. M. and MACSAI, M. S. (1981b) Role of chemotaxis in the association of motile bacteria with intestinal mucosa: In vivo studies. *Infect. Immun.* **34**: 234–240.

FUJITA, K. and FINKELSTEIN, R. A. (1972) Antitoxic immunity in experimental cholera: Comparison of immunity induced perorally and parenterally in mice. *J. Infect. Dis.* **125**: 647–655.

FÜRER, E., CRYZ, S. J., JR. and GERMANIER, R. (1983) Protection of piglets against neonatal colibacillosis based on antitoxic immunity. *Dev. Biol. Stand.* **53**: 161–167.

GEARY, S. J., MARCHLEWICZ, B. A. and FINKELSTEIN, R. A. (1982) Comparisons of heat-labile enterotoxins from porcine and human strains of *Escherichia coli*. *Infect. Immun.* **36**: 215–220.

GERMANIER, R., FÜRER, E., VARALLYAY, S. and INDERBITZEN, T. M. (1976) Preparation of a purified antigenic cholera toxoid. *Infect. Immun.* **13**: 1692–1698.

GIANNELLA, R. A. (1981) pathogenesis of acute bacterial diarrheal disorders. *A. Rev. Med.* **32**: 341–357.

GILL, D. M. (1978) Seven toxic peptides that cross cell membranes. In: *Bacterial Toxins and Cell Membranes*, pp. 291–332, JELJASZEWICZ, J. and WADSTRÖM, T. (eds) Academic Press, London.

GILL, D. M. (1982) Cholera toxin-catalyzed ADP-ribosylation of membrane proteins. In: *ADP Ribosylation Reactions Biology and Medicine*, pp. 593–621, HAYAISHI, O. and UEDA, K. (eds) Academic Press, New York.

GILL, D. M. and KING, C. A. (1975) The mechanism of action of cholera toxin in pigeon erythrocyte lysates. *J. biol. Chem.* **250**: 6424–6432.

GILL, D. M. and MEREN, R. (1978) ADP-ribosylation of membrane proteins catalyzed by cholera toxin: Basis of the activation of adenylate cyclase. *Proc. natn. Acad. Sci. U.S.A.* **75**: 3050–3054.

GILL, D. M. and RAPPAPORT, R. S. (1976) Origin of the enzymatically ative A$_1$ fragment of cholera toxin. *J. Infect. Dis.* **139**: 674–680.

GREENOUGH III, W. B., PIERCE, N. F. and VAUGHAN, M. (1970) Titration of cholera enterotoxin and antitoxin in isolated fat cells. *J. Infect. Dis.* **121** (Suppl.): S111–S113.

GUENTZEL, M. N. and BERRY, L. J. (1975) Motility as a virulence factor for *Vibrio cholerae*. *Infect. Immun.* **11**: 890–897.

HANNE, L. F. and FINKELSTEIN, R. A. (1982) Characterization and distribution of the hemagglutinins produced by *Vibrio cholerae*. *Infect. Immun.* **36**: 209–214.

HOLLENBERG, M. D., FISHMAN, P. H., BENNETT, V. and CUATRECASAS, P. (1974) Cholera toxin and cell growth: role of membrane gangliosides. *Proc. natn. Acad. Sci. U.S.A.* **71**: 4224–4228.

HOLMES, R. K., VASIL, M. L. and FINKELSTEIN, R. A. (1975) Studies on toxinogenesis in *Vibrio cholerae*. III. Characterization of nontoxinogenic mutants in vitro and in experimental animals. *J. clin. Invest.* **55**: 551–560.

HOLMGREN, J. (1973) Experimental studies on cholera immunization: the protective immunogenicity in rabbits of monomeric and polymeric crude exotoxin. *J. Med. Microbiol.* **6**: 363–370.

HOLMGREN, J. (1981) Actions of cholera toxin and the prevention and treatment of cholera. *Nature* **292**: 413–417.

HOLMGREN, J., LÖNNROTH, I., MANSSON, J.-E. and SVENNERHOLM, L. (1975) Interaction of cholera toxin and membrane G$_{M1}$ ganglioside of small intestine. *Proc. natn. Acad. Sci. U.S.A.* **72**: 2520–2524.

HOLMGREN, J., LÖNNROTH, I. and SVENNERHOLM, L. (1973) Fixation and inactivation of cholera toxin by G$_{M1}$ ganglioside. *Scand. J. Infect. Dis.* **5**: 77–78.

HONDA, T. and FINKELSTEIN, R. A. (1979) Selection and characteristics of a novel *Vibrio cholerae* mutant lacking the A (ADP-ribosylating) portion of the cholera enterotoxin. *Proc. natn. Acad. Sci. U.S.A.* **76**: 2052–2056.

JOÓ, I. (1974) Cholera vaccines. In *Cholera*, pp. 333–355, BARUA, D. and BURROWS, W. (eds) Saunders.

KAPER, J. B. and LEVINE, M. M. (1981) Cloned cholera enterotoxin genes in study and prevention of cholera. *Lancet* **88**: 1162–1163.

KLAPPER, D. G., FINKELSTEIN, R. A. and CAPRA, J. D. (1976) Subunit structure and N-terminal amino acid sequence of the three chains of cholera enterotoxin. *Immunochemistry* **13**: 605–611.

KUROSKY, A., MARKEL, D. E. and PETERSON, J. W. (1977a) Covalent structure of the β chain of cholera enterotoxin. *J. biol. Chem.* **252**: 7257–7264.

KUROSKY, A., MARKEL, D. E., PETERSON, J. W. and FITCH, W. M. (1977b) Primary structure of cholera toxin β-chain: A glycoprotein hormone analog? *Science* **195**: 2299–2301.

LAI, C.-Y. (1977) Determination of the primary structure of cholera toxin B subunit. *J. biol. Chem.* **252**: 7249–7256.

LAI, C.-Y. (1980) The chemistry and biology of cholera toxin. *CRC Crit. Rev. Biochem.* **9**: 171–206.

LEVINE, M. M., BLACK, R. E., CLEMENTS, M. L., CISNEROS, L., NALIN, D. R. and YOUNG, C. R. (1981) Duration of infection-derived immunity to cholera. *J. Infect. Dis.* **143**: 818–820.

LEVINE, M. M., BLACK, R. E., CLEMENTS, M. L., CISNEROS, L., SAAH, A., NALIN, D. R., GILL, D. M., CRAIG, J. P., YOUNG, C. R. and RISTAINO, P. (1982) The pathogenicity of nonenterotoxigenic *Vibrio cholerae* serogroup 01 Biotype El Tor isolated from sewage water in Brazil. *J. infect. Dis.* **145**: 296–299.

LEVINE, M. M., BLACK, R. E., CLEMENTS, M. L., YOUNG, C. R., LANATA, C., SEARS, S., HONDA, T. and FINKELSTEIN, R. A. (1983) Texas Star-SR: attenuated *Vibrio cholerae* oral vaccine candidate. *Dev. Biol. Stand.* **53**: 59–65.

LEVINE, H. and CUATRACASAS, P. (1981) An overview of toxin-receptor interactions. *Pharmac. Ther.* **12**: 167–207.

MARCHLEWICZ, B. A. and FINKELSTEIN, R. A. (1983) Immunologic differences among the cholera/coli family of enterotoxins. *Diag. Microbiol. Infect. Dis.* **1**: 129–138.

MEKALANOS, J. J., COLLIER, R. J. and ROMIG, W. R. (1978) Purification of cholera toxin and its subunits: new methods of preparation and the use of hypertoxinogenic mutants. *Infect. Immun.* **20**: 552–558.

MEKALANOS, J. J., COLLIER, R. J. and ROMIG, W. R. (1979) Enzymic activity of cholera toxin. II. Relationships to proteolytic processing, disulfide bond reduction, and subunit composition. *J. biol. Chem.* **254**: 5855–5861.

MEKALANOS, J. J., SWARTZ, D. J., PEARSON, G. D. N., HARFORD, N., GROYNE, F. and DE WILDE, M. (1983) Cholera toxin genes: nucleotide sequence, deletion analysis and vaccine development. *Nature* **306**: 551–557.

MORITA, A., TSAO, D. and KIM, Y. S. (1980) Identification of cholera toxin binding glycoproteins in rat intestinal microvillus membranes. *J. biol. Chem.* **255**: 2549–2553.

MOSLEY, W. H. (1969) The role of immunity in cholera. A review of epidemiological and serological studies. *Texas Rep. Biol. Med.* **27** (Suppl. 1): 227–241.

MOSS, J., FISHMAN, P. H., MANGANIELLO, V. C., VAUGHAN, M. and BRADY, R. O. (1976) Functional incorporation of ganglioside into intact cells: induction of choleragen responsiveness. *Proc. natn. Acad. Sci. U.S.A.* **73**: 1034–1037.

MOSS, J., RICHARDS, R. L., ALVING, C. R. and FISHMAN, P. H. (1977) Effect of A and B protomers of choleragen on release of trapped glucose from liposomes containing or lacking ganglioside G_{M1}. *J. biol. Chem.* **252**: 797–798.

MOSS, J. and VAUGHAN, M. (1979) Activation of adenylate cyclase by choleragen. *A. Rev. Biochem.* **48**: 581–600.

MOSS, J. and VAUGHAN, M. (1982) Mechanism of action of *Escherichia coli* heat-labile enterotoxin: activation of adenylate cyclase by ADP-ribosylation. In: *ADP Ribosylation Reactions Biology and Medicine*, pp 623–636, HAYAISHI, O. and UEDA, K. (eds) Academic Press, New York.

MUKERJEE, S. (1963) Preliminary studies on the development of a live oral vaccine for anti-cholera immunization. *Bull. WHO* **29**: 753–766.

NEILL, R. J., IVINS, B. E. and HOLMES, R. K. (1983) Synthesis and secretion of the plasmid-coded heat-labile enterotoxin of *Escherichia coli* in *Vibrio cholerae*. *Science* **221**: 289–291.

NELSON, E. T., CLEMENTS, J. D. and FINKELSTEIN, R. A. (1976) *Vibrio cholerae* adherence and colonization in experimental cholera: electron microscopic studies. *Infect. Immun.* **14**: 527–547.

NICHOLS, J. C., TAI, P.-C. and MURPHY, J. R. (1980) Cholera toxin is synthesized in precursor form on free polysomes in *Vibrio cholerae* 569B. *J. Bacteriol.* **144**: 518–523.

NORIKI, H. (1977) Evaluation of toxoid field trial in the Philippines. In: *Proceedings of the 12th Joint Conference U.S.–Japan Cooperative Medical Science Program, Symposium on Cholera*, Sapporo, 1976, pp. 302–310, FUKUMI, H. and ZINNAKA, Y. (eds) National Institute of Health, Tokyo, Japan.

NORTHRUP, R. S. and CHISARI, F. V. (1972) Response of monkeys to immunization with cholera toxoid, toxin, and vaccine: reversion of cholera toxoid. *J. Infect. Dis.* **125**: 471–479.

OHTOMO N. (1977) Safety and potency tests of cholera toxoid Lot II in animals and volunteers. In: *Proceedings of the 12th Joint Conference U.S.–Japan Cooperative Medical Science Program, Symposium on Cholera*, Sapporo, 1976, pp. 286–296, FUKUMI, H. and ZINNAKA, Y. (eds) National Institute of Health, Tokyo, Japan.

OHTOMO, N., MURAOKA, T. and KUDO, K. (1978) Observations on intracellular synthesis of cholera toxin subunits. In: *Proceedings of the 13th Joint Conference on Cholera*, Atlanta, Ga., 1977. U.S.–Japan Cooperative Medical Science Program DHEW Publication No. (NIH) 78–1590, pp. 413–423.

OUCHTERLONY, O. and HOLMGREN, J. (eds) (1980) *Cholera and Related Diarrheas*. Karger, Basel.

PEARSON, G. D. N. and MEKALANOS, J. J. (1982) Molecular cloning of *Vibrio cholerae* enterotoxin genes in *Escherichia coli* K-12. *Proc. natn. Acad. Sci. U.S.A.* **79**: 2976–2980.

PETERSON, J. W. (1979a) Synergistic protection against experimental cholera by immunization with cholera toxoid and vaccine. *Infect. Immun.* **26**: 528–533.

PETERSON, J. W. (1979b) Protection against experimental cholera by oral or parenteral immunization. *Infect. Immun.* **26**: 594–598.

PIERCE, N. F. (1973) Differential inhibitory effects of cholera toxoids and ganglioside on the enterotoxins of *Vibrio cholerae* and *Escherichia coli*. *J. exp. Med.* **137**: 1009–1023.

PIERCE, N. F., CRAY, W. C., JR and SACCI, J. B., JR. (1982) Oral immunization of dogs with purified cholera toxin, crude cholera toxin, or B subunit: evidence for synergistic protection by antitoxic and antibacterial mechanisms. *Infect. Immun.* **37**: 687–694.

PIERCE, N. F., CRAY, W. C., JR., SACCI, J. B., JR., CRAIG, J. P., GERMANIER, R. and FÜRER, E. (1983) Procholeragenoid: A safe and effective antigen for oral immunization against experimental cholera. *Infect. Immun.* **40**: 112–118.

POLLITZER, R. (1959) *Cholera*. World Health Organization.

RAPPAPORT, R. S. and BONDE, G. (1981) Development of a vaccine against experimental cholera and *Escherichia coli* diarrheal disease. *Infect. Immun.* **32**: 534–542.

RAPPAPORT, R. S., BONDE, G., McCANN, T., RUBIN, B. A. and TINT, H. (1974) Development of a purified cholera toxoid. II. Preparation of a stable, antigenic toxoid by reaction of purified toxin with glutaraldehyde. *Infect. Immun.* **9**: 304–317.

ROBERTSON, D. C., McDONELL, J. L. and DORNER, F. (1986) *E. coli* heat-labile enterotoxin(s). *Pharmac. Ther.* in press.

SANYAL, S. C. and MUKERJEE, S. (1969) Live oral cholera vaccine: report of a trial on human volunteer subjects. *Bull. WHO* **40**: 503–511.

SATTLER, J., WIEGANDT, H., STAERK, J., KRANZ, T., RONNEBERGER, H. J., SCHMIDTBERGER, R. and ZILG, H. (1975) Studies on the subunit structure of choleragen. *Eur. J. Biochem.* **57**: 309–316.

SCHAFER, D. E., LUST, W. D., SIRCAR, B. and GOLDBERG, N. D. (1970) Elevated concentration of adenosine 3′:5′-cyclic monophosphate in intestinal mucosa after treatment with cholera toxin. *Proc. natn. Acad. Sci.* **67**: 851–856.

SCIORTINO, C. V. and FINKELSTEIN, R. A. (1983) *Vibrio cholerae* expresses iron-regulated outer membrane proteins *in vivo*. *Infect. Immun.* **42**: 990–996.

SHARP, G. W. G. and HYNIE, S. (1971) Stimulation of intestinal adenyl cyclase by cholera toxin. *Nature* **229**: 266–269.

SIGLER, P. B., DRUYAN, M. E., KIEFER, H. C. and FINKELSTEIN, R. A. (1977) Cholera toxin crystals suitable for x-ray diffraction. *Science* **197**: 1277–1279.

SPICER, E. K., KAVANAUGH, W. M., DALLAS, W. S., FALKOW, S., KONIGSBERG, W. H. and SCHAFER, D. E. (1981) Sequence homologies between A subunits of *Escherichia coli* and *Vibrio cholerae* enterotoxins. *Proc. natn. Acad. Sci. U.S.A.* **78**: 50–54.

SPICER, E. K. and NOBLE, J. A. (1982) *Escherichia coli* heat-labile enterotoxin: Nucleotide sequence of the A subunit gene. *J. biol. Chem.* **257**: 5716–1521.

STEDMAN'S MEDICAL DICTIONARY (1972) 22nd Edition, Williams and Wilkins.

SVENNERHOLM, A.-M. and HOLMGREN, J. (1976) Synergistic protective effect in rabbits of immunization with *Vibrio cholerae* lipopolysaccharide and toxin/toxoid. *Infect. Immun.* **13**: 735–740.

SVENNERHOLM, A.-M., JERTBORN, M., GOTHEFORS, L., KARIM, A., SACK, D. A. and HOLMGREN, J. (1983) Current status of an oral B subunit whole cell cholera vaccine. *Dev. Biol. Stand.* **53**: 73–79.

THOMPSON, M. R. and IGLEWSKI, B. H. (1982) *Pseudomonas aeruginosa* toxin-A and exoenzyme-S. In: *ADP Ribosylation Reactions Biology and Medicine, Molecular Biology*: An International Series of Monographs and Textbooks, pp. 661–674, HAYAISHI, O. and UEDA, K. (eds) Academic Press.

TOSTESON, M. T., TOSTESON, D. C. and RUBNITZ, J. (1980) Cholera toxin interactions with lipid bilayers. *Acta Physiol. Scand. Suppl.* **481**: 21–25.

TSURU, S., MATSUGUCHI, M., OHTOMO, N., ZINNAKA, Y. and TAKEYA, K. (1982) Entrance of cholera enterotoxin subunits into cells. *J. gen. Microbiol.* **128**: 497–502.

UCHIDA, T. (1983) Diphtheria toxin. *Pharmac. Ther.* **19**: 107–122.

VAN HEYNINGEN, S. (1982) Cholera toxin (review). *Bioscience Rep.* **2**: 135–154.

VAN HEYNINGEN, W. E. and SEAL, J. R. (1983) *Cholera. The American Scientific Experience* 1947–1980. Westview Press, Boulder, Colorado.

VASIL, M. L., HOLMES, R. K. and FINKELSTEIN, R. A. (1974) Studies on toxinogenesis in *Vibrio cholerae*. II. An in vitro test for enterotoxin production. *Infect. Immun.* **9**: 195–197.

VASIL, M. L., HOLMES, R. K. and FINKELSTEIN, R. A. (1975) Conjugal transfer of a chromosomal gene determining production of enterotoxin in *Vibrio cholerae*. *Science* **187**: 849–850.

VAUGHAN, M., PIERCE, N. F. and GREENOUGH III, W. B. (1970) Stimulation of glycerol production in fat cells by cholera toxin. *Nature* **226**: 658–659.

WOODWARD, W. E., GILMAN, R. H., HORNICK, R. B., LIBONATI, J. P. and CASH, R. A. (1976) Efficacy of a live oral cholera vaccine in human volunteers. *Dev. Biol. Standard* **33**: 108–112.

WORLD HEALTH ORGANIZATION (1983) The management of diarrhoea and use of oral rehydration therapy: a joint WHO/UNICEF statement. World Health Organization. Geneva, pp. 1–25.

YANCEY, R. J., WILLIS, D. L. and BERRY, L. J. (1979) Flagella-induced immunity against experimental cholera in adult rabbits. *Infect. Immun.* **25**: 220–228.

CHAPTER 9

ENTEROTOXIGENIC DIARRHEA: MECHANISMS AND PROSPECTS FOR THERAPY

DON W. POWELL

Division of Digestive Diseases and Nutrition, Department of Medicine, University of North Carolina, Chapel Hill, North Carolina 27514, U.S.A.

1. INTRODUCTION

In the past decade, three evolving concepts have given hope for the development of effective antidiarrheal therapy. First has come the realization that diarrhea, at least that causing significant morbidity and mortality, is a disease of water and electrolyte metabolism and not a disease of altered intestinal motility (Phillips and Gaginella, 1977). Secondly, there is a growing understanding of the mechanisms of intestinal absorption and secretion (Binder, 1979; Field *et al.*, 1980; Janowitz and Sachar, 1979; Read, 1981). Lastly, there is new knowledge of how various agents promote intestinal water and electrolyte absorption or inhibit secretion (Powell and Field, 1980). Because much of the impetus for studies in this field comes from a keen appreciation for the mortality of diarrheal diseases in the Third World and because the bacterial enterotoxins have been so important to an understanding of electrolyte transport in the gut, it is only fitting that concepts of mechanism and prospects of therapy be discussed in a symposium on enterotoxins and enterotoxigenic bacteria. This article will briefly review mechanisms of intestinal secretion and discuss four promising categories of antisecretory drugs: neurotransmitters (modulators), calmodulin and calcium inhibitors, anti-inflammatory drugs, and opiates.

2. MECHANISMS OF INTESTINAL WATER AND ELECTROLYTE TRANSPORT

2.1. IONIC TRANSPORT MECHANISMS

While intestinal water and electrolyte absorption and secretion may occur simultaneously throughout the gut and in all parts of the mucosa, there is some evidence that absorption and secretion are separate processes occurring in different regions of the intestinal epithelium. Figure 1 assigns absorption to villous cells and secretion to the crypts. Water transport in any epithelium is largely due to osmotic gradients created by the active transport of electrolytes from one side of the epithelium to the other, therefore Na and Cl transport mechanisms are central to an understanding of intestinal secretion and enterotoxigenic diarrhea.

Both absorption and secretion are two-part processes: ions enter one cell border, usually by carrier mediated processes, and exit the opposite cell border, often by active transport. The Na ion is the one actively transported during water absorption, while Cl is the ion mediating intestinal secretion. During absorption, Na enters the cell from gut lumen either by itself, moving across the apical cell membrane by passive diffusion, or it enters the cell by processes that couple Na movement to nonelectrolytes, such as glucose or amino acid, or those that couple Na entry to Cl. Those entry mechanisms appear to be the rate-limiting step to water and electrolyte absorption; there is ample NaK-ATPase on the basolateral cell membrane to actively pump Na out of the cell. The Na is transported into the intercellular space, causing increases in the osmolality in this relatively constricted compartment resulting in the movement of water from lumen to intercellular space and then to blood.

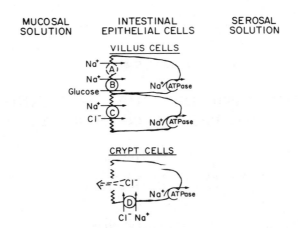

FIG. 1. Villous cell absorptive processes and crypt cell secretory mechanisms in the rabbit ileum. A, B, C and D are membrane processes transporting Na and Cl or glucose into the cell. The NaK-ATPase on the basolateral cell membrane transports Na out of the cell. Secretory stimuli inhibit coupled NaCl influx across the brush border (C) and allow Cl to be 'secreted' from the crypt cells.

The addition of glucose to Na solutions in the gut lumen stimulates Na and water absorption several fold. This occurs both as result of the Na–glucose coupled process and because the resulting bulk flow of water between and through the cells traps additional Na and Cl molecules in the flowing stream (a phenomenon called solvent drag). This glucose-mediated enhancement of Na and water absorption is the principle behind the glucose-containing oral replacement solution that has been so effective in rehydrating diarrheal victims in the Third World. However, oral glucose electrolyte solutions are not really antidiarrheals; stooling continues as they are administered. Instead, this form of therapy should be considered as resuscitation and, as such, should be the initial form of therapy. Antidiarrheal medications may be administered later after assurance that there will be a live patient to treat.

Secretory processes are, in some respects, the opposite of absorption. Coupled NaCl entry processes in the basolateral membrane increase the Cl concentration within the crypt cell to a level above electrochemical equilibrium. The Na entering with the Cl is recycled back across the basolateral membrane by the NaK-ATPase. Various secretory stimuli, via intracellular messengers such as cyclic nucleotides and calcium, increase the crypt cell apical membrane permeability to Cl, allowing it to exit the cell (be 'secreted'). This movement of Cl, and the Na that accompanies it, creates a blood to lumen flow of water.

2.2. INTRACELLULAR MEDIATORS

The major intracellular messengers of stimulus–secretion coupling in the gut, as in other organs, are cyclic nucleotides and calcium (Field et al., 1980). Recently, a role for metabolites of arachidonic acid—prostaglandins and leukotrienes—has been proposed (Cuthbert and Margolius, 1982; Manning et al., 1982; Musch et al., 1982, 1983). However, it is possible that these agents also ultimately promote secretion via the classic messengers. Table 1 correlates various bacterial enterotoxins with certain cyclic nucleotide messengers. Perhaps the large group of toxins listed as 'unknown' promote secretion by increasing intercellular calcium or arachidonic acid metabolites.

Figure 2a depicts the control of intestinal secretion by cyclic nucleotides. Cyclic AMP or cyclic GMP are synthesized from their appropriate nucleotide precursor upon stimulation of the respective cyclase. Adenylate and guanylate cyclase stimulation requires calcium and calmodulin as cofactors (Cheung, 1980). Cyclic nucleotides then act through one or possibly two routes: (1) they may activate membrane phosphorylating enzymes called protein kinases which then directly stimulate or inhibit the ion transport mechanisms; or (2) the cyclic nucleotides, perhaps through protein kinase action, may liberate calcium from intercellular reservoirs. Calcium may then act on the ion carriers via

TABLE 1. *Intracellular Messengers Coupling Exotoxins to Intestinal Secretion**

Cyclic AMP
Cholera enterotoxin (CT)
E. coli heat-labile enterotoxin (LT)
? *B. cereus* toxin
? *S. aureus* delta toxin

Cyclic GMP
E. coli heat-stable enterotoxin A (ST$_a$)
Yersinia enterotoxin
? *C. difficile* toxin

Unknown
E. coli ST$_b$
Staph enterotoxins
Shiga toxin
C. difficile cytotoxin
C. perfrigens enterotoxin
Other coliform enterotoxin

*Adapted from Gianella (1982)

calcium–calmodulin stimulated protein kinases. In either event, cyclic nucleotide action results in inhibition of Na absorption from the villus by reducing coupled NaCl entry across the brush border while it simultaneously increases the Cl permeability of crypt cell apical membranes, initiating Cl secretion.

Figure 2b illustrates another form in intracellular messenger-mediated secretion. This secretion is caused by agents, such as the neurotransmitters acetylcholine (ACh) and serotonin (5-HT), that allow 'gating' of calcium across the basolateral cell membrane. Recently Lundgren's laboratory has reported that neuronal inhibitors, such as tetrodotoxin and lidocaine, and ganglionic blockers, such as hexamethonium, inhibit a portion of cholera toxin stimulated intestinal secretion. He has proposed that bacterial enterotoxins might liberate 5-HT from enterochromaffin cells in the gut epithelium. The 5-HT might have secretory activity itself or might release ACh or other secretory peptides such as VIP from mucosal neurons (Cassuto *et al.*, 1981). Thus schemes of hormone or neurotransmitter-stimulated secretions as shown in Figs 2a and 2b could be part of enterotoxin-induced secretion as well.

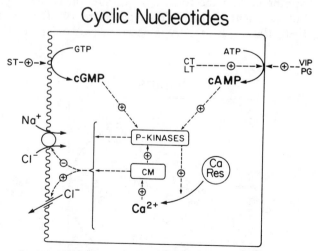

Cyclic Nucleotides

FIG. 2a. Cyclic nucleotide-stimulated secretory mechanisms. Increased intracellular levels of cyclic GMP via stimulation of guanylate cyclase by ST (*E. coli* ST$_a$ toxin and Yersinia enterotoxin) and of cyclic AMP via stimulation of adenylate cyclase by cholera toxin (CT), *E. coli* LT toxin (LT), vasoactive intestinal polypeptide (VIP), or prostaglandins (PG) cause secretion by: (a) stimulating cyclic nucleotide-dependent protein kinases, or (b) by releasing calcium from intracellular reservoirs and the formation of a calomodulin (CM) complex that stimulates calcium-dependent protein kinases.

Calcium

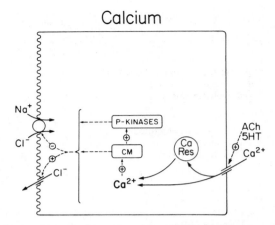

Fig. 2b. Calcium-stimulated intestinal secretion. Acetylcholine (ACh) and serotonin (5-HT) allow calcium gating across the basolateral cell membrane. Other agents (e.g. perhaps cyclic nucleotides) may release calcium from intracellular reservoirs. Increased intracellular levels of ionized calcium would then affect transport via calcium–calmodulin dependent kinases.

Figure 3 illustrates the most recent addition to the list of possible intracellular messengers—the prostaglandin and leukotriene metabolites of membrane-bound arachidonic acid. This mechanism may be more important in the diarrheas due to invasive bacteria because potent stimulants of this system are the kinins which are released during tissue damage and inflammation. Bradykinin (BK) and kallidin (LBK) are peptides formed by the action of tissue kallikrein on a_2-globulin precursors which are called kininogens. Recent studies have demonstrated kinin receptors on enterocyte basolateral cell membranes (Manning *et al.*, 1982). When activated, these initiate the arachidonic acid cascade to form the various prostaglandins (PG) and leukotrienes (LT) by the cyclo-oxygenase and lipoxygenase pathways, respectively (see Fig. 4). Bradykinin appears to affect intestinal electrolyte transport in the same way as stimulants that increase cellular levels of cyclic nucleotides and calcium. Since arachidonic acid metabolites are stimulants of adenylate cyclase, it is likely that cyclic nucleotides are involved in kinin-induced secretion. However, this remains to be proven. Because calcium is necessary for phospholipase activity, calcium and calmodulin certainly play a prominent role in this system. Another recent hypothesis germane to intestinal secretion is the suggestion that arachidonic acid metabolites might be involved in all forms of stimulus–secretion coupling (Marshall *et al.*, 1980, 1981). This theory is based in part on the fact that prostaglandin

Kinins

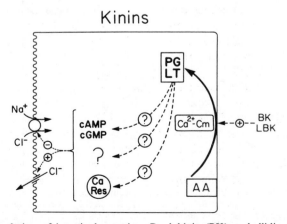

Fig. 3. Kinin stimulation of intestinal secretion. Bradykinin (BK) or kallidin (LBK) stimulate prostaglandin (PG) and leukotriene (LT) synthesis from membrane-bound arachidonic acid (AA) by a calcium–calmodulin (Ca^{2+}-Cm)-dependent process. PG and LT then alter transport either directly or via cyclic nucleotides or calcium.

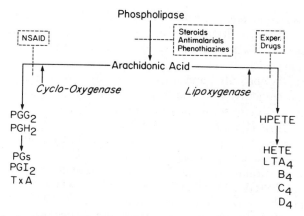

FIG. 4. Arachidonic acid metabolic pathway. Phospholipases release arachidonic acid (AA) from membrane-bound phosphoinositol. AA is then metabolized via the cyclo-oxygenase or lipo-xygenase pathways to various prostaglandins (PGs), prostacyclin (PGI_2), or thromboxane (TxA), or to various leukotrienes (LTA_4–D_4). The locus of inhibition by various drugs is shown in the dashed line boxes.

synthesis blockers inhibit pancreatic amylase secretion due to cyclic nucleotides and calcium, a finding that applies to intestinal secretion as well (see below). The most compelling evidence, however, is that of Marshall *et al.* (1980, 1981) who have shown a stoichiometric release of arachidonic acid from phosphoinositol after hormone stimulation of pancreatic amylase secretion.

3. POTENTIAL ANTISECRETORY AGENTS

The list of potential antisecretory agents is long and has been reviewed in detail before (Powell and Field, 1980). The reader is referred to this previous review for a discussion of some of the agents not covered here and for additional references. In this article, only four of the more promising categories of antisecretory agents are discussed and the bibliography on these updated.

3.1. NEUROTRANSMITTERS AND MODULATORS

One of the first agents shown to stimulate electrolyte absorption was epinephrine (Field and McColl, 1973). In rabbit ileum, this catecholamine alters electrolyte transport by stimulation of α_2-receptors (Chang *et al.*, 1982), however, β-receptors appear to be also involved in this response in the colon and perhaps in the human small intestine. α_2 Agonists, such as norepinephrine, clonidine, and oxymetazoline, and synthetic drugs with α agonist activity, such as lidamidine, have been shown to inhibit intestinal secretion stimulated by cholera toxin (Nakaki *et al.*, 1982), *E. coli* ST_a (Newsome *et al.*, 1981), and to reduce the watery diarrhea in patients with bronchogenic carcinoma (McArthur *et al.*, 1982). These agents have antisecretory activity by interacting with adrenergic receptors on the enterocyte. Neuromodulators, such as angiotensin II, that release α-adrenergic neurotransmitters from nerves in the gut, also stimulate intestinal absorption (Levens *et al.*, 1981).

Dopamine is another catecholamine with absorptive-stimulating (Donowitz *et al.*, 1982) and antisecretory (Donowitz *et al.*, 1983) activity. Although dopamine is not likely to be useful itself since it is not effective orally, similar activity has been found with bromocriptine, a dopamine agonist that can be given by mouth. Studies with both of these agents indicate that they stimulate α_2-receptors as well as specific dopamine receptors in the gut.

The neuropeptide somatostatin (SRIF) stimulates absorption and/or blocks the secretion induced by VIP, theophylline, cyclic AMP, and cholinergic drugs (Carter *et al.*, 1978; Dharmsathaphorn *et al.*, 1980; Guadalini *et al.*, 1980). SRIF has also been found to decrease the diarrhea due to pancreatic cholera (Ruskone *et al.*, 1982) and carcinoid syndrome (Dharmsathaphorn et al., 1980). It is possible that this peptide acts by releasing other absorptive neurotransmitters. If so, the transmitter released is probably not norepinephrine because SRIF's action is not blocked by α-adrenergic antagonists (Guadalini et al., 1980).

The mechanism of the absorptive and antisecretory effects of these agents remains unclear. Some of the studies listed above have shown inhibition of cyclic nucleotide synthesis, while others have not. In fact, there seems to be antisecretory activity in the face exogenously administered cyclic GMP (Carter et al., 1978; Newsome et al., 1981). Thus, while these agents may inhibit secretion by preventing the increase in intracellular cyclic nucleotides, they must also work at some step distal to this part of the secretory scheme. Interference with calcium gating or mobilization has been suggested as a possible locus of action for the catecholamines and SRIF (Powell and Field, 1980). However, the only reported studies of a calcium relationship are with dopamine (Donowitz et al., 1982). Dopamine was found to decrease total calcium content in rabbit ileum and to decrease ^{45}Ca influx across the basolateral cell membrane, changes in calcium metabolism that would stimulate Na and Cl absorption.

3.2. CALMODULIN AND CALCIUM 'INHIBITORS'

In view of the central role intracellular calcium plays in secretory processes, it is not surprising that drugs which alter calcium metabolism or transport might have antisecretory effects. The most widely studied of such drugs are the phenothiazines. Holmgren et al. (1978) were the first to show that phenothiazines would inhibit cyclic AMP-mediated intestinal secretion. This was confirmed by many others, and inhibition of cholera toxin and E. coli toxin-induced secretion, as well as other cyclic nucleotide and calcium-mediated secretory states, has been demonstrated (Abbey and Knoop, 1979; Ilundain and Naftalin, 1979; Lonnroth and Munck, 1980; Robins-Browne and Levine, 1981; Smith and Field, 1980). Phenothiazines have been found to be effective in the severe watery diarrhea caused by hormone-secreting tumors and that due to cholera vibrio (Donowitz et al., 1980; Islam et al., 1982; Rabbani et al., 1979, 1982). Controlled studies of cholera victims have shown a reduction in stool volume by as much as 50% in the first 24 hr after either oral or parental administration (Rabbani et al., 1979, 1982). The role of phenothiazines in cholera therapy remains to be defined, however, since their use seems to make little difference in clinical outcome except in those patients with severe diarrhea (Islam et al., 1982), and the single recognized side effect of phenothiazine, sedation, could interfere with oral rehydration therapy (Rabbani et al., 1982).

The mechanism of action of these neuroleptics remains to be determined. Chloropromazine and trifluoroparazine bind to calmodulin and inhibit most calcium–calmodulin dependent processes (Cheung, 1980). These lipid soluble agents also have a host of other actions on biological membranes, including 'membrane stabilization', which might interfere with calcium gating or mobilization. Thus these drugs could inhibit cyclic nucleotide production or degradation (calcium-dependent processes), or they could interfere with the protein kinases (Kuo et al., 1980) that phosphorylate gut cell membrane proteins (Taylor et al., 1981).

Other calcium 'inhibitors' that might be useful as antisecretory drugs are the antimaterials, such as chloroquine, and calcium-channel blockers, such as verapamil. Chloroquine, a drug with membrane stabilizing action, will inhibit cholera toxin- and theophylline-stimulated secretion in the rat ileum without altering cyclic AMP production (Fogel et al., 1982). Changes in calcium content and influx suggest that chloroquine might sequester intracellular calcium and thus interfere with stimulus secretion coupling. Unpublished studies by Donowitz's group with dantrolene, another calcium sequestering agent (Janjic et al., 1982), indicate that this drug has antisecretory effects. Alternatively, chloroquine might interfere with arachidonic acid metabolism as does a similar drug, mepacrine (see Fig. 4). Donowitz's group has also looked at the antisecretory effects of calcium-channel blockers. Verapamil has been shown to block secretion induced by calcium-gating drugs such as serotonin, but does not block cyclic nucleotide-induced secretion (Donowitz et al., 1980). Therefore it is unlikely that calcium-channel blockers will be effective against enterotoxin-produced secretion.

3.3. ANTI-INFLAMMATORY DRUGS

Both corticosteroid and nonsteroidal anti-inflammatory drugs (NSAIDs) have anti-secretory effects (Powell and Fields, 1980). Corticosteroids are thought to work by increasing NaK-ATPase activity in the colon (mineralo-corticoids) or in both small and large intestine (glucocorticoids). Although glucocorticoids are useful in the therapy of inflammatory bowel disease, their efficiency in acute diarrhea seems limited because it takes several days of administration before absorption is stimulated and because early in the course of drug action it may actually cause intestinal secretion (Tai et al., 1981).

NSAIDs appear more promising as antidiarrheals. In the early 1970s, indomethacin and acetylsalicyclic acid were shown to inhibit cholera toxin-induced secretion (Finch and Katz, 1972; Jacoby and Marshall, 1972). These effects were subsequently confirmed in Ussing chamber experiments with isolated gut (Farris et al., 1976; Smith et al., 1981). These drugs partially or completely reverse both cyclic nucleotide- and calcium-mediated secretion in experimental animals. In humans, indomethacin has been reported to inhibit secretory diarrheas due to villous adenoma (Steven et al., 1981) and to reduce the diarrheas due to turista (DuPont et al., 1977). Aspirin has been reported to reduce fluid loss in infants and children with infectious diarrhea (Burke et al., 1980).

The mechanism of the antisecretory effects of NSAIDs is uncertain. They decrease cholera toxin-stimulated cyclic AMP synthesis, but also block secretion stimulated by cyclic AMP itself (Farris et al., 1976; Smith et al., 1981). Both aspirin and indomethacin inhibit cyclic AMP-dependent protein kinases, and this could be the site of action that is distal to cyclic AMP production. Alternatively, if prostaglandin and lipoxygenase metabolites are involved with all types of stimulus–secretion coupling (see above), then blockade of the arachidonic acid cascade would be a likely locus of action. Since the conventional NSAIDs do not block the lipoxygenase pathway, it is possible that drugs that block both metabolic pathways may be more effective antisecretory agents. Synthesis of new lipoxygenase blockers is an area of intense interest by the pharmaceutical houses, so it is doubtful that we will have to wait long to find out. It also should be obvious that drugs that affect other parts of bradykinin pathways may also be useful as antisecretory drugs since kinin levels are elevated in inflammatory disease and kinins stimulate secretion.

3.4. OPIATES

A discussion of opiates as potential antidiarrheals is somewhat incongruous; these agents have been used for this purpose for several hundred years. What is new is the idea that opiates might have antidiarrheal activity by virtue of antisecretory effects rather than through actions on intestinal motility (Powell, 1981). Opiate derivatives such as codeine (Racusen et al., 1978; McKay et al., 1982; Powell, 1981), synthetic opiates such as loparamide (Sandhu et al., 1981), and endogenous opiates such as the enkephalins (Dobbins et al., 1980; McKay et al., 1981), all stimulate intestinal water and electrolyte absorption and inhibit the secretion induced by cyclic AMP and calcium. These effects are blocked by naloxone, indicating that opiate receptors are involved. An exciting idea is that the class of receptors involved with the antisecretory effect (δ-receptor) is different from that involved in motility (μ-receptor) (Kachur et al., 1980). This finding raises the intriguing possibility that opiates with antisecretory, but not antimotility, activity might be developed.

The mechanism of antidiarrheal action of opiates is even less certain than that of the other drugs mentioned in this article. Indeed, it is not even clear whether these drugs act directly on the enterocyte or by stimulating or inhibiting the release of other neurotransmitters that act on the enterocyte. The effect of opiates is blocked by tetrodotoxin, which suggests a neural intermediate (Dobbins et al., 1980). Attempts to locate opiate receptors on the enterocyte have failed (Binder et al., 1983). This has led Gaginella and

Wu to demonstrate that opiates inhibit the release of acetylcholine from gut neurons and to propose that this is the mechanism of opiate's antisecretory effect (Gaginella and Wu, 1983). Another possibility would be that opiates might actually stimulate release of some as yet unidentified absorptive neurotransmitter. Adrenergic antagonists do not block the opiate effect, therefore norepinephrine is not likely to be the absorptive transmitter. Opiates do not consistently alter cyclic nucleotide levels in the gut, so it has been suggested that they may have effects via calcium or membrane prostaglandin pathways. Recently, a preliminary report has suggested that loparamide might inhibit calcium–calmodulin processes (Merritt *et al.*, 1982), but this has not been reported for the other opiates. An understanding of the mechanism of opiates in the gut may allow the development of antidiarrheal opiates that are even more useful than those currently available.

4. SUMMARY AND CONCLUSIONS

Studies over the past decade have led to a rudimentary but working knowledge of intestinal electrolyte transport. Purification of bacterial exotoxins has allowed an understanding of how these agents stimulate cells. Coupled NaCl influx processes and chloride secretory mechanisms have been shown to be affected by exotoxin-stimulated increases in cyclic nucleotides, as well as by increases in intracellular calcium and arachidonic acid metabolites. Catecholamines, somatostatin, phenothiazines, nonsteroidal anti-inflammatory drugs, and opiates appear to be the most promising of the antisecretory drugs. While the mechanism of action of these agents remains to be determined, there is significant hope that effective antisecretory drugs will emerge in the near future.

REFERENCES

Abbey, D. M. and Knoop, F. C. (1979) Effect of chlorpromazine on the secretory activity of *Escherichia coli* heat-stable enterotoxin. *Infect. Immun.* **26:** 1000–1003.

Binder, H. J. (ed.) (1979) *Mechanisms of Intestinal Secretion*, Alan R. Liss, New York.

Binder, H. J., Reinprecht J., Dharmsathaphorn K. and Dobbins J. W. (1980) Intestinal peptide receptors. *Regulatory Peptides (Suppl.)* **1:** S10.

Burke, V., Gracey, M. and Suharyono, S. (1980) Reduction by aspirin of intestinal fluid-loss in acute childhood gastroenteritis. *Lancet* **i:** 1329–1330.

Carter, R. F., Bitar, K. N., Zfass, A. M. and Makhlouf, G. M. (1978) Inhibition of VIP-stimulated intestinal secretion and cyclic AMP production by somatostatin in the rat. *Gastroenterology* **74:** 726–730.

Cassuto, J., Jodal, M., Tuttle, R. and Lundgren, O. (1981) On the role of intramural nerves in the pathogenesis of cholera toxin-induced intestinal secretion. *Scand. J. Gastroent.* **16:** 377–384.

Chang, E. B., Field, M. and Miller, R. J. (1982) α_2-Adrenergic receptor regulation of ion transport in rabbit ileum. *Am. J. Physiol.* **242:** G237–G242.

Cheung, W. Y. (1980) Calmodulin plays a pivotal role in cellular regulation. *Science* **207:** 19–27.

Cuthbert, A. W. and Margolius, H. S. (1982) Kinins stimulate net chloride secretion by the rat colon. *Br. J. Pharmac.* **75:** 587–598.

Dharmsathaphorn, K., Sherwin, R. S., Cataland, S., *et al.*, (1980) Somatostatin inhibits diarrhea in the carcinoid syndrome. *Ann. intern. Med.* **90:** 68–69.

Dharmsathaphorn, K., Sherwin, R. S. and Dobbins, J. W. (1980) Somatostatin inhibits fluid secretion in the rat jejunum. *Gastroenterology* **78:** 1554–1558.

Dobbins, J., Racusen, L. and Binder, H. J. (1980) Effect of D-alanine methionine enkephalin amide on ion transport in rabbit ileum. *J. clin. Invest.* **66:** 19–28.

Donowitz, M., Asarkof, N. and Pike, G. (1980) Calcium dependence of serotinin-induced changes in rabbit ileal electrolyte transport. *J. clin. Invest.* **66:** 341–352.

Donowitz, M., Cusolito, S., Battisti, L., Fogel, R. and Sharp, G. W. G. (1982) Dopamine stimulation of active Na and Cl absorption in rabbit ileum. *J. clin. Invest.* **69:** 1008–1016.

Donowitz, M., Elta G., Battisti, L., Fogel, R. and Label-Schwartz, E. (1983) Effect of dopamine and bromocriptine on rat ileal and colonic transport: stimulation of absorption and reserval of cholera toxin-induced secretion. *Gastroenterology* **84:** 516–523.

Donowitz, M., Elta, G., Bloom, S. R. and Nathanson, L. (1980) Trifluoroparazine reversal of secretory diarrhea in pancreatic cholera. *Ann. intern. Med.* **93:** 284–285.

DuPont, H. L., Sullivan, P., Pickering, L. K., Haynes, G. and Ackerman, P. B. (1977) Symptomatic treatment of diarrhea with bismuth subsalicylate among students attending a Mexican university. *Gastroenterology* **73,** 715–718.

Farris, R. K., Tapper, E. J., Powell, D. W. and Morris, S. M. (1976) Effect of aspirin on normal and cholera toxin-stimulated intestinal electrolyte transport. *J. clin. Invest.* **57:** 916–924.

Field, M., Fordtran, J. S. and Schultz, S. G. (eds) (1980) *Secretory Diarrhea*, American Physiological Society, Bethesda, MD.

FIELD, M. and MCCOLL, I. (1973) Ion transport in rabbit ileal mucosa. III. Effects of catecholamines. *Am. J. Physiol.* **225**: 852–857.

FINCH, A. D. and KATZ, R. L. (1972) Prevention of cholera-induced intestinal secretion in the cat by aspirin. *Nature* **238**, 273–274.

FOGEL, R., SHARP, G. W. G. and DONOWITZ, M. (1982) Chloroquine stimulates absorption and inhibits secretion of ileal water and electrolytes. *Am. J. Physiol.* **243**: G117–G126.

GAGINELLA, T. S., RIMELE, T. J. and WIETECHA, M. (1983) Studies on rat intestinal epithelial cell receptors for serotonin and opiates. *J. Physiol.* **335**: 101–111.

GAGINELLA, T. S. and WU, Z. C. (1983) Enkephalin [D-Ala^2, D-Met^{5}NH$_2$] inhibits acetylcholine release from the submucosal plexus rat colon. *J. Pharm. pharmac.* **35**: 823–825.

GIANELLA, R. A. (1982) Effect of bacterial toxins on the intestine. In: *American Gastroenterological Association Postgraduate Course: Interaction of the intestine with its Environment*, Chicago.

GUADALINI, S., KACHUR, J. F., SMITH, P. L., MILLER, R. J. and FIELD, M. (1980) *In vitro* effects of somatostatin in ion transport in rabbit intestine. *Am. J. Physiol.* **238**: G67–G74.

HOLMGREN, J., LANGE S. and LONNROTH I. (1978) Reversal of cyclic AMP-mediated intestinal secretion in mice by chloropromazine. *Gastroenterology* **75**: 1103–1108.

ILUNDAIN, A. and NAFTALIN, R. J. (1979) Role of Ca^{2+}-dependent regulator protein in intestinal secretion. *Nature* **279**: 446–448.

ISLAM, M. R., SACK, D. A., HOLMGREN, J., BARDHAN, P. K. and RABBANI, G. H. (1982) use of chlorpromazine in the treatment of cholera and other severe acute watery diarrheal diseases. *Gastroenterology*. **82**: 1335–1340.

JACOBY, H. L. and MARSHALL, C. H. (1972) Antagonism of cholera enterotoxin by anti-inflammatory agents in the rat. *Nature* **235**: 163–165.

JANJIC, D., WOLLHEIM, C. B. and SHARP, G. W. G. (1982) Selective inhibition of glucose-stimulated insulin release by dantrolene. *Am. J. Physiol.* **243**: E59–E67.

JANOWITZ, H. D. and SACHAR, D. B. (eds.). (1979) *Frontiers of Knowledge in the Diarrheal Disease*. Projects in Health, Upper Montclair, NJ.

KACHUR, J. F., MILLER, R. J. and FIELD, M. (1980) Control of guinea pig intestinal electrolyte secretion by a delta-opiate receptor. *Proc. natn. Acad. Sci. U.S.A.* **77**: 2753–2756.

KUO, J. F., ANDERSSON, R. G. G., WISE, B. C., MACKERLOVA, L., SALOMONSSON, I., BRACKETT, N. L., KATOH, N., SHOJI, M. and WRENN, R. W. (1980) Calcium-dependent protein kinase: widespread occurrence in various tissues and phyla of the animal kingdom and comparison of effects of phospholipid, calmodulin, and trifluoroperazine. *Proc. natn. Acad. Sci. U.S.A.* **77**: 7039–7043.

LEVENS, N. R., PEACH, M. J., CAREY, R. M., POAT, J. A. and MUNDAY, K. A. (1981) Response of rat jejunum to angiotestin II: role of norepinephrine and prostaglandins. *Am. J. Physiol.* **240**: G17–G24.

LONNROTH, I. and MUNCK, B. G. (1980) Effect of chlorpromazine on ion transport induced by cholera toxin, cyclic AMP and cyclic GMP in isolated mucosa from hen intestine. *Acta. pharmac. toxicol.* **47**: 190–194.

MANNING, D. C., SNYDER, S. H., KACHUR, J. F., MILLER, R. J. and FIELD, M. (1982) Bradykinin receptor mediated chloride secretion in intestinal function. *Nature* **229**: 256–259.

MARSHALL, P. J., BOATMAN, D. E. and HOKIN, L. E. (1981) Direct demonstration of the formation of prostaglandin E$_2$ due to phosphatidylinositol breakdown associated with stimulation of enzyme secretion in the pancreas. *J. biol. Chem.* **256**: 844–847.

MARSHALL, P. J., DIXON, J. F. and HOKIN, L. E. (1980) Evidence for a role in stimulus-secretion coupling of prostaglandins derived from release of arachidonoyl residues as a result of phosphatidylinositol breakdown. *Proc. natn. Acad. Sci., U.S.A.* **77**: 3292–3296.

MCARTHUR, K. E., ANDERSON, D. S., DURBIN, T. E., ORLOFF, M. J. and DHARMSATHAPHORN, K. (1982) Clonidine and lidamidine to inhibit watery diarrhea in a patient with lung cancer. *Ann. intern. Med.* **96**: 323–325.

MCKAY, J. S., LINAKER, B. D., HIGGS, N. B. and TURNBERG, L. A. (1982) Studies of the antisecretory activity of morphine in rabbit ileum *in vitro*. *Gastroenterology* **82**: 243–247.

MCKAY, J. S., LINAKER, B. D. and TURNBERG, L. A. (1981) Influence of opiates on ion transport across rabbit ileal mucosa. *Gastroenterology* **80**: 279–284.

MERRITT, J. E., BROWN, B. L. and TOMLINSON, S. (1982) Loperamide and calmodulin. *Lancet* I: 283.

MUSCH, M. W., KACHUR, J. F., MILLER, R. J., FIELD, M. and STOFF, J. S. (1983) Bradykinin stimulated electrolyte secretion in rabbit and guinea pig intestine: involvement of arachidonic acid metabolites. *J. clin. Invest.* **71**: 1073–1083.

MUSCH, M. W., MILLER, R. J. and FIELD, M. (1982) Stimulation of colonic secretion by lipoxygenase metabolites of arachidonic acid. *Science* **217**: 1255–1256.

NAKAKI, T., NAKADATE, T., YAMAMOTO, S. and KATO, R. (1982) a_2-Adrenoceptors inhibit the cholera-toxin-induced intestinal fluid accumulation. *Arch. Pharmac.* **318**: 181–184.

NEWSOME, P. M., BURGESS, M. N., HOLMAN, G. D., MULLAN, N. A., RICHARDS, D. H. and SMITH, M. R. (1981) a_2-Adrenoceptors controlling intestinal secretion. *Biochem. Soc. Trans.* **9**: 413–414.

PHILLIPS, S. F. and GAGINELLA, T. S. (1977) Intestinal secretion as a mechanism in diarrheal disease, In: *Progress in Gastroenterology*, pp. 481–504, JERZY GLASS, G. B. (ed.) Grune & Stratton, New York.

POWELL, D. W. (1981) Muscle or mucosa: the site of action of antidiarrheal opiates? *Gastroenterology* **80**: 406–408.

POWELL, D. W. and FIELD, M. (1980) Pharmacological approaches to treatment of secretory diarrhea, In: *Secretory Diarrhea*, pp. 187–209, FIELD, M., FORDTRAN and SCHULTZ, S. G. (eds) American Physiological Society, Bethesda, MD.

RABBANI, G. H., GREENOUGH III, W. B., HOLMGREN, J. and KIRKWOOD, B. (1982) Controlled trial of chlorpromazine as antisecretory agent in patients with cholera hydrated intravenously. *Br. med. J.* **284**: 1361–1364.

RABBANI, G. H., GREENOUGH III, W. B., HOLMGREN, J. and LONNROTH, I. (1979) Chlorpromazine reduces fluid-loss in cholera. *Lancet* I: 410–412.

Racusen, L. C., Binder, H. J. and Dobbins, J. W. (1978) Effect of exogenous and endogenous opiate compounds on ion transport in rabbit ileum *in vitro*. *Gastroenterology* **74:** 1081.

Read, N. W. (ed.) (1981) *Clinical Research Reviews. Diarrhoea: New Insights*, Janssen Pharmaceutical, Marlow, England.

Robins-Browne, R. M. and Levine, M. M. (1981) Effect of chlorpromaxine on intestinal secretion mediated by *Escherichia coli* heat-stable enterotoxin and 8-Br-cyclic GMP in infant mice. *Gastroenterology* **80:** 321–326.

Ruskone, A., Rene, E., Chayvialle, J. A., Bonin, N., Pignal, F., Kremer, M., Bonfils, S. and Rambaud, J. C. (1982) Effect of somatostatin on diarrhea and on small intestinal water and electrolyte transport in a patient with pancreatic cholera. *Dig. Dis. Sci.* **27:** 459–466.

Sandhu, B. K., Tripp, J. H., Candy, D. C. A. and Harries, J. T. (1981) Loperamide: studies on its mechanism of action. *Gut* **22:** 658–662.

Smith, P. L., Blumberg, J. B., Stoff, J. S. and Field, M. (1981) Antisecretory effects of indomethacin on rabbit ileal mucosa *in vitro*. *Gastroenterology* **80:** 356–365.

Smith, P. L. and Field, M. (1980) *In vitro* antisecretory effects of trifluoroperazine and other neuroleptics in rabbit and human small intestine. *Gastroenterology* **78:** 1545–1553.

Steven, K., Lange, P., Bukhave, K. and Rask-Madsen, J. (1981) Prostaglandin E_2-mediated secretory diarrhea in villous adenoma of rectum: effect of treatment with indomethacin. *Gastroenterology* **80:** 1562–1566.

Tai, Y-H., Decker, R. A., Marnane, W. G., Charney, A. N. and Donowitz, M. (1981) Effects of methylprendisolone on electrolyte transport by *in vitro* rat ileum. *Am. J. Physiol.* **240:** G365–G370.

Taylor, L., Guerina, V. J., Donowitz, M., Cohen, M. and Sharp, G. W. G. (1981) Calcium and calmodulin-dependent protein phosphorylation in rabbit ileum. *FEBS Lett.* **131,** 322–324.

CHAPTER 10

THERMOSTABLE DIRECT HEMOLYSIN OF
VIBRIO PARAHAEMOLYTICUS

YOSHIFUMI TAKEDA

*Department of Bacterial Infection, The Institute of Medical Science, The University of Tokyo,
4–6–1 Shirokanedai Minato-ku, Tokyo 108, Japan*

1. INTRODUCTION

Vibrio parahaemolyticus was first isolated by Fujino and his coworkers (1953) from a case of food poisoning in Japan. It is one of the major causative agents of food poisoning, acute gastroenteritis; cases of food poisoning due to *V. parahaemolyticus* constitute about 20–30 % of all cases of food poisoning recorded during the last 20 years in Japan. Among the bacteria causing food poisoning in Japan, *V. parahaemolyticus* is the most frequently isolated, followed in decreasing order by *Staphylococcus*, *Salmonella*, *Escherichia coli* and *Clostridium botulinum*. (Miwatani and Takeda, 1976). Several outbreaks of food poisoning associated with *V. parahaemolyticus* and sporadic cases of *V. parahaemolyticus* infection have also been reported from the United States of America, European countries, Asian countries and elsewhere (Chatterjee *et al.*, 1970; Fujino *et al.*, 1974; Barker, 1974; Miwatani and Takeda, 1976; Blake *et al.*, 1980).

In epidemiological studies on *V. parahaemolyticus*, Kato and his coworkers (Kato *et al.*, 1965; Miyamoto *et al.*, 1969) at the Kanagawa Prefectural Public Health Laboratory discovered that strains isolated from the feces of patients caused hemolysis on special blood-agar, whereas strains isolated from vehicles of food poisoning were not hemolytic. Sakazaki *et al.* (1968) confirmed this by examining 3,370 cultures from various sources. Special blood-agar medium for measuring the hemolytic character of *V. parahaemolyticus* was developed by Wagatsuma (Wagatsuma, 1968; Miwatani and Takeda, 1976), and the hemolysis produced by *V. parahaemolyticus* on Wagatsuma's medium has been called the Kanagawa-phenomenon. Thus, it has been accepted that the Kanagawa-phenomenon is closely related to the enteropathogenicity of *V. parahaemolyticus*.

2. ENTEROPATHOGENICITY OF *V. PARAHAEMOLYTICUS*

The main symptoms of *V. parahaemolyticus* infection are diarrhea and abdominal pain. The diarrhea is either watery or bloody. Before demonstration of a close correlation between Kanagawa-phenomenon positive strains and human enteropathogenicity, several tests on the effect of oral administration of *V. parahaemolyticus* were reported. Takikawa (1958) demonstrated the enteropathogenicity of *V. parahaemolyticus* isolated from a case of food poisoning by feeding broth cultures of isolates to human volunteers. Aiso and Fujiwara (1963) also reported tests on the effect of oral administration of *V. parahaemolyticus* to human volunteers. In their tests, four strains—three isolated from the feces of patients and one from a shell fish—were given, and one of the three test strains isolated from human patients caused gastroenteritis in volunteers.

Sanyal *et al.* (1973) reported a case of *V. parahaemolyticus* infection in a laboratory worker, in which symptoms of gastroenteritis developed after accidental ingestion of 3×10^5 viable cells of a Kanagawa-phenomenon positive strain of *V. parahaemolyticus*. In contrast, ingestion of more than 10^9 cells of Kanagawa-phenomenon negative strains by human volunteers did not cause any symptoms (Sakazaki *et al.*, 1968).

Sanyal and Sen (1974) fed Kanagawa-phenomenon positive and negative strains of *V. parahaemolyticus* to human volunteers and found that administration of relatively large numbers of Kanagawa-phenomenon negative cells ($1-2 \times 10^{10}$) did not cause any symptoms of gastroenteritis, whereas administration of 2×10^5 to 3×10^7 cells of Kanagawa-phenomenon positive strains caused abdominal discomfort and diarrhea.

The ligated ileal loop test in rabbits has been used by several workers to test the enteropathogenicity of *V. parahaemolyticus* (Twedt and Brown, 1974; Ghosh *et al.*, 1974; Sakazaki *et al.*, 1974a,b; Zen-Yoji *et al.*, 1974; Brown *et al.*, 1977). Sakazaki *et al.* (1974a) reported that 14 of 16 Kanagawa-phenomenon positive strains, but only 7 of 32 Kanagawa-phenomenon negative strains gave positive results in this test. Twedt and Brown (1974) obtained similar results; namely, 23 of 25 Kanagawa-phenomenon positive and 2 of 10 Kanagawa-phenomenon negative strains gave positive reactions in the rabbit ileal loop test. Subsequent studies, however, indicated that some of the positive results reported previously were due to the presence of $1-3\%$ NaCl in the samples, which resulted in a false positive results in rabbit ileal loops (Johnson and Calia, 1976).

Honda *et al.* (1983) showed that antiserum against thermostable direct hemolysin did not neutralize positive reaction in the rabbit ileal loop test induced by a Kanagawa-phenomenon positive strain, suggesting that the positive reactions are induced not only by thermostable direct hemolysin (Zen-Yoji *et al.*, 1974) but also by other factor(s).

3. ISOLATION OF THERMOSTABLE DIRECT HEMOLYSIN

The hemolytic character of *V. parahaemolyticus* was observed by Fujino *et al.* (1953) when this bacterium was first isolated. Several kinds of hemolysins were reported (Kato *et al.*, 1965, 1966; Kawamura, 1967, Yanagase *et al.*, 1970; Fujino *et al.*, 1969; Zen-Yoji *et al.*, 1971; Miwatani *et al.*, 1972a), and attempts to isolate a hemolysin responsible for the Kanagawa-phenomenon have been made by several workers since epidemiological studies demonstrated a close correlation between Kanagawa-phenomenon positive strains and human enteropathogenicity (Kato *et al.*, 1965; Miyamoto *et al.*, 1969; Sakazaki *et al.*, 1968). Obara (1971) isolated a thermostable hemolysin from culture filtrates of Kanagawa-phenomenon positive strains and suggested that this hemolysin might be responsible for the Kanagawa-phenomenon. Zen-Yoji *et al.* (1971) isolated a thermostable hemolysin from a strain that induced the Kanagawa-phenomenon and proposed the name 'enteropathogenic toxin' for it (Zen-Yoji *et al.*, 1974, 1975). On the other hand, Sakurai *et al.* (1973) found that the hemolytic activity of the thermostable hemolysin produced by Kanagawa-phenomenon positive strains was not activated by adding lecithin, and thus proposed the name 'thermostable direct hemolysin' for it. This name has been adopted in this article.

Sakurai *et al.* (1974) studied the distribution of the thermostable direct hemolysin in various strains of *V. parahaemolyticus* by an immunodiffusion technique with antiserum against the purified thermostable direct hemolysin. They demonstrated that the thermostable direct hemolysin was produced by only Kanagawa-phenomenon positive strains, not Kanagawa-phenomenon negative strains. Immunological methods for detecting the production of the thermostable direct hemolysin by *V. parahaemolyticus* were developed by Ohta *et al.* (1979) and Honda *et al.* (1980). Ohta *et al.* (1979) developed a reverse passive hemagglutination technique using antiserum against the purified thermostable direct hemolysin. The method is very sensitive and can detect as little as 1 ng/ml of the thermostable direct hemolysin. A modified Elek test and an immuno-halo test using antiserum against the purified thermostable direct hemolysin were developed by Honda *et al.* (1980). Although the sensitivities of these methods were not as high as that of reversed passive hemagglutination, the methods were reported to be reproducible, and easier with regard to the procedure and reading of results than the routine method in Wagatsuma's medium. Enzyme-linked immunosorbent assay of the thermostable direct hemolysin was recently developed by Honda *et al.* (1985).

4. PURIFICATION OF THERMOSTABLE DIRECT HEMOLYSIN

Several workers have purified thermostable direct hemolysin from culture supernatants of Kanagawa-phenomenon positive strains of *V. parahaemolyticus* (Zen-Yoji *et al.*, 1971, 1974, 1975; Obara, 1971; Nikkawa *et al.*, 1972; Sakurai *et al.*, 1973; Honda *et al.*, 1976a; Miyamoto *et al.*, 1980; Cherwonogrodzky and Clark, 1982).

The procedure described by Honda *et al.* (1976a) was as follows: *V. parahaemolyticus* WP-1, a Kanagawa-phenomenon positive strain, was cultured in medium containing 30 g of sodium chloride, 10 g of peptone (Difco), 5 g of dibasic sodium phosphate and 5 g of glucose per liter in distilled water, at pH 7.6–7.8. After incubation at 37°C for about 15 hr with shaking, the culture supernatant was collected by centrifugation. Solid ammonium sulfate (35.1 g/100 ml) was then added and the resulting precipitate was dissolved in a small amount of 0.01 M phosphate buffer (Na_2HPO_4–KH_2PO_4, pH 7.0) and dialyzed overnight against the same buffer for use as crude hemolysin. Crude hemolysin from 11,500 ml of culture supernatant was applied to a DEAE-cellulose column (2.2 cm × 55 cm) equilibrated with 0.01 M phosphate buffer (pH 7.0). Material was eluted with about 1,000 ml of the same buffer containing 0.2 M NaCl and then 1,000 ml of a linear gradient of 0.2–1.0 M NaCl in the same buffer. Fractions containing hemolytic activity were concentrated to a small volume and applied to a hydroxylapatite column (2.2 cm × 35 cm) equilibrated with 0.1 M phosphate buffer (pH 7.0). The column was eluted with 500 ml of 0.1 M phosphate buffer (pH 7.0), and then with 800 ml of a linear gradient of 0.1–0.3 M phosphate buffer (pH 7.0). Fractions containing hemolytic activity were concentrated to a small volume and applied to a Sephadex G-200 column (2.2 cm × 55 cm) equilibrated with 0.01 M phosphate buffer (pH 7.0). The column was eluted with the same buffer. Fractions containing hemolytic activity were collected and concentrated and their homogeneity was examined by polyacrylamide gel disc electrophoresis, SDS-polyacrylamide gel disc electrophoresis and analytical ultracentrifugation. By both polyacrylamide gel disc electrophoresis and SDS-polyacrylamide gel disc electrophoresis, the preparation gave a single band staining with Coomassie brilliant blue. Moreover, on analytical ultracentrifugation it sedimented as a single symmetric peak (Honda *et al.*, 1976a). These results indicate that the preparation is highly purified. Typical results obtained during the purification are summarized in Table 1. About 7.4 mg of purified thermostable direct hemolysin was obtained from about 46 liters of culture supernatant with a yield of about 15.5% and 540-fold purification from the culture supernatant.

Purified thermostable direct hemolysin was also obtained by Zen-Yoji *et al.* (1974, 1975), Miyamoto *et al.* (1980) and Cherwonogrodzky and Clark (1982).

Takeda *et al.* (Takeda, Yutsudo and Miwatani, unpublished results) recently reported crystallization of the purified thermostable direct hemolysin, a typical crystal being presented in Fig. 1.

TABLE 1. *Purification of Thermostable Direct Hemolysin**

Fraction	Total volume (ml)	Total protein (mg)[†]	Total activity (HU)[‡]	Specific activity (HU/mg)	Relative activity	Yield (%)
Culture filtrate	46,000	25,760	223,744	8.7	(1.0)	100
Ammonium sulfate fraction	400	14,036	201,142	14.3	1.64	89.9
DEAE-cellulose column eluate	10.8	59.4	68,314	1,150.1	132.2	30.6
Hydroxylapatite column eluate	1.2	11.6	46,966	4,048.8	465.4	21.1
Sephadex G-200 column eluate	1.76	7.4	34,520	4,664.9	536.2	15.5

*From Honda *et al.* (1976a).

†Protein content was determined by the method of Lowry *et al.* (1951).

‡Hemolytic activity was determined as described by Honda *et al.* (1976a). One hemolytic unit (HU) was defined as the amount which gave $A_{540} = 0.5$.

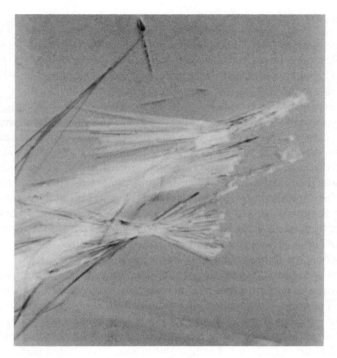

FIG. 1. A typical crystal of the thermostable direct hemolysin (Takeda,
Yutsudo and Miwatani, unpublished results).

5. SOME PHYSICOCHEMICAL PROPERTIES OF THE THERMOSTABLE DIRECT HEMOLYSIN

The purified thermostable direct hemolysin was free from phospholipid and carbohydrates. Its ultraviolet absorption spectrum was that of a typical protein, with maximal and minimal absorptions at 277 nm and 250 nm, respectively. Its pI was about 4.2. The hemolytic activity of the purified thermostable direct hemolysin was destroyed by pepsin or alpha chymotrypsin, but not by trypsin (Zen-Yoji et al., 1976). The molecular weight of the purified thermostable direct hemolysin was determined to be about 42,000 by gel filtration (Honda et al., 1976a; Miyamoto et al., 1980). Takeda et al. (1978) examined the molecular structure of the purified thermostable direct hemolysin by Triton X-100- and SDS-polyacrylamide gel disc electrophoreses. Although SDS-polyacrylamide gel disc electrophoresis showed that the molecular weight of the hemolysin was 21,000, Triton X-100-polyacrylamide gel disc electrophoresis indicated a value of 42,000. Moreover, when cross-linked with glutaraldehyde, it gave several bands at 21,000, 41,000, 63,000, 87,000, 108,000 and 130,000 on SDS-polyacrylamide gel disc electrophoresis. Thus it is concluded that the thermostable direct hemolysin is composed of two subunit molecules of approximately 21,000 daltons. The amino acid composition of the purified thermostable direct hemolysin was reported by Zen-Yoji et al. (1975), Honda et al. (1976a) and Miyamoto et al. (1980). In general their results, shown in Table 2, are in good agreement. Zen-Yoji et al. (1975) reported that the amino acid sequence of the N-terminal region of the thermostable direct hemolysin.

Recently, Kaper et al. (1984) and Taniguchi et al. (1985) cloned the gene encoding the thermostable direct hemolysin into pBR 322 vector in Escherichia coli, and Nishibuchi and Kaper (1985) determined the sequence of the structural gene. The identical nucleotide sequence was determined by Taniguchi and Mizuguchi (personal communication). Amino acid sequence of the thermostable direct hemolysin deduced from the nucleotide sequence (Nishibuchi and Kaper, 1985) is shown in Fig. 2.

TABLE 2. *Amino Acid Composition of the Purified Thermostable Direct Hemolysin*

Amino acid	Amino acid residue (%)*		
Lys	6.1†	5.7‡	6.1§
His	2.2	2.6	2.5
Arg	1.9	2.0	1.5
Asp	12.1	12.5	12.2
Thr	6.2	6.3	6.6
Ser	8.9	10.8	10.7
Glu	9.4	10.2	10.2
Pro	4.6	5.1	5.1
Gly	5.5	6.3	5.1
Ala	4.7	5.1	4.6
Cys	3.1	0.9	2.0
Val	12.0	10.8	11.7
Met	1.9	2.0	2.0
Ile	3.1	3.1	3.0
Leu	3.9	3.7	3.6
Tyr	6.2	5.4	5.6
Phe	6.6	6.3	7.1
Trp	1.6	1.4	0.5

*The total of individual amino acid residues is taken as 100.0%.
†Data from Honda *et al.* (1976a).
‡Data from Zen-Yoji *et al.* (1975).
§Data from Miyamoto *et al.* (1980).

```
1                                      10
Phe-Glu-Leu-Pro-Ser-Val-Pro-Phe-Pro-Ala-
11                                     20
Pro-Gly-Ser-Asp-Glu-Ile-Leu-Phe-Val-Val-
21                                     30
Arg-Asp-Thr-Thr-Phe-Asn-Thr-Gln-Ala-Pro-
31                                     40
Val-Asn-Val-Lys-Val-Ser-Asp-Phe-Trp-Thr-
41                                     50
Asn-Arg-Asn-Val-Lys-Arg-Lys-Pro-Tyr-Glu-
51                                     60
Asp-Val-Tyr-Gly-Gln-Ser-Val-Phe-Thr-Thr-
61                                     70
Ser-Gly-Thr-Lys-Trp-Leu-Thr-Ser-Tyr-Met-
71                                     80
Thr-Val-Asn-Ile-Asn-Asp-Lys-Asp-Tyr-Thr-
81                                     90
Met-Ala-Ala-Val-Ser-Gly-Tyr-Lys-Ser-Gly-
91                                     100
His-Ser-Ala-Val-Phe-Val-Lys-Ser-Gly-Gln-
101                                    110
Val-Gln-Leu-Gln-His-Ser-Tyr-Asn-Ser-Val-
111                                    120
Ala-Asn-Phe-Val-Gly-Glu-Asp-Glu-Gly-Ser-
121                                    130
Ile-Pro-Ser-Lys-Met-Tyr-Leu-Asp-Glu-Thr-
131                                    140
Pro-Glu-Tyr-Phe-Val-Asn-Val-Glu-Ala-Tyr-
141                                    150
Glu-Ser-Gly-Ser-Gly-Asn-Ile-Leu-Val-Met-
151                                    160
Cys-Ile-Ser-Asn-Lys-Glu-Ser-Phe-Phe-Glu-
161
Cys-Lys-His-Gln-Gln
```

FIG. 2. Amino acid sequence of the thermostable direct hemolysin deduced from the nucleotide sequence (Nishibuchi and Kaper, 1985).

Complete amino acid sequence of the thermostable direct hemolysin was also reported by Tsunasawa *et al.* (1983). The sequence was consisted of 165 amino acid residues, as in the sequence shown in Fig. 2, but there was disagreement on 7 of the residues.

6. HEAT STABILITY OF THE THERMOSTABLE DIRECT HEMOLYSIN AND ARRHENIUS EFFECT

The purified thermostable direct hemolysin was not inactivated by heating at 100°C for 10 min, and so was named thermostable direct hemolysin. However, the hemolytic activity of crude hemolysin of *V. parahaemolyticus* was partially inactivated by heating at around 60°C for 10 min (Miwatani *et al.*, 1972b). This peculiar characteristic of the hemolysin has been reported for staphylococcal alpha hemolysin and named the Arrhenius effect (Arbuthnott, 1970), since it was first described by Arrhenius as early as 1907. Takeda *et al.* (1974, 1975a) examined the mechanism of the Arrhenius effect of crude hemolysin from *V. parahaemolyticus*. They studied the effect of heat treatment on the hemolytic activities of various preparations of hemolysin and found that the degree of inactivation of the hemolysin, on heating at 60–70°C, decreased with increase in the purity of the preparation. This suggests that the crude hemolysin preparations contained some factor(s) that inactivated hemolysin.

By DEAE-cellulose column chromatography of the culture supernatant of *V. parahaemolyticus*, Takeda *et al.* (1975a) isolated a factor that inactivated the hemolytic activity of the purified thermostable direct hemolysin under certain experimental conditions. The isolated inactivating factor was mixed with the purified thermostable direct hemolysin and heated at various temperatures. Heating the mixtures at 50–60°C for 10 min resulted in significant loss of hemolytic activity, whereas heating at 80–90°C for 10 min did not cause loss of activity. The activity of the inactivating factor was enhanced by Na^+ and Mg^{2+}, but was not affected significantly by NH_4^+ or K^+. The factor showed maximal activity in the presence of more than 20 mM NaCl or $MgCl_2$. The factor was stable in the presence of more than 0.6 M NaCl. Its optimal pH for activity was about pH 8.0. The inactivating factor itself was heat labile. Thus, when the inactivating factor alone was heated at or above 60°C for 10 min and then mixed with the purified thermostable direct hemolysin and heated at 60°C, it caused scarcely any inactivation.

The Arrhenius effect of exotoxin A from *Pseudonomas aeruginosa* was demonstrated, and isolation of a similar inactivating factor was reported (Vasil *et al.*, 1976).

Zen-Yoji *et al.* (1975) reported that most of the hemolytic activity of the purified thermostable direct hemolysin was lost when the preparation was heated alone at 60°C for 30 min. This loss of hemolytic activity on heating purified thermostable direct hemolysin at 60°C without the inactivation factor was found to be due to aggregation of the hemolysin (Takeda *et al.*, 1975a) and thus was a distinct phenomenon from the Arrhenius effect of crude hemolysin.

7. HEMOLYTIC ACTIVITY OF THE THERMOSTABLE DIRECT HEMOLYSIN

The purified thermostable direct hemolysin shows various biological activities, such as hemolytic activity, cytotoxic activity on various cultured cells, and lethal toxicity in mice and rats. Zen-Yoji *et al.* (1971) studied the hemolytic activity on different kinds of erythrocytes and found that the hemolysin showed high hemolytic activity on erythrocytes of various species, its activity decreasing in the order: rat, dog, mouse, monkey, man, rabbit and guinea-pig. It had no activity on horse erythrocytes (Table 3). Sakurai *et al.* (1975a) studied the mechanism of hemolysis induced by the thermostable direct hemolysin and found that hemolysis varied with the temperature and it did not occur at low temperatures, but that binding of the thermostable direct hemolysin to human erythrocytes did occur at low temperatures (0–4°C). The binding was followed by lysis of the cells and it was stimulated by divalent cations, such as Ca^{2+}, Mn^{2+} and Mg^{2+}. Sakurai *et al.* (1975a) also studied the kinetics of inhibition of the hemolysis by antiserum against the purified thermostable direct hemolysin and concluded that the hemolysis is at least a two-step process involving the binding of the thermostable direct hemolysin and a subsequent steps(s). It is still uncertain whether the hemolysis involves some enzymic action on the cell membranes.

TABLE 3. *Hemolytic Activities of the Thermostable Direct Hemolysin on Erythrocytes from Various Species**

Source of erythrocytes	Reciprocal of titer of minimum hemolytic dose
Rat	10,240
Dog	5,120
Mouse	2,560
Monkey	2,560
Human	1,280
Rabbit	640
Guinea-pig	640
Chicken	160
Sheep	30
Horse	0

*From Zen-Yoji *et al.* (1971).

8. CYTOTOXICITY OF THE THERMOSTABLE DIRECT HEMOLYSIN

The thermostable direct hemolysin is cytotoxic to various cultured cells, such as HeLa cells (Sakazaki *et al.*, 1974a), L cells (Sakazaki *et al.*, 1974a), FL cells (Sakurai *et al.*, 1975b), neuroblastoma cells (Honda and Miwatani, personal communication), primary cultures of fetal mouse heat cells (Goshima *et al.*, 1978), and CCL-6 cells derived from human intestine (Takeda *et al.*, 1980). Sakurai *et al.* (1975b) studied the effect of the purified thermostable direct hemolysin on FL cells in detail. When 6.6×10^5 cells/ml were incubated with 5 μg/ml of the hemolysin at 37°C, death of the cells occurred after 20 min. In this experiment, survival of the cells was assayed by examining trypan blue staining of the cells or measuring release of alkaline phosphatase from the cells, both of which change in parallel with death of the cells.

It was found that morphological changes of microvilli of the cells occurred before death of the cells (Sakurai *et al.*, 1975b). Scanning electron microscopy of cells treated with the hemolysin showed that after 5 min of incubation the number of microvilli on the cell surface had decreased (Fig. 3b) relative to that on control cells (Fig. 3a) and that the shape of the microvilli also changed. After 10 min of incubation, few cells had died, but almost all the microvilli had disappeared (Fig. 3c). After 60 min of incubation, more than 95 % of the cells had died and marked degeneration of the cell surface was observed (Fig. 3d). Figure 4 shows electron micrograms of thin sections of cells treated with the hemolysin. The surface of control cells was covered with microvilli (Fig. 4a). When 6.6×10^5 cells per ml were treated with 5 μg/ml of the hemolysin at 37°C for 5 min, significant changes were observed in the shape of the microvilli, but no significant changes were observed in the cytoplasm of the cells (Fig. 4b). An electron micrograph showed that after 30 min of incubation the microvilli had disappeared, the cytoplasm had changed and the nucleus had disintegrated (Fig. 4c). After 60 min of incubation, complete degeneration of the cytoplasm was observed and no nuclei could be detected (Fig. 4d). Morphological changes of the microvilli were also observed on treatment of the cells with a sublethal amount of the hemolysin.

9. ENTEROTOXICITY OF THE THERMOSTABLE DIRECT HEMOLYSIN

Zen-Yoji *et al.* (1974) injected the purified thermostable direct hemolysin into ligated rabbit ileal loops. Injection of 100 μg of the hemolysin did not cause fluid accumulation. However, on injection of 500 μg of the hemolysin, turbid, bloody fluid accumulated in the loop and histopathological examination showed erosive lesions and desquamation of necrotic mucosa accompanied by marked neutrophil-infiltration into the intestinal wall. These changes are probably due to the cytotoxicity of the thermostable direct hemolysin described in the preceeding section.

Obara *et al.* (1974) and Miyamoto *et al.* (1980) studied the histopathological changes in the small intestine of suckling mice challenged orally with the purified thermostable direct hemolysin. On administration of 50 μg of the hemolysin by stomach tube to suckling mice of 5–6 days old, almost all the animals developed diarrhea and soon died. With a dose of 2.0–12.5 μg of the hemolysin, only some animals died while others suffered transiently from diarrhea and then recovered. The intestinal mucosa of animals with diarrhea, induced by challenge with a relatively small dose of the hemolysin, showed no destructive changes. However, light microscopic examination showed that the *lamina propria* was edematous. In ultrathin sections, intercellular junctions at interdigitations were seen to have been lost, and the resulting spaces between cells were greatly enlarged, suggesting fluid accumulation. With a large dose of the hemolysin, destructive changes were seen in parts of the intestinal mucosa

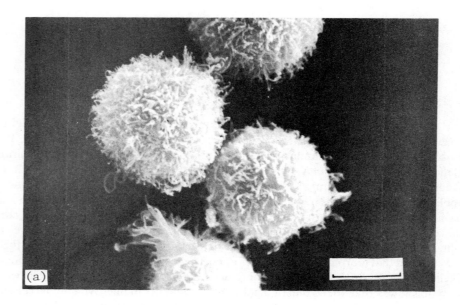

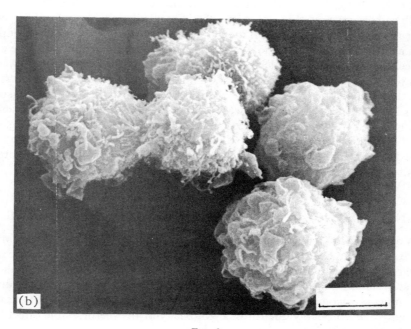

FIG. 3.

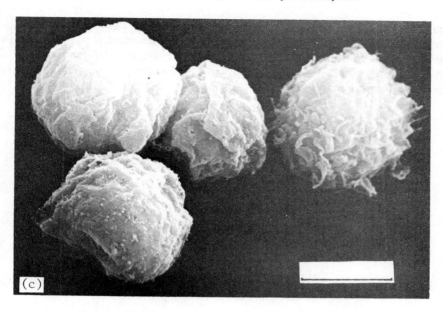

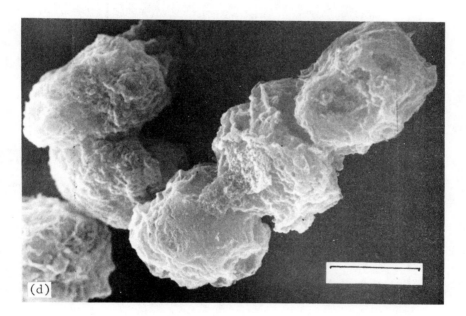

FIG. 3. Scanning electron micrograms of FL cells treated with the purified thermostable direct hemolysin (from Sakurai *et al.*, 1975b). A mixture of 5 μg of the hemolysin and FL cells (6.6×10^5) was incubated in 1 ml of Eagle's minimum essential medium at 37°C. (a) FL cells incubated at 37°C for 60 min in the absence of hemolysin; FL cells incubated with the hemolysin for (b) 5 min, (c) 10 min, and (d) 60 min. The bar represents 10 μm.

just before death of the animals. Ultrathin sections of small intestinal villi of an animal challenged with 25 μg of the hemolysin showed structural disturbance of the endoplasmic reticulum, and swollen mitochondria with indistinct cristae. Numerous vacuoles of various sizes were observed in the cytoplasm and the microvilli were disordered or had degenerated. In some epithelial cells the nucleus had become less electron-dense and showed degenerative changes. From these results, Obara *et al.* (1974) and Miyamoto *et al.* (1980) concluded that the purified thermostable direct hemolysin might be important in causing gastroenteritis in food poisoning due to *V. parahaemolyticus* in human patients.

Recent results by Honda *et al.* (1983), however, showed that fluid accumulation in the ligated rabbit ileal loop by living cells of a Kanagawa-phenomenon positive strain of *V. parahaemolyticus* was not inhibited by the antiserum against the thermostable direct hemolysin. This suggests that diarrheagenicity of *V. parahaemolyticus* cannot be explained solely by the thermostable direct hemolysin.

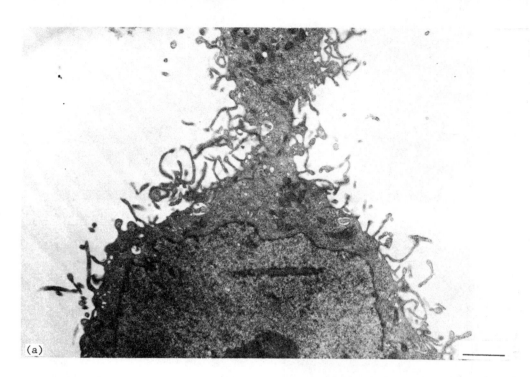

(a)

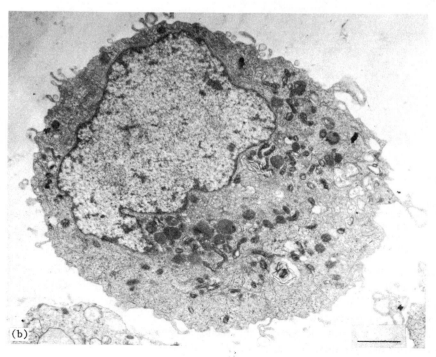

(b)

FIG. 4.

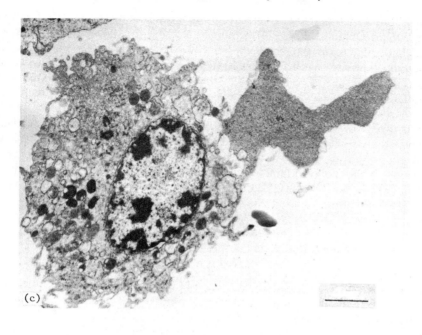

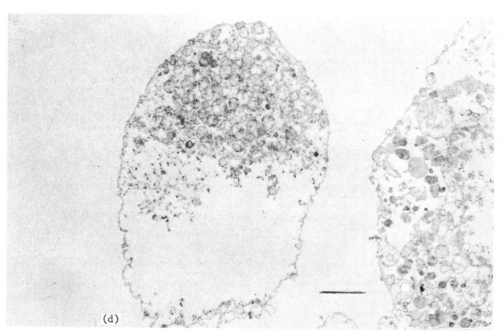

FIG. 4. Electron micrograms of thin sections of FL cells treated with the purified thermostable-direct hemolysin (from Sakurai *et al.*, 1975b). FL cells were treated with the hemolysin as described in Fig. 3. (a) Control cells: cell incubated with the hemolysin for (b) 5 min, (c) 30 min and (d) 60 min. The bar represents 1 μm.

10. LETHAL TOXICITY OF THE THERMOSTABLE DIRECT HEMOLYSIN

Fujino *et al.* (1953) reported the lethal toxicity of *V. parahaemolyticus* to mice and guinea-pigs in their paper on isolation of this organism. Several workers have attempted to isolate lethal toxin from *V. parahaemolyticus*. Kuriyama (1964) and Akehashi and Yoneda (1967) reported the existence of a toxic substance in cells of *V. parahaemolyticus*, whereas Ueyama *et al.* (1964) found a lethal toxin to mice in culture filtrates of this organism. Zen-Yoji *et al.* (1974, 1975) and Obara *et al.* (1974) demonstrated that the purified thermostable direct hemolysin had lethal toxicity to small experimental animals. Honda *et al.* (1976a) purified the lethal toxin extensively from culture filtrates of *V. parahaemolyticus* and found that this toxin was identical to the thermostable direct hemolysin. They fractionated culture supernatants of a Kanagawa-phenomenon positive strain of *V. parahaemolyticus* with ammonium sulfate and then purified it by successive column chromatographies on DEAE-cellulose, hydroxylapatite and Sephadex G-200. Each fraction was assayed for hemolytic activity and lethal activity to mice. Results showed that hemolytic activity and lethal toxicity did not dissociate during the purification procedure. Since the final preparation appeared homogeneous on both polyacrylamide gel disc electrophoresis and SDS-polyacrylamide gel disc electrophoresis, the thermostable direct hemolysin itself was concluded to be the lethal toxin produced in culture supernatants of *V. parahaemolyticus*.

11. CARDIOTOXICITY OF THE THERMOSTABLE DIRECT HEMOLYSIN

The purified lethal toxin killed various experimental animals, such as mice, rats and guinea-pigs. Rapid death of these experimental animals was observed with rather small doses of the toxin. Typical experimental results are shown in Table 4 (Honda *et al.*, 1976a,b). Intravenous injection of 5 μg of the purified thermostable direct hemolysin killed mice within 1 min and even 1 μg of the hemolysin killed mice within 20 min. Rapid death of rats was also observed; the average survival time after injection of 10 μg of the purified thermostable direct hemolysin was about 2 min. The hemolysin also had a lethal effect when injected intraperitoneally into mice and rats, although less than on intravenous injection.

Of the various bacterial toxins so far reported, streptolysin O (Halbert *et al.*, 1961; Halpern and Rahman, 1968), tetanolysin (Hardegree *et al.*, 1971) and hemolysin of *Listeria monocytogenes* (Kingdon and Sword, 1970) caused rapid death of animals on intravenous injection. Like these bacterial toxins, the thermostable direct hemolysin showed cardiotoxicity (Honda *et al.*, 1976b).

A rat weighing 445 g was injected intravenously with 15 μg of the purified thermostable direct hemolysin and its electroencephalogram and electrocardiogram were recorded

TABLE 4. *Lethal Activity of the Purified Thermostable Direct Hemolysin on Intravenous Injection into Mice and Rats**

Amount of the hemolysin injected (μg of protein per animal)	Survival time after injection (mean ± S.D.)
Mouse†	
10.0	35.5 ± 4.8 sec.
5.0	49.0 ± 8.4
2.5	561.2 ± 368.8
1.0	1121.5 ± 291.0
0.5	no death§
Rat‡	
25.0	1.87 ± 0.22 min.
10.0	2.15 ± 0.36
7.5	7.00 ± 1.53
5.0	180.00 ± 174.000
2.5	no death§

*From Honda *et al.* (1976a, b).
†ddO strain mice of 6 weeks old were used and each dose was tested on 10 mice.
‡Sprague–Dawley rats of 12–15 weeks old were used and each dose was tested on 5 rats.
§Observation continued for 24 hr.

simultaneously (Fig. 5). The electroencephalogram (lines III and IV in Fig. 5) did not change significantly after intravenous injection of the hemolysin. However, the electrocardiogram (line II in Fig. 5) showed a voltage increase after about 13 sec and the heart stopped beating after 33.5 sec. The electroencephalogram remained normal for 55 sec after this (until 80 sec after the injection).

The electrocardiograms from chest leads in a rat weighing 448 g after intravenous injection of 7.5 μg of toxin at zero time are shown in Fig. 6. About 15 sec after the injection, the P wave became wider and higher than normal, suggesting changes in conduction of intra-atrial impulses. About this time, the voltage of QRS increased and ST–T changed, suggesting changes in conduction of intra-ventricular impulses of electrical activation. After about 17–18 sec, the PQ intervals became longer, suggesting inhibition of atrio-ventricular conduction. Then after about 41 sec, the patterns showed change of the exciting foci in the ventricle and the heart rate decreased owing to reduced excitation of the heart muscle. Ventricular flutter developed after about 50 sec and the heart stopped after 148 sec.

The cardiotoxicity of the thermostable direct hemolysin was also demonstrated using cultured mouse heart cells (Honda *et al.*, 1976b). When ventricular tissue from the hearts of mouse fetuses of 14–16 days old were cultured in Eagle's minimum essential medium supplemented with 10% fetal bovine serum at 36°C under an atmosphere of 5% CO_2 and 95% air, the cells beat spontaneously and regularly. When $1-2 \times 10^5$ cells were seeded into gelatin-coated petri dishes (35 mm in diameter) and cultured for 1 day at 36°C, single isolated myocardial cells are obtained and these cells beat independently of each other at various rates of 10 to 260 beats/min (average, about 70 beats/min). The beating rhythms of most of the cells were regular and were maintained for at least 5 hr. When $1-1.5 \times 10^6$ cells were seeded into dishes, a large cluster of 2–4 mm in diameter containing more than 10^5 cells was obtained after cultivation for 1 day. All the myocardial cells in the cell cluster beat synchronously and regularly at 100–180 beats/min and this rate was maintained for at least 24 hr (Goshima, 1969, 1973).

The effect of the purified thermostable direct hemolysin on the beating of a cell cluster of cultured myocardial cells is shown in Fig. 7. On addition of 0.05 μg/ml of the hemolysin to the medium the beating increased slightly, but it returned to normal within 10 minutes (Fig. 7a). On addition of 0.1 μg/ml of the hemolysin, the beating was first rapidly stimulated and then stopped suddenly within one minute. Then, six minutes after the addition of the

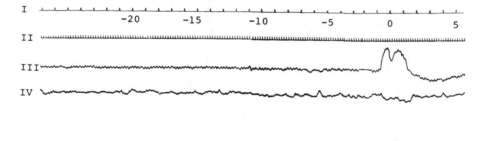

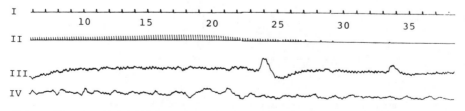

FIG. 5. Electroencephalograms of a rat injected with the purified thermostable direct hemolysin (from Honda *et al.*, 1976b). The hemolysin was injected at zero time. Line I, time in seconds; line II, electrocardiogram with a unipolar chest lead around the apex of the heart; line III, electroencephalogram with a lead from the hippocampal area; line IV, electroencephalogram with a lead from the motor area.

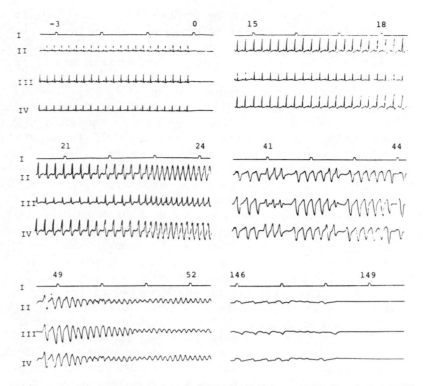

FIG. 6. Electrocardiograms of a rat injected with the purified thermostable direct hemolysin (from Honda *et al.*, 1976b). The hemolysin was injected at 0 time. Line I, time in seconds; line II, lead from a combination of electrodes in the right and left fore legs; line III, lead from a combination of electrodes in the right fore leg and left hind leg; line IV, lead from a combination of electrodes in the left fore leg and left hind leg.

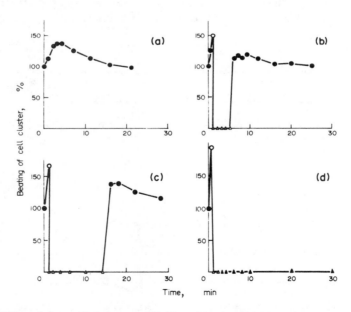

FIG. 7. Effect of the purified thermostable direct hemolysin on the beating of myocardial cell clusters cultured *in vitro*. (from Honda *et al.*, 1976b). Mouse heart cells were cultured and the amounts of the hemolysin indicated below were added to the medium at zero time. The beating of the cell clusters was expressed as a percentage of that observed in the absence of hemolysin. The concentrations of hemolysin in the medium were: (a) 0.05 μg/ml, (b) 0.1 μg/ml, (c) 0.2 μg/ml and (d) 1 μg/ml. ($\bullet$) Normal beating; (O) weaker beating; ($\triangle$) no beating but no cell disintegration; ($\blacktriangle$) disintegration of the cells.

hemolysin, the beating suddenly started again at the normal rate and remained unchanged during further observation (Fig. 7b). Similarly, on addition of 0.2 μg/ml of the toxin, the beating first increased, then stopped and then started again (Fig. 7c); but the interval between the time of stopping and of starting again was longer than that on addition of 0.1 μg/ml of the hemolysin. On addition of 1 μg/ml or more of the hemolysin per milliliters of medium, the beating also first increased and then stopped abruptly, and then almost all the cells rapidly disintegrated (Fig. 7d). Stimulation, stopping and recovery of the beating were observed repeatedly on repeated addition of the purified thermostable direct hemolysin to the medium (Fig. 8). It was concluded that the hemolysin added in the medium was somehow inactivated during the incubation and thus beating of the cells recovered after a short while.

The cardiotoxicity of the purified thermostable direct hemolysin was also demonstrated with single isolated myocardial cells (Goshima *et al.*, 1977). Two to five minutes after the addition of 0.05 μg/ml of the hemolysin, the number of cells beating rhythmically decreased and the number of cells showing irregular, faint fibrillatory movements increased. On further incubation, these cells regained their normal rhythmical beating. When 0.5 μg/ml of the hemolysin was added, morphological damage of the cells was observed and the numbers of quiescent cells and those showing irregular, faint fibrillatory movements increased. On further incubation, all these cells except those showing morphological damage regained their normal rhythmic beating. On addition of 2 μg/ml of the hemolysin, degeneration of most single isolated myocardial cells was observed. The thermostable direct hemolysin had a similar effect on cultured rat myocardial cells, but did not affect chick myocardial cells.

Goshima *et al.* (1978) studied the mechanism of cell degeneration by the thermostable direct hemolysin and found that mouse myocardial cells take up Ca^{2+} from the culture medium in the presence of the thermostable direct hemolysin, whereas chick myocardial cells under similar experimental conditions do not. From these results, they suggested that degeneration of mouse myocardial cells caused by the thermostable direct hemolysin is due to excess uptake of Ca^{2+} from the incubation medium.

Seyama *et al.* (1977) studied the action of the thermostable direct hemolysin on the sino— atrial (S–A) node and on cells of the right atrium of rabbits and found that reduction in membrane resistance and depolarization of the membrane, without any effect on the mechanism generating the action potential, were the major responses of both S–A nodal and atrial cells to the hemolysin. The depolarization seemed to be due to increase in conductance of Na^+.

12. MEMBRANE RECEPTOR OF THE THERMOSTABLE DIRECT HEMOLYSIN

One method for studying the membrane receptor(s) for bacterial toxin is to examine the inhibition of biological activities of the toxin by gangliosides. The membrane receptors of

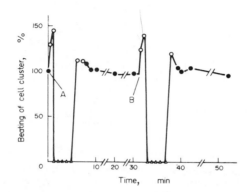

FIG. 8. Effect of repeated additions of the purified thermostable direct hemolysin to the medium on beating of myocardial cell clusters cultured *in vitro* (from Honda *et al.*, 1976b). The hemolysin was added successively at arrow A (0.1 μg/ml) and arrow B (0.1 μg/ml). Symbols are as for Fig. 7.

tetanus toxin (van Heyningen, 1959, van Heyningen and Miller, 1961), cholera enterotoxin (Holmgren et al., 1973) and Escherichia coli heat-labile enterotoxin (Holmgren, 1973) were determined in this way. Attempts to determine the membrane receptor for the thermostable direct hemolysin using gangliosides were reported by Takeda et al. (1975b, 1976). When the hemolysin was preincubated with G_{T1} and G_{D1a} gangliosides, its hemolytic activity was lost, whereas when it was preincubated with G_{M1} and G_{M2} gangliosides its hemolytic activity did not decrease (Fig. 9). Results also showed that treatment of gangliosides G_{T1} and G_{D1a} with neuraminidase abolished their inhibitory effects on the hemolytic activity of the hemolysin.

The thermostable direct hemolysin caused hemolysis of human erythrocytes, but not of horse erythrocytes. The results in Fig. 10 (Takeda et al., 1976) suggest that the different sensitivities of human and horse erythrocytes to the hemolysin are due to the absence of gangliosides G_{T1} and G_{D1a} in horse erythrocytes.

The lethal toxicity of the thermostable direct hemolysin was also lost on incubation with gangliosides G_{T1} and G_{D1a} (Takeda et al., 1976). As shown in Table 5, preincubation of the hemolysin with ganglioside G_{T1} significantly inhibited the lethal activity of the thermostable direct hemolysin on subsequent intravenous injection into mice. Ganglioside G_{D1a} had a similar inhibitory effect, although it was less inhibitory than ganglioside G_{T1}. Preincubation of the hemolysin with gangliosides G_{M1} and G_{M2} did not affect the lethal activity of the hemolysin.

From these results, it is concluded that the membrane receptors of the thermostable direct hemolysin are gangliosides G_{T1} and G_{D1a}, and that ganglioside G_{T1} binds the hemolysin more strongly than ganglioside G_{D1a}.

13. CLINICAL MANIFESTATIONS OF V. PARAHAEMOLYTICUS INFECTION AND THE THERMOSTABLE DIRECT HEMOLYSIN

The clinical symptoms of V. parahaemolyticus infection are diarrhea, abdominal pain, headache, vomiting, fever, general lassitude, chill, tenesmus and nausea. Of these, diarrhea and abdominal pain are the main symptoms (Table 6; Saito, 1967). The frequency of

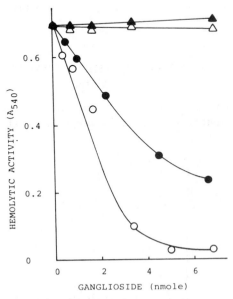

FIG. 9. Effects of various ganglioside components on the hemolytic activity of the purified thermostable direct hemolysin (from Takeda et al., 1976). The indicated amounts of the various ganglioside components were mixed with 5 μg (~0.12 nmol) of the purified hemolysin in 0.01 M Tris-hydrochloride buffer (pH 7.2) in a volume of 0.125 ml and incubated at 37°C for 30 min. Hemolytic activity was assayed after further incubation at 37°C for 30 min by measuring the absorbance at 540 nm. Symbols: (O) G_{T1}; (●) G_{D1a}; (△) G_{M1}; (▲) G_{M2}.

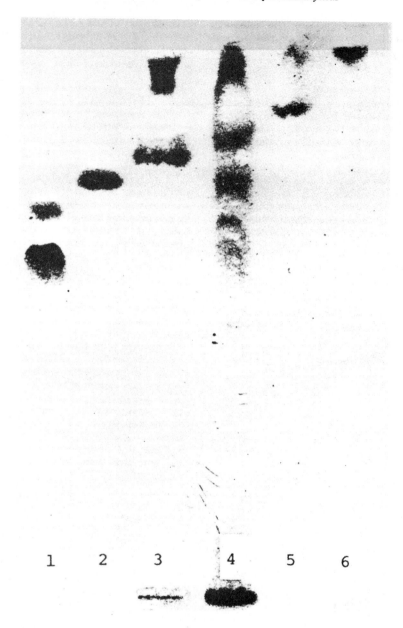

FIG. 10. Ganglioside compositions of horse and human erythrocyte membranes (from Takeda *et al.*, 1976). Membranes were prepared from erythrocytes in 400–500 ml of horse and human blood, and gangliosides were extracted from them. Ganglioside mixtures from horse and human erythrocyte membranes, containing about 15 μg of *N*-acetylneuraminic acid, were applied to a thin-layer plate and chromatographed and stained. G_{T1}, G_{D1a}, G_{M1} and G_{M2} gangliosides (Supelco, Inc.) were chromatographed as controls. (1) G_{T1}; (2) G_{D1a}; (3) ganglioside from horse erythrocyte membranes; (4) ganglioside from human erythrocyte membranes; (5) G_{M1}; (6) G_{M2}.

diarrhea is usually less than 10 times a day, but some cases show a frequence of more than 21 times a day (Table 7; Saito, 1967). The diarrhea is usually watery, but mucous and bloody discharges are also sometimes observed (Yanai *et al.*, 1981). Diarrhea or soft stools persist for 4–7 days or more.

Although there is no direct evidence that the thermostable direct hemolysin is a cause of diarrhea due to *V. parahaemolyticus* infection, several findings suggest that it is at least one of the major causes of diarrhea, as discussed in Section 9.

TABLE 5. *Effects of Various Gangliosides on the Lethal Activity of the Thermostable Direct Hemolysin after Intravenous Injection into Mice**

| Ganglioside | Survival time after hemolysin injection (mean ± S.D.)† | |
	25 nmol‡	50 nmol
G_{M1}	87 ± 10 sec.	88 ± 13 sec.
G_{M2}	81 ± 14	73 ± 3
G_{D1a}	360 ± 209	1,076 ± 187
G_{T1}	926 ± 239	no death§

*A 0.5 nmol portion of the hemolysin was incubated with the indicated amounts of gangliosides in 0.5 ml of 0.01 M Tris-hydrochloride buffer (pH 7.2) at 37°C for 30 min, and then a 0.1 nmol equivalent of the hemolysin (4.2 µg) was injected into each mouse intravenously. From Takeda et al. (1976).

†The hemolysin incubated without ganglioside killed mice in 76 ± 4 sec. Each group consisted of five mice. SD, Standard deviation.

‡Amount of ganglioside.

§Observation continued for 24 hr.

TABLE 6. *Symptoms of Food Poisoning due to V. parahaemolyticus**

Symptom	Number of patients (%)†
Diarrhea	2,293 (94.9)
Abdominal pain	2,073 (85.8)
Headache	962 (39.8)
Vomiting	860 (35.6)
Fever	847 (35.1)
General lassitude	709 (29.4)
Chill	551 (22.8)
Tenesmus	428 (17.7)
Nausea	15 (0.01)

*From Mizoguchi (1963).

†A total of 2,416 patients were examined.

TABLE 7. *Frequencies of Diarrhea in Patients with Food Poisoning due to V. parahaemolyticus**

Frequency	Number of patients†
1–5	255
6–10	144
11–20	48
≥21	28

*From Saito (1967).

†A total of 475 patients were examined.

Cardiovascular symptoms have not been claimed in *V. parahaemolyticus* infection. However, there are several reports indicating cardiovascular disturbances. Since thermostable direct hemolysin is cardiotoxic, it is assumed that the reported cardiovascular symptoms were due to the thermostable direct hemolysin produced by *V. parahaemolyticus*. Takikawa (1958) administered living cells of *V. parahaemolyticus* to a volunteer and observed a significant change in the blood pressure: the maximum blood pressure decreased to 77 mmHg on the first day of infection and returned to 136 mmHg after 4 days. Significant decrease in blood pressure in severe cases of food poisoning due to *V. parahaemolyticus* was also reported by Saito (1967). As shown in Table 8, low blood pressure was observed in patients in the first and second days of the disease.

Honda *et al.* (1976c) compared electrocardiograms of patients during acute gastroenteritis due to *V. parahaemolyticus* and after recovery. As shown in Fig. 11 the T wave was significantly lower during the disease than after recovery. The P wave also became wider and higher during the disease, especially in case 2, but was normal after recovery. Typical changes in electrocardiograms from chest leads of one of these patients are shown in Fig. 12.

TABLE 8. *Maximal Blood Pressure in Patients with Food Poisoning due to* V. parahaemolyticus*

Maximum blood pressure	Days after admission						
	1	2	3	4	5	6	≥7
	Number of patients†						
≥130	7	1				4	5
120–129	14	6	3	2	3	1	6
110–119	42	8	3	3	4	4	20
100–109	27	8	3	5	1	5	9
90–99	11	6		1	2	1	7
80–89	5	2					
70–79	4	1	1				
60–69							
50–59	1						
Total number of patients examined	111	32	10	11	9	15	47

*From Saito (1967).
†A total of 141 patients were examined.

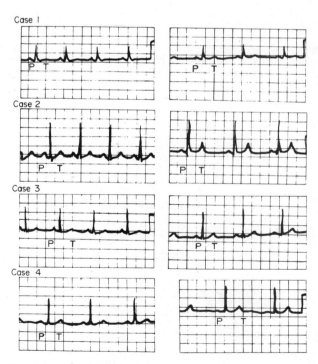

Case 1

Case 2

Case 3

Case 4

FIG. 11. Electrocardiograms (aVF) of patients with food poisoning due to *V. parahaemolyticus*: Comparison of records during and after the disease (from Honda *et al.*, 1976c). Left and right columns show records during and after the disease, respectively.

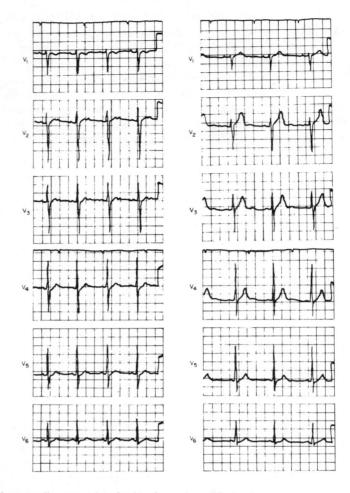

FIG. 12. Electrocardiograms (chest leads) of a patient suffering from severe diarrhea due to *V. parahaemolyticus* infection (from Honda *et al.*, 1976c). The antihemolysin titer was very high after the disease. Left and right columns show records during and after the disease, respectively.

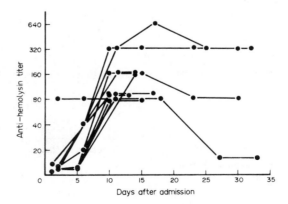

FIG. 13. Change of antihemolysin titers in the serum during food poisoning due to *V. parahaemolyticus* (from Miwatani *et al.*, 1976). Eleven typical cases with increased antihemolysin titers are shown. A total of 33 cases were examined and 16 cases showed no increase of antihemolysin titer.

Changes in the T wave are very clear during the disease, the T wave not only became lower but also became biphasic in the V_2 and V_3 leads.

Miwatani *et al.* (1976) examined the titers of antihemolysin (antibody against the thermostable direct hemolysin) and found that increase of the antihemolysin titer occurred on about 33 % of the patients. Typical cases showing increase of the antihemolysin titer are shown in Fig. 13. On the day of admission to hospital the titers were very low; increase in the titer began about 5 days after admission and reached a maximum after 10–15 days. Similar observations were reported by Miyamoto *et al.* (1980). From these data, it is concluded that the thermostable direct hemolysin produced by *V. parahaemolyticus* in the intestinal cavity is absorbed during the disease and circulates in the blood stream, and may, therefore, cause the electrocardiographic changes. In Japan during the last 19 years, 74 cases of death due to *V. parahaemolyticus* food poisoning have been reported. This figure represents about 32.3 % of all cases of death due to bacterial food poisoning. Many patients with *V. parahaemolyticus* infection died of cardiac insufficiency. Since there have been no histopathological studies on the effect of the thermostable direct hemolysin on cardiac tissues, it is difficult to conclude that these deaths were caused by the thermostable direct hemolysin. However, it is quite probable that the cardiotoxicity of the thermostable direct hemolysin is somehow related to death after *V. parahaemolyticus* infection.

REFERENCES

AISO, K. and FUJIWARA, K. (1963) Feeding tests of "pathogenic halophilic bacteria". *A. Rep. Inst. Food Microbiol. Chiba Univ.* **15**: 34–38.

AKEHASHI, H. and YONEDA, M. (1967) Toxins of *Vibrio parahaemolyticus* (in Japanese). In: *Vibrio parahaemolyticus II*, pp. 215–231, FUJINO, T. and FUKUMI, H. (eds). Naya Shoten, Tokyo.

ARBUTHNOTT, J. P. (1970) Staphylococcal (α-toxin. In: *Microbial Toxins Vol. 3*, pp. 189–236, MONTIE, T. C., KADIS, S. and AJL, S. J. (eds). Academic Press, New York.

BARKER, W. H. JR. (1974) *Vibrio parahaemolyticus* outbreak in the United States. In: *International Symposium on Vibrio parahaemolyticus*, pp. 47–52, FUJINO, T., SAKAGUCHI, G., SAKAZAKI, R. and TAKEDA, Y. (eds). Saikon Publ., Tokyo.

BLAKE, P. A., WEAVER, R. E. and HOLLIS, D. G. (1980) Diseases of humans (other than cholera) caused by vibrios. *Ann. Rev. Microbiol.* **34**: 341–367.

BROWN, D. F., SPAULDING, P. L. and TWEDT, R. M. (1977) Enteropathogenicity of *Vibrio parahemolyticus* in the ligated rabbit ileum. *Appl. Envir. Microbiol.* **33**: 10–14.

CHATTERJEE, B. D., GORBACH, S. L. and NEOGY, K. N. (1970) *Vibrio parahaemolyticus* and diarrhoea associated with non-cholera vibrios. *Bull. W. H. O.* **42**: 460–463.

CHERWONOGRODZKY, J. W. and CLARK, A. G. (1982) The purification of the Kanagawa haemolysin from *Vibrio parahaemolyticus*. *FEMS Microbiol. Lett.* **15**: 175–179.

FUJINO, T., MIWATANI, T., TAKEDA, Y. and TOMARU, A. (1969) A thermolabile direct hemolysin of *Vibrio parahaemolyticus*. *Biken J.* **12**: 145–148.

FUJINO, T., OKUNO, Y. NAKADA, D., AOYAMA, A., FUKAI, K., MUKAI, T. and UENO, T. (1953) On the bacteriological examination of shirasu food poisoning. *Med. J. Osaka Univ.* **4**: 299–304.

FUJINO, T., SAKAGUCHI, G., SAKAZAKI, R. and TAKEDA, Y. (eds). (1974) International Symposium on *Vibrio parahaemolyticus*. Saikon Publ., Tokyo.

GHOSH, A. K., GUHAMAZUMDER, D. N., BANERJEE, P. L., SENGUPTA, K. P., BOSE, A. K. and MAJUMDER, R. N. (1974) Studies on mechanism of pathogenicity of *Vibrio parahaemolyticus*. In: *International Symposium on Vibrio parahaemolyticus*, pp. 219–226, FUJINO, T. SAKAGUCHI, G., SAKAZAKI, R. and TAKEDA, Y. (eds). Saikon Publ., Tokyo.

GOSHIMA, K. (1969) Synchronized beating of embryonic mouse myocardial cells mediated by FL cells in monolayer culture. *Exp. Cell Res.* **58**: 420–426.

GOSHIMA, K. (1973) A study on the preservation of the beating rhythm of single myocardial cells *in vitro*. *Exp. Cell Res.* **80**: 432–438.

GOSHIMA, K., HONDA, T., HIRATA, M., KIKUCHI, K., TAKEDA, Y. and MIWATANI, T. (1977) Reversible stopping of spontaneous beating of myocardial cells *in vitro* by a toxin from *Vibrio parahaemolyticus*. *J. Mol. Cell. Cardiol.* **9**: 191–213.

GOSHIMA, K., OWARIBE, K., YAMANAKA, H. and YOSHINO, S. (1978) Requirement of calcium ions for cell degeneration with a toxin (vibriolysin) from *Vibrio parahaemolyticus*. *Infect. Immun.* **22**: 821–832.

HALBERT, S. P., BIRCHER, R. and DAHLE, E. (1961) The analysis of streptococcal infections. V. Cardiotoxicity of streptolysin O for rabbits *in vivo*. *J. Exp. Med.* **113**: 759–785.

HALPERN, B. N. and RAHMAN, S. (1968) Studies on the cardiotoxicity of streptolysin O. *Br. J. Pharmac. Chemother.* **32**: 441–452.

HARDEGREE, M. C., PALMER, A. E. and DUFFIN, N. (1971) Tetanolysin: *In-vivo* effects in animals. *J. Infect. Dis.* **123**: 51–60.

HOLMGREN, J. (1973) Comparison of the tissue receptors for *Vibrio cholerae* and *Escherichia coli* enterotoxins by means of gangliosides and natural cholera toxoid. *Infect. Immun.* **8**: 851–859.

HOLMGREN, J. LÖNNROTH, I. and SVENNERHOLM, L. (1973) Tissue receptor for cholera exotoxin: Postulated structure from studies with G_{M1} ganglioside and related glycolipids. *Infect. Immun.* **8**: 208–214.

HONDA, T., TAGA, S. TAKEDA, T., HASIBUAN, M. A., TAKEDA, Y. and MIWATANI, T. (1976a) Identification of lethal toxin with thermostable direct hemolysin produced by *Vibrio parahaemolyticus* and some physiocochemical properties of the purified toxin. *Infect. Immun.* **13**: 133–139.

HONDA, T., GOSHIMA, K., TAKEDA, Y., SUGINO, Y. and MIWATANI, T. (1976b) Demonstration of the cardiotoxicity of the thermostable direct hemolysin (lethal toxin) produced by *Vibrio parahaemolyticus*. *Infect. Immun.* **13**: 163–171.

HONDA, T., TAKEDA, Y., MIWATANI, T., KATO, K. and NIMURA, Y. (1976c) Clinical features of patients suffering from food poisoning due to *Vibrio parahaemolyticus*–especially on changes in electrocardiograms (in Japanese). *J. Jap. Ass. Infect. Dis.* **50**: 216–223.

HONDA, T., CHEARSKUL, S., TAKEDA, Y. and MIWATANI, T. (1980) Immunological methods for detection of Kanagawa-phenomenon of *Vibro parahaemolyticus*. *J. Clin. Microbiol.* **11**: 600–603.

HONDA, T., TAKEDA, Y., MIWATANI, T. and NAKAHARA, N. (1983) Failure of antisera to thermostable direct hemolysin and cholera enterotoxin to prevent accumulation of fluid caused by *Vibrio parahaemolyticus*. *J. Infect. Dis.* **147**: 779.

HONDA, T., YOH, M., KONGMUANG, U. and MIWATANI, T. (1985) Enzyme-linked immunosorbent assays for detection of thermostable direct hemolysin of *Vibrio parahaemolyticus*. *J. Clin. Microbiol.* **22**: 383–6.

JOHNSON, D. E. and CALIA, F. M. (1976) False-positive rabbit ileal loop reactions attributed to *Vibrio parahaemolyticus* broth filtrates. *J. Infect. Dis.* **133**: 436–440.

KAPER, J. B., CAMPEN, R. K., SEIDLER, R. J., BALDINI, M. M. and FALKOW, S. (1984) Cloning of the thermostable direct or Kanagawa phenomenon associated hemolysin of *Vibrio parahaemolyticus*. *Infect. Immun.* **45**: 290–292.

KATO, T., OBARA, Y., ICHINOE, H., NAGASHIMA, K., AKIYAMA, S., TAKIZAWA, K., MATSUSHIMA, A., YAMAI, S. and MIYAMOTO, Y. (1965) Grouping of *Vibrio parahaemolyticus* (biotype 1) by hemolytic reaction (in Japanese). *Shokuhin Eisei Kenkyu* **15**(8): 83–86.

KATO, T., OBARA, Y., ICHINOE, H., YAMAI, S., NAGASHIMA, K. and SAKAZAKI, R. (1966) Hemolytic activity and toxicity of *Vibrio parahaemolyticus* (in Japanese) *Jap. J. Bacteriol.* **21**: 442–443.

KAWAMURA, O. (1967) On the hemolytic character of *Vibrio parahaemolyticus* (in Japanese). In: *Vibrio parahaemolyticus II*, pp. 241–243, FUJINO, T. and FUKUMI, H. (eds). Naya Shoten, Tokyo.

KINGDON, G. C. and SWORD, C. P. (1970) Cardiotoxic and lethal effects of *Listeria monocytogenes* hemolysin. *Infect. Immun.* **1**: 373–379.

KURIYAMA, K. (1964) Biological and immunological studies on the DNA derived from *Vibrio parahaemolyticus*. 1. On the purification of the toxic fraction isolated from *Vibrio parahaemolyticus* (in Japanese). *Jap. J. Bacteriol.* **19**: 418–424.

LOWRY, O. H., ROSEBROUGH, J., FARR, A. L. and RANDALL, R. J. (1951) Protein measurement with the Folin phenol reagent. *J. Biol. Chem.* **193**: 265–275.

MIWATANI, T. and TAKEDA, Y. (1976) *Vibrio parahaemolyticus*—A causative bacterium of food poisoning. Saikon Publ., Tokyo.

MIWATANI, T., SAKURAI, J., YOSHIHARA, A. and TAKEDA, Y. (1972a) Isolation and partial purification of thermolabile direct hemolysin of *Vibrio parahaemolyticus*. *Biken J.* **15**: 61–66.

MIWATANI, T., TAKEDA, Y., SAKURAI, J., YOSHIHARA, A. and TAGA, S. (1972b) Effect of heat (Arrhenius effect) on crude hemolysin of *Vibrio parahaemolyticus*. *Infect. Immun.* **6**: 1031–1033.

MIWATANI, T., SAKURAI, J., TAKEDA, Y., SUGIYAMA, S. and ADACHI, T. (1976) Antibody titers against the thermostable direct hemolysin in sera of patients suffering from gastroenteritis due to *Vibrio parahaemolyticus* (in Japanese). *J. Jap. Ass. Infect. Dis.* **50**: 46–51.

MIYAMOTO, Y., KATO, T., OBARA, Y., AKIYAMA, S., TAKIZAWA, K. and YAMAI, S. (1969) *In vitro* hemolytic characteristic of *Vibrio parahaemolyticus:* its close correlation with human pathogenicity. *J. Bacteriol.* **100**: 1147–1149.

MIYAMOTO, Y., OBARA, Y., NIKKAWA, T., YAMAI, S., KATO, T., YAMADA, Y. and OHASHI, M. (1980) Simplified purification and biophysicochemical characteristics of Kanagawa phenomenon-associated hemolysin of *Vibrio parahaemolyticus*. *Infect. Immun.* **28**: 567–576.

MIZOGUCHI, T. (1963) Clinical features of food poisoning due to *Vibrio parahaemolyticus* (in Japanese). In: *Vibrio parahaemolyticus*, pp. 367–395, FUJINO, T. and FUKUMI, H. (eds). Isseido. Tokyo.

NIKKAWA, T., OBARA, Y., YAMAI, S. and MIYAMOTO, Y. (1972) Purification of a hemolysin from *Vibrio parahaemolyticus*. *Jap. J. Med. Sci. Biol.* **25**: 197–200.

NISHIBUCHI, M. and KAPER, J. B. (1985) Nucleotide sequence of the thermostable direct hemolysin gene of *Vibrio parahaemolyticus*. *J. Bacteriol.* **162**: 558–564.

OBARA, Y. (1971) Studies on hemolytic factors of *Vibrio parahaemolyticus*. *II*. The extraction of hemolysin and its properties (in Japanese). *J. Jap. Ass. Infect. Dis.* **45**: 392–398.

OBARA, Y., YAMAI, S., NIKKAWA, T., MIYAMOTO, Y., OHASHI, M. and SHIMADA, T. (1974) Histopathological changes in the small intestine of suckling mice challenged orally with purified hemolysin from *Vibrio parahaemolyticus*. In: *International Symposium on Vibrio parahaemolyticus*. pp. 253–257, FUJINO, T., SAKAGUCHI, G., SAKAZAKI, R. and TAKEDA, Y. (eds). Saikon Publ., Tokyo.

OHTA, K., KUDOH, Y., TSUNO, M., SAKAI, S., MARUYAMA, T., ITOH, T. and OHASHI, M. (1979) Development of a sensitive serological assay based on reversed passive hemagglutination for detection of enteropathogenic toxin (Kanagawa hemolysin) of *Vibrio parahaemolyticus*, and re-evaluation of the toxin producibility of isolates from various sources (in Japanese). *Jap. J. Bacteriol.* **34**: 837–846.

SAITO, M. (1967) Clinical features of gastroenteritis due to *Vibrio parahaemolyticus* (in Japanese). In: *Vibrio parahaemolyticus II*, pp. 295–310, FUJINO, T. and FUKUMI, H. (eds). Naya Shoten, Tokyo.

SAKAZAKI, R., TAMURA, K., KATO, T., OBARA, Y., YAMAL, S. and HOBO, K. (1968) Studies on the enteropathogenic, facultatively halophilic bacteria, *Vibrio parahaemolyticus*. *III*. Enteropathogenicity. *Jap. J. Med. Sci. Biol.* **21**: 325–331.

SAKAZAKI, R., TAMURA, K., NAKAMURA, A., KURATA, T., GHODA, A. and KAZUNO, Y. (1974a) Enteropathogenic activity of *Vibrio parahaemolyticus*. In: *International Symposium on Vibrio parahaemolyticus*, pp. 231–235, FUJINO, T., SAKAGUCHI, G., SAKAZAKI, R. and TAKEDA, Y. (eds). Saikon Publ., Tokyo.

SAKAZAKI, R., TAMURA, K., NAKAMURA, A., KURATA, T., GHODA, A. and KAZUNO, Y. (1974b) Studies on enteropathogenic activity of *Vibrio parahaemolyticus* using ligated gut loop model in rabbits. *Jap. J. Med. Sci. Biol.* **27**: 35–43.

SAKURAI, J., MATSUZAKI, A. and MIWATANI, T. (1973) Purification and characterization of thermostable direct hemolysin of *Vibrio parahaemolyticus*. *Infect. Immun.* **8**: 775–780.

SAKURAI, J., MATSUZAKI, A., TAKEDA, Y. and MIWATANI, T. (1974) Existence of two distinct hemolysins in *Vibrio parahaemolyticus*. *Infect. Immun.* **9**: 777–780.

SAKURAI, J., BAHAVAR, M. A., JINGUJI, Y. and MIWATANI, T. (1975a) Interaction of thermostable direct hemolysin of *Vibrio parahaemolyticus* with human erythrocytes. *Biken J.* **18**: 187–192

SAKURAI, J., HONDA, T., JINGUJI, Y., ARITA, M. and MIWATANI, T. (1975b) Cytotoxic effect of the thermostable direct hemolysin produced by *Vibrio parahaemolyticus* on FL cells. *Infect. Immun.* **13**: 876–883.

SANYAL, S. C., SIL, J. and SAKAZAKI, R. (1973) Laboratory infection by *Vibrio parahaemolyticus*. *J. Med. Microbiol.* **6**: 121–122.

SANYAL, S. C. and SEN, P. C. (1974) Human volunteer study on the pathogenicity of *Vibrio parahaemolyticus*. In: *International Symposium on Vibrio parahaemolyticus*, pp. 227–235, FUJINO, T., SAKAGUCHI, G., SAKAZAKI, R. and TAKEDA, Y. (eds). Saikon Publ., Tokyo.

SEYAMA, I., IRISAWA, H., HONDA, T., TAKEDA, Y. and MIWATANI, T. (1977) Effect of hemolysin produced by *Vibrio parahaemolyticus* on membrane conductance and mechanical tension of rabbit myocardium. *Jap. J. Physiol.* **27**: 43–56.

TAKEDA, Y., HORI, Y. and MIWATANI, T. (1974) Demonstration of a temperature-dependent inactivating factor of the thermostable direct hemolysin in *Vibrio parahaemolyticus*. *Infect. Immun.* **10**: 6–10.

TAKEDA, Y., HORI, Y., TAGA, S., SAKURAI, J. and MIWATANI, T. (1975a) Characterization of the temperature-dependent inactivating factor of the thermostable direct hemolysin in *Vibrio parahaemolyticus*. *Infect. Immun.* **12**: 449–454.

TAKEDA, Y., TAKEDA, T., HONDA, T., SAKURAI, J. OHTOMO, N. and MIWATANI, T. (1975b) Inhibition of hemolytic activity of the thermostable direct hemolysin of *Vibrio parahaemolyticus* by ganglioside. *Infect. Immun.* **12**: 931–933.

TAKEDA, Y., TAKEDA, T., HONDA, T. and MIWATANI, T. (1976) Inactivation of the biological activities of the thermostable direct hemolysin of *Vibrio parahaemolyticus* by ganglioside G_{T1}. *Infect. Immun.* **14**: 1–5.

TAKEDA, Y., TAGA, S. and MIWATANI, T. (1978) Evidence that thermostable direct hemolysin of *Vibrio parahaemolyticus* is composed of two subunits. *FEMS Microbiol. Lett.* **4**: 271–274.

TAKEDA, T., HONDA, T., TAKEDA, Y. and MIWATANI, T. (1980) Pathogenesis of *Vibrio parahaemolyticus*. In: *Natural Toxins*, EAKER, D. and WADSTROM, T. (eds). Pergamon Press, Oxford.

TAKIKAWA, I. (1958) Studies on pathogenic halophilic bacteria. *Yokohama Med. Bull.* **9**: 313–322.

TANIGUCHI, H., OHTA, H., OGAWA, M. and MIZUGUCHI, Y. (1985) Cloning and expression in *Escherichia coli* of *Vibrio parahaemolyticus* thermostable direct hemolysin and thermolabile hemolysin genes. *J. Bacteriol.* **162**: 510–515.

TSUNASAWA, S., SUGIHARA, A., MASAKI, T., NARITA, K., SAKIYAMA, F., TAKEDA, Y. and MIWATANI, T. (1983) The primary structure of a protein toxin, hemolysin, of *Vibrio parahaemolyticus* (in Japanese). *Seikagaku* **55**: 807.

TWEDT, R. M. and BROWN, D. F. (1974) Studies on the enteropathogenicity of *Vibrio parahaemolyticus* in the ligated rabbit ileum. In: *International Symposium on Vibrio parahaemolyticus*, pp. 211–217, FUJINO, T., SAKAGUCHI, G., SAKAZAKI, R. and TAKEDA, Y. (eds). Saikon Publ., Tokyo.

UEYAMA, T., BABA, T. and BITO, Y. (1964) Studies on the toxic substance of *Vibrio parahaemolyticus* (in Japanese). *Jap. J. Bacteriol.* **19**: 480–482.

VAN HEYNINGEN, W. E. (1959) The fixation of tetanus toxin by nervous tissue. *J. Gen. Microbiol.* **20**: 291–300.

VAN HEYNINGEN, W. E. and MILLER, P. A. (1961)The fixation of tetanus toxin by ganglioside. *J. Gen. Microbiol.* **24**: 107–119.

VASIL, M. L., LIU, P. V. and IGLEWSKI, B. H. (1976) Temperature-dependent inactivating factor of *Pseudomonas aeruginosa* exotoxin A. *Infect. Immun.* **13**: 1467–1472.

WAGATSUMA, S. (1968) On a medium for hemolytic reaction (in Japanese). *Media Circle* **13**: 159–162.

YANAGASE, Y., INOUE, K., OZAKI, M., OCHI, T., AMANO, T. and CHAZONO, M. (1970) Hemolysins and related enzymes of *Vibrio parahaemolyticus*. I. Identification and partial purification of enzymes. *Biken J.* **13**: 77–92.

YANAI, Y., KANDA, T., HASHIMOTO, S. ABE, H. and OGAWA, R. (1981) Bacteriological study of traveller's diarrhoea. (2) *Vibrio parahaemolyticus* strains isolated from patients with traveller's diarrhoea (in Japanese). *J. Jap. Ass. Infect. Dis.*, **55**: 701–708.

ZEN-YOJI, H., HITOKOTO, H., MOROZUMI, S. and LECLAIR, R. A. (1971) Purification and characterization of a hemolysin produced by *Vibrio parahaemolyticus*. *J. Infect. Dis.* **123**: 665–667.

ZEN-YOJI, H., KUDOH, Y., IGARASHI, H., OHTA, K. and FUKAI, K. (1974) Purification and identification of enteropathogenic toxins a and a' produced by *Vibrio parahaemolyticus* and their biological and pathological activities. In: *International Symposium on Vibrio parahaemolyticus*, pp. 237–243, FUJINO, T., SAKAGUCHI, G., SAKAZAKI, R. and TAKEDA, Y. (eds). Saikon Publ., Tokyo.

ZEN-YOJI, H., KUDOH, Y., IGARASHI, H., OHTA, K., FUKAI, K. and HOSHINO, T. (1975) An enteropathogenic toxin of *Vibrio parahaemolyticus*. In: *Proc. 1st Intersect. Conf. IAMS*, Vol. **4**, pp. 263–272. HASEGAWA, T. (ed). Science Council of Japan, Tokyo.

ZEN-YOJI, H., KUDOH, Y., IGARASHI, H., OHTA, K., FUKAI, K. and HOSHINO, T. (1976) Further studies on characterization and biological activities of an enteropathogenic toxin of *Vibrio parahaemolyticus*. In: *Animal, Plant and Microbial Toxins*, Vol. **1**, pp. 479–498, OHSAKA, A., HAYASHI, K. and SAWAI, Y. (eds). Plenum, New York.

CHAPTER 11

NAG VIBRIO TOXIN

S. C. SANYAL

*Department of Microbiology, Institute of Medical Sciences, Banaras Hindu University,
Varanasi-221005, India*

1. INTRODUCTION

The vibrios that have biochemical reactions similar to those of *Vibrio cholerae* and are not agglutinable by *V. cholerae* O-subgroup 1 antiserum have been designated cholera-like vibrios (Gardner and Venkatraman, 1935), noncholera vibrios or NCV (McIntyre *et al.*, 1965) and nonagglutinable or NAG vibrios (Felsenfeld, 1967). However, the ICSB Subcommittee on Taxonomy of Vibrios recommended that all these vibrios be included in the species *V. cholerae*, and the above vernacular names should not be used (Hugh and Feeley, 1972; Hugh and Sakazaki, 1975). The only taxonomic criterion distinguishing *V. cholerae* from the so-called NAG vibrios is the lack of an antigen. Based on somatic antigen, both the classical and *eltor* biotypes of *V. cholerae* are designated O-group 1. The NAG vibrios have so far been divided into 59 serovars as reported by Shimada and Sakazaki (1977), whereas 72 serovars had been recognized by Smith (WHO Scientific Working Group, 1980). The H antigen is common for all the serotypes of *V. cholerae* (Bhattacharya, 1975; Shimada and Sakazaki, 1977). An increasing number of strains have been isolated in recent years which are not typable within these schemes, necessitating their further extension.

The NAG vibrios have been found to be widely distributed in the environment. Little significance has been attached to the occurrence of these vibrios unless associated with disease in a nearby community. They have been isolated from sewage, surface and estuarine waters, seafoods, animals, poultry, cockroaches and tadpoles (Sack, 1973; Pulverer and Savchenko, 1973; Sanyal *et al.*, 1974; Singh *et al.*, 1975; Marwah *et al.*, 1975; Avtsyn *et al.*, 1976; Müller, 1978; Bisgaard *et al.*, 1978; WHO Scientific Working Group, 1980). The ecological studies carried out in the U.S.A. (Colwell *et al.*, 1977; Kaper *et al.*, 1979) and in West Germany (Müller, 1978) indicated that the habitats of these vibrios are natural bodies of water such as rivers, marshes, bays and coastal areas, with an optimal salinity limit in the range of 4–17%. By ribosomal RNA homology it was observed that *V. cholerae* is more closely related to the 'marine enterobacteria' than to 'terrestrial enterobacteria' (Baumann and Baumann, 1977), a finding readily understood if *V. cholerae* is indeed considered to be a natural inhabitant of the brackish water areas of the estuaries. Although doubts have been expressed about the capability of these free-living strains to cause disease in man (WHO Scientific Working Group, 1980). Bäck *et al.* (1974) reported cases of diarrheal and extraintestinal infections due to NAG vibrios where connection with the brackish water was a significant common feature.

2. ASSOCIATION OF THE NAG VIBRIOS WITH DIARRHEAL DISEASES IN MAN

2.1. INCIDENCE

Yajnik and Prasad (1954) reported the first outbreak caused by NAG vibrios on the occasion of a religious fair at Allahabad, India. Pollitzer (1959), while reviewing the various reports of isolation of the NAG vibrios, concluded that they are frequently implicated in sporadic cases and outbreaks of diarrhea in different geographical areas of the world. They have been isolated from stools of diarrheal patients from various countries, including Bangladesh (McIntyre *et al.*, 1965), Thailand (Gaines *et al.*, 1964), India (Chatterjee *et. al.*, 1972; Singh *et al.*, 1975), Iran and Saudi Arabia (Zafari *et al.*, 1973), Iraq (El-Shawi and Thewaini, 1969), Malaysia (Dutt *et al.*, 1971) and Hong Kong (WHO Scientific Working Group, 1980) in Asia; South Africa (Freiman *et al.*, 1977) and Sudan (WHO, 1969) in Africa; Czechoslovakia (Aldova *et al.*, 1968; Draśkovićová *et al.*, 1977), West Germany (Hoffler and Ko, 1977), Rumania (Nacescu and Cuifecu, 1978), Portugal (Blake *et al.*, 1977), Sweden (Bäck *et al.*, 1974), Bulgaria, Hungary, U.K. and U.S.S.R. (WHO Scientific Working Group, 1980) in Europe; Mexico and the U.S.A. (Hughes *et al.*, 1978) and Canada (Health and Welfare Canada, 1975) in North America; Brazil (WHO Scientific Working Group, 1980) in South America, and Australia (Dakin *et al.*, 1974). It is likely that in many countries infections by these vibrios go unrecognized because of inaccurate bacteriological techniques, which are aimed at detecting *V. cholerae* serotype 1 only. However, no large epidemic or pandemic like that caused by *V. cholerae* serotype 1 has yet been reported.

2.2. SEASONALITY

Little is known about the seasonality of NAG infections. Most infections occur in the warmer months in the U.S.A. (Hughes *et al.*, 1978) and in spring and summer in Bangladesh (WHO Scientific Working Group, 1980). Although the organisms are isolated throughout the year in Varanasi, India, maximum isolations take place during the months of May to September.

2.3. MODE OF TRANSMISSION AND INCUBATION PERIOD

Contaminated food and water is probably the exclusive mode of transmission. The incubation period in the reported outbreaks in Czechoslovakia and Australia were noted to be 20–30 hr and 5–37 hr respectively.

2.4. CLINICAL FEATURES

In India and Bangladesh, the classical home of cholera, the NAG vibrios have been associated with the 'full-blown cholera syndrome' (Lindenbaum *et al.*, 1965; Chatterjee *et al.*, 1972; Tiwari *et al.*, 1975). The clinical features of NAG diarrhea range from a cholera-like disease with rice-water stools to mild gastroenteritis (McIntyre *et al.*, 1965; Aldova *et al.*, 1968). It should be noted that the duration of diarrhea and the volume of fluid excreted and/or required for treatment is usually less than those of patients with severe forms of cholera. However, a detailed study of the clinical features is yet to be done.

2.5. ANTIBODY RESPONSE TO NAG VIBRIO INFECTIONS

McIntyre *et al.* (1965) observed up to 32-fold increase in serum agglutinating antibody titer on the sixth day of NAG diarrhea. However, the antibody response was less regular than that observed in infection with *V. cholerae* serotype 1. The WHO Scientific Working Group (1980) reported that, in Bangladesh, significant rises were observed in serum agglutinating titers against the homologous strain in patients excreting either toxigenic or nontoxigenic NAG vibrios, and significant antitoxin titer rises occurred in some patients with toxigenic isolates. The development of antibody specific for the infecting NAG vibrios and the failure to develop antibody against *V. cholerae* substantiate the specificity of the disease.

3. ASSOCIATION OF NAG VIBRIOS IN DISEASES OTHER THAN DIARRHEA

One very interesting feature of the NAG vibrios, unlike *V. cholerae* serotype 1, is its ability to cause diseases other than diarrhea. These vibrios have been reported from cases of septicemia and meningencephalitis (Fearington *et al.*, 1974; Prats *et al.*, 1975; Robins-Browne *et al.*, 1977). Bäck *et al.* (1974) described two cases of vibrio wound infections in Sweden. These vibrios were also isolated from acute appendicitis, acute cholecystitis, cholangitis, cellulitis, meningitis, otitis media, pneumonia, etc. (Hughes *et al.*, 1978). These reports indicate that the so-called NAG vibrios may possess invasive properties, in addition to their enteroxicity, like those of *V. parahaemolyticus*.

4. ENTEROTOXIGENICITY OF NAG VIBRIOS

Although the NAG vibrios were isolated from cases of diarrhea and various other sources, it is thought that not all these vibrios are enterotoxigenic. The general idea is that only those strains actually isolated from cases of diarrhea can produce an entero-toxin, and that others do not. The WHO Working Group (1980) reported that in a study in Bangladesh, patients yielding NAG vibrios that produced cholera-toxin like entero-toxin had more severe illnesses than those yielding nontoxic isolates. This would indicate that the NAG vibrios have not been studied extensively for their enterotoxigenicity. Further, the experimental models used for studying enterotoxin differ from laboratory to laboratory, although all the models used for detection of cholera and *E. coli* enterotoxins may not be suitable for NAG vibrio toxin. Moreover, there are no internationally accepted and standardized methods for measuring enterotoxicity. Factors like inoculum size, time of incubation, source of laboratory animals, choice of the model, and definition of a positive response, which can profoundly affect the observed results, may vary from laboratory to laboratory. Keeping these points in view, it would probably be convenient to discuss the enterotoxigenicity of the NAG vibrios according to the response obtained in various models.

4.1. RABBIT ILEAL LOOP MODEL

4.1.1. *Enterotoxicity of Live Cells*

Gupta *et al.* (1956) first demonstrated the enterotoxigenicity of the so-called NAG vibrios isolated from the Kumbh fair at Allahabad in 1954. However, they observed that the NAG strains isolated from patients, but not from water, caused accumulation of fluid in the experimental model of the ligated ileal loop of the adult albino rabbit, developed by De and Chatterjee (1953). Positive reactions with live cells of certain strains of NAG vibrios using the ileal loop test have also been recorded by many workers (Sil *et al.*, 1971; Zinnaka and Carpenter, 1972; Draśkovićová *et al.*, 1977; Robins-Browne *et al.*, 1977; Singh and Sanyal, 1978). The inocula of most of these experiments consisted of overnight peptone water cultures diluted in the same medium containing about 10^7–10^8 colony forming units (cfu). Observations were made 16–18 hr later. The volumes of intraluminal fluid and the lengths of the ligated loops were measured, and the volume/length ratio (ml/cm) was determined for each loop. The experiments were usually done in duplicate or triplicate in rabbits weighing 1–2 kg. Strain to strain and rabbit loop to rabbit loop variations were noted. Range of fluid accumulation varied from 0.2 to 1.92. Apparently the ability of NAG vibrios to produce fluid accumulation in rabbit loops was lower than that of *V. cholerae* serotype 1.

Fluid accumulations, in a similar range, with live cells of NAG vibrios were observed in this laboratory using 3–4 hr peptone water growths and inocula of 10^4–10^5 cfu and on observation at 6–8 hr after inoculation instead of 16–18 hr (Singh and Sanyal, 1978; Shanker *et al.*, 1982; Figs 1 and 2). No significant increase in fluid accumulation was

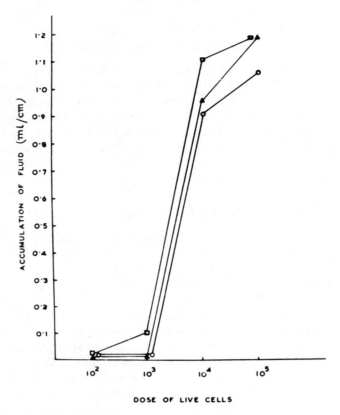

Fig. 1. Minimum infective dose of live cells of NAG vibrios for rabbit ileal loop reaction.

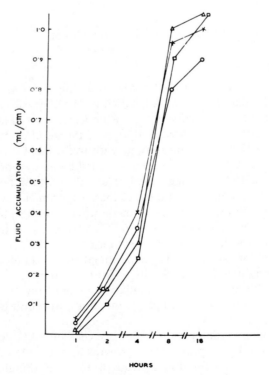

Fig. 2. Time course of fluid accumulation with NAG vibrios.

noted when the inoculum size was increased and there was no outpouring of fluid with an inoculum of less than 10^3 cfu. These studies indicate that an optimal bacterial population is essential for gut reaction. The amount of fluid accumulated also depends on the release of sufficient enterotoxin by the vibrios. The variation from strain to strain in the amounts of fluid accumulated in the loop was probably due to differences amongst them in the quantitative release of toxin. The NAG vibrios multiplied by about 10^4–10^5 within a 6 hr period in ileal loops, implying a capacity for colonization in the ileal loop mucosa, as has been observed by Spira *et al.* (1979).

4.1.2. *Enhancement of Enterotoxicity of NAG Vibrios by Ileal Loop Passage*

It was observed in this laboratory (Singh and Sanyal, 1978; Shanker *et al.*, 1982) that a group of strains, most of which were isolated from sources other than diarrheal patients, caused no fluid accumulation on repeated tests. One milliliter of a 3–4 hr peptone water culture of these strains, diluted 10^2–10^3 in saline, was injected into a loop. After 16–18 hr the contents of the loop were removed aseptically and cultured on nutrient agar. Five to six colonies were isolated each time, then cultured and inoculated into another loop until the strain gave a positive reaction. All the strains caused accumulation of fluid after only one or two passages (Table 1). A reduction of infective dose and increase in fluid outpouring was also noted after passage. These data indicate the potential enterotoxicity of these vibrios. It may be that a mechanism of repression and derepression is active in the toxin gene, which is chromosomal in the species of *V. cholerae* (Vasil *et al.*, 1975), depending on the microenvironment, or the toxic organisms may have been selected during passage from a mixed population (Annapurna and Sanyal, 1977).

4.1.3. *Enterotoxicity of Environmental Isolates*

While studying the enterotoxicity of the NAG vibrios Draśkovićová *et al.* (1977) obtained positive ileal loop reactions with strains isolated from surface waters along with those from diarrheal cases. Singh and Sanyal (1978), during their study of NAG vibrios from a community, observed that all the strains isolated from feces of healthy individuals, well and surface waters, and sewage and feces of domestic animals, caused accumulation of fluid in ligated rabbit gut loops. Some of the strains, however, needed one or two serial passages.

TABLE 1. *Enhancement of Enterotoxicity after Passage in Ileal Loops*

Strain	Source	Serotype	Average accumulation of fluid in ml/cm of loop		Number of passages
			Before passage*	After passage†	
345	Hand pump	17	0	1.3	1
768	Tap water	8	0	1.2	1
589	River Ganges	14	0	0.9	2
438	Sewage	5	0	1.2	1
4329	Healthy human	15	0	1.3	1
6054	Buffalo	36	0	1.2	1
3555	Cow	18	0	0.6	1
5429	Cow	NT‡	0	1.0	2
6072	Goat	40	0	1.2	2
4480	Cow	40	0	1.2	2
2514	Cow	18	0	1.0	1
6119	Buffalo	40	0	0.9	2
6113	Chicken	2	0	0.8	1

*Inocula ranged between 10^7–10^9 cfu.
†Inocula were 10^4–10^5 cfu.
‡Not typed.

4.1.4. *Enterotoxicity of cell-free culture filtrates*

Bhattacharya *et al.* (1971) first showed accumulation of fluid in ileal loops by cell-free culture filtrates of NAG vibrios. They inoculated 0.1 ml of 18 hr surface culture harvested in saline containing 10^{12} cfu/ml into 50 ml of medium (containing 2% peptone, Difco and 0.5% sodium chloride) in a 250 ml flask, incubated it for 8 hr in a shaker (120 oscillations/ min) at 37°C, centrifuged the culture at a low temperature, and filtered the supernatant through millipore membrane filter. A positive reaction in ileal loop was obtained after 18 hr; however, this occurred only with a 10-fold concentrated culture filtrate, but not

TABLE 2. *Ileal Loop Tests with Culture Filtrates of NAG Vibrios*

Number of culture filtrates	Range of fluid accumulation (ml/cm)*
44	0.5–0.9
13	1.0–1.5
2	1.6–2.0
Positive control (culture filtrate of *V. cholerae* 569B)	1.2–2.0
Negative control (BHIB)	0

*Culture filtrates of 11 strains were prepared after one or two passage(s) in ileal loops.

with unconcentrated preparations. Draśkovićová *et al.* (1977) also observed positive ileal loop reaction only with 5-fold concentrated culture filtrates prepared in a medium containing 3% peptone (Difco) and 0.5% yeast extract, with strains isolated from diarrheal cases and water. However, Ohashi *et al.* (1972) observed good accumulation of fluid at 18 hr after inoculation with original culture filtrate prepared in Casamino acids–yeast extract dialysate medium of Kusama and Craig (1970). Singh and Sanyal (1978) prepared culture filtrates with 30 NAG strains isolated from humans, animals and waters in Brain Heart Infusion Broth (BHIB, Difco), 24 of which caused fluid accumulation at 6 hr in ileal loops. The remaining six did so only when the culture filtrates were prepared with rabbit passaged strains. Shanker *et al.* (1982), while studying the enterotoxicity of the NAG strains belonging to all the known serovars, prepared culture filtrates with 59 strains—50 ml of BHIB contained in a 250 ml conical flask was inoculated with 1 ml of a 3–4 hr peptone water culture of the organism. The cultures, after incubation at 37°C in a shaking water bath, were centrifuged at 4°C for 30 min at 22,000 g. The supernatants were filtered through millipore filters of 0.45 μm average pore diameter and stored at 4°C. All the filtrates gave positive ileal loop reactions, the majority being comparable to that of *V. cholerae*, 569B. (Table 2).

4.2. INFANT RABBIT MODEL

Dutta *et al.* (1963), using the infant rabbit model as a test animal, examined the toxigenicity of NAG vibrios including those tested by Gupta *et al.* (1956). They found that these strains, at a dose of 10^6 cfu, caused typical choleraic diarrhea in this model, characterized by rice water stools, dehydration, anuria etc, only when they were passaged through rabbit gut, but not prior to that. However, McIntyre *et al.* (1965) demonstrated that NAG vibrios isolated from patients with diarrhea caused fluid outpouring in infant rabbits when inoculated with a dose of 4×10^2 cfu intraintestinally. Similar observations were also made by Sakazaki *et al.* (1967) in this experimental model using overnight broth cultures.

4.3. Skin Vascular Permeability Factor (PF)

Craig (1965) reported that a heat-labile factor in sterile filtrates of both cholera stools and young cultures of *V. cholerae* evokes induration and a prolonged increase in capillary permeability following intracutaneous injection in albino guinea-pigs and rabbits. He found this factor to be associated with the enterotoxin preparations from *V. cholerae*. Zinnaka and Carpenter (1972) reported that two NAG strains capable of causing fluid accumulation in ligated ileal loop, also produced a substance which gave rise to increased permeability of the small blood vessels of rabbit skin with a bluing diameter of about 8 mm. They observed that the skin permeability response was positive in tests with culture filtrates, but generally negative with their ileal loop fluid supernates, whereas in

TABLE 3. *Skin Permeability Tests with Culture Filtrates of NAG Vibrios**

Number of strains belonging to different serotypes	Bluing diameter (mm)
12	4–7
31	8–14
16	15–21

*Some of the culture filtrates caused necrosis at the site of injection.

V. cholerae serotype 1 both the tests were consistently positive. They explained this finding by a rapid and apparently irreversible binding of the toxin to the gut epithelial cells. Eight of the 41 NAG strains tested by Ohashi *et al.* (1972) elaborated PF and induration factor in culture filtrates when tested in guinea-pig skin. The most potent strain gave a bluing zone of nearly 10 mm in diameter at 1:200 dilution. Draśkovićová *et al.* (1977) reported the presence of PF and induration in all the 41 strains tested that were isolated from cases of diarrhea and surface waters. Robins-Browne *et al.* (1977) noted a bluing diameter of 24 mm with a strain of NAG vibrio isolated from blood of a Kwashiorkor patient with persistent fever. They used Syncase broth (Finkelstein *et al.*, 1966) culture filtrates, concentrated by dialysis and ultrafiltration through a Diaflow UM10 membrane (Amicon Corp.). In a recent study in this laboratory (Shanker *et al.*, 1982) it was observed that the 59 strains belonging to all the known serovars of the NAG vibrios elaborated induration and vascular permeability factor in their BHIB culture filtrates. The bluing zones ranged between 4–21 mm (Table 3). Strain to strain and animal to animal variations in elaboration of these factors were common features. The induration produced by culture filtrates of NAG vibrios was similar in appearance to that induced by *V. cholerae* 569B toxin, and it has been proved to be attributable to the increased permeability as shown by the indicator dye method. Studies on the dose–response relationship indicated that all the culture filtrates showed positive PF, up to a dilution of 1:16, and none showed any reaction at a dilution of 1:256 (Fig. 3). These data suggest that all the NAG vibrios produce the permeability factor although it appears to be less potent than that of *V. cholerae* serotype 1, which usually gives rise to a wider bluing diameter. These findings also indicate the possibility of PF being used as an alternative bioassay system for NAG enterotoxin.

4.3.1. *Hemorrhagic principle*

Ohashi *et al.* (1972) reported that culture filtrates of some NAG vibrio strains produce a concentric hemorrhagic spot at the site of injection into guinea-pig skin in permeability tests. With a larger dose, necrosis also developed at the central part of the lesion. They named this the hemorrhagic principle and observed similar reactions with culture

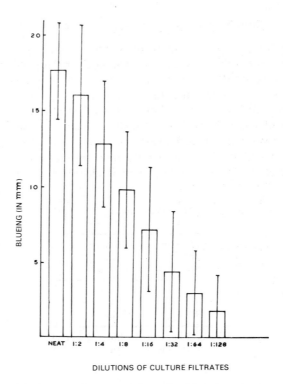

DILUTIONS OF CULTURE FILTRATES

FIG. 3. Dose–response relationship of PF of NAG vibrios.

filtrates of two *V. cholerae* strains. In some instances the hemorrhagic spot was formed in the bluing lesion, starting at the site of injection, suggesting the co-existence of the permeability factor and hemorrhagic principle. The hemorrhagic response in rabbit skin caused by NAG vibrios and *V. cholerae* serotype 1 was also noted by Draśkovićová *et al.* (1977) and Bisgaard *et al.* (1978). Variable degrees of dermonecrotic/hemorrhagic activities were observed in this laboratory in skin tests with some of the culture filtrates of NAG vibrios (Lahiri *et al.*, 1982; Shanker *et al.*, 1982, Fig. 4). Zinnaka and Carpenter (1972) correlated the hemorrhagic factor with proteinase activity. This factor is heat-labile, being inactivated at 65°C for 10 min but not at 56°C for 30 min; maximum activity

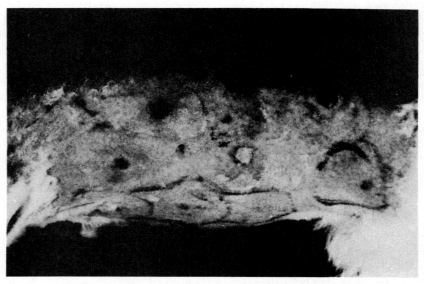

FIG. 4. Skin necrosis caused by culture filtrates of NAG vibrios.

is observed at pH 6.0–8.0 with gradual loss at lower and higher pH values and is also nondialyzable. It is not lyzed with red blood cells of human, horse, sheep, rabbit or chicken in the presence or absence of cysteine. This factor is neutralized with antitoxin to *V. cholerae* and *E. coli* LT, indicating their probable relatedness to enterotoxin (Lahiri *et al.*, 1982).

The fluid in the rabbit gut loop inoculated with live cells and culture filtrates of NAG vibrios was occasionally found to be mucous and bloody (Draśkovićová *et al.*, 1977; Ciznar *et al.*, 1977). However, other workers (Zinnaka and Carpenter, 1972; Ohashi *et al.*, 1972) observed clear or slightly pink fluid like that caused by *V. cholerae* 569B. In this laboratory we usually note the results after 6–8 hr of inoculation for the enterotoxicity test in rabbit ileal loop and do not normally encounter bloody fluid. Burrows (1968) had observed in cases of *V. cholerae* that 'at earlier points when the system is still physiological, the composition of the fluid closely resemble that of human rice water stool but in observations made more than 12 hr after inoculation the intraluminal fluid may contain cells and protein due to ischemic damage'. It need be noted here the term 'hemorrhagic principle' caused by NAG vibrio culture filtrate was coined only in relation to the skin test but not to the loop test.

4.4. SUCKLING MOUSE ASSAY

Ohashi *et al.* (1972) reported a lethal diarrhea in four-day old suckling mice challenged with culture filtrates of NAG vibrios. Ciznar *et al.* (1977) also reported a lethal effect on four-day old mice after intragastric inoculation. Mice were immobile shortly after injection, some had diarrhea and almost all of them died within 4 hr. No fluid accumulation was present at autopsy. The ratio of gut weight to mouse body weight were less than 0.07, which was considered negative by Dean *et al.* (1972) who suggested a ratio of 0.09 or higher as positive. We tested 14 strains of NAG vibrios belonging to different serotypes and observed the ratios to be always less than 0.08, indicating a negative result. It should be noted that the suckling mouse model had been found to be specific for heat-stable enterotoxins such as those of *E. coli* (Dean *et al.*, 1972) and *Plesiomonas shigelloides* (Sanyal *et al.*, 1980b) but not for a heat-labile enterotoxin such as cholera toxin which may stimulate dilatation of the intestine only at high concentrations. It is supposed that a sort of lethal factor produced *in vitro* by NAG vibrios is responsible for the infant mouse toxicity and lethal effect. These results are similar to those described for *V. parahaemolyticus* by Ohashi *et al.* (1972).

During their purification process of NAG vibrio enterotoxin, Ciźnár *et al.* (1977) obtained a fraction termed S_1 which was toxic for mice by i.v. injection. The toxicity was apparently due to the free endotoxin released in the medium. The S_1 fraction contained a high proportion of the LPS which was released during the exponential phase of growth. Regarding this property, the NAG vibrios revealed similarities to the Ogawa and Inaba strains of *V. cholerae* as described by Holmgren *et al.* (1971) and Pike and Chandler (1974).

4.5. TISSUE CULTURES

The Chinese hamster ovarian tissue culture assay is used to detect the enterotoxin of cholera and the heat-labile toxin of *E. coli* (Guerrant *et al.*, 1974). Robins-Browne *et al.* (1977) obtained positive results in this test with the Syncase broth filtrate of a NAG strain. The Y_1 mouse adrenal tumour cell culture has also been widely used for detection of cholera toxin and *E. coli* LT (Sack and Sack, 1975). Out of the 65 NAG isolates in the Chesapeake Bay, Kaper *et al.* (1979) observed positive results with 57 (88%) in Y_1 cell cultures. On the other hand, Bisgaard *et al.* (1978) noted that NAG vibrios induced a distinctive cytotoxic effect on Y_1 adrenal cells. Affected cells were round and many of them floated freely in the medium. The cytotoxic effect of the culture filtrate was destroyed by heating at 100°C for 15 min but was not neutralized by cholera antitoxin. It has been observed that these two cell cultures, although highly sensitive and yielding reproducible results for detection of enterotoxins of *V. cholerae* and *E. coli*, are not suitable for screening enterotoxin production by *A. hydrophila*, *P. shigelloides* Group F, and NAG vibrios which frequently elaborate cytotoxic substance(s) in the culture medium (Sanyal *et al.*, 1980a; Agarwal and Sanyal, 1981). However, in the case of *A. hydrophila*, when the enterotoxin was purified to electrophoretic homogeneity to give only an ileal loop positive reaction, but no hemolysis (Dubey *et al.*, 1980), it could cause rounding of Y_1 and elongation of CHO cell cultures as found with cholera enterotoxin (Sanyal *et al.*, 1980).

5. RELATIONSHIP BETWEEN PF AND ENTEROTOXIC FACTOR OF NAG VIBRIOS

NAG vibrio toxin contains both enterotoxic and vascular permeability factors like cholera toxin (Zinnaka and Carpenter, 1972; Ohashi *et al.*, 1972; Draśkovićová *et al.*, 1977; Ciźnár *et al.*, 1977). Recently it was observed in this laboratory that culture filtrates of all the strains belonging to the 59 serovars of NAG vibrios caused both accumulation of fluid in the rabbit gut loop as well as increased vascular permeability in the rabbit skin, like that of *V. cholerae* 569B (Shanker *et al.*, 1982). Mosley *et al.* (1970) put forth sufficient data to show that cholera enterotoxin and PF are two expressions of the same toxin molecule in a biological system. Both the activities are heat-labile, acid-labile, nondialyzable and neutralizable by the convalescent patients' sera (Craig, 1970; Mosley *et al.*, 1970). Finkelstein and LoSpalluto (1972) demonstrated the presence of both factors as a mixed crystallized form in purified cholera toxin. Similarly the PF and enterotoxicity of NAG vibrios are heat-labile, acid-labile, nondialyzable and neutralizable by convalescent patients' sera (Ghosh *et al.*, 1970; Zinnaka and Carpenter, 1972; Ohashi *et al.*, 1972; WHO Scientific Working Group, 1980; Shanker·*et al.*, 1982). Although available data indicate that these two factors may co-exist in NAG vibrio toxin, confirmation of the fact can only be done after complete purification of the toxin molecule.

6. PHYSICOCHEMICAL NATURE OF NAG ENTEROTOXIN

It was observed in this laboratory (Shanker *et al.*, 1982) that heating at 56°C for 30 min caused appreciable loss of activity of the culture filtrates with complete inactivation of enterotoxicity and PF at 60°C for 20 min or 65°C for 10 min. Similar observations were also made by Draśkovićová *et al.* (1977). However, some workers have reported complete loss of activity at 56°C for 30 min (Zinnaka and Carpenter, 1972; Ohashi *et al.*, 1972). The relative heat resistance observed by us may be due to the presence of organic matter in the medium which may protect the toxin molecule from the effect of heat. It is also possible that some other factors are associated with the toxin molecule (Zinnaka and Carpenter, 1972). In the time course experiments, following the method of Evans *et al.* (1973), fluid outpouring started after a lag period of about 2 hr, increasing rapidly thereafter up to 8 hr, and this was sustained up to 18 hr with slight increase (Fig. 2). This indicates that the enterotoxin of NAG vibrios is heat-labile, similar to that of *V. cholerae* serotype 1. The heat-labile nature of the enterotoxin is further substantiated by the observation of a negative suckling mouse assay (Shanker *et al.*, 1982).

The activity of cholera toxin has been shown by Kasai and Burrows (1966) to be present in the pH range 6.5–9.0. However, in this study with NAG vibrios the maximum activity of enterotoxin and PF was seen in the pH range of 6.0–8.0, with a decrease at higher and lower ph values (Fig. 5).

The NAG enterotoxin and PF can be precipitated by 70–90% saturation with ammonium sulfate, is nondialyzable, and is immunogenic (Zinnaka and Carpenter, 1972; Ohashi *et al.*, 1972).

Regarding the chemical nature of the NAG enterotoxin, Ghosh *et al.* (1970) suggested a combination of protein with the presence of an exopolysaccharide moiety. By am-

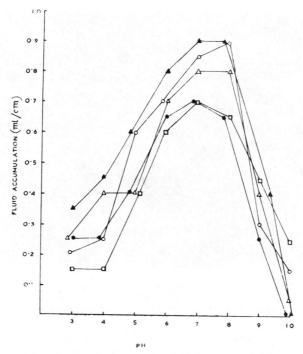

FIG. 5. Effect of pH on enterotoxicity of culture filtrates of NAG vibrios.

monium sulfate precipitation of the culture filtrate of NAG vibrios grown in a non-synthetic medium (1% peptone, Difco; 0.5% yeast extract and 0.5% sodium chloride, adjusted to pH 7.4) and fractionation on Sephadex G-100 column, Ciznar *et al.* (1977) obtained three fractions. The first fraction contained mainly polysaccharide which possessed no enterotoxic activity as measured by the fluid accumulation in the ligated rabbit ileal loop as well as no activity in the skin permeability test. However, it was toxic for mice on i.v. injection. The second fraction contained one antigenic protein and revealed four bands in the region of albumin migration in polyacrylamide electrophoresis. The size of the molecules from this fraction was estimated by the elution volume from the sephadex G-100 and polyacrylamide electrophoresis to be approximately 50,000–70,000 daltons. This fraction contained enterotoxic activity identical to that of the original filtrate, as evidenced by accumulation of fluid in ileal loop. The permeability and hemorrhagic factors co-existed in this fraction as proven by the rabbit skin test. Mouse lethal factor was also present in the moiety. This fraction also showed high proteolytic activity. The third fraction contained the highest amount of protein, which was same for all the strains tested, and this was attributed to that present in the culture medium.

7. RELATIONSHIP OF NAG VIBRIO TOXIN TO CHOLERA ENTEROTOXIN

Ghosh *et al.* (1970), by immunodiffusion and immunoelectrophoresis, showed that NAG vibrios isolated from cases of acute diarrhea possess toxin antigens similar to those of *V. cholerae* 569B and that they are equally immunogenic. As there was only a single precipitin band with both NAG vibrio and *V. cholerae* 569B whole cell lysates when they reacted with antiserum to cholera toxin, it was suggested that NAG toxin is almost identical to cholera toxin (Ghosh *et al.*, 1970; Zinnaka *et al.*, 1972). In a recent study in this laboratory (Lahiri *et al.*, 1982) 11 culture filtrates of different serotype strains of NAG vibrios gave identical reactions in immunodiffusion studies with cholera antitoxin, indicating their immunological identity with the enterotoxin of *V. cholerae* serotype 1 (Fig. 6). Some of the culture filtrates did not give any precipitin band with cholera

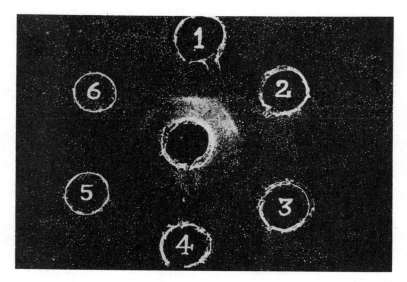

FIG. 6. Immunodiffusion showing reaction of identity between cholera antitoxin and NAG vibrio
toxin. Central well contains antitoxin to *V. cholerae* 569B; wells 1 and 2 contain cholera toxin;
and wells 2, 3, 5 and 6 contain culture filtrates of NAG vibrio serotypes 15, 16, 17 and 19.

antitoxin. These culture filtrates probably needed further concentration, because to
demonstrate immunologic relationships between cholera toxin and *E. coli* LT, by Ouchterlony technique, crude preparations must be concentrated (Clements and Finkelstein,
1979; Geary *et al.*, 1982).

Regarding biological activity, NAG toxin was shown to be similar to cholera toxin in
certain strains whereas in others the toxin was assumed to have more than one toxic
factor giving two-step neutralization with antiserum to cholera toxin (Zinnaka and
Carpenter, 1972). Daniel and Spira (1979), in a study to characterize the biological
activity of the NAG vibrios, showed that they produce a cholera-like toxin and give a
reaction of partial to complete identity with choleragen in neutralization with homologous or heterologous antisera. Similar results were obtained in this laboratory in a
study using culture filtrates of 50 strains belonging to different serotypes; complete
neutralization of enterotoxic activity in gut loop was observed in 31, and varying degrees
of partial neutralization were noted in others, when tested against cholera antitoxin
(Lahiri *et al.*, 1982). Identical observations were also made in tests for neutralization of
PF. The neutralizations of ileal loop activity and PF were proportional with serial
dilutions of cholera antitoxin (Fig. 7).

These data indicate that NAG vibrio toxin is similar to that of *V. cholerae*, both
biologically and immunologically.

It has been suggested that NAG vibrio enterotoxin is weaker than cholera enterotoxin
(Ohashi *et al.*, 1972; Ciznár *et al.*, 1977; Draskovicová *et al.*, 1977; Robins-Browne *et al.*,
1977). Daniel and Spira (1979) indicated that the NAG vibrios form a gradient that
ranges from a virulence character the same as the wild types of *V. cholerae* biotype *eltor*
to a point with no demonstrable biological activity, when tested for production of
cholera toxin or cholera toxin like toxin. The toxin production by NAG vibrios *in vitro*
may depend on many factors, as has been shown in a case of *V. cholerae* serotype 1
(Richardson 1969; Kusama and Craig, 1970). It may be assumed that several factors, as
yet poorly understood, influence the production of toxin in these vibrios *in vitro* and *in
vivo* (Zinnaka and Carpenter, 1972). In an interesting series of experiments Karuna-Sagar
et al. (1979) have demonstrated that metal ions, such as magnesium, iron, zinc, nickel,
manganese and copper, affect either the growth or the toxigenicity of *V. cholerae*.
However, magnesium and iron ions, in optimal concentrations, produced a remarkable
increase in toxigenicity. They found that metal ions affected the efficient utilization of
glycerol and amino acids which resulted in increased toxin synthesis. The study also

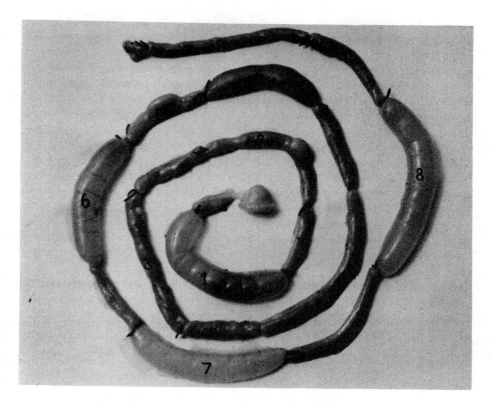

FIG. 7. Neutralization of culture filtrates of NAG vibrios with cholera antitoxin loop 1 (positive control): 0.5 ml of culture filtrate mixed with 0.5 ml of normal rabbit serum; loops 2–8: 0.5 ml of culture filtrate mixed with 0.5 ml of undiluted, 1:2, 1:4, 1:8, 1:16, 1:32 and 1:64 dilutions of antitoxin; loop 9: (negative control) 1 ml sterile BHIB.

showed that serine metabolism is closely allied to toxin synthesis. They did not observe any correlation between growth yields and toxin production. Very little is known about the conditions of optimal toxin yield by the NAG vibrios as no study has yet been conducted to delineate these factors. In all the studies carried out so far NAG vibrio toxin was produced in media used for production of cholera toxin.

Toxigenicity is a chromosomally mediated trait in *V. cholerae* serotype 1, toxin production being coded for by a bacterial gene (Vasil *et al.*, 1975). The phenomena of conjugation and transfer of sex factors P and V have been shown to occur in *V. cholerae* serotype 1 (Bhaskaran *et al.*, 1969). The NAG vibrios have been shown to contain V factor and can be induced with P plasmid by conjugation (Bhaskaran and Sinha, 1971). Sinha and Srivastava (1978) reported decreased production of toxin, leading to suppression of pathogenicity in *V. cholerae* when P and V plasmids were introduced. The cells harboring both P and V plasmids became attenuated and could not cause experimental cholera. Parallel data for NAG vibrios are lacking except for some tentative speculation.

8. RELATIONSHIP OF NAG VIBRIO TOXIN TO *E. COLI* LT

In a recent study in this laboratory (Lahiri *et al.*, 1982) 12 out of the 18 culture filtrates of NAG vibrios were completely neutralized, and the remaining only partially, when tested against antitoxin to *E. coli* LT. Skin reactivities were also neutralized in a similar way. Proportional neutralization was observed with serial dilutions of the antitoxin, indicating their biological relatedness to *E. coli* LT.

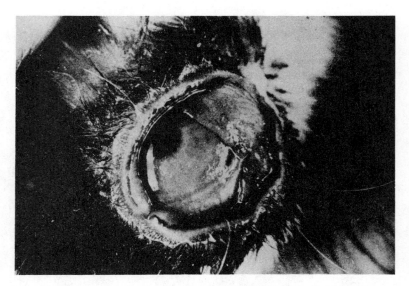

FIG. 8. Positive Sereny's test showing keratoconjunctivitis with live cells of *Shigella flexneri* 543.

In the immunodiffusion studies with culture filtrates of different serotype strains of NAG vibrios and antitoxin to *E. coli* LT, no precipitin band was formed and as such immunological identity between these toxins could not be confirmed.

9. INVASIVENESS OF THE NAG VIBRIOS

All the NAG vibrios so far yielded negative results in Sereny's test (1957) and did not produce keratoconjunctivitis in the guinea-pig or the rabbit eye on instillation of 10^6–10^7 cfu in 0.1 ml peptone water in the conjunctival sac and observed over a period of 72 hr (Robins-Browne *et al.*, 1977; Shanker *et al.*, 1982), whereas the positive control *S. flexneri* 543 did so consistently (Figs 8 and 9). Robins-Browne *et al.* (1977), however, demonstrated that a strain of NAG vibrio isolated from the blood of a Kwashiorkor patient with fever of unknown origin, invaded the ileal loop mucosa repeatedly. Cultures of peripheral venous blood, liver and spleen of two rabbits enterally infected with the

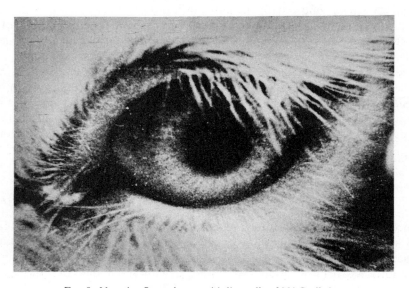

FIG. 9. Negative Sereny's test with live cells of NAG vibrios.

strain yielded the organism after 18 hr. The strain was negative in Sereny's test. Repeated tests for invasion of ileal loop with various strains of *V. cholerae* serotype 1 and a NAG vibrio isolated from the stool of a patient with diarrhea gave consistently negative results. The authors claimed that although there have been reports of septicemia or other extraintestinal infections as mentioned earlier theirs is the first *in vitro* demonstration of invasion. They also suggested that the presence of the organism in the peripheral blood was probably due to depressed host immunity associated with malnutrition compounded by the invasive capability of the strain. However, detailed studies both *in vitro* and *in vivo* are essential to prove the invasive capability of the NAG vibrios.

10. RELATIONSHIP OF SEROVARS OF NAG VIBRIOS TO THEIR ENTEROTOXIGENICITY

It was noted by various workers that there is no correlation between the serovar of a NAG strain and its ability to cause fluid accumulation in rabbit ileal loop or a positive Y_1 adrenal cell response (Singh and Sanyal, 1978; Bisgaard *et al.*, 1978; Kaper *et al.*, 1979). Recently, it was demonstrated in this laboratory (Shanker *et al.*, 1982) that strains belonging to all the known 59 serovars are enterotoxigenic in ileal loops of PF tests with occasional requirement of passage in ileal loop.

The observations that no correlation exists between the serotype of a strain and its enterotoxicity, coupled with the earlier observation by the same group of workers (Singh *et al.*, 1975) that there is no preponderance of particular serotypes either amongst humans or their environments emphasizes the importance of surveillance of these vibrios in all possible sources in a particular community. As it is quite probable that these strains are circulating between the environment ⇋ animal ⇋ man, the occurrence of such toxigenic/potential toxigenic vibrios constitute a health hazard for the community.

11. PROBABLE MODE OF ACTION OF THE NAG ENTEROTOXIN

11.1. Experimental Studies

Studies were carried out in this laboratory (Shanker *et al.*, 1982) in order to determine the possible mode of action of the NAG enterotoxin. The method was same as described earlier (Sanyal *et al.*, 1980a). Rabbits were pretreated with inhibitors of various mediators of enterotoxic activity. One rabbit without any drug was included to serve as control. Ileal loop tests were performed as usual with culture filtrates of two strains of NAG vibrios both on test and control animals which were sacrificed after 8 hr and the amount of fluid accumulated was measured.

11.1.1. *Drugs—Dosage and Route of Administration*

a) *Prostaglandin synthesis blockers.* Diclofenac sodium was administered (20 mg/kg of body weight i.p.) for two consecutive days and on the third day 3 hr prior to the experiment. Indomethacin was given 25 mg/kg i.p. on the first day and the following day 3 hr before the experiment.

b) *Prostaglandin receptor blocker.* SC 19220 20 mg/kg with 0.1% Tween-80 was given 2 hr prior to the experiment. The same volume of Tween-80 was used as control.

c) *5-hydroxytryptamine (5-HT) synthesis blocker.* p-chlorphenylalanine was injected 300 mg/kg i.p. for three consecutive days, the experiment being done on the fourth day.

d) *5-HT receptor blocker.* Methysergide 2 mg/kg was given i.p. 3 hr before the experiment.

e) *cAMP inhibitor.* Chlorpromazine (5 mg/kg of body weight) was administered i.m. 1 hr before the experiment.

11.2. RESULTS

No inhibition of fluid outpouring was observed in rabbits pretreated with PGs and 5-HT inhibitors. On the other hand, chlorpromazine, a cAMP inhibitor reduced the fluid outpouring by 60–70%. Chlorpromazine has been shown to block the diarrheagenic action of cholera toxin, *E. coli* LT (Lönnroth *et al.*, 1977; 1979) and *A. hydrophila* enterotoxin (Dubey *et al.*, 1980). It has been suggested that the cAMP level may be regulated by hormones such as 5-HT and PGs (Lönnroth *et al.*, 1977). In the present series of experiments, 5-HT and PG synthesis and receptor blockers did not cause any difference in the amount of fluid outpouring, suggesting that they are not involved in the reaction. Results with chlorpromazine suggest that enterotoxin of NAG vibrios may also act through mediation of cAMP as do the enterotoxins *V. cholerae* serotype 1, *E. coli* and *A. hydrophila*.

12. CONCLUDING REMARKS

Because of their ubiquitous nature there has been a tendency to underestimate the pathogenic importance of the so-called NAG vibrios. With the present state of knowledge obtained from clinical, epidemiological, and laboratory studies, it becomes imperative to give more attention to these vibrios than has been accorded in the past. Further, recent studies indicate that, as in the case of *V. cholerae* serotype 1, almost all the strains of the so-called NAG vibrios are toxigenic with the strain to strain variation being in the quantity of toxin released. However, comprehensive studies with a large number of freshly isolated strains are necessary in order to draw a definite conclusion regarding their enterotoxic character. Application of recently developed genetic techniques for analysis of toxin genes may also prove useful. A search for highly sensitive and reproducible new models for detection of enterotoxin in these vibrios is also necessary as the relatively new techniques, like CHO and Y_1 adrenal cell cultures, ELISA etc., which have proved to be very useful for *V. cholerae* and *E. coli* are not suitable for them as they produce substance(s) which are either cytotoxic or interfere with the test. To demonstrate their enterotoxicity we are, therefore, still completely dependent on the less sensitive but expensive and laborious classical rabbit ileal loop, infant rabbit or skin permeability models.

Very little is known about the optimal conditions of growth for enterotoxin production by the NAG vibrios. There is no report based on a systematic study of the kinetics of toxin production by them. Only a few incomplete attempts have been made to characterize the enterotoxic activities and purify the enterotoxin. Although data are available showing that a protein moiety is responsible for enterotoxic activity, the purification, determination of chemical structure, and delineation of its properties are essential for proper understanding of the pathogenesis of the disease, which is needed for formulating therapeutic and preventive measures. There are indications that NAG vibrio toxin is similar immunobiologically to cholera and *E. coli* LT, but further studies are required to elucidate the nature and extent of the relationship. Other heat-labile enterotoxins also need to be compared to explore the possibility of any similarity.

Little work has been done on the other extracellular and intracellular products of the NAG vibrios. We know only of the mice toxicity of the lipopolysaccharide liberated by the vibrios. Except for a few, we know nothing about the various enzymes elaborated by them and their roles in the toxic properties of the organism. The cytotoxin(s) need to be characterized. As these vibrios can occasionally cause extraintestinal infections and septicemic conditions, unlike *V. cholerae* serotype 1, the properties responsible for invasiveness need to be identified.

Preliminary studies indicate that the mode of action of NAG vibrio toxin may be mediated through cAMP. However, more studies need be done to reach a reasonable conclusion.

As almost everything is now known about the toxin of *V. cholerae* serotype 1 it should not be difficult to learn the details of the NAG vibrio toxin as well, following the methods used in cholera. However, it is to be noted that these vibrios may elaborate some substance(s) not usually encountered in *V. cholerae* serotype 1 and these need to be considered when characterizing the enterotoxin.

REFERENCES

AGARWAL, R. K. and SANYAL, S. C. (1981) Experimental studies on enteropathogenicity and pathogenesis of Group 'F' vibrio infections. *Zentbl. Bakt. ParasitKde., Abt. 1, Orig.* **A249**: 392–399.

ALDOVA, E., LAZNICKOVA, K., STEPANKOVA, E. and LIETAVA, J. (1968) Isolation of nonagglutinable vibrios from an enteritis outbreak in Czechoslovakia. *J. infect Dis.* **118**: 25–31.

ANNAPURNA, E. and SANYAL, S. C. (1977) Enterotoxicity of *Aeromonas hydrophila. J. med. Microbiol.* **10**: 317–323.

AVTSYN, A. P., SHAKHLAMOV, V. A., TRAGER, R. S., KALININA, N. A., BALYN, I. R., TIMASHKEVICH, T. B. and POLYAKEVA, G. P. (1976) NAG infections in tadpoles in *Rana temporaria. Bull. exp. Biol. Med. U.S.S.R.* **82**: 1045–1048.

BÄCK, E., LJUNGGREN and SMITH, H. JR. (1974) Noncholera vibrios in Sweden *Lancet* i: 723–724.

BAUMANN, P. and BAUMANN, L. (1977) Biology of marine enterobacteria: genera Beneckea and Photobacterium. *A. Rev. Microbiol.* **31**: 39–61.

BHASKARAN, K., DYER, P. Y. and ROGERS, G. E. (1969) Sex pili in *Vibrio cholerae. Aust. J. exp. Biol. med. Sci.* **47**: 647–650.

BHASKARAN, K. and SINHA, V. B. (1971) Transmissible plasmid factors and fertility inhibition in *Vibrio cholerae. J. gen. Microbiol.* **69**: 89–97.

BHATTACHARYA, F. K. (1975) *V. cholerae* flagellar antigens: A serodiagnostic test, functional implications of H reactivity and taxonimic importance of cross-reactions within the *Vibrio genus. Med. Microbiol. Immun.* **162**: 29–41.

BHATTACHARYA, S., BOSE, A. K. and GHOSH, A. K. (1971) Permeability and enterotoxic factors of non-agglutinating vibrios, *Vibrio alcaligenes,* and *Vibrio parahaemolyticus. Appl. Microbiol.* **22**: 1159–1161.

BISGAARD, M., SAKAZAKI, R. and SHIMADA, T. (1978) Prevalence of noncholera vibrios in cavum nasi and pharynx of ducks. *Acta path. microbiol. scand. Sect. B* **86**: 261–266.

BLAKE, P. A., ROSENBERG, M. L., COSTA, B. J., FERREIRA, P. S., GUIMARAES, C. L. and GANGAROSA, E. J. (1977) Cholera in Portugal: Modes of transmission. *Am. J. Epidem.* **105**: 337–343.

BURROWS W. (1968) Cholera toxins. *A. Rev. Microbiol.* **22**: 245–268.

CHATTERJEE, B. D., GORBACH, S. L. and NEOGY, K. N. (1972) Characteristics of noncholera vibrios isolated from patients with diarrhoea. *J. med. Microbiol.* **3**: 677–682.

CIŽNAR, I., DRAŚKOVIĆOVÁ, M., HOŚTACKA, A. and KAROLCEK, J. (1977) Partial purification and characterisation of the NAG vibrio enterotoxin. *Zentbl. Bakt. ParasitKde, Abt. 1, Orig.* **A239**: 493–503.

CLEMENTS, J. D. and FINKELSTEIN, R. A. (1979) Isolation and characterization of homogenous heat-labile enterotoxins with high specific activity from *Escherichia coli* cultures. *Infect. Immun.* **24**: 760–769.

COLWELL, R. R., KAPER, J. and JOSEPH, S. W. (1977) *Vibrio cholerae, Vibrio parahaemolyticus* and other *Vibrios*: Occurrence and distribution in Chesapeake Bay. *Science* **198**: 394–396.

CRAIG, J. P. (1965) A permeability factor (toxin) found in cholera stools and culture filtrates and its neutralisation by convalescent sera. *Nature* **207**: 614–616.

CRAIG, J. P. (1970) Some observations on neutralisation of cholera vascular permeability factor *in vivo. J. infect. Dis.* **121** (Suppl): 100–110.

DAKIN, W. P. H., HOWELL, D. J., SUTTON, R. G. A., O'KEEFE, M. F. and THOMAS, P. (1974) Gastroenteritis due to non-agglutinable (non-cholera) vibrios. *Med. J. Aust.* **2**: 487–490.

DANIEL, R. R. and SPIRA, W. M. (1979) Biotype clusters formed on the basis of virulence characters in Non-O Group 1 *Vibrio cholerae. Abst. 15th Joint Conf. on Cholera,* p. 21. The U.S.–Japan Cooperative Medical Science Programme.

DE, S. N. and CHATTERJEE, D. N. (1953) An experimental study on the mechanism of action of *Vibrio cholerae* on the intestinal mucous membranes. *J. Path. Bact.* **66**: 559–562.

DEAN, A. G., CHING, Y. C., WILLIAMS, R. G. and HARDEN, L. B. (1972) Test for *Escherichia coli* enterotoxin using infant mice. *J. infect. Dis.* **125**: 407–411.

DRAŚKOVIĆOVÁ, M., KAROLCEK, J. and WINKLER, D. (1977) Experimental toxigenicity of NAG vibrios. *Zentbl. Bakt. ParasitKde., ***A237**: 65–71.

DUBEY, R. S., SANYAL, S. C. and MALHOTRA, O. P. (1980) Purification of *Aeromonas hydrophila* enterotoxin and its mode of action in experimental model. In: *Natural Toxins,* pp. 259–268, EAKER, D. and WADSTRÖM, T. (eds). Pergamon Press, Oxford.

DUTT, A. K., ALWI, S. and VELAUTHAN, T. (1971) A shellfish-borne cholera outbreak in Malaysia. *Trans. R. Soc. trop. Med. Hyg.* **65**: 815–818.

DUTTA, N. K., PAUSE, M. V. and JHALA, H. I. (1963) Choleragenic property of certain strains of *eltor,* NAG and water vibrios confirmed experimentally. *Br. med. J.* **1**: 1200–1203.

EL-SHAWI, N. and THEWAINI (1969) Non-agglutinable vibrios isolated in the 1966 epidemic cholera in Iraq. *Bull. Wld Hlth Org.* **40**: 163–166.

EVANS, D. G., EVANS, D. J. JR. and PIERCE, N. F. (1973) Differences in the response of rabbit small intestine to heat-labile and heat-stable enterotoxins of *Escherichia coli. Infect. Immun.* **7**: 873–880.

FEARINGTON, E. L., RAND, C. H. JR., MEWBORN, A. and WILKERSON, J. (1974) Non-cholera *Vibrio* septicimia and meningoencephalitis. *Ann. intern. Med.* **81**: 401.

FINKELSTEIN, R. A., ATTHASAMPUNNA, P., CHULASAMAYA, M. and CHARUMMETHEE, P. (1966) Pathogenesis of experimental cholera: Biologic activities of purified procholeragen A. *J. Immun.* **96**: 440–449.

FINKELSTEIN, R. A. and LOSPALLUTO, J. J. (1972) Crystalline cholera toxin and toxoid. *Science* **175**: 529–530.

FREIMAN, I., HARTMEN, E., KASSEL, H., ROBINS-BROWNE, R. M., SCHOUB, B. D., KOORNHOF, H. J., LAEATSAS, G. and PROZESKY, O. W. (1977) A microbiological study of gastroenteritis in black infants. *S. Afr. med. J.* **52**: 261–265.

FELSENFELD, O. (1967) *The Cholera Problem*, p. 165. Warren H. Green, St. Louis.

GAINES, S., DUANGMANI, C., NOYES, H. E. and OCCENO, T. (1964) Occurrence of nonagglutinable vibrios in diarrhoea patients in Bangkok, Thailand. *J. Microbiol. Soc. Thailand* **8–10**: 6–17.

GARDNER, A. D. and VENKATRAMAN, K. V. (1935) The antigen of the cholera group of vibrios. *J. Hyg.* **35**: 262–282.

GEARY, S. J., MARCHLEWICZ, B. A. and FINKELSTEIN, R. A. (1982) Comparison of heat-labile enterotoxins from porcine and human strains of *Escherichia coli Infect. Immun.* **36**: 215–220.

GHOSH, A. K., DE, S. P. and MUKERJEE, S. (1970) Immunogenic studies on NAG vibrios with particular reference to toxigenicity. *Annls Inst. Pasteur* **118**: 41–48.

GUERRANT, R. L., BRUNTON, L. L., SCHNAITMAN, T. C., REBHUN, L. I. and GILMAN, A. G. (1974) Cyclic adenosine monophosphate and alteration of Chinese hamster ovary cell morphology: a rapid sensitive *in vitro* assay for the enterotoxin of *Vibrio cholerae* and *Escherichia coli*. *Infect. Immun.* **10**: 320–327.

GUPTA, N. P., GUPTA, S. P., MANGLIK, U. S., PRASAD, B. G. and YAJNIK, B. S. (1956) Investigations into the nature of vibrio strains isolated from the epidemic of gastroenteritis in Kumbh Fair at Allahabad in 1954. *Indian J. med. Sci.* **10**: 781.

HEALTH AND WELFARE CANADA (1975) Noncholera vibrio importation. *Can. Dis. week. Rep.* **1–17**: 65–68.

HÖFFLER, U. and KO, H. L. (1977) Gastroenteritiden durch NAG—Vibrionen. *Dt. Äratebl* **74**: 1077–1080.

HOLMGREN, J., LÖNNROTH, J. and OUCHTERLONY, O. (1971) Immunochemical studies of two cholera toxin-containing standard culture filtrate preparations of *V. cholerae*. *Infect Immun.* **3**: 747–755.

HUGH, R. and FEELEY, J. C. (1972) Report (1966–70) of the Subcommittee on Taxonomy of Vibrios to the International Committee on Nomanclature of Bacteria. *Int. J. syst. Bact.* **22**: 123–124.

HUGH, R. and SAKAZAKI, R. (1975) International Committee on Systematic Bacteriology, Subcommittee on Taxonomy of Vibrios, Minutes of the closed meeting, 3 September, 1974. *Int. J. syst. Bact.* **25**: 389–391.

HUGHES, J. M., HOLLIS, D. G., GANGAROSA, E. J. and WEAVER, R. E. (1978) Noncholera vibrio infections in the United States, Clinical, epidemiological and laboratory features. *Ann. Intern. Med.* **88**: 602–606.

KAPER, J., LOCKMAN, H., COLWELL, R. R. and JOSEPH, S. W. (1979) Ecology, serology and enterotoxin production of *Vibrio cholerae* in Chesapeake Bay. *Appl. envir. Microbiol.* **37**: 91–103.

KARUNA-SAGAR, I., NAGESH, C. N. and BHAT, J. V. (1979) Effect of metal ions on the production of permeability factor of 569B strain of *V. cholerae*. *Indian J. med. Res.* **69**: 18–25.

KASAI, G. J. and BURROWS, W. (1966) The titration of cholera toxin and antitoxin in the rabbit ileal loop. *J. infect. Dis.* **116**: 606–614.

KUSAMA, H. and CRAIG, J. P. (1970) Production of biologically active substances by two strains of *Vibrio cholerae*. *Infect. Immun.* **1**: 80–87.

LAHIRI, A., AGARWAL, R. K. and SANYAL, S. C. (1982) Biological Similarity of Enterotoxins of *Vibrio cholerae* serotypes other than 1 to cholera toxin and *Escherichia* Heat-labile *Enterotoxin*, *J. med. Microbiol.* **15**: 429–440.

LINDENBAUM, J., GREENOUGH, W. B. (III), BENENSON, A. S., OSEASOHN, R., RIZVI, S. and SAAD, A. (1965) Non-vibrio cholera. *Lancet* i: 1081–1083.

LÖNROTH, I., ANDREU, B., LANGE, S., MARTINSSEN, K. and HOLMGREN, J. (1979) Chlorpromazine reverses diarrhoea in piglets caused by enteroxigenic *Escherichia coli*. *Infect. Immun.* **24**, 900–905.

LÖNNROTH, I., HOLMGREN, J. and LANGE, S. (1977) Chlorpromazine inhibits cholera toxin-induced intestinal hypersecretion. *Med. Biol. (Helsinki).* **55**: 126–129.

MARWAH, S. M., TIWARI, I. C., SINGH, S. J., SANYAL, S. C., SEN, P. C., RAO, N. S. N. and SARAN, M. (1975) Epidemiological studies on cholera in non-endemic regions with special reference to the problem of carrier state during epidemic and non-epidemic period. *Indian J. prev. soc. Med.* **6**: 326–337.

MCINTYRE, O. R., FEELEY, J. C., GREENHOUGH W. B. III, BENENSON A. S., HASSAN, S. I., and SAAD, A. (1965) Diarrhea caused by noncholera vibrios. *Am. J. trop. Med. Hyg.* **14**: 412–418.

MOSLEY, W. H., AZIE, K. M. and Ahmed, A. (1970) Serological evidence for the identity of the vascular permeability factor and ileal loop toxin of *Vibrio cholerae*. *J. infect. Dis.* **121**: 243–250.

MÜLLER, H. E. (1978) Occurrence and ecology of NAG vibrios in surface waters. *Zentbl. Bakt. ParasitKde., Abt. I., Orig.* **B167**: 272–284.

NACESCU, N. and CUIFECU, C. (1978) Serotypes of NAG vibrios isolated from clinical and environmental sources. *Zentbl. Bakt. ParasitKde., Abt. I., Orig.* **A240**: 334–338.

OHASHI, M., SHIMADA, T. and FUKUMI, H. (1972) *In vitro* production of enterotoxin and haemorrhagic principle by *V. cholerae* NAG. *Jap. J. med. Sci. Biol.* **25**: 179–194.

PIKE, R. M. and CHANDLER, C. H. (1974) The spontaneous release of somatic antigen from *V. cholerae*. *J. Gen. Microbiol.* **81**: 59–67.

POLLITZER, R. (1959) *Cholera* (Monograph series No. 43) Wld Hlth Org., Geneva.

PRATS, G. B., MIRELIS, R. P. and VERGER, G. (1975) Non-cholera vibrio septicimia and meningoencephalitis. *Ann. intern. Med.* **82**: 848–849.

PULVERER, K. YU and SAVCHENKO, B. I. (1973) On infection with vibrios and the possibility of a carrier state in oriental (*Blatta orientalis*) and common (*Blatella germenica* L) Cockroaches. *Medskaya Parazit* **42**: 683–686.

RICHARDSON, S. H. (1969) Factors influencing *in vitro* skin permeability factor production by *Vibrio cholerae J. Bact.* **100**: 27–34.

ROBINS-BROWNE, R. M., STILL, C. S., ISSAESON, M., KNORNHOF, H. I., APPELBAUM, P. L. and SCRAGG, J. N. (1977)

Pathogenic mechanisms of a nonagglutinable *Vibrio cholerae* strain: demonstration of invasive and entero-toxigenic properties. *Infect. Immun.* **18**: 542–545.

SACK, D. A. and SACK, R. B. (1975) Test for enterotoxigenic *Escherichia coli* using Y₁ adrenal cells in mini-culture. *Infect. Immun.* **11**: 334–336.

SACK, R. B. (1973) A search for canine carriers of *Vibrio. J. infect. Dis.* **127**: 709–712.

SAKAZAKI, R., GOMEZ, C. Z. and SEBALD, M. (1967) Taxonomical studies of the so-called NAG vibrios. *Jap. J. med. Sci. Biol.* **20**: 265–280.

SANYAL, S. C., DUBEY, R. S. and ANNAPURNA, E. (1980a) Enteropathogenicity and pathogenesis of *Aeromonas hydrophila* in experimental models. In *Sympsoum on Diarrhoeal Diseases*, pp. 39–51, GUHA MASUMDAR, D. N., CHAKRABORTY, A. K., DE, S. and KIRAN KUMAR, A. (eds). Proceedings National Conference on Communicable Diseases held in A.I.I.H. & P.H. Calcutta-73 December 8–10, 1978.

SANYAL, S. C., SARASWATHI, B. and SHARMA, P. (1980b) Enteropathogenicity of *Plesiomonas shigelloides. J. med. Microbiol.* **13**, 401–409.

SANYAL, S. C., SINGH, S. J., TIWARI, I. C., SEN, P. C. MARWAH, S. M., HAZARIKA, U. R., SINGH, H., SHIMADA, T. and SAKAZAKI, R. (1974) Role of household animals in maintenance of cholera infection in a community. *J. infect. Dis.* **130**: 575–579.

SERENY, B. (1957) Experimental keratoconjunctivitis in Shigellosa. *Acta. microbiol. hung.* **4**: 367–376.

SHANKER, P., AGARWAL, R. K. and SANYAL, S. C. (1982), Experimental studies on enteropathogenicity of *Vibrio cholerae* serotypes other than 1. *Zentbl. Bakt. ParasitKde., Abt I., Orig.* **A252**: 514–524.

SHIMADA, T. and SAKAZAKI, R. (1977) Additional serovars and inter-O antigenic relationships of *V. cholerae. Jap. J. med. Sci. Biol.* **30**: 275–277.

SIL, J., SANYAL, S. C., DATTA, N. K. and MUKERJEE, S. (1971) Animal pathogenicity of nonagglutinable vibrios and the problem of immunization. *ICMR Technical Report Series No. 9* pp. 125–128.

SINGH, S. J. and SANYAL, S. C. (1978) Enterotoxicity of the so-called NAG vibrios. *Ann. Soc. belge. Méd. trop.* **58**, 133–140.

SINGH, S. J., SANYAL, S. C., SEN, P. C., TIWARI, I. C., MARWAH, S. M., SINGH, H., SHIMADA, T. and SAKAZAKI, R. (1975) studies on the bacteriology of cholera infection in Varanasi. *Indian J. med. Res.* **63**: 1089–1097.

SINHA, V. B. and SRIVASTAVA, B. S. (1978) Plasmid induced loss of virulence in *V. cholerae. Nature* **276**: 708–709.

SPIRA, W. M., DANIEL, R. R., AHMED, Q. S., HUQ, A., YUSUF, A. and SACK, D. A. (1979) Clinical features and pathogenicity of O group 1, non-agglutinable *Vibrio cholerae* and other vibrios isolated from cases of diarrhoea in Dacca, Bangladesh. In: *Symposium on Cholera*, pp. 137–153, TAKEYA, K. and ZINNAKA, Y. (eds). *U.S.–Japan Cooperative Medical Science Program*, Karatsu, 1978.

TAKEYA, K. and ZINNAKA, Y. (eds). *U.S.–Japan Cooperative Medical Science Program*, Karatsu, 1978.

TIWARI I. C., SANYAL, S. C., MARWAH, S. M., SINGH, S. J., SEN, P. C. and SINGH, H. (1975) An outbreak of cholera *eltor* in Varanasi. *Indian J. prev. Soc. Med.* **6**: 95–99.

VASIL, M., HOLMES, R. K. and FINKELSTEIN, R. A. (1975) Conjugal transfer of a chromosomal gene determining production of enterotoxin in *V. cholerae. Science* **187**: 849–850.

WORLD HEALTH ORGANIZATION (1969) Outbreak of gastroenteritis by nonagglutinable (NAG) vibrios. *Wkly epidem. Rec.* **44**: 10.

WHO SCIENTIFIC WORKING GROUP (1980) Cholera and other vibrio-associated diarrhoeas. *Bull. Wld Hlth Org.* **58**: 353–374.

YAJNIK, B. S. and PRASAD, B. G. (1954) A note on vibrios isolated in Kumbh Fair, Allahabad. *Indian med. Gaz.* **89**: 341–349.

ZAFARI, Y., ZARIFI, A. Z., RAHMANZADEH, S. and FAKHAR, N. (1973) Diarrhoea caused by non-agglutinable *Vibrio cholerae* (non-cholera vibrio). *Lancet* **ii**: 429–430.

ZINNAKA, Y. and CARPENTER, C. C. J. (1972) An enterotoxin produced by noncholera vibrios. *Johns Hopkins med. J.* **131**: 403–411.

ZINNAKA, Y., FUKUOYOSHI, S. and OKAMURA, Y. (1972) Some observations on the NAG vibrio toxin. *Proc. 8th Joint Conf. Cholera Panel*, p. 116. The U.S.–Japan Cooperative Medical Science Programme, NIH, Tokyo.

CHAPTER 12

SALMONELLA TOXINS

JOHNNY W. PETERSON, Ph. D.

*Professor Department of Microbiology, The University of Texas Medical Branch
Galveston, Texas 77550*

1. INTRODUCTION

Salmonella are gram negative, facultative anaerobic bacilli that have been clearly associated with intestinal and extraintestinal infections of man and animals. The majority of salmonellae are animal pathogens that only incidently infect humans, because of contamination of animal products (e.g., poultry, eggs, etc.) used for food. An exception to this generalization is *Salmonella typhi*, a strict human pathogen and etiologic agent of typhoid fever. When *Salmonella* colonize the intestinal tract, diarrheal disease may ensue. The toxic factors that contribute to the pathogenesis of these intestinal infections are the subject of this review; however, it is important to note that salmonellae are invasive bacterial pathogens that may disseminate from the intestinal lumen to virtually any tissue site. Because *Salmonella* toxins were only recently discovered, their role, if any, in systemic infections is unknown, but their action in the intestine has received considerable attention.

Despite a longstanding association of *Salmonella* and systemic disease, information pertaining to their pathogenic mechanism is limited. For purpose of discussion, the pathogenesis of salmonellosis can be divided into several phases based on progression of the disease process. Initially, colonization of the intestinal mucosa must occur and may involve adherence factors (e.g., pili), chemotaxis, and motility. Some studies have associated epithelial cell invasion capacity with virulence, but it is unclear whether *Salmonella* toxins exert their ultimate effect on the intestinal mucosa before or after tissue invasion. Factors that facilitate entry of salmonellae into cells and contribute to their survival after phagocytosis are also unknown. The reason(s) are unclear why many salmonellae are restricted to intestinal tissue and cause a self-limiting form of gastroenteritis while other strains may progress to systemic disease. Recent experimental data indicate that during intestinal colonization, salmonellae form at least two protein toxins that may contribute to the pathogenic mechanism in the intestine. The *Salmonella* enterotoxin is a cholera toxin-like enterotoxin which activates adenylate cyclase causing an elevation in mucosal cyclic adenosine monophosphate (cyclic AMP) concentration. The enterotoxin appears to be responsible for the hypersecretion of fluid and electrolytes from the intestinal epithelium. In addition, a recently described *Salmonella* cytotoxin, that inhibits ^{3}H-leucine incorporation in intestinal epithelial cells and causes detachment of cultured cell monolayers, may contribute to the tissue damage occurring in the intestinal mucosa during salmonellosis. This review will attempt to summarize the characteristics of the enterotoxin and the cytotoxin as well as to evaluate their potential significance in diarrheal disease mediated by *Salmonella*.

2. CLINICAL FORMS OF *SALMONELLA* INFECTIONS

Salmonella species cause two basic forms of clinical disease: gastroenteritis and enteric fever. *Salmonella* gastroenteritis is a type of 'food poisoning' that is usually characterized by the abrupt onset of nausea, fever, vomiting, diarrhea, and abdominal cramps 8–24 hr after consumption of contaminated food or water. Although the infection results in considerable discomfort for the patient, *Salmonella* gastroenteritis usually is a self-limiting infection for which antibiotics are contraindicated. In this form of the infection, *Salmonella* bacilli colonize the small intestine and penetrate the columnar epithelial cells of the intestinal villi. Although the focus of infection extends to the lamina propria, dissemination of the bacilli to the blood stream rarely occurs.

The second form of *Salmonella* infection is enteric fever which connotes a disease with greater systemic involvement. The clinical symptoms of enteric fever are typified by those of typhoid fever, which is caused specifically by *S. typhi*. Many strains of *Salmonella*, however, cause typhoid-like enteric fever. In enteric fevers, *Salmonella* become disseminated via the lymphatic vessels and phagocytic cells to the bloodstream after penetration of the small intestinal epithelium. Practically any organ can become infected resulting in serious sequelae. Unlike the treatment of gastroenteritis, enteric fevers require appropriate antibiotic therapy (i.e., chloramphenicol, ampicillin, etc.).

3. PATHOGENESIS OF SALMONELLOSIS: *SALMONELLA* EXOTOXINS

Salmonella Enterotoxins—The *Salmonella* enterotoxin is similar to the heat-labile enterotoxins from several other enteric bacilli (e.g., *Vibrio cholerae* and *Esherichia coli*) in that several types of biological activities are demonstrable. Because the enterotoxin elevates cyclic AMP levels, it may affect vascular permeability when injected into rabbit skin as well as elicit fluid secretion in the small intestine. Stimulatory effects of the enterotoxin on the adenylate cyclase system may also be demonstrated in cultured cells (e.g., Chinese hamster ovary cell elongation). Because of the exquisite sensitivity of the rabbit skin permeability test (Craig, 1965), much of the initial work on the *Salmonella* enterotoxin was performed using this model. Intestinal loop assay methods were later pursued to validate that the toxin indeed possessed enterotoxic activity. The cell culture methods have provided a convenient and inexpensive technique for measuring the effects of the toxin on cyclic AMP levels. The latter procedures are also less variable than the responses of experimental animals, many of which are not immunologic virgins relative to the cholera toxin family of enterotoxins.

Permeability Factor Activity—Sandefur and Peterson (1976a) demonstrated two skin permeability factors (PF) in culture filtrates of *Salmonella typhimurium* using a modification of the skin permeability test for cholera toxin described by Craig (1965) and Craig *et al.* (1972). Visualization of the skin permeability reaction was enhanced by i.v. injection of Pontamine sky blue dye (bluing). A rapid-acting permeability factor (rapid PF), produced optimally in brain heart infusion broth at 37°C, was found in numerous *Salmonella* species. This factor had a critical bluing time of 1 hr after completion of skin testing, was heat stable at 100°C for at least 4 hr, and was reported to have no associated induration, although soft, spongy edema was noted later with more concentrated preparations. The second factor was delayed in onset, appearing in 18–24 hr as an area of firm induration accompanied by bluing. The delayed factor was heat-labile, being completely destroyed within 30 min at 75°C. The induration response observed at 18 hr was indistinguishable from the skin permeability reactions of cholera toxin and *E. coli* heat-labile enterotoxin (LT). The delayed induration response was not observed when unconcentrated crude culture filtrates were tested unless the preparations were first chromatographed on Sephadex G-100. Both early and delayed PF's were estimated to have a molecular weight of at least 90,000. Further, the delayed PF appeared to have an isoelectric point of 4.3–4.8, compared to 6.8 for cholera toxin, and was resistant to most proteolytic enzymes (Peterson and Sandefur, 1979). The *Salmonella* delayed PF was further observed to compete with cholera toxin for binding sites on rabbit intestinal mucosa (Peterson and Sandefur, 1979). Cholera toxin and heat-labile *E. coli* toxin are known to bind to G_{M1} ganglioside (Donta and Viner, 1975; Kwan and Wishnow, 1974; van Heyningen *et al.*, 1971). We have found that the *Salmonella* delayed PF activity was also blocked by preincubation with G_{M1} ganglioside (Peterson and Sandefur, 1979); therefore, cholera toxin, heat-labile *E. coli* toxin, and *Salmonella* enterotoxin appear to share the property of attachment to this tissue receptor.

Sandefur and Peterson (1976b) reported that partially purified, delayed PF from *Salmonella typhimurium* (986) culture filtrates elongated Chinese hamster ovary (CHO) cells in a manner identical to that of cholera toxin. Moreover, both the delayed PF activity and the CHO elongation activity could be neutralized by monospecific antisera to cholera toxin but not by preimmunization sera. Peterson and Sandefur (1979) were also able to protect rabbits against *Salmonella*-induced fluid exsorption by immunizing them with procholeragenoid, a heat-aggregated derivative of cholera toxin. This indirect toxoid vaccination approach strongly indicated an integral role of this cholera toxin-like toxin in the pathogenesis of salmonellosis.

Peterson and Sandefur (1979) confirmed their earlier report of a delayed PF from culture filtrates and showed that toxin production was not limited to a single isolate. In addition, they found that the delayed PF was progressively inactivated by overnight exposure to extremes in pH (< 6.0 and > 8.0) at 4°C. The delayed PF activity was unaffected by various proteolytic enzymes, including pronase, protease, trypsin, pepsin, and carboxypeptidase. Chromatography on columns of Sephadex G-100 and G-150 confirmed the molecular weight to be approximately 90,000 d. The isoelectric point of the delayed PF from the two *Salmonella* isolates (2000 and 986) was always in a range of pH 4.3 to 4.8.

Since *Salmonella* toxin (formerly referred to as delayed PF or CHO elongation factor) resembled cholera toxin, Peterson and Sandefur (1979) found that partially purified *Salmonella* toxin would compete with ^{125}I-labeled cholera toxin for binding sites on guinea pig intestinal homogenates. Purified GM_1 ganglioside also completely inactivated the vascular permeability factor activity. Other gangliosides (GT_1, GD1a, and mixed gangliosides without GM_1) had no effect on the biological activity of *Salmonella* toxin. Because of these studies, it was concluded that GM_1 ganglioside was the likely receptor for this toxin.

The delayed permeability factor activity of *Salmonella* culture filtrates was confirmed and extended by Kuhn *et al.* (1978). These investigators examined culture filtrates from 378 *Salmonella* isolates from Germany representing 21 different serotypes. Among them, filtrates from 205 strains of 15 serotypes yielded positive PF responses. Like the delayed PF described above (Peterson and Sandefur, 1979; Sandefur and Peterson, 1976a,b), the PF examined in the study by Kuhn *et al.* (1978) was heat-labile resulting in complete inactivation within 10 minutes at 100°C. Importantly, this *Salmonella* PF was neutralized by antiserum to cholera toxin B subunit. The characteristics of the toxin described by Kuhn *et al.* (1978) are essentially the same as those reported by Sandefur and Peterson (Peterson and Sandefur, 1979; Sandefur and Peterson, 1976a,b). Jiwa (1981a,b) observed positive vascular permeability responses with cell free, culture filtrates from 29 of 40 *Salmonella* (11 serotypes) isolated in Sweden. This delayed PF was described as heat-labile (80°, 30 minutes), neutralized by goat antiserum to cholera toxin, and inactivated by purified GM_1 ganglioside. Therefore, the characteristics of this *Salmonella* toxin are comparable to those presented previously (Kuhn *et al.*, 1978; Peterson and Sandefur, 1979; Sandefur and Peterson, 1976a,b). Further, Caprioli *et al.* (1981, 1982a,b) identified and partially purified a vascular permeability and enterotoxic factor from culture filtrates of *Salmonella wien*. The toxin also caused elongation of CHO cells. Two peaks of activity were detected in fractions from a Biogel A 1.5 m column; the first was resistant to heating at 75°C for 30 minutes while the second was heat labile.

Intestinal Fluid Secretory Activity—Taylor and Wilkins (1961) reported that live cultures of many *Salmonella* evoked fluid accumulation responses in intestinal loops of adult rabbits. Early attempts to demonstrate enterotoxin activity in culture filtrates, cell extracts, and concentrated loop fluids were unsuccessful (Giannella, 1973 and 1979). In contrast, Sakazaki *et al.* (1974a,b) later reported that culture filtrates from 11 of 13 strains yielded positive responses in the rabbit ligated loop model.

Koupal and Deibel (1975) reported that culture supernatants of *Salmonella enteritidis* yielded reproducible fluid accumulation results in the suckling mouse model of Dean *et al.* (1972). Since the culture supernatant preparations tested in this study apparently were not filter sterilized, the observations could have resulted from the presence of residual viable cells. This could explain why the 'enterotoxic' activity was associated with heavy, cell-wall fragment fractions rather than with soluble fractions. Responses in this model have not been confirmed by later studies (Jiwa, 1981a,b; Peterson, 1980).

Thapliyal and Singh (1978) described cell-free, enterotoxic activity of *Salmonella weltevreden* culture filtrates using the rabbit intestinal loop method. Only the larger volumes of Syncase culture filtrates (5 and 9 ml) elicited a fluid response; three ml volumes yielded no fluid accumulation. Partial purification of the enterotoxin was achieved by precipitation with 80% $(NH_4)_2SO_4$. Further characterization of the enterotoxin from *Salmonella weltevreden*, a commonly isolated strain in India, was reported by Thapliyal and Singh (1979).

Kuhn *et al.* (1978) reported several strains of *Salmonella* whose culture filtrates evoked fluid accumulation responses in both the suckling mouse test of Giannella (1976) and the rabbit intestinal loop test (De and Chatterje, 1953). The enterotoxic activity was heat labile, being destroyed in 10 minutes at $100°C$. Sedlock *et al.* (1978) also described enterotoxic activity in filtrates of an isolate of *Salmonella typhimurium*. By washing the small intestinal lumen of adult rabbits with Ringer's solution or a solution of PBS containing sodium citrate and N-acetylcysteine prior to ligation of loops, fluid responses were larger and more rabbits responded to both *Salmonella* infection and *Salmonella* culture filtrates.

Jiwa (1981) and Jiwa and Mansson (1983) compared several *in vivo* and *in vitro* tests for enterotoxic activity of *Salmonella* filtrates including the rabbit intestinal loop test and the suckling mouse assay. He found that 17 of 19 cell-free culture filtrates of various *Salmonella* serotypes yielded positive fluid accumulation responses in the rabbit intestinal loop test, but only 2 of 27 *Salmonella* filtrates yielded a positive suckling mouse test. He reported a high degree of correlation between the rabbit intestinal loop assay, the CHO cell assay (Sakazaki *et al.*, 1974), the adrenal cell assay (Jiwa, 1981b), and the rabbit skin permeability assay (Sandefur and Peterson, 1976a).

In an attempt to prove that the *Salmonella* enterotoxin truly exerted its biological effect on the adenylate cyclase system during the course of experimental *Salmonella* infection, Peterson *et al.* (1983) isolated epithelial cells from normal as well as infected intestinal loops challenged with live *Salmonella*. The crypt epithelial cells and to some extent the lamina propria cells contained elevated levels of cyclic AMP. This was in contrast to *Vibrio cholerae* infected loops where only the epithelial cells contained higher concentrations of cyclic AMP. Just as importantly, isolated epithelial cells from normal rabbit intestine responded *in vitro* after exposure to a cell-free lysate of *Salmonella*. These epithelial cells treated with crude *Salmonella* enterotoxin displayed marked increases in cyclic AMP content compared to untreated epithelial cells. These data provide additional supportive evidence for an integral role of *Salmonella* enterotoxin in the pathogenesis of salmonellosis.

Tissue Culture Cell Activity—Sandefur and Peterson (1976b) first reported that Chinese hamster ovary cells were elongated by cell free, culture filtrates of *Salmonella typhimurium*. The observation has since been confirmed by Jiwa (1981b) and Caprioli *et al.* (1982a,b). Using the CHO elongation assay, Molina and Peterson (1980) observed that the concentration of *Salmonella* toxin in culture filtrates could be increased by adding mitomycin C to growing cultures of various *Salmonella* isolates. The physical characteristics of the *Salmonella* toxin were the same as those observed previously with the rabbit skin and in CHO cell assays (Peterson and Sandefur, 1979; Sandefur and Peterson, 1976a,b). The addition of mitomycin C enabled these investigators to determine that the best toxin production was obtained in media such as casaminoacid-yeast extract (CYE) broth and syncase with glucose instead of sucrose, while complex media such as BHI and HI yielded very little toxin.

Peterson *et al.* (1981) later found that mitomycin C caused extensive bacterial cell lysis by inducing temperate bacteriophage. Such induction provided a convenient technique for release of *Salmonella* toxin, which in this study was measured by a modification of the CHO cell assay. Nozawa *et al.* (1978) had reported that cholera toxin and *E. coli* LT increased the adhesiveness of CHO cells and reduced the number of 'floating' cells in the medium above the monolayer. The CHO floating cell assay allows the use of a Coulter counter to count the number of unattached or 'floating' cells in the tissue culture well. Standard dilutions of purified cholera toxin, ranging from 10 pg to 1 ng yield a linear response, thus reducing the subjectivity of the CHO elongation assay and increasing assay sensitivity.

An ELISA for quantitation of *Salmonella* toxin using specifically purified, cholera antitoxin was developed by Houston *et al.* (1982) and Peterson *et al.* (1981). Comparisons were made between results obtained with this rapid serological procedure and those with the CHO floating cell assay. Using the CHO floating cell assay, as well as the ELISA, *Salmonella* toxin was measured directly in sonicated cell preparations from a variety of *Salmonella* species. The characteristics of the *Salmonella* toxin detected by the CHO floating cell assay and the ELISA were essentially the same as those reported earlier (i.e., pI = 4.3–4.8; molecular weight = 110,000; and heat-labile biological activity).

A chemically-defined culture medium for production of *Salmonella* toxin was recently reported by Koo and Peterson (1981). They observed that the 'supplemented M-9' medium yielded about 80 % as much toxin as CYE medium, as measured by the CHO floating cell assay. Ingredients of the 'supplemented M-9' medium that stimulated toxin production were Mn^{++}, biotin, riboflavin, glycerol, histidine, glutamic acid, arginine, serine, and lysine. Additional nutritional studies with fermenter grown CYE cultures of *Salmonella* have recently been completed (Koo and Peterson, 1982). While CYE broth is somewhat superior to the chemically defined 'supplemented M-9' medium, most of the *Salmonella* toxin in 'supplemented M-9' cultures remains associated with the bacterial cells; CYE medium ordinarily results in release of at least 50 % of the toxin into the culture medium.

Finally, Kuhn *et al.* (1978) and Fumarola *et al.* (1977a, b) have employed a novel cell assay involving enterotoxin-mediated inhibition of platelet aggregation to measure enterotoxic activity of various *Salmonella* strains. Kuhn *et al.* (1978) have shown that the method correlates well with vascular permeability factor activity and fluid exsorption in the intestinal loop test.

Little is known about the genetic basis for *Salmonella* toxin production; however, Houston *et al.* (1981) showed that temperate bacteriophage were not responsible. No association could be made between the presence of temperate phage and *Salmonella* toxin production. Likewise, lysogenic conversion did not alter toxin-producing capacity. Kuhn *et al.* (1978) transferred plasmid pIE342, the only known plasmid of *Salmonella typhimurium* strain IE 705, to several *Escherichia coli* and *Salmonella* species, but toxin production was not altered in the recipient *Salmonella* or detected in the recipient *E. coli*. Support for the contention that plasmids may not be the genetic locus for *Salmonella* toxin synthesis was also derived by C. W. Houston (personal communication), who has found two strains of *Salmonella* (Q1, M206) that possessed no detectable plasmids, but each produced toxin. Cisek *et al.* (1981) also presented evidence that the enterotoxin gene in *Salmonella* may be located on the chromosome. They observed a weak reaction between chromosomal digests and a radiolabeled *E. coli* toxin gene probe. The results were preliminary, however, because of some uncertainty about specificity of the probe. Therefore, presumptive data suggest that the *Salmonella* toxin gene may be located on the chromosome.

The first report on the purification of *Salmonella* enterotoxin to apparent homogeneity was made recently by Finkelstein *et al.* (1983). Using affinity chromatography with a column of Agarose A-5m (Bio Rad), the protein toxin was purified from cell lysates of *Salmonella typhimurium* W-118-2. SDS-PAGE analysis revealed two subunits A and B. The *Salmonella* A subunit migrated similar to the A subunit of cholera toxin while the *Salmonella* B subunit monomer more closely resembled the B subunit of *E. coli* LT (human) than cholera toxin B subunit. Ouchterlony analysis showed that the antigenic composition of *Salmonella* enterotoxin most closely resembled *E. coli* LT (human).

Salmonella Cytotoxin—The earliest description of a heat-labile cytotoxic factor produced by *Salmonella* was reported by Mesrobeanu *et al.* (1960, 1962). Using human embryonic cells and KB tumor cells, cytopathic effects (i.e., morphological alterations and reduction in cell number) were observed when the cells were exposed to partially purified neurotoxin preparations from both *Salmonella* and *Shigella*. The heat-labile neurotoxin of *Salmonella* was reported by Mesrobeanu *et al.* (1961). The *Salmonella* neurotoxin was so named because it induced limb paralysis, convulsions, diarrhea, hypothermia, and death following injection into rabbits. Other publications (Marx and Mesrobeanu, 1964; Mesrobeanu *et al.*, 1973).

relating to *Salmonella* neurotoxin have been reviewed elsewhere (Mesrobeanu and Mesrobeanu, 1971; Mesrobeanu *et al.*, 1966).

Ketyi *et al.* (1979) described a *Shigella dysenteriae* 1-like cytotoxic enterotoxin produced by *Salmonella thompson*, *Salmonella kapemba* and *Salmonella enteritidis*. In this study, the *Salmonella* cytotoxin was neutralized by antiserum to *Shigella dystenteriae* 1 toxin but to a lesser degree than the homologous toxin. Koo and Peterson (1983) recently reported that cell-free, dialyzed sonic extracts from several *Salmonella* serotypes contained a heat-labile cytotoxin that caused extensive detachment of intact Vero cells. Using a modification of the cell detachment assay of Gentry and Dalrymple (1980), undiluted sonic extracts of *Salmonella* exhibited 20–50% cell detachment. Upon dilution, a linear, dose-related cytotoxic effect was observed. Heating at 100°C for 30 minutes destroyed much but not all of the cytotoxic factor. Although cell detachment was not apparent until 48 hr, progressive inhibition of Vero cell protein synthesis began 1–2 hr after exposure. Attempts to demonstrate neutralization of the *Salmonella* cytotoxin with antisera to Shiga toxin have not been successful (F. C. W. Koo and J. W. Peterson—unpublished observations). It is possible that this heat-labile cytotoxin, inhibiting protein synthesis, is related to the *Salmonella* cytotoxin/neurotoxin described by Mesrobeanu *et al.* (1960, 1961 and 1962) and the *Shigella*-like *Salmonella* cytotoxin reported by Ketyi *et al.* (1979). Considering the cellular damage apparent in the small intestinal mucosa during experimental salmonellosis (Giannella, 1979; Madge, 1974), it seems reasonable to postulate that the cytotoxic factor(s) mentioned above may participate in the pathogenesis of salmonellosis. Baloda *et al.* (1983) also recently noted a cytotoxic effect in CHO cells treated with culture filtrates from 2 of 10 strains of *Salmonella*. The authors pointed out that such cytotoxic factors could disguise biological effects caused by enterotoxins in the Y1 adrenal and Chinese hamster ovary cell assays.

Proving that any toxin is important in the pathogenesis of a microbial infection and requires more than mere detection of the toxic activity in extracts or filtrates of that pathogen. Convincing proof must be sought by demonstrating that a related biological effect occurs during the disease. With regard to the *Salmonella* cytotoxin, Koo *et al.* (1984) recently demonstrated that small intestinal epithelial cells, isolated from rabbit intestinal loops challenged with live *Salmonella*, exhibited markedly reduced rates of protein synthesis. In addition, epithelial cells isolated from normal rabbit small intestine exhibited reduced rates of protein synthesis when exposed *in vitro* to *Salmonella enteritidis* cell lysate, previously shown to inhibit protein synthesis in Vero cells *in vitro* (Koo and Peterson, 1983). The rate of protein synthesis in the underlying lamina propria cells from *Salmonella*-infected intestinal loops compared to normal controls, was unaffected. Based on these experiments, there is little doubt that the *Salmonella* cytotoxin inhibits protein synthesis in epithelial cells of the intestinal mucosa during experimental salmonellosis. It is likely that the inability of the epithelial cells to synthesize protein constitutes an important mechanism of epithelial cell damage (Madge, 1974) observed during salmonellosis. The precise sequence of events whereby both the enterotoxin and cytotoxin interact with the intestinal mucosa remains to be determined.

4. GENERAL DISCUSSION

Based upon recent research described above, it is now apparent that *Salmonella* species elaborate an enterotoxin and a cytotoxin. The full significance of these toxins in human disease is not yet clear, but their involvement in the pathogenesis of experimental salmonellosis is convincing (Koo and Peterson, 1983; Peterson *et al.*, 1983). The studies indicate that the enterotoxin affects fluid transport in the small intestine by perturbing the adenylate cyclase system. In contrast, the cytotoxin appears to be a lethal toxin capable of affecting intestinal cell viability and causing tissue damage.

The relationship between bacterial invasion and toxin production is virtually unknown. It is also unclear if the *Salmonella* toxins are elaborated by the bacteria prior to or after the entry into the epithelial cells. The toxins are produced in relatively low concentrations by

Salmonella, which might affect the efficiency of toxin delivery to the cells. On the other hand, invasion of the epithelial cells by *Salmonella* could be a more efficient toxin delivery mechanism. Once inside the intestinal epithelial cells, production of even trace amounts of these toxins could have a marked effect on fluid and electrolyte transport as well as cell viability. Continued study of the basic pathogenic mechanism of salmonellosis may eventually lead to the development of effective modes of prophylaxis and/or treatment.

REFERENCES

BALODA, S. B., FARIS, A., KROVACEK, K. and WADSTROM, T. (1983) Cytotonic enterotoxins and cytotoxic factors produced by *Salmonella enteritidis* and *Salmonella typhimurium*. *Toxicon* **21**: 785–795.

CAPRIOLI, A., D'AGNOLO, G., FALBO, V., RODA, L. G. and TOMASI, M. (1981) Detection of a skin permeability factor in culture filtrates of *Salmonella wien* isolated from man. *Microbiol.* **4**: 261–270.

CAPRIOLI, A., D'AGNOLO, G., FALBO, V., RODA, L. G. and TOMASI, M. (1982a) Isolation of *Salmonella wien* heat-labile enterotoxin. *Toxicon* **20**: 254 (abstract).

CAPRIOLI, A., D'AGNOLO, G., FALBO, V., RODA, L. G. and TOMASI, M. (1982b) Isolation of *Salmonella wien* heat-labile enterotoxin. *Microbiol.* **5**: 1–10.

CISEK, L., KAZIC, T. and BENSON, C. E. (1981) Detection of enterotoxin-like gene in pathogenic *Salmonella*. Conference of Research Workers in Animal Disease (Abstracts of the 62nd annual meeting, Nov., 1981).

CRAIG, J. P. (1965) A permeability factor (toxin) found in cholera stools and culture filtrates and its neutralization by convalescent cholera sera. *Nature (London)* **207**: 614–616.

CRAIG, J. P., EICHNER, E. R. and HORNICK, R. B. (1972) Cutaneous responses to cholera toxin in man. I. Responses in immunized American males. *J. Infect. Dis.* **125**: 203–215.

DE, S. N. and CHATTERJE, D. N. (1953) An experimental study of the mechanism of action of *Vibrio cholerae* on the intestinal mucous membrane. *J. Pathol. Bacteriol.* **46**: 559–562.

DEAN, A. G., CHING, Y. C., WILLIAMS, R. G. and HARDER, L. B. (1972) Test for *Escherichia coli* enterotoxin using infant mice: application in a study of diarrhea in children in Honolulu. *J. Infect. Dis.* **125**: 407–411.

DONTA, S. T. and VINER, J. P. (1975) Inhibition of the steroidogenic effects of cholera and heat-labile *Escherichia coli* enterotoxins by G_{M1} ganglioside: Evidence for a similar receptor site for the two toxins. *Infect. Immun.* **11**: 982–985.

FINKELSTEIN, R. A., MARCHLEWICZ, B. A., MCDONALD, R. J. and BASEMAN–FINKELSTEIN, M. (1983) Isolation and characterization of a cholera-related enterotoxin from *Salmonella typhimurium*. *FEMS Microbiology Letters* **17**: 239–241.

FUMAROLA, D., MIRAGLIOTTA, G., PALMA, R. and PANARO, A. (1977a) Experimental contribution to the study of enterotoxigenic activity of some *Salmonella typhimurium* strains: Investigations with the model of the platelet aggregation by ADP. *Ann. Sclavo.* **19**: 1243–1247.

FUMAROLA, D., MIRAGLIOTTA, G., PALMA, R. and PANARO, A. (1977b) Experimental study of enterotoxic activity in some strains of *Salmonella typhimurium*: Observations on the model of ADP-induced platelet aggregation. G. Batteriol. *Virol. Immunol.* **70**: 28–33.

GENTRY, M. K. and DALRYMPLE, J. M. (1980) Quantitative microtiter cytotoxicity for *Shigella* toxin. *J. Clin. Microbiol.* **12**: 361–366.

GIANNELLA, R. A. (1973) Cholera-like diarrhea in salmonellosis. *Lancet* I (7813): 1185–1186.

GIANNELLA, R. A. (1976) Suckling mouse model for detection of heat stable *E. coli* enterotoxin: Characteristics of the model. *Infect. Immun.* **14**: 95–99.

GIANNELLA, R. A. (1979) Importance of the intestinal inflammatory reaction in *Salmonella*-mediated intestinal secretion. *Infect. Immun.* **23**: 140–145.

HOUSTON, C. W., DAVIS, C. P. and PETERSON, J. W. (1982) *Salmonella* toxin synthesis is unrelated to the presence of temperate bacteriophages. *Infect. Immun.* **35**: 749–751.

HOUSTON, C. W., KOO, F. C. W. and PETERSON, J. W. (1981) Characterization of *Salmonella* toxin released by mitomycin C-treated cells. *Infect. Immun.* **32**: 916–926.

JIWA, S. F. H. (1981a) Enterotoxigenic bacteria from clinical alimental and environmental sources: Studies on enterotoxic factors and surface properties with particular reference to *Salmonella* and *Aeromonas*. In: Doctoral Thesis, Swedish Univ. of Agri. Sci. Uppsala.

JIWA, S. F. H. (1981b) Probing for enterotoxigenicity among the salmonellae: An evaluation of biological assays. *J. Clin. Microbiol.* **14**: 463–472.

JIWA, S. F. H. and MANSSON, I. (1983) Hemagglutinating and hydrophobic surface properties of salmonellae producing enterotoxin neutralized by cholera anti-toxin. *Vet. Microbiol.* **8**: 443–458.

KETYI, I., PACSA, S., EMODY, L., VERTENYI, A., KOCSIS, B. and KUCH, B. (1979) *Shigella dysenteriae* 1-like cytotoxic enterotoxins produced by *Salmonella* strains. *Acta Microbiol. Acad. Sci. Hung.* **26**: 217–223.

KOO, F. C. W. and PETERSON, J. W. (1983) Cell-free extracts of *Salmonella* inhibit protein synthesis and cause cytotoxicity in eukaryotic cells. *Toxicon* **21**: 309–320.

KOO, F. C. W. and PETERSON, J. W. (1981) The influence of nutritional factors on synthesis of *Salmonella* toxin. *J. Food Safety* **3**: 215–232.

KOO, F. C. W. and PETERSON, J. W. (1982) Effects of cultural conditions on the synthesis of *Salmonella* toxin. *J. Food Safety* **5**: 61–71.

KOO, F. C. W., PETERSON, J. W., HOUSTON, C. W. and MOLINA, N. C. (1984) Pathogenesis of experimental salmonellosis: inhibition of protein synthesis by cytotoxin. *Infect. Immun.* **43**: 181–188.

KOUPAL, L. R. and DEIBEL, R. H. (1975) Assay, characterization, and localization of an enterotoxin produced by *Salmonella. Infect. Immun.* **11**: 14–22.

KUHN, H., TSCHAPE, H. and RISCHE, H. (1978) Enterotoxigenicity among salmonellae—A prospective analysis for a surveillance programme. *Zbl. Bakt. Hyg. I. Abt. Orig.* **A240:** 171–183.

KWAN, C. N. and WISHNOW, R. M. (1974) *Escherichia coli* enterotoxin-induced steroidogenesis in cultured adrenal tumor cells. *Infect. Immun.* **10:** 146–151.

MADGE, D. S. (1974) Scanning electron microscopy of normal and diseased mouse small intestinal mucosa. *J. de Microscopie* **20:** 45–50.

MARX, A. and MESROBEANU, L. (1964) Contribution a l-etude de la constitution en acides amines des neurotoxines de *S. typhimurium*. *Arch. Roum de Pathol. exper. et de Microbiologie*. **23:** 573–580.

MESROBEANU, L., BUTUR, D. and MOVILEANU, D. (1973) Toxines microbiennes et contact intercellulaire in vitro. Endotoxines thermostable et thermolabile de *Salmonella typhimurium* "S". *Arch. Roum. de Pathol. exper. et de Microbiologie* **32:** 245–253.

MESROBEANU, I., GEORGESCO, M., JEREMIA, T., PAPAZIAN, E., DRAGHICI, D. and MESROBEANU, L. (1960) Action des toxines microbiennes sur les cultures de tissus: I. Action cytotoxique des endotoxines glucido-lipidiques. *Arch. Roum. de Pathol. exper. et de Microbiologie*. **19:** 345–354.

MESROBEANU, L. and MESROBEANU, I. (1971) *Salmonella typhimurium* and *Escherichia coli* neurotoxins. In: *Microbial Toxins*, vol. IIA. S. KADIS, T. C. MONTIE and S. J. AJL, editors. Academic Press, New York, pp. 301–336.

MESROBEANU, I., MESROBEANU, L., GEORGESCO, M., DRAGHICI, D., ALAMITA, E. and IEREMIA, T. (1962) Action des toxines microbiennes sur les cultures de tissus. II. Action cytotoxique es endotoxines thermolabiles (neurotoxines) des germes gram-negatifs. *Arch. Roum. de Pathol. exper. et de Microbiologie*. **21:** 19–30.

MESROBEANU, I., MESROBEANU, L. and MITRICA, N. (1961) Endotoxines thermolabiles (neurotoxins) des germes gram negatifs. I. Les neurotoxines du bacille typhimurium "S" et "R". *Arch. Roum. de Pathol. exper. et de Microbiologie*. **20:** 399–423.

MESROBEANU, L., MESROBEANU, I. and MITRICA, N. (1966) The neurotoxins of gram-negative bacteria: The thermolabile endotoxin. *Ann. N.Y. Acad. Sci.* **133:** 685–699.

MOLINA, N. C. and PETERSON, J. W. (1980) Cholera toxin-like toxin released by *Salmonella* species in the presence of mitomycin C. *Infect. Immun.* **30:** 224–230.

NOZAWA, R. T., YOKOTA, T. and KUWAHARA, S. (1978) Assay method for *Vibrio cholerae* and *Escherichia coli* enterotoxins by automated counting of floating Chinese ovary cells in culture medium. *J. Clin. Microb.* **7:** 479–485.

PETERSON, J. W. (1980) Salmonella toxin. *Pharmac. Ther.* **11:** 719–724.

PETERSON, J. W., HOUSTON, C. W. and KOO, F. C. W. (1981) Influence of cultural conditions on mitomycin C-mediated bacteriophage induction and release of *Salmonella* toxin. *Infect. Immun.* **32:** 232–242.

PETERSON, J. W., MOLINA, N. C., HOUSTON, C. W. and FADER, R. C. (1983) Elevated cAMP in intestinal epithelial cells during experimental cholera and salmonellosis. *Toxicon* **21:** 761–775.

PETERSON, J. W. and SANDEFUR, P. D. (1979) Evidence of a role for permeability factors in the pathogenesis of salmonellosis. *Amer. J. Clin. Nutrition.* **32:** 197–209.

SAKAZAKI, R., TAMURA, K., NAKAMURA, A. and KURATA, T. (1974a) Enteropathogenic and enterotoxigenic activities on ligated gut loops in rabbits of *Salmonella* and some other enterobacteria isolated from human patients with diarrhea. *Japan. J. Med. Sci. Biol.* **27:** 45–48.

SAKAZAKI, R., TAMURA, K., NAKAMURA, A., KURATA, T., GOHDA, A. and TAKDUCHI, S. (1974b) Enteropathogenicity and enterotoxigenicity of human enteropathogenic *Escherichia coli*. *Japan. J. Med. Sci. Biol.* **27:** 19–33.

SANDEFUR, P. D. and PETERSON, J. W. (1976a) Isolation of skin permeability factors from culture filtrates of *Salmonella typhimurium*. *Infect. Immun.* **14:** 671–679.

SANDEFUR, P. D. and PETERSON, J. W. (1976b) Neutralization of *Salmonella* toxin induced elongation of Chinese hamster ovary cells by cholera antitoxin. *Infect. Immun.* **15:** 988–992.

SEDLOCK, D. M., KOUPAL, L. R. and DEIBEL, R. H. (1978) Production and partial purification of *Salmonella* enterotoxin. *Infect. Immun.* **20:** 375–380.

TAYLOR, J. and WILKINS, M. P. (1961) The effect of *Salmonella* and *Shigella* on ligated loops of rabbit gut. *Indian J. Med. Res.* **49:** 544–549.

THAPLIYAL, D. C. and SINGH, I. P. (1978) Enterotoxic activity of *Salmonella weltevreden* culture filtrates. *Indian J. Exp. Biol.* **16:** 396–398.

THAPLIYAL, D. C. and SINGH, I. P. (1979) Partial characterization of *Salmonella weltevreden* enterotoxin. *Indian J. Exp. Biol.* **17:** 528–530.

VAN HEYNINGEN, W. E., CARPENTER, C. C. J., PIERCE, N. F. and GREENOUGH, W. B. III. (1971) Deactivation of cholera toxin by ganglioside. *J. Infect. Dis.* **125:** 415–418.

CHAPTER 13

SHIGELLA TOXIN(S): DESCRIPTION AND ROLE IN DIARRHEA AND DYSENTERY

GERALD T. KEUSCH, ARTHUR DONOHUE-ROLFE and MARY JACEWICZ

Department of Medicine, Division of Geographic Medicine, Tufts University School of Medicine,
136 Harrison Avenue, Boston, MA 02111, U.S.A.

1. INTRODUCTION

The interest in soluble toxins from *Shigellae* has risen and fallen more than once in the 80 years since *S. dysenteriae* 1 was reported to produce a toxin ("Shiga toxin") (Conradi, 1903). Debate has continued to center on whether or not the toxic activity might be involved in pathogenesis of any part of the disease syndrome produced by the micro-organism itself. After 50 years of study, the answer seemed to be "no" (Engley, 1952). However, in 1970 the first clear and relevant gastrointestinal effect of Shiga toxin was reported (Keusch *et al.*, 1970), stimulating the current surge in interest and investigation. The accompanying suggestion that an enterotoxin might be involved in pathogenesis of *Shigella* diarrhea or dysentery was received with great scepticism by workers in the field (Gemski *et al.*, 1972), although this has dramatically changed in the past decade. Indeed, a role for toxin or toxins in pathogenesis of both major *Shigella* intestinal syndromes, diarrhea and dysentery, is now not only plausible, but also very likely (Keusch, 1976, 1978; O'Brien *et al.*, 1979). Beyond the role of toxin in pathogenesis and the implications for therapeutic or prophylactic interventions for this important human illness, basic questions in the realm of microbial physiology and genetics, cell biology, and biochemistry are now being asked about regulation of toxin production, receptor and cellular uptake mechanisms, and mode of action of the toxin(s).

This review will summarize nearly eight decades of work on *Shigella* toxins, but will concentrate on the phenomenal productivity of the most recent 10 years.

2. CLINICAL AND EPIDEMIOLOGICAL ASPECTS OF *SHIGELLA* INFECTIONS

Shigellosis is an acute infectious enteritis afflicting only humans and, on occasion, sub-human primates. (Good *et al.*, 1969; Keusch, 1979a; Mulder, 1971). This narrow host range is a consequence of the fact that the causative organisms are exceedingly host adapted to the higher primates, although the basis for this selectivity is not understood. There are four *Shigella* species (*S. dysenteriae, S. flexneri, S. boydii* and *S. sonnei*) and multiple strains within species, distinguished on the basis of antigenic characteristics or by colicin typing. All four species appear to be capable of causing two distinct, major intestinal presentations, watery diarrhea of mild–moderate severity or dysentery (Keusch, 1979a; Rout *et al.*, 1975). The latter, which is the basis for the common designation of shigellosis as bacillary dysentery, is usually a much more severe clinical syndrome manifested by frequent passage of bloody, mucus containing stool, with waves of intense abdominal cramps and tenesmus. *Shigella dysenteriae* 1 tends to cause the most severe illness, *S. sonnei* tends to be more mild, while *S. flexneri* or *S. boydii* can be either severe or mild (Keusch, 1979a). These two clinical pictures are attributable to involvement of anatomically distant parts of the gastrointestinal tract, the proximal small bowel in the case of diarrhea, and the colon in the case of dysentery (Keusch, 1978, 1979a; Rout *et al.*, 1975). Furthermore, whereas microbial invasion has clearly occurred in the dysenteric colon (Formal *et al.*, 1965a, 1966) (bacillary dysentery actually representing an acute inflammatory invasive bacterial colitis), the affected proximal small bowel appears to be histologically intact and free of invading bacteria (Rout *et al.*, 1975). The role of toxin in these clinical expressions of shigellosis will be described in Section 7.

The infection occurs worldwide (Keusch, 1981a). In developing countries *Shigella* account for 5–20% of the acute diarrheal diseases of childhood (Behforouz *et al.*, 1977; Feldman *et al.*, 1970; Gordon *et al.*, 1964, 1965; Hansen *et al.*, 1978; Higgins *et al.*, 1955; Kourany *et al.*, 1971; Levine, 1979; Mata, 1978). In highland Mayan Indian infants in Guatemala the incidence rate may reach 1900 cases per 1000 children per year in the third year of life (Mata, 1978). In contrast, in the United States, the incidence of *Shigella* infection in the under five year old population is estimated to be 0.27/1000 per year, but this varies according to socio-economic and environmental factors (Keusch, 1982; Rosenberg *et al.*, 1976). In certain high risk populations, such as institutionalized retarded children, rates as high as 370/1000 per year may be recorded ('asylum dysentery') (DuPont *et al.*, 1970; Keusch, 1982).

The infection readily spreads among individuals living at close quarters (Gordon *et al.*, 1964; Hardy and Watt, 1948; Weissman *et al.*, 1974), as in households, in part because the inoculum size needed to initiate infection can be as few as 200 or less organisms (DuPont *et al.*, 1969; Levine *et al.*, 1973). It is for this reason that institutionalized retarded or psychiatric patients are at such great risk since it is difficult to control fecal contamination in the environment. The route of transmission is a circle from stool to the mouth and back to stool (Keusch, 1979a, 1982). Clinical cases may excrete 10^5–10^8 organisms/g of feces, and even convalescent carriers have in excess of 10^2 shigellas per gram (Dale and Mata, 1968). The fecal–oral route may deviate through food or water, on occasion carried there by flies, and this may initiate common source outbreaks (Black *et al.*, 1978; Donadio and Gangarosa, 1969). Such acute epidemics have been described in households, towns, or other defined populations such as in hospitals or aboard ships (Keusch, 1982). Recently, spread via venereal contact among homosexuals has also been documented (Dritz *et al.*, 1977; Mildvan *et al.*, 1977).

3. HISTORICAL REVIEW

3.1. THE FIRST 50 YEARS, 1900–1950

The early history of study of *Shigella* toxin can be viewed as a rapid initial explosion of knowledge followed by a long period of confusion regarding the number of toxins produced and their properties. Three major points emerge from this work. First, that *S. dysenteriae* Type 1, apparently unique among the species, produces a toxin causing a characteristic limb paresis–paralysis lethal effect. Second, that this neurotoxin activity is distinct from lipopolysaccharide endotoxin. Third, that parenteral injection of large amounts of endotoxin in experimental animals causes intestinal lesions, including edema, hemorrhage and mucosal damage. This last observation led to the concept of an enterotoxin (or endo-enterotoxin), and the early literature is crowded with reports of neurotoxin and enterotoxin, sometimes separable and sometimes not. An overview, with the perspective of the intervening years, offers an explanation; the preparations of toxin(s) employed were, in general, grossly contaminated with massive quantities of lipopolysaccharide. In the following review, we will not refer to endo-enterotoxin or enterotoxin in the context of the original description, for it is now obvious and widely accepted that this is a false and unphysiological concept. Rather, we will refer simply to endotoxin or lipopolysaccharide (LPS), in order to distinguish this bacterial cell wall component from the recently described protein enterotoxin which does appear to be relevant to the disease. In undertaking this review, we have read the original papers cited, in order to avoid the errors inherent in relying upon secondary sources.

The causative agent of bacillary dysentery was conclusively identified by Shiga in 1898 in his report of a severe epidemic in Japan in 1896, during which a mortality rate of 24%

was observed in nearly 90,000 cases. Shiga found a distinct gram-negative rod to be involved, and in recognition of this feat, the genus was ultimately named after him; the prototype organism *S. dysenteriae* Type 1, is often called Shiga's bacillus. This discovery was rapidly followed by isolation of the same organism in different parts of the world (Flexner, 1900; Kruse, 1900). It required an additional 40 years, however, to sort out the microbiology and to define and characterize the four species and multiple types now included in the genus *Shigella*: *S. dysenteriae, S. flexneri, S. boydii* and *S. sonnei*.

In 1900, Flexner reported that live cultures of Shiga bacillus produce an inflammatory infiltrate at the site of injection in mice and guinea pigs and in the peritoneal cavity, as well as pleuropericarditis, inflammation of serous vessels in subcutaneous tissues, with scattered small hemorrhages, splenomegaly, swelling, congestion, or hemorrhage of lymph nodes, renal and adrenal gland congestion, and inflammation of the gut which was filled with a glutinous secretion. Mice were more sensitive than guinea pigs; death occurred much earlier (1–2 days) in the former species, and a lower inoculum (but not quantified) would suffice. In the guinea pigs, small intestine serosal exudates, dilation of blood vessels, ecchymoses of the wall, swelling and hyperemia of Peyers patches, with eventual sloughing ("shaven beard" appearance) were noted and the lumen also contained a soft glutinous matter.

However, cultures killed by heating at 60°C for 15–20 min were also toxic. Injection of dead cultures into guinea pigs (dose not stated) produced fever, symptoms of "intoxication" within a few hours, and death shortly thereafter. Injection of heat killed bouillon culture subcutaneously into a goat led to self limited diarrhea and induration at the injection site. A second dose one week later resulted in death within 24 hr. On the basis of these experiments, Flexner (1900) concluded that shigellosis was due to "a toxic agent rather than to an infection *per se*." In spite of the prophetic ideas which came out of this work neither model employed is satisfactory for study of shigellosis, and it seems clear now that the toxic agent referred to is undoubtedly endotoxin. Whether or not neurotoxin or the protein enterotoxin were present as well and contributed to the pathology is uncertain. This is, however, the first report of any possible Shiga toxin that we are aware of.

In 1903 Neisser and Shiga found that intravenous administration of filtered extracts of heat killed bacteria was fatal to rabbits in two days. In the same year Conradi (1903) demonstrated the presence of a toxin in autolysates of 18 hr cultures of Shiga bacillus; intravenous injection into rabbits caused paralysis, diarrhea and collapse, with death in 48 hr. Intraperitoneal injection into guinea pigs caused a fall in temperature and fatal collapse, but no neurological signs. In spite of difference in size, the lethal dose in both cases was about 0.1 ml. Autopsy of the guinea pigs showed congestion and hemorrhage of the intestine, consistent with effects of parenteral injection of large doses of endotoxin. The symptoms in rabbits suggested the presence of a "neurotoxic" factor in the extract as well. Because of this description, the toxic factor was named neurotoxin and Conradi is generally given credit for its discovery.

These results were quickly confirmed and extended by Vaillard and Dopter (1903) and Dopter (1905a,b) who described lesions in the central nervous system of rabbits injected subcutaneously with 24 hr broth cultures of the organism. Autopsy of the brain and spinal cord revealed chromatolysis of neurons in the anterior horn, with small interstitial hemorrhages and focal necrosis of the gray matter. In 1904 Rosenthal clearly described the clinical symptoms caused by Shiga toxin, including paresis, first of the fore limbs then spreading to the hind limbs, with accompanying hypothermia frequently with diarrhea, dehydration, and death in 24–48 hr. Pathological examination showed dilatation of the large intestine with hemorrhagic infiltrations and necrosis of the gut, hyperemia of the small intestine, and the presence in the lumen of mucoid secretions, sometimes mixed with blood.

Todd in 1904 compared the effects of intravenous injection of aged (4–6 week old) alkaline broth culture supernatants in different animals. He concluded that horses and rabbits were more susceptible to the material than guinea pigs, rats and mice. His preparation was stable at room temperature for 4·5 months, was destroyed by heating at 80°C for 1 hr, and could be precipitated by ammonium sulfate, and therefore was probably a protein.

Todd (1904) also noted that *Shigella paradysenteriae* Flexner (*Shigella flexneri*) filtrates caused diarrhea but not paralysis, the first indication that neurotoxin production differs among members of the genus.

Krauss and Dorr (1905) found a soluble toxin in broth or saline filtrates of Shiga bacilli which was fatal to rabbits, but not to guinea pigs, eliciting neutralizing antibody. An insoluble toxin (LPS) was also found, present only in the bacterial cell body, which was fatal to both species.

Thus, within five years of the initial observation of Flexner, various workers demonstrated that Shiga bacillus produced a soluble, antigenic, protein toxin, precipitable by ammonium sulfate and destroyed by heating, causing delayed onset neurologic symptoms and death in rabbits but not guinea pigs. In addition it was shown that bacterial endotoxin was present, producing fever or hypothermia in a few hours (effects of LPS known to be species, dose, and time dependent), with hyperemia, hemorrhage and necrosis of various parenchymal organs and death.

Over the next 15 years various authors confirmed these findings but argued whether one or two toxins were present (Bessau, 1911; Flexner and Sweet, 1906; Horimi, 1913; Olitsky and Kligler, 1920; Pfeiffer and Ungermann, 1909). Pfeiffer and Ungermann (1909) stated clearly that Shiga bacillus produced an exotoxin causing neurotoxic symptoms in rabbits, and endotoxin which caused hypothermia, peritoneal exudation and death in guinea pigs. Two years later, Bessau (1911) added the observation that antitoxin produced against the neurotoxin would neutralize its nervous system toxicity but had no effect on the intestinal symptoms produced in animals injected with endotoxin. In spite of this early work, the argument was not resolved until the studies of Olitsky and Kligler (1920). They showed that neurotoxin was obtained from filtrates of 1–3 day old cultures, before much autolysis of the organisms had taken place; that the yield was increased by aeration of the culture; and confirmed that the toxin was a heat labile protein that could be neutralized by antitoxin. No intestinal symptoms or lesions were produced by intravenous injection in rabbits. Neurotoxin-free endotoxin was prepared from aged cultures in which extensive autolysis had taken place, removing neurotoxin with antitoxin. This material was heat stable and caused intestinal lesions without neurotoxic symptoms upon parenteral administration in rabbits. McCartney and Olitsky (1923) confirmed and extended the latter observations, obtaining neurotoxin-free endotoxin by growing the organisms anaerobically. Autolysis of cells yielded an intestinal toxin which had no effect on the central nervous system of rabbits.

Most studies showed that systemic injection of neurotoxin did not affect the gut. Robertson (1922), however, suggested that his exotoxin preparation had a secondary action on the intestine through inhibition of peristalsis, which he noted prior to the passage of mucus or desquamated epithelial debris. The reigning confusion (Barg, 1932; Boroff, 1949; Boroff and Macri, 1949; Kanai, 1922; Okell and Blake, 1930; Waaler, 1936) concerning intestinal manifestations was largely because of the failure to separate the protein toxin and LPS. An additional source of confusion is related to the convention in toxin nomenclature to refer to *exotoxin* as substances secreted or released in soluble form into the growth medium, whereas *endotoxins* were associated with and extracted from the bacillary cell bodies. Okell and Blake (1930), for example, demonstrated that neurotoxin remained intracellular during bacterial growth and was released upon autolysis. They concluded that *S. dysenteriae* 1 produced one toxin which they called an endotoxin, although it resembled classical exotoxins in many of its properties. Indeed, Shiga neurotoxin, like a number of bacterial toxins, is associated with the cell during early growth (see Section 4.7). Topography is now an unimportant criterion in classification; the contemporary distinction is based upon chemical nature of the toxin, whether protein or lipopolysaccharide.

Boivin and Mesrobeanu (1937a–f) finally separated the neuro- and endo-toxins by means of chemical fractionation. The protein neurotoxin was precipitated by trichloro-acetic acid, was produced by both rough (R) and smooth (S) variants, was heat and trypsin labile and did not precipitate in antisera raised against either whole R or S organisms. No neurotoxin was found in *Shigella flexneri* filtrates. Endotoxin was isolated by extraction of trichloroacetic acid treated filtrates with ethanol or acetone. The extracted material caused intestinal lesions in mice following parenteral injection, was precipitated by anti-S antiserum, and upon acid hydrolysis yielded a protein, fatty acids, and a polysaccharide. It was produced by S strains only. Horses immunized with endo-toxin from different shigellas produced species specific agglutinins and precipitating anti-bodies which protected mice against challenge by endotoxin and live bacteria, but not against neurotoxin; immunization with neurotoxin gave rise to antibody with high anti-toxic titers, but no activity against endotoxin or live bacteria.

The work was independently confirmed by Haas (1937, 1938) and Morgan *et al.* (1937, 1940, 1943). The latter group immunized human volunteers with the complete somatic antigen. The subjects produced specific agglutinins which protected mice against an intraperitoneal dose of 50 million live toxigenic organisms in mucin. Olitzki and colla-borators (Olitzki and Leibowitz, 1935, Olitzki and Avinery, 1937; Olitzki *et al.*, 1937; Tal, 1950; Tal and Olitzki, 1948) showed that antigenic fractions inducing immunity to LPS or live S-bacterial challenge also induced effects known to be due to endotoxin, including hyperglycemia, leukopenia and hypothermia, but no neurotoxicity. They also found that intravenous injection of the S variant heated at 50°C for 30 min into rabbits produced diarrhea, intestinal hemorrhages, and paresis, followed by death (Koch and Olitzki, 1946; Olitzki and Koch, 1943; Olitzki *et al.*, 1943, Olitzki and Bichowsky, 1946). Injection of organisms heated to 100°C for 30 min gave rise to intestinal symptoms only. Similar experiments with the R variants showed that only the heat labile neurotoxin was produced. Reversion of R to S variants through serial culture was associated with return of the ability of the organism to cause intestinal lesions.

By 1950, then, it was known that *Shigella dysenteriae* Type 1 produced a potent protein toxin in addition to the lipopolysaccharide endotoxin and something was known about their distinct properties. However, the role of the protein toxin in the pathogenesis of dysentery and its mechanism of action were open to question. Indeed it seemed that LPS was more important, while the few early reports suggesting enterotoxic activity of the protein toxin and its production by other *Shigella* species were somewhat inconclu-sive and largely ignored. For example, Ecker and Wolpaw (1930) observed the effect of *Shigella dysenteriae* culture filtrates on small intestinal pouches *in vivo*. They found changes in tone and amplitude of contractions, which correlated with the intensity of the neurotoxic symptoms induced. Direct observation of the intestine under oil revealed increased contraction in the longitudinal muscles and increased motor activity of the colon and cecum. Istrati (1938) found gelatinous edema and congestion of the cecum, with injection and edema of the intestinal walls, at autopsy of rabbits with typical CNS symptoms following intravenous injection of neurotoxin prepared from a rough Shiga strain by the method of Boivin (1937c). Steabben (1943) also noted hemorrhagic patches along the whole length of the mucous surface of the cecum in rabbits dying after intra-dermal administration of toxin prepared from a rough Shiga strain. In these studies, toxin was applied indirectly rather than directly to the intestine, or the likelihood of contamination of toxin by endotoxin made the results difficult to interpret. The possi-bility that the enterotoxin effect might be primarily local and measurable by direct application of neurotoxin to the intestinal mucosa, however, was not fully examined until 1972 (Keusch *et al.*, 1972a,b).

There are a few early reports on neurotoxin production by species other than *Shigella dysenteriae* 1. Thjøtta and Sundt (1921) reported that intravenous injection of broth filtrates of a 7-day culture of *Shigella sonnei* into rabbits resulted in paresis of the hind legs after 2–3 days, followed by recovery. Administration of *S. sonnei* endotoxin gave rise to bloody diarrhea without paresis in rabbits, and enterocolitis in mice. Boivin and Mesrobeanu (1937f) also mention in one of their papers, the isolation of a protein toxin from *Shigella schmitzii* (*Shigella dysenteriae* Type 2) by Buchwald, which caused paralysis in mice and rabbits.

3.2. THE SECOND 20 YEARS, 1950–1970

During these two decades there was little scientific interest in Shiga toxin. Nevertheless a number of significant observations were reported. Of major importance, in our opinion, was the work of van Heyningen and Gladstone (1953a) who, with relatively simple methods, achieved a 500–600-fold purification of neurotoxin, and showed that it was one of the most potent of the bacterial toxins. This toxin was subsequently found to be relatively impure, giving rise to multiple bands on polyacrylamide gel electrophoresis, and to exhibit cytotoxin and enterotoxin activities as well. Bridgewater *et al.* (1955) and Howard (1955) examined its neurotoxic properties and independently concluded that Shiga toxin was not neuronotropic but was primarily a vascular toxin acting in the brain and spinal cord, with neurological symptoms a secondary consequence (see Section 6.1).

Vicari *et al.* (1960) proved that neurotoxin was also cytotoxic to cells in tissue culture when they described effects on KB, monkey kidney, and human liver cells. In a dose-dependent fashion, and within a few hours of contact with neurotoxin, the cell membranes became thickened, large eosinophilic granules appeared until the cytoplasm was completely destroyed, the nucleus became pyknotic and the cell died. These effects were neutralized by specific antisera. The amount of toxin required for destruction of 50% of the cells was 3700-fold less than that required for production of 50% lethal effects in intraperitoneally injected mice. Mesrobeanu *et al.* (1962) confirmed the action of Shiga toxin on mammalian cells in culture, and demonstrated a dose related detachment of monolayers from the culture dish surface. It was proposed that neurotoxin might exert its action through this cytotoxic property.

In 1965, Arm *et al.* showed that injection of live *Shigella flexneri* into ligated rabbit ileal loops caused an enterotoxin-like fluid response, although no cell free enterotoxin could be isolated from the organism. Viewed in retrospect the investigative road seems clear on the basis of all of these observations. They had only to be conceptually linked for progress to occur.

3.3. THE PAST DECADE, 1970–1980

Two factors stimulated the experiments that first conclusively demonstrated enterotoxic activity of Shiga toxin in 1970 (Keusch *et al.*, 1970, 1972a,b). The first was the proof that clinical cholera was due to the action of a heat labile protein toxin elaborated by the causative organism, *Vibrio cholerae*, and the characterization of model systems for its study in the laboratory which provided the precedent for a gram-negative bacterial toxin in pathogenesis of diarrheal disease (Finkelstein, 1973). The second event was the occurrence in 1969–71 of a massive epidemic of diarrhea and dysentery in Mexico and Central America due to *S. dysenteriae* 1, after several decades of dormancy as a pathogen in the region (Mata *et al.*, 1970). This provided fresh isolates of highly virulent organisms, and an opportunity to observe the clinical presentation of the disease. When the experiments were done, Keusch *et al.* (1970, 1972a) found that the epidemic *Shigella* strain produced an enterotoxin *in vitro* which was active in ligated rabbit ileal loops and they suggested that it might cause the diarrhea and/or dysentery of shigellosis. Following this report, interest in Shiga toxin suddenly surged and much progress has been made in a relatively short time.

In addition to the discovery of enterotoxin, a major finding in the past decade has been that other *Shigella* species are also toxigenic (Keusch and Jacewicz, 1977a; O'Brien *et al.*, 1977). The failure to previously detect protein toxins in *S. flexneri* or *S. sonnei* with methods adequate for *S. dysenteriae* 1 is related to the fact that the former produce much smaller quantities than the latter strain. Also, animal experiments and flocculation assays, which provided the only means of detection previously available, require relatively large amounts of toxin. Thus it was necessary to develop a more sensitive method before toxin production by other species could be shown.

Gemski *et al.* (1972) and Keusch, Jacewicz and Hirschman (1972c) solved this problem by developing cytotoxicity assays employing HeLa cells in culture. The latter group devised a quantitative microassay based on toxin related cell detachment from mono-layer cultures. By a modification of the test, antibody could be detected, and serum toxin neutralizing antibody was demonstrated for the first time in patients with *Shigella* infec-tions due to *S. dysenteriae* 1, *S. flexneri*, and *S. sonnei*, but not in controls (Keusch and Jacewicz, 1973). Using these assay techniques Keusch and Jacewicz (1977a) showed the production by *Shigella flexneri* 2a and *S. sonnei* of a cell-free cytotoxin which was neutralized by *S. dysenteriae* 1 antitoxin, and the development of serum antibodies in human patients during the course of *S. sonnei* and *S. flexneri* infections which neutralized *S. dysenteriae* 1 exotoxin. O'Brien *et al.* (1977) also found a cytotoxin in *Shigella flexneri* 2a, serologically related to *S. dysenteriae* 1 toxin, with neurotoxic and enterotoxic proper-ties as well.

4. PRODUCTION

4.1. STRAINS

Both smooth and rough cell variants of *S. dysenteriae* 1 have been shown to produce neuro-, cyto- and enterotoxin (Boivin and Mesrobeanu, 1937f; Keusch and Jacewicz, 1975; Koch and Olitzki, 1946). Toxin activity was initially not detected in cell free preparations derived from other *Shigella* species suggesting that production of toxin was unique to the Shiga bacillus (Engley, 1952). More recently, however, it has been demon-strated that both *S. flexneri* and *S. sonnei* produce these same toxins (Keusch and Jacew-icz, 1977a; O'Brien *et al.*, 1977). However, the biological activity produced, per milligram (dry weight) of bacterial cell pellet, by these latter two species in liquid culture is at least 1000-fold less than that produced under identical conditions by *S. dysenteriae* 1 (O'Brien *et al.*, 1977). The toxin yields from *S. boydii* are not reported.

4.2. IRON REGULATION

Similar to diphtheria toxin formation, the production of toxin in *Shigella* strains is iron dependent. Dubos and Geiger (1946) deferrated medium by calcium phosphate precipi-tation. They found that adding Fe^{3+} back to the growth medium resulted in a marked inhibition of neurotoxin production with no effect on cell growth. This relationship between neurotoxin production *in vitro* and iron content of the medium was confirmed and extended by van Heyningen and Gladstone (1953b). Using repeated calcium phos-phate precipitations they were able to reduce the basal iron content in their medium to 0.05 μg/ml. By adding back small increments of Fe^{3+}, they found the optimal iron content to be 0.1–0.15 μg/ml. Above this level marked reduction in neurotoxin produc-tion per organism, was observed, whereas below this concentration bacterial growth was inhibited. The highest yield of toxin per unit volume of culture was obtained when iron concentration was in the range of 0.1–0.15 μg/ml. Recently we have examined the re-lationship between the level of iron in the medium and the level of cytotoxin activity found in lysates derived from stationary phase *S. dysenteriae* 1 grown in shake culture. Increasing the iron levels 10-fold above optimum resulted in an approximately 80-fold reduction in cytotoxin levels (Table 1). Over the range studied (0.1–1 μg Fe/ml) no effect on cell growth was observed.

The biochemical mechanism by which medium iron concentration exerts control over toxin production is not known. Furthermore it is also not known why toxin is under iron control. An obvious speculation is that the toxin protein actually plays an active role in iron uptake, either by acting as an iron binding siderophore and/or via its toxic proper-ties preventing the *Shigella* infected host from withholding growth essential iron (Wein-

TABLE 1. *Effect of Medium Iron Content on Bacterial Growth and Toxin Production*

Iron (Fe^{2+}) (μg/ml)	Growth (OD_{600})	Cytotoxicity (TC_{50}/ml)
0.1	4.14	1.25×10^5
0.2	4.06	4.75×10^4
0.4	4.15	1.00×10^4
1.0	3.99	1.60×10^3

berg, 1978). Both phenolate enterochelin and hydroxamate siderophores have been shown to be secreted by both *S. boydii* and *S. sonnei* strains (Perry and San Clemente, 1979), and Moore *et al.* (1980) have recently reported that *S. dysenteriae* 1 and *S. flexneri* can be used to absorb an enterochelin specific immunoglobulin from human serum that is responsible for iron-reversible bacteriostasis of *Salmonella typhimurium* in heat inactivated serum. The latter observation indicates the presence of an enterochelin related siderophore on the cell surface of *S. dysenteriae* 1 and *S. flexneri* that might play a role in iron homeostasis.

4.3. GROWTH MEDIUM

A variety of culture media have been used for *S. dysenteriae* 1 toxin production. Peptone broth (Keusch *et al.*, 1972a); a modified syncase medium (O'Brien *et al.*, 1977); N Z amine medium (McIver *et al.*, 1975); meat infusion broth (Olitsky ard Kligler, 1970); and CCY medium (van Heyningen and Gladstone, 1953a) are some of those used successfully in recent studies.

No systematic study has been made of the effect of different growth media on neurotoxin production or yield. Deferration of high iron containing medium before use improves toxin production (Dubos and Geiger, 1946; Keusch *et al.*, 1976a; Keusch and Jacewicz, 1977a), however it is not known whether at equivalent iron levels toxin production varies significantly from one medium to the next. We have recently compared the cytotoxin yields of *S. dysenteriae* culture grown in either N Z amine, Casamino acid-yeast extract (CYE), or a modified syncase, all adjusted to an iron concentration of 0.1 μg/ml. *S. dysenteriae* 1 produced nearly identical levels of cytotoxin activity in the three media.

4.4. AEROBIC GROWTH

In 1904, Rosenthal found that anaerobic conditions diminish the yield of "Shiga bacillus poison". Olitsky and Kligler (1920) reported that aerobic conditions favored neurotoxin production while anaerobiasis suppressed it. McCartney and Olitsky (1923) also found that aerobic conditions decreased the incubation time for neurotoxin production in broth filtrates.

Dubos, Hoberman and Pierce (1942) and Olitzki and Bichowsky (1946) made similar observations, and throughout the literature it is reported that high yields of neurotoxin are obtained from 24 hr cultures on solid media, where aeration is maximal, whereas prolonged growth (for at least one week) is usually required for good toxin production in stationary liquid media. Dubos and Geiger (1946) confirmed these observations when they obtained their most toxic preparations in broth which had been agitated vigorously or aerated with stirring throughout the culture period, and to which fumaric acid had been added to encourage aerobic metabolism.

4.5. MEDIUM pH

There is very little information on the effect of altering medium pH on Shiga toxin production. Olitsky and Kligler (1920) reported that neurotoxin was produced only after the organisms reached the alkaline phase of growth. Dubos and Geiger (1946), however, noted that increased toxin production at alkaline pH may be due to removal of organic iron via precipitation from the medium. They were able to obtain high neurotoxin yields from cultures in deferrated neutral broth.

4.6. Mitomycin-C Induction

Takeda and his coworkers (1979), in their study of a *Shigella* toxin that produces morphological changes in Chinese hamster ovary (CHO) cells, found that in some *Shigella* strains the addition of mitomycin-C (1 μg/ml of culture) greatly increased the CHO cell activity in the culture filtrates. Strains from all four *Shigella* species showed mitomycin related increases in yield of the toxin. It is unclear what effect, if any, the addition of mitomycin had on the induction or release of neurotoxin. The molecular basis for this observation is unknown.

4.7. Release of Toxin

It is apparent that under normal culture conditions *Shigella* toxin is a cell associated protein. Little toxicity is present in culture cell-free supernatants during the exponential phase of growth. Only in early to late stationary growth phase do significant levels of toxic activity appear in the medium. McIver *et al.* (1975) found only cell associated toxin in the first 8 hr of fermenter culture of *S. dysenteriae* 1. Thereafter, toxin was present in medium supernatant, through four cycles of growth in the fermenter. Presumably release of toxin during stationary phase is due either to bacterial autolysis or to leakage of toxin from its cellular compartment.

Toxin can be released from the bacterial cell by either mechanical disruption (O'Brien *et al.*, 1980), by alkaline extraction of heat inactivated bacteria (van Heyningen and Gladstone, 1953a), or by polymyxin B extraction (Griffin *et al.*, 1978). Our results with polymyxin B extraction shows release of more than 90% of the total cytotoxin activity but less than 5% of the total cellular protein, suggesting that the toxin may be present in the periplasmic space. What role the toxin might play in the periplasm is not known, but since regulation of toxin production is coupled to iron levels it is possible that it functions in iron uptake.

5. CHARACTERIZATION AND PURIFICATION OF TOXINS

5.1. Characterization

Flexner and Sweet (1906) first discovered that the rabbit lethal neurotoxic activity found in crude Shiga preparations was heat labile (81°C for 60 min). The heat lability of neurotoxin, enterotoxin, and cytotoxin activities has been confirmed and reported by many groups (Keusch *et al.*, 1972a, 1972c; Olitsky and Kligler, 1920). The cytotoxin activity of Shiga toxin is sensitive to extensive degradation by trypsin, chymotrypsin, papain and protease (Keusch *et al.*, 1976a). In contrast, limited proteolysis with trypsin or chymotrypsin appears to activate cytotoxin, as determined by assay in cell free protein synthesis systems derived from rabbit reticulocytes or in a wheatgerm/globin mRNA system (Brown *et al.*, 1980a). Neurotoxin has been reported to be pronase sensitive and trypsin resistant (Keusch *et al.*, 1972a).

Enterotoxin activity in the ligated rabbit ileal loop is also activated at alkaline pH (Keusch *et al.*, 1972a) while the cytotoxin activity is stable over a fairly broad pH range (Table 2). The instability of toxin at a pH above 9.0 (Dubos and Geiger, 1946) raises serious questions about the efficacy of the van Heyningen and Gladstone (1953a) procedure which utilizes extraction at pH 11. Even though impressive toxicity is recovered, the amount obtained by this procedure may reflect only a small proportion of the starting cell associated activity, unless a protective effect is exerted in the crude preparation.

TABLE 2. *Effect of pH stability of Shigella Cytotoxin*

pH*	Cytotoxicity	
	% Mortality	% of Control†
4.5	30.5	71
5.0	30.0	70
5.5	40.7	95
6.0	43.3	101
6.5	42.8	100
7.0	42.8	100
7.5	43.0	100
8.0	41.4	97
8.5	40.4	94
9.0	39.5	92
9.5	10.2	24

* Incubation period was 2 hr at 37°C. After incubation toxin samples were neutralized before measuring HeLa cytotoxicity.

† % mortality at experimental pH ÷ % mortality at pH 7.0.

5.2. PURIFICATION

Crude shigella toxin preparations can thus be obtained by one of three general methods: the van Heyningen and Gladstone (1953a) extraction of heat killed stationary phase cells at high pH; concentration of the spent supernatant medium, either by ammonium sulphate precipitation or by pressure dialysis through a membrane filter (Keusch et al., 1972a; Takeda et al., 1977); or lysis of washed exponential phase cells by either sonic disruption or by passage through a French pressure cell (Brown et al., 1980a; O'Brien et al., 1980). We have recently utilized polymyxin B, 2 mg/ml for 2 min at 37°C, for initial toxin extraction. This accomplishes an immediate 30–40-fold purification over crude French press lysates.

The further purification of toxin from these crude preparations has been hampered by two technical problems. First, under the culture conditions so far employed and with the *Shigella* strains thus far investigated, toxin protein is present in extremely low amounts (McIver et al., 1975). Secondly, there is a high background of nontoxic contaminating proteins in the preparations. The first problem can be overcome by either increasing the amount of starting material, using large fermenters for toxin production, or by amplifying the detection of minor protein components by iodination. The second problem requires use of a variety of chromatographic and electrophoretic techniques which separate proteins by size, charge, or other properties.

Van Heyningen and Gladstone (1953a) in 1953 achieved substantial purification of crude toxin obtained by the alkaline lysis method by means of a series of cycles of dialysis against distilled water, which precipitates the toxin, followed by solution of the precipitate in saline. The final preparation was purified 500–600-fold compared to the crude material, measured by mouse killing and by flocculation with antisera (van Heyningen and Gladstone, 1953c). This toxin moved a single band on simple paper electrophoresis (van Heyningen and Gladstone, 1953a), with molecular weight estimated by ultracentrifugation to be 82,000 daltons (dal) (Baldwin, 1953). Polyacrylamide gel electrophoresis of the van Heyningen–Gladstone toxin reveals a multiplicity of protein bands (Fig. 1), indicating the lack of purity of this preparation, although some denaturation undoubtedly occurred during the 25 years of freezer storage of the toxin. Nonetheless, the vintage van Heyningen–Gladstone preparation contained potent neurotoxin, cytotoxin, and enterotoxin activity (Keusch and Jacewicz, 1975).

In studying the relationship between the three toxicities Keusch and Jacewicz (1975) and McIver et al. (1975) found two regions of cytotoxic activity by isoelectric focusing of crude toxin. One peak with pI 7.2 contained neurotoxin, cytotoxin, and enterotoxin activity. The second peak focused at pI 6.0; only cytotoxin activity was detected. When

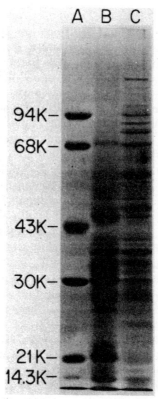

FIG. 1. Sodium dodecyl sulfate–polyacrylamide gel electrophoresis of Shiga toxin preparations. All samples were reduced and heated in denaturing buffer containing 2% SDS and 0.7 M 2-mercaptoethanol before application to an 11% polyacrylamide slab gel. (A) Molecular weight markers. (B) 1953 van Heyningen–Gladstone Shiga toxin preparation. (C) French press lysate of *S. dysenteriae* 1 (strain 60R). The molecular weight markers used were phosphorylase-B (94,000) bovine serum albumin (68,000), ovalbumin (43,000) carbonic anhydrase (30,000) soybean trypsin inhibitor (21,000) and lysozyme (14,300).

acrylamide gels used for isoelectric focusing were stained for protein one faintly staining band in the pI 7.2 region was seen (McIver *et al.*, 1975). Elution of the pI 7.2 toxin and subsequent electrophoresis in polyacrylamide (McIver *et al.*, 1975) gave a molecular weight of 72,000 dal for the major protein component of the pI 7.2 region. The evidence that this 72,000 dal protein represents in fact one toxin molecule having enterotoxin, neurotoxin, and cytotoxin activity is circumstantial. It is certainly possible that the toxin activity is really in one or more minor component(s) in the pI 7.2 region that are not detectable by protein staining with Coomassie blue dye.

Keusch and Jacewicz (1977b) have described a cytotoxin receptor on HeLa cells which appears to involve $\beta 1 \rightarrow 4$ linked *N*-acetyl-D-glucosamine oligomers. Keusch *et al.* (1977) then reported that both cytotoxicity and neurotoxicity were retained on columns containing chitin oligosaccharides attached to Sepharose-4B. The toxin activity was released by elution with 1 M NaCl and had a specific activity about 1000-fold greater than the starting material. Olsnes and Eiklid (1980) have recently purified a *Shigella* cytotoxin, in part taking advantage of the toxin affinity for *N*-acetyl-D-glucosamine oligomers. These investigators reported that 60% of the applied cytotoxin activity was bound to a column of acid treated chitin. The activity, measured by its effect on protein synthesis in HeLa cell monolayers exposed to toxin for 20 hr, was eluted with 1 M NaCl. However, by analysis of the specific activity the chitin column step provided only a 15-fold purification. Olsnes and Eiklid (1980) radioiodinated the toxin eluted from chitin. Adding unlabeled protein to prevent nonspecific absorption, the partially purified preparation was then applied to a DE52 column and the bound material was eluted with a linear NaCl gradient. Toxin eluted between 0.1 and 0.2 M NaCl; these fractions were subsequently pooled and subjected to sucrose gradient centrifugation and the peak of toxin activity was analyzed by SDS polyacrylamide electrophoresis. Two major bands corresponding to molecular weights of 30,500 and 11,000 dal were found. The iodinated purified toxin was run in polyacrylamide gels without SDS and on gel filtration columns. In both cases the radioactivity corresponded well with the toxic activity, strongly suggesting that the iodinated material indeed represents toxin. Additional studies by Olsnes and Eiklid (1980) to determine the subunit composition of the native toxin molecule are difficult to assess at this time. Crosslinking the toxin subunits by glutaraldehyde treatment gave a broad distribution of bands in SDS–PAGE. At high glutaraldehyde concentrations most of the labeled material was found in the 60,000 to 70,000 dal region, although molecular weight bands as high as 90,000 dal were also observed. On IEF both the ^{125}I radioactivity and toxicity showed a broad distribution between pI 5.9 and 6.8.

Utilizing an antibody affinity column O'Brien et al. (1980) have reported a 200-fold purification of Shiga toxin from whole cell lysates. Rabbit antitoxin was made by injecting animals with cytotoxin eluted from a non-denaturing polyacrylamide gel. The antitoxin gamma globulin fraction, precipitated with 40% ammonium sulfate, was coupled to cyanogen bromide activated Sepharose-4B. Passage of S. dysenteriae 1 concentrated cell lysates through the column resulted in the binding of a small amount of protein, which was then eluted with high salt containing buffer. The eluted material had neurotoxic (rabbit lethal), enterotoxic and cytotoxic activity. On gel filtration the ^{125}I-labeled affinity column eluate revealed two peaks; peak I, 32,000 dal and peak II, 4–7,000 dal. Peak I had greater than 90% of the cytotoxin activity, was neuro- and entero-toxic, and migrated as a single band on non-denaturing polyacrylamide gels. On SDS–PAGE three major bands, 33,000, 29,000 and 4–7000 dal were identified. Peak II had a very small degree of toxicity, which may be explainable by a small degree of peak I contamination. On SDS–PAGE a 4–7000 dal band was found. A small amount of 4–7000 dalton material could also be generated by treatment of peak I material with 8 M urea followed by chromatography on a gel filtration column. The authors concluded that the three major biological activities of Shiga toxin are found in a 33,000 dal complex which is dissociable into 29,000 and 4–7000 dal fragments. O'Brien et al. (1980) were unable to determine the subunit structure of native toxin due to the high salt conditions employed in their purification scheme.

Takeda and his coworkers (1977, 1979) report that they have separated and purified the neurotoxin and a distinct toxin that causes morphological changes in CHO cells. When crude toxin preparations were applied to a diethylaminoethyl-cellulose column and eluted in stepwise fashion with 0.2 M and 0.9 M NaCl, two toxin fractions were found: fraction I which eluted with 0.2 M NaCl and had neurotoxin activity with little CHO cell activity; and fraction II which eluted with 0.9 M NaCl and contained the CHO cell toxin. Fraction I, obtained from a culture of S. dysenteriae 1, was subsequently chromatographed on columns of CM-cellulose, hydroxylapatite, and Sephadex G-200. Fraction II, obtained from a culture of S. sonnei, was subsequently chromatographed on columns of hydroxylapatite, DEAE-Sephadex A-50 and Sephadex G-100. The final purified preparations each gave one major band on acrylamide gel, both with and without SDS. The molecular weights of the neurotoxin (Fraction I) and CHO factor (Fraction II) were 31,000 and 20,000 dal respectively. Unfortunately Takeda and his co-workers do not report the activity of their fractions in the standard Shiga enterotoxin and cytotoxin assays. Separation of two cytotoxic components has been reported by other workers (Keusch and Jacewicz, 1975; McIver et al., 1975; O'Brien et al., 1977). Takeda et al. (1977, 1979) do not mention specific activities of either neurotoxin or CHO factor, thus making comparisons to either the Olsnes and Eiklid (1980) or O'Brien et al. (1980) purification difficult.

Studies in our own laboratory, purifying cytotoxin by a five step sequence—Polymyxin B extraction of the bacterial cell biomass from broth culture, 50% $(NH_4)_2SO_4$ precipitation, Sephadex G-150 chromatography, Blue-Sepharose column chromatography and

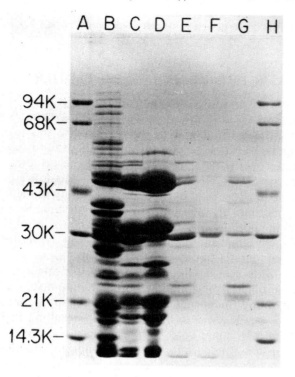

Fɪɢ. 2. Sodium dodecyl sulfate–polyacrylamide gel electrophoresis of fractions during purification of *S. dysenteriae* 1 cytotoxin. All samples were reduced and heated in denaturing buffer containing 2% SDS and 0.7 ᴍ 2-mercaptoethanol before application to an 11% polyacrylamide slab gel. (A) and (H), molecular weight markers. (B) Polymyxin-B toxin extract. (C) Pooled cytotoxic fractions after G-150 sephadex column chromatography. (D) Flow through material not retained on blue sepharose column. (E) Cytotoxic fraction which eluted with 0.5 ᴍ NaCl from the same blue sepharose column. (F) Peak cytotoxic fraction obtained from E by passage through a DE52 column and elution with an NaCl gradient. (G) Fraction which eluted from the DE52 column at a NaCl concentration greater than 0.2 ᴍ at which the peak cytotoxic fraction is removed. The molecular weight markers used were phosphorylase-B (94,000), bovine serum albumin (68,000), ovalbumin (43,000), carbonic anhydrase (30,000), soybean trypsin inhibitor (21,000) and lysozyme (14,300).

elution with 0.5 ᴍ NaCl, and DE-52 ion exchange chromatography with salt elution—gives a single region of bioactivity on nonreducing polyacrylamide gel electrophoresis and two major peaks on SDS–PAGE at 30,000 and approximately 11,000 dal (Fig. 2).

A consistent finding, then, in all of these purifications is a component migrating similarly on SDS–PAGE as an approximately 30,000 dal polypeptide (A. Donohue-Rolfe and G. T. Keusch, unpublished; O'Brien *et al.*, 1980; Olsnes and Eiklid, 1980). In addition, a smaller molecular weight component has been detected but the assigned molecular weight differs from laboratory to laboratory, and further work is needed to identify this component.

The molecular weight of native toxin is uncertain. Gel filtration of crude toxin preparations (Keusch *et al.*, 1972a), polyacrylamide gel electrophoresis of partially purified toxin (McIver *et al.*, 1975) and sucrose gradient centrifugation of a highly purified preparation (Olsnes and Eiklid, 1980) indicate the molecular weight of native Shiga toxin to be between 64,000 and 72,000 dal. Based on preliminary crosslinking studies, Olsnes and Eiklid (1980) postulate that native toxin may be composed of a large approximately 30,000 dal subunit and a cluster of 4 or 5 small 7–11,000 dal subunits. Such a model would be consistent with the A–B structure of other toxins (Keusch, 1979b) where the larger molecular weight biologically active A-subunit is associated with a cluster of smaller B-subunits involved in receptor binding. Both Takeda and O'Brien and their co-workers found toxin biological activity in a component of 31,000–33,000 dal. The presence of toxin activity in a 30,000–33,000 dal. component suggests that the association of a cluster of smaller subunits with the larger subunit may not be necessary for activity in intact cell systems.

6. PHYSIOLOGICAL PROPERTIES

For the first half century of study of Shiga toxin, the 'enterotoxic' properties associated with parenteral injection of heat killed organisms or cell free extracts were believed to be due to endotoxin, and indeed numerous reports referred to this toxic activity as endo-enterotoxin. Looking back at these studies and the methods of toxin preparation employing either aged culture supernatants, in which autolysis occurred naturally, or prepared autolysates of the bacteria, it is obvious that enormous quantities of endotoxin were in all the "toxins" administered to experimental animals. Many of the symptoms described, including fever, hypothermia, hypotension, shock and intestinal hemorrhage are consistent with overwhelming endotoxemia. Even the "protein" toxin preparations of that era most certainly contained significant quantities of endotoxin. Nevertheless, it was possible to ascribe the delayed paresis–paralysis–lethal toxicity to a protein product of the bacillus on the basis of its heat lability, susceptibility to proteolytic enzymes, failure of production under anaerobiasis, precipitation with ammonium sulfate, and stoichiometric neutralization by antibody, independent of its agglutination titer for whole smooth organisms. This toxin was believed to be neurotropic, resulting in hemorrhages in the central nervous system and spinal cord with secondary neurological symptoms. When the more purified neurotoxin preparation of van Heyningen and Gladstone (1953a) was tested in cell culture in 1960, a cytotoxic effect was found which appeared to explain the *in vivo* effects of neurotoxin (Vicari *et al.*, 1960).

During the next decade many studies demonstrated the *in vivo* invasive abilities of *Shigella* species in the gastrointestinal tract, and correlated this property with virulence of the organism and its ability to cause dysentery (Formal *et al.*, 1963, 1965a,b, 1966). Because other endotoxin containing organisms did not cause dysentery, the concept of an endo-enterotoxin was lain to rest. Since then, the demonstration of similarity in the basic structure of endotoxin on all gram-negative rods, particularly the toxic lipid A portion of the molecule, and its lack of effect in the gut lumen (Keusch *et al.*, 1972a) have confirmed this judgement.

The stage was thus set for the demonstration in 1970 (Keusch *et al.*, 1970, 1972a) that *Shigella* neurotoxin had an enterotoxin action on gut epithelium. Many studies since then have indeed shown that a purified protein product of *Shigella dysenteriae* 1, *S. flexneri*, and *S. sonnei* are neurotoxic, cytotoxic, and enterotoxic (Binder and Whiting, 1977; Brown *et al.*, 1980a,b; Charney *et al.*, 1976; Donowitz *et al.*, 1975; Flores *et al.*, 1974; Gemski *et al.*, 1972; Keusch and Jacewicz, 1975, 1977a,b; Keusch *et al.*, 1976a; Levine *et al.*, 1973; McIver *et al.*, 1975; O'Brien *et al.*, 1977, 1980; Steinberg *et al.*, 1975; Takeda, *et al.*, 1977, 1979; Thompson *et al.*, 1976). These three properties will be discussed separately, although it is still not certain if they are due to one, two or three distinct toxins.

6.1. NEUROTOXIN

As previously described (Section 3) the ability of cell free extracts of *S. dysenteriae* 1 to cause limb paresis, paralysis, and death in experimental animals has long been known (Conradi, 1903). Accordingly, this activity has been called Shiga neurotoxin ever since its discovery. Studies in animals have shown a remarkable variation (> 10,000-fold) in sensitivity to the lethal action of neurotoxin, as summarized in Table 3 (Boivin, 1940; Cavanagh *et al.*, 1956; Koch and Olitzki, 1946; Todd, 1904). In the very sensitive rabbit, a characteristic progression of symptoms occurs, the timing and duration being affected by the dose of toxin (Flexner and Sweet, 1906). Following an i.v. dose of one or two times the LD_{50}, the animal appears well for about 48 hr when forelimb paresis first becomes apparent (van Heyningen, 1971). The muscle weakness causes the forelimbs to splay out

TABLE 3. *Lethal Dose of* Shigella *Neurotoxin for Several Animal Species**

Species	Relative Dose/kg body weight
Rabbit	1
Rhesus monkey	5
Hamster	40
Mouse	700
Rat	5000
Guinea Pig	>10,000

* Adapted from Cavanagh *et al.* (1956).

and the animal has some difficulty in moving about. This increases in severity over the next 24–28 hr, begins to affect the hind limbs, and progresses to paralysis. By then, the rabbit is obviously sick, prostrated, usually with loss of muscle tone so that the head cannot be held up, although sometimes there is opisthotonus. Depending on the dose, the animal may die or recover in a few days, usually with no sign of residual paresis. In the mouse, flaccid paralysis also occurs although in this species it characteristically appears first in the hind limbs (Branham and Carlin, 1948; Gemski *et al.*, 1972). No paralysis is noted in hamsters, and instead bilateral pleural effusions associated with congestion and pulmonary edema have been described (Cavanagh *et al.*, 1956). Minimal pathology of the gastrointestinal tract is noted in the rat (see below), with no CNS lesions, while the guinea pig appears to be totally resistant (Cavanagh *et al.*, 1956; van Heyningen, 1971).

Many studies have been performed in the highly sensitive rabbit to assess the nature of the neurotoxin effect. Dopter (1905a,b) first observed pathology in the nervous system involving chromatolysis of the anterior horn cells in the spinal cord along with focal hemorrhages. One year later, Flexner and Sweet (1906) reported hemorrhages in the brain and softening of gray matter in the spinal cord. Using the more purified neurotoxin preparation of van Heyningen and Gladstone (1953a) Bridgewater *et al.* (1955) conducted a detailed study of the effects of a dose $2 \times LD_{50}$ given by the intravenous route. Macroscopic changes in spinal cord were found in animals sacrificed at the height of intoxication. Particularly in the cervical enlargement, but also in the lumbar area, the cord was swollen, with marked softening of gray matter and extensive punctate hemorrhages, and sparing of white matter. By serial study of toxin treated animals, Bridgewater *et al.* (1955) demonstrated capillary and venular hemorrhages after 24 hr, before any clinical signs of intoxication were present. At this time neurons in the cervical bulb region were unaffected. By 48 hr, vascular abnormalities were pronounced and there were early signs of degeneration of the large motor neurons of the anterior horn, but still in the absence of neurological signs. Both histologic changes and clinical symptoms increased in parallel over the next 48 hr as the gray matter region was replaced by necrotic debris of neurons, glial cells, and the vasculature, and death ensued shortly thereafter. From these studies Bridgewater *et al.* (1955) concluded that neurotoxin was actually not a neurotropic toxin but rather caused damage to vascular endothelium with secondary changes in spinal cord. Indeed the studies suggested a predilection for blood vessels of the cervical enlargement of the cord. This was supported by the results of unilateral injection of toxin into one vertebral artery, in which sharply localized lesions restricted to the cervical enlargement region were found only on the injected side.

Similar conclusions were reached by Howard (1955) from comparative studies of intraperitoneal vs intravenous injection to mice or rabbits. In both species the LD_{50} by the intravenous route was significantly less than intraperitoneally.

Rǎsková and Vaněček (1958) later reported that intracerebral injection of 1–10 μg of Shiga neurotoxin into the left ventricle of the brain of unanesthetized cats produced behavioral changes after a latent period of 3–4 hr. The animals became unusually quiet and docile and were thoroughly uninterested in their surroundings. Coordination of the fore and hind limbs was impaired, respiration was rapid, there was a tremor of the head and they became photophobic. These signs progressed to stupor and death within 24 hr and mimicked the effects produced by intraventricular injection of 5-hydroxytryptamine. Rásková and Vanĕček therefore suggested that the neurotoxin might function as a serotonin releaser in its biological action. Masek, Smetana and Rásková (1961) then reported that, consistent with this hypothesis, intracerebral injection of toxin into mice resulted in depletion of norepinephrine and serotonin in brain, reaching a nadir (50% decrease) at 48 hr post injection.

This suggests that neurotoxicity could be a consequence of the local action of serotonin upon blood vessels in the neuraxis. Stulc (1966, 1967) therefore studied the effect of neurotoxin on the permeability of the blood–brain barrier in mice, employing various tracers to measure the integrity of this physiological function. In the first study (Stulc, 1966) carrier-free sodium orthophosphate-^{32}P was used to indicate permeability. The tracer was given intravenously at various times after $4 \times LD_{50}$ of toxin were administered; one hour later the brain–plasma radioactivity ratio and the specific activity of brain organic and inorganic phosphorus fractions were determined. By 24 hr post toxin, penetration of radioactive orthophosphate was significantly increased, peaking at 36 hr, and returning to control by 60 hr, in parallel with the development of lesions. At the peak, the specific activity of both organic and inorganic phosphate fractions was increased in intoxicated animals as compared to controls, with no change in the ratio of specific activities of the two fractions. This suggests an increase in permeability rather than an acceleration in turnover of brain organic phosphorus. When the experiments were repeated in rats, a species quite resistant to neurotoxic effects, the rate of entry of orthophosphate-^{32}P did not increase in the toxin treated group, and in fact actually appeared to decrease. In a second study Stulc (1967) examined the effects of toxin on water and electrolyte content of brain, determined the ^{51}Cr-labeled erythrocyte space, and measured entry into brain of ^{131}I-albumin and ^{14}C-sucrose from the blood. No changes in the brain parenchymal content of Na, K, or water were found, indicating integrity of the permeability barrier of brain cells. No significant abnormalities were detected in the ^{51}Cr-erythrocyte space, used to measure the residual blood content of the intoxicated brain, or the sucrose space, a marker for a rapidly equilibrating pericapillary space. In contrast, the entry of ^{131}I-albumin into brain, a marker of the blood–brain barrier itself, increased by about 100% in intoxicated mice. Expansion in the ^{131}I-albumin space that is unaccompanied by a parallel increase in the erythrocyte space is evidence for a selective increased permeability of brain capillaries. This would also be consistent with the absence of hemorrhages in toxin treated mice.

Does neurotoxin cause intestinal lesions? Penner and Bernheim (1960) reported that intracerebral injection of Shiga neurotoxin directly into the third ventricle of dogs resulted in gastrointestinal lesions. Congestion and petechial hemorrhages were found in stomach, duodenum, terminal ileum, and the middle third of the colon, with sparing of intervening segments. Lesions were most profound in the colon, in which gross hemorrhage occurred. They hypothesized that intestinal lesions in shigellosis might be a consequence of centrally acting neurotoxin disturbing "integrative mechanisms which regulate homeostasis". However, the toxin preparation employed in these studies was described as a polysaccharide–protein complex that had only modest neurotoxin activity (LD_{50} for mice of 80 μg) but was highly pyrogenic at a dose of 0.002 μg i.v. Thus it is likely that this preparation contained considerable quantities of endotoxin.

However it is not outrageous to postulate a role for neurotoxin in the pathophysiology of the intestinal disease, although not through a central nervous system action. As a speculation, local serotonin release in the gastrointestinal tract could mediate at least some of the intestinal effects of clinical shigellosis and/or those resulting from inoculation of toxin. Serotonin is present in high concentrations throughout the gastrointestinal tract in the myenteric plexus and in the mucosa primarily in enterochromaffin cells and to a lesser extent in neurons (Gross and Sturke, 1975). Enteric neurons contain tryptophan hydroxylase, the enzyme involved in serotonin biosynthesis, and a serotonin-binding protein. It is thought that serotonin causes the intestinal hypermotility of the carcinoid syndrome (Phillips, 1972), and serotonin administration causes increased intestinal motility (Bülbring and Lin, 1958; Misiewicz *et al.*, 1966). Shigellosis is also characterized by intense waves of abdominal cramping due to exaggerated peristalsis (Keusch, 1979a). Interestingly, as early as 1922 Luccini reported that Shiga bacillus culture filtrates increased tone and motility of isolated intestinal preparations of animals, whereas still higher doses inhibited tone and motility, (cited by Ecker and Wolpaw, 1930). However, this activity was stable after heating at 75°C for 1 hr. Four years later, Tadokoro and Suga found that perfusion of isolated rabbit intestine with small doses of a toxic culture filtrate stimulated peristalsis while larger doses caused paralysis (cited by Ecker and Wolpaw, 1930). This activity was also resistant to heating at 85°C for 1 hr, suggesting that it might be related to the presence of LPS.

In 1930 Ecker and Wolpaw reported that culture filtrates of Shiga bacillus caused acute lethal reactions within an hour or so of intravenous administration. With lower doses, animals survived the acute reaction and developed typical signs of neurotoxicity after 48 hr. Heating the preparation to 100°C for up to 30 min did not alter the acute reaction; thus it is certain that the preparation contained overwhelming quantities of endotoxin, but it clearly had the protein neurotoxin in it as well. When this toxin was applied to small intestinal mucosa in surgically created pouches *in situ*, preparations that caused diarrhea in intact rabbits also resulted in a rise in tone of longitudinal muscles and increased amplitude of contraction. Filtrates giving rise to severe neurotoxicity caused the most dramatic rise in tone but a decrease in amplitude of contractions. There was some variation in effect of filtrates according to the strain of organism employed to prepare the toxin. In four animals, colonic mucosa, examined by direct observation under oil, revealed "increased activity of the lower colon, with marked propulsion."

Recently, studies on the effect of Shiga toxin on myoelectric activity of ligated rabbit ileal loops perfused with toxin for 8 hr have been reported (Mathias *et al.*, 1980). This toxin preparation would be expected to be primarily protein in nature, with minor endotoxin contamination, however no fluid was produced in these loops within the 8 hr experiment. Increases were noted in both migrating action potential complexes (MAPC), which reflects the activity of single isolated ring contractions, and repetitive bursts of action potential (RBAP), which are multiple simultaneous ring contractions which may or may not propagate for short distances.

Other loops in the same animals were infected with toxigenic *Shigella dysenteriae* 1 which either were invasive (strain 3818-T) or noninvasive (strain 3818-0). The results of infection or toxin infusion were similar. Increases in MAPC occurred, but these were not as prominent as noted with toxigenic *E. coli* infection in the same model (Burns *et al.*, 1978). The most striking abnormality was an increase in RBAP, which has been associated with inflammatory lesions produced by invasive *E. coli* infection in the same model (Burns *et al.*, 1980), or perfusion with a cytotoxic enterotoxin produced by *Clostridium perfringens* (Justus *et al.*, 1980). In addition to the changes in infected or perfused loops, proximal unmanipulated gut showed similar but less intense changes in myoelectric activity, even though separated from the treated loops by an intervening segment of bowel. An effect at a distance could be due to absorption and circulation of toxin, activation of a neural reflex arc, or release of a hormone or mediator molecule such as serotonin.

Other attributes of serotonin are of interest in speculating about pathogenesis of *Shigella* diarrhea. The molecule has recently been shown to have effects on water and electrolyte transport that might underlie the diarrhea of the carcinoid syndrome, independently and in addition to altered motility (Donowitz *et al.*, 1979). The direct action of serotonin as an intestinal serotogogue through inhibition of neutral NaCl absorption in rabbits has been demonstrated. This effect occurs *in vitro* only from serotonin bathing the serosal surface of the gut or, *in vivo* in the blood and is in contrast to the motility effects of the molecule when applied to the mucosal surface. Although unproven, the secretory effects of serotonin are likely to be due to the serotonin pool in the enterochromaffin cells, while the motor effects could be secondary to myenteric plexus pool. Intestinal secretion in response to *Shigella* toxins will be extensively discussed in Section 6.3.

6.2. CYTOTOXIN

In 1960, Vicari *et al.*, reported that Shiga toxin was lethal to KB, human liver, and monkey kidney cells *in vitro*. Within an hour, there was visible thickening of the plasma membrane and transparency of the cytoplasm, as observed by light microscopy. With time, large eosinophilic granules appeared in the cytoplasm and degenerative nuclear changes were noted. Ultimately, the cells appeared swollen, filled with cytoplasmic granules surrounding a pyknotic nucleus. This destructive process was time and dose dependent, and it was neutralizable in stoichiometric fashion by antitoxin within the first 5 min of incubation of cells with toxin. After that, neutralization was no longer possible, indicating rapid and irreversible fixation of toxin to the cells. This was accompanied by consumption of bioactivity from the medium supernatant. Mesrobeanu (1962) soon confirmed that Shiga toxin was cytotoxic to KB cells and to human embryonic cells, noting massive detachment of cells from the monolayer.

At the suggestion of Dr. Samuel B. Formal we began intensive study of the cytotoxic properties of Shiga toxin in 1972. Employing a microquantitative assay (Keusch *et al.*, 1972c), developed to measure toxin induced detachment of cells from confluent monolayers, the basic observations of Vicari *et al.* (1960) and Mesrobeanu (1962) were quickly verified. Cytotoxicity followed a log–linear dose–response curve (Fig. 3), occurred after a latent period of several hours, the duration of which was also dose related (Fig. 4), was neutralizable by antitoxin but only when added prior to or shortly after toxin, and toxin was consumed from the supernatant medium concomitant with its bioactivity (Keusch 1973; Keusch and Jacewicz, 1977b). No toxin was removed from the medium overlying resistant cell lines (Y-1 adrenal or W1-38 lung fibroblasts) (Fig. 5), suggesting that sensitive, but not resistant, cells might possess a specific cell surface toxin-binding receptor (Keusch and Jacewicz, 1977b).

Binding of toxin to HeLa or rat liver cells does in fact appear to be the first step in cytotoxicity; this is mediated by a cell surface receptor containing oligomeric *N*-acetyl-D-

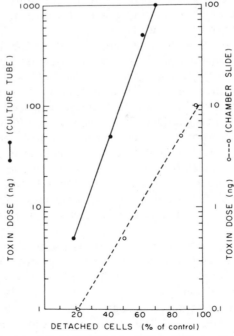

FIG. 3. Dose–response curve of *S. dysenteriae* 1 toxin assayed by a cytotoxicity assay in HeLa cells. Dilutions of toxin were incubated overnight on HeLa cell monolayers and the percentage of cells detaching from the glass surface was determined in roller tubes (●) or in micro tissue culture chambers (○). This was accomplished by vigorously washing the monolayer to remove nonadherent and poorly adherent cells, removing the firmly attached cells with 0.25% trypsin, and counting them in a Neubauer bright line hemocytometer. (From Keusch *et al.*, 1972c.)

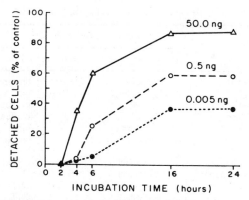

FIG. 4. Assay of *S. dysenteriae* 1 cytotoxin in HeLa cells, performed as described in Fig. 3, with 0.01, 1, and 100 50% lethal doses of toxin. Note the dose related lag period, the subsequent steep rise in cell detachment, and the plateau between 16–24 hr of incubation. (From Keusch *et al.*, 1972c).

glucosamine (Keusch and Jacewicz, 1977b). Three lines of evidence support this contention (Table 4). In the first place, enzyme treatment of HeLa cells reduces cell sensitivity to cytotoxin in cells exposed to proteolytic enzymes or lysozyme, but not various other glycosidases (Keusch and Jacewicz, 1977b). This suggests that the receptor is a glycoprotein containing a lysozyme sensitive substrate. Secondly, in competitive inhibition studies with soluble mono- or oligo-saccharide haptens, of 28 hapten inhibitors tested only the lysozyme substrates of *N*-acetyl-D-glucosamine oligomers of 3 or 4 units in length (chitotriose or tetraose) were effective inhibitors of toxicity (Keusch and Jacewicz, 1977b). Thirdly, the sugar binding protein (lectin) wheat germ agglutinin (WGA), which has specificity for chitotriose, is effective in blocking cytotoxin action, whereas lectins with different specificity, including phytohemagglutinin (PHA) and concanavalin-A (Con-A), were not (Keusch and Jacewicz, 1977b). These data collectively indicate that the presence of specific sugar containing receptors is necessary for cytotoxicity to occur and that the receptor contains a chitotriose-like moiety.

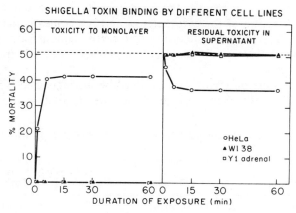

FIG. 5. Binding of *S. dysenteriae* 1 cytotoxin to HeLa, WI-38 and Y-1 adrenal cells. Toxin was incubated on monolayers for varying periods of 1–60 min at which time the toxin containing medium was removed by aspiration. The monolayer was washed and incubated overnight in fresh toxin free medium for assay as in Fig. 3 (left panel). Five minutes of incubation of one 50% tissue culture lethal dose of toxin with HeLa cells produced as much cytotoxicity as a 60 min contact period, amounting to about 84% of the toxicity obtained with overnight incubation. There was no detectable cytotoxicity for WI-38 or Y-1 adrenal cells. When the aspirated toxin containing supernatant was applied to fresh HeLa monolayers (*right panel*), there was no reduction in bioactivity of medium aspirated from WI-38 or Y-1 adrenal cells. However, there was a significant reduction in bioactivity in the medium overlaying the sensitive HeLa cell, inversely related to the direct cytotoxicity observed on the monolayer itself. (From Keusch and Jacewicz, 1977b).

TABLE 4. *Properties of the* Shigella *Toxin Receptor*

	Test System	
Treatment	Intact HeLa cells	Rat liver cell membranes
Pronase	NT*	↓ binding
Trypsin	↓ binding	↓ binding
Neuraminidase	No effect	No effect
Galactose Oxidase	No effect	No effect
β-galactosidase	↑ binding	↑ binding
Lysozyme	↓ binding	↓ binding
Ganglioside	No effect	No effect
N-acetyl-D-glucosamine	No effect	NT
Chitobiose	No effect	NT
Chitotriose	↓ binding	NT
Chitotetraose	↓ binding	NT
PHA	No effect	No effect
Con-A	No effect	No effect
WGA	↓ binding	↓ binding

* NT = Not tested.

HeLa cell lethality of Shiga toxin is also decreased when incubation is carried out at 4°C, suggesting that an active process is involved in the intoxication process (Keusch, 1973). Investigation of the effects of metabolic inhibitors of glycolysis, oxidative phosphorylation, the electron transport chain, and protein synthesis on toxin activity (Table 5), are consistent with this contention. At low, non lethal concentrations, these various inhibitors all reduce Shiga toxin effects on HeLa cells and result in increased recovery of toxin in the supernatant. Of the active processes which might be affected by both energy and protein synthesis inhibitors, we consider endocytosis to be the most likely, requiring energy for the internalization process and protein synthesis for turnover of surface membrane.

The possible involvement of endocytosis for uptake of biologically active cytotoxin has been studied by means of inhibitors of microfilament, microtubule, and lysosomal function (Table 6), because these cellular components are intimately involved in the endocytic process. Each of the drugs employed significantly reduces bioactivity of cytotoxin, indicating that normal function of the cytoskeleton and lysosomes is necessary for toxin to cause HeLa cell death. While such data do not directly demonstrate endocytic uptake of toxin, they do indicate that membrane and cytoplasmic organelle motility are required for cytotoxicity to occur.

There are two types of endocytosis which must be distinguished (Fig. 6). Nonselective (fluid phase) endocytosis is a characteristic of many cell types that continuously pinch off

TABLE 5. *Effects of Metabolic Inhibitors on* Shigella *Cytotoxin Activity in HeLa Cells*

		Cytotoxicity Assay*	
Inhibitor	Dose (Time)	Cell mortality	Medium toxicity
Fluoride	10^{-3} M (90 min)	−71%	+41%
Iodacetate	5×10^{-9} M (90 min)	−48%	+36%
Cyanide	5×10^{-6} M (60 min)	−80%	+34%
DNP	10^{-5} M (60 min)	−49%	+26%
Antimycin A	5×10^{-9} M (90 min)	−58%	+31%
Oligomycin	0.05 μg/ml (60 min)	−87%	+31%
Puromycin	0.005 μg/ml (90 min)	−73%	+39%
Cycloheximide	0.1 μg/ml (60 min)	−56%	+23%
Actomycin D	0.0005 μg/ml (60 min)	−46%	+26%

*Change in cell mortality and residual toxin activity in medium supernatant from inhibitor heated monolayers compared to control.

TABLE 6. *Effects of Microfilament and Microtubule Inhibitors and Lysosomotropic Drugs on* Shigella *Cytotoxin Activity in HeLa Cells*

Inhibitor	Concentration	Percent inhibition of cytotoxin
Cytochalasin-B	50 μg/ml	40.2 $\pm$ 5.2
Colchicine	0.5 μg/ml	43.1 $\pm$ 4.1
Chloroquine HCl	2×10^{-6} M	28.9 $\pm$ 5.5
Hydrocortisone	100 mg/ml	50.6 $\pm$ 7.9

endocytic vesicles and as a consequence imbibe extracellular fluid (and whatever is in it). The general fate of macromolecules taken up by this mechanism is degradation due to the action of enzymes contained in primary lysosomes, deposited into the endocytic vesicle during its fusion with a primary lysosome (Silverstein *et al.*, 1977). Thus endocytosis may be involved in cellular nutrition or perhaps in recycling of substrate building blocks for a variety of anabolic processes. Receptor-mediated endocytosis is, in contrast, selective (Goldstein *et al.*, 1979). The selectivity results from the specificity of the recep-

ENDOCYTIC MECHANISMS

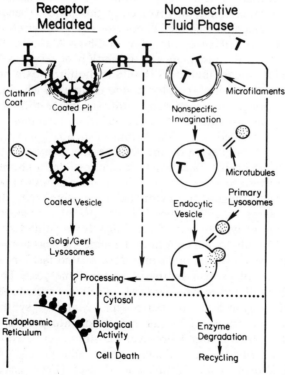

FIG. 6. Schematic representation of the two distinct mechanisms of endocytosis. *Right side*: Nonselective fluid phase endocytosis. The cell membrane is constantly invaginating to form cytoplasmic (endocytic) vesicles, involving microfilaments and expenditure of energy, and inbibing extracellular medium in the process along with any macromolecules present such as toxin, T. Fusion with primary lysosomes occurs, involving microtubules, and the lysosomal enzymatic contents are dumped into the fused vesicle. Degradation of the ingested molecule then follows. *Left side*: Selective receptor-mediated endocytosis. Ligands such as T bind to specific cell surface receptors, R, and cluster at specialized clathrin coated sites on the membrane called coated pits. These invaginate to form vesicles and fuse with lysosomes, also requiring energy, microfilament and microtubule function. The fate of the clathrin coated vesicle appears to be different from the noncoated vesicle, and may process, activate, and deliver biologically active macromolecules to their intracellular locus of action. In the case of the toxin, this is the cytoplasmic ribosome which is inhibited in protein synthesis, leading to cell death.

TABLE 7. *Effects of Transglutaminase Inhibitors on* Shigella *Cytotoxin Activity in HeLa cells*

Agent	Concentration (mM)	Toxicity	Antibody rescue
NH$_4$Cl	18	↓↓↓*	↓↓↓↓
Methylamine	50	0	↓↓↓
Ethylamine	100	0	↓
Propylamine	50	0	↓
Butylamine	50	0	↓
Dansylcadaverine	5	↓	↓↓↓
Bacitracin	0.1	↓	↓↓
Putrescine	1	↓↓	↓↓↓

*↓ = 10–20% ↓ in toxicity.
↓↓ = 20–40% ↓ in toxicity.
↓↓↓ = 40–60% ↓ in toxicity.
↓↓↓↓ = >60% ↓ in toxicity.

tor–ligand interaction, and involves specialized regions of the cell membrane known as coated pits that possess a coating of a distinctive protein, clathrin. These clathrin coated regions occupy less than 1% of the total cell membrane surface (Goldstein *et al.*, 1979). Macromolecules taken up by such a mechanism may be processed to an active form within the lysosome and directed to distinctive sites within the cell where they exert their biological function. Recent evidence suggests that membrane cross-linking, regulated by the enzyme transglutaminase, may be involved in this process because transglutaminase inhibitors also inhibit receptor-mediated endocytosis (Davies *et al.*, 1980; Maxfield *et al.*, 1979). These agents also reduce cytotoxicity of Shiga toxin to HeLa cells (Table 7) (Keusch, 1981). If this is a consequence of inhibition of receptor-mediated internalization of toxin, transglutaminase inhibitors should immobilize toxin on the cell surface and permit antitoxin neutralization of receptor-bound toxin even when untreated, intoxicated control cells can no longer be rescued by antitoxin. Since this period of time is only 5–10 min of incubation, we studied the ability of transglutaminase inhibitors to permit antibody rescue of intoxicated cells after 30 min of incubation with toxin and inhibitor. Each agent permitted some degree of antibody rescue, demonstrating that they indeed act to retain toxin on the cell surface where it is accessible to antibody. Failure of direct protection may be related to reversible inhibition of transglutaminase.

Several lines of study suggest that cytotoxicity correlates with an action of toxin on cellular protein synthesis. In 1976 (Keusch *et al.*, 1976b) we reported that treatment of human peripheral blood lymphocytes with Shiga toxin inhibited the burst in protein synthesis stimulated by phytohemagglutinin. Leucine incorporation by lymphocyte lines in long term culture was also inhibited in a dose related fashion, suggesting that Shiga toxin was an inhibitor of protein synthesis. In the same year, Thompson *et al.* (1976) found that the toxin inhibited protein synthesis in cell-free systems derived from rat liver, including both polyuridylic acid directed polyphenylalanine synthesis and endogenous mRNA directed incorporation of labeled amino acids into polypeptides. No effect upon amino-acylation of tRNA was found, however transfer of activated amino acid to nascent polypeptide chains on ribosomes was significantly reduced. Osato *et al.* (1979), Olsnes and Eiklid (1980), Brown *et al.* (1980b), and Keusch (1981) have since reported that nanogram quantities of toxin inhibit amino acid incorporation by intact embryonic human "intestinal epithelial" cells (HIE) or HeLa cells. Brown *et al.* (1980b) and Keusch (1981) also found no effect upon uridine incorporation into TCA precipitable material at a time when leucine incorporation was inhibited by 50–60%. Brown *et al.* (1980b) also observed that inhibition of thymidine incorporation paralleled the decrease in protein synthesis. They also could find no alteration in α-aminoisobutyric acid uptake or on intracellular potassium release at the time of inhibition of leucine incorporation, indicating that the effect is primarily on protein synthesis and not on amino acid uptake or cell viability. Both Olsnes and Eiklid (1980) and Keusch *et al.* (1981) have found that inhibition of protein synthesis occurs in HeLa cell lines sensitive to the cytotoxic action of

Shiga toxin, but not in lines resistant to its cytotoxic effect. In the latter studies leucine incorporation decreased after 2 hr, but uridine incorporation remained normal for at least 4 hr. HeLa cell morphology by scanning or transmission electron microscopy remained unaltered during this period of time (Fig. 7) and cell destruction and detachment were not found until after 6 hr of incubation. Thus, inhibition of protein synthesis may be the first biochemical effect noted during the intoxication process of HeLa cells and therefore may be the specific mechanism underlying cytotoxicity. This sequence is already known to be true for diphtheria toxin and pseudomonas exotoxin A, and for the lectins abrin and ricin (Gill, 1978). Brown *et al.* (1980b) found four cytotoxic protein bands in purified Shiga toxin, separable by polyacrylamide gel electrophoresis, and each of these was a potent inhibitor of protein and DNA synthesis. Olenick and Wolfe (1980) have also reported that Shiga toxin in high concentration inhibits polyuridylic acid directed polyphenylalanine synthesis in cell free prokaryotic protein synthesis systems derived from *E. coli* or *S. dysenteriae* 1, apparently by preventing attachment of polyuridylic acid to toxin treated ribosomes. While this observation supports the concept that toxin is an inhibitor of protein synthesis, the specific mechanisms in the prokaryotic system may be entirely different from those involved in eukaryotic ribosomes. Indeed, Brown *et al.* (1980a) suggest, on the basis of studies in a rabbit reticulocyte or wheat germ system, that toxin inhibits elongation of nascent peptide chains.

If Shiga cytotoxin is an inhibitor of protein synthesis and it gains access to the cell interior by means of a receptor-mediated endocytic process (Keusch, 1981), then toxin must still move from inside of the endocytic vesicle to the cytoplasm where it can finally reach its target, the ribosome (Fig. 8). How is this accomplished? Based on the inhibitory effects of the lysosomotropic agents, chloroquine and steriods, we postulate that an intralysosomal processing step may occur to facilitate release of active toxin to the cytoplasm. We propose a speculative working model in which limited proteolytic digestion at acid pH may occur within the fused endocytic vesicle, exposing a "signal sequence-like" region of the molecule to initiate translocation of toxin to the cytoplasm. This mechanism is analogous to the Blobel–Sabatini model (Blobel and Sabatini, 1971; Blobel and Dobberstein, 1975) for the transport of export proteins from endoplasmic reticulum to the cell exterior, except in the reverse direction. The signal sequence is a discrete portion of the polypeptide chain of a number of transported proteins, consisting of short-lived 15–30 amino acid segments that control the movement of the protein through the membrane, and are cleaved off the final exported molecule. The presence in Shiga toxin of a hidden or internal signal sequence, exposed by partial digestion within the vesicle, thus permitting the functional toxic moiety to escape to the cytoplasm, would explain why receptor mediated endocytosis was required for passage through the plasma membrane of the susceptible cell. While this hypothesis is purely speculative, it has a rationale in biological fact, and is both a plausible and testable mechanism for the ultimate disposition of imported proteins with intracellular loci of action. Brown *et al.* (1980a) have suggested that native *Shigella* toxin must, in fact, be cleaved in order to activate it, consistent with the concept presented above.

Recently Hale and Formal (1980) have presented evidence that bacterial infection of HeLa cells leads to cell death due to intracellular production of cytotoxin. Invasive, toxigenic strains promptly inhibit HeLa cell protein synthesis whereas invasive nontoxigenic *Salmonella typhimurium* W118 does not. When Henle 407 cells, which are resistant to exogenous toxin, were studied the invasive toxigenic *Shigella* strains inhibited protein synthesis as well, suggesting that Henle 407 cells lack a receptor for toxin or a functional translocation mechanism which bacterial invasion and intracellular toxin production circumvents.

6.3. ENTEROTOXIN

The revival in interest in Shiga toxins was sparked by the report of Keusch *et al.* (1970, 1972a) that *S. dysenteriae* 1 produces a cell-free, heat labile toxin which causes fluid accumulation within the lumen of *in vivo* ligated segments of rabbit ileum. Prior to this, virtually all references to enterotoxin activity in Shiga toxin were to hemorrhagic intestinal lesions following parenteral injection of lipopolysaccharide endotoxin. In occasional reports, there was a hint that the neurotoxin also caused enteric lesions, but these were generally overshadowed by the neurological presentation and did not really reproduce characteristics of the disease. The question, *does it or doesn't it?*, seemed to be settled in 1953 when Branham and associates reported their studies on the effects of administration

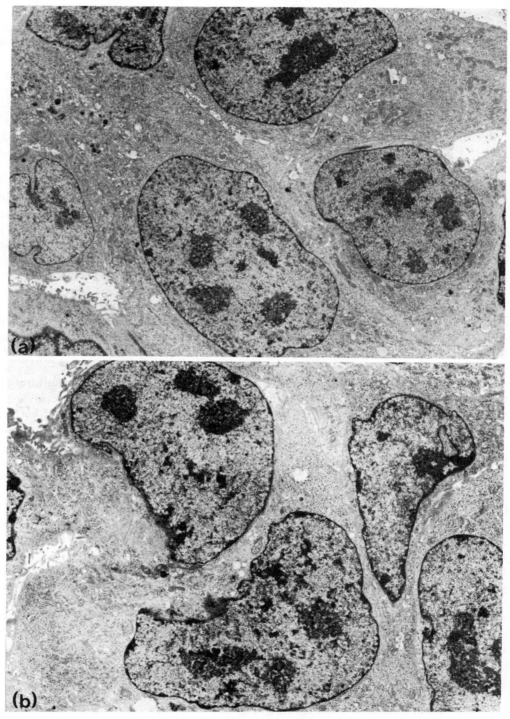

FIG. 7. (see facing page)

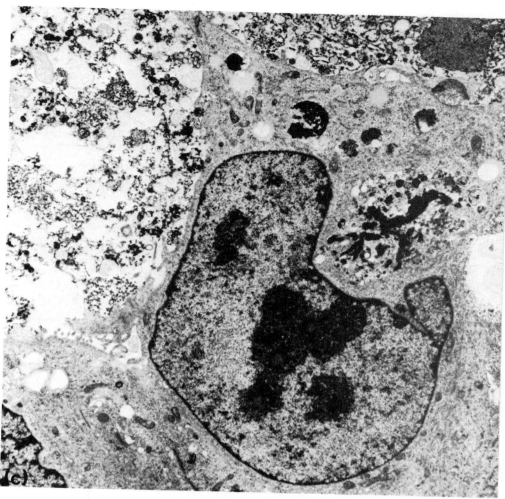

FIG. 7. Transmission electron micrographs (×4500) of HeLa cells grown on plastic petri dishes (a) Control cells exposed to medium for 6 h. (b) Cells exposed to one 50% lethal dose of toxin for 6 hr. There were no significant morphologic alterations in the toxin treated monolayers at this time. (c) 24 hr of intoxication (×6300) reveals extensive cellular damage, including the debris of dead and degenerated cells, and evidence of toxicity to intact cells remaining on the monolayer, such as the cytoplasmic inclusions seen in this cell. (Electron microscopy performed by Dr. David Philips, Rockefeller University, N.Y.).

of large doses of crude toxin preparations, containing both neurotoxin and endotoxin, either *per os* or directly into surgically constructed pouches of terminal ileum and ascending colon (Branham *et al.*, 1953). They found that no intestinal symptoms resulted from toxin given by either route, even though the animals developed neurotoxin neutralizing antibodies active in a mouse protection assay or capable of protecting the animal itself from later lethal challenge with intravenous toxin. Branham *et al.* (1953) concluded that Shiga toxin "is completely innocuous when in contact with the normal intestinal mucosa."

In contrast, Keusch *et al.* (1972a,b) found that partially purified neurotoxin preparations from 3% peptone broth culture supernatants, fractionated over polymeric Amicon membranes graded to retain molecules greater than 50,000 daltons in molecular weight and then chromatographed on a Sephadex G-150 column, caused positive responses in ligated rabbit ileal loops (Fig. 9). The major endotoxin fraction A, identified by the limulus lysate gelation reaction, was devoid of any effects on the loops. The neurotoxin fraction, however, caused two major effects. First, loops became distended with fluid, significant accumulation occurring by 6 hr of inoculation. The fluid was higher

MODEL MECHANISM FOR EXIT OF BIOLOGICALLY ACTIVE
MACROMOLECULES FROM ENDOCYTIC VESICLES

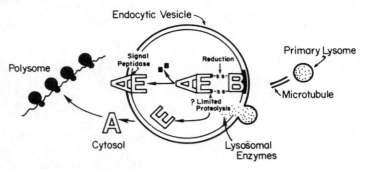

FIG. 8. Speculative model for activation and transmembrane transport of biologically active macromolecules across endocytic vesicles. The toxin molecule is represented by the symbols AE–B, in which AE is the biologically active subunit, B is the receptor binding subunit, and the two are held together by disulfide bonds. The model depicts the B subunit still attached to the membrane which is now at the internal face of the cytoplasmic vesicle following invagination of the cell surface. Lysosomal fusion occurs and the AE unit is processed (? reduction, ? limited proteolysis) to expose an entry (E) domain to facilitate translocation of the A subunit to the cytosol and its target, the ribosome. One mechanism to accomplish this would be for the E domain to function as a signal sequence, as in the translocation of export proteins, and the scheme depicts a signal peptidase clipping off the signal sequence as the A subunit passes through the membrane of the vesicle.

in potassium, chloride and protein content than that produced in response to cholera toxin but still was an isotonic transudate and not an exudate (Keusch *et al.*, 1972a). Secondly, the toxin resulted in striking histologic abnormalities of the mucosa (Keusch *et al.*, 1972b). By one hour of contact, focal changes consisting of mucus discharge from goblet cells and altered tinctorial qualities of individual epithelial cells at the apex and mid villous portion of the villi, with an increase in cellularity of the lamina propria, were apparent. These changes intensified with time, and by six hours, there was definite

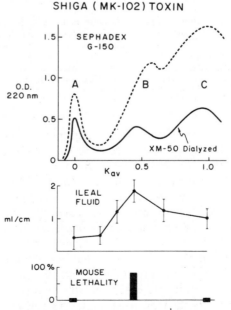

FIG. 9. Partial purification of *S. dysenteriae* 1 toxin by Sephadex G-150 chromatography and membrane filtration on Amicon XM-50 membranes. Fraction A contained the biologically active LPS endotoxin, and was devoid of enterotoxicity (secretory response in rabbit ileal loops) or neurotoxicity (mouse lethality). These biological properties were present in fraction B, along with cytotoxin (HeLa cell lethal toxin). (From Keusch *et al.*, 1972a).

shortening of villi, decreased villus to crypt ratio, extrusion of individual or small clumps of degenerating epithelial cells, disarray of the epithelial cell layer in general, focal micro-ulcers where necrotic cells had fallen off, and large numbers of lymphocytes in the lamina propria as well as transmigrating through the epithelium. The brush border was thinned out in places, the epithelium, particularly near the villous tip, was cuboidal with nuclear debris scattered about, and many inflammatory cells were present in the bowel lumen. Companion loops in the same animal inoculated with cholera toxin remained histologically normal, although an even greater fluid volume response was evoked. Cell-free neurotoxin thus induced the two principal manifestations of clinical shigellosis, accumulation of fluid and acute enteritis, in an intestinal model and the current concept of Shiga enterotoxin was born.

Further evidence for the enterotoxin effect of neurotoxin-containing preparations from *S. dysenteriae* 1, and an important nuance concerning tissue and perhaps host species specificity, were provided by studies of jejunal perfusion of toxin in rabbits. Steinberg *et al.* (1975) demonstrated that Shiga toxin caused a fluid response in rabbit jejunum that, at maximum doses, equalled the secretory rate for cholera toxin induced secretion, with identical protein content, and no histologic change in mucosa over a five hour period of study. This study showed that toxin induced fluid secretion could be independent of cytotoxic effects on gut mucosa, and that distinct portions of the small bowel responded in individual fashion to the biologically active fractions in the toxin preparation.

These observations suggest an explanation for the failure of neurotoxin to exert a grossly detectable effect on rhesus monkey ileum or ascending colon in the studies of Branham *et al.* (1953), that the tissue may be unresponsive to toxin rather than a lack of enterotoxin effect of the preparation. This site specificity is consistent with observations of Rout *et al.* (1975) who induced disease in *Macaca mulatta* monkeys with viable *S. flexneri* 2a. Infection was accompanied by net jejunal secretion of sodium, chloride and water and either decreased absorption or net secretion in colon, but without change in ileal transport. Of great interest, while the colonic abnormalities were accompanied by bacterial invasion and morphologic damage, no invasion of or histologic damage to either jejunum or ileum was found, although large numbers of organisms were found in the lumen. The combination of lumenal colonization, normal morphology, and net iso-tonic water and electrolyte secretion is certainly highly suggestive of an enterotoxin action on rhesus monkey jejunum. That this secretion was not secondary to the invasive inflammatory colitis was shown by Kinsey *et al.* (1976) who inoculated the same *Shigella* strain directly into the cecum of monkeys. While typical colonic lesions and the dysen-tery syndrome were produced, there was no evidence of jejunal secretion nor watery diarrhea in the animals. Since this specific isolate has been shown to produce Shiga toxin, its failure to induce ileal transport or histologic abnormalities is a strong indication of the lack of sensitivity of the tissue to toxin effects. Branham *et al.* (1953) apparently had the misfortune to choose the wrong end of the small bowel to study. The species specific response of different portions of the gut also explains the ability of the same *S. flexneri* 2a, or *S. dysenteriae* 1 strains to cause invasive acute enteritis in rabbit or guinea-pig ileum (Arm *et al.*, 1965; LaBrec *et al.*, 1964) but not in rhesus monkey ileum (Rout *et al.*, 1975).

The secretory effect of Shiga toxin in rabbit ileum was confirmed by Donowitz, Keusch and Binder (1975) in *in vitro* studies of stripped ileal mucosa mounted in a Ussing chamber following a five hour exposure to toxin *in vivo*. Net sodium secretion was present in toxin treated mucosa, although short-circuit current (I_{sc}) was not altered from control. The tissue remained responsive to the changes in I_{sc} normally caused by either dibutyryl cyclic AMP or theophylline. However, the response to glucose was significantly diminished in the toxin treated tissue. That impairment in glucose stimu-lated increases in I_{sc} is related to a defect in sugar transport, and not to uncoupling of glucose and sodium transport, was shown by Binder and Whiting (1977). They found that addition of 30 mM 3-*O*-methylglucose to both mucosal and serosal bathing solutions of rabbit ileum, treated with toxin and placed in lucite chambers as above, induced a smaller increment in I_{sc} and potential difference in toxin exposed as compared to control tissue. Influx of either galactose or L-alanine was reduced by 40–50%, providing convincing evidence of defects in hexose and amino acid transport in *Shigella* toxin treated rabbit ileum, and suggesting a correlation with the histologic evidence of cytotoxicity to epithelial cells in this tissue. Neither of these indications of mucosal damage is present in cholera toxin treated rabbit ileum.

Employing an *in vivo* closed loop technique in Sprague–Dawley rats, Donowitz and Binder (1976) failed to find an effect of Shiga toxin on cecal morphology or transport of water and electrolyte whereas cholera toxin induced net secretion of water and sodium and an increase in mucosal cyclic AMP, without histologic damage in the same system. This failure of Shiga toxin to affect colonic tissue in the rat is consistent with its lack of effect on the colonic portion of isolated *in situ* rhesus monkey ileo–colonic pouches, previously reported by Branham *et al.* (1953).

The mechanism of action of enterotoxin is not clear. Because Shiga toxin is choleralike in causing isotonic fluid accumulation without histologic damage in rabbit jejunum, several studies have investigated the possibility that Shiga toxin is a stimulator of adenylate cyclase. Flores *et al.* (1974) exposed rabbit ileal segments for 4 or 6 hr *in vivo* to Shiga or cholera toxin, and then measured fluid production and adenylate cyclase and phosphodiesterase activity, as well as cyclic AMP levels, in homogenized mucosal scrapings. Both toxins caused significant fluid secretion but only cholera toxin activated adenylate cyclase and increased mucosal cyclic AMP levels. Donowitz *et al.* (1975) were also unable to document any change in cyclic AMP in mucosal scrapings of rabbit ileum exposed for either 1 or 5 hr *in vivo* to Shiga toxin.

In contrast, Charney *et al.* (1976) showed activation of adenylate cyclase in Shiga toxin treated rabbit ileum, but only when the substrate concentration of ATP was raised 10-fold above the concentration usually employed in the cyclase assay. No effect on Na:K-ATP'ase activity was observed. Paulk *et al.* (1977) also reported that Shiga toxin causes an increase in mucosal cyclic AMP in perfused rabbit jejunum, however this was detected only after 6 hr of incubation, long after fluid secretion was significantly increased. Because of these temporal relationships between cAMP and secretion, Paulk *et al.* (1977) concluded that increased cAMP has nothing to do with the secretion. However in simultaneous studies employing cholera toxin, the rise in cAMP levels did not preceed the onset of secretion, and indeed statistically significant increases did not occur until 2 hr after significant secretion was documented. It seems unreasonable, therefore, to draw any conclusions as to the relevance of the changes in cAMP levels to the action of Shiga toxin based on the temporal sequence in these studies, for by the same criteria one would be forced to conclude that cholera toxin is not exerting its influence via the activation of adenylate cyclase as well. The question as to whether or not Shiga toxin is a cyclase activator thus remains unanswered. Moreover, no studies have been reported on possible effects on guanylate cyclase.

Certain studies in cell culture systems may provide some clues to cyclase activation. Cholera toxin activates adenylate cyclase in many cells *in vitro*, for example the Y-1 mouse adrenal tumor cell in continuous culture (Donta *et al.*, 1973) and the rat epididymal fat cell (Greenough *et al.*, 1970). These respond to the resulting increase in intracellular cAMP levels by, respectively, increasing steroid production and release or increasing lipolytic activity with release of glycerol, biochemical changes which are easily monitored and are frequently used to detect cholera enterotoxin. Studies with Shiga toxin in these cell systems have been negative (Keusch and Donta, 1975). This may be because the cells lack appropriate receptors for Shiga toxin or because the toxin does not, in fact, activate the cyclase enzyme.

Another cell type responsive to cholera toxin *in vitro* is the chinese hamster ovary (CHO) cell, in which alterations in gross morphology (elongation) occur when cAMP levels rise (Guerrant *et al.*, 1974). Takeda *et al.* (1977, 1979) have reported finding a cell free product of *S. dysenteriae* 1, distinct from the cytotoxin, that induces the elongation response. These toxins were isolated from culture supernatants by ammonium sulfate precipitation (56%), and chromatography on DEAE–cellulose, eluting with 0.01 M phosphate buffer (pH 7.0) in low (0.2 M) or high (0.9 M) NaCl and designated fractions I and II, respectively. Fraction I contained all of the mouse lethal activity (neurotoxin) whereas fraction II caused elongation of CHO cells. Further purification of fraction II on BioGel-A-5m and hydroxylapatite yielded a fraction causing significant CHO cell elongation in concentrations of 100 ng/ml or greater. In comparison to cholera toxin, the Shiga product was about 1000-fold less active.

The same group (Takeda *et al.*, 1979) has subsequently reported isolation of the CHO cell factor from *S. flexneri*, *S. boydii* and *S. sonnei*. However, adenylate cyclase activity or cAMP levels in these cells have not been reported and the significance of the observation for the enterotoxin activity of *Shigella* toxin(s) remains unknown.

Ketyi and colleagues (1978a) in Hungary have recently reported finding a heat stable enterotoxin in *Shigella flexneri* strains with characteristics similar to the ST enterotoxin of *E. coli*. This is a provocative finding because the assay for ST, intestinal fluid production in suckling mice, appears to be dependent upon activation of guanylate cyclase and increased intracellular levels of cyclic GMP. Ketyi *et al.* (1978a) found that ultrasonic lysates of two strains of *S. flexneri* 3a and one *S. flexneri* 4b strain produced positive mouse tests, with bowel to body weight ratios equal to or greater than 0.093 (a strongly positive response in this test). The two *S. flexneri* 3a strains were also said to be positive in the rabbit ileal loop test at 4 hr, but not after 20 hr of incubation, a characteristic of *E. coli* ST as well. However, results from only 6 loops were reported, only 4/6 were positive, and the activity was barely detectable (total loop weight − empty weight/empty weight of 1.2). Unlike the small molecular weight ST, the *S. flexneri* 3a ST activity chromatographed on Sephadex G-100 similar to high molecular weight *E. coli* heat labile toxin, with an estimated molecular weight of 100,000 for the *Shigella* product. It was nondialyzable, stable to heat at 100°C for 30 min, and resistant to pH 1.0 for 90 min. No CHO activity was present. Antisera raised in rabbits to Sephadex G-100 purified fractions neutralized the suckling mouse positive material, as did antisera against an LT/ST positive strain of *E. coli* (B7A) (Ketyi *et al.*, 1978b). The *Shigella* ST antiserum also neutralized the CHO cell activity of *E. coli* LT from B7A and an LT-only strain, 263, suggesting antigenic resemblance to both ST and LT of *E. coli*. The same authors have also reported finding both ST activity and cytotoxicity for a human amniotic cell line (AV-3) in the same Sephadex G-100 fraction of a cell lysate or alkaline pH extraction (according to van Heyningen and Gladstone, 1953a) of the *S. flexneri* 2a strain studied by Keusch and Jacewicz (1977a) and O'Brien *et al.* (1977). These materials were not very active, however, requiring around 1 mg of lyophilized toxin to cause positive reactions in the above tests.

While the validity or significance of the observations of Ketyi *et al.* (1978a,b) cannot really be interpreted from the studies reported to date, the data do hint at the presence of a heat stable toxin active in the suckling mouse, which might indicate the presence of an activator of guanylate cyclase (Field *et al.*, 1978). Further work is clearly required to sort this out.

7. RELEVANCE TO DISEASE

What is the possible relationship of these various toxic activities of the genus *Shigella* to the disease they cause? The discussion to follow will offer our speculations based on the data available and present understanding of the pathogenesis of other toxin-mediated enteric infections. It should be stressed, however, that these concepts, while rational and reasonable, are as yet unproven and require additional work to fill in the remaining gaps in knowledge.

As indicated earlier in this paper, shigellosis involves two distinct regions of the intestine, the proximal small bowel and the colon, resulting in two distinct intestinal disease syndromes, watery diarrhea and dysentery, respectively (Keusch, 1978). The capacity of the organism to invade intestinal eipthelial cells of the colon and to multiply therein has been shown to be a critical virulence factor for the shigellas in experimental infections in humans and in a model infection in rhesus monkeys (Formal et al., 1965; Gemski et al., 1972; Levine et al., 1973; Gemski and Formal, 1975; Rout et al., 1975). In the monkey, watery diarrhea is correlated with secretion of water and electrolytes in the proximal jejunum, even though bacterial invasion does not occur (Rout et al., 1975). The presence of organisms in the lumen at the site of secretion, and the lack of any alteration in jejunal transport of fluid when organisms are inoculated directly into the cecum (Kinsey et al., 1976), indicates the likelihood of a local effect of the lumenal population of bacteria, such as production of enterotoxin. It is not clear why toxigenic noninvasive colonial mutants of virulent Shigellae are totally avirulent, causing neither watery diarrhea nor dysentery, unless the change from invasive to noninvasive also effects their ability to colonize in the anterior bowel. At the present time there is no more reasonable suggestion for the pathogenesis of the jejunal transport abnormalities and the resulting watery diarrhea than the action of the enterotoxin (Keusch, 1976, 1978, 1979a, b). The mechanism by which this toxin causes fluid secretion is not yet known, but might conceivably involve either cyclic-AMP or cyclic-GMP, or possibly even serotonin release. Further work is needed to clarify these possibilities, which will be facilitated by the availability of highly purified toxin fractions. In this noninvasive proximal bowel phase of the disease, we believe that toxin produced in the lumen most likely binds to an intestinal cell surface receptor, such as the glycoprotein receptor described on the HeLa cell. This is not yet known, but is under active investigation in our laboratory. Following binding, toxin could be translocated to the cell interior to activate cyclase enzymes or to reach the serotonin responsive basal membrane. Whether or not a receptor mediated endocytic process might be involved, as it appears to be in the HeLa cell cytotoxicity system, or some other transport mechanism is employed also remains an open question.

The dysentery syndrome is clearly initiated by invasion of colonic epithelial cells by shigellas, followed by intracellular multiplication (Gemski and Formal, 1975; Kinsey et al., 1976). The evidence available at this time indicates that colonic epithelium is insensitive to exogenous toxin (Donowitz and Binder, 1976), however if the events following invasion of HeLa or Henle 407 cells in vitro (Hale and Formal, 1980) is a model for events in the colonic cell, then intracellular production of cytotoxin, resulting in prompt inhibition of cellular protein synthesis could in turn lead to epithelial cell death and initiate the inflammatory colitis that follows invasion and multiplication of the organisms. Invasion, in this hypothesis, is a mechanism to deliver cytotoxin to the susceptible intracellular target, the ribosomal protein synthetic mechanism. In support of this concept is the development of cytotoxin neutralizing antibodies in the course of clinical disease (Keusch and Jacewicz, 1973; Keusch et al., 1976a; Keusch and Jacewicz, 1977a). Whether or not the enterotoxic activity would act intracellularly in the colon is problematic for cell damage due to the cytotoxin alone could account for the decreased absorption or net secretion of water and electrolytes found in the dysenteric colon. Motor abnormalities of the gut, clinically manifested as waves of cramps and tenesmus, could be secondary to the inflammation per se or due to toxin acting on enteric neurons or enterochromaffin cells to locally release serotonin (Donowitz et al., 1979). Shigellosis, then, could be considered as part cholera, part carcinoid and part colitis. It is no wonder that patients are so dreadfully uncomfortable with the disease, often feeling that they would prefer death to dysentery (Keusch, 1979a) and why military campaigns throughout history have sometimes been decided more by dysentery than military leadership or strength (Gear, 1944).

What then is the relevance of neurotoxin? It was thought at one time that neurotoxin could be the cause of the frequent seizures in young children with the disease (Barrett-Connor and Connor, 1970; Keusch, 1979a). This became untenable when only S. dysenteriae 1 could be shown to produce neurotoxin while all species caused convulsions. However, we now in fact know that all species produce the neurotoxin, and the hypothesis is actually tenable. However, the seizures occur almost exclusively in young children in association with high fever, and have the epidemiological characteristics of febrile seizures (Keusch, 1979a; Keusch, 1981). We view the classical neurotoxin activity (the paresis–paralysis–death triad following parenteral administration of toxin) as an artifact of experimental manipulation of the host. This does not mean that these manifestations may not be a consequence of cytotoxicity, with a strong specificity for certain endothelial cells in the central nervous system. But we do suggest that it does not happen in the natural disease in which bacteria in the gastrointestinal tract are the agents of illness.

8. CONCLUSIONS

The genus *Shigella* produces a protein toxin with neurotoxic, cytotoxic and enterotoxic properties. Toxin production is regulated in part by iron concentration in the medium and is produced under aerobic conditions. The toxin appears to be a periplasmic protein, but its role in the life of the organism is unknown.

Under appropriate conditions, small quantities of toxin are made. The holotoxin has a molecular weight of approximately 72,000 daltons and contains a 30,000 dalton subunit. Other estimates of molecular weight and the presence of smaller 4–7000 or 11,000 dalton fragments or subunits have also been reported. The precise size, structure and composition of toxin are not yet certain.

Toxin antigen is made *in vivo* during shigellosis in humans and serum neutralizing antibodies may be readily detected. We believe toxin plays a crucial role in pathogenesis of both jejunal (watery diarrhea) and colonic (dysenteric) phases of the illness. The mechanism by which it causes intestinal secretion or cell death is under active investigation.

Acknowledgement—This work was supported by Grant AI 16242 from the National Institute of Allergy and Infectious Diseases, N.I.H., Bethesda, MD, and by the Rockefeller Foundation, New York.

REFERENCES

ARM, H. G., FLOYD, T. M., FABER, J. E. and HAYES, J. R. (1965) Use of ligated segments of rabbit small intestine in experimental shigellosis. *J. Bact.* **89**: 803–809.

BALDWIN, R. L. (1953) The neurotoxin of *Shigella shigae*. 2. Examination of the toxin in the oil turbine ultracentrifuge. *Br. J. exp. Pathl.* **34**: 217–220.

BARG, G. S. (1932) Zur Characteristik der Wirkung des Dysenterietoxins. *Z. Immunitatasforsch.* **74**: 372–379.

BARRETT-CONNOR, E. and CONNOR, J. D. (1970) Extraintestinal manifestations of shigellosis. *Am. J. Gastro.* **53**: 234–245.

BEHFOROUZ, N. C., AMIRHAKIMI, G. H. and GETTNER, S. M. (1977) Enteric pathogens in infants and children in Shiraz, Iran. A study of their incidences and infectious drug resistance. *Pahlavi. med. J.* **8**: 157–180.

BESSAU, G. (1911) Ueber die Dysenteriegifte und ihrer Antikörper. *Zentbl. Bakt. ParasitKde. Abt. I, Orig.* **57**: 27–56.

BINDER, H. J. and WHITING, D. S. (1977) Inhibition of small-intestinal sugar and amino acid transport by the enterotoxin of *Shigella dysenteriae* 1. *Infect. Immun.* **16**: 510–512.

BLACK, R. E., CRAUM, G. F. and BLAKE, P. A. (1978) Epidemiology of common-source outbreaks of shigellosis in the United States, 1961–1975. *Am. J. Epidemiol.* **108**: 47–52.

BLOBEL, G. and SABATINI, D. D. (1971) Ribosome-membrane interaction in eukaryotic cells. In: *Biomembranes,* pp. 193–195, MANSON, L. A. (ed). Plenum Press, New York.

BLOBEL, G. and DOBBERSTEIN, B. (1975) Transfer of proteins across membranes. Presence of proteolytically processed and unprocessed nascent immunoglobulin light chains in membrane-bound ribosomes of murine myeloma. *J. Cell Biol.* **67**: 835–857.

BOIVIN, A. (1940) Action comparée des deux toxines du bacille de Shiga sur diverses espèces animales. *C.r. Soc. Biol.* **133**: 232–255.

BOIVIN, A. and MESROBEANU, L. (1937a) Recherches sur les toxines des bacilles dysentériques. Sur la nature et sur les propritétés biologiques des principes toxiques susceptibles de se rencontrer dans les filtrats des cultures sur bouillon du bacille de Shiga. *C.r. Soc. Biol.* **124**: 442–444.

BOIVIN, A. and MESROBEANU, L. (1937b) Recherches sur les toxines des bacilles dysentériques. Sur les principes toxiques du bacille de Flexner. *C.r. Soc. Biol.* **124**: 1078–1081.

BOIVIN, A. and MESROBEANU, L. (1937c) Recherches sur les toxines des bacilles dysenteriques. Sur le pouvoir protecteur antitoxique des sérums obtenus en injectant à l'animal l'endotoxine-antigène O du bacille de Shiga et du bacille de Flexner. *C.r. Soc. Biol.* **125**: 796–799.

BOIVIN, A. and MESROBEANU, L. (1937d) Recherches sur les toxines des bacilles dysentériques. Sur l'existence d'un principe toxique thermolabile et neurotrope dans les corps bactériens du Bacille de Shiga. *C.r. Soc. Biol.* **126**: 222–225.

BOIVIN, A. and MESROBEANU, L. (1937e) Recherches sur les toxines des bacilles dysentériques; sur l'identité entre la toxine thermolabile de Shiga et l'exotoxine présente dans les filtrates des cultures sur bouillon de la même bactérie. *C.r. Soc. Biol.* **126**: 323–325.

BOIVIN, A. and MESROBEANU, L. (1937f) Recherches sur les toxines du bacille dysentérique. Sur la signification des toxines produites par le bacille de Shiga et par le bacille de Flexner. *C.r. Soc. Biol.* **126**: 652–655.

BOROFF, D. A. (1949) Study on toxins and antigens of *Shigella dysenteriae* 1. Toxicity and antigenicity of whole organisms and various fractions of *Shigella dysenteriae*. *J. Bact.* **57**: 617–632.

BOROFF, D. A. and MACRI, B. P. (1949) Study of toxins and antigens of *Shigella dysenteriae*. II. Active protection of rabbits with whole organisms and fractions of *Shigella dysenteriae*. *J. Bact.* **58**: 387–394.

BRANHAM, S. E. and CARLIN, S. A. (1984) Studies with *Shigella dysenteriae* (SHIGA) 1. Infection and toxin action in mice. *J. infect. Dis.* **83**: 60–65.

BRANHAM, S. E., DACK, G. M. and RIGGS, D. B. (1953) Studies with *Shigella dysenteriae* (SHIGA) IV. Immunological reactions in monkeys to the toxins in isolated intestinal pouches. *J. Immunol.* **70**: 103–113.

BRIDGEWATER, F. A. J., MORGAN, R. S., ROWSON, K. E. K. and PAYLING-WRIGHT, G. (1955) The neurotoxin of *Shigella shigae*. Morphological and functional lesions produced in the central nervous system of rabbits. *Br. J. exp. Path.* **36**: 447–453.

BROWN, J. E., USSERY, M. A., LEPPLA, S. H. and ROTHMAN, S. W. (1980a) Inhibition of protein synthesis by Shiga toxin. Activation of the toxin and inhibition of peptide elongation. *FEBS Lett.* **117**: 84–88.

BROWN, J. E., ROTHMAN, S. W. and DOCTOR, B. P. (1980b) Inhibition of protein synthesis in intact HeLa cells by *Shigella dysenteriae* 1 toxin. *Infect. Immun.* **29**: 98–107.

BÜLBRING, E. and LIN, R. C. Y. (1958) The effect of intraluminal application of 5-hydroxytryptamine and 5-hydroxytryptophan on peristalsis; the local production of 5-HT and its release in relation to intraluminal pressure and propulsive activity. *J. Physiol.* **140**: 381–407.

BURNS, T. W., MATHIAS, J. R., CARLSON, G. M., MARTIN, J. L. and SHIELDS, R. P. (1978) Effect of toxigenic *Escherichia coli* on myoelectric activity of small intestine. *Am. J. Physiol.* **235**: E311–E315.

BURNS, T. W., MATHIAS, J. R., MARTIN, J. L., CARLSON, G. M. and SHIELDS, R. P. (1980) Alteration of myoelectric activity of small intestine by invasive *Escherichia coli*. *Am. J. Physiol.* **238**: G57–G62.

CAVANAGH, J. B., HOWARD, J. G. and WHITBY, J. L. (1956) The neurotoxin of *Shigella shigae*; a comparative study of the effects produced in various laboratory animals. *Br. J. exp. Path.* **37**: 272–278.

CHARNEY, A. N., GOTS, R. E., FORMAL, S. B. and GIANNELLA, R. A. (1976) Activation of intestinal adenylate cyclase by *Shigella dysenteriae* 1 enterotoxin. *Gastroenterology* **70**: 1085–1090.

CONRADI, H. (1903) Über lösliche, durch aseptische Autolyse erhaltene Giftstoffe von Ruhr- und Typhusbazillen. *Dt. med. Wschr.* **20**: 26–28.

DALE, D. C. and MATA, L. J. (1968) Studies of diarrheal disease in Central America. XI. Intestinal bacterial flora in malnourished children with shigellosis. *Am. J. trop. Med.* **17**: 397–403.

DAVIES, P. J. A., DAVIES, D. R., LEVITZKI, A., MAXFIELD, F. R., MILHAUD, P., WILLINGHAM, M. C. and PASTAN, I. H. (1980) Transglutaminase is essential in receptor-mediated endocytosis of α2-macroglobulin and polypeptide hormones. *Nature* **283**: 162–167.

DONADIO, J. and GANGAROSA, E. (1969) Foodborne shigellosis. *J. infect. Dis.* **119**: 666–668.

DONOWITZ, M. and BINDER, H. J. (1976) Effect of enterotoxins of *Vibrio cholerae*, *Escherichia coli*, and *Shigella dysenteriae* Type 1 on fluid and electrolyte transport in colon. *J. infect. Dis.* **134**: 135–143.

DONOWITZ, M., KEUSCH, G. T. and BINDER, H. J. (1975) Effect of *Shigella* enterotoxin on electrolyte transport in rabbit ileum. *Gastroenterology* **69**: 1230–1237.

DONOWITZ, M., CHARNEY, A. N. and TAI, Y. H. (1979) A comprehensive picture of serotonin-induced ileal secretion. In: *Mechanisms of Intestinal Secretion*, pp. 217–230, BINDER, H. (ed). A. R. Liss, New York.

DONTA, S. T., KING, M. and SLOPER, K. (1973) Induction of steroidogenesis in tissue culture by cholera enterotoxin. *Nature (New Biol)* **243**: 246–247.

DOPTER, C. (1905a) Effets expérimentaux de la toxine dysentérique sur le système nerveux central. *C.r. Soc. Biol.* **58**: 400–402.

DOPTER, C. (1905b) Effets expérimantaux de la toxine dysentérique sur le système nerveux. *Ann. Inst. Pasteur* **19**: 353–366.

DRITZ, S. K., AINSWORTH, T. E., GARRARD, W. F., BACK, A., PALMER, R. D., BOUCHER, L. A. and RIVER, E. (1977) Patterns of sexually transmitted enteric diseases in a city. *Lancet* **2**: 3–4.

DUBOS, R. J., and GEIGER, J. W. (1946) Preparation and properties of Shiga toxin and toxoid. *J. exp. Med.* **84**: 143–156.

DUBOS, R. J., HOBERMAN, H. D. and PIERCE, C. (1942) Some factors affecting the toxicity of cultures of *Shigella dysenteriae*. *Proc. natn. Acad. Sci. U.S.A.* **28**: 453–458.

DUPONT, H. L., HORNICK, R. B., DAWKINS, A. T., SNYDER, M. J. and FORMAL, S. B. (1969) The response of man to virulent *Shigella flexneri* 2a. *J. infect. Dis.* **119**: 296–299.

DUPONT, H. L., GANGAROSA, E. J., RELLER, L. B., WOODWARD, W. E., ARMSTRONG, R. W., HAMMOND, J., GLASER, K. and MORRIS, G. K. (1970) Shigellosis in custodial institutions. *Am. J. Epidemiol.* **92**: 172–179.

ECKER, E. E. and WOLPAW, B. J. (1930) The effect of certain toxic substances in bacterial cultures on the movement of the intestine. *Archs Path.* **10**: 407–416.

ENGLEY, F. B., JR (1952) The neurotoxin of *Shigella dysenteriae* (SHIGA) *Bact. Rev.* **16**: 153–178.

FELDMAN, R. A., BHAT, P. and KAMATH, K. R. (1970) Infection and disease in a group of South Indian families. IV. Bacteriologic methods and a report of the frequency of enteric bacterial infection in preschool children. *Am. J. Epidemiol.* **92**: 367–375.

FIELD, M., GRAF, L. H., LAIRD, W. J. and SMITH, P. L. (1978) Heat stable enterotoxin of *Escherichia coli*: in vitro effects on guanylate cyclase activity, cyclic GMP concentration, and ion transport in small intestine. *Proc. natn. Acad. Sci. U.S.A.* **75**: 2800–2804.

FINKELSTEIN, R. A. (1973) Cholera. CRC *Crit. Rev. Microbiol.* **2**: 553–623.

FLEXNER, S. (1900) On the etiology of tropical dysentery. *Bull. Johns Hopkins Hosp.* **11**: 231–242.

FLEXNER, S. and SWEET, J. E. (1906) The pathogenesis of experimental colitis, and the relation of colitis in animals and man. *J. exp. Med.* **8**: 514–535.

FLORES, J., GRADY, G. F., McIVER, J., WITKUM, P., BECKMAN, B. and SHARP, G. W. G. (1974) Comparison of the effects of enterotoxins of *Shigella dysenteriae* and *Vibrio cholerae* on the adenylate cyclase system of the rabbit ileum. *J. infect. Dis.* **130**: 374–379.

FORMAL, S. B., ABRAMS, G. D., SCHNEIDER, H. and SPRINZ, H. (1963) Experimental *Shigella* infections VI. Role of the small intestine in an experimental infection in guinea-pigs. *J. Bact.* **85:** 119–125.

FORMAL, S. B., LABREC, E. H. and SCHNEIDER, H. (1965a) Pathogenesis of bacillary dysentery in laboratory animals. *Fed. Proc.* **24:** 29–34.

FORMAL, S. B., LABREC, E. H., KENT, T. H. and FALKOW, S. (1965b) Abortive intestinal infection with an *Escherichia coli–Shigella flexneri* hybrid strain. *J. Bacteriol.* **89:** 1374–1382.

FORMAL, S. B., KENT, T. H., AUSTIN, S. and LABREC, E. H. (1966) Fluorescent-antibody and histological study of vaccinated and control monkeys challenged with *Shigella flexneri*. *J. Bact.* **91:** 2368–2376.

GEAR, H. S. (1944) Hygiene aspects of the El Alamein victory, 1942. *Br. med. J.* **1:** 383–387.

GEMSKI, P., Jr and FORMAL, S. B. (1975) Shigellosis: an invasive infection of the gastrointestinal tract. In: *Microbiology 1975.* pp. 165–169, SCHLESSINGER, D. (ed). Am. Soc. Microbiol., Wash. DC.

GEMSKI, P., Jr, TAKEUCHI, A., WASHINGTON, O. and FORMAL, S. B. (1972) Shigellosis due to *Shigella dysenteriae* 1: Relative importance of mucosal invasion versus toxin production in pathogenesis. *J. infect. Dis.* **126:** 523–530.

GILL, D. M. (1978) Seven toxic peptides that cross cell membranes. In: *Bacterial Toxins and Cell Membranes,* pp. 291–332, JELJASZEWICZ, J. and WADSTROM, T. (eds). Academic Press, New York.

GOLDSTEIN, J. L., ANDERSON, R. G. W. and BROWN, M. S. (1979) Coated pits, coated vesicles and receptor mediated endocytosis. *Nature* **279:** 679–685.

GOOD, R. C., MAY, B. D. and KAWATOMARI, T. (1969) Enteric pathogens in monkeys. *J. Bact.* **97:** 1048–1055.

GORDON, J. E., GUZMAN, M. A., ASCOLI, W. and SCRIMSHAW, N. S. (1964) Acute diarrheal disease in less developed countries. 2. Patterns of epidemiological behavior in rural Guatemalan villages. *Bull. W.H.O.* **31:** 9–20.

GORDON, J. E. (1964) Acute diarrheal disease. *Am. J. med. Sci.* **248:** 345–365.

GORDON, J. E., ASCOLI, W., PIERCE, V., GUZMAN, M. A. and MATA, L. J. (1965) Studies of diarrheal disease in Central America. VI. An epidemic of diarrhea in a Guatemalan highland village, with a component due to *Shigella dysenteriae* type 1. *Am. J. trop. Med. Hyg.* **14:** 404–411.

GREENOUGH, W. B. III., PIERCE, N. F. and VAUGHAN, M. (1970) Titration of cholera enterotoxin and antitoxin in isolated fat cells. *J. infect. Dis.* **121:** S111–S113.

GRIFFIN, D. E., GEMSKI, P. and DOCTOR, B. P. (1978) The release of *Shigella dysenteriae* 1 toxin by polymyxin B. *Abstr. A. Meet. Am. Soc. Microbiol.* p. 21.

GROSS, K. B. and STURKE, P. D. (1975) Concentration of serotonin in intestine and factors affecting its release. *Proc Soc. exp. Biol. Med.* **148:** 1261–1264.

GUERRANT, R. L., BRUNTON, L. L., SCHNAITMAN, T. C., REBHUN, I. I. and GILMAN, A. G. (1974) Cyclic adenosine monophosphate and alteration of Chinese hamster ovary cell morphology: a rapid sensitive *in vitro* assay for enterotoxins of *Vibrio cholerae* and *Escherichia coli*. *Infect. Immun.* **10:** 320–327.

HAAS, R. (1937) Uber Exo- und Endotoxine von Shiga-bazillen. *Z. Immunitätsforsch.* **91:** 254–272.

HAAS, R. (1938) Uber Exo- und Endotoxine der Dysenterie-bazillen. II. Weitere Studien über Endotoxine von Shiga- und Flexner-Ruhrbazillen. *Z. Immunitätsforsch.* **92:** 355–381.

HALE, T. L. and FORMAL, S. B. (1980) Cytotoxicity of *Shigella dysenteriae* 1 for cultured mammalian cells. *Am. J. clin. Nutr.* **33:** 2485–2490.

HANSEN, D. P., KAMINSKI, R. B., BAGG, L. R., KAPIKIAN, A. Z., SLACK, R. C. and SACK, D. A. (1978) New and old agents in diarrhea: A prospective study of an indigenous adult African population. *Am. J. trop. Med. Hyg.* **27:** 609–615.

HARDY, A. V. and WATT, J. (1948) Studies of the acute diarrheal diseases. XVIII. Epidemiology. *Publ. Hlth Rep.* **63:** 363–378.

HIGGINS, A. R., FLOYD, T. M. and KADER, M. A. (1955) Studies in shigellosis. II. Observations on incidence and etiology of diarrheal disease in Egyptian village children. *Am. J. trop. Med. Hyg.* **4:** 271–280.

HORIMI, K. (1913) Ueber die pathogenen Wirkungen der Dysenterie Toxine. *Zentbl. Bakt. ParasitKde., Abt. I, Orig.* **68:** 342–358.

HOWARD, J. G. (1955) Observations on the intoxication produced in mice and rabbits by the neurotoxin of *Shigella shigae*. *Br. J. exp. Path.* **36:** 439–446.

ISTRATI, G. (1938) Action neurotrope et entérotrope de la toxine protéique thermolabile du bacille de Shiga. Action entérotrope de l'antigène glucido-lipidique du bacille de Shiga "S". *C.r. Soc. Biol.* **129:** 1010–1013.

JUSTUS, P. G., CARLSON, G. M., MARTIN, J. M., FORMAL, S. and SHIELDS, R. P. (1980) The myoelectric activity of the small intestine in response to *Clostridium perfringens* A enterotoxin and *Clostridium difficile* culture filtrate. In: *Gastrointestinal Motility*, pp. 379–386, CHRISTENSEN, J. (ed). Raven Press, New York.

KANAI, S. (1922) Further experimental studies on immunization against *S. dysenteriae* (Shiga) and its toxins. *Br. J. exp. Path.* **3:** 158–172.

KÉTYI, I., MALOVICS, I., VERTÉNYI, A., KONTROHR, T., PÁCSA, S. and KUCH, B. (1978a) Heat-stable enterotoxin produced by *Shigella flexneri*. *Acta microbiol. hung.* **25:** 165–171.

KÉTYI, I., VERTÉNYI, A., PÁCSA, S. and KOCSIS, B. (1978b) Enterotoxin production by *Shigella flexneri* type 2A, Strain No. M42–43. *Acta microbiol. hung.* **25:** 319–325.

KEUSCH, G. T. (1973) Pathogenesis of *Shigella* diarrhea. III. Effects of *Shigella* enterotoxin in cell culture. *Trans. N.Y. Acad. Sci.* **35:** 51–58.

KEUSCH, G. T. (1976) Bacterial toxins as virulence factors: Shiga bacillus dysentery viewed as a toxinosis. *Mt Sinai J. Med.* **43:** 33–41.

KEUSCH, G. T. (1978) Ecological control of the bacterial diarrheas: a scientific strategy. *Am. J. clin. Nutr.* **31:** 2208–2218.

KEUSCH, G. T. (1979a) Shigella infections. *Clin. Gastro.* **8:** 645–662.

KESUCH, G. T. (1979b) Specific membrane receptors: Pathogenetic and therapeutic implications in infectious diseases. *Rev. infect. Dis.* **1:** 517–529.

KEUSCH, G. T. (1981) Receptor mediated endocytosis of shigella cytotoxin. In: *Receptor Mediated Binding and*

Internalization of Toxins and Hormones, pp. 95–105, MIDDLEBROOK, J. and KOHN, L. (eds). Academic Press, New York.

KEUSCH, G. T. (1982) Shigellosis. In: *Bacterial Infections of Humans: Epidemiology and Control*. In press, EVANS, A. S. and FELDMAN, H. (eds). Plenum Press, New York.

KEUSCH, G. T. and DONTA, S. T. (1975) Classification of enterotoxins on the basis of activity in cell culture. *J. infect. Dis.* **131**: 58–63.

KEUSCH, G. T. and JACEWICZ, M. (1973) Serum enterotoxin-neutralizing antibody in human shigellosis. *Nature (New Biol.)* **241**: 31–32.

KEUSCH, G. T. and JACEWICZ, M. (1975) The pathogenesis of shigella diarrhea. V. Relationship of Shiga enterotoxin neurotoxin and cytotoxin. *J. infect. Dis.* **131**: S33–S39.

KEUSCH, G. T. and JACEWICZ, M. (1977a) Pathogenesis of shigella diarrhea. VI. Toxin and antitoxin in *S. flexneri* and *S. sonnei* infections in humans. *J. infect. Dis.* **135**: 552–556.

KEUSCH, G. T. and JACEWICZ, M. (1977b) Pathogenesis of shigella diarrhea VII. Evidence for a cell membrane toxin receptor involving $\beta 1 \rightarrow 4$-Linked *N*-Acetyl-D-Glucosamine oligomers. *J. exp. Med.* **146**: 535–546.

KEUSCH, G. T., MATA, L. J. and GRADY, G. F. (1970) Shigella enterotoxin: Isolation and characterization. *Clin. Res.* **18**: 442.

KEUSCH, G. T., GRADY, G. F., MATA, L. J. and McIVER, J. (1972a) The pathogenesis of *Shigella* diarrhea. I. Enterotoxin production by *Shigella dysenteriae* 1. *J. clin. Invest.* **51**: 1212–1218.

KEUSCH, G. T., GRADY, G. F., TAKEUCHI, A. and SPRINZ, H. (1972b) The pathogenesis of *Shigella* diarrhea. II. Enterotoxin induced acute enteritis in the rabbit ileum. *J. infect. Dis.* **126**: 92–95.

KEUSCH, G. T., JACEWICZ, M. and HIRSCHMAN, Z. (1972c) Quantitative microassay in cell culture for enterotoxin of *Shigella dysenteriae* 1. *J. infect. Dis.* **125**: 539–541.

KEUSCH, G. T., JACEWICZ, M., LEVINE, M. M., HORNICK, R. B. and KOCHWA, S. (1976a) Pathogenesis of *Shigella* diarrhea. Serum anticytotoxin antibody response produced by toxigenic and non-toxigenic *Shigella dysenteriae* 1. *J. clin. Invest.* **57**: 194–202.

KEUSCH, G. T., PAPENHAUSEN, P. R. and JACEWICZ, M. (1976b) Comparison of shigella and cholera toxin effects using lymphocytes as target cells. *Clin. Res.* **24**: 287A.

KEUSCH, G. T., PARIKH, I. and JACEWICZ, M. (1977) Affinity chromatography purification of shigella toxin (ST) on a sepharose–chitin column. *Clin. Res.* **25**: 490A.

KEUSCH, G. T., JACEWICZ, M. and PEREIRA, M. (1981) Alterations in surface determinants correlates with resistance of cloned HeLa cells to *Shigella* toxin. *Clin. Res.* **29**: 533A.

KINSEY, M. D., FORMAL, S. B., DAMMIN, G. J. and GIANNELLA, R. A. (1976) Fluid and electrolyte transport in rhesus monkeys challenged intracecally with *Shigella flexneri* 2a. *Infect. Immun.* **14**: 368–371.

KOCH, P. K. and OLITZKI, L. (1946) The action of dysentery toxins on different laboratory animals. *Exp. med. Surg.* **4**: 54–68.

KOURANY, M., VASQUEZ, M. A. and MATA, L. J. (1971) Prevalence of pathogenic enteric bacteria in children of 31 Panamanian communities. *Am. J. trop. Med. Hyg.* **20**: 608–615.

KRAUSS, R. and DÖRR, R. (1905) Ueber experimentelle Therapie der Dysenterie. *Wien klin. Wschr.* **18**: 1077–1079.

KRUSE, W. (1900) Ueber die Ruhr als Volkskrankheit und ihrer Erreger. *Dt. med. Wschr.* **26**: 637–639.

LABREC, E. H., SCHNEIDER, H., MAGNANI, T. J. and FORMAL, S. B. (1964) Epithelial cell penetration is an essential step in the pathogenesis of bacillary dysentery. *J. Bact.* **88**: 1503–1518.

LEVINE, M. M. (1979) *Shigella* and *Salmonella* diarrhoeal disease. *Trop. Doctor* **9**: 4–9.

LEVINE, M. M., DuPONT, H. L., FORMAL, S. B., HORNICK R. B., TAKEUCHI, A., GANGAROSA, E. J., SNYDER, M. J. and LIBONATI, J. P. (1973) Pathogenesis of *Shigella dysenteriae* 1 (Shiga) dysentery. *J. infect. Dis.* **127**: 261–270.

MAŠEK, K., SMETANA, R., and RAŠKOVÁ, H. (1961) Depletion of catecholamines by *Shigella shigae* toxin in the mouse brain. *Biochem. Pharmac.* **8**: 8–9.

MATA, L. J. (1978) *The children of Santa Maria Cauqué: A prospective field study of health and growth*. The M.I.T. Press, Cambridge, MA.

MATA, L. J., GANGAROSA, E. J., CÁCERES, A., PERERA, D. R. and MEJICANOS, J. L. (1970) Epidemic Shiga bacillus dysentery in Central America. I. Etiologic investigations in Guatemala, 1969. *J. infect. Dis.* **122**: 170–180.

MATHIAS, J. R., CARLSON, G. M., MARTIN, J. L., SHIELDS, R. P. and FORMAL, S. (1980) *Shigella dysenteriae* 1 enterotoxin: proposed role in pathogenesis of shigellosis. *Am. J. Physiol.* **329**: G382–G386.

MAXFIELD, F. R., WILLINGHAM, M. C., DAVIES, P. J. A. and PASTAN, I. (1979) Amines inhibit the clustering of α_2-macroglobulin and EGF on the fibroblast cell surface. *Nature* **277**: 661–663.

McCARTNEY, J. E. and OLITSKY, P. K. (1923) Separations of the toxins of bacillus dysenteriae Shiga. *J. exp. Med.* **37**: 767–779.

McIVER, J., GRADY, G. F. and KEUSCH, G. T. (1975) Production and characterization of exotoxin(s) of *Shigella dysenteriae* Type 1. *J. infect. Dis.* **131**: 559–566.

MESROBEANU, I., MESROBEANU, L., GEORGESCO, M., DRĂGHICI, D., ALĂMITA, L. and LEREMIA, T. (1962) Action des toxines microbiennes sur les cultures de tissus. III. Action cytotoxique des endotoxines thermolabiles (neurotoxines) des germes gram-négatifs. *Archs roum. Path. exp. Microbiol.* **21**: 19–30.

MILDVAN, D., GELB, A. M. and WILLIAM, D. (1977) Venereal transmission of enteric pathogens in male homosexuals. Two case reports. *J. Am. med. Ass.* **238**: 1387–1389.

MISIEWICZ, J. J., WALLER, S. L. and EISNER, M. (1966) Motor responses of human gastrointestinal tract to 5-hydroxytryptamine *in vivo* and *in vitro*. *Gut* **7**: 208–216.

MOORE, D. G., YANCEY, R. J., LANKFORD, C. E. and EARHART, C. F. (1980) Bacteriostatic enterochelin-specific immunoglobulin from normal human serum. *Infect. Immun.* **27**: 418–423.

MORGAN, W. T. J. (1937) Studies in immunochemistry. II. The isolation and properties of a specific antigenic substance from *B. dysenteriae* (Shiga). *Biochem. J.* **31**: 2003–2021.

MORGAN, W. T. J. and PARTRIDGE, S. M. (1940) Studies in immunochemistry. 4. The fractionation and nature of antigenic material isolated from *Bact. Dysenteriae* (Shiga). *Biochem. J.* **34**: 169–191.

MORGAN, W. T. J. and SCHUTZE, H. (1943) Prophylactic inoculation with the O antigen of *Bact. Shigae. Lancet* ii: 284–285.

MULDER, J. B. (1971) Shigellosis in nonhuman primates: A review. *Lab. Animal Sci.* **21**: 734–738.

NEISSER, M. and SHIGA, K. (1903) Ueber freie receptoren von typhus- und dysenterie-bazillen und über das dysenterie-toxin. *Dt. med. Wschr.* **29**: 61–62.

O'BRIEN, A. D., THOMPSON, M. R., GEMSKI, P., DOCTOR, B. P. and FORMAL, S. B. (1977) Biological properties of *Shigella flexneri* 2A toxin and its serological relationship to *Shigella dysenteriae* 1 toxin. *Infect. Immun.* **15**: 796–798.

O'BRIEN, A. D., GENTRY M. K., THOMPSON, M. R., DOCTOR, B. P., GEMSKI, P. and FORMAL, S. B. (1979) Shigellosis and *Escherichia coli* diarrhea: relative importance of invasive and toxigenic mechanisms. *Am. J. clin. Nutr.* **32**: 229–233.

O'BRIEN, A. D., LaVECK, G. D., GRIFFIN, D. E. and THOMPSON, M. R. (1980) Characterization of *Shigella dysenteriae* 1 (Shiga) toxin purified by anti-shiga toxin affinity chromatography. *Infect. Immun.* **30**: 170–179.

OKELL, C. C. and BLAKE, A. V. (1930) Dysentery toxin (Shiga): notes on its preparation with a discussion of its position as an endotoxin. *J. Path. Bact.* **33**: 57–63.

OLENICK, J. G. and WOLFE, A. D. (1980) Shigella toxin inhibition of binding and translocation of polyuridylic acid by *Escherichia coli* ribosomes. *J. Bact.* **141**: 1246–1250.

OLITSKY, P. K. and KLIGLER, I. J. (1920) Toxins and antitoxins of *Bacillus dysenteriae* Shiga. *J. exp. Med.* **31**: 19–33.

OLITZKI, L. and LEIBOWITZ, J. (1935) Toxicity and antigenic properties of different fractions of *B. dysenteriae* (Shiga). *Br. J. exp. Path.* **16**: 523–531.

OLITZKI, L. and AVINERY, S. (1937) The hypothermic factor of *B. dysenteriae* Shiga. *Br. J. exp. Path.* **18**: 316–321.

OLITZKI, L. and KOCH, P. K. (1943) Production of potent toxins by *Shigella dysenteriae* (Shiga) in a synthetic medium. *Nature* **151**: 334.

OLITZKI, L. and BICHOWSKY, L. (1946) The preparation of a potent toxin of *Shigella dysenteriae* (Shiga) on a semi-synthetic medium and its use for the preparation of an alum-precipitated toxoid. *J. Immun.* **52**: 293–300.

OLITZKI, L., LEIBOWITZ, J. and BERMAN, M. (1937) Further investigations on the chemistry, toxicity and other biological properties of different fractions of dysentery bacteria. *Br. J. exp. Path.* **18**: 305–316.

OLITZKI, L., BENDERSKY, J. and KOCH, P. K. (1943) Studies on the toxins of *Shigella dysenteriae* (Shiga). *J. Immun.* **46**: 71–82.

OLSNES, S. and EIKLID, K. (1980) Isolation and characterization of *Shigella shigae* cytotoxin. *J. biol. Chem.* **255**: 284–289.

OSATO, M. S., BRAWNER, T. A. and HENTGES, D. J. (1979) *In vitro* inhibition of DNA, RNA, and protein synthesis by *Shigella dysenteriae* type 1 enterotoxin. *Am. J. clin. Nutr.* **32**: 268.

PAULK, H. T., CARDAMONE, A. O., GOTTERRER, G. S. and HENDRIX, T. R. (1977) Secretory and cyclic AMP (cAMP) responses to shigella enterotoxin (ST) and cholera enterotoxin (CT). *Gastroenterology* **72**: 1164.

PENNER, A. and BERNHEIM, A. I. (1960) Studies in the pathogenesis of experimental dysentery intoxication. Production of lesions by introduction of toxin into the cerebral ventricles. *J. exp. Med.* **111**: 145–153.

PERRY, R. D. and SAN CLEMENTE, C. L. (1979) Siderophore synthesis in *Klebsiella pneumonia* and *Shigella sonnei* during iron deficiency. *J. Bact.* **140**: 1129–1132.

PFEIFFER, R. and UNGERMANN, E. (1909) Zur Antitoxinfrage bei der Dysenterie. *Zentbl. Bakt. ParasitKde., Abt. I, Orig.* **50**: 534–541.

PHILLIPS, S. F. (1972) Diarrhea: a current view of the pathophysiology. *Gastroenterology* **63**: 495–518.

RAŠKOVÁ, H. and VANĚČEK, J. (1958) Action of the *Shigella shigae* toxin after intracerebral injection. *Nature* **181**: 1129–1130.

ROBERTSON, R. C. (1922) The toxins of *B. dysenteriae* Shiga. *Br. med. J.* **2**: 729–730.

ROSENBERG, M. L., WEISSMAN, J. B., GANGAROSA, E. J., RELLER, L. B. and BEASLEY, R. P. (1976) Shigellosis in the United States: ten year review of nationwide surveillance. *Am. J. Epidemiol.* **104**: 543–551.

ROSENTHAL, L., (1904) Das Dysenterietoxin (auf natüreichem wege gewonnen) *Dt. med. Wschr.* **30**: 235.

ROUT, W. R., FORMAL, S. B., GIANNELLA, R. A. and DAMMIN, G. J. (1975) Pathophysiology of shigella diarrhea in the Rhesus monkey: intestinal transport, morphological, and bacteriological studies. *Gastroenterology* **68**: 270–278.

SHIGA, K. (1898) Ueber den Dysenteriebacillus (*Bacillus dysenteriae*) *Zentbl. Bakt. ParasitKde., Abt. I, Orig.* **24**: 817–824.

SILVERSTEIN, S. C., STEINMAN, R. M. and COHN, Z. A. (1977) Endocytosis. *A. Rev. Biochem.* **46**: 669–722.

STEABBEN, D. A. (1943) A study on bacteriological lines of the antigens derived from *Bact. dysenteriae* Shiga and of their antisera in protective tests against the living organisms. *J. Hyg.* **43**: 83–95.

STEINBERG, S. E., BANWELL, J. G., YARDLEY, J. H., KEUSCH, G. T. and HENDRIX, T. R. (1975) Comparison of secretory and histological effects of shigella and cholera enterotoxins in rabbit jejunum. *Gastroenterology* **68**: 309–317.

ŠTULC, J. (1966) The influence of exotoxin *Shigella shigae* on the blood–brain barrier permeability to inorganic phosphate. *Life Sci.* **5**: 1801–1808.

ŠTULC, J. (1967) Site of *Shigella* exotoxin activity in mouse brain. *Am. J. Physiol.* **213**: 1053–1055.

TAKEDA, Y., OKAMOTO, K. and MIWATANI, T. (1977) Toxin from the culture filtrate of *Shigella dysenteriae* that causes morphological changes in Chinese hamster ovary cells and is distinct from the neurotoxin. *Infect. Immun.* **18**: 546–548.

TAKEDA, Y., OKAMOTO, K. and MIWATANI, T. (1979) Mitomycin C stimulates production of a toxin in shigella species that causes morphological changes in Chinese hamster ovary cells. *Infect. Immun.* **23**: 178–180.

TAL, C. (1950) Differences in toxicity of the S- and R-variants of *Shigella dysenteriae*. *J. Immun.* **65**: 221–227.

TAL, C. and OLITZKI, L. (1948) The toxic and antigenic properties of fractions prepared from the complete antigen of Shigella dysenteriae. *J. Immun.* **58**: 337–348.

THJØTTA, T. and SUNDT, O. F. (1921) Toxins of *Bact. dysenteriae*, Group III. *J. Bact.* **6**: 501–509.

THOMPSON, M. R., STEINBERG, M. S., GEMSKI, P., FORMAL, S. B. and DOCTOR, B. P. (1976) Inhibition of *in vitro* protein synthesis by *Shigella dysenteriae* 1 toxin. *Biochem. biophys. Res. Commun.* **71**: 783–788.

TODD, C. (1904) On a dysentery toxin and antitoxin. *J. Hyg.* **4**: 480–494.

VAILLARD, L. and DOPTER, C. (1903) La dysenterie epidemique. *Ann. Inst. Pasteur* **17**: 463–491.

VAN HEYNINGEN, W. E. (1971) The exotoxin of *Shigella dysenteriae* In: *Microbial toxins*, Vol. **IIA**, pp. 255–269, KADIS, S., MONTIE, T. C., AJL, S. J. (eds). Academic Press, N.Y.

VAN HEYNINGEN, W. E. and GLADSTONE, G. P. (1953a) The neurotoxin of *Shigella dysenteriae* 1. Production, purification and properties of the toxin. *Br. J. exp. Path.* **34**: 202–216.

VAN HEYNINGEN, W. E. and GLADSTONE, G. P. (1953b) The neurotoxin of *Shigella shigae*. 3. The effect of iron on production of the toxin. *Br. J. exp. Path.* **34**: 221–229.

VAN HEYNINGEN, W. E. and GLADSTONE, G. P. (1953c) The neurotoxin of *Shigella shigae* 4. A semi-micro method for the flocculation assay of the toxin. *Br. J. exp. Path.* **34**: 230–231.

VICARI, G., OLITZKI, A. L. and OLITZKI, Z. (1960) The action of the thermolabile toxin of *Shigella dysenteriae* on cells cultivated *in vitro*. *Br. J. exp. Path.* **41**: 179–189.

WAALER, E. (1936) Studies on the toxin production of the Shiga bacilli. *J. exp. Med.* **63**: 1–15.

WEINBERG, E. D. (1978) Iron and infection. *Microbiol. Rev.* **42**: 45–66.

WEISSMAN, J. B., SCHMERLER, A., WEILER, P., FILICE, G., GODBEY, N. and HANSEN, I. (1974) The role of preschool children and day-care centers in the spread of shigellosis in the community. *J. Pediatr.* **84**: 797–802.

CHAPTER 14

PROPERTIES AND PHARMACOLOGICAL ACTION OF PLAGUE MURINE TOXIN

THOMAS C. MONTIE

Department of Microbiology, University of Tennessee, Knoxville, Tenn. 37916, U.S.A.

1. INTRODUCTION

The disease, plague, described ominously throughout history as the black death is caused by *Yersinia pestis* (formerly *Pasteurella pestis*). Although, seemingly not a problem in the modern industrial world, a number of cases appear in the Western United States annually. Wild rodents, rats, mice, squirrels and prairie dogs harbor the disease organism in a quiescent or semi-quiescent form. It is spread commonly by the flea from rodents to humans generally during epizootics. The epizootics so frequently noted to precede pandemics in historical accounts are significant in the spread of disease.

Bubonic plague is primarily a disease of rats and other rodents that is accidentally conveyed to man by fleas. Since fleas prefer the blood of rats, it is probable that they turn to man only when rats are scarce. An outbreak of plague in man tends to follow directly the epidemic decimation of plague diseased rats. Transmission of the disease to man via the flea, is an accidental phenomenon, since the flea is primarily searching for blood and regurgitates the bacilli which have accumulated in its digestive system.

The most common form of the disease in humans is bubonic plague, which in addition to fever and malaise is characterized by the enlargement of regional lymph nodes (buboes) at the site of bacterial cell proliferation. Another form, septicemic plague, is characterized by massive invasion of the blood stream from lymph nodes, resulting usually in toxemic death after 18 h to 3 days. A rarer, but more virulent, and fatal form of plague is the pneumonic form. Bacteria colonize in the lungs in this case and may be spread among humans by the coughing up of sputum and blood due to congested air passages.

The relationship of specific toxic entities in evoking the disease remains obscure. The high potency for rodents of protein murine toxin, which is the subject of this paper, would certainly contribute to lethality in infected animals during epizootics.

One can speculate that the survival value for the microorganism may be enhanced by production of murine toxin. This may occur because the toxin promotes the death of rodents resulting in increased feeding areas for fleas, therefore insuring a continuous spread and migration of toxigenic plague bacillus to other wild reservoirs. As a consequence the disease cycle continues uninterrupted. It is quite likely that in addition to the murine toxin, the endotoxin (Butler and Moller, 1977), purified by Albizo and Surgalla (1970), together with other bacterial cellular components (Brubaker 1972), is important in the overall disease syndrome in humans (Brubaker, 1972, Butler and Moller, 1977).

Our work has been concerned primarily with the protein murine toxin of *Y. pestis*. In this discussion we will introduce the subject by pointing up key features of the protein structure. This will be followed by a brief historical outline of experiments attempting to identify the biochemical activity of the toxin. Finally some apparently misleading conclusions with respect to toxin action on mitochondrial respiration are properly corrected by more recent studies emphasizing the likely role of the toxin as a β-adrenergic blocking agent. The latter investigations will be the major focus of this review.

2. COMPOSITION AND CHEMISTRY

In one sense, classifying plague murine toxin as an exotoxin is a misnomer, since evidence indicates that toxin is located in the envelope (membrane) of the bacterial cell and is not released until cellular autolysis occurs. This does not imply that it is an endotoxin, since typical lipopolysaccharide components are not associated with purified murine toxin.

Two highly purified murine toxin proteins have been isolated and designated toxins A and B (Montie and Ajl, 1970). The molecular weight of toxin A (240,000) is twice that of toxin B (120,000), and this is reflected in the sedimentation constants, 10.9S and 7.6S, respectively. Their properties are similar enough to suggest that both toxin components originate from a common structure in the $Y.\ pestis$ cytoplasmic membrane. It is interesting in this regard that 50 per cent of the toxin residues are hydrophobic amino acids. An anatomical origin in the membrane may be significant in explaining protein amino acid composition and hydrophobic properties which, in turn, may be revealing in interpretation of modes of toxin binding on and penetration into receptor cells. Both toxin proteins have a high content of acidic amino acids. Of greater significance (to be discussed below) is the low content of cysteine residues, 1/12,000 mol wt. Toxin B exhibits a 33 per cent lower level in tryptophan content compared with A. This difference can be accounted for by the presence of an unlike polypeptide chain (12,000 mol wt) occurring in each toxin, and probably contributing to the higher specific toxic activity associated with the A protein. A like chain identified by phenol-urea gel electrophoresis in both toxins, and no doubt representing the identical tryptic peptides observed in fingerprint comparisons of the two proteins probably accounts for toxicity of the A and B molecules. Both toxins A and B are polymeric proteins containing 5 or 10 subunits (24,000 mol wt), each subunit being composed of two chains of 12,000 (S value in sodium dodecyl sulfate [SDS] = 1.7).

An interesting aspect of these studies has been experiments concerned with detergent dissociation of the protein (Montie and Montie, 1971). High concentrations (0.5–1.0%) of SDS dissociate toxin to biologically active subunits or chains (24,000 to 12,000) with toxicity equivalent to the original polymer. Therefore, only a 12,000 unit may be needed for penetration and disruption of host-cell function. The requirement for only a portion of toxin polymer to exercise the *coup de grâce* to the cell seems to be more common in biology than previously realized. It appears, for example, that the diphtheria and cholera toxins exhibit such properties. Mechanisms for dissociation of aggregates may exist at the host-cell surface and involve chemical or enzymatic reactions with surface components.

If toxin is dissolved in 0.1% SDS, intermediate size oligomers are formed (2.5S). Treatment with 0.05% SDS causes little to no dissociation, but toxin is chemically perturbed. Addition of 0.05% detergent, although not affecting toxicity or quarternary structure, apparently alters tertiary structure so that certain active site probes can be utilized effectively (Montie and Montie 1973). Experiments conducted with toxin A perturbed with 0.05% SDS documented the essentiality of —SH groups and tryptophan residues for toxic activity. Toxin was titrated with Ag^+ and Hg^{2+} and, at equivalent metal concentrations to —SH group, toxicity was significantly reduced. Further evidence was obtained for the importance of —SH groups as follows: (i) detoxification and quenching of fluorescence occurred with fluorscein mercuric acetate (a specific reagent for —SH residues); (ii) competition of Ag^+ with fluorescein mercuric acetate showed specificity of Ag^+ for —SH; (iii) quenching of tryptophan fluorescence emission occurred by mercaptide bond formation; (iv) a Hg-cysteine complex was isolated and identified after toxin degradation. Evidence obtained for the involvement of tryptophan in the essential toxic site is as follows: (i) binding of Hg^{2+} directly to toxin tryptophan residue indicated by the appearance of a different spectrum peak at 298 nm; (ii) suggestive evidence for Hg^{2+} bound to tryptophan in an isolated tryptic peptide; (iii) quenching of tryptophan fluorescence by mercaptide formation suggestive of proximity of tryptophan to essential —SH site; (iv) inhibition of toxin A biosynthesis (and possibly toxin B activity) by the addition of tryptophan analogues to growing cells.

In summary, we view the essential toxin site as containing a single —SH group adjacent to a tryptophan residue. Heavy metals are bound to the —SH by a covalent bond and interact weakly with the tryptophan residue. It is now possible to modify toxicity in a rather subtle, but selective, manner. Eventually, this approach can be used to understand the interaction between toxin and receptor site in the host cell.

3. METABOLIC ACTIVITY AND MODE OF ACTION

The effect of partially purified toxin on mitochondrial respiration of heart and liver cells was studied over the period 1958–1966 (Kadis and Ajl, 1970). These results can be summarized briefly in the following statements. Toxin has been shown to inhibit oxygen uptake in the presence of a number of Krebs cycle acids. The blocked step was identified as the reduced nicotinamide adenine dinucleotide-coenzyme Q reductase activity of the electron transport system. In addition, toxin induced mitochondrial swelling and altered the ability of mitochondria to accumulate Ca^{2+} and inorganic phosphate. It was also shown that heart mitochondria of rats were susceptible, whereas heart mitochondria of rabbits, a resistant species, were resistant. The latter experiment, together with the observation that intoxicated rats exhibited an alteration in the electrocardiogram, suggested to these investigators (Kadis and Ajl, 1970) that animals died from heart failure because of mitochondrial malfunction. A disturbing fact, however, has been the high concentrations of toxin needed to block respiration, 0.5–2.0 mg/ml of mitochondrial suspension compared with 0.5–3.0 per mouse required for lethality.

In a related report, Hildebrand et al. (1966), using a relatively pure preparation of toxin did not find heart failure to be directly involved. Their data indicated that circulatory failure following peripheral vascular collapse was the lethal event which led to heart failure.

The inconsistency reflected by these reports suggested the possibility that a primary site of lethal action was not yet identified. This idea prompted a re-examination of toxin effects on the whole animal so that no possible mechanism of action would be arbitrarily excluded.

One of the first clues to the mode of action of toxin came when Wennerstrom observed that mice that were fasted, made diabetic, or placed at an ambient temperature of 37° were less susceptible to toxin (Wennerstrom et al., 1977). On the other hand, mice put on a fat-free diet or placed at a lowered ambient temperature showed increased susceptibility to toxin. The addition of cAMP, glucagon or cortisone partially decreased toxicity. Toxin partially blocked the effect of epinephrine on fatty acid mobilization and capacity to induce hyperglycemia.

These results, particularly the effects on carbohydrate metabolism, at first suggested to us the possibility that toxin was in some way increasing the insulin level. By use of a radio-insulin, antibody titration however it was demonstrated that plasma immunoreactive insulin was not elevated after challenge with toxin. A second theory was suggested that toxin itself was acting as an 'insulin-like' molecule, but, results from repeated experiments with fat cells in vitro showed no stimulation by toxin of glucose incorporation into fat cells. Later experiments indicated a more direct action of toxin on the β-adrenergic system (Brown and Montie, 1977).

Schar and Meyer (1956) using crude toxin preparations had noted that the clotting time of mouse blood obtained from toxemic mice was at least doubled. These authors further reported peripheral vascular collapse implicating serotonin as a possible agent inducing the shock syndrome. Since mast cell degranulation can be blocked by increasing cAMP the effects of toxin on this system were investigated. Wennerstrom (1973) found no evidence for a role of the plasma clotting mechanism in toxicosis. Three results indicated that toxin was not working via this mechanism. First, no increase in serotonin could be found in intoxicated rats or mice when measured by a fluorometric method. (Garattini and Valzelli, 1965). An indirect measurement of heparin release (a product of degranulation along with serotonin) from mast cells, i.e., plasma clotting time, failed to reveal any abnormalities in clotting time in toxin challenged mice or rats. Addition of reserpine, which is known to deplete serotonin levels in vivo (Wennerstrom, 1973), failed to alter toxin lethal activity further negating a role for serotonin in the intoxication process.

An important point which emerged from these early studies, was that all of the conditions which obviated toxin activity are also conditions which raise the level of cAMP in cells and subsequently lead to the mobilization of energy substrates. In fact, as mentioned above, addition of dibutyryl cAMP directly modified the lethal effects of toxin.

A series of studies were undertaken in my laboratory to clarify the above mechanism (Brown and Montie, 1977, Brown, 1976). To test the involvement of cAMP, attempts were made to artificially lower the cAMP level in mice using cAMP antiserum. The antiserum was injected at two h intervals beginning at time zero when toxin was injected at the level of 1 LD_{50}. Lethality was increased to 100 per cent in antiserum treated animals from 38 per cent lethality in controls. Thus, neutralization of cAMP (i.e. lowered cAMP levels) correlated with increased toxicity.

A direct approach to demonstrate the effect of toxin on the adenylate cyclase system in the whole animal involved utilization of sublethal doses of cholera toxin. It is well established that cholera toxin permanently activates adenylate cyclase. Apparently, this occurs by potentiating the activating effects of GTP via ADP ribosylation of the presumed GTP sensitive, nucleotide regulatory component (Rodbell 1980, Gill and Meren 1978) and inhibiting GTP hydrolysis (Cassel, and Selinger 1977). Plague toxin (1–2 LD_{50}) was injected i.m. followed immediately by i.p. injection of cholera toxin. Cholera toxin provided 73 per cent protection from 2 LD_{50} and complete protection from 1 LD_{50} of plague toxin. There was also a 50 per cent increase in time of death in animals receiving cholera toxin. These data indicated that: (1) the adenylate cyclase system is functional in plague toxin treated animals, and (2) that the site of toxin action is prior to the stimulation of adenylate cyclase. Exploration of the latter hypothesis produced evidence consistent with an inhibition site for toxin at a hormone receptor.

The effects of selected hormones on lethality were examined using epinephrine or glucagon. Glucagon provided up to 71 per cent protection from lethality and an increase of up to 60 per cent in mean time of death in toxin challenged mice. Epinephrine injected under the same experimental conditions, on the other hand, provided only minor protection and no evidence for an alteration in time until death. Controls injected with heated toxin were unaffected.

Results from preliminary experiments led us to suggest that toxin could inhibit epinephrine-induced mobilization of glucose and fatty acids (Wennerstrom, et. al., 1977). In confirmation, and to further understand the physiological and metabolic activity of plague toxin, mobilization of free fatty acids (FFA) from triglycerides was measured in hormone-stimulated mice (Brown and Montie, 1977). Increased FFA in the blood correlates with increased cAMP stimulation of lipase catabolic activities. The results indicated that toxin is capable of blocking the metabolic activity of epinephrine, but not of glucagon. Levels of FFA in epinephrine-stimulated cells were reduced 35 per cent equivalent to nearly 100 per cent blockage of epinephrine stimulated levels. Glucagon-induced mobilization was unaffected by toxin. Toxin lowered the FFA level of unstimulated animals by 16 per cent. On the other hand, endotoxin isolated from *Yersinia pestis* showed a stimulation of endogenous FFA levels. To assess the significance of toxin block of epinephrine mobilization as a *primary* reaction, attempts were made to determine the earliest time at which toxin inhibition of FFA could be measured. The first detectable block ocurred 75 min after the injection of toxin and increased in a linear manner for 2 hr. Since a metabolic defect could be indentified which preceded symptoms and lethality by two to 4 hr we maintain that this reflects a primary event leading to a sequence of metabolic reactions capable of causing death.

Further evidence supporting the importance of the epinephrine block in lethality was provided by experiments in which a killing curve of titrated toxins was compared to the effects on epinephrine block of FFA mobilization (Fig. 1). It is apparent from these data that a strong correlation exists between the dose required for lethality and the dose necessary for a block of FFA.

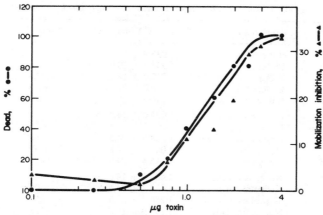

FIG. 1. Correlation between lethality and blockage of epinephrine-mobilized FFA. Mice were injected i.p with graded doses of toxin. At 2 h postinjection, one group of mice for each dosage was treated with 10 μg of epinephrine and bled after 10 min, and the plasma FFAs were estimated. A second group of mice for each dosage remained untreated for the determination of percent lethality. Symbols: ●, per cent lethality; ▲, per cent inhibition of epinephrine-induced mobilization of FFA. (From Brown, S. D. and Montie, T. C. (1977), Inf. Immun.)

We reasoned if toxin were capable of blocking the epinephrine response then it should be theoretically possible to circumvent the blocked step by injection of cAMP. Injection of cAMP into mice increased lipolysis up to 35 per cent when it was injected $1\frac{1}{2}$ hr post toxin injection. Toxin had almost no effect, in blocking this response.

If the early block of FFA mobilization is correlated with a lethal event(s), then it should be possible to by-pass the blocked step not only with cAMP, but also with catabolite products which result from increased cAMP activity. This prediction was validated. Injection of palmitic acid provided up to 60 per cent protection. Similar experiments were conducted to determine the effect of a variety of saturated fatty acids on lethality. Protection increased with increasing chain length from C_8 to C_{18}. Acids with chains of C_{11} and C_{18} gave maximum protection, from 50 to 60 per cent. The unsaturated acids oleic and linoleic (C_{18}) were not as protective (30–40 per cent under the same conditions). Butyric acid was completely ineffective.

Other energy yielding compounds gave results similar to those with the fatty acids. A variety of tricarboxylic and organic acids gave up to 60 per cent protection from lethality (e.g., citrate), and up to 98 per cent increase in mean time of death. In other experiments glucose was capable of providing 40 per cent protection. Adenosine triphosphate and NADH + H^+, although not directly modifying lethality, increased the mean time of death up to 100 per cent.

Fortuitous events contributed to our further understanding of the effects of plague toxin on metabolism. These early observations (Wennerstrom et al., 1977) added a segment of information which provided a reasonable explanation connecting early metabolic aberrations discussed above with lethal events. During the onset of these studies, it was observed that mice placed at ambient temperatures from 30–35°, because of a temporary absence of appropriate cooling of the laboratory, were not as susceptible to the toxin as mice held below that temperature. The experiments pointing to a block in catecholamine activity stimulated a more careful investigation of the apparent importance of adrenergic response and rodent body temperature. Mice were fasted for 4 hr at 4, 17, 25 or 37°. The mice were then injected with 1 LD_{50} of toxin (at 23°) and returned to their respective temperatures. A striking correlation between ambient temperature of incubation and susceptibility was evident. In mice placed at 5° toxin caused death of 100 per cent, 80 per cent at 17°, 40 per cent at 25° and at 37° all mice survived. These results indicate that mice challenged with plague toxin are unable to generate sufficient heat to maintain critical body temperature. The hypothesis was further substantiated by measuring the capacity of toxin to block FFA mobilization by epinephrine at various

TABLE 1. *Comparison of toxin to beta-adrenergic blocking agents*[a]

Challenge	Treatment	Plasma FFA (μeq/liter)	Change (%)	P
Buffer	Buffer	935.9 ± 12.8		
Ht toxin	Buffer	948.7 ± 20.9	−1.4	NS[b]
Toxin	Buffer	717.9 ± 14.8	−23.3	0.01
DCI	Buffer	1,000.0 ± 20.1	+6.8	NS
PROP	Buffer	846.2 ± 20.1	−9.6	0.05
Buffer	Dopamine	1,025.6 ± 14.8		
Ht toxin	Dopamine	1,000.0 + 20.1	−2.5	NS
Toxin	Dopamine	1,038.5 ± 24.5	+1.3	NS
DCI	Dopamine	1,089.7 ± 14.8	+6.3	NS
PROP	Dopamine	1,115.4 ± 24.5	+8.8	NS
Buffer	Norepinephrine	1,487.2 ± 14.8		
Ht toxin	Norepinephrine	1,474.3 ± 24.5	−0.8	NS
Toxin	Norepinephrine	1,256.4 ± 20.9	−15.5	0.01
DCI	Norepinephrine	1,294.9 ± 12.8	−12.9	0.01
PROP	Norepinephrine	1,320.5 ± 12.8	−11.2	0.01
Buffer	Epinephrine	1,641.3 ± 14.8		
Ht toxin	Epinephrine	1,628.2 ± 24.5	−0.8	NS
Toxin	Epinephrine	1,320.5 ± 12.8	−19.5	0.001
DCI	Epinephrine	1,448.7 ± 12.8	−11.7	0.01
PROP	Epinephrine	1,448.7 ± 12.8	−11.7	0.01
Buffer	Isoproterenol	1,807.7 ± 12.8		
Ht toxin	Isoproterenol	1,787.5 ± 51.5	−1.1	NS
Toxin	Isoproterenol	1,128.2 ± 14.8	−37.6	0.001
DCI	Isoproterenol	1,410.3 ± 20.9	−22.0	0.001
PROP	Isoproterenol	1,192.3 ± 12.8	−34.0	0.001

[a]Mice were treated i.p with either 0.1 ml of buffer, 3 μg of toxin, 3 μg of Ht toxin, 0.5 mg of dichloroisoproterenol (DCI), or 5.0 mg of propranolol (PROP). After 2 h, the mice were injected with buffer, 10 μg of dopamine, 10 μg of norepinephrine, 10 μg of isoproterenol. After 10 min the mice were bled and processed for FFA.
[b]NS, not significant.
(From Brown, S. D. and Montie, T. C. (1977) *Inf. Immun.*)

temperatures (Brown and Montie, 1977). It was found that mobilization was blocked at 5° and 25°, but not at 37°. This would explain the lack of lethality at 37°.

Catecholamine stimulation of β-adrenergic receptors results in an activation of adenylate cyclase, with a corresponding increase in cAMP leading to release of FFA. The blockade of FFA mobilization by the toxin suggested it was acting in a manner similar to that of known β-adrenergic blocking agents. This concept was tested by comparing the effects of toxin to those of known β-blockers. The results are shown in Table 1. Toxin exceeded the activity of the known blockers, dichloroiosproterenol (DCI) and propranolol (PROP), when injected two h preceding the addition of either dopamine, norepinephrine, epinephrine or isoproterenol (those compounds stimulated FFA levels 10, 60, 75 and 93 per cent respectively). By examining the pattern of responses of the β-blockers to each agonist, it became apparent that the relative effectiveness of the standard antagonists to each agonist paralleled the response elicited by toxin.

4. SUMMARY AND DISCUSSION

The proposed pharmacological mode of action of plague murine toxin can best be depicted by reference to Fig. 2. Metabolic blocking of the β-adrenergic receptor by the toxin, possibly through —SH and tryptophan interactions, is indicated. It is interesting to note in a recent publication by Vauquelin *et al.* (1979) that evidence exists for a requirement for essential disulfide bonds for maximum activation of B_1-adrenergic receptor sites. Any agent that reduces these bonds including SH reagents will cause a block of agonist binding. Both agonists and antagonists will protect the binding sites of a radiolabeled antagonist against inactivation by dithiothreitol. It may be that toxin acts to disrupt these disulfide bonds because an unblocked —SH is required for maximum

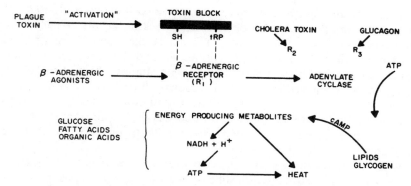

FIG. 2. Proposed action of plague murine toxin and the relation of the β-adrenergic block to subsequent metabolism. Separate receptors are R_1, R_2 and R_3.

toxicity (Montie and Montie, 1973). These groups may be implicated in reduction at the receptor site. A number of cells have been tested for their susceptibility to dithiothreitol. For example, C_6 glioma cells, rat liver membranes and avian erythrocytes are susceptible, but frog erythrocytes are not. Such differences in susceptibility could explain the selective action of toxin for rodents.

Explanation of the toxin effect by proposing a direct block of the β-adrenergic receptor is likely from results of a variety of experiments. A series of agonists was incapable of stimulating FFA production in intoxicated animals. Toxin blocked both endogenous and exogenous mobilization of fatty acids by epinephrine. Epinephrine was ineffective in reversing toxicity. In experiments with the compounds cortisone, glucagon, and cholera protection against toxin was evident, emphasizing that toxin was acting prior to adenylate cyclase, and that the cyclase system was not altered. Both cAMP and glucagon by-passed the toxin block and protected against both toxicity and metabolic inhibition of FFA increases. The capacity of compounds such as cholera toxin and glucagon to reverse metabolic activities of toxin is consistent with many studies pointing to separate receptors for these compounds. The concept of an early block mediated by toxin is substantiated by the results showing that cAMP–induced metabolites reversed toxicity. Variation in the degree of protection provided by a given catabolite presumably is a function of degree of accumulation in certain tissues, penetration into critical cell sites, and specific energy generating capacity. An irreversible impairment of respiration by toxin as suggested previously (Kadis and Ajl, 1970) does not explain the observed results, since compounds capable of stimulating respiration and energy production successfully by-pass the β-adrenergic block.

A terminal consequence of a blocked β-adrenergic system is the inability of an animal to generate adequate heat (Fig. 2). Decreased thermogenesis in a cold environment can result in hypothermia and death. This is precisely what was observed. Lowering of ambient temperature of intoxicated mice caused increased lethality which was correlated with decreased FFA levels. Therefore, inhibited thermogenesis and a net loss of body heat provides a very plausible explanation of toxin lethal effects. Beta- blockers would adversely affect peripheral vasculature (vasodilation) and cardiac function, as well as adipose tissue lipolysis. These effects could well be working in concert to compromise the animal.

It has been conclusively demonstrated that the effects of catecholamines on FFA mobilization are mediated through beta-adrenergic receptors (Fain, 1967, Fain et al., 1966). Adrenergic blocking agents, defined as drugs capable of antagonizing the effects of adrenergic amines, are capable of modifying the responses produced by catecholamines. Dichloroisoproterenol (Powell and Slater, 1958) and propranolol (Wilson and Theclen, 1967) were found to selectively and specifically block beta-adrenergic responses. Although dopamine and dopamine antagonists are considered β-adrenergic receptors they are rather in a separate class. These receptors are specific for separate tissues, for example, certain brain regions and renal vasculature (Lefkowitz et al., 1976). All of the responses to toxin are characteristic of known β-blocking agents. When the toxin was compared directly with two of these agents (Table) 1), the results were strikingly apparent. The toxin exceeded the abilities of propranolol and dichloroisoproterenol to block FFA mobilization induced by a variety of adrenergic amines. None of the agents, including.toxin, significantly affected the minimal response elicited by dopamine. Of particular interest is the observation by Fain (1970) that propranolol markedly inhibited catecholamine-induced lipolysis, but had no effect on lipolysis due to db-cAMP. Identical results are observed for the plague murine toxin. These results strongly document the role of the toxin as a β-adrenergic blocking agent.

Studies with certain blocking agents provide an analogy to plague toxin effects. Experiments have shown that treatment with dibenzyline during cold exposure leads to hypothermia and death (Leduc, 1961). Moreover, in regard to species specificity of plague murine toxin for mice and rats, it has been shown that dibenzyline inhibits the epinephrine response in rats (Schwartz, 1962), but not in dogs (Maling et al., 1964), cats (J. T. Elder, 1965) or humans (Pilkington et al., 1962). Butoxamine, on the other hand, blocks the hyperglycemic effect of catecholamines in dogs (Salvador, 1965; Salvador, et al., 1966) and rats (Salvador et al., 1966), but not in humans (Hunninghake, 1966). Thus, it can be surmised that the species specificity exhibited by the plague murine toxin is entirely consistent with its role as an adrenergic antagonist.

Numerous attempts have been made to examine the effect of plague murine toxin as a beta blocking agent in vitro by using fat cells (data not shown). No consistent effects have been observed, even though the cells were both actively responding to hormones and metabolizing. A likely explanation is that the toxin requires activation in the animal to a form that can interact with fat cells. Biological activation of beta-adrenergic antagonists has precedence. Butoxamine inhibited the metabolic effects of epinephrine in vivo (Salvador et al., 1965), yet this β-blocker consistently failed to produce any observable activity in isolated fat cells (Fain et al., 1966). Activation of bacterial toxins by dissociated reduction and proteolytic fragmentation is an established phenomenon for clostridium toxin types E and B (Dasgupta and Sugiyama, 1976), diphtheria toxin (Collier, 1975), and cholera toxin (Gill and King, 1975). We have previously discussed that plague murine can be dissociated to active subunits of 12,000 to 24,000 daltons and that even low concentrations (0.01% of sodium dodecyl sulfate (Montie and Montie, 1971) initiated a subtle conformational change, exposing buried sulfhydryl groups (Montie and Montie, 1973). It is entirely possible then that the plague murine toxin may be biologically activated in a manner similar to botulinum toxin or known adrenergic antagonists.

An important feature of the metabolic evidence discussed above relates to the fact that these experiments were performed with physiological doses of toxin ($1–2\,LD_{50}$'s). Such levels are capable furthermore of being released from Y. pestis organisms and circulated in the diseased animal. From all the evidence therefore the only plausible mechanism of action proposed is that toxin interferes with the reception of β-adrenergic agonists.

Acknowledgements—This research was supported by NIH Biomedical Grants from The University of Tennessee, a Training Grant from NIH in Infectious Diseases, and the National Science Foundation (1969–1972).

REFERENCES

ALBIZO J. M. and SURGALLA M. J. (1970). Isolation and biological characterization of Pasteurella pestis endotoxin. Infect. Immun. 2: 229–336.

BROWN S. D. (1976). Beta-adrenergic blocking activity of Yersinia pestis murine toxin, Ph.D. dissertation, Univ. of Tenn. 86 pgs.

BROWN S. D. and MONTIE, T. C. (1977). Beta-adrenergic blocking activity of Yersinia pestis. Inf. Immun. 18: 85–93.

BRUBAKER, R. R. (1972). The genus Yersinia: biochemistry and genetics of virulence. Curr. Top. Microbiol. Immunol. 57: 111–158.

BUTLER, T. AND MOLLER G. (1977). Mitogenic response of mouse spleen cells and gelation of limulus lysate by lipopolysaccharide of Yersinia pestis and evidence for neutralization of the lipopolysaccharide of Yersinia pestis and evidence for neutralization of the lipopolysaccharide by polymyxin B. Inf. Immun. 18: 400–404.

CASSEL, D. AND SELINGER, Z. (1977). Mechanism of adenylate cyclase activation by cholera toxin: inhibition of GTP hydrolysis at the regulatory site. Proc. Natl. Acad. Sci., U.S.A. 74: 3307–3311.

COLLIER, R. J. (1975). Diphtherie toxin: mode of action and structure. *Bacteriol Rev.* 39: 54–85.

DASGUPTA, B. R., and SUGIYAMA (1976). Molecular forms of neurotoxins in proteolytic Clostridium botulinum type B cultures. *Infect. Immun.* 14: 680–686.

ELDERE, J. T. (1965). Antagonism and Potentiation of Epinepheine-Induced Hyperglycemia. *Fed. Proc.* 24: 150.

FAIN, J. N. (1967). Adrenergic blockage of hormone-induced lipolysis in isolated fat cells. *Ann. N. Y. Acad. Sci.* 139: 870–890.

FAIN, J. N. (1970). Dihydroergotamine, propranolol and the beta adrenergic receptors of fat cells. *Fed. Proc.* 29: 1402–1407.

FAIN, J. N. GALLON D. J., and KOVACEV V. P. (1966). Effects of drugs on the lipolytic action of hormones in isolated fat cells. *Mol. Pharmacol.* 2: 237–247.

GARRATTINI S. and VALZELLI, L. (1965). *Serotonin.* Elsevier Co., New York.

GILL, M. D. and KING, C. A. (1975). The mechanism of action of cholera toxin in pigeon erythrocytes lysates. *J. Biol. Chem.* 250: 6424–6432.

GILL, D. M. and MEREN, R. (1978). ADP-ribosylation of membrane proteins catalyzed by cholera toxin: basis of the activation of adenylate cyclase. *Proc. Natl. Acad. Sci.* 75: 3050–3054.

HILDEBRAND, G. J., NG, J., VON METZ, E. K. and EISLER, D. M. (1966). Studies on the mechanism of circulatory failure induced in rates by *Pasteurella pestis* murine toxin. *J. Infect. Dis.* 116: 615–629.

HUNNINGHAKE, D. B., AZARNOFF, D L. and WAXMAN, D. (1966). The effect of butoxamine on catecholamine-induced metabolic changes in humans. *Clin. Pharmacol. Ther.* 7: 470–476.

KADIS, S. and AJL, S. J. (1970). Site and mode of action of murine toxin of *Pasteurella pestis,* p. 39–67. *In* MONTIE, T. C. KADIS, S., AND AJL, S. J. (eds), Microbial toxins, Vol. 3. Academic Press Inc., New York.

LEDUC, J. (1961). Catecholamine production and release in exposure to cold. *Acta Physiol. Scand.* 53: 183S, 1.

LEFKOWITZ, R. J., LIMBIRD, L. E., MUKHERJEE, C. and CARON, M. G. (1976). The β-adrenergic receptor and adenylate cyclase. *Biochem. Biophys. Acta.* 457: 1–39.

MALING, H. M., WILLIAMS M. A., HIGHMAN, B. GORBUS, J. and HUNTER, J. (1964). Influence of phenoxy-benzamine and isopropylmethoxamine (BW61–43) on cardiovascular metabolic, and histopathologic effects of norepinephrine infusion in dogs. "Naunyn-Schmiedeberg's *Arch. Exp. Pathol. Pharmakol.*" 248: 52–72.

MONTIE, T. C. and AJL, S. J. (1971). Nature and synthesis of murine toxins of *Pasteurella pestis,* p. 1–37. *In* MONTIE, T. C., KADIS, S., and AJL, S. J. (eds), Microbial toxins, Vol. 3. Academic Press Inc., New York.

MONTIE, T. C. and MONTIE, D. C. (1971). Protein toxins of *Pasteurella pestis.* Subunit composition and acid binding. *Biochemistry* 70: 2094–2100.

MONTIE, T. C. and MONTIE, D. C. (1973). Selective detoxification of murine toxin from *Yersinia pestis.* Reaction of heavy metals with essential sulfhydryl and tryptophan residues. *Biochemistry,* 12: 4958–4965.

PILKINGTON, T. R. E., LOWE, R. D., ROBINSON, B. F. and TITTERINGTON, E. (1962). Effect of adrenergic blockage on glucose and fatty acid metabolism in man. *Lancet,* ii: 316–317.

POWELL, L. E. and SLATER, I. H. (1958). Blocking of inhibitory adrenergic receptors by a dichloro analog of isoproterenol. *J. Pharmacol.* 122: 480–489.

RODBELL, M. (1980). The role of hormone receptors and GTP-regulatory proteins in membrane transduction. *Nature,* 284: 17–22.

SALVADOR, R. A., APRIL S. A. and LEMBERGER (1966). Blockade by Butoxamine of the Catecholamine-Induced elevation of blood glucose and lactic-Acid. *Fed. Proc.* 25: 500.

SALVADOR, R. A., COLVILLE, K. I., and BURNS, J. J. (1965). Adrenergic mechanisms and lipid mobilization. *Ann. N. Y. Acad. Sci.* 131: 113–118.

SCHAR, M. and MEYER, K. F. (1956). Studies on immunization against plague. XV. The pathophysiologic action of the toxin of *Pasteurella pestis* in experimental animals. *Schweiz. Z. Pthol. Bakteriol.* 19: 51–70.

SCHWARTZ, N. B. (1962). Effect of dibenzynine on the metabolic actions of epinephrine and thyroxine. *Am. J. Physiol.* 302: 525–531.

VAUGUELIN, G., BOTTARI, S., KANOREK, L. and STROSBERG, A. D. (1979). Evidence for essential disulfide bonds in β_1-adrenergic receptors of turkey erythrocyte membranes. *J. Biol. Chem.* 254: 4462–4469.

WENNERSTROM, D. E. (1973). *Yensinia pestis* murine toxin: a study of its activity, Ph.D. dissertation, Univ. of Tenn., 61 pgs.

WENNERSTROM, D. E., BROWN, S. D. and MONTIE, T. C. (1977). Altered lethality of murine toxin from *Yersinia pestis* under various metabolic conditions. *Proc. Soc. Exp. Biol. Med.* 154: 78–81.

WILSON, W. B. and THECLEN, E. O. (1967). Beta-adrenergic blocking drugs as physiological tools in clinical medicine. *Ann. N. Y. Acad. Sci.* 139: 981–996.

CHAPTER 15

TOXIC FACTORS ASSOCIATED WITH
LEGIONELLA ORGANISMS

KENNETH. W. HEDLUND

*Division of Communicable Disease and Immunology, Walter Reed Army Institute of Research,
Washington, D.C. 20307*

1. INTRODUCTION

Unlike the standard introduction for the review of well recognized microbial toxins which may have been studied for decades, this introduction will first attempt to orient the reader with our present understanding about the spectrum of disease caused by infection with the *Legionella* organisms and then present the early rationale for postulating the existence of a toxin or toxins. There have been a variety of suspected bacterial toxic components. We are in the present position of evaluating the contributory role of each.

At the outset the reader should understand that the term *Legionella pneumophila* applies to the causative agent of the fatal outbreak of pneumonia that occurred among American Legion conventioneers in Philadelphia in the summer of 1976. In the mid-1980s other gram-negative organisms genetically distinct by DNA homology studies but phenotypically similar to *L. pneumophila* were given the genus name *Legionella* for "operational purposes" by Brenner *et al.* (1980) and this will be developed in greater detail later.

2. THE "NEW PNEUMONIA" AGENTS: CLINICAL ASPECTS THAT LED TO THE CONCEPT OF TOXIN

It is apparent that laboratories once primarily concerned with the recognition of the etiologic agent of Legionnaires' disease must now by necessity be able to recognize and study the ever expanding spectrum of "new pneumonia" agents. These "new pneumonias" have been clinical entities for years. As Weinstein (1980) has noted the only new feature is the identification of their specific etiologic agents, a group of gram-negative bacilli. A great debt is owed to both Fraser *et al.* (1977) and McDade *et al.* (1977) who were the first to isolate and identify the causative agent of Legionnaires' disease only six months after the 1976 Philadelphia outbreak. Their pioneering discovery and demonstration of the relationship between this previously unrecognized gram-negative bacteria and the illness caused by it have expanded medical horizons. Two clinical entities are now recognized as being caused by *L. pneumophila*. The first is the intensely studied pneumonic form of the illness called Legionnaires' disease which may involve patients ranging from 3 to 82 years of age. The initial symptoms are nondescriptive headaches, myalgias and general malaise. In one or two days there is a rapid temperature rise associated with chills. A moderate nonproductive cough is frequently present and the symptoms progress to include chest pain, abdominal pain, vomiting and mental confusion. Diarrhea is seen in approximately one-sixth of the patients and may precede other symptoms. The clinical course of this rapidly progressive

In conducting the research described in this report, the investigators adhered to the "Guide for the Care and Use of Laboratory Animals," as promulgated by the Committee on Care and Use of Laboratory Animals of the Institute of Laboratory Animal Resources, National Research Council. The facilities are fully accredited by the American Association for Accreditation of Laboratory Animal Care.

The views of the authors do not purport to reflect the positions of the Department of the Army or the Department of Defence.

fulminant pneumonia can be followed by chest x-rays that initially show patchy infiltrates that may have an interstitial or consolidated appearance which typically, in the untreated case, progress to a unilateral or bilateral nodular consolidation. Laboratory data may reveal both hepatic and renal compromise. Death is associated with respiratory failure or shock.

The second form of recognized legionellosis, as the collective term for diseases caused by *L. pneumophila* agents, has come to be termed, "Pontiac Fever". In July and early August 1968 an epidemic of acute febrile illness occurred which affected 144 people including 95 % of the employee staff in a County Health Department building in Pontiac, Michigan. Glick *et al.* (1978) described this syndrome as a relatively uniform self-limiting illness which sometimes began quite abruptly but more often was marked by progressive malaise, diffuse myalgias, and headaches. Usually the complete syndrome appeared within six hours. Localized muscle pains, dizziness, cough, nausea and mental confusion were common. Diarrhea was reported in 15 % of the patients. Respiratory symptoms were not significant although 57 % complained of a dry cough. This acute nonpulmonic form of legionellosis tended to last 2–5 days and there have been no reported deaths.

Although clinical attention was focused primarily on the pulmonic component of Legionnaires' disease it was the multisystem involvement of lungs, kidneys and central nervous system in certain Legionnaires' disease patients that led Friedman (1978) to postulate a bacterial toxin. At the same time and for an entirely different reason Winn *et al.* (1978), also postulated that a bacterial toxin might be elaborated by the *Legionella* organism to explain the histopathologic findings of lysis of inflammatory exudate cells and the infarct-like necrosis seen in alveolar walls in lung tissue obtained from a study of 14 patients who had died in the 1977 Vermont outbreak. Fraser *et al.* (1979) noted that what determined whether *L. pneumophila* causes Legionnaires' disease or Pontiac fever is entirely unknown. He suggested that Pontiac fever might be the result of a large dose of nontoxigenic organisms. At the time he made that suggestion, no *L. pneumophila* toxins were recognized. In early 1979 there was only one known serotype of *L. pneumophila*. At the time of this writing there are nine *L. pneumophila* serotypes which can be shown to be genetically related by DNA homology procedures. It is precisely this coupling of new technologic advances with heightened clinical awareness that led to an unprecedented explosion of information about previously unrecognized gram-negative bacteria which can cause both pulmonic and nonpulmonic illness. In addition to the increase in the numbers of known serotypes of *L. pneumophila*, there has also been the discovery and rediscovery of other gram-negative *Legionella*-like organisms capable of causing human disease. Pasculle *et al.* (1980) noted that certain of the newly recognized gram-negative bacteria are serologically and genetically distinct from *L. pneumophila*, but phenotypically resemble this organism in the type of pneumonic illness they cause, in growth requirements and in abundance of cellular branched chain fatty acids. Brenner *et al.* (1980) offered a tentative solution in classifying the newly recognized pneumonia agents. While recognizing that ideally a genus should contain a group of genetically and phenotypically related species, when both criteria cannot be met, phenotypic relatedness should take precedence to ensure that the genus designation is of practical value. Under this convention in addition to *L. pneumophila*, twenty one additional *Legionella* species have been included in this ever growing list since 1981.

3. POTENTIAL CANDIDATE TOXINS

Clinical speculations about the pathogenesis of Legionnaires' disease and the possibility of toxins preceded the offering of potential toxin candidates by a different group of scientists. The first classic candidate to have been considered in this gram-negative infection was of course the endotoxin lipopolysaccharide (LPS). Fumarola (1978) published a short letter stating that *L. pneumophila* organisms, then termed Legionnaires' disease agent, were limulus lysate-positive. Miragliotta (*et al.*, 1982), a coworker of Fumarola, subsequently published on the *in vitro* generation of procoagulant activity (tissue factor) when *Legionella* organisms undergo prolonged incubation with pure mononuclear cell suspensions. However Wong *et al.* (1979) have convincingly demonstrated that while indeed there is limulus lysate gelating activity, the "endotoxicity" detected by *in vitro* and *in vivo* biological assays seemed to be different from the classic endotoxicity associated with gram-negative organisms. With endotoxins from *Salmonella, Klebsiella, Escherichia*, and other gram-negative species, the limulus lysate test is 10–20 times more sensitive than the rabbit pyrogen test (Wong *et al.*, 1977; Ronneberger, 1977). There was a greater than 1000-fold difference between these two tests observed with *L. pneumophila*. In addition to their low pyrogenicity, *L. pneumophila* organisms were also found to be very weak in inducing hepatin-precipitable protein and Schwartzman reactions in rabbits. Endotoxicity was of a lower order as measured by Dactinomycin potentiation or polymyxin B inhibition. The author (Hedlund, unpublished data) has given as much as $15\,\mu g$ of 2-keto-3-deoxyoctonate (KDO) containing *L. pneumophila* LPS to AKR/J mice without lethal effect.

Baine *et al.* (1979a) were the first to suggest that an enzymatic exotoxin-like activity was associated with *L. pneumophila* organisms based on hemolysis of guinea pig red blood cells incubated in the presence of allantoic fluid in which *L. pneumophila* had grown. Later Baine *et al.* (1979b) also noted hemolytic activity in plasma and urine from *L. pneumophila*-infected rabbits. Unfortunately a direct connection could not be made, and Baine cautioned that indeed the hemolytic activity in the filtrate of allantoic fluid might not be due to the presence of bacterial hemolysins, inasmuch as normal allantoic fluid spontaneously developed hemolytic activity in the absence of contact with a healthy embryo.

Müller (1980) has shown that at least four strains of *L. pneumophila* could degrade α_1-acid glycoprotein, α_1-chymotrysin, β-lipoprotein, β-IgE-globulin and α_2-glycoprotein. He suggested that the pathogenic action of *L. pneumophila* might be due to the proteolytic activities, since the degraded proteins either belonged to the acute phase protein group or, as is the case with β-lipoproteins, were involved with nonspecific resistance against infection.

Berdal and Fossum (1982) demonstrated proteinase production was particularly high in strains of *L. pneumophila* and much lower in the other species. They concluded that these proteinases could be pathogenicity factors.

Friedman *et al.* (1980) demonstrated that culture filtrates of *L. pneumophila* were cytotoxic for Chinese hamster ovary cells. The cytotoxin was methanol-soluble, heat-stable and stable from pH 5–8. The cytotoxin was sensitive to pronase and papain and insensitive to trypsin. Friedman suggested that it was a small polypeptide, but large enough to be retained by a dialysis membrane with a molecular weight cut-off of 1000.

In contrast to a cytotoxin released by *L. pneumophila* under proper culture conditions, Katz *et al.* (1980) reported that macrophage monolayers obtained from guinea pigs, mice or rats were rapidly lysed on incubation with ten virulent *L. pneumophila* organisms per cell. Washed *L. pneumophila* caused destruction of 50% of mouse peritoneal macrophage monolayers after 4 hr incubation, when assessed by trypan blue exclusion, along with light and electron microscopy. They found that opsonization enhanced by specific antisera increased monolayer toxicity to greater than 95% in 4 hr. Phagocytic inhibition by cytochalasin-D and lidocaine caused a marked decrease in monolayer lysis. Supernatants of virulent *L. pneumophila* suspensions, and ultraviolet or heat-killed *L. pneumophila* were not toxic to macrophage monolayers. The rapid time course suggested that while viable organisms were necessary for macrophage destruction, intracellular replication was not. Katz therefore felt that the data were not consistent with the action of a preformed soluble toxin, but suggested intracellular release of a toxin as a basis for the observed macrophage toxicity.

Hedlund *et al.* (1979) initially demonstrated that *L. pneumophila* were lethal for AKR/J mice. Later Hedlund and Larson (1981) showed that cell-free sonicates of the same organism were also lethal when injected i.p. into AKR/J mice. Acid partition of this crude toxin preparation followed by gel filtration and preparative isotachophoresis of the resultant supernatant material yielded a 3,400 molecular weight toxin. At the time when these preliminary experiments on *L. pneumophila* toxin purification were being done, the other new genetically distinct *Legionella* agents were being recognized. It now was a simple matter to extend these findings and techniques to the new members of the *Legionella* family. Representatives of all the known *Legionella* species were kindly provided by both

Dr. Pasculle of the University of Pittsburgh School of Medicine, Pennsylvania, and the Center for Disease Control in Atlanta, Georgia. These organisms were subjected to the identical cultural, harvesting and toxin separation procedures that were used on *L. pneumophila* and previously reported (Hedlund and Larson, 1981). We drew attention to the fact that cell-free acid supernatants of sonicated *L. pneumophila* and the genetically distinct *L. micdadei* (Pittsburgh pneumonia agent) were lethal for AKR/J mice. We reported that both contained 3,400 molecular weight proteins which were antigenically identical. These extended studies demonstrate that *L. pneumophila* serotype I shares a common toxic low molecular weight antigen with all other genetically distinct *Legionella* species (Fig. 1).

Attempts were made to find *in vitro* correlates to the AKR/J animal lethality studies that might shed some light on pathogenic mechanisms. New Zealand BWJM mouse macrophages were grown for 48 hr in culture flasks containing Eagles Minimal Essential Medium/Nonessential amino acids medium with 10% fetal calf serum, 1% penicillin–streptomycin and 1% sodium pyruvate; incubation was at $37°C$. Cells were removed from the growth surface by gently rolling glass beads across them. The suspension had a cell count of 6.4×10^5 cells/ml with a viability of 95%. The control sample contained 1.0 ml of cell suspension and 0.5 ml of preparative isotachophoresis elution buffer (H_3PO_4 Tris, pH 7.04). The treated sample contained 1.0 ml of an identical cell suspension and 0.5 ml of the isolated isotachophoretic peak derived from *L. pneumophila* organisms. The samples were incubated in tightly capped 5-ml Falcon plastic tubes at $37°C$. Viabilities were determined by the standard trypan blue exclusion method. The results are shown in Fig. 2. It is apparent that within 4 hr the number of viable toxin-treated macrophages dropped to less than one-half of the control levels.

Another demonstration of *Legionella*'s toxic impact on cells normally involved in antimicrobial defense is provided by chemiluminescence (CL) studies by Hedlund (1981b). Basically polymorphonuclear leukocytes (PMN) emit CL after phagocytosis of certain opsonized particles, like bacteria. Light emission can be detected and quantitated in a liquid

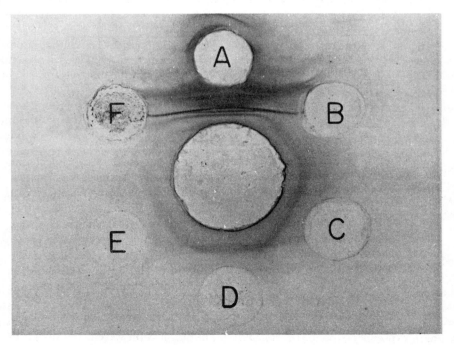

FIG. 1. The common *Legionella* toxin demonstrated by a line of identity connecting various *Legionella* species sources. A. *L. pneumophila*; B. *L. micdadei*; C. *L. bozemanii*; D. *L. dumoffii*; and E. *L. gormanii*; F. *E. coli* acid supernatant. Center well contains antibodies from *L. pneumophila*-immunized goat previously absorbed with *E. coli/pseudomonas* acid supernatant material.

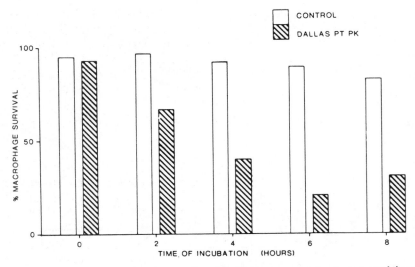

Fig. 2. Survival of mouse macrophages. Cross-hatched areas refer to *L. pneumophila* toxin challenged cells.

scintillation counter and appears to result from the ground state of electronically excited carbonyl groups, thought to be generated during singlet oxygen-mediated oxidation of the phagocytized substrate; one of the earliest studies by Stevens and Young (1976) demonstrated a correlation between resistance of certain strains of *E. coli* to opsonization and decreased *in vitro* killing, oxygen consumption, visual phagocytosis and CL responses of human granulocytes. Grebner *et al.* (1976) demonstrated parallel relationships between phagocytosis and CL under a variety of conditions designed to alter opsonization of bacteria. This led authors to the conclusion that the biochemical processes that control phagocytosis and CL may be closely related or interdependent. In addition to phagocytosis, Allen *et al.* (1974) also established the relationship of CL measurements resultant from superoxide anions and singlet molecular oxygen and the microbicidal activity of PMN. As noted by Trush *et al.* (1978) the CL response of phagocytic cells is dependent on cell metabolism and the measurement of CL represents a potentially useful index to assess the effects of pharmacologically toxic agents on phagocytic cells. To study the effects of *Legionella* toxin on CL, preparative isotachophore peaks obtained from *L. pneumophila* (Washington strain, serotype I) and *L. micdadei* were passed over an anion exchange column and two separate peaks were obtained (Fig. 3).

Similar bifid peaks could be obtained from the other *Legionella* species. CL techniques previously described by McCarthy *et al.* (1980), but specifically adapted to use human PMN as well as rat PMN were used to test the toxicity of the *Legionella* toxins. The results are shown in Fig. 4. It can be clearly seen that second peak consistently inhibits the CL activity of the PMN. Further evidence that *L. pneumophila* does indeed produce a toxin which depresses the oxidative metabolism of human polymorphonuclear leucocytes with the attendant sequelae has been subsequently been provided and expanded upon by the supporting work of Friedman *et al.* (1982) and Lochner *et al.* (1985).

The next question that arose was how readily can these "*in vitro*" similarities of antigenicity, molecular weight, toxic functions be translated into *in vivo* models? Could animals immunized with *L. pneumophila* be protected against a lethal challenge from genetically distinct *L. micdadei*? The following set of experiments were set up using the Washington strain serotype I, *L. pneumophila* and *L. micdadei* (Pittsburgh pneumonia agent) obtained from Dr. Pasculle. DNA homology studies were performed to document their genetic distinctness (Pasculle *et al.*, 1980). Using sublethal aliquots of acid supernatant material from both species of *Legionella* obtained by method previously described (Hedlund and Larson, 1981), AKR/J mice were inoculated and then boosted 28 days later. After 10 days

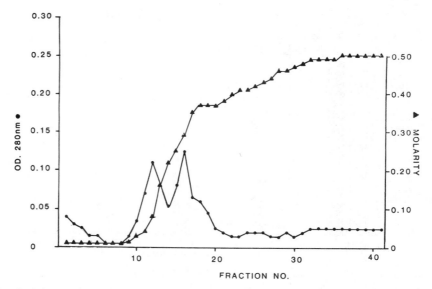

FIG. 3. Anion exchange separation of *Legionella pneumophila* of preparative tachophore peak. Only the second peak affected chemiluminescence.

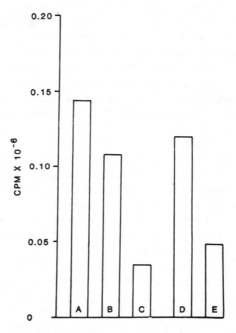

FIG. 4. Effect of *Legionella* toxin on PMN chemiluminescence. Column A is the bovine serum albumin control. B and C are 0.8-μg aliquots of the first and second anion exchange *L. micdadei* peaks. D and E are 0.8-μg aliquots of similar *L. pneumophila* anion exchange peaks.

they were challenged with either a lethal dose of viable *L. pneumophila* or *L. micdadei* or a lethal dose of acid supernatant material from the respective organisms. Nonimmunized mice were included for the appropriate lethal challenge controls. Results are shown in Table 1.

Animals immunized with *L. pneumophila* acid supernatant and challenged with a lethal inoculum of viable *L. pneumophila* or *L. micdadei* organisms are protected, as are animals given a lethal inoculation of *L. pneumophila* or *L. micdadei* acid supernatant. This cross-protection by a previously demonstrated single shared antigen was also confirmed when animals were immunized with *L. micdadei* acid supernatant and challenged with a lethal

TABLE 1. *Effect of Immunization of AKR/J Mice with* Legionella *Toxin*

Challenged	Survivors Total		Nonimmune
	Immune		
	L. pneumophila	*L. micdadei*	
1. *L. pneumophila* (A.S.*)	6/6		0/6
2. *L. pneumophila* (whole)	6/6		0/6
3. *L. micdadei* (whole)	6/6		1/6
1. *L. micdadei* (A.S.*)		6/6	0/6
2. *L. micdadei* (whole)		6/6	0/6
3. *L. pneumophila* (whole)		4/6	0/6

* Acid supernatant.

concentration of either viable *L. micdadei* or *L. pneumophila* organisms or their acid supernatants. Studies using *L. pneumophila* preparative tachophore peaks which contain the single shared, common antigen were used to protect animals with the same effectiveness as the acid supernatant preprations, although in this low molecular weight form they are probably less efficient as an antigen and harder to obtain.

4. SUMMARY

This is a chapter on *Legionella* toxins that is still being written. It originally started as a review based just on *L. pneumophila* at a time before the operational designations *L. micdadei*, *F. dumoffii*, *F. gormanii* and *L. bozemanii* were even suggested. The role of *Legionella* lipopolysaccharides with their limited expression of classic endotoxicity as well as the role of the various enzyme components found are still being evaluated, but appear to be of limited impact. The role of the various proteolytic enzymes described by both Muller (1980) and Berdal and Fossum (1982) may also play a role in the diseases caused by these recently recognized gram negative organisms.

At present there are no amino acid analysis studies, no receptor site studies, and no molecular mechanism of action analyses, but we still are in early times. What we do know is that there is a low molecular weight protein of approximately 3,400 daltons which can be isolated after disruption of the intact organism. This single common toxic moiety is shared by *L. pneumophila* serotype I and *L. micdadei*, *F. dumoffii*, *L. bozemanii* and *F. gormanii*. The toxin is capable of killing mouse macrophages and suppressing the oxidative metabolism of rat and human polymorphonuclear leukocytes. This induced depressed metabolic state has been associated with impaired phagocytic and bactericidal activity.

Whether or not this low molecular weight protein is an intact toxin or simply a biologically active piece of the parent molecule is not known at this time. The low molecular weight supernatant cytotoxin described by Friedman *et al.* (1980) and the intracellular cytotoxin of Katz *et al.* (1980) which have been associated in *L. pneumophila* may well be related to the common *Legionella* toxin described by Hedlund and Larson (1981) and expanded upon here.

REFERENCES

ALLEN, R. C., YEVICH, S. J., ORTH, R. W. and STEELE, R. H. (1974) The superoxide anion and singlet molecular oxygen: their role in the microbicidal activity of the polymorphonuclear leukocyte. *Biochem. Biophys. Res. Commun.* **60**: 909–917.

BAINE, W. B., RASHEED, J. K., MACKEL, D. C., BOPP, C. A., WELLS, J. G. and KAUFMANN, A. F. (1979a) Exotoxin activity associated with the Legionnaires' disease bacterium. *J. Clin. Microbiol.* **9**: 453–456.

BAINE, W. B., RASHEED, J. K., MACA, H. W. and KAUFMANN, A. F. (1979b) Hemolytic activity of plasma and urine from rabbits experimentally infected with *Legionella pneumophila*. *Rev. Infect. Dis.* **1**: 912–917.

BERDAL, B. P. and FOSSUM, K. (1982) Occurrence and immunogenicity of proteinases from *Legionella* species. *Eur. J. Clin. Microbiol.* **1**(1) 7–11.

BRENNER, D. J., STEIGERWALT, A. G., GORMAN, G. W., WEAVER, R. E., FEELEY, J. C., CORDES, L. G., WILKINSON, H. W., PATTON, C., THOMSON, B. M. and LEWALLEN SASSEVILLE, K. R. (1980) *Legionella hozemanii* sp. nov. and

Legionella dumoffii sp. nov.: classification of two additional species of *Legionella* associated with human pneumonia. *Curr. Microbiol.* **4**: 111–116.

FRASER, D. W., TSAI, T. R., ORENSTEIN, W., PARKIN, W. E., BEECHAM, H. J., SHARRAR, R. B., HARRIS, J., MALLISON, G. F., MARTIN, S. M., McDADE, J. E. SHEPARD, C. C., BRACHMAN, P. S. and the Field Investigation Team. (1977) Legionnaires' disease. Description of an epidemic of pneumonia. *New Engl. J. Med.* **297**: 1189–1197.

FRASER, D. W., DEUBNER, D. C., HILL, D. L. and GILLIAM, D. K. (1979). Nonpneumonic, short-incubation-period legionellosis (Pontiac fever) in men who cleaned a steam turbine condenser. *Science* **205**: 690–691.

FRIEDMAN, H. M. (1978) Legionnaires' disease in non-Legionnaires. A report of five cases. *Ann. Intern. Med.* **88**: 294–302.

FRIEDMAN, R. L., IGLEWSKI, B. H. and MILLER, R. D. (1980) Identification of a cytoxin produced by *Legionnella pneumophila. Infect. Immun.* **29**: 271–274.

FRIEDMAN, R. L., LOCHNER, J. E., BIGLEY, R. H. and IGLEWSKI, B. H. (1982) The effects of *Legionella pneumophila* toxin on oxidative processes and bacterial killing of human polymorphonuclear leucocytes. *J. Infect. Dis.* **146**: 328–334.

FUMAROLA, D. (1978) Legionnaires' disease agent and Limulus endotoxin assay. *Boll. Ist. Sieroter. Milan* **57**: 680–681.

GLICK, T. H., GREGG, M. B., BERMAN, B., MALLISON, G., RHODES, W. W., JR. and KASSANOFF, I. (1978) Pontiac fever. An epidemic of unknown etiology in a health department. I. Clinical and epidemiologic aspects. *Am. J. Epidemiol.* **107**: 149–160.

GREBNER, J. V., MILLS, E. L., GRAY, B. H. and QUIE, P. G. (1976) Comparison of phagocytic and chemiluminescence response of human polymorphonuclear neutrophils. *J. Lab. Clin. Med.* **89**: 153–159.

HEDLUND, K. W., McGANN, V. G., COPELAND, D. S., LITTLE, S. F. and ALLEN, R. G. (1979) Immunologic protection against Legionnaires' disease bacterium in the AKR/J mouse. *Ann. Intern. Med.* **90**: 676–679.

HEDLUND, K. W. and LARSON, R. (1981a) *Legionella pneumophila* toxin, isolation and purification. In: *Analytical Isotachophoresis*, pp. 81–89. EVERAERTS, F. M. (ed). Proceedings of the 2nd International Symposium on Isotachophoresis, 1980. Elsevier, Amsterdam.

HEDLUND, K. W. (1981b) Legionella Toxin. *Pharmac. Ther.* **15**: 123–130.

KATZ, L., ELLIOT, J., JOHNSON, W. and PESANTI, E. (1980) Macrophage toxicity of *Legionella pneumophila*. In: Proceedings of the 17th Annual National Meeting of the Reticuloendothelial Society, pp. 2a, abstract 9.

LOCHNER, J. E., BIGLEY, R. H. and IGLEWSKI, B. H. (1985) Defective Triggering of Polymorphonuclear Leucocyte Oxidative Metabolism by *Legionella pneumophila* Toxin. *J. Infect. Dis.* **151**: 42–46.

McCARTHY, J. P., BODROGHY, R. S., JAHRLING, P. B. and SOBOCINSKI, P. Z. (1980) Differential alterations in host peripheral polymorphonuclear leukocyte chemiluminescence during the course of bacterial and viral infections. *Infect. Immun.* **30**: 824–831.

McDADE, J. E., SHEPARD, C. C., FRASER, D. W., TSAI, T. R., REDUS, M. A., DOWDLE, W. R. and the Laboratory Investigation Team. (1977) Legionnaires' disease. Isolation of a bacterium and demonstration of its role in other respiratory disease. *New Engl. J. Med.* **297**: 1197–1203.

MIRAGLIOTTA, G., SEMERARO, N., MARCUCCIO, L. and FUMAROLA, D. (1982) *Legionella pneumophila* and related organisms induce the generation of procoagulant activity by peripheral mononuclear cells *in vitro Infection* (10) 215–218.

MÜLLER, H. E. (1980) Proteolytic action of *Legionella pneumophila* on human serum proteins. *Infect. Immun.* **27**: 51–53.

PASCULLE, A. W., FEELEY, J. C., GIBSON, Z. J., CORDES, L. G., MYEROWITZ, R. L., PATTON, C. M., GORMAN, G. W. CARMACK, C. L., EZZELL, J. W. and DOWLING, J. N. (1980) Pittsburgh pneumonia agent: direct isolation from human lung tissue. *J. Infect. Dis.* **141**: 727–732.

RONNEBERGER, H. J. (1977) Comparison of the pyrogen tests in rabbits and with limulus lysate. *Dev. Biol. Stand.* **34**: 27–32.

STEVENS, P. and YOUNG, L. S. (1976) Rapid detection of opsonophagocytic defects of human leucocytes to clinically isolated *E. coli* by chemiluminescence. *Fed. Proc.* **35**: 738.

TRUSH, M. A., WILSON, M. E. and VAN DYKE, K. (1978) The generation of chemiluminescence (CL) by phagocytic cells. *Methods Enzymol.* **LVII**: 462–494.

WEINSTEIN, L. (1980) The "new" pneumonias: the doctor's dilemma. *Ann. Intern. Med.* **92**: 559–561.

WINN, W. C. JR., GLAVIN, F. L., PERL, D. P., KELLER, J. L., ANDRES, T. L., BROWN, T. M., COFFIN, C. M., SENSECQUA, J. E., ROMAN, L. N. and CRAIGHEAD, J. E. (1978) The pathology of Legionnaires' disease. Fourteen fatal cases from the 1977 outbreak in Vermont. *Archs Pathol. Lab. Med.* **102**: 344–350.

WONG, K. H., BARRERO, O., SUTTON, MAY, J., HOCHSTEIN, D. H., ROBBINS, J. B., PARKMAN, P. D. and SELIGMANN, E. B. (1977) Standardization and control of meningococcal vaccines, group A and group C polysaccharides. *J. Biol. Stand.* **5**: 197–215.

WONG, K. H., MOSS, C. W., HOCHSTEIN, D. H., ARKO, R. J. and SCHALLA, W. O. (1979) "Endotoxicity" of the Legionnaires' disease bacterium, *Ann. Intern. Med.* **90**: 624–627.

CHAPTER 16

AEROMONAS TOXINS

Åsa Ljungh* and Torkel Wadström†

Department of Clinical Microbiology, Karolinska Hospital, S-10401 Stockholm
†*Department of Bacteriology and Epizootology, Swedish University of Agricultural Sciences,
College of Veterinary Medicine, Biomedicum, PO Box 583, S-75123 Uppsala, Sweden*

ABSTRACT

Aeromonas hydrophila (fam. *Vibrionaceae*), now recognized as a primary human pathogen, produces enzymes like proteases and phospholipases and several toxins during growth, some of which may act as virulence factors. Two toxins, alpha- and beta-haemolysin are membrane damaging. Alpha-haemolysin induces leakage of i.c. large molecular weight markers (> 200.000 D) in human embryonic lung fibroblasts whereas beta-haemolysin induces irreversible damage with exit of small molecules (< 1000 D). Most strains also produce a heat-labile enterotoxin which is separable from the membrane damaging toxins. It induces cytotonic changes in adrenal Y1 cells, fluid accumulation in rabbit intestine and increase skin permeability in rabbit skin. It further induces steroidogenesis in adrenal cells and increase the i.c. cAMP of adrenal cells and intestinal cells. However, it does not seem to be immunologically related to cholera toxin or *E. coli* LT enterotoxin, and does not bind to the same cell membrane receptor, G_{M1}.

1. INTRODUCTION

Aeromonas hydrophila is a member of the family Vibrionaceae and is universally distributed in aquatic and terrestrial environments. It was early recognized as a pathogen for cold-blooded animals (Sanarelli, 1891). Its role as a human pathogen has become increasingly evident over the past years (Caselitz, 1966; von Graevenitz and Mensch, 1968; Davis *et al.*, 1978; Trust and Chipman, 1979). A wide variety of clinical manifestations has been reported in both healthy and immunologically compromised hosts as recently reviewed (Davis *et al.*, 1978; Trust and Chipman, 1979). The incidence of healthy faecal carriers of *A. hydrophila* is low (Lautrop, 1961; von Graevenitz and Zinterhofer, 1970; Gracey *et al.*, 1982; Millership *et al.*, 1983). Nosocomial spread through dialysis fluids and hospital water supplies has been reported (Bulger and Sherris, 1966; Meeks, 1963). *A. hydrophila* has been suggested as a good indicator of the relative pollution of fresh water (Seidler *et al.*, 1980).

Seasonal variation has been reported both from Australia and U.S.A. with peak incidence of Aeromonas-induced diarrhoeal disease as well as higher rates of isolation of *A. hydrophila* in water during the summer and low during the winter (Gracey *et al.*, 1982; Kaper *et al.*, 1981a).

2. DESCRIPTION OF AEROMONADS

The taxonomy of Aeromonas is being currently reevaluated. The classification of Popoff and Véron (1976) identifies three species: *A. hydrophila*, *A. sobria* and *A. salmonicida*. Aeromonas species are gram negative, oxidase-positive, facultative anaerobic rods, most of them motile by a polar flagellum (Manual of Determinative Bacteriology, 1974). They are resistant to the vibriostatic agent O/129 and to novobiocin as well as to penicillin and ampicillin. Biochemical characteristics of *A. hydrophila* and *A. sobria* are listed in Table 1.

---

* Present Address: Stockholm County Council Central Microbiological Laboratory, PO Box 177, S-101 22 Stockholm.

TABLE 1. *Biochemical characteristics of* Aeromonas hydrophila *and* Aeromonas sobria[a]

Characteristics	A. hydrophila[b]	A. sobria[b]
Oxidase	+	+
Catalase	+	+
O/129 sensitivity[c]	−	−
Lecithinase	variable	variable
Casein hydrolysis	+	+
Gelatin liquefaction	+	+
Hydrogen sulfide from cystein	variable	+
Indole	+	+
Voges-Proskauer	variable	variable
O/F medium	+/+	+/+
Fermentation of lactose	variable[d]	variable[d]
Gas from glucose	variable	+
Fermentation of salicin	+	−
Esculin hydrolysis	+	−
L-Arginine dihydrolase	+	+
L-Lysine decarboxylase	−	−
L-Ornithine decarboxylase	−	−
Growth without added NaCl	+	+
Growth in 7.5% NaCl	−	−

[a]From Buchanan and Gibbons (1974), and Popoff and Véron (1976).
[b]DNA base ratio 57–63% G + C.
[c]2,4-diamino-6,7-diisopropylpteridine.
[d]The organism can be lactose-fermenting, late lactose-fermenting or non-lactose-fermenting (Trust and Chipman, 1979).

The incidence of Aeromonads in clinical specimens is certainly underestimated since isolates are easily misdiagnosed as *Escherichia coli, Serratia marcescens* or other members of Enterobacteriaceae (Washington, 1973; Neilson, 1978; Trust and Chipman, 1979). Selective media based on the resistance to antibiotics such as novobiocin or ampicillin and the production of extracellular enzymes such as deoxyribonuclease (DNase) have been developed (Shotts and Rimler, 1973; von Graevenitz and Zinterhofer, 1970).

Unlike most other gram negative organisms, Aeromonas species and Vibrio species produce a range of extracellular enzymes and toxins (Table 2, Liu, 1961; Caselitz, 1966). The extracellular protein profiles of *A. hydrophila* and *A. sobria* are similar, though elastase production is rarely seen in *A. sobria* (Popoff and Véron, 1976).

Aeromonas salmonicida does not grow at temperatures exceeding 21°C and is considered pathogenic only for poikilothermic animals. *A. salmonicida* also produces extracellular proteins (Liu, 1961; Caselitz, 1966). *A. hydrophila* and *A. salmonicida* both produce a protease (Dahle, 1971), and hemolysins of these two species have been suggested to be antigenically related (Karlsson, 1964). Two hemolytic activities have been described in *A. salmonicida* (Titball and Munn, 1981). This presentation will, however, only deal with toxins of the closely related species *A. hydrophila* and *A. sobria*.

3. CYTOLYTIC TOXINS

Hemorrhage is a conspicuous feature of Aeromonas induced infections, which are often referred to as 'red sore disease' and 'red leg disease' in some ectothermic animals, and soft tissue Aeromonas infections in humans may be indistinguishable from infections caused by *Streptococcus pyogenes* (Hanson *et al.*, 1977; Rigney *et al.*, 1978). These clinical observations, combined with the fact that the vast majority of strains are hemolytic on blood agar, indicate that hemolysin may be an important virulence factor in the pathogenesis of *A. hydrophila* infections. Caselitz (1966) suggested that *A. hydrophila* produced two hemolysins, and the presence of two distinct hemolysins was studied by our group (Wadström *et al.*, 1976; Ljungh *et al.*, 1978) and by Boulanger *et al.* (1977). The hemolysin that is released from cells during the late stationary growth phase was first studied by Wretlind *et al.* (1971, 1973) and will be referred to as α-hemolysin. The second hemolysin, which is released towards the end

TABLE 2. *Extracellular Enzymes and Toxins Produced by Aeromonas hydrophila*

Extracellular enzyme and toxin[a]	Optimal culture temperature	Time of culture	Molecular weight	Isoelectric point		References
Endopeptidase[b]	20–30°C	12 hr	29,000	~3	Heat-labile, dermonecrotic, nonhemolytic	Prescott *et al.* (1971) Foster and Hanna (1974) Prescott *et al.* (1971)
Zinc aminopeptidase[b]	20–30°C	12 hr	29,500	~3	Heat stable. Binds 2 g zinc per mol	
Proteinase A[b,c]	30°C	60–80 hr	22,100	—	Heat stable, pH optimum 7.9	Dahle (1971)
Proteinase B[b,c]	30°C	60–80 hr	43,600	—	Heat-labile, pH optimum 9.0	Dahle (1971)
Phosphatide acylhydrolase and Glycerophospholipid:cholesterol acyltransferase	30°C	10 hr	high	—	Non hemolytic. Produced by Aeromonads and Vibrios	McIntyre and Buckley (1978) McIntyre *et al.* (1979)
Sphingomyelinase	20°C	30 hr	—	—		T. Malmquist (unpubl.)
Staphylolytic enzyme	—	8 hr	—	~10	Mg-dependent	Coles and Gilbo (1967)
α-hemolysin	20°C	48–60 hr	65,000	4.8	Heat-labile, dermonecrotic, cytolytic	Wretlind *et al.* (1971, 1973)
β-hemolysin	37°C	20 hr	50–51,000	5.3–5.5 and 4.2	Heat-labile, dermonecrotic, cytolytic, resistant to proteolytic enzymes	Bernheimer and Avigad (1974) Bernheimer *et al.* (1975) Ljungh *et al.* (1978) Buckley *et al.* (1981)
Enterotoxin	37°C	12–18 hr	15–20,000	4.0–5.7	Heat-labile, cytotonic, antigenically unrelated to cholera toxin	Wadström *et al.* (1976) Annapurna and Sanyal (1977)
Leucocidin	32°C	24–72 hr	—	2.8, 5.0	Heat-labile, pronase sensitive Hot-cold lysis	Scholz *et al.* (1974)

[a] Strains of *A. hydrophila* also produce elastase (Scharmann, 1972), lipase, deoxyribonuclease and ribonuclease (Nord *et al.*, 1975), lecithinase (T. Malmquist, unpublished), phosphatases (Wretlind *et al.*, 1973) and fibrinolysin (Caselitz, 1966), but these proteins have not been further characterized.

[b] The production is controlled by multiple substances, e.g. peptides and short chain amines.

[c] The production of both proteinases is stimulated by Fe^{2+} and Co^{2+}.

of the logarithmic growth phase, is probably identical with the cytolytic toxin called aerolysin by Bernheimer (Bernheimer and Avigad, 1974; Bernheimer *et al.*, 1975) and 'cytotoxic protein' by us (Wadström *et al.*, 1976; Ljungh *et al.*, 1978); it will be referred to here as β-hemolysin.

3.1. ALPHA-HEMOLYSIN

The α-hemolysin is formed in various complex media. The yield is higher at $22°C$ than at $30°C$ and seems to be repressed at $37°C$ (Wretlind *et al.*, 1973; Ljungh *et al.*, 1981). The production is stimulated by zinc ions (1.8 mg/ml) and suppressed by iron (0.5 mg/ml) (Riddle *et al.*, 1981). The toxin was not released or activated by disruption of the cells in the logarithmic phase of growth (Wretlind *et al.*, 1973). Crude hemolysin is stable between pH 3.5 and 9.5 at room temperature and is inactivated by heating at $56°C$ for 10 min (Ljungh *et al.*, 1978). The isoelectric point is 5.2 (± 0.1) (Ljungh *et al.*, 1981). The yield is low ($\sim 1\%$) and the toxin is fairly unstable after isoelectric focusing. Partially purified hemolysin is destroyed by several proteolytic enzymes and is inactivated by DTT and zinc ions (Ljungh *et al.*, 1981). Less than 25% of the hemolytic activity is recovered after incubation with urea (4M) and much activity is lost on freezing and thawing the preparations.

Alpha-hemolysin was found to be dermonecrotic in the rabbit skin and to be lethal for mice as well as for rabbits (Wretlind *et al.*, 1971). The sensitivity of erythrocytes from a variety of animal species was determined; rat erythrocytes were found to be the most sensitive species and sheep the least (Ljungh *et al.*, 1978). A zone of incomplete hemolysis develops in ox blood agar (Boulanger *et al.*, 1977).

Alpha-hemolysin was also found to be cytotoxic to HeLa cells and human embryonic lung fibroblasts (Wretlind *et al.*, 1971). The morphological alterations were rounding of the cells and fading of the nuclei (Fig. 1a). Cytolytic toxins were classified according to the damage to the membranes of human lung fibroblasts as measured by leakage of intracellular markers of three different sizes (Thelestam and Möllby, 1975). Alpha-hemolysin induced release of all three markers, i.e. the functional holes were large (Table 3, Thelestam and Möllby, 1979). These changes in morphology and membrane permeability were, however, reversible if the cells were resuspended in fresh medium (Thelestam and Ljungh, 1981). Alpha-hemolysin did not induce cytotoxic alterations in cell cultures at $0-4°C$, nor did it bind to the fibroblast membrane at $0°C$ (Thelestam and Ljungh, 1981). The cytotoxic effect was dose-dependent and temperature-dependent with maximal effect at $37°C$. The action of α-hemolysin seems to be restricted to the membrane and may be of enzymatic character.

3.2. BETA-HEMOLYSIN

In the course of studying cytolytic toxins, Bernheimer and Avigad (1974) purified a heat-labile toxin from *A. hydrophila* which they called 'aerolysin'. It appeared in the logarithmic phase of growth and the production was stimulated in the presence of RNA. A complex medium was used and the culture was harvested after 24 hr at $37°C$ for production on a preparative scale. Partial purification was achieved by salt fractionation, dialysis and Sephadex G-100 gel chromatography, or by ultrafiltration, isoelectric focusing, and Biogel P-60 chromatography, and the molecular weight was estimated to be 50,000–51,000 (Bernheimer and Avigad, 1974; Ljungh *et al.*, 1981; Buckley *et al.*, 1981). The isoelectric points are 5.5 and 4.2 (± 0.1), or 5.56 and 5.39 (Ljungh *et al.*, 1981; Buckley *et al.*, 1981).

The hemolytic activity is abolished after heating at $50°C$ for 1 hr at pH 7 or at $37°C$ at pH 8.2 (Bernheimer and Avigad, 1974). It is not restored after further heating at $80°$ and $100°C$ (so called Arrhenius effect) as is the case with, for example, the hemolysins of *Vibrio parahaemolyticus* and *Staphylococcus aureus* (Takeda *et al.*, 1975; McCartney and Arbuthnott, 1978; Å. Ljungh, unpublished). Partially purified β-hemolysin is stable at room temperature between pH 4 and 9. This hemolysin was reported to be remarkably stable towards destruction by proteolytic enzymes—no inactivation was recorded after 1 hr at room temperature in the presence of Pronase, trypsin or subtilisin, and a curious observation was that papain seemed to stabilize the toxin against the partial inactivation that takes place

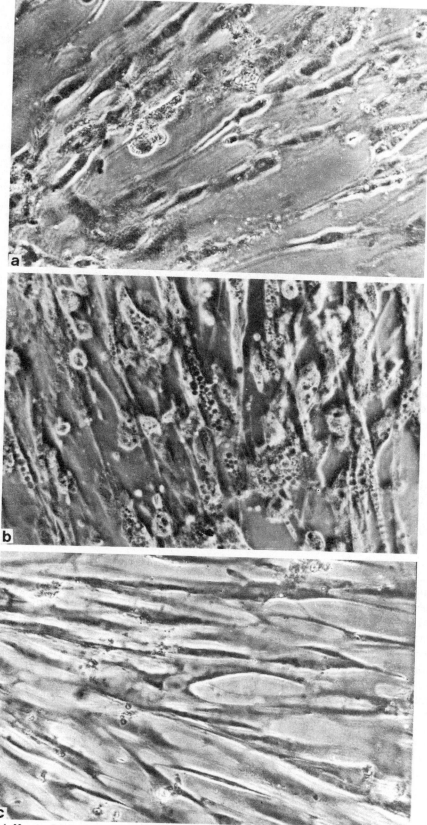

Fig. 1. Human Diploid Lung Fibroblasts Exposed to Aeromonas Hemolysins. (a) Cells incubated with 4 hemolytic units of α-hemolysin for 1 hr. The cells become rounded and the nuclei invisible. (b) Cells incubated with 2 hemolytic units of β-hemolysins for 1 hr. The cytoplasms fill with vacuoles. (c) Cells incubated with phosphate buffered saline. Negative control.

TABLE 3. *Effect of Aeromonas Hemolysins in Relation to other Cytolytic Toxins in Human Diploid Lung Fibroblasts*[d]

Cytolytic toxin	ED_{50} ratio nucleotide/ α-aminoisobutyric acid	ED_{50} ratio RNA/ α-aminoisobutyric acid
α-hemolysin (*A. hydrophila*)	15	26
δ-toxin (*S. aureus*)[a]	10	70
β-hemolysin (*A. hydrophila*)	6	> 40[c]
θ-toxin (*Cl. perfringens*)[b]	8	31
Streptolysin O[b]	7	> 50[c]

[a] McCartney and Arbuthnott, 1978.

[b] Smyth and Duncan, 1978.

[c] This figure was designated as exceeding the obtained quotient as it was not possible to release as much as 50% of the RNA label.

[d] Toxins were classified according to their ability to induce leakage of three cytoplasmic markers: α-aminoisobutyric acid (mol. wt. 103), nucleotides (mol. wt. < 1000) and RNA (mol. wt. > 200,000). The effective dose releasing 50% of the label, ED_{50}, was obtained by extrapolation from the dose–response curves with the markers. Characterization of toxins is based upon the two ratios of ED_{50}. The ratios for Aeromonas α-hemolysin and staphylococcal δ-toxin resemble each other, and the ratios for Aeromonas β-hemolysin and the oxygen-labile hemolysins streptolysin O and *Clostridium perfringens* θ-toxin after 30 min exposure to the fibroblasts. These toxins were all classified among the group of cytolysins that are thought to interact with specific receptor molecules in the cell membrane, thus inducing membrane lesions of limited size (Thelestam and Möllby, 1975, 1979).

with natural toxin (Bernheimer and Avigad, 1974). Our preparation of β-hemolysin was, however, inactivated by other proteolytic enzymes, such as subtilisin, papain and chymotrypsin (Ljungh et al., 1978).

Phospholipids and lipids were not found to inactivate the toxin, and hot-cold lysis was not observed (Bernheimer et al., 1975; Ljungh et al., 1978). Purified aerolysin exerted both phospholipase A and C-like activity, most of which was contamination (Bernheimer et al., 1975). One minor fraction of phospholipase C was similar to the hemolysin in charge and molecular weight and could not be separated from the toxin. Purified β-hemolysin was not found to have phospholipase C-like activity (Å. Ljungh and G. Blomquist, unpublished).

Buckley et al. (1981) reported that hemolysis was inhibited in the presence of ferrous ions, cysteine and DTT. However, in contrast to the finding of Avigad and Bernheimer (1976) hemolysis was not inhibited by zinc ions.

Beta-hemolysin is lethal to mice, rats and rabbits (Ljungh et al., 1978). It is dermonecrotic in rabbit skin, inducing capillary bleeding, induration and necrosis (~ 1.1 µg). In the rabbit intestinal loop test, high doses of the toxin (~ 25 µg) cause accumulation of small amounts of sanguinolent fluid (< 0.2 ml/cm) which is considered a negative test result (Ljungh and Kronevi, 1982; Söderlind and Möllby, 1978). The electrolyte content of this fluid is quite different from the fluid accumulated in response to cholera toxin (Table 4, Steinberg et al., 1975). The fluid leaks from damaged intestinal cells in which the albumin and calcium contents are quite high. This is consistent with the histopathological investigation of the intestine, which shows hemorrhagic enteritis with pronounced congestion throughout the intestinal wall (Ljungh and Kronevi, 1982).

TABLE 4. *Electrolyte and Albumin Content of Fluid Accumulated as a Response to Cholera Toxin, Aeromonas Enterotoxin and Aeromonas β-Hemolysin in Rabbit Intestinal Loops*

Toxin	Na^+ mEkv	Ca^{2+} mEkv	HCO_3^- mEkv	Cl^- mEkv	Albumin g/l
Cholera toxin (crude)	138	1.5	42	84	10
Aeromonas enterotoxin	138	1.6	29	89	10
β-hemolysin	125	2.1	3	89	47
NaCl	150	0.98	42	77	3

Purified β-hemolysin failed to induce steroidogenesis in adrenal Y1 cells (Fig. 2) and did not cause an increase in intracellular cyclic adenosin 3′5′-monophosphate (cAMP) content of the cells (Ljungh *et al.*, 1982a,b).

Erythrocytes from different animal species differ in their sensitivities to lysis by β-hemolysin. Rat erythrocytes were found to be the most sensitive, and sheep the least. With the exception of ox, cat and horse erythrocytes, this correlated with the erythrocyte membrane content of phosphatidyl choline (Bernheimer *et al.*, 1975). The erythrocyte spectra for α- and β-hemolysins are not identical (Ljungh *et al.*, 1978). A zone of clear hemolysis develops in blood agar after about 7 hr of incubation at room temperature (Ljungh *et al.*, 1981).

Bernheimer *et al.* (1975) have studied the interaction between erythrocyte membranes and hemolysin in a system of membranes from osmotically lysed erythrocytes of different species. The capacity of membranes to inhibit lysis by aerolysin was a function of the sensitivity to hemolysin-induced lysis of erythrocytes from the same animal species and was also related to binding of the toxin to the cells. Toxin binding was independent of ambient temperature and occurred at 0–37°C. Protease and neuraminidase treatment of membranes as well as inhibition studies with saccharides and ganglioside preparations failed to provide conclusive evidence that cell surface glycoconjugates are involved as cell receptors for *Aeromonas* β-hemolysin (Bernheimer *et al.*, 1975). However, incubation of β-hemolysin with crude gangliosides (bovine type II and III, Sigma Chemical Co.) was found to decrease the hemolytic activity significantly (Ljungh *et al.*, 1981). This is interesting in view of the recent elegant studies showing that the neuraminidase-sensitive ganglioside G_{T1} is the membrane receptor for the thermostable hemolysin of *V. parahemolyticus* (Takeda *et al.*, 1976) and that ganglioside G_{M2} is the membrane receptor for *Clostridium perfringens* type C cytolytic δ-toxin (Alouf *et al.*, 1979).

Pretreatment of the erythrocyte membranes with phospholipase C or proteases decreased the number of available binding sites (Bernheimer *et al.*, 1975). Incubation with human glycophorin did not affect the hemolytic activity (Bernheimer and Avigad, 1980). However, rat and mouse erythrocyte membranes were shown to contain a glycoprotein receptor for β-hemolysin, analogous to human glycophorin (Howard and Buckley, 1982).

Beta-hemolysin is cytoxic to a wide variety of tissue culture cells, such as HeLa cells, green monkey kidney cells, human diploid lung fibroblasts, adrenal Y1 cells and Chinese Hamster Ovary (CHO) cells (Ljungh *et al.*, 1978). Hitherto no cells have been found to be resistant to

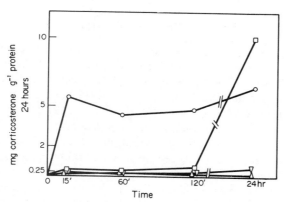

FIG. 2. Steroidogenesis in Adrenal Y1 Cells Exposed to Enterotoxins. Adrenal Y1 cells cultured in holes with 3 cm diameter were incubated with crude cholera toxin (20 loop units, □), partially purified *Aeromonas* enterotoxin (16 loop units, ○), purified β-hemolysin (32 hemolytic units, △) and plain Ham's medium (▽). Samples were drawn at different time intervals and steroids were extracted with diethylether. Quantitation was performed with antiserum B21-42 to corticosterone (Endocrine Sciences, Tarzana, Canada) and results are expressed as mg corticosterone g^{-1} protein and 24 hr. Because the antibody crossreacted with other steroids, mainly deoxycortisone ($\sim 45\%$) and progesterone ($\sim 60\%$), the recorded increase in corticosterone is interpreted as production of corticosteroids. Thus, it can be seen that *Aeromonas* enterotoxin induced steroidogenesis with a short lag phase but did not reach as high levels as cholera toxin. β-hemolysin had no steroidogenic effect.

this toxin. Beta-hemolysin is also toxic to leucocytes and could be identical to the leucocidin described by Scholz *et al.* (1974) and Ljungh *et al.* (1978). The morphological alterations are similar in these different cells; the cytoplasms fill with vacuoles and the nuclei become clearly visible (Fig. 1b). The sensitivity of the cells to β-hemolysin is pronounced, e.g. adrenal Y1 cells are about one hundred times more sensitive than rabbit erythrocytes (Ljungh *et al.*, 1981).

In ^{3}H and ^{14}C-labelled lung fibroblasts, β-hemolysin induced leakage of the low molecular weight markers but not of the high molecular weight marker (Table 3, Thelestam and Möllby, 1979). The functional holes are thus smaller than those induced by Aeromonas α-hemolysin. No reversibility of the changes in membrane permeability is observed with β-hemolysin (Thelestam and Ljungh, 1981). Results obtained in this cell system are in good agreement with data reported by Bernheimer *et al.* (1975). Thus, toxin binds rapidly to the fibroblasts at temperatures between 0° and 37°C, but the release of markers is only observed around 37°C. Pretreatment of the fibroblasts with neuraminidase does not affect the subsequent binding of the toxin. The hemolytic activity is inhibited by zinc ions but is unaffected by magnesium ions, while calcium ions potentiate the activity (Ljungh, 1981).

Antibodies to α-hemolysin or β-hemolysin neutralize both hemolysins. Whether this is due to cross-contamination or represents an antigenic relationship is under study. Immuno-gel diffusion studies of the two hemolysins cannot exclude partial identity between them (Ljungh *et al.*, 1981). Alpha- and beta-hemolysins have several characteristics in common and one might even speculate that the phospholipase, which according to Bernheimer was similar to aerolysin in charge and molecular weight, is α-hemolysin. No antagonism but a possible synergism between the two hemolysins is noted in blood agar (Ljungh *et al.*, 1981).

There are also several characteristics that β-hemolysin shares in common with the thermostable hemolysin of *V. parahemolyticus* (Miwatani and Takeda, 1976): (1) induction of clear hemolysis in ox and rabbit blood agar; (2) induction of similar morphological alterations in tissue culture cells; (3) binding to cell surfaces not temperature dependent (0–37°C); (4) stimulation of hemolytic activity by calcium ions; (5) partial inactivation of hemolytic activity by crude gangliosides, and finally (6) the antiserum to *V. parahemolyticus* hemolysin partially neutralizes both hemolysins of *A. hydrophila*, indicating an antigenic relationship as well (Ljungh, 1981).

However, crossed immunoelectrophoresis with β-hemolysin and *V. parahemolyticus* hemolysin and their respective antisera so far failed to reveal immunological relationship (Y. Takeda and A. Ljungh, unpublished).

4. ENTEROTOXIN

For decades *A. hydrophila* was isolated from patients with acute diarrhoeal disease, but its role as an intestinal pathogen was questioned (Lautrop, 1961; Martinez–Silva *et al.*, 1961; Fukaya *et al.*, 1962; Rosner, 1964; Mohieldin *et al.*, 1966; Buck *et al.*, 1970; von Graevenitz and Zinterhofer, 1970; Helm and Stille, 1970; Sack *et al.*, 1971; Chatterjee and Neogy, 1972; Bhat *et al.*, 1974; Chatterjee *et al.*, 1976; Gurwith and Williams, 1977; Samb *et al.*, 1977; Rahman and Willoughby, 1980; Echeverria *et al.*, 1981; Champsaur *et al.*, 1982; Pitarangsi *et al.*, 1982; Gracey *et al.*, 1982). Enteropathogenicity in strains of *A. hydrophila* was first demonstrated by Indian researchers who injected whole cells into ligated rabbit intestinal loops (Sanyal *et al.*, 1975). The presence of an extracellular heat-labile enterotoxin was shown independently by our group and the Indian group (Wadström *et al.*, 1976; Annapurna and Sanyal, 1977). Enterotoxigenic *A. hydrophila* has been isolated from fish (Boulanger *et al.*, 1977), pigs (Dobrescu, 1978) and dogs (P. Olsson, K. Krovacek and T. Wadström, unpublished) as well as from divers of the Anacostia river (Seidler *et al.*, 1980).

Aeromonas enterotoxin induces fluid accumulation in the rabbit intestinal loop, as well as in rat and mouse loops (Ljungh and Kronevi, 1982). Like cholera toxin, it gives a positive rabbit skin test (Craig, 1965), though the dermonecrosis of the hemolysins can occlude the increased capillary permeability and induration caused by enterotoxin (Ljungh *et al.*, 1977; Dubey and Sanyal, 1978). Recently, however, the skin permeability factor was reported to be separable from the loop active factor (Dubey *et al.*, 1980). After purification by acetone fractionation, salt precipitation, DEAE Sephadex and CM cellulose chromatography, these two factors appeared as two separate protein fractions in polyacrylamide gel electrophoresis.

The enterotoxin is produced in various complex media and appears in the culture fluid during the late logarithmic phase of growth (Wadström *et al.*, 1976). The isoelectric point is 4.0–5.7, and the molecular weight estimated to 15,000–20,000 (Ljungh *et al.*, 1978). The toxin is stable between pH 4.5 and 10 and was reported to be more active at alkaline pH (Dubey and Sanyal, 1978). Partially purified enterotoxin is stable at heating at 56°C for 10 min (Dubey and Sanyal, 1978; Ljungh *et al.*, 1978). It is destroyed by papain, but more than 75 % of the activity remains after incubation with trypsin or pronase (Ljungh *et al.*, 1981).

The titer of enterotoxin in *A. hydrophila* gradually decreases, and this may explain why Donta and Haddow (1978) were unable to detect enterotoxin production in enterotoxigenic strains. Strains that had lost their enterotoxigenicity become enterotoxigenic after passage through rabbit instestinal loops twice or more (Annapurna and Sanyal, 1977). This was described earlier for vibrios (Dutta *et al.*, 1963). Whether this is a result of a selection process or due to the presence of specific growth factors in the intestine is not known. It was recently claimed that all strains of *A. hydrophila* are enterotoxigenic (Annapurna and Sanyal, 1977). Our data support this because environmental strains that did not produce detectable amounts of enterotoxin upon initial testing, became enterotoxigenic after repeated passage (Ljungh and Kronevi, 1982).

Plasmids have not been detected in enterotoxigenic strains of *A. hydrophila* (Cumberbatch *et al.*, 1979; Å. Ljungh and M. Popoff, unpublished data). These findings support the hypothesis that enterotoxin production in Aeromonas is under chromosomal control as in *V. cholerae* (Finkelstein, 1973; Vasil *et al.*, 1975).

Keusch and Donta (1975) classified enterotoxins as cytotonic or cytotoxic on the basis of their activity in adrenal Y1 and HeLa cells. Cholera toxin and *E. coli* heat labile (LT) toxins are representative of cytotonic enterotoxins, i.e. toxins that cause typical rounding of adrenal Y1 cells and induce steroidogenesis in these cells (Donta *et al.*, 1973, 1974; Finkelstein, 1976). *Cl. perfringens* and Shigella enterotoxins are cytotoxic to HeLa cells and without morphological or steroidogenic effect in adrenal Y1 cells. They are representative of the cytotoxic enterotoxins.

Whether Aeromonas enterotoxin is a cytotonic or cytotoxic enterotoxin is a matter of dispute. We earlier claimed that it is cytotonic (Ljungh *et al.*, 1977; Ljungh, 1981; Ljungh *et al.*, 1982a,b), but this has been disputed (Donta and Haddow, 1978; Cumberbatch *et al.*, 1979; Hoštacká *et al.*, 1982). These authors, however, did not try to separate the enterotoxin from hemolytic activity or to neutralize the hemolysins. The membrane damage recorded with ^{51}Cr-labelled HeLa cells in the study by Cumberbatch *et al.* (1979) correlates well with our data on the effect of β-hemolysin in the ^{3}H and ^{14}C-labelled fibroblasts (Thelestam and Ljungh, 1981).

The majority of strains of *A. hydrophila*, regardless of the source of isolation, produce cytolytic toxins that occlude enterotoxic activity in cell tests such as the adrenal Y1 and CHO cell tests (Ljungh *et al.*, 1977, 1978). The sensitivity of adrenal Y1 cells to β-hemolysin is about 100-times greater than the hemolysin test with rabbit erythrocytes (Wretlind *et al.*, 1971; Ljungh *et al.*, 1981). As a result of the greater heat stability of crude enterotoxin, the hemolysins can be selectively inactivated by heating the crude culture supernatant at 56°C for 10 min. The hemolysins can also be neutralized by specific antisera (Wretlind *et al.*, 1971). The failure by Cumberbatch *et al.* (1979) to heat inactivate the hemolysins in several samples may be attributed to the presence of more heat stable cytolytic toxins or to a low titer of enterotoxin in the strains investigated. Even after inactivation of hemolysins, however, the enterotoxin seldom causes rounding of more than 50 % of the cells (Fig. 3). The sensitivity of adrenal Y1 cells to Aeromonas enterotoxin is thus lower than that for *E. coli* LT and cholera toxin (Donta *et al.*, 1974; Finkelstein, 1973) and the cell test is only about four times more sensitive than the rabbit intestinal loop test (Ljungh *et al.*, 1981). The use of the cell test alone to detect enterotoxic activity will give too low an incidence of enterotoxigenic strains of *A. hydrophila*, as recently discussed for other bacteria as well (Tenney *et al.*, 1979). Treatment of adrenal Y1 cells with β-glucosidase (from almonds, Sigma) or β-galactosidase (*E. coli*,

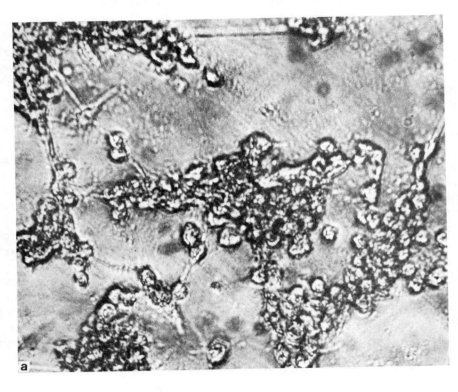

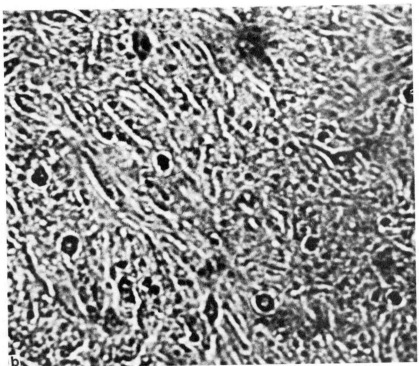

FIG. 3. Adrenal Y1 Cells Exposed to Aeromonas Enterotoxin. (a) Partially purified Aeromonas enterotoxin (1 loop unit) was incubated with adrenal Y1 cells overnight at 37°C. Typical rounding of about 50% of the cells is noted. (b) Negative control. Cells incubated with phosphate buffered saline.

Sigma) increased the sensitivity of the cells to Aeromonas enterotoxin and 75 % of the cells were changed (Ljungh *et al.*, 1981).

Aeromonas enterotoxin induces steroidogenesis in adrenal Y1 cells with a shorter lag phase than cholera toxin does, and to a suboptimal level (Fig. 2, Ljungh *et al.*, 1982a,b). Likewise, the intracellular cyclic adenosine monophosphate (cAMP) content of the cells was increased, whereas the cyclic guanosine monophosphate (cGMP) content was unchanged (Ljungh *et al.*, 1982a). Aeromonas enterotoxin was recently shown to increase the cAMP content of rabbit intestinal cells threefold (Dubey *et al.*, 1980).

Prostaglandin inhibitors such as indomethacin and phenylbutazone, known to inhibit cholera toxin-induced fluid accumulation in experimental models (Finck and Katz, 1972; Jacoby and Marshall, 1972; Bennett, 1976), did not reduce fluid accumulated as a response to Aeromonas enterotoxin in rabbit intestinal loops (Dubey *et al.*, 1980; Ljungh and Kronevi, 1982). Chlorpromazine, which was shown to inhibit both cholera toxin. *E. coli* heat-labile (LT) and heat-stable (ST) induced fluid secretion in mice but at another site than the prostaglandin inhibitors (Abbey and Knoop, 1979), was found to inhibit about 40 % of the accumulated intestinal fluid in Aeromonas exposed mice and rats (Ljungh and Kronevi, 1982). Thus, as Aeromonas enterotoxin induces steroidogenesis and rounding in adrenal Y1 cells without toxic manifestations, which purified hemolysins do not, the enterotoxin should be included among the cytotonic enterotoxins. Furthermore, some of these findings support the hypothesis that the adenylate cyclase-cAMP pathway is involved in Aeromonas induced diarrhoea.

Cholera toxin and *E. coli* LT are antigenically related (Holmgren *et al.*, 1973; Smith and Sack, 1973) and seem to share a common tissue receptor, G_{M1} (Holmgren, 1973; Pierce, 1973; King and van Heyningen, 1975). One might have expected that the enterotoxins of the related species *A. hydrophila* and *Vibrio cholerae* would exhibit similar antigenic relationship. Cross neutralization experiments in rabbit intestinal loops, rabbit skin, and in adrenal Y1 cell tests have, however failed to demonstrate any antigenic relationship between cholera toxin or *E. coli* LT and Aeromonas enterotoxin (Ljungh *et al.*, 1977, 1982a). Furthermore, Aeromonas enterotoxin did not bind in G_{M1}-ELISA, coagglutination test with antiserum to human *E. coli* LT (detection limit 5 ng *E. coli* LT) was negative with enterotoxin as well as with freshly isolated Aeromonas strains, and Kaper *et al.* (1981b) did not find *E. coli* LT-like genes with a DNA probe in enterotoxigenic strains of *A. hydrophila*. Immunogel diffusion studies indicated a reaction of non-identity between Aeromonas enterotoxin and the A and B subunits of cholera toxin (Clements and Finkelstein, 1978; Ljungh, 1981).

Likewise, Boulanger *et al.* (1977) and Champsaur *et al.* (1982) reported that cholera antitoxin did not neutralize Aeromonas-induced fluid accumulation in rabbit intestinal loop test, whereas Dobrescu (1978) was able to neutralize the Aeromonas enterotoxin with anti-*E. coli* LT in adrenal Y1 cell test. In a recent study, prior incubation of Aeromonas enterotoxin with cholera antitoxin did not inhibit fluid accumulation in the suckling mouse model, whereas fluid secretion was inhibited in rats immunized with cholera toxin when challenged with heated (100°C) samples of Aeromonas enterotoxin in an intestinal perfusion model (James *et al.*, 1982).

Crude gangliosides (bovine type II and III, Sigma) did not inhibit the activity of Aeromonas enterotoxin in any of the three test systems used (Ljungh *et al.*, 1977, 1982a). The tissue receptor is thus probably not a ganglioside. Cholera toxin binds rapidly to adrenal Y1 cells (Donta, 1974), which Aeromonas enterotoxin does not, as indicated by the non-induction of steroidogeneis when the cells were washed after 5 min incubation with Aeromonas toxin (Ljungh *et al.*, 1982a,b).

The delay in the onset of fluid accumulation in the rabbit intestinal loop is much shorter after exposure to Aeromonas enterotoxin than to cholera toxin and is similar to *E. coli* ST (Ljungh and Kronevi, 1982). Analysis of the loop content for electrolytes and albumin shows no significant difference between data obtained for cholera toxin and Aeromonas enterotoxin (Table 4, Steinberg *et al.*, 1975; Ljungh and Kronevi, 1982). Intestines exposed to the two enterotoxins for six hours show no mucosal damage (Fig. 4, Polotsky *et al.*, 1977; Annapurna and Sanyal, 1977). These findings are also consistent with the hypothesis that intestinal

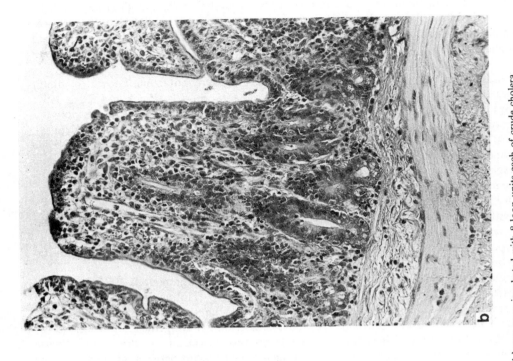

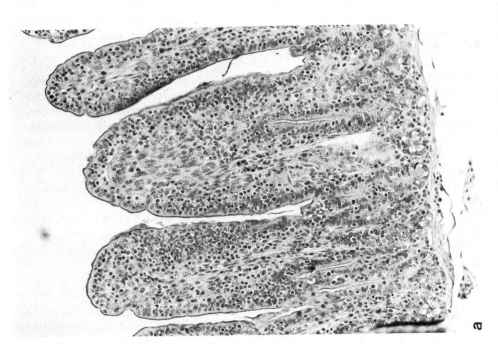

FIG. 4. Rabbit Intestinal Loop Exposed to Enterotoxins. Rabbit intestinal loops were incubated with 8 loop units each of crude cholera toxin and Aeromonas enterotoxin for 6 hr. Fluid had accumulated at 1 ml/cm of loop. No mucosal damage is noted in either the loop exposed to cholera toxin (a) or to Aeromonas enterotoxin (b).

secretion as a response to Aeromonas enterotoxin is mediated by the adenylate cyclase-cAMP pathway.

5. OTHER TOXINS

The presence of a heat-stable enterotoxin giving positive suckling mouse test (Dean *et al.*, 1972) has been reported earlier (Boulanger *et al.*, 1977). The toxin has, however not been further characterized. Nor has that heat-stable secretagogue described by James *et al.* (1982) been further studied. The suckling mouse model was found unsuitable for Aeromonas enterotoxin by us and others (Ljungh *et al.*, 1981; Cumberbatch *et al.*, 1979; Champsaur *et al.*, 1982) because cytolytic toxins are likely to interfere. However, others find the model useful (Jánossy and Tarján, 1980; Burke *et al.*, 1981).

Fibrinolysin and leucocidin may be potential virulence factors (Table 2, Caselitz, 1966; Scholz *et al.*, 1974). They have, however, not been further characterized. Much of the data reported for the leucocidin also fits for β-hemolysin.

It was recently stated that most of the strains of both Aeromonas and Vibrio species produce phospholipase and cholesterol transferase which are *per se* not hemolytic (McIntyre and Buckley, 1978; McIntyre *et al.*, 1979). Bernheimer *et al.* (1975) has described both phospholipase A and C-like activity in *A. hydrophila*, both of which were similar to aerolysin in charge and molecular weight. Recently, both sphingomyelinase and lecithinase activity were detected in strains of *A. hydrophila* (T. Malmquist and A. Ljungh, unpublished). The sphingomyelinase appeared in the stationary phase and was dependent on magnesium ions. The lecithinase showed a pronounced biphasic production curve, with maximum yield in the late logarithmic phase of growth. These phospholipases await further characterization as well as definition of their pathogenetic role.

Aeromonas species produce a cell-associated endotoxin (lipopolysaccharide), which has been suggested to enhance infections in frogs (Rigney *et al.*, 1978). It is probably of low toxicity for vertebrates, but it has not been extensively studied.

Proteolytic activity in strains of *A. hydrophila* was recognized early (Dahle, 1971). The production of protease was later shown to be stimulated in the presence of zinc ions and inhibited by ferric ions (Riddle *et al.*, 1981). The activity of protease was unaffected by these ions. Buckley *et al.* (1981), however, reported complete inhibition of proteolytic activity in the presence of zinc, ferrous and ferric ions. An interesting correlation was made between production of elastase and staphylolytic enzyme and virulence of *A. hydrophila* for fish (Hsu *et al.*, 1981). Elastase is well established as a virulence factor in *Pseudomonas aeruginosa* (Pavlovskis and Wretlind, 1979). In another recent study on experimental infections in fish, extracellular heat-labile products of *A. hydrophila* induced lesions but extracellular products from a protease-negative mutant of the same strain were more toxic (Allan and Stevenson, 1981). This indicates that either protease is not a virulence factor, or that virulence factor(s) are inactivated by protease in crude culture fluids. These data indicate that protease(s) may well be involved in the pathogenesis of Aeromonas-induced infections, the details of which remain to be elucidated.

6. GENERAL DISCUSSION

The correlation between the cytolytic toxins, particularly β-hemolysin, and extra-intestinal infections (often with necrosis of muscular tissue) is well established (Caselitz, 1966). It is also without doubt that Aeromonas enterotoxin evokes intestinal fluid secretion in rabbit loops. Attempts to induce experimental diarrhoea in rabbits, guinea pigs, hamsters and rats have so far failed even after elimination of parts of the resident intestinal flora by prior antibiotic treatment as well as neutralization of gastric pH and slowing of intestinal motility (Ljungh and Kronevi, 1982). Some of the animals died, presumably after resorption of hemolysins. Thus, though the enterotoxin is proposed as a major virulence factor in the pathogenesis of intestinal *A. hydrophila* infections, the lack of direct correlation between diarrhoea and enterotoxin indicates that additional virulence factors have to be considered.

In enterotoxigenic *E. coli* (ETEC) diarrhoea, adhesins of pilus nature on the bacterial surface that probably cause species-specific intestinal colonization have been described, which hemagglutinate erythrocytes of different animal species with characteristic patterns (Wadström *et al.*, 1979). In our collection of strains of *A. hydrophila*, the majority of strains hemagglutinate one or several species of erythrocytes and are fimbriated (Å. Ljungh, unpublished). This could reflect the presence of different surface antigens. In EM studies, various kinds of fimbriae and fimbriae-like structures on the surface of *A. hydrophila* were visualized (Freer *et al.*, 1978). Five different patterns of hemagglutination were described and correlated with the presence of pili and bacterial surface outer membrane proteins (Atkinson and Trust, 1980). These studies were recently extended to a typing scheme based on patterns of agglutination with erythrocytes and yeast cells (Adams *et al.*, 1983).

The toxins discussed in this chapter will have to be purified before their mode of action can be elaborated (Wadström, 1978). Purification work has been hampered by the complexity of the extracellular protein profile of Aeromonas and also by the instability of several of these toxins during purification procedures. The low sensitivity of adrenal Y1 cells to Aeromonas enterotoxin necessitated the adoption of the rabbit intestinal loop test as the basic test system, as the rabbit skin test also suffers from interference by cytolytic toxins. A more simple test system, preferably an *in vitro* system which permits quantitation, would facilitate further studies on this new enterotoxin.

ACKNOWLEDGEMENTS

We thank Dr Trevor Trust for providing us with unpublished data, and Drs T. Malmquist, Monica Thelestam and Bengt Wretlind for stimulating discussions. The authors' investigations have been supported by a grant from the Swedish Medical Research Council (16x-4723).

REFERENCES

ABBEY, D. M. and KNOOP, F. C. (1979) Effect of chlorpromazine on the secretory activity of *Escherichia coli* heat-stable enterotoxin. *Infect. Immun.* **26:** 1000–1002.

ADAMS, D., ATKINSON, H. M. and WOODS, W. H. (1983) *Aeromonas hydrophila* typing scheme based on patterns of agglutination with erythrocytes and yeast cells. *J. Clin. Microbiol.* **17:** 422–427.

ALLAN, B. J. and STEVENSON, R. M. W. (1981) Extracellular virulence factors of *Aeromonas hydrophila* in fish infections. *Can. J. Microbiol.* **27:** 1114–1122.

ALOUF, J. E., TIXIER, G. and KERAMBRUN, A. (1979) Purification and properties of *Clostridium perfringens* type C delta toxin. *Toxicon* **17** (Suppl. No. 1): 1.

ANNAPURNA, E. and SANYAL, S. C. (1977) Enterotoxicity of *Aeromonas hydrophila*. *J. Med. Microbiol.* **10:** 317–323.

ATKINSON, H. M. and TRUST, T. J. (1980) Hemagglutination properties and adherence ability of *Aeromonas hydrophila*. *Infect. Immun.* **27:** 938–946.

AVIGAD, L. S. and BERNHEIMER, A. W. (1976) Inhibition by Zinc of hemolysis induced by bacterial and other cytolytic agents. *Infect. Immun.* **13:** 1378–1381.

BENNETT, A. (1976) The relationship of prostaglandins to cholera. *Prostaglandins* **11:** 425–430.

BERNHEIMER, A. W. and AVIGAD, L. S. (1974) Partial characterization of aerolysin, a lytic exotoxin from *Aeromonas hydrophila*. *Infect. Immun.* **9:** 1016–1021.

BERNHEIMER, A. W., AVIGAD, L. S. and AVIGAD, G. (1975) Interactions between aerolysin, erythrocytes and erythrocyte membranes. *Infect. Immun.* **11:** 1312–1319.

BERNHEIMER, A. W. and AVIGAD, L. S. (1980) Inhibition of bacterial and other cytolysins by glycophorin. *FEMS Microbiol. Letters* **9:** 15–19.

BHAT, P., SHANIAKI MARI, S. and RAJAN, D. (1974) The characterization and significance of *Plesiomonas shigelloides* and *Aeromonas hydrophila* isolated from an epidemic of diarrhoea. *Indian J. Med. Res.* **62:** 1051–1060.

BOULANGER, Y., LALLIER, E. and COUSINEAU, G. (1977) Isolation of an enterotoxigenic Aeromonas from fish. *Can. J. Microbiol.* **23:** 1161–1164.

BUCHANAN, R. E. and GIBBONS, N. E. (1974) *Bergey's Manual of Determinative Bacteriology*, (8th edn) Williams and Wilkins, Baltimore.

BUCK, A. A., ANDERSON, R. I., SASAKI, T. T. and KAWATA, K. (1970) *Health and Disease in Chad, Epidemiology, Culture and Environment in Five Villages.* Johns Hopkins Press, Baltimore.

BUCKLEY, J. T., HALASA, L. N., LUND, K. D. and McINTYRE, S. M. (1981) Purification and some properties of the hemolytic toxin aerolysin. *Can. J. Biochem.* **59:** 430–435.

BULGER, R. J. and SHERRIS, J. C. (1966) The clinical significance of *Aeromonas hydrophila*. Report of two cases. *Archs Intern. Med.* **118:** 562–564.

BURKE, V., ROBINSON, J., BERRY, R. J. and GRACEY, M. (1981) Detection of enterotoxins of *Aeromonas hydrophila* by a suckling mouse test. *J. Med. Microbiol.* **14:** 401–408.

CASELITZ, F. H. (1966) *Pseudomonas-Aeromonas und ihre humanmedizinische Bedeutung.* VEB Gustav Fischer Verlag, Jena.

CHAMPSAUR, H., ANDREMONT, A., MATHIEU, D., ROTTMAN, E. and AUZEPY, P. (1982) Cholera-like illness due to *Aeromonas sobria*. *J. Infect. Dis.* **145**: 248–254.

CHATTERJEE, B. D. and NEOGY, K. N. (1972) Studies on Aeromonas and Plesiomonas species isolated from cases of choleraic diarrhoea. *Indian J. Med. Res.* **60**: 520–524.

CHATTERJEE, B. D., DE, P. K., SEN, T. and MISRA, I. B. (1976) Cholera syndrome in Bengal. *Lancet* I: 317.

CLEMENTS, J. D. and FINKELSTEIN, R. A. (1978) Immunological crossreactivity between a heat-labile enterotoxin(s) of *Escherichia coli* and subunits of *Vibrio cholerae* enterotoxin. *Infect. Immun.* **21**: 1036–1039.

COLES, N. W. and GILBO, C. M. (1967) Lysis of *Staphylococcus aureus* by culture supernatant fluids of a species of Aeromonas. *J. Bact.* **93**: 1193–1194.

CRAIG, J. P. (1965) A permeability factor (toxin) found in cholera stools and culture filtrates and its neutralization by convalescent cholera sera. *Nature (London)* **207**: 614–616.

CUMBERBATCH, N., GURWITH, M. J., LANGSTON, C., SACK, R. B. and BRUNTON, J. L. (1979) Cytotoxic enterotoxin produced by *Aeromonas hydrophila*: relationship of toxigenic isolates to diarrhoeal disease. *Infect. Immun.* **23**: 829–837.

DAHLE, H. K. (1971) The purification and some properties of two Aeromonas proteinases. *Acta Path. Microbiol. Scand. Sect.* B **79**: 726–738.

DAVIS, W. A., KANE, J. G. and GARAGUI, V. F. (1978) Human Aeromonas infection: A review of the literature and a case report of endocarditis. *Medicine* **57**: 267–277.

DEAN, A. G., CHING, Y. C., WILLIAMS, R. G. and HARDEN, L. B. (1972) Test for *Escherichia coli* enterotoxin using infant mice: Application in a study of diarrhoea in children in Honolulu. *J. Infect. Dis.* **125**: 407–411.

DOBRESCU, L. (1978) Enterotoxigenic *Aeromonas hydrophila* from a case of piglet diarrhoea. *Zentbl. Vet. Med.* B, **25**: 713–718.

DONTA, S. T. (1974) Differentiation between the steroidogenic effects of cholera enterotoxin and adrenocorticotropin through use of a mutant adrenal cell line. *J. Infect. Dis.* **129**: 728–731.

DONTA, S. T. and HADDOW, A. D. (1978) Cytotoxic activity of *Aeromonas hydrophila*. *Infect. Immun.* **21**: 989–993.

DONTA, S. T., KING, M. and SLOPER, K. (1973) Induction of steroidogenesis in tissue culture by cholera enterotoxin. *Nature* **243**: 246–247.

DONTA, S. T., MOON, H. W. and WHIPP, S. C. (1974) Detection of heat-labile *Escherichia coli* enterotoxin with the use of adrenal cells in tissue culture. *Science* **183**: 334–336.

DUBEY, R. S. and SANYAL, S. C. (1978) Enterotoxicity of *Aeromonas hydrophila*: Skin responses and *in vivo* neutralisation. *Zentbl. Bakt. Hyg. I. Abt. Orig. A.* **242**: 487–499.

DUBEY, R. S., SANYAL, S. C. and MALHOTRA, O. P. (1980) Purification of *Aeromonas hydrophila* enterotoxin and its mode of action in experimental model. In: *Animal, Plant and Microbial Toxins*, pp. 259–268, EAKER, D. and WADSTRÖM, T. (eds). Proceedings of the International Symposium held in Uppsala, 1979, Pergamon Press, Oxford.

DUTTA, N. K., PANSE, M. V. and JHALA, H. I. (1963) Choleragenic property of certain strains of ElTor, nonagglutinable and water vibrios confirmed experimentally. *Br. Med. J.* **1**: 1200–1203.

ECHEVERRIA, P., BLACKLOW, N. R., SANFORD, L. B. and CUKOR, G. G. (1981) A study of travelers' diarrhoea among American Peace Corps volunteers in rural Thailand. *J. Infect. Dis.* **143**: 767–771.

FINCK, A. D. and KATZ, R. L. (1972) Prevention of cholera induced intestinal secretion in the cat by aspirin. *Nature* **238**: 273–274.

FINKELSTEIN, R. A. (1973) Cholera. *CRC Critical Rev. Microbiol.* **2**: 553–623.

FINKELSTEIN, R. A. (1976) Progress in the study of cholera and related enterotoxins. In: *Mechanisms in Bacterial Toxinology*, pp. 53–84, BERNHEIMER, A. W. (ed). John Wiley, New York.

FOSTER, B. G. and HANNA, M. O. (1974) Toxic properties of *Aeromonas proteolytica*. *Can. J. Microbiol.* **20**: 1403–1409.

FREER, J. H., ELLIS, A., WADSTRÖM, T. and SMYTH, C. J. (1978) Occurrence of fimbriae among enterotoxigenic intestinal bacteria isolated from cases of human infantile diarrhoea. *FEMS Microbiol. Lett.* **3**: 277–281.

FUKAYA, K., NAKAMURA, S., TAKAYAMA, H. and SUKAZAK, R. (1962) Isolation of Aeromonas from two cases of acute diarrhoea *J. Jap. Ass. Infect. Dis.* **36**: 8–10.

GRACEY, M., BURKE, V. and ROBINSON, J. (1982) Aeromonas-associated gastroenteritis. *Lancet* ii: 1304–1306.

VON GRAEVENITZ, A. and MENSCH, A. H. (1968) The genus Aeromonas in human bacteriology. *New Engl. J. Med.* **178**: 245–249.

VON GRAEVENITZ, A. and ZINTERHOFER, L. (1970) The detection of *Aeromonas hydrophila* in stool specimens. *Health Lab. Sci.* **7**: 124–127.

GURWITH, M. J. and WILLIAMS, T. W. (1977) Gastroenteritis in children: a two-year review in Mannitoba. I. Etiology. *J. Infect. Dis.* **136**: 239–247.

HANSON, P. G., STANDRIDGE, J., JARETT, F. and MAKI, D. G. (1977) Fresh-water wound infection due to *Aeromonas hydrophila*. *J. Am. Med. Assoc.* **238**: 1053–1054.

HELM, E. P. and STILLE, W. (1970) Akute Enteritis durch *Aeromonas hydrophila*. *Dtsch. Med. Wschr.* **95**: 18–23.

HOLMGREN, J. (1973) Comparison of the tissue receptors for *Vibrio cholerae* and *Escherichia coli* enterotoxins by means of gangliosides and natural cholera toxoid. *Infect. Immun.* **3**: 747–755.

HOLMGREN, J. SÖDERLIND, O. and WADSTRÖM, T. (1973) Cross-reactivity between heat-labile enterotoxins of *Vibrio cholerae* and *Escherichia coli* in neutralisation tests in rabbit ileum and skin. *Acta. Path. Microbiol. Scand. Sect.* B **81**: 757–762.

HOŠTACKÀ, A. ČIŽNÁR, I., KORYCH, B. and KAROLČEK, J. (1982) Toxic factors of *Aeromonas hydrophila* and *Plesiomonas shigelloides*. *Zentbl. Bakt. Hyg., I. Abt. Orig. A.* **252**: 525–534.

HOWARD, S. P. and BUCKLEY, J. T. (1982) Membrane glycoprotein receptor and holeforming properties of a cytolytic protein toxin. *Biochemistry* **21**: 1662–1667.

HSU, T. C. WALTMAN, W. D. and SHOTTS, E. B. (1981) Correlation of extracellular enzymatic activity and biochemical characteristics with regard to virulence of *Aeromonas hydrophila*. In: *Develop. Biol. Standard.* **49**: pp. 101–111. ANDERSON, D. P. and HENNESSEN, W. (eds) S. Karger, Basel.

JACOBY, H. I. and MARSHALL, C. H. (1972) Antagonism of cholera enterotoxin by antiinflammatory agents in the rat. *Nature* **235**: 163–165.

JAMES, C., DIBLEY, M., BURKE, V., ROBINSON, J. and GRACEY, M. (1982) Immunological cross-reactivity of enterotoxins of *Aeromonas hydrophila* and cholera toxin. *Clin. Exp. Immunol.* **47:** 34–42.

JÁNOSSY, G. and TARJÁN, V. (1980) Enterotoxigenicity of Aeromonas strains in suckling mice. *Acta Microbiol. Acad. Sci. Hung.* **27:** 63–69.

KAPER, J. B., LOCKMAN, H. and COLWELL, R. R. (1981a) *Aeromonas hydrophila*: Ecology and toxigenicity of isolates from an estuary. *J. Appl. Bacteriol.* **50:** 359–377.

KAPER, J. B., MOSELEY, S. L. and FALKOW, S. (1981b) Molecular characterization of environmental and nontoxigenic strains of *Vibrio cholerae*. *Infect. Immun.* **32:** 661–668.

KARLSSON, K. A. (1964) Serologische Studien von *Aeromonas salmonicida*. *Zentbl. Bakt. ParasitKde I. Orig.* **194:** 73–80.

KEUSCH, G. T. and DONTA, S. T. (1975) Classification of enterotoxins on the basis of activity in cell culture. *J. Infect. Dis.* **131:** 58–63.

KING, C. A. and VAN HEYNINGEN, W. E. (1975) Evidence for the complex nature of the ganglioside receptor for cholera toxin. *J. Infect. Dis.* **131:** 643–648.

LAUTROP, H. (1961) *Aeromonas hydrophila* isolated from human faeces and its possible pathological significance. *Acta. Path. Microbiol. Scand.* **51** (Suppl. 144): 299–301.

LIU, P. V. (1961) Observations on the specificities of extracellular antigens of the genera Aeromonas and Serratia. *J. Gen. Microbiol.* **24:** 145–153.

LJUNGH, Å. (1981) *Aeromonas hydrophila*—A study on three extracellular toxins. PhD Diss. Karolinska Institute, Stockholm.

LJUNGH, Å., ENEROTH, P. and WADSTRÖM, T. (1982a) Cytotoxic enterotoxin from *Aeromonas hydrophila*. *Toxicon* **20:** 787–794.

LJUNGH, Å., ENEROTH, P. and WADSTRÖM, T. (1982b) Steroid secretion in adrenal Y1 cells exposed to *Aeromonas hydrophila* enterotoxin. *FEMS Microbiol. Letts.* **15:** 141–144.

LJUNGH, Å. and KRONEVI, T. (1982) *Aeromonas hydrophila* toxins—Intestinal fluid accumulation and mucosal injury in animal models. *Toxicon* **20:** 397–402.

LJUNGH, Å., POPOFF, M. and WADSTRÖM, T. (1977) *Aeromonas hydrophila* in acute diarrhoeal disease: Detection of enterotoxin and biotyping of strains. *J. Clin. Microbiol.* **6:** 96–100.

LJUNGH, Å., WRETLIND, B. and MÖLLBY, R. (1981) Separation and characterization of three extracellular toxins from *Aeromonas hydrophila*. *Acta. Path. Microbiol Scand. Sect. B.* **89:** 387–397.

LJUNGH, Å., WRETLIND, B. and WADSTRÖM, T. (1978) Evidence for enterotoxin and two cytolytic toxins in human isolates of *Aeromonas hydrophila*. In: *Toxins: Animal, Plant and Microbial*, pp. 947–960, ROSENBERG, P. (ed). Proceedings of the International symposium held in San José, 1976. Pergamon Press, Oxford.

MARTINEZ–SILVA, R., GUZMANN–URREGO, G. and CASELITZ, F. H. (1961) On the problem of the significance of Aeromonas strains in enteritis in infants. *Z. Tropenmed. Parasitol.* **12:** 445–453.

MCCARTNEY, A. C. and ARBUTHNOTT, J. P. (1978) Mode of action of membrane damaging toxins produced by Staphylococci. In: *Bacterial Toxins and Cell Membranes*, pp. 89–127. JELJASZEWICZ, J. and WADSTRÖM, T. (eds). Academic Press, London.

MCINTYRE, S. and BUCKLEY, J. T. (1978) Presence of glycerophospholipid: cholesterol acyltransferase and phospholipase in culture supernatant of *Aeromonas hydrophila*. *J. Bact.* **117:** 402–407.

MCINTYRE, S. TRUST, T. J. and BUCKLEY, J. T. (1979) Distribution of glycerophospholipid: cholesterol acyltransferase in selected bacterial species. *J. Bact.* **139:** 132–136.

MEEKS, M. V. (1963) The genus Aeromonas: Methods for identification. *Am. J. med. Tech.* **29:** 361–378.

MILLERSHIP, S. E., CURNOW, S. R. and CHATTOPADHYAY, B. (1983) Faecal carriage rate of *Aeromonas hydrophila*. *J. clin. Pathol.* **36:** 920–923.

MIWATANI, T. and TAKEDA, Y. (1976) *Vibrio parahaemolyticus. A causative bacterium of food poisoning*. Saikon publ., Tokyo.

MOHIELDIN, M. S., GABR, M., EL–HEFNY, A., MAHMOUD, S. S. and ABDALLAH, A. (1966) Bacteriological and clinical studies in infantile diarrhoea. *J. trop. Pediatrics* **11:** 88–93.

NEILSON, A. H. (1978) The occurrence of Aeromonads in activated sludge: Isolation of *Aeromonas sobria* and its possible confusion with *Escherichia coli*. *J. appl. Bact.* **44:** 259–264.

NORD, C. E., SJÖBERG, L., WADSTRÖM, T. and WRETLIND, B. (1975) Characterization of three aeromonads and nine pseudomonas species by extracellular enzymes and haemolysins. *Med. Microbiol. Immunol.* **161:** 79–87.

PAVLOVSKIS, O. R. and WRETLIND, B. (1979) Assessment of protease (elastase) as a *Pseudomonas aeruginosa* virulence factor in experimental mouse burn infection. *Infect. Immun.* **24:** 181–187.

PIERCE, N. E. (1973) Differential inhibitory effects of cholera toxoids and ganglioside on the enterotoxins of *Vibrio cholerae* and *Escherichia coli*. *J. exp. Med.* **137:** 1009–1023.

PITARANGSI, C., ECHEVERRIA, P., EHITMIRE, R., TIRAPAT, C., FORMAL, S., DAMMIN, G. J. and TINGTALAPONG, M. (1982) Enteropathogenicity of *Aeromonas hydrophila* and *Plesiomonas shigelloides*: Prevalence among individuals with and without diarrhoea in Thailand. *Infect. Immun.* **35:** 666–673.

POLOTSKY, Y. E., DRAGUNSKAYA, E. M., SAMOTRELSKY, A. Y., VASSER, N. R., EFREMOV, V. E., SNIGIREVSKAYA, E. S. and SELIVERSTOVA, V. G. (1977) Interaction of *Vibrio cholerae* EITor and gut mucosa in ligated rabbit ileal loop experiment. *Med. Biol.* **55:** 130–140.

POPOFF, M. and VÉRON, M. (1976) A taxonomic study of the *Aeromonas hydrophila–Aeromonas punctata* group. *J. gen. Microbiol.* **94:** 11–22.

PRESCOTT, J. M., WILKES, S. H., WAGNER, F. W., and WILSON, K. J. (1971) Aeromonas aminopeptidase. Improved isolation and some physical properties. *J. biol. Chem.* **246:** 1756–1764.

RAHMAN, S. A. F. M. and WILLOUGHBY, J. M. T. (1980) Dysentery-like syndrome associated with *Aeromonas hydrophila*. *Br. med. J.* **281:** 976.

RIDDLE, L. M., GRAHAM, T. E. and AMBORSKI, R. L. (1981) Medium for the accumulation of extracellular hemolysin and protease by *Aeromonas hydrophila*. *Infect. Immun.* **33:** 728–733.

RIGNEY, M. M., ZILINSKY, J. W. and ROUF, M. A. (1978) Pathogenicity of *Aeromonas hydrophila* in red leg disease in frogs. *Curr. Microbiol.* **1:** 175–179.

ROSNER, R. (1964) *Aeromonas hydrophila* as the etiological agent in a case of severe gastroenteritis. *Am. J. clin. Pathol.* **42**: 402–404.

SACK, R. B., GORBACH, S. L., BANWELL, J. G., JACOBS, B., CHATTERJEE, B. D. and MITRA, R. C. (1971) Enterotoxigenic *Escherichia coli* isolated from patients with severe cholera-like disease. *J. infect. Dis.* **123**: 378–385.

SAMB, A., CHIRON, J.-P., DENIS, F., SOW, A., DIOP, E. H. I. and DIOP MAR, I. (1977) Syndrome cholériformes à *Aeromonas hydrophila*. Deux cas. *Nouv. Presse méd.* **6**: 2520.

SANARELLI, G. (1891) Uber einen Mikroorganismsus des Wassers, welches für Tiere mit veränderlicher und constanter Temperatur pathogen ist. *Zentbl. Bakt. Parasitkde* **19**: 193–199.

SANYAL, S. C., SINGH, S. J. and SEN, B. C. (1975) Enteropathogenicity of *Aeromonas hydrophila* and *Plesiomonas shigelloides*. *J. med. Microbiol.* **8**: 195–199.

SCHARMANN, W. (1972) Vorkommen von Elastase bei Pseudomonas und Aeromonas. *Zentbl. Bakt. Hyg.*, I Abt. Orig. A. **220**: 435–442.

SCHOLZ, D., SCHARMANN, W. and BLOBEL, H. (1974) Leucocidic substances from *Aeromonas hydrophila*. *Zbl. Bakt. Hyg.*, I. Abt. Orig. A. **228**: 312–316.

SEIDLER, R. J., ALLAN, D. A., LOCKMAN, H., COLWELL, R. R., JOSEPH, S. W. and DAILY, O. P. (1980) Isolation, enumeration and characterization of Aeromonas from polluted waters encountered in diving operations. *Appl. envir. Microbiol.* **39**: 1010–1018.

SHOTTS, JR. I. B. and RIMLER, R. (1973) Medium for the isolation of *Aeromonas hydrophila Appl. Microbiol.* **26**: 550–553.

SMITH, N. W. and SACK, R. B. (1973) Immunologic cross-reactions of enterotoxins from *Escherichia coli* and *Vibrio cholerae*. *J. infect. Dis.* **127**: 164–170.

SMYTH, C. J. and DUNCAN, J. L. (1978) Thiol-activated (Oxygen-labile) cytolysins. In: *Bacterial Toxins and Cell Membranes*, pp. 129–183. JELJASZEWICZ, J. and WADSTRÖM, T. (eds). Academic Press, London.

STEINBERG, S. E., BANWELL, J. G., YARDLEY, J. H., KEUSCH, G. T. and HENDRIZ, T. R. (1975) Comparison of secretory and histological effects of Shigella and cholera enterotoxins in rabbit jejunum. *Gastroenterology* **68**: 309–317.

SÖDERLIND, O. and MÖLLBY, R. (1978) Studies on *Escherichia coli* in pigs. V. Determination of enterotoxicity and frequency of O groups and K88 antigen in strains from 200 piglets with neonatal diarrhoea. *Zentbl. Vet. Med. B* **25**: 719–728.

TAKEDA, Y., HORI, Y., TAGA, S., SAKURAI, J. and MIWATANI, T. (1975) Characterization of the temperature-dependent inactivating factor of the thermostable direct hemolysin in *Vibrio parahaemolyticus*. *Infect. Immun.* **12**: 449–454.

TAKEDA, Y., TAKEDA, T., HONDA, T. and MIWATANI, T. (1976) Inactivation of the biological activities of the thermostable direct hemolysin of *Vibrio parahaemolyticus* by ganglioside G_{T1}. *Infect. Immun.* **14**: 1–5.

TENNEY, J. H., SMITH, T. F. and WASHINGTON, J. A. II (1979) Sensitivity, precision and accuracy of the Y1 adrenal cell enterotoxin assay. *J. clin. Microbiol.* **9**: 197–199.

THELESTAM, M. and MÖLLBY, R. (1975) Sensitive assay for detection of toxin-induced damage to the cytoplasmic membrane of human diploid fibroblasts. *Infect. Immun.* **12**: 225–232.

THELESTAM, M. and MÖLLBY, R. (1979) Classification of microbial, plant and animal cytolysins based on their membrane-damaging effects on human fibroblasts. *Biochim. biophys. Acta.* **557**: 156–169.

THELESTAM, M. and LJUNGH, Å. (1981) Membrane damaging and cytotoxic effects on human fibroblasts by the two hemolysins from *Aeromonas hydrophila*. *Infect. Immun.* **34**: 949–957.

TITBALL, R. W. and MUNN, C. B. (1981) Evidence for two haemolytic activities from *Aeromonas salmonicida*. *FEMS Microbiol. Letts* **12**: 27–30.

TRUST, T. J. and CHIPMAN, D. C. (1979) Clinical involvement of *Aeromonas hydrophila*. *Can. med. Assoc. J.* **120**: 942–947.

VASIL, M. L., HOLMES, R. K. and FINKELSTEIN, R. A. (1975) Conjugal transfer of a chromosomal gene determining production of enterotoxin in *Vibrio cholerae*. *Science* **187**: 849–850.

WADSTRÖM, T. (1978) Advances in the purification of some bacterial protein toxins. In: *Bacterial Toxins and Cell Membranes*, pp. 9–57, JELJASZEWICZ, J. and WADSTRÖM T. (eds). Academic Press, London.

WADSTRÖM, T., LJUNGH, Å. and WRETLIND, B. (1976) Enterotoxin, haemolysin and cytotoxic protein in *Aeromonas hydrophila* from human infections. *Acta path. microbiol. scand.* Sect. B. **84**: 112–114.

WADSTRÖM, T., SMYTH, C. J., FARIS, A. and FREER, J. (1979) Hydrophobic and hemagglutinating properties of enterotoxigenic *Escherichia coli* with different colonizing factors: K88 antigen, K99 antigen, colonization factor antigen and adherence factor. In: *Proceedings of the Second International Symposium on Neonatal Diarrhoea, VIDO*, pp. 29–55, ACRES, S. (ed) Stuart Bundle Press, Saskatoon.

WASHINGTON, J. A. II (1973) The role of *Aeromonas hydrophila* in clinical infections. In: *Infectious Disease Reviews*, pp. 75–86. HOLLOWAY, W. J. (ed). Futura Publ., New York.

WRETLIND, B., MÖLLBY, R. and WADSTRÖM, T. (1971) Separation of two hemolysins from *Aeromonas hydrophila* by isoelectric focusing. *Infect. Immun.* **4**: 503–505.

WRETLIND, B., HEDÉN, L. and WADSTRÖM, T. (1973) Formation of extracellular haemolysin by *Aeromonas hydrophila* in relation to protease and staphylolytic enzyme. *J. gen. Microbiol.* **78**: 57–65.

CHAPTER 17

ENDOTOXINS OF GRAM-NEGATIVE BACTERIA

Otto Lüderitz*, Chris Galanos* and Ernst Th. Rietschel†

*Max-Planck-Institut für Immunbiologie, D-78 Freiburg, F.R.G.
†Forschungsinstitut Borstel, D-2061 Borstel, F.R.G.

1. INTRODUCTION

Characteristic symptoms of infections caused by gram-negative bacteria such as *Salmonella*, *E. coli*, *Shigella*, are fever, headache, changes in white blood cell counts and blood pressure, diarrhoea, and in severe cases the infection may lead to shock and death. It is well known that these effects of gram-negative pathogens are not dependent on bacterial viability: they can equally be elicited by the injection of killed cells. The active principle participating in the induction of these toxic effects resides in the cell envelope of gram-negative bacteria and has been termed *endo*toxin because of its tight association with the cell wall (the *exo*toxins, in contrast, are released by the bacteria into the environment).

Chemically, the endotoxins are lipopolysaccharides. They form a huge class of macromolecules which is unique to gram-negative bacteria. Lipopolysaccharides are endowed with a great compositional and structural diversity, but they all express typical endotoxic activities.

Some of the characteristic properties of lipopolysaccharides are illustrated in Fig. 1–4. Figure 1a shows a thin section electron micrograph of a *Veillonella* cell (Bladen and Mergenhagen, 1964). The three layers forming the cell envelope and surrounding the cytoplasm can be recognized (PM, plasma or inner membrane; SM, solid membrane, peptidoglycan; OM, outer membrane). After treatment of the bacteria with phenol/water, the cells are devoid of the outer membrane (Fig. 1b), indicating that the components of the outer membrane have been solubilized in the solvent. The lipopolysaccharide is found, in addition to proteins, phospholipids and nucleic acid, among the extracted compounds and can be prepared in a purified form after some steps of fractionation. The endotoxic lipopolysaccharides represent the surface O antigens of the gram-negative bacterial cells. This is illustrated in Fig. 2. Ferritin-labelled anti-O antibodies against *S. typhimurium*, obtained by immunization with heat-killed bacteria or with lipopolysaccharide, were incubated with homologous cells. The electron micrograph shows a thin layer of densely packed specific ferritin conjugates close to the outer membrane indicating the surface location of lipopolysaccharide (Mühlradt et al., 1973).

Lipopolysaccharides often represent specific receptor sites for bacteriophages. Figure 3 shows the electron micrograph of a phenol/water-extracted lipopolysaccharide (from *S. minnesota* Ra), which due to the lipophilic character of these amphiphile molecules is aggregated to long micellar filaments. The lipopolysaccharide had been incubated with a phage (Felix O-1) for which it functions as a receptor. The phages, attached to the lipopolysaccharide, are present as ghosts, the tails being contracted and the heads being empty. In an analogous way the phages would react with the complete bacterial cell carrying this lipopolysaccharide on its surface (Lindberg, 1977).

Figure 4 shows some characteristic *in vivo* effects of endotoxic lipopolysaccharide. A dose of 1.0 μg lipopolysaccharide from *S. abortus equi* injected intravenously into an adult person induces fever and typical changes in white blood cell counts with leucopenia and leucocytosis. The injection of a corresponding amount of bacteria would induce the same effects (Westphal, 1960).

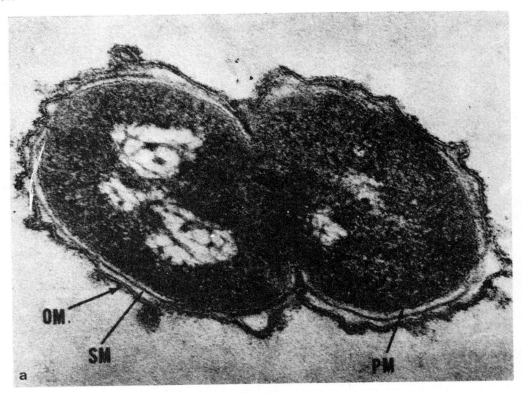

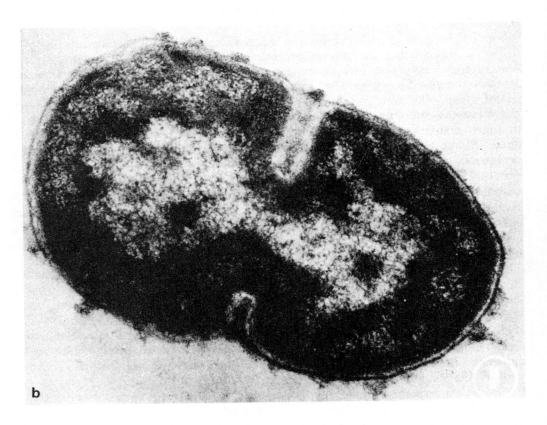

Fig. 1. Electron micrograph (∼ 60,000 × magnification) of *Veillonella* bacteria before (a) and after (b) extraction with phenol/water. OM, outer membrane; SM, solid membrane (peptidoglycan); PM plasma (inner) membrane. (Bladen and Mergenhagen, 1964).

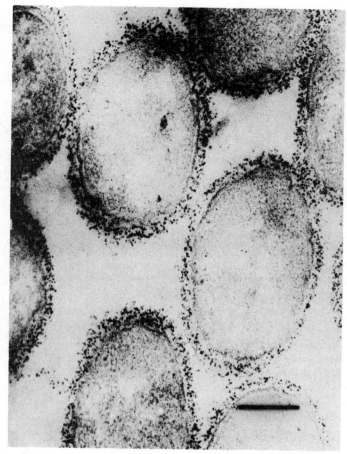

FIG. 2. Electron micrograph (~80,000× magnification) of *S. typhimurium* cells after interaction with ferritin-labelled anti-lipopolysaccharide antibodies (Mühlradt *et al.*, 1973).

Figures 1–4 show that the lipopolysaccharide is anchored to the bacterial surface. It has been demonstrated that lipopolysaccharide is exclusively located in the outer leaflet of the outer membrane, together with proteins, while the inner leaflet contains phospholipids and proteins (Nikaido and Nakae, 1979). This exposed position allows the lipopolysaccharide to communicate with the environment. Immunization with bacterial cells leads to the formation of anti-O antibodies which are directed against, and can react with, lipopolysaccharide present on the cell. The phenol/water-extraction procedure (Westphal *et al.*, 1952) has proven to be universally applicable to gram-negative bacteria yielding lipopolysaccharide of high purity and full biological activity as endotoxin, O antigen, and phage receptor. It should be mentioned that for the isolation of lipopolysaccharides expressing a high lipophilic character (i.e. those from R form strains) the recently developed phenol/chloroform/petroleum ether- (PCP-) extraction method is preferrable (Galanos *et al.*, 1969).

A considerable number of reviews on different aspects of endotoxin research have recently appeared dealing with the following topics: structure, biosynthesis, and genetics of lipopolysaccharides (Galanos *et al.*, 1977a, Rietschel *et al.*, 1981a, Lüderitz *et al.*, 1981, Mäkelä and Stocker, 1981); their action as phage receptors (Lindberg, 1977, Braun and Hantke, 1981); the assembly and organization of the outer membrane (Nikaido and Nakae, 1979, Osborn *et al.*, 1980, Osborn, 1979, Osborn and Wu, 1980); the role of lipopolysaccharide in bacterial virulence and infection (Mäkelä *et al.*, 1973, Shands, 1975, McCabe *et al.*, 1977, Smith *et al.*, 1980, Rietschel *et al.*, 1982); the effects of endotoxin and mechanisms of its action (Galanos *et al.*, 1977a, Rietschel *et al.*, 1981a, Lüderitz *et al.*,

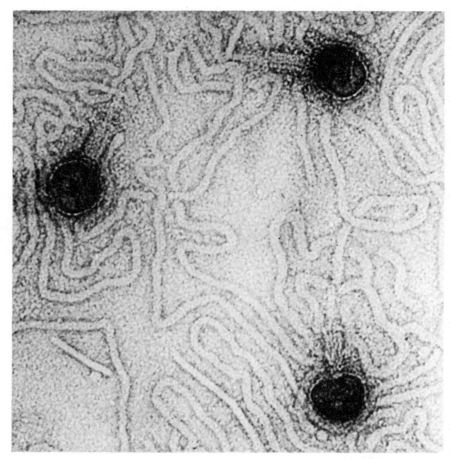

Fig. 3. Electron micrograph (~400,000× magnification) of *Salmonella Ra* mutant lipopolysaccharide after incubation with Felix 0–1 phages (Lindberg, 1967).

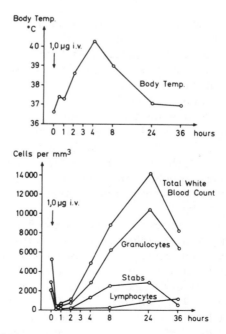

Fig. 4. Changes in the body temperature (a) and white blood cell counts (b) following the injection of 1 μg of *Salmonella* lipopolysaccharide into man. (1) Total number of leucocytes; (2) granulocytes; (3) stabs; (4) lymphocytes.

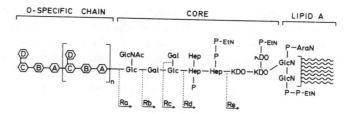

FIG. 5. General structure of a *Salmonella* lipopolysaccharide. A–D, sugar residues; Glc, D-glucose; Gal, D-galactose; GlcN, D-glucosamine; GlcNAc, N-acetyl-D-glucosamine; Hep, L-glycero-D-*manno*-heptose; KDO, 2-keto-3-deoxy-D-*manno*-octonate; AraN, 4-amino-L-arabinose; P, phosphate; EtN, ethanolamine; ∿, hydroxy- and nonhydroxy fatty acids. Ra to Re, indicated are incomplete R form lipopolysaccharides.

1981, Kadis *et al.*, 1971, Kass and Wolff, 1973, Schlessinger, 1977, Berry, 1977, Kabir *et al.*, 1978, Morrison and Ulevitch, 1978, Bradley, 1979).

2. CHEMICAL STRUCTURE OF LIPOPOLYSACCHARIDES

Figure 5 shows a schematic representation of the structure of a *Salmonella* lipopolysaccharide. It contains a lipid region, the lipid A, and a covalently bound hydrophilic heteropolysaccharide chain, often being branched, which is subdivided into the core and the O-specific chain.

2.1. O-Specific Chains

The O chains are made up by a sequence of identical oligosaccharides, the repeating units (e.g. a tetrasaccharide as shown in Fig. 5). In rare cases, O chains may represent a homopolysaccharide, such as a mannan or a galactan. Each serotype among the group of gram-negative bacteria is characterized by a unique structure of the O-specific chain. Consequently, there exists a great diversity in lipopolysaccharide structure and composition. Studies on O-specific chains have revealed many new sugar classes as well as unusual sugar derivatives.

Due to the methodological advances made in polysaccharide analyses, about 70 O-chain structures have been elucidated in the last decade, including O chains from *Salmonella*, *E. coli*, *Shigella*, *Yersinia*, and others (reviewed by Lüderitz *et al.*, 1981).

The average length of O chains varies from one species to another. A recent investigation by SDS–polyacrylamide–gel electrophoresis of the lipopolysaccharide of *S. typhimurium* revealed an average length of 7–10 repeating units. But a high degree of heterogeneity was seen (Palva and Mäkelä, 1980). About 60% of the molecules were devoid of O chains and contained only core-lipid A. About 30% of the molecules contained O chains with between 20 and 30 repeating units, and about 10% had an intermediate or greater length. Similar results were obtained with *E. coli* 0111 (Goldman and Leive, 1980). A further reason for the often observed heterogeneity of O chains is given by a frequently incomplete substitution of the main chain by sugar branches (e.g. D in Fig. 5) or by sugar substituents (e.g. acetyl or acetal groups) (Wright and Kanegasaki, 1971).

2.2. The Core

Core structures express less diversity than O chains. The core shown on Fig. 5 is probably common to all *Salmonella* and it has been identified also in species of other *Enterobacteriaceae*. It contains a lipid A-distal branched oligosaccharide containing the common sugars *N*-acetyl-D-glucosamine, D-glucose, and D-galactose, and a lipid A—proximal branched oligosaccharide containing the core-specific sugars, L-glycero-D-mannoheptose (L,D-Hep, Hep) and 2-keto-3-deoxy-D-mannooctonate (KDO, dOclA).

The O chain is linked to the subterminal glucose residue; the reducing KDO group forms the link to lipid A. Heptose and KDO residues are substituted by phosphate, phosphoryl-, and pyrophosphoryl-ethanolamine groups (Lehmann et al., 1971). Together with the carboxyl groups of KDO, these confer negative charge to the molecule, which is neutralized by a mixture of cations, including metal ions and polyamines. These cations are always present in original lipopolysaccharide preparations (Galanos and Lüderitz, 1975).

The potential physiological functions of the highly charged inner core region for the translocation and integration of lipopolysaccharides into the outer membrane, as well as for conferring stability to the outer membrane through cation-mediated ionic linkages between lipopolysaccharide molecules and to proteins, has been discussed recently by Schindler and Osborn (1979).

In addition to the *Salmonella* core, 5 further core types have been identified in *Enterobacteriaceae* and their structure evaluated, i.e., the coli 1 to 4 core types and the *E. coli* K-12 core. They occur in *E. coli*, *Shigella*, *Arizona* and other enterobacterial serotypes. In their structural make-up these core types resemble the *Salmonella* core; they differ, however, with regard to the structure of the hexose region (reviewed by Lüderitz et al., 1981).

Core types other than those of the family of *Enterobacteriaceae* have been occasionally studied and their structures are quite distinct from that of the *Salmonella* core. Heptose and/or KDO may be missing and unusual constituents have been identified (e.g. d-glycero-D-mannoheptose, fructose, amino acids) (Wilkinson, 1977).

Structural, biosynthetic, and genetic investigations of the core region of *Salmonella* lipopolysaccharides became feasible when it was recognized that the so-called R mutants, which had long been known to bacteriologists as being devoid of O antigenicity, are defective in lipopolysaccharide biosynthesis (Lüderitz et al., 1966b). Two main groups of R mutants can be distinguished. As indicated on Fig. 5, Ra mutants, often with a mutation in the *rfb*-locus, are defective in O chain biosynthesis and, therefore, produce complete core linked to lipid A. Rb to Re mutants, often with a mutation in the *rfa*-locus, are defective in core biosynthesis and, therefore, produce a more or less complete fragment of the core depending on the blocked biosynthetic step. In Fig. 5 only the structures of Ra, Rb, and Re lipopolysaccharides are indicated. Today, the whole series comprises 12 defective *Salmonella* lipopolysaccharides which represent most of the theoretically possible intermediates of the core-lipid A biosynthesis (for KDO-defective mutants see below). Many of the respective mutants have been characterized with regard to their biosynthetic defects (Osborn and Rothfield, 1971), genetics (Stocker and Mäkelä, 1971), antigenic properties (Nixdorff and Schlecht, 1972) and phage pattern (Wilkinson et al., 1972).

Similar series of R mutants have been isolated from *E. coli*, *Shigella*, *Proteus* and others and their lipopolysaccharides studied (Jann and Westphal, 1975).

2.3. LIPID A

Figure 6 shows the structure proposed for *Salmonella* lipid A. It contains a β1,6-linked D-glucosamine disaccharide, which is substituted by two phosphate groups, one in ester

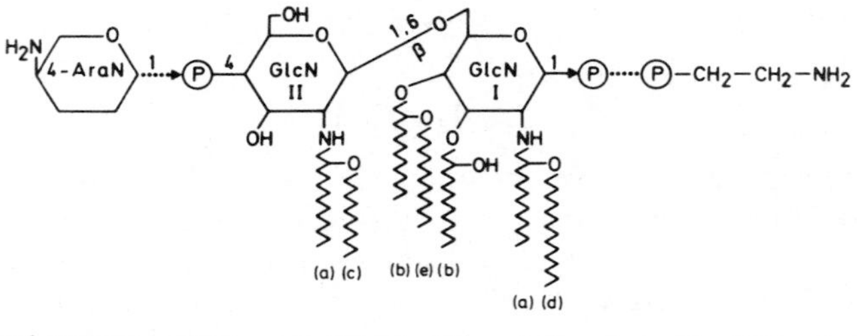

FIG. 6. Proposed structure of *Salmonella* lipid A. Abbreviations as in Fig. 5. For designations a–e and other details see text.

linkage at position 4 of glucosamine II, the other one occupying the glycosidic hydroxyl group of glucosamine I. The phosphorylated glucosamine disaccharide is termed the lipid A backbone. Both phosphate groups are substituted partially (indicated by dotted linkages) by polar head groups, 4-amino-4-deoxy-L-arabinose (at glucosamine II) and phosphorylethanolamine (at glucosamine 1), respectively. In the complete lipopolysaccharide the terminal KDO residue of the core is linked to the hydroxyl group at position 3 of glucosamine II (Gmeiner *et al.*, 1969, 1971; Hase and Rietschel, 1976, 1977; Mühlradt *et al.*, 1977).

The lipophilic character of the molecule is provided by 7 moles of fatty acids which are bound to the backbone: 4 moles of D-3-hydroxytetradecanoic (3-OH-14:0, β-hydroxy-myristic acid; a,b of Fig. 6), and about 1 mole of each dodecanoic (12:0, lauric acid; c of Fig. 6), tetradecanoic (14:0, myristic acid; e of Fig. 6), and hexadecanoic (16:0; palmitic acid; d of Fig. 6). It has recently been found that a variable fraction of tetradecanoic acid is replaced by L-2-hydroxytetradecanoic acid (2-OH-14:0, α-hydroxymyristic acid (not shown in Fig. 6) (Rietschel *et al.*, 1972, Bryn and Rietschel, 1978). Our present knowledge (reviewed by Rietschel *et al.*, 1981) of the distribution of the fatty acids on the molecule suggests that only the 3-hydroxy fatty acids are bound directly to the backbone, 2 moles (a of Fig. 6) to the amino groups in amide linkage, and 2 moles (b of Fig. 6) to available hydroxyl groups of the disaccharide in ester linkage (available are the hydroxyl groups at positions 3 and 4 of glucosamine I, and 6 of glucosamine II). In Fig. 6 the two ester-linked hydroxy fatty acids have been arbitrarily linked to positions 3 and 4 of glucosamine I, but it is very possible that in lipid A the distribution of the hydroxy fatty acids over the glucosamine residues is random and therefore more balanced.

The non-hydroxylated fatty acids substitute hydroxyl groups of the hydroxylated fatty acids: 12:0 and 16:0 (c and d of Fig. 6) being bound to the amide-linked (a of Fig. 6), and 14:0 (d of Fig. 6) to the ester-linked 3-OH-14:0 (b of Fig. 6) (H.-W. Wollenweber, K. Broady, O. Lüderitz and E. Th. Rietschel, unpublished). In Fig. 6, 14:0 is arbitrarily attached to one 3-OH-14:0, but a distribution over both is equally possible. The polar head groups are not substituted by fatty acids and their amino groups are free.

Similarly to the other regions of the lipopolysaccharide molecule, lipid A is endowed with a certain degree of microheterogeneity, e.g. due to incomplete substitutions by polar head groups, possibly also due to a random distribution of fatty acids.

Investigations in various laboratories have also shown that lipid A's, obtained from different bacterial genera, to some extent, express variability (reviewed by Rietschel *et al.*, 1981). A common, nonvariable structural element of lipid A's of different origin, however, is the diphosphorylated β1,6-linked glucosamine disaccharide, the lipid A backbone (Fig. 7; A, B and C = hydrogen). A certain variability is seen with respect to the number and nature of head groups and backbone substituents (Table 1). The simplest lipid A structure encountered so far is expressed by the lipid A of *E. coli* K-12 (Rosner *et al.*, 1979a,b,c), where the backbone is only, and furthermore incompletely (about 50%), substituted by one phosphate group (position B of Fig. 7). Substituents of other lipid A's include 4-amino-L-arabinose (position A), phosphorylethanolamine, D-glucosamine, and D-arabinose (position B), and D-glucosamine (position C). The nature of the fatty acids (R and C of Fig. 7) varies with respect to chain length (C_{10} to C_{20}), branching (iso, ante-iso),

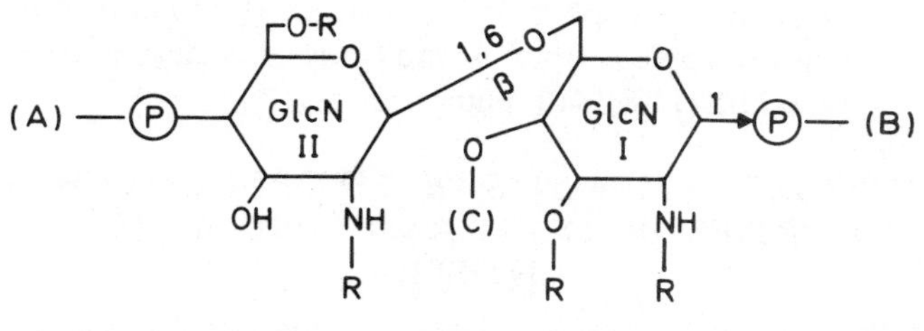

FIG. 7. General structure of lipid A's. (A), (B) and (C) substituents of the lipid A backbone; R (and in most cases C) = fatty acid residues.

TABLE 1. *Nature of Substituents of Lipid A Phosphate Groups
The Polar Head Groups*

Lipid A	Substituent of Phosphate Groups at		Reference
	GlcN II	GlcN I	
Escherichia coli K-12	—	P	Rosner *et al.* (1979a,b,c)
Vibrio cholerae	—	PETN*	Broady *et al.* (1981)
Yersinia enterocolitica	L-4-AraN	—	Jensen (1980)
Proteus mirabilis	L-4-AraN*	—	Z. Sidorczyk and E. Th. Rietschel, unpublished data.
Salmonella minnesota	L-4-AraN	PETN	Rietschel *et al.* (1977); Mühlradt *et al.* (1977)
Chromobacterium violaceum	L-4-AraN*	D-GlcN*	Hase and Rietschel (1977)
Rhodospirillum tenue	L-4-AraN*	D-Ara(f)*	Tharanathan *et al.* (1978)

The C4-position of the phosphate group at GlcN II is established only in *Salmonella* (Gmeiner *et al.*, 1971), and *E. coli* K-12 (Rosner *et al.*, 1979a).

L-4-AraN: 4-amino-4-deoxy-L-arabinose: P: phosphate, PETN: phosphorylethanolamine; D-GlcN: 2-amino-2-deoxy-D-glucose; D-Ara(f): D-arabinofuranoside.

*Complete substitution.

and hydroxylation (2- and 3-hydroxy fatty acids). Without exception, however, the amino groups of the backbone are substituted by D-3-hydroxy fatty acids. As in *Salmonella* lipid A, the head groups are not substituted by acyl residues.

Some groups of bacteria have been encountered, the lipid A component of which is devoid of the otherwise common backbone structure, such as *Rhodopseudomonas viridis, Rh. palustris, Rh. sulfoviridis* (Weckesser *et al.*, 1979) and *Pseudomonas diminuta, Ps. vesicularis* (Wilkinson and Taylor, 1978). In these cases, lipid A is represented by a N-acylated 2,3-diamino-2,3-dideoxy-D-glucose structure (3-amino-D-glucosamine), which is not phosphorylated. Neither the lipopolysaccharide nor the free lipid A of these species exhibit endotoxic activities (see below).

2.4. LIPID A PRECURSOR MOLECULES

For a long time Re lipopolysaccharides represented the most incomplete structures isolated from R mutants. It turned out that R mutants with a defect deeper than Re were not viable, indicating that the KDO-lipid A structure represents the minimum requirement for bacterial viability. Only recently, a number of conditional *Salmonella* mutants have been isolated, most of them being defective in the synthesis of KDO (Osborn *et al.*, 1974; Osborn, 1979; Lehmann *et al.*, 1977). At 30°C these mutants synthesize KDO and lipopolysaccharide, and exhibit normal growth. After shifting the culture to 40°C, KDO and lipopolysaccharide synthesis stops, and after one generation growth ceases. After this time, at non-permissive conditions, the bacteria were found to contain incomplete lipid A molecules. Their structural investigation revealed that one product (precursor 1) contains the *Salmonella* lipid A backbone substituted by 4 moles of 3-OH-14:0, 2 moles being present in amide linkage, and two in ester linkage, i.e. in the same way as in lipid A (Lehmann 1977; Rick *et al.*, 1977). A second precursor molecule (precursor II) was isolated and identified to contain, in addition, the two *Salmonella*-specific polar head groups, 4-aminoarabinose and phosphorylethanolamine (Lehmann *et al.*, 1978). Precursors I and II represent incomplete lipid A molecules because of the absence of the non-hydroxylated fatty acids, 12:0, 14:0, and 16:0.

3. IMMUNODETERMINANTS OF LIPOPOLYSACCHARIDES, PROPERTIES OF O-, R-, AND LIPID A-SPECIFIC ANTISERA

Lipopolysaccharides contain a great number of antigenic determinants located along the polysaccharide chain. Most of them, however, are not or only poorly expressed in the

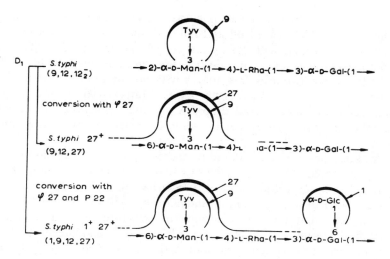

Fig. 8. Chemical structure and serological specificity (O factors) of the O chain of *S. typhi* lipopolysaccharide, and the modifications induced by converting phage $\varphi 27$ and P22 (Nghiem and Staub, 1975). The lines indicate the determinant groups, their thick parts the respective immunodominant sugars, and the numbers the O factors (Lüderitz *et al.*, 1966a).

complete molecule. In S form lipopolysaccharides, the immunodeterminants of the O-specific chain, the O factors, are expressed. They are determined by distinct, often overlapping, structures on the O-specific chain (Lüderitz *et al.*, 1971). That sugar constituent of an O factor (or an immunodeterminant, in general), which is best adapted to the specific site of the respective antibody as determined by serological inhibition tests, has been termed immunodominant (Lüderitz *et al.*, 1966a). It may occupy a terminal or internal position of the chain. Together with neighboring sugar residues it forms the immunodeterminant structure (O factor). This is shown in Fig. 8.

It should be mentioned that in the last decade a number of O factor structures of pathogens have been chemically synthesized. Coupled to protein carriers, they are used for producing highly specific and high titer O factor antisera which serve for diagnostic purposes and passive immunization (Svenungsson and Lindberg, 1978; Josephson and Bundle, 1979).

Figure 8 gives two examples of lipopolysaccharide modifications induced through genes linked to infective phages (Nghiem and Staub, 1975). In a first step, lysogenic conversion of *S. typhi* (O factors 9, 12) by phage 27 leads to a new linkage of galactose to mannose with the appearance of the new O factor 27. In a second step, infection with phage P22 results in the attachment of a new glucose residue which determines the new O factor 1.

In Ra to Re mutant lipopolysaccharides, which are devoid of O chains, previously cryptic immunodeterminants are exposed (Ruschmann and Niebuhr, 1972; Nixdorff and Schlecht, 1972). In general, the respective nonreducing terminal sugars of the different R lipopolysaccharides act as the immunodominants. They are different for the different types of R form lipopolysaccharides, which therefore exhibit distinct serological specificities, and thus can be classified serologically, as can the respective mutants. Pure antibodies with high specificity for the different R types have been prepared with the aid of R-oligosaccharide carrier immunogens and immunoabsorbants (Nixdorff *et al.*, 1975).

Antibodies against lipid A (Galanos *et al.*, 1971b, 1977b) are not induced on immunization with S or R form lipopolysaccharides. Immunodeterminant structures are, however, exposed in free lipid A, which can be obtained (devoid of all core sugars) by mild acid hydrolysis of lipopolysaccharides (see below). Free lipid A exhibits strong antigenic properties, but as such it represents a poor immunogen. For the production of anti-lipid A antisera (in rabbits) several methods have been developed to render free lipid A immunogenic: exposure of free lipid A on bacterial cells by treatment of Re mutants with mild acid whereby KDO is cleaved off and internal free lipid A is exposed on the cell surface, which is then coated with an excess of external free lipid A (Galanos et al., 1971b; 1977b); incorporation of free lipid A into liposomes (Schuster et al., 1979; Banerji and Alving, 1979); complexation of free lipid A with bovine serum albumin (Gorbach et al., 1979); exposure of free lipid A on erythrocytes (Mattsby-Baltzer and Kaijser, 1979); coupling of antigenically active degraded lipid A (i.e. after removal of the ester- and part of the amide-linked fatty acids) to a protein carrier (C. Galanos and Nerker, unpublished data).

Anti-lipid A antibodies are detected and measured by the passive hemolysis test using sheep erythrocytes coated with free or alkali-treated free lipid A (Galanos et al., 1971b). An enzyme-linked immunosorbant assay (ELISA) has also been described (Jay, 1978; Mattsby-Baltzer and Kaijser, 1979; Fink and Kozak, 1980; Fink and Galanos, 1981). Many results indicate that the immunodominant structure of lipid A comprizes the linkage region of glucosamine and amide-bound fatty acid, and precursor I containing this region, is antigenically as active as lipid A (Lüderitz et al., 1973; Galanos et al., 1977b). This region must be cryptic in lipopolysaccharides since lipopolysaccharides neither react with nor induce lipid A antibodies.

Many animal species respond readily to the injection of lipid A immunogen with the production of anti-lipid A antibodies (Galanos et al., 1971b). Mice, however, fail to give an antibody response. They will respond under special conditions only. Two injections of lipid A-coated cells at an interval of 3 to 4 weeks will lead to high titer antisera in all mouse strains tested, including the lipopolysaccharide-nonresponder strain C3H/HeJ (Freudenberg, 1977; Galanos et al., 1971b).

Many animal species and humans (but not mice) often contain natural antibodies cross-reacting with free lipid A, the level of which may be increased in gram-negative infections, especially of the urinary tract (Galanos et al., 1977b; Blake et al., 1980; Westenfelder et al., 1977a,b). This indicates that in higher organisms determinant structures of lipid A must become sufficiently exposed to express immunogenicity.

As expected from their structural similarities, lipid A's from many bacterial groups exhibit complete (or partial) cross reactions (Galanos et al., 1977a; Rietschel et al., 1981a). Exceptions have been found with the group of lipid A's not containing the otherwise common glucosamine backbone (such as Rh. viridis, see above). These lipid A's express their own specificity (Galanos et al., 1977a).

Unlike anti-O antibodies, the anti-R and anti-lipid A antibodies are directed against structures common to lipopolysaccharides of different origin, the latter moreover against the toxic moiety of the lipopolysaccharide molecule. Many groups, therefore, have investigated potential biological properties of these antibodies in different systems. Several investigators have independently shown that immunization with R mutant bacteria induces cross protection against infection by a variety of pathogens (McCabe et al., 1977; Diena et al., 1978; Ziegler et al., 1979). Anti-lipid A antisera have been shown to exhibit opsonizing effects leading to enhanced intraperitoneal phagocytosis of E. coli 0111 (Galanos et al., 1977c), clearance from the circulation of S. enteritidis, and protection against infection with S. typhimurium (M. Parant and Ch. Galanos, unpublished data; Galanos et al., 1977c).

In several laboratories, anti-endotoxin effects of lipid A antiserum have been demonstrated. Lipid A antiserum prevents the local Shwartzman reaction in rabbits (Rietschel et al., 1975, Rietschel and Galanos, 1977) and the abortive effect in pregnant mice (F. Rioux-Darrieulat et al., 1978) provoked by lipopolysaccharide or free lipid A. Under special conditions, the lipopolysaccharide- or lipid A-induced fever response in rabbits is suppressed by anti-lipid A serum (Rietschel and Galanos, 1977; Rietschel et al., 1975; Galanos et al., 1977c).

Beneficial and damaging effects of lipid A antiserum in the pathogenesis of kidney inflammation have been demonstrated and, more generally, the possible involvement of an interaction of lipid A antibodies with cell-fixed endotoxin (free lipid A) in the mediation of some endotoxic effects has been discussed (Westenfelder *et al.*, 1975, 1977*a,b*, 1978).

4. LIPID A, THE ENDOTOXIC PRINCIPLE OF LIPOPOLYSACCHARIDES

It was of general importance when it was found that the incomplete lipopolysaccharides (Ra to Re of Fig. 5) of R mutants all exhibit equal endotoxic activity indistinguishable from that of wild type complete lipopolysaccharides (Lüderitz *et al.*, 1966a). This showed that the innermost part of lipopolysaccharides, i.e., $(KDO)_3$-lipid A must contain the endotoxic principle, and that the polysaccharide is not essential. It was then found that even KDO can be missing. Free lipid A, devoid of all core sugars, can be obtained by mild acid hydrolysis of S and R form lipopolysaccharides. This treatment cleaves the KDO linkages and free lipid A is liberated. When it was achieved to solubilize free lipid A in water, either by coupling to bovine serum albumin (Galanos *et al.*, 1972), or by conversion to the uniform triethylammonium salt form (Galanos and Lüderitz, 1975), it became possible to demonstrate its activity in many biological test systems. Table 2 lists the effects that have been shown to be exhibited by free lipid A.

It must be emphasized that free lipid A is released by mild acid treatment only from those lipopolysaccharides in which the linkage of the polysaccharide chain to lipid A is mediated by a sugar unit whose glycosidic linkage is acid-labile, e.g. the ketosidic linkage of KDO. Other lipopolysaccharides need more drastic conditions of hydrolysis, and in

TABLE 2. *Biological Activities Exhibited by Free Lipid A*

Activity	Reference
Pyrogenicity	Galanos *et al.* (1972); Rietschel *et al.* (1973)
Lethal Toxicity in Mice	Galanos *et al.* (1972)
Leucopenia, Leucocytosis	O. Westphal and C. Galanos, unpublished data.
Local Shwartzman Reaction	Rietschel and Galanos (1977).
Bone Marrow Necrosis	Galanos *et al.* (1972); Yoshida *et al.* (1972).
Embryonic Bone Resorption	Hausmann *et al.* (1975).
Complement Activation	Galanos *et al.* (1971a).
Depression of Blood Pressure	Westenfelder *et al.* (1975).
Platelet Aggregation	
Hageman Factor Activation	Morrison and Cochrane (1974).
Induction of Plasminogen Activator	Gordon *et al.* (1974)
Limulus Lysate Gelation	Yin *et al.* (1972)
Toxicity Enhanced by BCG and Adrenalectomy	Galanos *et al.* (1977b); M. Parant and C. Galanos, unpublished data.
Enhanced dermal Reactivity to Epinephrine	Neter *et al.* (1960)
Induction of nonspecific Resistance to Infection	M. Parant and C. Galanos, unpublished data
Induction of Tolerance to Endotoxin	Greer and Rietschel (1978a), Rietschel *et al.* (1973).
Induction of Early Refractory State to Temperature Change	Greer and Rietschel (1978a)
Adjuvance Activity	Andreesen (1974)
Mitogenic Activity for Cells	Andersson *et al.* (1973); Bona *et al.* (1975); Peavy *et al.* (1973); Rosenstreich *et al.* (1973); Janossy *et al.* (1973).
Macrophage Activation	Alexander and Evans (1971)
Induction of Colony Stimulating Factor	Apte *et al.* (1975); Urbaschek *et al.* (1980)
Induction of IgG Synthesis in New-Born Mice	Kolb *et al.* (1976)
Induction of Prostaglandin Synthesis	Dey *et al.* (1974), Rietschel *et al.*, 1980
Induction of Interferon Production	Schiller *et al.* (1976)
Induction of Tumor-Necrotizing Factor	C. Galanos, unpublished data
Induction of Mouse Liver Pyruvate Kinase	Smith and Snyder (1975)
Type C RNA Virus Release from Mouse Spleen Cells	Phillips *et al.* (1976)
Helper Activity for Friend Spleen Focus-Forming Virus in Mice	Steeves and Grundke-Iqbal (1976)
Inhibition of Phosphoenolpyruvate Carboxykinase	G. Hewlett and E. Th. Rietschel, unpublished data
Hypothermia in Mice	Greer and Rietschel (1978a,b)

these cases either degraded free lipid A or lipid A still linked to polysaccharide fragments are obtained (see Wilkinson, 1977).

4.1. PHYSICOCHEMICAL AND STRUCTURAL PREREQUISITES OF BIOLOGICAL ACTIVITIES

Lipopolysaccharides are amphiphiles. Due to their amphipathic character, they form micellar aggregates. Furthermore, their amphoteric character allows the formation of intermolecular cation- and polyamine-mediated ionic linkages which, depending on the nature of ions, may increase aggregation. Conversion of lipopolysaccharides into uniform salt forms after electrodialysis (Galanos and Lüderitz, 1975), has offered the possibility of investigating the influence of different cations on the degree of aggregation, and of studying the effect of aggregation on biological activities of lipopolysaccharides (Galanos, 1975; Galanos et al., 1979b). As seen from Table 3, S. abortus equi lipopolysaccharide expresses different degrees of aggregation (represented by sedimentation coefficients) depending on the nature of the cation neutralizing the negative charge. Furthermore, individual biological activities change with the state of aggregation, some increasing (lethal toxicity in rats, clearance from the blood, complement interaction, affinity to erythrocytes), others decreasing (lethal toxicity for mice, pyrogenicity) with increasing sedimentation coefficients, and others being independent (mitogenicity, Limulus lysate gelation).

The pronounced dependance of biological effects of endotoxins on their physical state has to be considered when lipopolysaccharides of different origin are being compared biologically. The standardized S. abortus equi lipopolysaccharide preparation described recently (Galanos et al., 1979a), which is available in a uniform salt form (sodium salt) as a highly purified preparation devoid of detectable amounts of proteins and other contaminants, should be useful as a reference compound in such investigations.

Comparative biological studies have been performed on Salmonella free lipid A and defined chemical degradation products thereof; on incomplete lipid A (lipid A precursor I); as well as on free lipid A's of different origin which are structurally distinct from Salmonella lipid A (see Table 1) and the respective parent lipopolysaccharides, in order to reveal structure/activity relationships (Lüderitz et al., 1978; Galanos et al., 1977a; Rietschel et al., 1981a).

These studies have shown that different endotoxic effects are separable in that different preparations exhibit selectively only some of the activities tested (lipid A antigenicity, complement reactivity, mitogenicity, Limulus lysate gelation, lethal toxicity, pyrogeni-

TABLE 3. *Sedimentation Coefficients and Biological Activities of the Lipopolysaccharide of* S. Abortus Equi *in Different Salt Forms*

S. abortus equi LPS Salt Form	Sedimentation coefficient (S)	Biological Activities with Increasing Sedimentation Coefficient		
		Increasing	Decreasing	Unchanged
Triethylamine	(9.3)	Lethal Toxicity (rat)	Lethal Toxocity (mouse)	Mitogenicity
Ethanolamine	(64)	Rate of Clearance from the Blood	Pyrogenicity (rabbit)	Limulus Lysate Gelation
Pyridin	(72)			
Sodium	(105)	Interaction with Complement		
Potassium	(135)			
Putrescine	(230)	Affinity to Red Blood Cells		
Calcium	partly insoluble			

city). The expression of these activities, therefore, must be linked to different qualities such as substructures or conformations of lipid A.

It became obvious that the various polar head groups detected in lipid A's (see Table 1) are not essential for biological activities and can be lacking. In fact, there are indications that substituents of the lipid A backbone such as the glucosamine residue of *Rh. tenue*, and even in some cases the O chain-core polysaccharide, may cause some inhibition in the expression of some biological effects (Rietschel *et al.*, 1981a). The phosphate groups of the backbone certainly play an indirect role for activity in that they mediate solubility of lipid A in water, and in that sense they are essential.

The smallest lipid A substructure tested and still endowed with endotoxic activities is the lipid A precursor I. Compared to *Salmonella* lipid A, it lacks the polar head groups and the non-hydroxylated fatty acids. It exhibits antigenicity, mitogenicity, lethal toxicity, and to some degree pyrogenicity and Limulus activity. The completely O-deacylated free lipid A, although still expressing antigenicity and mitogenicity, is devoid of typical endotoxin activities. Therefore, the structure important for endotoxicity is linked to the acylated lipid A backbone. Presently, we do not know whether the lipophilic character of the fatty acids *per se*, or their specific nature as 3-hydroxy fatty acids and their D-configuration as well as their positions are of importance.

Several approaches of chemically synthesizing lipid A and lipid A analogues are presently conducted in different laboratories (Inage *et al.*, 1980a,b; 1981; Kiso *et al.*, 1981a,b). With their help, many of the still open questions will be attacked.

Those lipid A's not containing the glucosamine backbone, but 3-amino-glucosamine instead, as well as the corresponding lipopolysaccharides, were found to be endotoxically inactive (*Rh. viridis*, *Rh. palustris*). Only complement and, in one case, Limulus gelation activities were expressed (Galanos *et al.*, 1977a).

5. MODE OF ACTION AND THE FATE OF LIPOPOLYSACCHARIDES IN EXPERIMENTAL ANIMALS

Many endotoxic activities are induced by mediators of host origin (Schlessinger, 1980). Lipopolysaccharides exert their actions in most instances because the higher animal reacts with the production of such mediators as endogenous pyrogen (Murphy *et al.*, 1980; tumor necrotizing factor (Carswell *et al.*, 1975; Männel *et al.*, 1980); superoxide anion (Pabst and Johnston, 1980); colony stimulating factor (Apte *et al.*, 1975; Nowotny *et al.*, 1975; Urbascheck *et al.*, 1980; Moore *et al.*, 1980); interferon (Youngner *et al.*, 1973); interleukin-1 (Rosenstreich and Wilton, 1975; Mizel *et al.*, 1978); glucocorticoid antagonizing factor (Berry *et al.*, 1977); plasminogen activator (Gordon *et al.*, 1974); prostaglandins (Rietschel *et al.*, 1980); histamine and serotonin (Urbascheck and Forssmann, 1980); and activated hormonal and enzymatic systems and others (for literature see Berry, 1977; Morrison and Ulevitch, 1978; Bradley, 1979, Schlessinger, 1980). Humoral systems and target cells of the host thus make endotoxin such an active biological principle. Lipopolysaccharide contains the very structures that act as biological signals for the subsequent activation or release of the many endogenous mediators which are finally responsible for the various effects of endotoxin *in vivo*.

One early target of lipolysaccharide after i.v. administration is the complement system. It has been demonstrated that, both *in vitro* and *in vivo*, a high degree of aggregation of lipopolysaccharide is required for the interaction with complement (Galanos and Lüderitz, 1976; see also Table 3). Lipopolysaccharide-induced complement activation is, however, not related to the toxic effects of endoxin. Thus the lipopolysaccharide of *Rh. viridis* exhibits high anti-complementary activity *in vivo* without causing toxic effects and, *vice versa*, lipopolysaccharides in the triethlamine form are highly toxic without causing complement inactivation (Freudenberg and Galanos, 1978; Mathison *et al.*, 1980).

Skarnes (1968) was the first to identify lipopolysaccharide complexes formed with plasma lipoprotein. Recently, lipopolysaccharide complexes with rat high density lipoprotein (HDL) have been identified (Mathison and Ulevitch, 1979; Ulevitch et al., 1979; Freudenberg et al., 1980a), which are formed within 3 min of lipopolysaccharide administration. The binding to HDL leads to a reduction of the rate of lipopolysaccharide clearance from the blood. Complex formation occurs with high affinity and it is mediated by lipid A. An important biological consequence of the interaction of endotoxin with HDL is the prevention of random adherence of lipopolysaccharide to cells and tissues, ensuring a more specific transport to organs of clearance (Freudenberg et al., 1980c).

It was first shown by Braude (1964) that endotoxin is cleared mainly into the liver, and to some extent, the spleen. Recent immuno-histochemical methods have been applied to study the kinetics of the distribution of Salmonella S- and Re-form lipopolysaccharides in the rat. In agreement with previous studies it was found (Freudenberg et al., 1980b; Ramadori et al., 1979) that the first cellular target for the S form lipopolysaccharide was macrophages, mainly Kupffer cells of the liver, and to a minor extent granulocytes. Two to three days after injection, however, a redistribution of the lipopolysaccharide in the liver was observed, and at this time the hepatocytes became strongly endotoxin-positive. When Re form lipopolysaccharides were used, they were also found to be distributed mainly in the liver, but the distribution was different from that of the S form. In addition to macrophages and granulocytes, a large proportion of the lipopolysaccharide was also found throughout the experiment in association with hepatocytes. In contrast, the lung was free of tissue-bound endotoxin during the first hours after injection. A large amount of endotoxin-positive cells appeared, however, after several hours. It is possible that these cells originate from the liver and/or spleen and are excreted through the lung (Freudenberg et al., 1980b).

There are a number of indications that the liver is an important organ of endotoxin excretion. In rabbits, high levels of lipopolysaccharides labelled with ^{125}J were detected in the gall bladder (Mathison and Ulevitch, 1979), and after injection of ^{14}C, ^3H-lipopolysaccharide, about 60% of the label was found in the feces of rats collected for up to 3 weeks (Kleine, 1981).

A number of endoxotin effects such as fever (Feldberg, 1975), early hypotension (Parrat and Sturges, 1977), shock (Fletcher and Ramwell, 1978), and abortion (Skarnes and Harper, 1972), can be suppressed by acetylsalicylic acid (aspirin) or indomethacin, i.e. drugs, which are inhibitors of prostaglandin biosynthesis. Furthermore, certain members of the prostaglandin family induce typical endotoxic reactions. These observations have led to the hypothesis that prostaglandins may represent mediators of lipopolysaccharide effects. In fact, macrophages could be identified as the cell type which, on incubation with lipopolysaccharide, would be stimulated to synthesis and excretion of prostaglandins of the E_2 and $F_{2\alpha}$ type (for reviews see Rietschel et al., 1980, 1981a, 1982).

Three lines of evidence exist indicating that macrophages are indeed the source of prostaglandins mediating lipopolysaccharide effects in vivo. The mouse strain C3H/HeJ, which is genetically resistant to a number of endotoxin effects including lethality (lipopolysaccharide nonresponder), harbours macrophages that cannot be stimulated by lipopolysaccharide to secrete PGE_2 and $F_{2\alpha}$ (Wahl et al., 1979; Rietschel et al., 1980). Macrophages from mice rendered tolerant (nonresponsive to endotoxin) by administration of sublethal doses of endotoxin are completely refractory to the action of lipopolysaccharide and do not secrete prostaglandins (Schade and Rietschel, 1980). Rats and mice fed with a diet devoid of essential fatty acids (precursors of prostaglandin biosynthesis) are highly resistant to lipopolysaccharide lethality (Cook et al., 1979; K. Tanamoto, U. Schade and E. Th. Rietschel, unpublished results).

These results are consistent with the hypothesis that macrophage-derived prostaglandins play a role in the mediation of endotoxin effects. Most results have been obtained with mouse macrophages from the peritoneum, or derived from the bone marrow. Preliminary observations show also that Kupffer cells (rat) and alveolar macrophages (rabbit) are stimulated by lipopolysaccharide to release prostaglandins E_2 and $F_{2\alpha}$ (Bhatnagar K. Decker, U. Schade, E. Th. Rietschel unpublished data).

6. CONCLUDING REMARKS

The main structural features of lipopolysaccharides have been elucidated. Presently, there are no indications that constituents or structural peculiarities have escaped detection, although this possibility cannot be fully excluded. The comparative chemical and biological investigation of natural and chemically synthesized lipid A will finally prove whether the proposed structure of *Salmonella* lipid A is correct and includes the toxophore groups. The synthesis of defined lipid A partial structures would then be of importance to elucidate structure/activity relationships and the mode of endotoxin actions, and to attack in a sophisticated way the possibilities to dissociate desirable and unwanted endotoxin effects, a goal that has accompanied the history of endotoxin research.

As mentioned before, endotoxin acts through the activation of a considerable number of mediators, each exhibiting a selective specific activity. The functioning of these complex biological systems obviously depends on various factors, including general genetic and individual conditions of the host. It is known that there are great species differences with regard to the sensitivity or resistance to one and the same lipopolysaccharide preparation. Rabbits, dogs, horses or humans are highly sensitive; mice, rats and guinea pigs are generally of medium sensitivity, and certain primates such as baboons or vervets are highly insensitive. The susceptibility of humans and baboons to endotoxin pyrogenicity differs by a factor of more than $1:100,000$. The mouse strain C3H/HeJ has been found to be largely resistant to endotoxin activities. For experiments to be comparable and reproducible the use of genetically controlled animal material is, therefore, indispensable. Species differences in the susceptibility may also allow a more detailed insight into the endogenous conditions that make lipopolysaccharide in certain species, like man, so highly active and inactive in others. The fact that very small amounts of lipopolysaccharide are active in sensitive species is one of the reasons for the difficulty to follow its fate *in vivo* by the usual radiolabelling techniques, making highly sensitive tests for endotoxin studies so urgent.

Several experimental models exist by which the natural sensitivity of animals towards lipopolysaccharide (endotoxin) may be increased. Examples are adrenalectomy, treatment with bacillus Calmette-Guerin (BCG), actinomycin D, ,lead tetraacetate, α-amanitin (Schlievert *et al.*, 1978), galactosamine (Galanos *et al.*, 1979c) or antigen–antibody complexes (Galanos, 1979).

These few comments are intended to emphasize that the standarization of experimental conditions, especially in endotoxin research, is of great importance. This is true for the genetic and individual (hormonal, pharmacological, immunological) make-up of the "biological substrate" of lipopolysaccharide and for the lipopolysaccharide preparation as well.

REFERENCES

ALEXANDER, P. and EVANS, R. (1971) Endotoxin and double stranded RNA render macrophages cytotoxic. *Nature (New Biology)* 232: 76–78.

ANDERSSON, J., MELCHERS, F., GALANOS, C. and LÜDERITZ, O. (1973) The mitogenic effect of lipopolysaccharide on bone marrow-derived mouse lymphocytes. Lipid A as the mitogenic part of the molecule. *J. exp. Med.* 137: 943–953.

ANDREESEN, R. (1974) Untersuchungen zur Adjuvansaktivität und Mitogenität von Lipopolysacchariden. Ph. D. Thesis, Universität Freiburg.

APTE, R. N., GALANOS, C. and PLUZNIK, D. V. (1975) Lipid A, the active part of bacterial endotoxins in inducing serum colony stimulating activity and macrophage progenitor cells. *J. cell. Physiol.* 87: 71–78.

BANERJI, E. and ALVING, C. R. (1979) Lipid A from endotoxin: antigenic activities of purified fractions in liposomes. *J. Immun.* 123: 2558–2562.

BERRY, L. J. (1977) Bacterial toxins. *Critical Rev. Toxicol.* 5: 239–318.

BERRY, L. J., MOORE, R. N., GOODRUM, K. J. and COUCH, R. E. JR. (1977) Cellular requirements for enzyme inhibition by endotoxin in mice. In: *Microbiology—1977*, pp. 321–325, SCHLESSINGER, D. (ed). Am. Soc. Microbiol., Washington, D. C.

BLADEN, H. A. and MERGENHAGEN, ST. E. (1964) Ultrastructure of *Veillonella* and morphological correlation of an outer membrane with particles associated with endotoxic activity. *J. Bact.* 88: 1482–1492.

BLAKE, D., HAMLYN, A. N., PROCTOR, S. and WARDLE, E. N. (1980) Anti-endotoxin (anti-lipid A) antibodies. *Experientia* **36**: 254–255.

BONA, C., DAMAIS, C., GALANOS, C. and CHEDID, L. (1975) The mitogenic activity of lipopolysaccharides on lymphocytes in culture. II. Comparative study in five mammalian species. In: *Gram-Negative Bacterial Infections and Mode of Endotoxin Actions*, pp. 182–189, URBASCHEK, B., URBASCHEK, R. and NETER, E. (eds). Springer, New York.

BRADLEY, S. G. (1979) Cellular and molecular mechanism of action of bacterial endotoxins. *A. Rev. Microbiol.* **33**: 67–94.

BRAUDE, A. J. (1964) Absorption, distribution and elimination of endotoxins and their derivatives. In: *Bacterial Endotoxins*, pp. 98–109, LANDY, M. and BRAUN, W. (eds.). Rutgers Univ. Press, New Brunswick, N.J.

BRAUN, V. and HANTKE, K. (1981) Bacterial cell surface receptors. In: *Organization of Prokaryotic Cell Membranes*, Vol. **2**, GOSH, B. K. (ed). CRC Press, Florida.

BROADY, K. W., RIETSCHEL, E. TH. and LÜDERITZ, O. (1981) The chemical structure of the lipid A component of lipopolysaccharides from *Vibro cholerae*. *Eur. J. Biochem.* **115**: 463–468.

BRYN, K. and RIETSCHEL, E. TH. (1978) L-2-hydroxytetradecanoic acid as a constituent of *Salmonella* lipopolysaccharides (lipid A). *Eur. J. Biochem.* **86**: 311–315.

CARSWELL, E. A., OLD, L. J., KASSEL, R. L., GREEN, S., FIORE, N. and WILLIAMSON, B. (1975) An endotoxin-induced serum factor that causes tumor necrosis. *Proc. natn. Acad. Sci. U.S.A.* **72**: 3666–3670.

COOK, J. A., WISE, W. C. and CALLIHAN, C. (1979) Resistance to endotoxin shock by rat deficient in essential fatty acids. *Fedn Proc.* **38**: 1261.

DEY, P. K., FELDBERG, W. and WENDLANDT, S. (1974) Lipid A and prostaglandin. *J. Physiol., London* **239**: 102–103.

DIENA, B. B., ASHTON, F. E., RYAN, A., WALLACE, R. and PERRY, M. B. (1978) The lipopolysaccharide (R type) as a common antigen of *Neisseria gonorrhoeae*. I. Immunizing properties. *Can. J. Microbiol.* **23**: 117–123.

FELDBERG, W. (1975) Body temperature and fever: changes in our views during the last decade. *Proc. R. Soc. London B.* **191**: 199–229.

FINK, P. C. and KOZAK, J. (1980) Determination of free lipid A by enzyme-immunoassay (ELISA). *Fresenius, Z. Analyt, Chem.* **301**: 117–118.

FINK, P. C. and GALANOS, C. (1981) Determination of anti-lipid A and lipid A by enzyme immunoassay. *Immunology* **158**: 380–390.

FLETCHER, J. R. and RAMWELL, P. W. (1978) *E. coli* endotoxin shock in the baboon: Treatment with lidocaine oder indomethacin. In: *Advances Prostaglandin Thromboxin Research*, Vol. **3**, pp. 183–192, GALLI, C., GALLI, G. and PORCELLATI, G. (eds). Raven Press, New York.

FREUDENBERG, M. (1977) Specific immune responses of different animals to lipid A. *Acta microbiol. hung.* **24**: 166–167.

FREUDENBERG, M. and GALANOS, C. (1978) Interaction of lipopolysaccharides and lipid A with complement in rats and its relation to endotoxicity. *Infect. Immun.* **19**: 875–882.

FREUDENBERG, M., BØG-HANSEN, T. C., BACK, U. and GALANOS, C. (1980a) Interaction of LPS with plasma high-density lipoprotein in rats. *Infect. Immun.* **28**: 373–380.

FREUDENBERG, M., FREUDENBERG, N. and GALANOS, C. (1980b) Studies on the distribution of endotoxin in rats. *FEMS Symposion on Microbial Envelopes* Abstract 123.

FREUDENBERG, M. A., BØG-HANSE, T. C., BACK, U., JIRILLO, E. and GALANOS, C. (1980c) Interaction of lipopolysaccharides with plasma high density lipoprotein in rats. In: *Natural Toxins*, pp. 349–354, EAKER, D. and WADSTRÖM, T. (eds.). Pergamon Press, Oxford, New York.

GALANOS, C. (1975) Physical state and biological activity of lipopolysaccharides. Toxicity and immunogenicity of the lipid A component. *Z. Immun. Forsch.* **149**: 214–229.

GALANOS, C. (1979) Biological properties of lipopolysaccharides (LPS) and lipid A. *Toxicon Suppl.* 1, **17**: 53.

GALANOS, C. and LÜDERITZ, Q. (1975) Electrodialysis of lipopolysaccharides and their conversion to uniform salt forms. *Eur. J. Biochem.* **54**: 603–610.

GALANOS, C. and LÜDERITZ, O. (1976) The role of the physical state of lipopolysaccharides in the interaction with complement. *Eur. J. Biochem.* **65**: 403–408.

GALANOS, C., LÜDERITZ, O. and WESTPHAL, O. (1969) A new method for the extraction of R lipopolysaccharides. *Eur. J. Biochem.* **9**: 245–249.

GALANOS, C., RIETSCHEL, E. TH., LÜDERITZ, O. and WESTPHAL, O. (1971a) Interaction of lipopolysaccharides and lipid A with complement. *Eur. J. Biochem.* **19**: 143–152.

GALANOS, C., LÜDERITZ, O. and WESTPHAL, O. (1971b) Preparation and properties of antisera against the lipid A component of bacterial lipopolysaccharides. *Eur. J. Biochem.* **24**: 116–122.

GALANOS, C., RIETSCHEL, E. TH., LÜDERITZ, O., WESTPHAL, O., KIM, B. and WATSON, D. W. (1972) Biological activities of lipid A complexed with bovine-serum albumin. *Eur. J. Biochem.* **31**: 230–233.

GALANOS, C., ROPPEL, J., WECKESSER, J., RIETSCHEL, E. TH. and MAYER, H. (1977a) Biological activities of LPS and lipid A from *Rhodospirillaceae*. *Infect. Immun.* **16**: 407–412.

GALANOS, C., FREUDENBERG, M., HASE, S., JAY, F. and RUSCHMANN, E. (1977b) Biological activities and immunological properties of lipid A. In: *Microbiology—1977*, pp. 269–276, SCHLESSINGER, D. (ed.) Amer. Soc. Microbiol., Washington, D.C.

GALANOS, G., LÜDERITZ, O., RIETSCHEL, E. TH. and WESTPHAL, O. (1977c) Newer aspects of the chemistry and biology of bacterial lipopolysaccharides, with special reference to their lipid A component. In: *International Review of Biochemistry*: Biochemistry of lipids II, Vol. **14**, 239–335, GOODWIN, T. W. (ed). University Press, Baltimore.

GALANOS, C., LÜDERITZ, O. and WESTPHAL, O. (1979a) Preparation and properties of a standardized lipopolysaccharide from *Salmonella abortus equi*. *Zbl. Bakt. Hyg., I. Abt. Orig. A* **243**: 225–244.

GALANOS, C., FREUDENBERG, M., LÜDERITZ, O., RIETSCHEL, E. TH. and WESTPHAL, O. (1979b) Chemical, physicochemical, and biological properties of bacterial lipopolysaccharides. In: *Biomedical Applications of the Horseshoe Crab (Limulidae)*, pp. 321–332, COHEN, E. (ed). A. R. Liss, New York.

GALANOS, C., FREUDENBERG, M. A. and REUTTER, W. (1979c) Galactosamine-induced sensitization to the lethal effects of endotoxin. *Proc. natn. Acad. Sci. U.S.A.* **76**: 5939–5943.

GMEINER, J., LÜDERITZ, O. and WESTPHAL, O. (1969) Biochemical studies on lipopolysaccharides of Salmonella R mutants 6. Investigations on the structure of the lipid A component. *Eur. J. Biochem.* **7**: 370–379.

GMEINER, J., SIMON, M. and LÜDERITZ, O. (1971) The linkage of phosphate groups and of 2-keto-3-deoxyocto-nate to the lipid A component in a *Salmonella minnesota* lipopolysaccharide. *Eur. J. Biochem.* **21**: 355–356.

GOLDMAN, R. C. and LEIVE, L. (1980) Heterogeneity of antigenic-side-chain length in LPS from *E. coli* 0111 and *S. typhimurium* LT2. *Eur. J. Biochem.* **107,** 145–153.

GORBACH, C. I., KRASIKOVA, I. N., LUKYANOV, P. A., RAZMAKHNINA, O. Y., SOLOV'EVA, T. F. and OVODOV, Y. S. (1979) Structural studies on the immunodominant group of lipid A from lipopolysaccharide of *Yersinia pseudotuberculosis. Eur. J. Biochem.* **98**: 83–86.

GORDON, S., UNKELESS, J. C. and COHN, Z. A. (1974) Induction of macrophage plasminogen activator by endotoxin stimulation and phagocytosis; evidence for a 2 stage process. *J. exp. Med.* **140**: 995–1010.

GREER, G. G. and RIETSCHEL, E. TH. (1978a) Lipid A-induced tolerance and hyperreactivity to hypothemia in mice. *Infect. Immun.* **19**: 357–368.

GREER, G. G. and RIETSCHEL, E. TH. (1978b) Inverse relationship between the susceptibility of lipopolysac-charide (lipid A)-pretreated mice to the hypothermic and lethal effect of lipopolysaccharide. *Infect. Immun.* **20**: 366–374.

HASE, S. and RIETSCHEL, E. TH. (1976) Isolation and analysis of the lipid A backbone. Lipid A structure of lipopolysaccharides from various bacterial groups. *Eur. J. Biochem.* **63**: 101–107.

HASE, S. and RIETSCHEL, E. TH. (1977) The chemical structure of the lipid A component of lipopolysaccharides from *Chromobacterium violaceum* NCTC 9694. *Eur. J. Biochem.* **75**; 23–34.

HAUSMANN, E., LÜDERITZ, O., KNOX, K. and WEINFELD, N. (1975) Structural requirements for bone resorption by endotoxin and lipoteichoic acid. *J. dent. Res.* **54**: B94–B99.

INAGE, M., CHAKI, H., KUSUMOTO, S., SHIBA, T., TAI, A., NAKAHATA, M., HARADA, T. and IZUMI, Y. (1980a) Chemical synthesis of bidephospho lipid A of *Salmonella* endotoxin. *Chemistry Lett.* (Japan): 1373–1376.

INAGE, M., CHAKI, H., KUSUMOTO, S. and SHIBA, T. (1980b) Synthesis of lipopolysaccharide corresponding to fundamental structure of *Salmonella*-type lipid A. *Tetrahedron Lett.* **21**: 3889–3892.

INAGE, M., CHAKI, H., KUSUMOTO, S. and SHIBA, T. (1981) Chemical synthesis of phosphorylated fundamental structure of lipid A. *Tetrahedron Lett.* **22**: 2281–2284.

JANN, K. and WESTPHAL, O. (1975) Microbial polysaccharides. In: *The Antigens*, Vol. **III,** pp. 1–125, SELA, M. (ed). Academic Press, New York.

JANOSSY, H., HUMPHREY, J. H., PEPYS, M. B. and GREAVES, M. F. (1973) Complement independence of stimu-lation of mouse splenic B lymphocytes by mitrogens. *Nature (New Biol.)* **245**: 108–112.

JAY, F. A. (1978) Gram-negative lipopolysaccharide. Characterization of the immunodeterminant structure of lipid A. Ph.D. Thesis. University of Surrey, Guildford, England.

JENSEN, M. (1980) Strukturanalyse der Lipoid A Komponente von Lipopolysacchariden aus *Yersinia enterocoli-tica.* Ph. D. Thesis, Universität Freiburg.

JOSEPHSON, S. and BUNDLE, D. R. (1979) Artificial carbohydrate antigens: the synthesis of the tetrasaccharide repeating unit of *Shigella flexneri* O antigen. *Can. J. Chem.* **57**: 3073–3097.

KABIN, S., ROSENSTREICH, D. L. and MERGENHAGEN, S. E. (1978) Bacterial endotoxins and cell membranes. In: *Bacterial Toxins and Cell Membranes*, pp. 59–87, JELIJASZEWICZ, J. and WADSTRÖM, T. (eds). Academic Press, New York and London.

KADIS, S., WEINBAUM, G. and AJL, S. J. (eds.) (1971) Bacterial Endotoxins. In: *Microbial Toxins*, Vol. V, pp. 1–507, Academic Press, New York, London.

KASS, E. H. and WOLFF, S. M. (eds.) (1973) *Bacterial Lipopolysaccharides, the Chemistry, Biology and Clinical Significance of Endotoxins*, pp. 1–304, University of Chicago Press, Chicago.

KISO, M., NISHIGUCHI, H., MURASE, S. and HASEGAWA, A. (1981a) A convenient synthesis of 2-deoxy-2-(D-3-hydroxytetradecanoyl-amino)-D-glucose: diastereoisomers of the monomeric lipid A component of the bacterial lipopolysaccharide. *Carboh. Res.* **88**: C5–C9.

KISO, M., NISHIGUCHI, H., NISHIHORI, K. and HASEGAWA, A. (1981b) Synthesis of β-D-(1-6)linked disaccharides of N-fatty acylated 2-amino-2-deoxy-D-glucose: an approach to the lipid A component of the bacterial lipopolysaccharide. *Carboh. Res.* **88**: C10–C13.

KLEINE, B. (1981) Das Schicksal von bakteriellem Lipopolysaccharid *in vivo*. Untersuchungen zur Ausscheidung von Lipopolysaccharide durch Meerkatzen und Ratten. Ph.D. Thesis, Universität Freiburg.

KOLB, C., DI PAULI, R. and WEILER, E. (1976) Induction of IgG in young nude mice by lipid A or thymus grafts. *J. exp. Med.* **144**: 1031–1036.

LEHMANN, V. (1977) Isolation, purification and properties of an intermediate in 3-deoxy-D-*manno*-octulosonic acid–lipid A biosynthesis. *Eur. J. Biochem.* **75**: 257–266.

LEHMANN, V., LÜDERITZ, O. and WESTPHAL, O. (1971) The linkage of pyrophosphorylethanolamine to heptose in the core of *Salmonella minnesota* lipopolysaccharide. *Eur. J. Biochem.* **21**: 339–347.

LEHMANN, V., RUPPRECHT, E. and OSBORN, M. J. (1977) Isolation of mutants conditionally blocked in the biosynthesis of the 3-deoxy-D-*manno*-octulosonic acid–Lipid A part of lipopolysaccharides derived from *Salmonella typhimurium. Eur. J. Biochem.* **76**: 41–49.

LEHMANN, V., REDMOND, J., EGAN, A. and MINNER, I. (1978) The acceptor for polar head groups of the lipid A component of *Salmonella* lipopolysaccharides. *Eur. J. Biochem.* **86**: 487–496.

LINDBERG, A. A. (1967) Studies of a receptor for Felix 0-1 phage in *Salmonella minesota. J. gen. Microbiol.* **48**: 225–233.

LINDBERG, A. A. (1977) Bacterial surface carbohydrates and bacteriophage adsorption. In: *Surface Carbo-hydrates of the Prokaryotic Cell*, pp. 289–356. SUTHERLAND, I. (ed). Academic Press, London, New York.

LÜDERITZ, O., STAUB, A. M. and WESTPHAL, O. (1966a) Immunochemistry of O and R antigens of *Salmonella* and related *Enterobacteriaceae. Bact. Rev.* **30**: 192–255.

LÜDERITZ, O., GALANOS, C., RISSE, H. J., RUSCHMANN, E., SCHLECHT, S., SCHMIDT, G., SCHULTE-HOLTHAUSEN,

H., Wheat, R., Westphal, O. and Schlosshardt, J. (1966b) Structural relationships of *Salmonella* O and R antigens. *Ann. N.Y. Acad. Sci.* **133**: 349–374.

Lüderitz, O., Westphal, O., Staub, A. M. and Nikaido, H. (1971) Isolation and chemical and immunological characterization of bacterial lipopolysaccharides. In: *Microbial Toxins*, pp. 145–233, Weinbaum G., Kadis, S. and Ajl, S. J. (eds). Vol. IV, Bacterial Endotoxins, Academic Press, New York, London.

Lüderitz, O., Galanos, C., Lehmann, V., Nurminen, M., Rietschel, E. Th., Rosenfelder, G., Simon, M. and Westphal, O. (1973) Lipid A: Chemical structure and biological activity. *J. infect. Dis.* **128**: (suppl.) S17-S29.

Lüderitz, O., Galanos, C., Lehmann, V., Mayer, H., Rietschel, E. Th. and Weckesser, J. (1978) Chemical structure and biological activities of lipid A's from various bacterial families. *Naturwissenschaften* **65**: 578–585.

Lüderitz, O., Freudenberg, M. A., Galanos, Ch., Lehmann, V., Rietschel, E. Th., Shaw, D. H. (1981) Lipopolysaccharides of gram-negative bacteria. In: *Microbial Membrane Lipids*, Razin, S. and Rottem, S. (eds). Current Topics in Membranes and Transport. Academic Press, New York.

Mäkelä, P. H. and Stocker, B. A. D. (1981) Genetics of the bacterial cell surface. In: *Genetics as a Tool in Microbiology*, Glover, S. (ed). 31st. Symp. Soc. Gen. Microbiol., Cambridge University Press, Cambridge.

Mäkelä, P. H., Valtonen, V. V. and Valtonen, M. (1973) Role of O-antigen (lipopolysaccharide) factors in the virulence of *Salmonella*. *J. infect. Dis.* **128**: S81–S85.

Männel, D. N., Moore, R. N. and Mergenhagen, S. E. (1980) Endotoxin-induced tumor cytotoxic factor. In: *Microbiology—1980*, pp. 141–143, Schlessinger, D. (ed). Am. Soc. Microbiol., Washington, D.C.

Mathison, J. C. and Ulevitch, R. J. (1979) The clearance, tissue distribution and cellular localisation of intravenously injected lipopolysaccharides in rabbits. *J. Immun.* **123**: 2133–2143.

Mathison, J. C., Ulevitch, R. J., Flechter, J. R. and Cochrane, C. G. (1980) The distribution of lipopolysaccharides in normocomplementemic and C3-depleted rabbits and Rhesus monkeys. *Am. J. Path.* **101**: 245–262.

Mattsby-Baltzer, I. and Kaijser, B. (1979) Lipid A and anti-lipid A. *Infect. Immun.* **23**: 758–763.

McCabe, W. R. Bruins, Sc. C., Graven, D. E. and Johns, M. (1977) Cross-reactive antigens: their potential for immunization-induced immunity to gram-negative bacteria. *J. infect. Dis.* **136**: 161–166.

McCabe, W. R., Johns, M. A., Craven, D. E. and Bruins, S. C. (1977) Clinical implications of enterobacterial antigens. In: *Microbiology—1977*, pp. 293–297. Schlessinger, D. (ed). Am. Soc. Microbiol., Washington, D.C.

Mizel, S. B., Oppenheim, J. J. and Rosenstreich, D. L. (1978). Characterization of lymphocyte-activating factor (LAF) produced by a macrophage cell line, P388D$_1$. II. Biochemical characterization of LAF induced by activated T cells and LPS. *J. Immun.* **120**: 1504–1514.

Moore, R. N., Steeg, P. S., Männel, D. N. and Mergenhagen, St. E. (1980) Role of lipopolysaccharide in regulating colony-stimulating factor-dependent macrophage proliferation *in vitro*. *Infec. Immun.* **30**: 797–804.

Morrison, D. C. and Cochrane, Ch. G. (1974) Direct evidence for Hageman factor (factor XII) activation by bacterial lipopolysaccharides (endotoxins). *J. exp. Med.* **140**: 797–811.

Morrison, D. C. and Ulevitch, R. J. (1978) The effects of bacterial endotoxins on host mediation systems. *Am. J. Path.* **93**: 526–618.

Mühlradt, P. F., Menzel, J., Golecki, J. R. and Speth, V. (1973) Outer membrane of *Salmonella*. Sites of export of newly synthesized lipopolysaccharide on the bacterial surface. *Eur. J. Biochem.* **35**: 471–481.

Mühlradt, P. F., Wray, V. and Lehman, V. (1977) A ^{31}P-nuclear-magnetic-resonance study of the phosphate groups in lipopolysaccharide and lipid A from *Salmonella*. *Eur. J. Biochem.* **81**: 193–203.

Murphy, P., Hanson, D. F., Simon, P. L., Willoughby, W. F. and Windle, B. E. (1980) Properties of two distinct endogenous pyrogens secreted by rabbit macrophages. In: *Microbiology—1980*, pp. 158–161, Schlessinger, D. (ed). Am. Soc. Microbiol., Washington, D.C.

Neter, E., Anzi, H., Gorzynski, E. A., Nowotny, A. and Westphal, O. (1960) Effects of the lipid A component of *E. coli* endotoxin on dermal reactivity of rabbits to epinephrine. *Proc. Soc. exp. Biol. Med.* **103**: 783–786.

Nghiem, H. O. and Staub, A. M. (1975) Molecular immunological heterogeneity of the *Salmonella zuerich* (1,9,23,(46),27) cell-wall polysaccharides. *Carboh. Res.* **40**: 153–169.

Nikaido, H. and Nakae, T. (1979) The outer membrane of gram-negative bacteria. In: *Advances in Microbiology and Physiology*, Vol. **20**, pp. 163–250, Rose, A. H. and Morris, I. G. (ed). Academic Press, London.

Nixdorff, K. K. and Schlecht, S. (1972) Heterogeneity of the hemagglutinin responses to *Salmonella minnesota* R-antigens in rabbits. *J. gen. Microbiol.* **71**: 425–440.

Nixdorff, K. K., Schlecht, S., Rüde, E. and Westphal, O. (1975) Immunological responses to *Salmonella* R antigens. The bacterial cell and the protein edestin as carriers for R oligosaccharide determinants. *Immunology* **29**: 87–102.

Nowotny, A., Behling, U. H. and Chang, H. L. (1975) Relation of structure to function in bacterial endotoxins. VIII. Biological activities in a polysaccharide-rich fraction. *J. Immun.* **115**: 199–203.

Osborn, M. J. (1979) Biosynthesis and assembly of the lipopolysaccharide of the outer membrane. In: *Bacterial Outer Membranes*, pp. 15–34. Inouye, M. (ed). Wiley Interscience, New York.

Osborn, M. J. and Rothfield, L. I. (1971) Biosynthesis of the core region of lipopolysaccharides. In: *Microbial Toxins*, Vol IV, Bacterial Endotoxins, pp. 331–350, Weinbaum, G., Kadis, S. and Ajl S. J. (eds). Academic Press, New York and London.

Osborn, M. J. and Wu, H. C. P. (1980) Proteins of the outer membrane of gram-negative bacteria. *A. Rev. Microbiol.* **34**: 369–422.

Osborn, M. J., Rick, P. D., Lehmann, V., Rupprecht, E. and Singh, M. (1974) Structure and biogenesis of the cell envelope of gram-negative bacteria. *Ann. N.Y. Acad. Sci.* **235**: 52–65.

Osborn, M. J., Rick, P. D. and Rasmussen, N. S. (1980) Mechanism of assembly of the outer membrane of

Salmonella typhimurium. Translocation and integration of an incomplete mutant lipid A into the outer membrane. *J. biol. Chem.* **255:** 4246–4251.

PABST, M. J. and JOHNSTON, R. B. (1980) Increased production of superoxide anion by macrophages exposed *in vitro* to muramyl dipeptide or lipopolysaccharide. *J. exp. Med.* **151:** 101–114.

PALVA, E. T. and MÄKELÄ, P. H. (1980) Lipopolysaccharide heterogeneity in *Salmonella typhimurium* analyzed by sodium dodecylsulfate-polyacrylamide gel electrophoresis. *Eur. J. Biochem.* **107:** 137–143.

PARRATT, J. R. and STURGESS, R. M. (1977) Evidence that prostaglandin release mediates pulonary vasoconstriction induced by *E. coli* endotoxin. *J. Physiol., Lond.* **246:** 79–80.

PEAVY, D. L., SHANDS, J. W. and ADLER, W. H. (1973) Mitogenicity of bacterial endotoxins: characterization of the mitogenic principle. *J. Immun.* **11:** 352–357.

PHILLIPS, S. M., STEPHENSON, J. R., GREENBUGER, J. S., LANE, P. E. and AARONSON, S. A. (1976) Release of xenotropic type CRNA virus in response to lipopolysaccharide: Activity of lipid A portion upon B lymphocytes. *J. Immun.* **116:** 1123–1128.

RAMADORI, G., GALANOS, C., HOPF, V. and MEYER ZUM BÜSCHENFELDE, K. (1979) *In vitro* and *in vivo* reactivity of lipopolysaccharides and lipid A with parenchymal and non-parenchymal liver cells in mice. In: *The Reticuloendothelial System and the Pathogenesis of Liver Disease*, pp. 285–294. LIEHR, H. and GRÜN, M. (eds). Elsevier/North-Holland, Amsterdam.

RICK, D. P., FUNG, L. W. M., HO, CH. and OSBORN, M. J. (1977) Lipid A mutants of *Salmonella typhimurium.* Purification and characterization of a lipid A precursor produced by a mutant in 3-deoxy-D-*mannooctulo-sonate*-8-phosphate synthetase. *J. biol. Chem.* **252:** 4904–4912.

RIETSCHEL, E. TH. and GALANOS, C. (1977) Lipid A antiserum-mediated protection against lipopolysaccharide- and lipid A-induced fever and skin necrosis. *Infect. Immun.* **15:** 34–49.

RIETSCHEL, E. TH., GALANOS, C. and LÜDERITZ, O. (1975) Structure, endotoxicity and immunogenicity of the lipid A component of bacterial lipopolysaccharides. In: *Microbiology—1975*, pp. 307–314, SCHLESSINGER, D. (ed). Am. Soc. Microbiol., Washington, D.C.

RIETSCHEL, E. TH., GALANOS, C., LÜDERITZ, O. and WESTPHAL, O. (1981) Chemical structure, physiological function and biological activity of lipopolysaccharides and lipid A. In: *Immunopharmacology*. WEBB, D. R. (ed). Marcel Decker, New York.

RIETSCHEL, E. TH., GOTTERT, H., LÜDERITZ, O. and WESTPHAL, O. (1972) Nature and linkages of the fatty acids present in the lipid A component of *Salmonella lipopolysaccharides. Eur. J. Biochem.* **28:** 166–173.

RIETSCHEL, E. TH., HASE, S., KING, M.-T., REDMOND, J. and LEHMANN, V. (1977) Chemical structure of lipid A. In: *Microbiology—1977*, pp. 262–268, SCHLESSINGER, D. (ed). Am. Soc. Microbiol., Washington, D.C.

RIETSCHEL, E. TH., SCHADE, U., LÜDERITZ, O., FISCHER, H. and PESKAR, B. A. (1980) Prostaglandins in endotoxicosis. In: *Microbiology—1980*, pp. 66–72, SCHLESSINGER, D. (ed). Am. Soc. Microbiol., Washington, D.C.

RIETSCHEL, E. TH., KIM, Y. B., WATSON, D. W., GALANOS, C., LÜDERITZ, O. and WESTPHAL, O. (1973) Pyrogenicity and immunogenicity of lipid A complexed with bovine serum albumin or human serum albumin. *Infect. Immun.* **8:** 173–177.

RIETSCHEL, E. TH., SCHADE, U., JENSEN, M., WOLLENWEBER, H.-W., LÜDERITZ, O. and GREISMAN, S. G. (1982) Bacterial endotoxins: chemical structure, biological activity, and role in septicaemia. *Scand. J. Infect. Dis.,* S**31:** 8–21.

RIOUX-DARRIEULAT, F., PARANT, M. and CHEDID, L. (1978) Prevention of endotoxin-induced abortion by treatment of mice with antisera. *J. Infect. Dis.* **137:** 7–13.

ROSENSTREICH, D. L. and WILTON, J. M. (1975) The mechanism of action of macrophages in the activation of T-lymphocytes *in vitro* by antigens and mitogens. In: *Proceedings of the 9th Leukocyte Culture Conference*, pp. 113–132. ROSENTHAL, A. S. (ed). Academic Press, New York.

ROSENSTREICH, D. L., NOWOTNY, A., CHUSED, T. and MERGENHAGEN, S. E. (1973) *In vitro* transformation of mouse bone-marrow-derived (B) lymphocytes induced by the lipid component of endotoxin. *Infect. Immun.* **8:** 406–411.

ROSNER, M. R., TANG, J. Y., BARZILAY, I. and KHORANA, H. G. (1979a) Structure of the LPS from an *E. coli* heptose-less mutant. I. Chemical degradations and identification of products. *J. biol. Chem.* **254:** 5904–5917.

ROSNER, M. R., KHORANA, H. G. and SATTERTHWAIT, A. C. (1979b) The structure of lipopolysaccharide from a heptose-less mutant of *E. coli* K-12. II. The application of ^{31}P NMR spectroscopy. *J. biol. Chem.* **254:** 5918–5925.

ROSNER, M. R., VERRET, R. C. and KHORANA, H. G. (1979c) The structure of LPS from an *E. coli* heptoseless mutant. III. Two fatty acyl amidases from *Dictyiostelium discoideum* and their action on LPS derivatives. *J. biol. Chem.* **254:** 5926–5933.

RUSCHMANN, E. and NIEBUHR, C. (1972) Bestimmung der Antigen-Faktoren des Kernpolysaccharids von *S. minnesota*- und *S. ruiru*-R-Mutanten. *Zbl. Bakt. Hyg., I. Abt. Orig. A* **222:** 326–341.

SCHADE, U. and RIETSCHEL, E., TH. (1980) Difference in lipopolysaccharide-induced prostaglandin release and phagocytosis capacity of peritoneal macrophages from LPS-hyperreactive and tolerant mice. In: *Natural Toxins*, pp. 271–277, EAKER, D. and WADSTRÖM, T. (eds). Pergamon Press, New York.

SCHILLER, J. G., RIBOVITCH, R., FEINGOLD, D. S. and YOUNGNER, J. (1976) Interferon production in mice by components of *Salmonella minnesota* R595 lipid A. *Infect. Immun.* **14:** 586–589.

SCHINDLER, M. and OSBORN, M. J. (1979) Interaction of divalent cations and polymyxin B with lipopolysaccharide. *Biochem.* **18:** 4425–4430.

SCHLESSINGER, D. (ed.) (1977) In: *Microbiology—1977·* Part IV: Bacterial Antigens and Host Response. pp. 219–326, Am. Soc. Microbiol., Washington, D.C.

SCHLESSINGER, D. (ed.) (1980) *Microbiology—1980,* Part I: Endogenous Mediators in Host Responses to Bacterial Endotoxins, pp. 1–170. Am. Soc. Microbiol., Washington, D.C.

SCHLIEVERT, P. M. and WATSON, D. W. (1978) Group A streptococcal pyrogenic endotoxin: Pyrogenicity, alteration of blood brain barrier, and separation of sites for pyrogenicity and enhancement of lethal endotoxin shock. *Infect. Immun.* **21:** 753–763.

SCHUSTER, B. G., NEIDIG, M., ALVING, B. M. and ALVING, C. R. (1979) Production of antibodies against phosphocholine, phosphatidylcholine, sphingomyelin, and lipid A by injection of liposomes containing lipid A. *J. Immun.* **122**: 900–905.

SHANDS, J. W. (1975) Endotoxin as a pathogenic mediator of gram-negative infection. In: *Microbiology—1975*, pp. 330–335, SCHLESSINGER, D. (ed). Am. Soc. Microbiol., Washington D.C.

SKARNES, R. C. (1968) *In vivo* interaction of endotoxin with a plasma lipoprotein having esterase activity. *J. Bact.* **95**: 2031–2034.

SKARNES, R. C. and HARPER, M. J. K. (1972) Relationship between endotoxin-induced abortion and the synthesis of prostaglandin F. *Prostaglandins* **1**: 191–203.

SMITH, H., SKEHEL, J. J. and TURNER, M. J. (eds.) (1980) *Life Sciences Research Report: The Molecular Basis of Microbial Pathogenicity*, pp. 1–359. Verlag Chemie, Weinheim, Deerfield, Basel.

SMITH, S. M. and SNYDER, I. S. (1975) Effect of LPS and lipid A on mouse liver pyruvate kinase activity. *Infect. Immun.* **12**: 993–998.

STEEVES, R. A. and GRUNDKE-IQBAL, I. (1976) Bacterial LPS as helper factors for Friend spleen focus-forming virus in mice. *J. natn. Cancer Inst.* **56**: 541–546.

STOCKER, B. A. D. and MÄKELÄ, P. H. (1971) Genetic aspects of biosynthesis and structure of *Salmonella* lipopolysaccharide. In: *Microbial Toxins*, Vol. IV, Bacterial Toxins, pp. 369–438, WEINBAUM, G., KADIS, S. and AJL, S. J. (eds). Academic Press, New York and London.

SVENUNGSSON, B. and LINDBERG, A. A. (1978) Identification of *Salmonella* bacteria by coagglutination, using antibodies against synthetic disaccharide-protein antigens 02, 04 and 09, adsorbed to protein A-containing *Staphylococci*. *Acta path. microbiol. scand. Sect. B.* **86**: 283–290.

THARANATHAN, R. N., WECKESSER, J. and MAYER, H. (1978) Structural studies on the D-arabinose-containing lipid A from *Rhodospirillum tenue* 2761. *Eur. J. Biochem.* **84**: 385–394.

ULEVITCH, R. J., JOHNSTON, A. R. and WEINSTEIN, D. V. (1979) New function of high density lipoproteins, their participation in intravascular reactions of bacterial lipopolysaccharides. *J. Clin. Invest.* **64**: 1516–1524.

URBASCHECK, B. and FORSSMANN, W. G. (1980) The endothelial cell of the microvascular bed as a target of endotoxin activities. In: *The Reticuloendothelial System and the Pathogenesis of Liver Disease*, pp. 401–407, LIEHR, H. and GRÜN, M. (eds). Elsevier/North Holland, Amsterdam.

URBASCHECK, R. M., SHADDUK, R. H., BONA, C. and MERGENHAGEN, S. E. (1980) Colony-stimulating factor in nonspecific resistance and in increased susceptibility to endotoxin. In: *Microbiology—1980*, pp. 115–119, SCHLESSINGER, D. (ed). Am. Soc. Microbiol., Washington, D.C.

WAHL, L. M., ROSENSTREICH, D. L., GLODE, L. M., SANDBERG, A. L. and MERGENHAGEN, S. E. (1979) Defective prostaglandin synthesis by C3H/HeJ mouse macrophages stimulated with endotoxin preparations. *Infect. Immun.* **23**: 8–13.

WECKESSER, J., DREWS, G. and MAYER, H. (1979) Lipopolysaccharides of photosynthetic prokaryotes. *Ann. Rev. Microbiol.* **33**: 215–239.

WESTENFELDER, M., GALANOS, C. and MADSEN, P. O. (1975) Experimental lipid A-induced nephritis in the dog. *Invest. Urology* **12**: 337–345.

WESTENFELDER, M., GALANOS, C., MADSEN, P. O. and MARGET, W. (1977a) Pathological activities of lipid A: Experimental studies in relation to chronic pyelonephritis. In: *Microbiology—1977*, pp. 277–279, SCHLESSINGER, D. (ed). Am. Soc. Microbiol., Washington, D.C.

WESTENFELDER, M., GALANOS, C., WITHÖFT, A. and LANG, G. (1977b) Vorkommen, Bedeutung und klinische Konsequenz der Lipoid A-Antikörper-Titer bei Patienten mit Harnwegsinfekt. *Infect.* **5**: 144–148.

WESTENFELDER, M., GALANOS, C. and MARGET, W. (1978) Role of antibodies to lipid A in nephritis induced by lipid A: A possible mechanism in the pathogenesis of chronic pyelonephritis. In: *Infections of the Urinary Tract*, pp. 100–104, KASS, E. H. and BRUMFITT, W. (eds). University of Chicago Press, Chicago.

WESTPHAL, O. (1960) Récentes recherches sur la chimie et la biologie des endotoxines des bactéries a gram-négatif. *Ann. Inst. Pasteur* **98**: 789–813.

WESTPHAL, C., LÜDERITZ, O. and BISTER, F. (1952) Über die Extraktion von Bakterien mit Phenol/Wasser. *Z. Naturf.* **7b**: 148–155.

WILKINSON, R. G., GEMSKI, P. and STOCKER, B. A. D. (1972) Non-smooth mutants of *Salmonella typhimurium*: Differentiation by phage sensitivity and genetic mapping. *J. gen. Microbiol.* **70**: 527–554.

WILKINSON, S. G. (1977) Composition and structure of bacterial lipopolysaccharides. In: *Surface Carbohydrates of the Prokaryotic Cell*, pp. 97–175. SUTHERLAND, I. (ed). Academic Press, London and New York.

WILKINSON, S. G. and TAYLOR, D. P. (1978) Occurrence of 2,3-diamino-2,3-dideoxy-D-glucose in lipid A from lipopolysaccharide of *Pseudomonas diminuta*. *J. gen. Microbiol.* **109**: 367–370.

WRIGHT, A. and KANEGASAKI, S. (1971) Molecular aspects of lipopolysaccharides. *Physiol. Rev.* **51**: 748–784.

YIN, E. T., GALANOS, C., KINSKY, S., BRADSHAW, R. A., WESSLER, S., LÜDERITZ, O. and SARMIENTO, M. E. (1972) Picrogram-sensitive assay for endotoxin: gelation of Limulus polyphemus blood cell lysate induced by purified lipopolysaccharides and lipid A from gram-negative bacteria. *Biochim. biophys. Acta* **261**: 284–289.

YOSHIDA, M., RIETSCHEL, E. TH., GALANOS, C., HIRATA, M., LÜDERITZ, O. and WESTPHAL, O. (1972) Hemorrhage and necrosis in the bone marrow by lipid A. *Jap. J. med. Sci. Biol.* **25**: 238–242.

YOUNGNER, J. S., FEINGOLD, D. S. and CHEN, J. K. (1973) Involvement of a chemical moiety of bacterial lipopolysaccharide in production of interferon in animals. *J. infect. Dis.* **128**: (Suppl.) 219–225.

ZIEGLER, E. J., MCCUTCHAN, J. A. and BRAUDE, A. I. (1979) Treatment of gram-negative bacteria with antiserum to core glycolipid. I. The experimental basis of immunity to endotoxin. *Eur. J. Cancer* **15**: 71–76.

CHAPTER 18

BORDETELLA PERTUSSIS TOXINS

A. C. Wardlaw and R. Parton

Microbiology Department, Glasgow University, Glasgow, G116NU, Scotland

ABSTRACT

Bordetella pertussis produces three distinct toxins: a heat-labile, dermonecrotizing toxin, a lipopolysaccharide endotoxin and a toxic substance variously known as pertussigen, pertussis toxin, histamine-sensitizing factor, leukocytosis-promoting factor and islets-activating protein. Circumstantial evidence suggests that this latter toxin may be the factor principally responsible for the paroxysmal cough in whooping cough. Pertussigen and endotoxin are probably the main contributors to the toxicity of pertussis vaccine. Pertussigen (m.w. 117,000) has an A–B subunit structure, the A component being an ADP-ribosylating enzyme which affects the activity of adenylate cyclase in target cells.

1. INTRODUCTORY OVERVIEW OF *B. PERTUSSIS* TOXINS

1.1. THE THREE PRINCIPAL TOXINS

Under suitable cultural conditions all freshly-isolated strains, and also all undegraded laboratory strains of *B. pertussis* so far investigated, consistently produce three principal toxins: the heat-labile, or dermonecrotizing toxin (HLT): the lipopolysaccharide (LPS) endotoxin; and a third substance which is variously known as histamine-sensitizing factor (HSF), leukocytosis-promoting factor or lymphocytosis-promoting factor (LPF), LPF-Hemagglutinin (LPF-HA), islets-activating protein (IAP), pertussigen (Munoz, 1976) and pertussis toxin (Pittman, 1979). For convenience, brevity and avoidance of ambiguity within the context of this article, the third substance will be referred to as pertussigen, despite certain unresolved discrepancies in its characterization.

For general reviews of whooping cough and its pathogenesis, and on the biologically-active substances produced by *B. pertussis*, see the articles by Pittman (1970, 1979) Munoz (1963a, 1971), Olson (1975), Morse (1976), Munoz and Bergman (1977), Manclark and Hill (1979) and Wardlaw and Parton (1983).

1.2. LOCATION

At least two of the principal toxins are primarily cell-associated, the HLT being a cytoplasmic component while the LPS is located in the cell envelope. Pertussigen in actively growing cultures is found in both cell and supernate fractions (Sato *et al.*, 1974; E. O. Idigbe, personal comm.). In old cultures and with certain strains of *B. pertussis*, all three toxins may be released to a considerable extent into the surrounding medium, although some of each remains with the cells.

1.3. GROWTH OF CULTURES AND PRODUCTION OF TOXINS

The production of HLT and pertussigen during the growth of *B. pertussis* is strongly influenced by culture conditions, and the levels of both of these toxins can be manipulated in a controlled fashion by particular changes in medium composition and incubation temperature. For example, replacing the NaCl in Hornibrook medium with $MgSO_4$ causes a reversible phenotypic alteration known as *antigenic modulation*. During this process, both the pertussigen (i.e. HSF, LPF and mouse-protective activities) and HLT contents of the bacteria fall by 85–95 % (Parton and Wardlaw, 1975; Wardlaw *et al.*, 1976; Livey *et al.*, 1978; Idigbe *et al.*, 1981). The relatively nontoxic, $MgSO_4$-grown cells are referred to as C-mode, while those from NaCl medium are designated X-mode. C-mode cells can also be produced by cultivation on X-mode media but at an incubation temperature of 28°C in place of the usual 35–37° (Lacey, 1960). The possibility of changes in LPS during antigenic modulation has so far received little attention.

Loss of pertussigen and to some extent of HLT, can be induced by growth in various media in which the usual trace amounts of nicotinic acid or nicotinamide (1–5 μg/ml) are replaced by 500 μg/ml nicotinic acid (Pusztai and Joó, 1967; Wardlaw *et al.*, 1976). Curiously, a similar high level of nicotinamide does not do this. Both the X-mode to C-mode change and that induced by high nicotinic acid, by virtue of their reversibility, are to be distinguished from another type of variation exhibited by *B. pertussis*, namely *phase variation* (Leslie and Gardner, 1931; Kasuga *et al.*, 1953).

This latter type of variation involves more permanent, genetic changes in the organism. Freshly isolated, and undegraded laboratory strains of *B. pertussis* are designated as Phase I and, as indicated, contain HLT, LPS and pertussigen. On prolonged subculture, variant (Phase IV or rough) strains may appear which lack HLT (Kasuga *et al.*, 1954) and HSF (pertussigen) (Kind, 1953; Aprile, 1972). Phase variation bears some relation to the smooth-to-rough variation in *Enterobacteriaceae* in that it may involve loss of virulence and of antigenic determinants from the LPS (Kasuga *et al.*, 1953, 1954; Aprile and Wardlaw, 1973).

For additional information on the growth requirements and cultivation of *B. pertussis*, see Rowatt (1957), Stainer and Scholte (1971) and Parker (1976).

1.4. OTHER BIOLOGICALLY-ACTIVE SUBSTANCES

In addition to the three principal toxins of *B. pertussis*, a variety of other biologically-active substances have been described. Cultures on Bordet–Gengou agar show zones of hemolysis (Lautrop, 1960) presumably due to an excreted hemolysin, but the toxic potential of this hypothetical factor is unkown. Kuwajima (1978) reported a heat-stable neurotoxin but this awaits confirmation and characterisation.

A polymorphonuclear leukocyte-inhibitory factor (PIF) was partially purified by Utsumi *et al.* (1978). In that this factor inhibited the chemotactic and phagocytic activities of leukocytes, it might be described as a toxin although it was not grossly cytotoxic to leukocytes, as judged by trypan blue exclusion and respirometer measurements. Perhaps 'aggressin' would be a more appropriate term. PIF was 75 % inactivated during 30 min at 56°C but was distinct from HLT in fractionation behaviour and in its resistance to trypsin and pronase. Its chemical nature remains to be determined. In a later paper, Imagawa *et al.* (1980) suggested that PIF may be the same as LPF. Benjamin *et al.* (1981) described an 80°C-labile factor in pertussis vaccine that affected various aspects of marcophage function. An effect on liver microsomal enzyme activity, also due to an 80°C-labile component of pertussis vaccine, was reported by Williams *et al.* (1980).

An unusual feature of *B. pertussis* is the production of large amounts of extracellular adenylate cyclase (Hewlett and Wolff, 1976). In a recent report, Confer and Eaton (1982) suggested that this enzyme may act as an aggressin by impairing the antibacterial activity of phagocytes. Yet another potential aggressin, the tracheal cytotoxin (TCT) was described by Goldman *et al.* (1982). This substance was released into the supernate of log-phase cultures and appeared to originate from the peptidoglycan component of the cell envelope. It inhibited DNA synthesis in cultured hamster tracheal cells and caused loss of ciliary activity and had a marked cytopathic effect in the ciliated epithelium of hamster tracheal organ cultures.

B. pertussis produces several other components which may be important in the pathogenesis of disease and immunity, but not through toxicity. These include the heat-labile agglutinogens (Preston, 1963) that determine the serotype of the organism, and the filamentous hemagglutinin (F-HA) which may play a role in attachment of the bacteria to cilia in the host respiratory tract (Sato *et al.*, 1979). A confusing feature of the filamentous appendages on the surface of *B. pertussis* is that the structures identified as fimbriae appear to carry agglutinogen 2 and not F-HA (Ashworth *et al.*, 1982). There is some evidence that immune responses to both F-HA and to the agglutinogens may contribute to immunity in experimental *B. pertussis* infections of the mouse and in human whooping cough respectively.

1.5. POTENTIAL FOR INTERACTION

Until recently, most of the experimental work on HLT and on the activities now attributed to pertussigen was done with crude materials such as whole cells, lysates obtained by physical methods of disintegration or detergent extraction or, at best, with only partially-purified toxins. Thus, inevitably there are some uncertainties in attributing to one specific substance any toxic or other pathophysiological activity that may be exhibited by mixtures. This difficulty may become especially acute when endotoxin, with its diverse pharmacological activities, is also present—as is almost certain in extracts or fractions from *B. pertussis* cultures. An example of the complications that may arise was described by Kurokawa *et al.* (1978a) who showed that the slope of the leukocytosis dose-response curve of LPF was significantly altered by endotoxin. Therefore, although there is good evidence that *B. pertussis* has three principal toxins, it may be unwise to pursue the accurate quantitation of some of the pathophysiological activities until the possible role of endotoxin as a cofactor, particularly with pertussigen, has been explored with rigorously-purified materials.

1.6. CLINICAL SIGNIFICANCE

Of necessity, most of the experimental observations on *B. pertussis* toxins have been made in laboratory animals rather than man. However, there are certain clinical signs in whooping cough which can usefully be discussed within the context of current knowledge of the toxins. Likewise, the toxic reactions produced by pertussis vaccine in the human infant merit discussion in the light of what is known about the three principal toxins. The plan for the rest of this article is therefore to review the information on the three *B. pertussis* toxins individually and then to apply this to the clinically important considerations of the role of the toxins in pathogenesis and immunity in whooping cough and in the toxicity of pertussis vaccines.

2. THE LIPOPOLYSACCHARIDE ENDOTOXIN

2.1. GENERAL FEATURES

Like all Gram-negative bacteria, *B. pertussis* possesses in its cell envelope a lipopolysaccharide (LPS) endotoxin with the characteristic chemical, immunological and pharmacological properties of this class of substance. Since LPS endotoxins are reviewed elsewhere (Lüderitz *et al.*, 1981), we shall deal here only with the particular and unusual features of *B. pertussis* LPS and not discuss the properties of LPS in general.

2.2. CHEMISTRY

LPS has been extracted from several strains of *B. pertussis* by the hot phenol/water method (Westphal *et al.*, 1952) and purified by ultracentrifugation (MacLennan, 1960; Kasai, 1966; Nakase *et al.*, 1970; Aprile and Wardlaw, 1973; Finger *et al.*, 1976; Le Dur *et al.*, 1978, 1980). The yield from different strains was in the range of 6–34 mg/g dry weight of bacteria.

One of the most distinctive features of *B. pertussis* endotoxin is that it contains two chemically distinct LPS which have been designated LPS-I and LPS-II (Le Dur *et al.*, 1980).

These LPS, present in the ratio 2 : 3 were seen as two distinct peaks on a hydroxylapatite column eluted with increasing sodium phosphate solutions containing 0.1 % w/v sodium dodecyl sulfate. Such a column permitted separation of LPS-I and LPS-II on a preparative scale. The presence of two LPS was demonstrated in a number of *B. pertussis* strains including one Phase IV strain. Under the same conditions, endotoxins from *Escherichia coli*, *Salmonella typhimurium* and *Shigella flexneri* were eluted as single peaks.

Chemical analysis of *B. pertussis* endotoxin revealed two different polysaccharides (PS-I and PS-II) and two different lipids (Lipid A and Lipid X). Lipid A, the major lipid component (23 % of the endotoxin), is analogous to the Lipid A of enterobacterial endotoxin (Le Dur *et al.*, 1978). Its main components were esterified phosphate, glucosamine, tetradecanoic acid, 3-hydroxytetradecanoic acid and 3-hydroxydecanoic acid. Lipid X made up only about 2 % of the endotoxin and was reported to contain the unusual fatty acids 2-methyl-3-hydroxydecanoic acid and 2-methyl-2-hydroxytetradecanoic acid in addition to those found in Lipid A (Haeffner *et al.*, 1977). However these unusual fatty acids could not be detected by Kawai and Moribayashi (1982).

PS-I and PS-II were each bound to Lipid A to give LPS-I and LPS-II respectively, but the position of Lipid X in the endotoxin complex was not determined. PS-I was bound to Lipid A through a single molecule of non-phosphorylated KDO (3-deoxy-2-octulosonic acid). It had a molecular weight of approximately 2,800 and contained the branched trisaccharide 7-*O*-(α-D-glucosaminyl-2-*O*-(β-D-glucuronyl)-L-*glycero*-D-mannoheptose (Chaby *et al.*, 1977). PS-II had a molecular weight of approximately 3,600 and was bound to Lipid A through a single molecule of phosphorylated KDO. The difference in phosphate content of LPS-I and LPS-II was probably responsible for their different chromatographic behavior on hydroxylapatite (Le Dur *et al.*, 1980). Another branched trisaccharide containing D-glucose, D-glucosamine and 2-amino-2-deoxy-D-galacturonic acid also has been isolated from both polysaccharide moieties of *B. pertussis* endotoxin (Moreau *et al.*, 1982).

Despite containing two chemically-distinct LPS molecules, the endotoxin of Le Dur *et al.* (1978) gave a single precipitin line in immunodiffusion tests with mouse antisera against whole *B. pertussis* cells. Aprile and Wardlaw (1973) however, using rabbit antisera to whole cells found evidence for two immunologically distinct types of LPS in some *B. pertussis* strains. They concluded that the LPS of *B. pertussis* strain 18334, a routine vaccine strain, possessed five different antigenic determinants distributed over two non-cross reacting LPS molecules. Strain 134, the Pillemer vaccine strain, had only two determinants on a single type of LPS molecule as did strain 11615, a Phase IV organism. Clearly, a more detailed characterization of the chemical composition and antigenic structure of LPS from a wider range of *B. pertussis* strains is desirable.

2.3. ENDOTOXIC PROPERTIES

B. pertussis LPS exhibits the characteristic range of endotoxic properties, notably toxicity, pyrogenicity, Shwartzman reactivity, adjuvanticity and enhancement of non-specific resistance to infection (Farthing, 1961; Nakase *et al.*, 1970; Ayme *et al.*, 1980). Typical activities are shown in Table 1. There appeared to be no significant differences between LPS-I and LPS-II in any of the biological parameters examined (Le Dur *et al.*, 1980).

When properties of the purified polysaccharide and lipid fractions were investigated, the adjuvant and resistance-enhancing properties were found in the lipid moieties. Lipid X was toxic, pyrogenic and Shwartzman-reactive, whereas the Lipid A had lost these activities. It seems that the selective destruction of the effectors of these activities had taken place during preparation of the Lipid A, since a glycolipid fraction from which the Lipid A was derived, and which was devoid of Lipid X, had normal endotoxic activities (Ayme *et al.*, 1980).

Another unusual activity of *B. pertussis* LPS was its mitogenic effect on spleen cells of C3H/HeJ mice which are resistant to the mitogenic effect of LPS from certain Enterobacteriaceae. However, this particular activity was also found in LPS from *Brucella abortus* and *Proteus mirabilis*. PS-I and PS-II were the active fractions of *B. pertussis* LPS for this particular mitogenic effect (Girard *et al.*, 1981).

TABLE 1. *Biological Activities of* B. pertussis *LPS*

Test	Result
Mouse weight-gain (18–20 g mice)	Maximum dose that yielded a zero change in body weight 24 hr after injection was 1.07 μg.
Pyrogenicity in rabbits	2 μg/kg gave a maximum average temperature elevation of 2.0°C.
Local Shwartzman reaction in rabbits	Positive with sensitizing doses in the range 12.5 to 200 μg.
Induction, in mice, of non-specific resistance to infection with *Salmonella typhi, Escherichia coli, Klebsiella pneumoniae, Pseudomonas aeruginosa* and *Staphylococcus aureus* (3 day interval between LPS and challenge)	LPS doses in the range 12.5 to 200 μg afforded significant protection against all challenges. Strongest protection was induced against *K. pneumoniae* and weakest against *P. aeruginosa.*
Induction, in mice, of non-specific resistance to Semliki Forest (250 LD_{50}) and encephalomyocarditis (1.7 LD_{50}) viruses (24 hr interval between LPS and challenge)	200 μg was fully protective; lower doses not reported
Adjuvant activity for influenza virus vaccine in mice	2.5-fold enhancement of level of serum antiviral hemagglutinin.

(From data of Ayme *et al.*, 1980).

3. THE HEAT-LABILE TOXIN

3.1. OPERATIONAL DEFINITION

Cells of *B. pertussis* freshly harvested from suitable solid or liquid media are dermonecrotizing and lethal when injected into mice, rabbits or guinea-pigs. When such cells are heated for 30 min at 56°C, all of the dermonecrotizing and a large part of the lethal toxicity are destroyed. The factor inactivated in this way is defined operationally as the heat-labile, or dermonecrotizing toxin, or HLT. It was first demonstrated by Bordet and Gengou (1909), the original discoverers of *B. pertussis*, as the causative agent of whooping cough.

Since highly purified HLT has been produced by only two groups of investigators (Onoue *et al.*, 1963; Nakase *et al.*, 1969), most of the observations on this substance are based on the difference in activity of crude preparations, such as whole cells, lysates or partially purified toxin, before and after heating at 56°C.

3.2. INSTABILITY

The characteristic instability of HLT has been a major obstacle to its purification. Crude preparations of the protein show the following losses of activity at different temperatures: 100% within 10 min at 56°C; 95% after 9 hr at 40°C; 95% after 2 days at 37°C; 50% after 1 week at 4°C (Munoz, 1971). At −20°C, the crude toxin appears to be stable for at least one year (Livey and Wardlaw, 1984).

HLT is rapidly inactivated by exposure to various chemicals, notably formaldehyde, phenol, chloroform, alcohol and toluene. It is destroyed by trypsin but not by DNase or RNase. It is difficult to purify chromatographically, apparently because of poor or unreliable recovery from many of the commonly-used column-packing materials. It can however be fractionated, without serious loss, by ammonium sulfate precipitation and by gel-filtration at 4°C (Livey and Wardlaw, 1984).

3.3. PRODUCTION AND PURIFICATION

There appears to be no uniquely potent strain of *B. pertussis* for maximizing HLT production, and different authors have used various strains. In recent studies, Livey and Wardlaw (1984) found the Pillemer strain 134 to be at least as active a producer of HLT as the strain Maeno that had been used by Nakase *et al.* (1969), the authors who have produced the purest toxin so far. Whole cells of strain 134 were also as toxic as any of the 201 strains isolated by Spasojević (1977) from patients in Belgrade during the years 1954 to 1975.

As already described above (Section 1.3) HLT production is adversely affected by X to C-modulation and by phase variation of *B. pertussis*. In addition, too vigorous an aeration and too high a pH during the growth of cultures may yield cells with a low content of HLT (Lane, 1968). With strain 134, there was little difference in HLT content between cells harvested from Bordet–Gengou medium and from Hornibrook medium (Livey and Wardlaw, 1984). Unlike the production of diphtheria and some other bacterial toxins, HLT synthesis was not affected by the iron concentration in the medium (Livey and Wardlaw, 1984). A worthwhile increase in toxicity was obtained in a modified Stainer and Scholte (1971) medium by altering the amounts of glutamate and proline (Stainer, 1979). The toxin has an intracellular location and does not appear to be secreted into the culture medium by actively-growing cells. The peak of toxin production occurs before the onset of the stationary phase (Cowell *et al.*, 1979).

References to early attempts to purify HLT may be found in Munoz (1971), Onoue *et al.* (1963) and Nakase *et al.* (1969). Since only the last two groups of investigators appear to have obtained highly purified HLT, we shall disregard the earlier work. Both groups of investigators obtained final products with a minimal dermonecrotizing dose for the guinea-pig of 0.01 μg (Table 2). The mouse LD_{50} of the preparation of Onoue *et al.* (1963) was 16.5 μg/kg body weight. With both these and earlier papers it is impossible to deduce information on the overall yield of final product as a percentage of the starting material. Livey and Wardlaw (1984) who attempted to repeat the DEAE-cellulose procedure described by Nakase *et al.* (1969) and earlier workers found the yield to be extremely poor.

The final purified toxin of Nakase *et al.* (1969) gave a single line on gel diffusion against a *B. pertussis* 'anti-phase I' serum as well as against a specific anti-HLT serum. It was free from detectable amounts of hemagglutinin, agglutinogens and HSF.

3.4. CHEMISTRY

The highly purified HLT of Nakase *et al.* (1969) was homogeneous by electrophoresis, ultracentrifugation and Ouchterlony diffusion tests. It had the very low sedimentation value of 1.4S, which does not agree with the behavior of HLT in crude preparations subjected to gel filtration. Here the HLT exhibited an apparent molecular weight of around 89,000 (Livey and Wardlaw, 1984). However, Nakase *et al.* (1969) suggested that HLT might have the capacity to combine with other proteins, thereby giving an apparent increase in molecular weight.

TABLE 2. *Purification of HLT: Brief Particulars From the Two Papers That Describe the Most Active Purified Preparations.*

Authors	*B. pertussis* strain and growth medium	Method of cell disruption	Main steps in purification after high-speed centrifugation	Toxicity of final product
Onoue *et al.* (1963)	Sakurayashiki; charcoal–agar + casamino acids	grinding at 3°C with glass powder in a mortar	1. Absorption/elution on calcium phosphate 2. ammonium sulphate precipitation 3. potassium phosphate precipitation 4. DEAE-cellulose chromatography	g.p. M.N.D.* = 0.01 μg mouse LD_{50} = 16.5 μg/kg
Nakase *et al.* (1969)	Maeno; modified charcoal–agar	sonic oscillator	1. DEAE-cellulose chromatography 2. ammonium sulphate precipitation 3. preparative acrylamide-gel electrophoresis	g.p. M.N.D. = 0.01 μg

*Guinea-pig minimal necrotizing dose.

Nakase's purified HLT contained 14.6%N and 1.4% reducing sugar, identified as probably mannose. There was no detectable lipid or phosphorous, and acid hydrolysis revealed no unusual features in the amino acid composition. To date there has been no independent confirmation of this work.

3.5. IMMUNOLOGICAL PROPERTIES

For many years after its discovery in 1909, HLT was considered to be nonantigenic. However in the 1940's several groups of investigators showed that crude, formalin-detoxified HLT induced, both in children and in experimental animals, antibodies that neutralized the dermonecrotizing and lethal activities (see Munoz, 1971). It is possible that the poor antigenicity of the active toxin is due to its toxic action on spleen and lymph nodes. The intracellular location of HLT within the bacterium is also unfavorable for stimulation of antibody production. A combination of these factors may explain why human pertussis convalescent sera lack neutralizing antibody to HLT (Evans and Maitland, 1939; Cravitz and Williams, 1946).

HLT appears not to function as a protective antigen in experimental *B. pertussis* infections of mice (Munoz, 1971). However, most of the work was done with impure HLT and is not definitive. The most direct evidence was provided by Nakase *et al.* (1969) who reported (without giving data) that 1 mg of purified formalin-detoxified, alum-precipitated HLT failed to protect mice against intracerebral challenge with 200 LD_{50} of the standard 18–323 strain of *B. pertussis*. However, these authors did not state whether the mice that had been subjected to immunization actually possessed detectable levels of anti-HLT in their serum. Therefore the failure of HLT to act as a protective antigen in the mouse might be due to absence of antibody production under the conditions of immunization. The question of HLT being able to function as a protective antigen in the mouse or child should therefore be regarded as unanswered.

Perhaps the most notable immunological feature of *B. pertussis* HLT is that apparently indistinguishable toxins are produced by *B. parapertussis* and *B. bronchiseptica* (see Munoz, 1971). In rabbits and guinea-pigs all three toxins showed quantitatively similar neutralization of their dermonecrotizing and lethal toxicities by *B. pertussis* anti-HLT (Evans, 1940). Clearly it would be desirable for this work to be confirmed with purified HLT from each of the three species.

3.6. TOXIC ACTIVITIES

The mode of action of HLT is not known, and most of the activities attributed to it were observed with preparations which would be expected to contain LPS and pertussigen. The highly purified HLT of Nakase *et al.* (1969) was dermonecrotizing in guinea-pigs and lethal to mice. When animals of both species were injected with HLT i.v. or i.p. (dose not specified) there was 'significant necrosis, hemorrhage, congestion and degeneration in liver, spleen and kidney'. Injection of one guinea-pig minimal skin dose i.v. into mice caused retardation of the normal rate of weight gain and also induced a significant leukocytosis.

Returning to crude HLT, the toxin is dermonecrotizing in sheep, pigs and chickens in addition to rabbits and guinea-pigs (Munoz, 1971). Some recent investigators (Cowell *et al.*, 1979) have favored the suckling mouse (Katsampes *et al.*, 1942; Kurokawa *et al.*, 1969) as a sensitive recipient for detecting HLT activity. Typically, a single 25–50 μl dose of test material was injected s.c. in the nape of the neck and dermonecrotic lesions scored on a scale from 0 to 4 + after 18–20 hr, or their diameters measured at 48 hr. Figure 1 presents dose–response regressions of the dermonecrotizing activity of HLT in the suckling mouse, rabbit and guinea-pig.

A notable effect of i.v.-injected, partially purified HLT in mice is atrophy of the spleen (Wood, 1940), an activity described as 'lienotoxicity' (Iida and Okonogi, 1971). In a typical experiment the average spleen weight of mice injected with the HLT-containing preparation declined from 51 to 13 mg within seven days. The severely atrophied spleen was grey-yellow in color and on histological examination showed general fibrosis, with virtual absence of lymphocytes. Although the HLT preparation used for this work was not pure, the lienotoxic effect is probably attributable to HLT itself since it was lost after heating at 56°C for 10 min. The HLT of *B. bronchiseptica* which is apparently indistinguishable from that of *B. pertussis* may be the factor responsible for nasal turbinate atrophy in pigs (Goodnow, 1980).

Crude HLT has been found harmful to organ tissue cultures (Felton *et al.*, 1954) and to HeLa cells (Angela *et al.*, 1962) and it would be of interest to see if pure toxin also produces cytopathic effects *in vitro*. An example of the difficulty that faces the reviewer is provided by Střižova and Trlifajová (1964) who reported that certain tissue culture cells, notably primary mouse embryo and KB cells, were extremely sensitive to the cytopathic effect of *B. pertussis* saline extract. However, the activity persisted after heating the extract for 30 min at 56°C and was only destroyed by 60 min at 56°C or 30 min at 75°C. The relationship of this activity to HLT or to other *B. pertussis* components is therefore obscure. Some effects of live *B. pertussis* on mammalian cell and organ cultures are reported later (Section 5).

4. PERTUSSIGEN OR PERTUSSIS TOXIN

4.1. Problems of Identity and Nomenclature

Pertussigen is the component of *B. pertussis* which has been most extensively investigated and which appears to be unique to this bacterial species. It is probably of major importance in the pathogenesis of whooping cough although its exact role in the disease remains to be defined. At present, there is a confusion of nomenclature which compounds the difficulty in deciding whether present evidence adequately supports the single-factor idea that is implicit in the name pertussigen; alternatively whether the activities attributed to it reside in more than one substance. We believe that, on balance, there is sufficient evidence for the pertussigen concept, but with reservation that some aspects may require modification as the purified substance is investigated more thoroughly.

The notion that the histamine-sensitizing factor (HSF), mouse-protective antigen (MPA) and heat-labile adjuvant (HLAd) represent different activities of the same substance was propounded in the 'Unitarian Hypothesis' of Levine and Pieroni (1966) and supported by other investigators. In 1976, Munoz proposed the term 'pertussigen' for a substance in *B. pertussis* which sensitized mice to histamine, induced leukocytosis, stimulated IgE production, accelerated induction of experimental allergic encephalomyelitis, and protected mice against intracranial challenge with live *B. pertussis*. Two years later, Yajima *et al.* (1978a,b) described the purification from *B. pertussis* culture supernate of a substance which they designated islets-activating protein (IAP). This protein, of apparent molecular weight 77,000, had HSF, LPF and IgE-adjuvant activities (Mizushima *et al.*, 1979) in addition to its

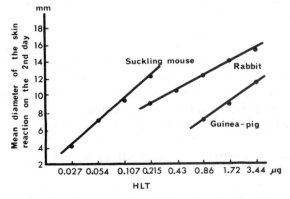

Fig. 1. Comparative dermonecrotizing activities of HLT in the suckling mouse, the rabbit and the guinea-pig. The doses shown were injected in volumes of 100 μl into rabbits and guinea-pigs and 25 μl into suckling mice. (From Kurokawa *et al.* (1969) *Japan, J. med. Sci. Biol.* **22**: 293–307; reproduced with the permission of the authors and the Japanese Journal of Medical Science and Biology.)

sensitizing effect on the insulin-secreting B-cells of the pancreas. These Japanese authors did not use the word pertussigen in their papers (Yajima *et al.*, 1978a,b; Mizushima *et al.*, 1979) and, indeed, did not claim any identity between IAP and the other factors. Nevertheless, IAP was reported to have a similar molecular weight to LPF (M.W. 67,000–73,000) purified by Morse and Morse (1976) and shown by them to have HSF activity and to cause resistance to epinephrine-induced hyperglycemia—an effect which was also found with IAP (Yajima *et al.*, 1978b). Independently, Lehrer *et al.* (1974) had obtained partially-purified HSF with a molecular weight of approximately 90,000 and with LPF and adjuvant activities.

Yet another activity of this versatile substance was discovered by Arai and Sato (1976) who found that partially purified LPF, which had hemagglutinating (HA) activity for chicken erythrocytes, could be separated into two protein components both with HA activity: the fimbrial hemagglutinin (F-HA) and the leukocytosis-promoting factor hemagglutinin (LPF-HA). Later, Irons and MacLennan (1979a,b) established that the HA activity of F-HA was inhibited by cholesterol, while that of LPF-HA was inhibited by sialoproteins, notably haptoglobin from human serum. This latter property led to an affinity-chromatography method for the purification of LPF-HA (i.e. pertussigen) in good yield. These authors also showed that goose erythrocytes were more sensitive to HA than those from the chicken.

Finally, to this list of activities of pertussigen must be added its *in vitro* mitogenicity for mouse lymphocytes which was exhibited by the LPF of Morse (1977a) at concentrations below 1 μg/ml.

A summary of these principal activities of pertussigen is given in Table 3. The late-appearing toxicity factor refers to the behavior of pertussigen (LPF) in the mouse weight-gain test (see Section 6.2). Protective antigen activity is discussed in more detail below (Section 4.6.5).

Linked to considerations of the nature and identity of pertussigen are various questions of nomenclature. Pittman (1979) recently advanced the hypothesis that whooping cough should be regarded as an exotoxin disease in which the substance with HSF/LPF/IAP activities is responsible for the harmful effects of the bacteria and for the induction of the prolonged immunity that follows infection. On this basis she suggested that the primary pathogenic component of the organism should be called 'pertussis toxin', by analogy with the classical exotoxin diseases, diphtheria and tetanus. However, to avoid ambiguity in this article where two other toxins of *B. pertussis* are discussed, we propose to use 'pertussigen'.

In presenting a supporting case for the pertussigen concept, we have so far ignored a considerable body of apparently contrary evidence. Most of this has emerged from studies with whole-cell pertussis vaccine or crude extracts, rather than with purified preparations. As an example may be cited the data of Cameron (1967) who assayed 20 batches of pertussis vaccine for HSF and MPA and found little correlation between the two activities. Similar lack of correlation between HSF and MPA activities in vaccines or cell-extracts, particularly after heat or chemical treatment, has been reported by Pittman (1951b; 1975), Dolby (1958),

TABLE 3. *The Main Activities Attributed to Pertussigen (Munoz and Bergman, 1979a)*

Activity	Abbreviation
Histamine-sensitizing factor	HSF
Leukocytosis (or lymphocytosis) promoting factor	LPF
Islets-activating protein	IAP
Heat-labile (80°C) adjuvant	HLAd
Mouse-protective antigen (intracerebral challenge test)	MPA
Late-appearing toxicity factor	—
Mitogenicity	—
Hemagglutinin (sensitive to inhibition by sialoproteins)	LPF-HA

Preston and Garrity (1967), Nagel (1970), Morse and Bray (1969) and Ishida *et al.* (1979). Lack of correlation between HSF and LPF activities was reported by Ishida *et al.* (1979) and Idigbe *et al.* (1981). Among the possibilities for reconciling these findings with the pertussigen concepts are:

(1) the state of dispersion of the preparation may have a differential effect on the quantitative expression of the various biological activities;

(2) there may be more than one *B. pertussis* component with mouse-protective activity;

(3) there may be a differential modulating effect of endotoxin on the expression of the various activities (Section 1.5);

(4) there may be changes analogous to toxoiding which may affect the pharmacological activity of the toxin but not its antigenicity.

With the present evidence, further speculation is unlikely to be fruitful, and the consolidation or modification of the pertussigen concept will only emerge from the thorough investigation of purified materials.

4.2. INFLUENCE OF STRAIN AND CULTURE CONDITIONS

There has been no uniquely favored strain of *B. pertussis* to provide starting material for the preparation of pertussigen. Only a very few strains, such as 'Tohama' have been used by more than a single group of investigators. It is, of course, essential that the culture should be a Phase I and X-mode (Section 1.3).

There appear to have been few systematic studies on the effect of medium composition on pertussigen synthesis, except in connection with antigenic modulation where both the ionic and vitamin content of the medium may greatly affect the final cell content of this factor (Section 1.3). Of more practical importance for maximizing pertussigen production are the observations of Stainer (1979) who showed that varying the concentration of glutamate and proline had a marked influence on the yield of MPA and HSF. The time of harvest was also an important variable, maximum levels of MPA and HSF generally being obtained in late-logarithmic phase rather than in stationary phase cultures.

As will be seen below, most methods for purifying pertussigen start with culture supernates rather than with whole cells, even though the latter may contain a considerable part of the active material. This is because the disadvantage of discarding the cell-associated pertussigen is outweighed by the convenience of having a soluble starting material that is relatively uncontaminated with other cellular components. It is also advantageous to have all components of the growth medium as low-molecular weight and dialyzable substances (Morse and Bray, 1969). An important practical point that requires further research is to define the cultural conditions that maximize the release of pertussigen from cells without gross lysis.

4.3. EXAMPLES OF METHODS FOR PURIFICATION

The purification of pertussigen will be discussed on the basis that we are dealing with a single entity that has been given different names by different investigators and four examples are now presented.

4.3.1. *Lymphocytosis-Promoting Factor (Morse and Morse, 1976)*

B. pertussis strain NIH 114 (3779 B) was grown in a casein hydrolysate medium for 5 days, thiomersal added to 0.02 %, and after 24 hr at 4°C the cells removed by centrifugation. The supernate was treated with ammonium sulfate to 90 % saturation at pH 6.4 and the precipitate collected. After washing with water and saline, it was dissolved in high ionic strength pH 10 Tris–NaCl buffer and ultracentrifuged on a cesium chloride gradient. The final step in purification was gel-filtration of Sephadex G-150. No data on yield were reported but there was a 25–40 fold increase in specific activity over the culture supernate.

4.3.2. *Islets-Activating Protein (Yajima et al., 1978a)*

B. pertussis strain Tohama, Phase I, was grown in a modified Cohen and Wheeler medium for 48 hr at 37°C, and the cells killed by adding thiomersal and heating at 56°C for 30 min. The culture was then centrifuged and the supernate saved as starting material for purification. The subsequent steps were: (1) adsorption on to hydroxyapatite at pH 6.0; (2) elution with high ionic strength pH 7.0 phosphate buffer; (3) chromatography on Sepharose CL-6B; (4) chromatography on concanavalin A–Sepharose; and (5) gel-filtration on Biogel P-100. The final yield of IAP was 17 % of that in the culture supernate and there was a specific purification of 1350-fold. Further particulars on yield and purity are given in Table 4.

4.3.3. *Lymphocytosis-Promoting Factor Hemagglutinin (Irons and MacLennan, 1979a,b)*

B. pertussis strain 'Tohama' was grown in a modified Cohen and Wheeler medium and the cells collected by centrifugation. Unlike the above cited methods, the starting material was cell paste rather than culture supernate. The cells were disintegrated mechanically in a Dyno-Mill and the clarified extracts precipitated with ammonium sulfate. The active fraction was applied to a column of Sepharose 4B to which had been coupled human haptoglobin. The haptoglobin–Sepharose constituted a highly specific and effective affinity-column to which the LPF-HA became attached. The active material was then eluted from the column by high ionic strength, pH 10 buffer and the eluate brought to pH 8 and concentrated. The overall purification was about 1000-fold over the supernate from Dyno-Mill treatment.

4.3.4. *Pertussigen (Munoz et al., 1981b)*

In a recent paper, Munoz et al., (1981b) described the preparation of crystalline pertussigen from *B. pertussis* strain 3779 BL_2S_4 grown in Stainer and Scholte (1971) medium. Organisms were killed with thiomersal, removed by centrifugation and the culture supernate used as starting material. The main steps in purification were: (1) precipitation with $ZnCl_2$ at pH 6.5; (2) extraction of the precipitate with Na_2HPO_4; (3) dialysis against 5 mM Tris HCl buffer (pH 8) followed by collection of the precipitate; (4) extraction of this precipitate with sodium pyrophosphate; (5) chromatography on Sepharose CL-6B; (6) chromatography on Bio-Gel A.5; (7) concentration by ultrafiltration; and (8) crystallization of pertussigen during 2–3 weeks at 2–5°C. The overall yield of pertussigen was less than 1.8 mg from 20 l of culture.

4.4. Physicochemical and Chemical Properties

4.4.1. *Molecular Structure*

The main difficulty in providing a satisfactory tabulation of the physicochemical properties of pertussigen is that Munoz's preparations which carry this name are the least-well characterized, while the IAP of Yajima et al. (1978a,b) and the LPF of Morse and Morse

TABLE 4. *Yield and Specific Activity During the Purification of IAP*

Stage	Total protein (mg)	Total activity (units × 10^{-6})	Specific activity (units/µg)	Yield (%)	Purification
Supernatant of culture medium	22,000	14	0.64	100	1
Hydroxyapatite	15.2	5.9	386	42	610
CM-Sepharose	7.5	4.8	642	34	1010
Con A-Sepharose	5.0	3.8	760	27	1200
Biogel P-100	2.8	2.4	858	17	1350

From Yajima et al. (1978a). *J. Biochem.* (*Tokyo*) **83**: 295–303; reproduced with the permission of the authors and the Japanese Biochemical Society.

(1976) and of Irons and MacLennan (1979a,b) are not claimed by any of these authors to be the same as Munoz's pertussigen. A further obstacle is that the various independent groups of investigators, although working more or less contemporaneously, do not appear to have examined each other's purification methods or final products, or to have submitted their own preparations to independent evaluation.

Information on the molecular weight and polypeptide composition of pertussigen reported by various investigators since 1974 is summarized in Table 5. Further discussion on the molecular structure will be restricted to the data of Tamura et al., (1982) who worked with material purified by the procedure of Yajima et al., (1978a).

The purified toxin could be dissociated, by heating in SDS and urea, into five dissimilar polypeptides designated S-1 (mol. wt. 28,000), S-2 (23,000), S-3 (22,000), S-4 (11,700) and S-5 (9,300) all of which are required for biological activity in vivo. The molar ratio of these polypeptides in native IAP was found to be 1:1:1:2:1 and the mol. wt. of 117,000, estimated by sedimentation equilibrium, was similar to the mol. wt. of 106,000 calculated by summation. Differences between these and previous estimates of molecular weights and sub-unit structure were explained by differences in the analytical methods used. In 5M urea, the native toxin dissociated into 4 components: S-1, S-5 and two dimers (S-2, S-4) and (S-3, S-4). On the basis of molecular weight, amino acid composition and isoelectric point, S-2 and S-3 were similar and hence the two dimers were similar. The binding sites for haptoglobin were shown to reside on these dimers. The smallest polypeptide, S-5 (C-subunit) was required to connect the two dimers to give a pentamer. The authors concluded that the structure of IAP conformed to the A-B model which has been proposed for several bacterial toxins with the ability to penetrate plasma membranes and to catalyze ADP-ribosylation of certain proteins (see Section 4.7). The pentamer is the B (binding) subunit and the largest polypeptide, S-1, is the A (active) component.

4.4.2. Stability

Taking islets-activating ability as the index of pertussigen activity, it appears from Yajima et al., (1978b) that purified IAP is a fairly stable protein. When adjusted to a series of pH values and held for 24 hr at 4°C, it retained full activity within the pH range 4–10, but was inactivated outside of this range. When adjusted to pH 7.0 and exposed to different temperatures for 15 min it was fully stable up to 50°C, but was rapidly inactivated at 60°C and above.

These data for purified IAP may be compared with the stability of the other activities of pertussigen when it is present in intact cells or sonic lysates of B. pertussis. In these crude preparations, HSF and mouse-protective antigen (MPA) were only slightly inactivated at pH 3.0 and 10.0 during 1 hr at 20°C (Jakus et al., 1968). In regard to temperature stability of crude preparations, HSF, LPF and MPA are generally regarded as stable during heating for

TABLE 5. *Physiochemical Properties of Pertussigen and of Otherwise Designated Substances Assumed in This Chapter to be the Same as Pertussigen*

Reference	Authors' designation of substance	Molecular weight ($\times 10^{-3}$)	Molecular weight of component polypeptides ($\times 10^{-3}$)				
Lehrer et al. (1974)	HSF	90					
Arai and Sato (1976)	Hemagglutinin	107, 103,	10 13	20 26			
	LPF	30 (by different methods)	minor bands	major bands			
Morse and Morse (1976)	LPF	67–73.6	13.4 17.4	19.3 23.5			
Yajima et al. (1978a)	IAP	77	12 20 25 (in ratio 1:2:1)				
Irons and MacLennan (1979a,b)	LPF-HA		12.6 21.1 22.4 27.2				
Munoz et al. (1981a,b)	Pertussigen	98–102*					
Tamura et al. (1982)	IAP	106–117	9.3 11.7 22 23 28 (in ratio 1:2:1:1:1)				

*Munoz (personal comm).

30 min at 56°C and not fully inactivated until the temperature is raised to 80°C. In thiomersal-containing pertussis vaccines stored at 4°C, HSF, LPF and MPA activities retain their activities for many years. The purified LPF of Arai and Sato (1976) was relatively resistant to attack by papain.

4.5. BIOLOGICAL ACTIVITIES—GENERAL

4.5.1. *Comparative Overview*

Table 6 summarizes the biological activity data reported by six groups of investigators who have obtained pertussigen at levels of purity ranging from moderate (Lehrer *et al.*, 1974) to high (Yajima *et al.*, 1978b) and using a variety of names for the material investigated. Before attempting to assess these data, certain points should be noted: (1) a variety of strains of mice and rats were used by the different investigators and since this is known to influence greatly certain tests, notably that for HSF, it is difficult in most cases to compare the data vertically down each column; (2) in no instance was an international or other reference preparation used, and therefore the various end-point values have no common basis of comparison; (3) the various biological tests were performed in ways that differed significantly in experimental details such as route of injection and time of sampling or challenge; and (4) there is inherently poor precision in most of the bioassay systems, and in very few instances were 95% confidence limits or other indexes of precision provided. Nevertheless certain general conclusions about the biological properties of these preparations seem justifiable:

Toxicity	The LD_{50} for mice was about 4 μg (or perhaps as low as 0.5 μg) (Munoz *et al.*, 1981a).
Histamine sensitization	Pertussigen was active (in mice) in doses of the order or 0.01 μg, of even lower, in suitably sensitive animals.
Leukocytosis promotion	Doses in the order of 0.02 μg induced significant leukocytosis in mice.
Islets activation	0.02 μg per rat produced a significant promotion of insulin release in response to glucose loading.
Attentuation of epinephrine-induced hyperglycemia	Doses around 1 μg per rat or 0.02 μg per mouse were active.
Adjuvant activity	Pertussigen had adjuvant activity in various systems at doses in the range 0.01 to 1 μg.
Mouse protection (intracerebral challenge)	Munoz *et al.* (1981a) reported PD_{50} values of purified pertussigen in the range 1–2 μg per mouse, but Irons and MacLennan (1979a) found LPF-HA to be non-protective at up to 4 μg per mouse and toxic at higher doses.
Hemagglutination	2000–8000 HA units/mg were reported by several investigators who used chicken erythrocytes. Irons and MacLennan (1979a) found goose erythrocytes to be considerably more sensitive.

4.5.2. *Toxoiding*

Munoz *et al.* (1981a,b) reported the successful conversion of pertussigen to an immunogenic toxoid by treatment with 0.05% (w/v) glutaraldehyde in 20 mM sodium phosphate buffer (pH 7.6) containing 0.5 M NaCl for 2 hr at room temperature. The reaction was stopped by addition of lysine and subsequent dialysis against phosphate buffered saline containing lysine. The pertussigen toxoid was active as protective antigen ($PD_{50} = 1.7 \mu$g) in the intracerebral mouse protection test but was not histamine-sensitizing. An earlier formalin-detoxified preparation of LPF-HA made by Sato *et al.* (1979) was inactive as a mouse-protective antigen. Several years previous to this, Munoz and Hestekin (1966) reported that mouse-protective antigen and HSF were inactivated by formalin at 37°C, the

TABLE 6. *Biological Properties of Pertussigen and of Otherwise Designated Substance Assumed in This Chapter to be the Same as Pertussigen*

Reference	Authors' name of substance	Toxicity (LD$_{50}$)	Histamine sensitization (HSD$_{50}$)	Leukocytosis promotion[a]	Islet activation (μg/rat)	Attenuation of epinephrine hyperglycemia	Adjuvant (μg)	Mouse protection (intracerebral challenge)	HA units/mg (chicken erythrocytes)
Lehrer et al. (1974)	HSF		0.06						
Arai and Sato (1976)	Hemagglutinin LPF		0.02	0.025					7×10^3
Morse and Morse (1976)	LPF	4	0.01	0.02		0.02			2×10^3
Yajima et al. (1978a,b)	IAP		0.8	0.5	0.02[b]	0.02	1.0[d]		
Irons and MacLennan (1979a,b)	LPF–HA	4	0.04	0.02				>4[f]	8×10^3 (1.2×10^5)[h]
Munoz et al. (1981a)	Pertussigen	0.5	0.0005	0.008	0.002[c]		0.0001[e]	1.7[g]	5.3 ± 10^3

Except where otherwise indicated, data are given as μg protein per mouse. Where authors quote a range of values, only that representing the highest activity is cited.

[a] Different authors use different criteria for leukocytosis. The data given are the doses in μg per mouse that induced a significant, or highly-significant, elevation in white-cell count above the baseline.

[b] Dose that doubled the insulin-secretory response at 15 min. after 0.2 g glucose per 100 g body weight in fasted animals.

[c] Dose that significantly increased secretion of insulin due to glucose load.

[d] Dose per kg in Wistar rats that exhibited significant adjuvant activity in stimulating IgE antibodies to DNP-ascaris antigen.

[e] Dose per mouse that exhibited significant adjuvant activity in stimulating IgE antibodies to ovalbumin.

[f] The preparation was non-protective at doses up to 4 μg and was toxic at this and higher doses.

[g] Value for pertussigen toxoided with glutaraldehyde.

[h] HA titre with goose erythrocytes.

latter more rapidly. Working with crude extracts of *B. pertussis*, Matsui and Kuwajima (1959) reported that formalin-treatment eliminated HSF activity but gave the preparation the ability to inhibit histamine-sensitization by a second dose of HSF-containing vaccine.

4.5.3. *Neutralization by Antisera*

Purified pertussigen (designated by various names) gave a single line of antigen–antibody precipitate in gel-diffusion tests (Morse and Morse, 1976; Irons and MacLennan, 1979a,b; Ui *et al.*, 1979; Munoz *et al.*, 1981b). In addition, several of the biological activities were neutralized *in vitro* by antisera against either crude or purified extracts. Such neutralization was noted for histamine sensitization (Maitland *et al.*, 1955; Lehrer *et al.*, 1975a), leukocytosis-promotion (Sato *et al.*, 1974, 1981; Morse and Morse, 1976) and attenuation of epinephrine hyperglycemia (Morse and Morse 1976). According to Lehrer *et al.* (1975a), adjuvant activity for hemagglutinating antibodies to sheep erythrocytes was not abolished by prior admixture with antiserum, whereas the adjuvant effect for IgE antibody production was. Several of the above authors remarked that if the HSF, LPF etc., is located on an intact bacterial cell or large cell-wall fragment, the apparent neutralizing effect of a polyspecific antiserum may be due to antibodies directed against various surface components of the bacterium and not necessarily against pertussigen itself.

Lehrer (1979) explored the time-course of neutralization of purified HSF by antiserum injected at various times *after* the administration of the HSF, both injections being given i.v. With a time interval of 4 hr between the injections, the HSF activity was still almost completely (91 %) neutralized by antiserum; with an 8 hr interval, it was 75 % neutralized; but with a 24 hr interval, the antiserum had no effect. This indicated that even after 8 hr, HSF was not irreversibly bound to receptor sites in the mouse.

4.6. INDIVIDUAL BIOLOGICAL ACTIVITIES

The various biological activities attributed to pertussigen will now be described in terms of phenomenology. The possible underlying molecular mechanisms of action of the substance will be discussed later (Section 4.7). Data relating to human responses are presented in Sections 5.3 and 6.3.

4.6.1. *Histamine Sensitization*

Parfentjev and Goodline (1948) were the first to show that pertussis vaccine injected i.p. into mice made the animals hypersensitive to a subsequent injection of histamine. Normally, mice are relatively insusceptible to i.p. challenge with histamine, the LD_{50} being in the range 344–844 (or higher) mg base/kg body weight (Munoz and Bergman, 1968). If, however, the animals have received pertussis vaccine a few days previously, the LD_{50} of histamine drops by about 50-fold. The substance in *B. pertussis* cells responsible for this effect was designated histamine-sensitizing factor (HSF) by Maitland *et al.* (1955). Later work showed that HSF activity was absent from the related organisms *B. parapertussis* and *B. bronchiseptica* (Ross *et al.*, 1969) and from other bacteria (Munoz and Bergman, 1968). There is, however, the exception that endotoxin from various Gram-negative organisms, including *Bordetella* species, may sensitize mice to a challenge dose of histamine given 90 min later. After 24 hr, the sensitization had disappeared (Bergman and Munoz, 1977). Also, *Corynebacterium parvum* and related organisms were histamine sensitizing in mice (Adlam, 1973). However, HSF differs from endotoxin and from *C. parvum* in the time-course of the sensitization, in thermolability and in the small dose of purified HSF (pertussigen) needed.

HSF is present only in Phase I, X-mode *B. pertussis*, and is lost, or greatly diminished, during phase variation and antigenic modulation (Section 1.3). In liquid media it is found both cell-associated and in supernates, particularly in old cultures. HSF activity is one of the cardinal properties of pertussigen. Since highly purified pertussigen has become available only recently, most of the pharmacological observations relating to histamine sensitization have been made with whole-cell pertussis vaccine or crude extracts of the organism. For access to the earlier literature, see Munoz and Bergman (1968), Munoz (1971) and Morse (1976).

Animal species vary greatly in sensitization by HSF. The majority of work has been done with the mouse, a species that is normally resistant to the lethal toxicity of histamine ($LD_{50} = 344 - 844$ mg base/kg). The rabbit and guinea-pig, which are already highly sensitive to histamine ($LD_{50} = 2.3$ and 0.9 mg base/kg, respectively), do not become more sensitive after injection of pertussis vaccine; if anything, they actually become more resistant (Stronk and Pittman, 1955; Munoz and Bergman, 1968). The rat and the chicken behave similarly to the mouse but are less responsive to HSF.

In mice, there are great variations between different strains in their responsiveness to HSF, even although the LD_{50} of histamine alone in non-pertussis-treated animals does not vary much. In a list of 31 mouse strains compiled by Munoz and Bergman (1968), 12 strains were histamine-sensitizable by HSF, 17 were unresponsive and 2 gave a questionable result. Manclark et al. (1975), starting with an outbred strain of mouse of Swiss–Webster ancestry, developed two sublines of greatly differing sensitivity. After 14 generations of selections for both HSF-responsiveness and unresponsiveness, there was a 10-fold difference in the LD_{50} sensitizing dose of pertussis vaccine. During this selection process there were only trival changes in the LD_{50} of histamine itself in unvaccinated animals.

In an investigation of the inheritance of HSF-responsiveness in inbred strains of mice, Wardlaw (1970) found that F1-hybrids, obtained by crossing various sensitive strains with nonsensitive strains, were sensitive. This indicated that HSF-responsiveness was dominant over HSF-unresponsiveness. The character was not sex-linked and, from results with F2 and backcross animals, appeared to be inherited unifactorially, a conclusion which was later contested (Ovary and Caiazza, 1975). Nevertheless, it does appear that small genetic differences may determine responsiveness, since mice of a given designated strain, but obtained from different suppliers, may be either HSF-responsive or not (Munoz and Bergman, 1968). In contrast, Vaz et al. (1977) failed to demonstrate a clear pattern of inheritance of HSF-susceptibility in mice, although they showed that different strains varied in sensitivity to challenge with vasoactive amines before B. pertussis treatment and in resistance to acute hypovolemic shock afterwards. Most strains of mice which appear to be HSF-unresponsive when tested with a histamine challenge, exhibit some degree of HSF-responsiveness when challenged with a mixture of histamine and serotonin (Munoz and Bergman, 1968).

In addition to genetic factors, the sensitivity of mice to HSF is affected by the age and sex of the animal and by environmental stress (Munoz and Bergman, 1968). In general, old mice (more than seven weeks of age) are considerably more sensitizable than weanlings (three-week old) and females better responders than males. Stress during shipment from the supplier to the laboratory may cause histamine sensitization without administration of pertussis vaccine. The route of injection of vaccine also affects the mouse response. The i.p. route is commonly used because of its convenience when dealing with large numbers of animals. However, the i.v. route may give more rapid sensitization and may induce a significant response to a lower dose of vaccine or purified pertussigen than is attainable i.p. The s.c. route is poor for induction of sensitization. Whole-cell vaccines given i.p. produce an increasing sensitization to histamine which reaches a plateau around 4–5 days, and then gradually diminishes for the next 3–4 weeks. By the i.v. route, soluble preparations of pertussigen induce sensitization within 90 min, show a peak at one day and thereafter decline, but with some degree of sensitization persisting for up to 80 days. Histamine-sensitization may also be induced by the respiratory infection of mice with B. pertussis (Pittman, 1951a; Pittman et al., 1980) or by intracranial injection of vaccine (Munoz and Bergman, 1968).

HSF sensitizes mice to challenges with agents other than histamine, e.g. serotonin, bradykinin, methacholine, anoxia, cold shock, X-irradiation and endotoxin (Munoz and Bergman, 1968). Thus endotoxin is not only capable of sensitizing mice to histamine, but HSF sensitizes mice to the lethal effect of endotoxin. Figure 2 summarizes the time-course of

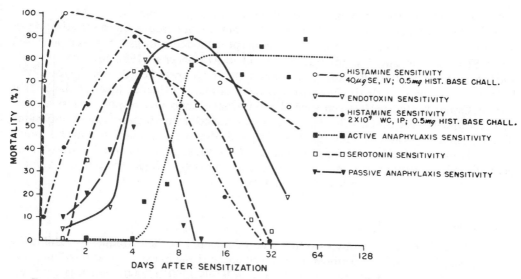

FIG. 2. Time-course of sensitization of mice by pertussis vaccine (WC) or saline extract (SE) to the lethal effect of various challenges. (From Munoz and Bergman (1968) *Bact. Rev.* **32**: 103–126; reproduced with the permission of the authors and the American Society for Microbiology.)

sensitization of mice to a variety of challenges after administration of HSF either as *B. pertussis* whole cells or saline extract. Points particularly to note are that (1) with a histamine challenge, saline extract given i.v. produced peak sensitization at 1 day; whereas (2) with whole cells given i.p., the peak was at 4 days; (3) sensitivity to serotonin challenge after whole cells i.p. was also at 4 days, but (4) with endotoxin challenge the peak sensitivity was at 8 days. The active and passive anaphylactic sensitization shown in this figure are discussed later in Section 4.6.4.

The state of dispersion, or solubility, of the pertussigen preparation has a significant influence on its HSF activity. For example, we have commonly observed a two-fold increase in HSF activity when *B. pertussis* cells are disrupted mechanically. With purified pertussigen, Munoz and his colleagues have reported HSD_{50} values from as high as 260 ng/mouse (Munoz *et al.*, 1978) to as low as 0.5 ng/mouse (Arai and Munoz, 1981). The former high value was with pertussigen extracted from acetone-treated cells while the latter was with pertussigen purified from culture supernates.

HSF activity is conveniently assayed by injecting groups of mice i.p. with graded doses of the test preparations, in 2-, 3-, 4- or 5-fold dilutions, and then challenging the animals 3, 4 or 5 days later with a constant i.p. dose of histamine (e.g. 1.8 mg base/20 g mouse), usually as the dihydrochloride or diphosphate. This dose should be confirmed as being nonlethal in untreated mice, or mice given diluent on the day when the test animals received their sensitizing injection. Dead and surviving animals are counted 2–4 hr after histamine challenge and the percentage mortality recorded. A standard vaccine, or other source of HSF, should be run in parallel with the test preparations to permit evaluation of the potency relative to the standard, instead of simply in terms of HSD_{50}, i.e. the dose of the preparation which causes a 50% mortality after histamine challenge. There is a linear relationship between log dose of vaccine, or extract, and the probit of the mortality. This permits applications of standard statistical methods for analysis of variance and estimation of relative potency and 95% confidence limits. Pittman (1975) and Kurokawa *et al* (1978a) have reported on the HSF activity of the United States' and Japanese Standard Pertussis Vaccine relative to the Netherlands' Standard.

As an alternative to observing mortality or time of death after histamine challenge of pertussis vaccine-treated mice, Ishida *et al.* (1978) have proposed the measurement of rectal temperature 30 min after histamine challenge. This hypothermia method was reported to be 20–30 times more sensitive than observing mortality, but has not been confirmed by other investigators.

The mechanism of histamine sensitization in mice has been the subject of much investigation and speculation (e.g. Munoz, 1971) but is still obscure. Since sensitization of mice to histamine could be induced by β-adrenoceptor-blocking drugs it has been proposed that HSF acts by producing β-adrenoceptor blockade (Fishel et al., 1962; Szentivanyi et al., 1963; Townley et al., 1967; Bergman and Munoz, 1968). Later studies (Section 4.7) however, have negated this hypothesis. Nevertheless there is ample evidence (Section 4.6.3) that certain tissues of the pertussigen-treated mouse have abnormal responsiveness to epinephrine and it is also noteworthy that the changes induced by pertussigen can be duplicated by adrenalectomy (Table 7). Thus, the role of altered adrenoceptor function in the histamine sensitivity induced by HSF remains to be clarified. Further speculation on the contribution of altered adrenoceptor function to other aspects of pathophysiological responses produced by pertussigen is presented below (Section 4.7).

4.6.2. Leukocytosis Promotion

As early as 1897, Frölich observed that whooping cough patients frequently exhibited a striking lymphocytosis, the peripheral white cell count rising in extreme cases (Munoz and Bergman, 1977) to 175,000 per mm^3 (c.f. normal levels 7000–11,000). Much later, Sauer (1933) noted the occurrence of lymphocytosis in children injected with pertussis vaccine, and Tuta (1937) detected a similar response in rabbits. The substance responsible for these effects has been designated leukocytosis-promoting factor and lymphocytosis-promoting factor, both names being applicable and abbreviated to LPF, since the blood counts of lymphocytes and polymorphonuclear (PMN) leukocytes are substantially increased. Our knowledge of this factor is largely due to the investigations of Morse and his coworkers (1965–1977b), Arai and Sato (1976) and Irons and MacLennan (1979a,b).

A response to LPF has been demonstrated in a remarkably broad range of vertebrate species including lampreys, pigs, calves, sheep, rabbits, guinea-pigs, rats, mice, monkeys and man (Olson, 1975). Of these, the mouse has been by far the most extensively studied. The marked effects of mouse age and strain, seen with HSF, do not seem to have their counterparts in LPF-responsiveness.

Induction of leukocytosis in mice occurs most rapidly and fully if the B. pertussis cells or soluble preparation is injected i.v. A less substantial response follows i.p. injection, while the s.c. route is ineffective. Peak leukocytosis occurs between the second and fourth day after i.v. injection (Fig. 3) and declines to normal values after 2–3 weeks, i.e. more rapidly than the decline in histamine sensitization. Sublethal pulmonary infection of mice with B. pertussis induced leukocytosis that lasted for at least 5 weeks (Pittman et al., 1980). Such mice however, were carrying the live organisms for 2–3 weeks, or longer, which provided a prolonged stimulus.

At the height of the leukocytosis response in mice, about 60–70 % of the cells were mature-appearing, small lymphocytes—both T-cells and B-cells, the former predominating but the relative increase in B-lymphocytes being greater (Morse and Morse, 1976). Most of the rest

TABLE 7. *Similarities of Response Between Adrenalectomized and Bordetella pertussis-Treated Mice*

Feature	Adrenal-ectomized	B. pertussis-treated
Histamine shock	+	+
Endotoxin shock	+	+
Anaphylactic shock	+	+
Cold stress	+	+
Susceptibility to EAE	+	+
Effect on sugar and fat metabolism	+	+
Effect on permeability of capillaries	+	+
Adjuvant action	+(?)	+

(From Munoz and Bergman (1979a) and reproduced with the permission of the authors.)

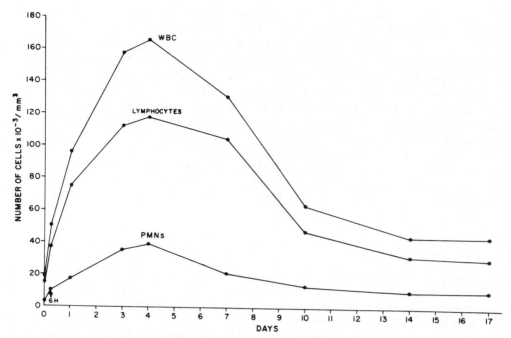

FIG. 3. Time-course of the leukocytosis response in mice after the i.v. injection of 0.5 μg purified LPF. (From Morse, S. I. and Morse, J. H. (1976) *J. exp. Med.* **143**: 1483–1502; reproduced with the permission of Dr. Jane H. Morse and the Journal of Experimental Medicine.)

were PMN leukocytes, but there was also a relative increase in the numbers of large lymphocytes and monocytes. Eosinophils and basophils remained rare on blood films throughout the period of leukocytosis. A slight eosinophilia in rats and mice given pertussis vaccine was reported by Terpstra *et al.* (1979).

Morse and Riester (1967a) investigated the mechanism of leukocytosis by injecting mice with tritiated thymidine—a total of 16 injections at 4-hourly intervals—starting 30 min after i.v. injection of pertussis vaccine or physiological saline. Autoradiography was then applied to blood films made at intervals to detect growing and dividing cells that had incorporated radioactive label into their nuclei. The results with small and medium lymphocytes and with PMN leukocytes were different: the lymphocytes, in pertussis vaccine-treated animals exhibited the same small percentage of labelled cells as in normal animals throughout the period of lymphocytosis, despite the 10-fold increase in blood lymphocyte count. This meant that the new lymphocytes in the blood stream had not arisen from recent cell division but had been released into the blood compartment from extravascular sites and then had failed to leave. The PMN leukocytes, on the other hand, which showed at 3 days a 15–30 fold elevation in count, exhibited a high percentage of tritium-labelling, indicating active proliferation of myeloid elements. In addition, there was release of mature (and therefore unlabelled) PMN leukocytes from tissue reserves.

The mechanism of retention of lymphocytes in the blood stream of pertussis vaccine-treated mice was investigated by transfusion of lymphocytes labelled *in vitro* with tritiated uridine. These experiments showed that the lymphocytosis was due to a blockade in the normal traffic of these cells between the blood and the lymphatic compartments. Thus lymphocytes that had entered the blood had a diminished capacity to leave via the postcapillary venules in lymph nodes. The main cause of the lymphocytosis appeared to be a change in the lymphocytes themselves rather than in the vascular endothelium (Morse and Barron, 1970). Additional evidence for the lymphocytosis being a consequence of interruption of the normal 'traffic' of these cells was provided by observations on the through-put of lymphocytes in the cannulated thoracic duct of pertussis vaccine-treated animals. Here, both concentration of lymphocytes and the through-put over 24 hr were actually *less* than in normal animals, despite the treated animals having a 10-fold higher-than-normal level of lymphocytes in the blood stream (Morse and Riester, 1967b). The exact nature of the change induced by LPF on the lymphocyte remains to be elucidated.

The assay of LPF activity of pertussis vaccine or cell-extracts is complicated by endotoxin also having an effect on the white-cell count in the blood. However, the peak leukocytosis (Fig. 4) after purified endotoxin (LPS) occurs 24 hr after i.p. injection, whereas that produced by endotoxin-free LPF is at 3–4 days (Kurokawa *et al.*, 1978a). Thus, by making the white-cell counts on day 3 or 4 postinjection, the interference by endotoxin in the LPF assay was minimized. Kurokawa *et al.* (1978a) showed that there was a linear relationship between the log-dose of LPF injected and the leukocytosis response expressed as log-ratio of leukocyte count in the experimental group over the control group. This permitted a parallel-line assay to be performed, but with the complication that purified LPF and whole-cell vaccine gave linear dose–response regressions but of different slopes. This meant that different reference preparations for purified LPF and for LPF in a whole-cell vaccine would have to be established.

4.6.3. *Islets Activation*

In 1936, Regan and Tolstoouhov observed that children with whooping cough tended to have blood-glucose concentrations that were lower than normal (see Table 11). This hypoglycemic tendency extended into convalescence, despite the children taking and retaining food and often gaining weight. Hypoglycemia in rabbits injected with a lethal dose of *B. pertussis* crude extract was reported by Oddy and Evans (1940). It was preceded by marked hyperglycemia. Much more recently, Pittman *et al.* (1980) reported that mice with a respiratory-tract infection of *B. pertussis* were, between day 10 and day 33 postinfection, significantly hypoglycemic compared with controls, even though they had free access to food at all times. It seems likely that hypoglycemia associated with *B. pertussis* infection is due to a pertussigen-induced change in the pancreatic B-cells that leads to hypersecretion of insulin in response to various insulin-releasing stimuli.

A single i.p. injection of pertussis vaccine into rats and mice caused marked elevation of plasma insulin, as measured by radioimmunoassay, which persisted for at least 17 days in the mouse and beyond 24 days in the rat (Gulbenkian *et al.*, 1968). Peak levels of plasma insulin were observed at post-injection day 3 in the rat and day 7 in the mouse (Table 8). As with histamine sensitization and lymphocytosis promotion, hyperinsulinemia induction by

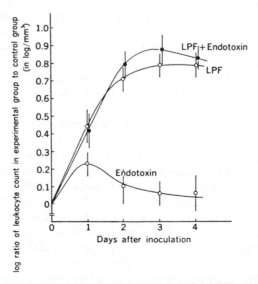

Fig. 4. The time-course of leukocytosis after endotoxin and after LPF and after a mixture of the two. Each circle represents the mean of 5 mice and the vertical line the confidence interval of the mean. (From Kurokawa *et al.* (1978a) *Jap. J. med. Sci. Biol.* **31**: 91–103; reproduced with the permission of the authors and the Japanese Journal of Medical Science and Biology.)

TABLE 8. *Time-Course of Insulin Changes in the Plasma of Normal and Pertussis-Vaccinated (PV) Rats and Mice*

Rats

Days post-PV		1	3	5	12	18	24
Plasma insulin	Control	52 ± 24.9	180 ± 16.1	77 ± 6.1	111 ± 25.2	130 ± 24.1	68 ± 24.1
μU/ml	PV	361 ± 85.7	649 ± 82.6	429 ± 56.9	253 ± 53.4	382 ± 30.2	221 ± 55.3

Mice

Days post-PV		1	3	7	9	14	17	21
Plasma insulin	Control	34 ± 4.6	13 ± 10.5	20 ± 7.0	19 ± 13.7	7 ± 2.4	15 ± 5	11 ± 6.2
μU/ml	PV	75 ± 17.7	126 ± 20.1	228 ± 40.7	168 ± 9.9	102 ± 53.7	57 ± 16.3	26 ± 17.8

There were 4–6 rats or 10 mice on each day. The figures after ± are standard errors.
(From Gulbenkian *et al.* (1968) *Endocrinology* **83**: 885–892; reproduced with permission of the authors and of The Endocrine Society; copyright Williams & Wilkins, Baltimore.)

pertussis vaccine was much less effective by the s.c. route than by the i.v. or i.p. routes (**B. L. Furman** and **A. C. Wardlaw**, unpublished observations).

The time-course of hyperinsulinemia in the rat was the same as that for the attenuation of epinephrine-induced hyperglycemia, suggesting that the latter phenomenon was related to hypersecretion of insulin (Tabachnick and Gulbenkian, 1969). Indeed, pretreatment of rats with pertussis vaccine was shown to *reverse* the insulin response to epinephrine—in normal rats, epinephrine caused a slight fall in plasma insulin, whereas in *B. pertussis*-treated rats it caused an enormous rise (Table 9).

A puzzling feature of pertussis-vaccinated or -infected mice or rats is the apparent coexistence of relatively mild hypoglycemia and very marked hyperinsulinemia. A solution to this paradox was proposed by Furman *et al.* (1981) who showed that although freely-fed, *B. pertussis*-treated mice were mildly, but significantly, hypoglycemic relative to controls, the plasma insulin levels were not chronically elevated. However, if ether anesthesia was given to the animals at the time of withdrawing blood (as was done in earlier investigations), there was a rapid and massive increase of plasma insulin concentration, so that the blood sample exhibited simultaneous mild hypoglycemia with marked hyperinsulinemia (Table 10). If on the other hand, blood was obtained rapidly by decapitation without anesthetic, the mild

TABLE 9. *Effect of Epinephrine on Levels of Glucose and Insulin in the Plasma of Normal and Pertussis-Vaccinated (PV) Rats*

Treatment	Plasma glucose (mg/100 ml)	Plasma insulin (μU/ml)
Normal	124 (110–133)	47 (23–71)
Normal + Epinephrine	280 (258–302)	26 (4–50)
PV	126 (117–136)	163 (111–215)
PV + Epinephrine	193 (170–216)	757 (242–1271)

There were ten rats per group. Epinephrine was injected s.c. at 2 mg/kg 30 min before bleeding. The figures in brackets are 95% confidence limits.

(From Gulbenkian *et al.* (1968) *Endocrinology* **83**: 885–892; reproduced with permission of the authors and of The Endocrine Society; copyright Williams & Wilkins, Baltimore.)

TABLE 10. *Serum IRI and Glucose Concentrations in Mice Exposed to* B. pertussis *by Infection or Vaccination and Bled in Three Different Ways*

Method of bleeding	*B. pertussis* treatment	No. of mice	IRI μU/ml: geometric mean, significance level* (and 95% CL)	Glucose mg/100 ml: arithmetic mean, significance level* (and 95% CL)
Ether plus heart puncture	nil	144	31 (27,35)	196 (191, 201)
	infection	102	78 + + (68, 89)	164 + + (159, 169)
	vaccine	45	145 + + (114,184)	129 + + (119,140)
Decapitation without anesthetic	nil	114	33 (29, 37)	193 (189, 197)
	infection	72	34 NS (28, 41)	139 + + (127, 138)
	vaccine	56	37 NS (33, 42)	144 + + (139, 149)
Ether plus decapitation	nil	198	33 (30, 36)	206 (203, 209)
	vaccine	198	148 + + (138, 159)	152 + + (149, 155)

* In the *t*-test, comparing each pertussis treatment with the nil group in each method of bleeding: NS = not significant ($P > 5\%$); + = significant ($5\% \geqslant P > 1\%$); + + = highly significant ($P \leqslant 1\%$).

(From Furman *et al.* (1981) *Br. J. Exp. Path.*; reproduced with the permission of the senior author and the editor of the British Journal of Experimental Pathology).

hypoglycemia was the same but the hyperinsulinemia failed to appear (Table 10). Furman *et al.*, (1981) suggested that: (1) pertussigen acts on the pancreas so as to alter the response of the islet B-cells to epinephrine. This alteration consists in epinephrine having an insulin-releasing instead of an insulin-retaining effect; (2) ether is known to cause release of endogenous epinephrine, therefore (3) the pertussis-treated mouse, when bled under ether-anesthesia, yields a hyperinsulinemic plasma, whereas without the ether there is no release of epinephrine and the B-cells, in turn, do not secrete additional insulin. Ether was not the only anesthetic to exhibit the insulin-releasing effect, for trichloroethylene and pentobarbitone were also active.

Changes similar to those seen with pertussis vaccine were also observed with highly purified IAP (Yajima *et al.*, 1978b). Figure 5 shows that peak responses in rats developed in a dose-dependent manner between days 3 and 10 post injection and persisted for up to 60 days. In order to elicit hyperinsulinemia in the IAP-treated rat, glucose was injected i.p. shortly before withdrawal of blood for insulin analysis. This procedure provided the basis of the assay of IAP (Yajima *et al.*, 1978b) now to be described.

Male rats of the Wistar strain were injected i.v. with graded doses of the preparation containing IAP. Three days later (the last 20 hr of which were with fasting) the animals were given a uniform insulin-releasing, i.p. challenge of 200 mg glucose/100 g body weight. Blood samples (0.1 ml) were taken from a tail vein immediately before the glucose injection and then exactly 15 min afterwards. The concentrations of glucose and insulin in the two blood specimens were determined. Note that because the insulin was assayed by a radioim-munoassay technique, it was referred to as immuno-reactive insulin (IRI). This designation is because the assay does not distinguish between pro-insulin (the storage form of the hormone) and insulin, the former having a much lower biological activity than insulin itself. However there is no evidence that the IRI measured in the IAP assay is, from its hypoglycemic effect, other than active insulin although this question does not appear to have been explored.

From the two blood specimens from each rat, a value ΔG was calculated for the difference in glucose concentrations (mg/100 ml), and a value ΔIRI for the difference in insulin concentration (μU/ml). Then a ratio $R = \Delta$IRI$/\Delta G$ was calculated for each rat. This ratio expressed the extent of hyperinsulinemia per unit increase in plasma glucose, consequential to the glucose loading. Mean values of R were obtained for groups of animals that had been

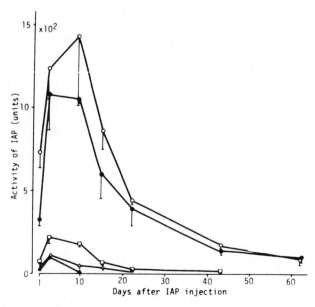

FIG. 5. The time-course of islet activation in rats after i.v. injection of doses of IAP ranging from 8 ng to 2 μg. The dose of IAP was: (▲) 8 ng; (△) 32 ng; (□) 125 ng; (●) 1 μg; (○) 2 μg. Each point with a vertical line shows the mean ± SEM from three animals. (From Yajima *et al.* (1978b) *J. Biochem.* (Tokyo) **83**: 305–312; reproduced with the permission of the authors and through the courtesy of the Japanese Biochemical Society.)

initially injected with a test preparation (R_t) and for control animals injected with saline (R_c) on day zero. The unit of IAP activity was then defined by

$$1 \text{ IAP unit} = \frac{R_t - R_c}{R_c} \times 100.$$

According to this definition, 100 IAP units correspond to the activity that doubles the insulin-secretory response to a given degree of hyperglycemia. The log-dose–response curve of IAP in rats is shown in Fig. 6.

As part of their investigation of glucose and IRI changes in IAP-treated rats, Yajima *et al.* (1978b) showed that the attenuation of epinephrine-induced hyperglycemia previously reported with rats given whole-cell vaccine (Gulbenkian *et al.*, 1968) and mice given purified LPF (Morse and Morse, 1976), was also demonstrable with purified IAP. The strong correlation between the IAP activity and inhibition of epinephrine hyperglycemia is shown in Fig. 7.

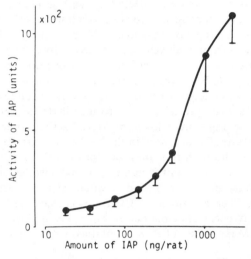

FIG. 6. Dose-response curve of purified IAP injected into rats. The unit of IAP activity is described in the text. (From Yajima *et al.* (1978a) *J. Biochem.* (Tokyo) **83**: 295–303; reproduced with the permission of the authors and through the courtesy of the Japanese Biochemical Society.)

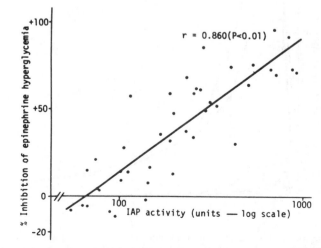

FIG. 7. The strong positive correlation between inhibition of epinephrine hyperglycemia in rats and IAP activity. (From Yajima *et al.* (1978b) *J. Biochem.* (Tokyo) **83**: 305–312; reproduced with the permission of the authors and through the courtesy of the Japanese Biochemical Society.)

The conclusion, from tests in the whole animal, that IAP acts on the islet B-cells of the pancreas was strengthened by experiments on the rate of insulin secretion by the isolated perfused organ *in vitro* (Katada and Ui, 1977a). The pancreas was taken from normal rats and from animals injected i.v. with pertussis vaccine several days previously. By releasing additional IRI into the perfusate, both types of pancreas responded to the following insulin secretagogues: glucose, arginine, sulfonylureas and 3-isobutyl-1-methylxanthine (IBMX). With each agent, however, the 'pertussis' pancreas released significantly more IRI than the normal one. A particularly dramatic difference was seen with epinephrine which in the normal pancreas caused a decline in insulin secretion, but in a 'pertussis' pancreas caused an enhancement.

Evidence that the IAP-induced modification of B-cell function was not mediated by direct automatic fiber innervation of the cell was provided by Katada and Ui (1980b). These authors showed that rats rendered diabetic with streptozotocin and then intraportally transfused with islets isolated by the collagenase digestion method, responded to IAP, administered subsequently, in a manner similar to normal animals.

Further experiments were performed by the same authors (Katada and Ui, 1979) with isolated islets *in vitro*, a system which facilitated analysis of the *B. pertussis*-induced changes in terms of adrenoceptor function. An unstimulated normal islet secreted insulin continuously but at a very slow rate; addition of glucose greatly promoted this process, whereas epinephrine, through its predominantly α-adrenoceptor effect, inhibited it. Epinephrine also attenuated the stimulatory effect of glucose. In contrast, the islet from a pertussis-vaccine or IAP-treated animal behaved as if the α-adrenoceptor function was absent. Thus epinephrine, through its β-stimulatory properties *augmented* the promotional effect of glucose and was no longer susceptible to inhibition by phentolamine. The effect of IAP did not seem to be by direct blockade of the α-adrenoceptor itself but by alteration in the pathway of intracellular events that would normally follow α-adrenoceptor stimulation. A schematic representation of the effect of pertussis treatment on insulin secretion by the islet B-cell is shown Fig. 8.

A prime feature of IAP action on the pancreas is its slowness in producing the altered responsiveness to insulin secretagogues. IAP had no immediate effect on insulin secretion when added to the fluid perfusing a normal pancreas *in vitro* and, in order to obtain an altered pancreas, it was necessary to have injected the donor animal with IAP or vaccine about three days previously (Katada and Ui, 1977a). Similar results were obtained with isolated islets, except that since these cells could be kept in culture, it was possible to show that exposure to IAP *in vitro* did cause a partial development of the characteristic abnormal response to epinephrine (Katada and Ui, 1979).

Although pretreatment of rats with pertussis vaccine or purified IAP altered the insulin-secretagogue responsiveness of the pancreas, there was little evidence of gross damage to the organ three days later (Katada and Ui, 1979). Thus between the pancreases of normal and IAP-treated rats, there were no significant differences in net weight of tissue, total extractable insulin, extractable insulin per islet and number of islets per pancreas.

In addition to enhancing the secretion of insulin, IAP also enhanced the release of glucagon. This was demonstrated both with perfused pancreas from normal and IAP-pretreated rats (Narimiya *et al.*, 1980) and with isolated islets treated with IAP *in vitro* (Nielsen, *et al.*, 1980). On the other hand, IAP pretreatment was shown to *diminish* the stimulatory effect of norepinephrine on glucagon secretion by the isolated perfused pancreas of normal and diabetic rats (Toyota *et al.*, 1978).

Purified IAP was shown to have a beneficial effect in spontaneously diabetic mice (Okamoto *et al.*, 1980) and rats (Toyota *et al.*, 1978) and in ordinary rats that had been made diabetic with streptozotocin (Katada and Ui, 1977b). The normalization of glucose-tolerance by IAP treatment of spontaneously-diabetic rats is shown in Fig. 9. A notable feature of this normalization was its persistence for up to 35 days. The antigenicity of IAP is, however, likely to limit its usefulness in the long-term treatment of diabetes (Toyota *et al.*, 1980). These latter authors found that purified IAP at i.v. doses of 0.5 and 1.0 μg/kg was well tolerated by six healthy human volunteers and was also pharmacologically active. Thus on day 4 post injection, peak plasma IRI in response to oral glucose loading was significantly elevated over

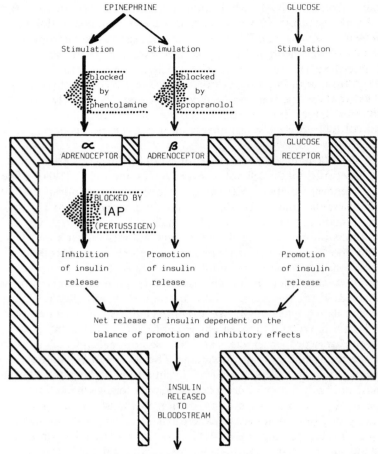

FIG. 8. Schematic diagram of the insulin-secreting islet B-cell showing α and β-adrenoceptors, the glucose receptor, the effect of stimulation by epinephrine and glucose and the postulated location of the functional lesion caused by IAP.

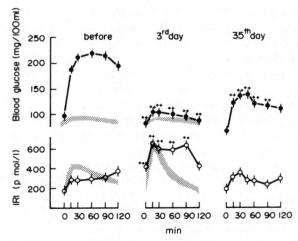

FIG. 9. Ability of IAP to normalize the glucose-tolerance curve of spontaneously diabetic rats. The values are presented as the mean of 7 experiments ± SEM. **$P < 0.01$ vs the value before IAP-injection. The dotted shadow shows the results of six normal rats before and after IAP-injection. (From Toyota *et al.* (1978) *Diabetologia* **14**: 319–323; reproduced with the permission of the authors and of Springer-Verlag New York.

the pre-injection value. This abnormal responsiveness was still detectable at 60 days. The volunteers developed antibodies to IAP which were detectable by allergic skin tests, although specific IgE was not found by radio-allergosorbent test (RAST). However, there was abundant evidence of IgG production to the IAP, and the authors cautioned against anaphylaxis in patients injected with this substance.

An additional report concerning the potential exploitation of the metabolic actions of pertussis vaccine in the treatment of diabetes came from Dhar *et al.* (1975). These authors gave pertussis vaccine (2 ml i.m.) to 20 patients with maturity-onset diabetes and who had developed partial or full insulin-resistance i.e. were not properly controlled by 100 or > 200 units of insulin per day, respectively. Within a few days, eight of the patients were being controlled with less than 100 units of insulin per day and only four remained with a requirement of > 200. Although the beneficial effect lasted in the majority of patients only for a few weeks, it was considered of potential value for insulin-resistant diabetics in certain specific circumstances, e.g. in the treatment of severe infections and as a preparation for surgery.

It is difficult to explain the beneficial effects of the vaccine in these patients in terms of the insulinotropic effect of IAP. It is possible that pertussis vaccine had additionally some effect on insulin sensitivity and, indeed, it was shown by Lane (1969) that pertussis vaccine markedly augmented the sensitivity of mice to the lethal/convulsant effects of insulin.

4.6.4. *Adjuvanticity*

Whole-cell pertussis vaccine is noted for several distinct kinds of immunopotentiating activities (Finger, 1975). These include: (1) enhancement of serum antibody titers to various antigens; (2) production of hyperacute experimental autoallergic encephalomyelitis (HEAE); and (3) production of anaphylactic sensitivity in mice and rats. For reviews see also Pittman (1957), Olson (1975) and Morse (1976). An adjuvant effect on cell-mediated immunity has been shown (Athanassiades, 1977), and the successful application of pertussis vaccine in the immunotherapy of mammary tumors in mice has been reported (Likhite, 1974). The converse effect of enhancement of tumor growth by pertussis vaccine in mice has also been noted (Hirano *et al.*, 1967).

Undoubtedly, some of the adjuvant activity of *B. pertussis* is due to the LPS (Section 2.3) but this does not account for all of it. Pieroni and Levine (1966) showed that heating pertussis vaccine at 100°C for 40 min abolished its adjuvant activity for tetanus toxoid in mice. Indeed, the heated vaccine had a partial immunosuppressive effect on the toxoid, but this might be due to different routes of injection having been used (i.p. vaccine, s.c. toxoid). From the evidence of heat-lability and other data, Levine and Pieroni (1966) put forward the idea that HSF, protective antigen and heat-labile adjuvant activity were due to one and the same substance, i.e. that which is identified in this article as pertussigen.

More direct support for the view that pertussigen could act as an adjuvant was provided by studies with X-mode and C-mode *B. pertussis* vaccines, both of which contain LPS, but the latter lack pertussigen (Section 1.3). Figure 10 shows that in two quite different systems— induction of HEAE to guinea-pig spinal cord in Lewis rats, and of reaginic antibodies to ovalbumin in mice—the C-mode vaccine had only slight adjuvant activity, while the X-mode vaccine had pronounced dose-dependent adjuvant effects (Wardlaw *et al.*, 1979; Wardlaw and Parton, 1979). The residual adjuvant activity in the C-mode vaccine was probably due to LPS.

In addition to the above studies with whole-cell vaccines, pertussigen preparations in various states of purity were shown to have adjuvant activity in the following systems: stimulation of IgE antibodies to ovalbumin in mice (Lehrer *et al.*, 1975b, 1976; Munoz *et al.*, 1978) and to DNP-ascaris in rats (Mizushima *et al.*, 1979); and induction of HEAE with guinea-pig spinal cord in Lewis rats (Levine *et al.*, 1966; Bergman *et al.*, 1978).

In contrast to the foregoing, pertussigen has been shown to exert an immunosuppressive effect under certain conditions. For example, the *in vitro* IgM plaque-forming-cell response of mouse spleen cells to sheep erythrocytes was strongly inhibited by mitogenic doses of LPF (Suzuki *et al.*, 1978). A similar inhibition was found in the living mouse, (Asakawa, 1969) when

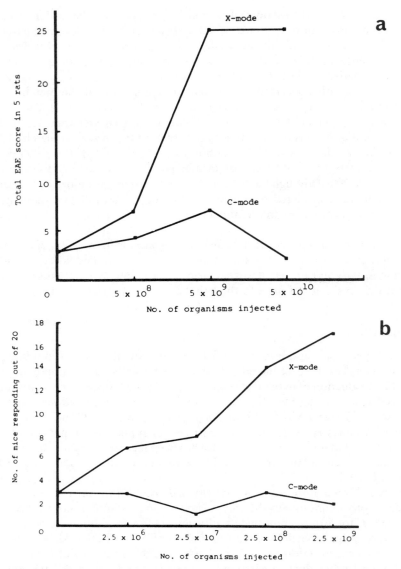

FIG. 10. Comparative adjuvant activities of X-mode and C-mode pertussis vaccines (a) for induction of HEAE to guinea-pig spinal cord in Lewis rats; (b) for promotion IgE antibodies to ovalbumin in mice. In both systems the dose of antigen was kept constant and the amount of pertussis vaccine (expressed as number of organisms) was varied. The dose of antigen was 25 mg in (a) and 200 μg in (b). IgE was assayed on 21-day sera by passive cutaneous anaphylaxis with a 48 hr interval between sensitization and challenge. (After Wardlaw and Parton, 1979.)

LPF was injected several days before the injection of antigen (tetanus toxoid or sheep erythrocytes).

Although many studies have attempted to unravel the mechanism of adjuvant activity of whole-cell pertussis vaccine (reviewed by Finger, 1975), few similar studies have been done with purified pertussigen, and its mode of adjuvant action is poorly understood. Finger, (1975) considered that adjuvancy, as a general phenomenon, depends on 'cytotoxic activity which initially functions as a nonspecific proliferative impulse'. In this context the mitogenic activity of LPF for murine T-lymphocytes may be significant (Section 4.6.6), although there is no evidence for mitogenicity *in vivo* (Kong and Morse, 1977a). On the other hand, Morse (1976) speculated that IgE-antibody response might be regulated by a suppressor population of lymphocytes. Thus the disruption of normal recirculation of these cells due to LPF activity may lead to loss of suppressor control.

Further insights into the regulation of IgE production by pertussis vaccine, and involving macrophages and helper T-cells, have been reported by Hirashima *et al.* (1981).

Lehrer *et al.* (1975b) emphasized the complex interplay of factors that may influence IgE antibody production, e.g. the genetic capabilities of the host, the dose, type and relative timing of administration of adjuvant and antigen, and of removal of sera.

Some insight into the mechanism of induction of HEAE was recently provided by Bergman *et al.* (1978) who emphasized that the hyperacute form of EAE that develops in rats injected with pertussigen and guinea-pig spinal cord differed histologically from the EAE occurring after giving spinal cord in complete Freund's adjuvant. The former was characterized by a neutrophil infiltrate with deposition of fibrin, whereas the latter showed a mainly mononuclear cell infiltrate. Bergman *et al.* (1978) noted that in HEAE there was an increase in vascular permeability of capillaries in the spinal cord associated with the ascending paralysis. They suggested that the paralysis in HEAE is therefore due to edema. It seems likely that the pertussigen also had an adjuvant effect on the encephalitogenic antigen in guinea-pig spinal cord, perhaps inducing a cellular hypersensitivity. Serum antibodies to the neuroantigen were easily detected but did not passively transfer HEAE.

One of the earliest adjuvant activities demonstrated for pertussis vaccine was its anaphylactic sensitizing effect in mice (Malkiel and Hargis, 1952). Ordinarily the mouse does not become sensitive to anaphylactic shock after a single dose of a soluble protein antigen. However, if the antigen is mixed with pertussis vaccine, a dramatic change occurs whereby a subsequent i.v. challenge dose of the homologous antigen generally proves fatal. The overall reaction appears to be due to a combination of reaginic antibody production plus sensitization to the endogenous vasoactive amines released by the antigen–antibody reaction at the time of challenge. The onset of shock sensitivity is not until 7 days after the initial injection and remains demonstrable for at least 70 days (Fig. 2). Anaphylactic sensitivity to ovalbumin was passively transferred to mice by i.v. administration of homologous, semi-purified IgG_1, but not IgE antibodies to ovalbumin (J. J. Munoz and R. K. Bergman, unpublished observations).

B. pertussis cells could not be replaced by other bacteria or by endotoxin for induction of anaphylactic sensitization (Finger, 1975), which suggests that pertussigen was playing an essential role. It may be noted, however, that complete Freund's adjuvant also had the capacity to induce anaphylactic sensitization of mice to ovalbumin, but the effect was associated with much higher levels circulating antibody (Munoz, 1963b).

4.6.5. *Mouse Protection*

The whooping-cough immunization field-trials conducted by the Medical Research Council (1951, 1956, 1959) in Great Britain yielded two important results: (1) pertussis vaccines in use at that time varied greatly in protective immunizing potency, and (2) there was a strong correlation between the protective efficacy of a vaccine in children and its protective potency in the intracerebral mouse-protection test (IC-MPT). This test, which had been described by Kendrick *et al.*, (1947) and others, therefore became accepted as the standard method for assaying the mouse-protective antigen (MPA) content of pertussis vaccines and also of extracts and biochemical fractions of the bacillus. Subsequently a vast research effort in many countries was directed at purifying the MPA with the IC-MPT being used to monitor the protective activity. To date, this approach has not yielded a homogeneous preparation of MPA, although certain useful conclusions have emerged: MPA tends to parallel or resemble HSF in being subject to loss from cultures by phase variation and antigenic modulation (Wardlaw *et al.*, 1976, Wardlaw and Parton, 1979); both activities have similar sensitivities to heat, trypsin and various injurious chemicals (Levine and Pieroni, 1966; Wardlaw and Jakus, 1966; Jakus *et al.*, 1968) and they tend to occur in the same biochemical fractions during purification procedures (Levine and Pieroni, 1966; Munoz *et al.*, 1978). However, for exceptions to the above, see Section 4.1.

Meanwhile, a different research approach has yielded purified HSF and LPF which some investigators have found active in the IC-MPT. Unfortunately not all of the purified preparations of pertussigen, e.g. the IAP of Yajima and coworkers (1978a,b) appear to have been assayed for mouse-protective activity. Munoz and coworkers consistently reported MPA in their preparations of pertussigen (Munoz, 1976; Munoz and Bergman, 1977, 1979a,b; Munoz et al., 1981b). In the last-cited reference, the PD_{50} (50% protective dose) of purified pertussigen in the IC-MPT was $1.4\,\mu g$/mouse. Pertussigen which had been detoxified with glutaraldehyde had a PD_{50} of $1.7\,\mu g$ although in a subsequent article (Munoz and Arai, 1982), crystalline pertussigen was lethal for mice at a dose of $0.5\,\mu g$. On the other hand, the LPF-HA of Irons and MacLennan (1979a) which in this chapter is taken to be the same as pertussigen, was found by these authors to be nonprotective at the highest levels ($4\,\mu g$/mouse) permitted by the toxicity of the material. For further discussion of MPA see Section 5.

4.6.6. Other Activities

A variety of other activities is attributable to pertussigen, notably induction of hypoproteinemia and enhancement of vascular permeability in skin and striated muscle, toxicity (systemic and local), in vitro mitogenicity of lymphocytes, and a potentially useful in vitro metabolic assay—the release of glycerol from adipocytes.

Hypoproteinemia in mice was observed in blood samples taken between 1 and 14 days after i.v. injection of B. pertussis extract (Bergman and Munoz, 1969). Whereas the plasma protein concentration in normal mice was $6.20 \pm 0.06\,g/100\,ml$, it was $5.19 \pm 0.079\,g/ml$ in the treated animals. The reduction was due mainly to loss of albumin. Although the mechanism of the effect was not examined in detail, it seems likely to be related to the increase in vascular permeability produced by pertussigen in skin (Bergman and Munoz, 1975) and skeletal muscle (Munoz et al., 1981a). These latter reactions may be likened to a localized HSF test in that a sublethal challenge dose of histamine, or another vasoactive substance, is injected into skin or muscle at the same time as i.v. Evans Blue, and local permeability changes measured. Bergman and Munoz (1975) suggested that there is an alteration in the vascular bed, or the physiological mechanisms that regulate the vascular bed, to make blood vessels more susceptible to the permeability-inducing effects of histamine and serotonin, and less responsive to the palliative effects of catecholamines. Since the hypoproteinemia did not require a challenge injection of histamine or other substance for its manifestation, there is the implication that the blood vessels of the pertussigen-treated mouse are leaky towards albumin through the action of endogenous stimuli.

The in vitro mitogenicity of LPF for mouse lymphocytes was described by Kong and Morse (1977a,b) and Suzuki et al. (1978). The mitogen was somewhat more active than the phytohemagglutinin of Phaseolus vulgaris but slightly less stimulatory than concanavalinA. The target cells for the B. pertussis mitogen where the T-lymphocytes which were induced to incorporate ^{3}H-thymidine during three days of in vitro culture. The target cells were obtained from the spleen or lymph nodes of normal mice but not from the thymus, whose cells were unresponsive. Human blood lymphocytes were also responsive. The mitogenic response of the T-cells required the presence of helper B-lymphocytes in the culture (Ho et al., 1979). This requirement of a B helper-cell for stimulation of T-lymphocytes is unique to pertussigen and is not exhibited by other mitogens. A curious feature of the mitogenic activity was its sharp dosage optimum—around $0.5\,\mu g/0.25\,ml$ culture containing 5×10^5 lymph node cells (Kong and Morse, 1977a). This feature may explain the apparent lack of mitogenic activity in vivo.

The T-lymphocytes stimulated by in vitro exposure to LPF were cytotoxic for syngeneic and allogeneic tumour cells and for allogeneic and semisyngeneic normal cells, but not for syngeneic normal cells (Morse et al., 1979). Recently a new lymphocyte mitogen from B. pertussis was described by Ho et al. (1981). It differed from LPF in inducing the proliferation of human and murine B-lymphocytes and having no effect on T-cells.

Of potential importance as a rapid in vitro assay for pertussigen is the adipocyte/glycerol-release procedure recently described by Endoh et al. (1980) based on earlier observations of Gulbenkian et al. (1968). Suspensions of adipocytes from rat epididymal fat pads were mixed with purified HSF and incubated for 3 hr at $37°C$, after which glycerol released into the medium was assayed enzymatically. The dose–response curves for glycerol release from rat adipocytes and the HSF and LPF activities of the same preparation in mice is shown in Fig. 11. It will be noted that the *in vitro* adipocyte assay was more sensitive on a nanogram per tube basis than the HSF or LPF tests on a nanogram per mouse basis.

Later, Endoh and Nakase (1982) reported that mouse adipocytes could not replace those from the rat and also that anti-HSF serum neutralized the glycerol-releasing activity of HSF on the rat cells.

Another potentially useful *in vitro* assay for pertussigen is the clumping of Chinese hamster ovary (CHO) cells as described by Hewlett *et al.*, (1982).

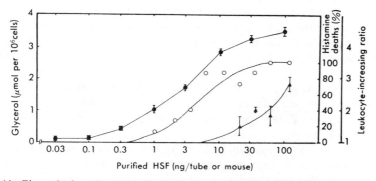

FIG. 11. Glycerol release from rat adipocytes as an *in vitro* assay for purified HSF. Dose response curves of purified HSF with respect to its ability to induce a glycerol-releasing response in rat adipocytes (●), and its histamine-sensitizing activity (○), and leukocytosis-promoting activity (▲), in mice (adipocytes: 1.8×10^5 cells/ml). (From Endoh *et al.* (1980) *Microbiol. Immunol.* **24**: 887–890; reproduced with the permission of the authors and of Microbiology and Immunology.)

4.7. MOLECULAR BASIS OF ACTIVITY

The title of the section should not imply that the molecular basis of pertussigen activity is properly understood, but only that an attempt will be made to summarize present information. As detailed above (Section 4.4.1), pertussigen is a protein of molecular weight around 117,000 and consisting of several subunits, all of which appear to be required for biological activity *in vivo*. It has the capacity to interact with a wide variety of cell types including lymphocytes, neutrophils, macrophages, adipocytes, pancreatic islet B-cells and heart cells. The HSF and HEAE-adjuvant activities probably depend, at least in part, on interaction with capillary endolethelial or other cells associated with blood vessels. Although the nature of the receptor(s) on these diverse cell types has not been defined, it seems likely to be a sialoprotein, from the high affinity of LPF-HA for haptoglobin, ceruloplasmin and fetuin and from the hemagglutination-inhibition activity of *N*-acetyl neuraminic acid (Irons and MacLennan, 1979a; Askelöf *et al.*, 1982).

Having combined with its receptor, which seems to take place very rapidly, at least on islet B-cells (Katada and Ui, 1980a), pertussigen is still neutralizable by antiserum for up to several hours. This is suggested by the results of Lehrer (1979) in respect of HSF activity, and of Katada and Ui (1980a) for interaction of IAP with pancreatic islets. The subsequent resistance to neutralization by antibody implies irreversible insertion of pertussigen into the cell membrane. Thereafter it may take from several hours to several days for its maximum effect to develop. Certainly in the whole animal, the peaks of histamine sensitization, leukocytosis and islet activation are usually between three and seven days after injection. The exact nature of the changes that occur within the various cells during this time is obscure although the end-results are readily detected: i.e. the lymphocyte *in vitro* is stimulated to incorporate ³H-thymidine and to divide; the lymphocyte *in vivo* appears impaired in its capacity to pass through post capillary venules; the adipocyte shows accelerated release of glycerol *in vitro*; the islet B-cell exhibits enhanced release of insulin in response to secretagogues; cells of the vascular endothelium when exposed to histamine permit an exaggerated loss of plasma from the blood stream, resulting in fatal hemoconcentration;

blood vessels supplying the spinal cord of an animal given neuroantigen plus pertussigen become leaky, giving rise to edema and fibrin deposition in proximity to nerve tissue and causing an ascending paralysis.

As noted in Table 7, the pertussis-treated mouse shows many similarities to the adrenalectomized animal, except that the latter has no central store of epinephrine to release, whereas the former shows functional abnormalities of response to epinephrine from either endogenous or exogenous sources. In regard to histamine sensitivity and resistance to epinephrine-mediated hyperglycemia, the pertussis-treated mouse resembles the normal mouse that has been given a β-adrenoceptor blocking drug. This gave rise to the widely quoted hypothesis (Fishel et al., 1962; Szentivanyi et al., 1963) that pertussis vaccine produced β-adrenoceptor blockade. Subsequent work, however, has revealed that the effects are more complex than initially envisaged, and the actual blockade of the β-adrenoceptor by B. pertussis is no longer accepted. Several lines of evidence have contributed to this rejection, most notably:

(1) In relation to insulin secretion in either the whole animal (Sumi and Ui, 1975), the isolated perfused pancreas (Katada and Ui, 1977a) or the isolated islets (Katada and Ui, 1979), pretreatment with IAP, far from producing a functional β-blockade, was shown to enhance β-adrenoceptor responsiveness.

(2) In relation to cAMP-accumulation by human lymphocytes (Parker and Morse, 1973), a process that is promoted by β-agonists, pretreatment with B. pertussis fractions caused the β-agonist to be less effective and therefore gave the superficial appearance of induction of β-blockade. However, the pertussis vaccine pretreatment also caused loss of responsiveness to prostaglandin E, and to methacholine, neither of which act on β-adrenoceptors. Therefore the apparent β-blockading effect of pertussis vaccine could not be at the β-receptor itself but must have been at some other point in the complex processes that regulate the level of cAMP.

(3) The actual numbers of β-adrenoceptors on cell membranes (rat reticulocytes) was measured directly with the specific β-receptor-binding agent, iodohydroxybenzylpindolol (Hewlett et al., 1978) and there was no difference between membranes from normal and pertussis vaccine-treated animals.

(4) Children with whooping cough responded favorably to salbutamol, a β-adrenoceptor agonist, by having fewer paroxysms per 24 hr than a control group (Badr-el-Din et al., 1976a). This result is contrary to what would be expected if pertussigen released during infection were to produce β-blockade. Moreover the dose of salbutamol which gave the ameliorating effect was quite normal, whereas if the children had been β-blockaded, one might have expected that the dose would have to be increased several fold for benefit. Nevertheless the authors of the report seem to regard their observations as supporting the β-blockade hypothesis. Subsequently there were conflicting reports on the value of salbutamol in the treatment of pertussis (Linnemann, 1979).

There is abundant evidence that what we refer to as pertussigen modified the responsiveness of various cells and tissues to adrenergic and other agents, and that the adenylate cyclase system is affected (Parker and Morse, 1973; Ortez et al., 1975; Krzanowski et al., 1976; Ortez, 1977; Lee, 1977; Hewlett et al., 1982).

Detailed investigations of the mode of action of IAP at the molecular level have been made by Ui and Katada (1978) and by Katada and Ui (1979; 1980a,b; 1981a,b) with pancreatic islets in vitro. In islets from IAP-treated rats, marked changes in cAMP turnover and calcium movements across the cell membrane and within the cell were demonstrated. With rat heart cells (Hazeki and Ui, 1981), C_6 glioma cells (Katada et al., 1982) and canine thyroid slices (Katori and Yamashita (1982), a similar enhancement of cAMP accumulation was noted. The toxin (IAP) caused enhancement of β-adrenergic-receptor-mediated stimulation of adenylate cyclase and the attenuation of α-receptor-mediated, and of other types of receptor-mediated inhibition of the enzyme. The authors concluded that these effects were due to some modification of the coupling mechanism whereby membrane receptors are linked to adenylate cyclase.

The latest reports have shown that IAP catalyzes the transfer of the ADP-ribose moiety of NAD to a protein of molecular weight 41,000 in the membrane of C_6 glioma cells and of other cell types (Katada and Ui, 1982a, b; Kurose *et al.*, 1983; Murayama and Ui, 1983; Murayama *et al.*, 1983). This protein is one of the subunits of the guanine nucleotide regulatory protein (N_i) which is responsible for inhibition of adenylate cyclase. IAP-catalyzed modification of this subunit was responsible for the uncoupling of the N_i receptor–adenylate cyclase system and for the enhancement of receptor-mediated and GTP-dependent activation of adenylate cyclase. Thus, although IAP resembles cholera toxin in its ADP-ribosylation of guanine nucleotide-binding proteins, their modes and sites of action are clearly distinguishable. ADP-ribosylation of N_i in islet cell membranes would readily explain the effect of IAP on insulin secretory responses of islets (Ui, pers. comm.).

The work of Tamura *et al.*, (1982) has shown that IAP, like cholera and certain other bacterial toxins, has an A–B subunit structure with an A(enzymically-active) component and a B(cell surface-binding) component (Section 4.4.1). The lag time which precedes any demonstrable effect of the toxin on intact cells (Katada and Ui, 1980a) is the time required for the A component (S-1 polypeptide) to traverse the cell membrane. In broken cell preparations the A subunit was as effective as the native toxin in its ADP-ribosylating activity. In the absence of cellular components, however, the A component, but not IAP, hydrolysed NAD to ADP-ribose and nicotinamide. It has been suggested that the A component is released from the whole toxin and activated by 'processing' enzymes within the cell membrane (Katada *et al.*, 1983).

In addition to its role in enabling the A-protomer to reach its site of action, the B-oligomer of IAP alone has demonstrable biological activities. Tamura *et al.*, (1983) showed that purified B-oligomer stimulated mitosis of lymphocytes and caused enhancement of glucose oxidation in adipocytes, presumably as a result of the cross-linking of binding proteins on the cell surface. The authors suggested that the B-oligomer plays an important role in the lymphocytosis-promoting, hemagglutinating and adjuvant activities of IAP.

The extent to which the ADP-ribosylating activity of the A component and the mitogenic effect of the B component can account for the various *in vivo* and *in vitro* effects of pertussigen should be an exciting field for future investigations. In addition, as suggested by Katada and Ui (1981a, b) and Murayama and Ui (1983) IAP (pertussigen) may prove to be a valuable probe in gaining a better understanding of the mechanism of interaction between membrane receptors and the adenylate cyclase system.

5. ROLE OF THE TOXINS IN *B. PERTUSSIS* INFECTIONS

Although man is the only species subject to natural infection with *B. pertussis*, respiratory-tract infections can be established experimentally in other species, notably the mouse, rabbit (Preston *et al.*, 1980), marmoset (Stanbridge and Preston, 1974) and Taiwan monkey (Huang *et al.*, 1962). However, in none of these species, except the last-mentioned, has it been possible to establish the paroxysmal coughing syndrome that is characteristic of pertussis in the human. The most widely used of the various experimental infections is the intracerebral infection of mice which forms part of the pertussis-vaccine potency test. In man, the causative role of *B. pertussis* in whooping cough was established experimentally by MacDonald and MacDonald (1933) who deliberately infected children with *B. pertussis* and then followed the time-course and clinical signs of the subsequent disease.

In addition to infection experiments in the whole animal, there is a considerably body of work on the infection of vertebrate cell and organ cultures with *B. pertussis*. The embryonated hen's egg has also been used in this context (Gallavan and Goodpasture, 1937). Most of these studies have been concerned with tissue tropism and attachment phenomena, although various cytopathic effects have also been observed (Holt, 1972; Iida and Ajiki, 1974, 1975; Matsuyama, 1977; Muse *et al.*, 1977). Among the most significant of these effects are ciliostasis and expulsion of ciliated epithelial cells from hamster tracheal organ cultures (Collier *et al.*, 1977; Muse *et al.*, 1979; Goldman *et al.*, 1982). At present, however, there is little information which permits discussion of the observed changes in terms of the recognized toxins of *B. pertussis*. Therefore the accounts which follow are restricted to *B. pertussis* infections in mouse and in man because these are the only two species where particular toxins can be implicated in some of the pathophysiological changes.

5.1. INTRACEREBRAL INFECTION OF MICE

The intracerebral route for infecting mice with *B. pertussis* is a required feature of the mouse protection test as used routinely to standardize the immunizing potency of pertussis vaccine. Much effort has been expended in unravelling the mechanism of the test, but the role of the three main toxins of *B. pertussis* is still only partly defined.

Relatively few strains of *B. pertussis*, such as strain No. 18-323, are able to establish in mice a fatal cerebral infection from a small inoculum (Standfast, 1958a). Berenbaum *et al.* (1960) showed that the organisms did not invade the brain substance but appeared to remain localized on the ciliated epithelial cells that form the ependymal lining of the ventricles. Here the bacteria multiplied at a steady rate for several days or until a count of around 10^5 cells per brain was reached. At this point there was a change in permeability of the blood–brain barrier which allowed antibodies (if present) and perhaps cellular defences to gain access to the bacteria. Thereafter, an adequately vaccinated (or passively protected) mouse showed a rapidly declining brain count of viable *B. pertussis* and the animal survived. However, in an unprotected animal, the bacteria continued to multiply unchecked until a count of about 10^8–10^9 per brain was reached, whereupon death ensued (Standfast and Dolby, 1961). The cardinal features of the fatal intracerebral infection are thus the initial lodgment of bacteria on ciliated ependymal cells, the unchecked bacterial multiplication, the failure of normal host defences to intervene after the blood–brain barrier becomes permeable, and eventual death due to the toxic burden of *B. pertussis* cells in the brain.

The role of individual virulence factors in the overall infectious process is difficult to define. Strain 18-323 does not appear to be unusual in its content of the three main toxins or in its rate of growth, at least *in vitro*. Its high intracerebral virulence for mice is so far unexplained although there is a suggestion (Adams and Hopewell, 1970) that ability to evade phagocytosis by local brain macrophages may be important. Strain 18-323 was unusually insusceptible to nicotinic acid modulation (Pusztai and Joó, 1967), a property which may help to maintain the virulent phenotype *in vivo*.

Mice can be protected against otherwise fatal intracerebral infection by previous administration of vaccine made from Phase I *B. pertussis* which has been killed by heating at 56°C or by treatment with formaldehyde or thiomersal. Circumstantial evidence points to pertussigen being the protective antigen in such vaccines, since the HLT is destroyed by the 56°C-treatment, and the LPS can be ruled out because boiled vaccine is essentially nonprotective. More compellingly, highly purified pertussigen after conversion to toxoid, functions as a protective antigen against intracerebral infection (Munoz *et al.*, 1981a,b). Caution should, however, be exercised in assuming that pertussigen is necessarily the *only* component of the bacillus that is capable of protecting mice against intracerebral infection. In particular, the filamentous haemagglutinin (F-HA) has been found to function as a protective antigen by some investigators (Arai and Sato, 1976; Irons and MacLennan, 1979a; Sato *et al.*, 1979). However, Munoz *et al.* (1981b) claimed that this activity was dependent on the F-HA being contaminated with pertussigen.

Previously Nakase and Doi (1979) had found that mixtures of F-HA and LPF, neither of which alone had protective activity, gave significant protection against intracerebral infection. This has been confirmed by Robinson and Irons (1983) who also showed that LPF, in non-protective amounts enhanced the protective activity of different antigenic preparations of *B. pertussis* and other *Bordetella* species. The protective activity of F-HA alone appears to depend on the test conditions (Cowell *et al.*, 1982; Sato *et al.*, 1982).

Although with ordinary vaccines, neither HLT nor LPS seem to function as protective antigens in the IC-MPT, it is likely that they contribute to the death of the unprotected animal. HLT is the main source of toxicity in laboratory cultures of *B. pertussis* and might therefore be presumed also to be the major source of toxicity *in vivo*. Thus, it is possible that mice with high levels of circulating anti-HLT might be afforded some protection against intracerebral challenge, but this awaits experimental demonstration.

5.2. RESPIRATORY INFECTION OF MICE

Two types of experimental respiratory infection—lethal and sublethal—may be established in the mouse by using, respectively, either a large (10^7) or small (10^5) infecting dose of *B. pertussis* strain 18-323 (Dolby *et al.*, 1961). However, the lethal respiratory infection of the mouse fell into disfavor after Standfast's (1958b) demonstration that the protective activity of pertussis vaccines, assayed with this type of challenge, did not correlate with protection of children. Also the protective antigen in this system was stable to boiling, which suggests that it may be LPS-an antigen which is not credited with much importance for protection in man.

In contrast, the *sublethal* respiratory infection of mice with *B. pertussis* has recently attracted new attention as a convenient model for studying some aspects of pertussis in man (Pittman *et al.*, 1980; Sato *et al.*, 1980; 1982). Although the sublethally-infected mice do not cough, they exhibit some of the other features of the human disease, notably its sublethality, the leukocytosis, disturbance of carbohydrate metabolism and histamine sensitization, the time-course of which parallels the onset and duration of the paroxysmal coughing phase of human pertussis (Pittman *et al.*, 1980).

All three of the principal toxins of *B. pertussis* appear to play a role during respiratory infection of the mouse. To the pertussigen may be attributed the leukocytosis, histamine sensitization and alterations in blood levels of glucose and insulin secretagogue responsiveness; to the LPS may be attributed the hypothermia—a known effect of this substance in mice (Prashker and Wardlaw, 1971); and to the HLT may, possibly, be attributed the spleen atrophy (Iida and Okonogi, 1971). Antibodies against both pertussigen and F-HA were capable of protecting mice against respiratory infection (Sato *et al.*, 1981). As antibodies to the purified toxins become available, it should be possible to define more clearly the roles of HLT, LPS and pertussigen in both respiratory and cerebral infections of the mouse.

5.3. PERTUSSIS IN MAN

The general information on whooping cough that now follows is available in more detail in the reviews by Pittman (1970, 1979), Olson (1975), Linnemann (1979), Walker *et al.* (1981) and Jenkinson and Pepper (1982). Here the discussion will be focused on the possible roles of the *B. pertussis* toxins in the various stages of the human disease.

5.3.1. *Incubation and Catarrhal Stages*

Pertussis in the human subject starts with the aerial transmission of the organism from the respiratory tract of an infected individual to that of the new host. There the organism lodges and multiplies between the cilia of the epithelial cells during the incubation phase of the disease which is variably between 6 and 20 days, commonly around 7 days. All ages of man are susceptible to infection with *B. pertussis* but the disease is only life-threatening in the very young infant. Whooping cough is one of the most highly communicable of the common childhood diseases.

The filamentous haemagglutinin (F-HA) of the organism has been suggested as the factor involved in adhesion to the respiratory epithelial cells (Pittman, 1979) and therefore local, secretory antibodies against F-HA may prevent infection of man since, experimentally, anti-F-HA is protective in the mouse (Sato *et al.*, 1982).

The infection then progresses to the second, catarrhal, stage which may give no hint of being little more than an ordinary cold or catarr. Thus, there is likely to be slight fever, rhinorrhea, occasional sneezing and mild cough, edema of the eyelids and congestion and watering of the conjunctiva. It is difficult to attribute these signs to any particular toxin of the organism and probably the response is nonspecific since many other infectious agents produce similar effects.

5.3.2. *Paroxysmal Coughing Stage*

After one to two weeks in the catarrhal stage, the disease enters the paroxysmal coughing stage when, for the first time, the true nature of the illness may be suspected. Indeed the uncontrollable coughing paroxysms are the essence of pertussis and the name itself means 'of a severe cough'. In addition to the characteristic 'whoop' which a majority of infant cases exhibit at some time, the paroxysmal cough in pertussis is notable because of other striking features:

(1) The onset of the paroxysmal coughing stage is usually associated with the rapid disappearance of the live organisms from the patient (which creates obvious problems in diagnosis). However, the pertinent point here is that paroxysmal coughing does not occur throughout the period of the infection (Pittman, 1970) but, once started, may last for several months during most of which time the patient is noninfectious. This lends support to the hypothesis (Pittman, 1979) that pertussis is primarily a bacterial intoxication, analogous to diphtheria and tetanus, i.e. a disease in which localized, and noninvasive proliferation of bacilli provides a source from which toxin is dispersed, causing pathophysiological changes which may be remote from the site of infection and which may persist long after the live bacilli have been eliminated.

(2) Once the paroxysmal coughing stage has been reached, antipertussis serum is of little benefit and there is no accepted antitussive drug. Salbutamol (Peltola and Michelsson, 1982) and prednisolone (Zoumboulakis *et al.*, 1973; Barrie, 1982) have been found beneficial, particularly for severe cases, but possible side effects may limit their routine use.

Antibiotics may hasten the elimination of the bacteria and prevent secondary infection but they do not halt the paroxysmal coughing stage once it has been entered although they may shorten it. These observations support the Pittman hypothesis since they are consonant with toxin–receptor interaction.

(3) Usually in pertussis there is a substantially elevated white cell count in the blood, with the predominant cells being normal mature lymphocytes. The fact that these are mature cells and that the patient does not show signs of lymphoid hyperplasia indicates that the lymphocytosis is not due to the manufacture of new cells but rather to the abnormal retention of preexisting cells within the blood compartment. In short, the pertussis patient bears in this respect, a striking resemblance to the mouse injected with pertussigen and suggests that although in the human disease the bacteria may be noninvasive, pertussigen is released into the circulation. Whether this occurs continuously during the growth of the organisms in the respiratory tract or whether it takes place in a short period around the time of immune elimination of the bacteria is not known.

(4) There may be significant changes in blood chemistry during pertussis. Regan and Tolstoouhov (1936) reported (Table 11) that the average pH and the inorganic phosphate and glucose concentrations in pertussis cases were below the normal range of values, while uric acid was elevated. It would be highly desirable to have independent support for these observations, especially as one recent group of investigators (Badr-el-Din *et al.*, 1976b) found no significant difference in fasting blood glucose levels between ten children with pertussis and ten normal individuals. However, these investigators showed that the hyperglycemic response to epinephrine was strongly attenuated in the children with pertussis (Table 12) compared with controls. Moreover, the difference was still detectable five months after recovery and suggests that the IAP activity was involved.

(5) Children in the paroxysmal coughing stage exhibited increased sensitivity to histamine administered by iontophoresis (Sanyal, 1960).

(6) In patients recovered from pertussis, paroxysmal coughing may recur with succeeding respiratory tract infections (Olson, 1975) for as long as two years after the attack of whooping cough. This supports the idea of a long-lasting alteration of neurological function produced by a diffusible toxin of the organism.

TABLE 11. *Changes in Blood Chemistry in Whooping Cough Patients Reported by Regan and Tolstoouhov (1936)*

Blood component or activity*	Range of values in normal individuals	Data from whooping cough patients	
		No. of determinations	Average value (and range)
pH	7.35–7.45	43	7.27 (6.95–7.45)
Inorganic phosphate	4–5	74	2.5 (0.7–5.5)
Uric acid	2–3	25	3.4 (2.4–6.5)
Glucose	70–120	41	63 (35–80)

*In addition, calcium, CO_2, urea and creatinine were determined but the averages for whooping cough patients were within the normal ranges.

†Except pH which was determined on blood, values are mg/100 ml of plasma. Samples were taken before breakfast.

TABLE 12. *Attenuation of Epinephrine-Induced Hyperglycemia in Children with Pertussis, Compared with Normal Children*

Children	No. of cases	Maximum % rise in blood glucose ($\pm$S.D.) after subcutaneous epinephrine†
Normal	24	67.0 $\pm$ 11.5
Pertussis		
5–7 days*	7	29.4 $\pm$ 6.8
10–14 days*	7	23.1 $\pm$ 16.9
21–30 days*	11	21.9 $\pm$ 9.4
5 months after recovery	6	48.7 $\pm$ 16.9

*Duration of coughing.

†Capillary blood glucose determined after 10 h fasting, then epinephrine injected subcutaneously and blood samples taken for glucose determination at 30, 60, 90 and 120 min after injection. The dose of 1:1000 solution of epinephrine in children weighing <19, 19–30 and >30 kg was 0.1, 0.15 and 0.2 ml respectively.

(From Badr-el-Din *et al.* (1976) *J. Trop. Med. Hyg.* **79**: 213–217; reproduced with the permission of the authors and The London School of Hygiene and Tropical Medicine.)

5.3.3. *Pathophysiology of the Paroxysmal Cough*

Perhaps the central enigma in pertussis is the nature of the pathophysiological changes that underlie the paroxysmal cough. As Olson (1975) pointed out, local irritation due to the local inflammatory disease and locally-acting toxins may provide the primary stimulus to coughing. But this does not explain the special features of the pertussis cough, notably its onset, apparently around the time of rapid bacterial elimination, its refractoriness to antitussives, its persistence long into the postinfection period and its reactivation by unrelated succeeding infections. A major obstacle to experimental investigation is the complete lack of a satisfactory animal model. For although a variety of mammalian species can support a respiratory tract infection with *B. pertussis* and may develop catarrh and a mild cough, none exhibits the characteristic and sustained postinfection paroxysmal coughing syndrome of pertussis in man. Pittman (1970, 1979) considers that the basis of the cough is some kind of enzymatic, hormonal or pharmacological alteration in neurological function, which is slow in recovery, and that 'pertussis toxin' (i.e. pertussigen) is the responsible bacterial component. While subscribing to this view, we also note the unresolved inconsistency pointed out by Olson (1975) that whooping cough, usually in a milder form, may also be caused by *B. parapertussis* and *B. bronchiseptica*, neither of which species contained pertussigen (Ross *et al.*, 1969). There is also the problem that viruses may produce a pertussis-like syndrome (Olson, 1975; Linnemann, 1979).

5.3.4. *Complications*

In Britain and other countries with good standards of health care, the mortality rate from pertussis has declined dramatically in the last hundred years. Whereas in 1871 the mortality rate from whooping cough in England and Wales was 1000 per million children under age 15 years, in 1971 it was 3 per million (Reports, 1981). It seems unlikely that the organism itself has declined in virulence to this extent, since in some of the developing countries today, pertussis may be responsible for about 2 % of the deaths that occur among infants and pre-school children (Mahieu *et al.*, 1978; Cook, 1979). Improved nutrition, housing and access to intensive-care facilities in hospitals together with widespread use of pertussis vaccine and antibiotics all appear to have contributed to the reduced morbidity and mortality in the developed countries.

However, despite its low mortality rate in developed countries, pertussis continues to give concern. Not only is the violent and uncontrollable paroxysmal cough distressing for both parent and child, but in a significant proportion (around 10 %) of cases in a recent epidemic, hospitalization was needed (Miller and Fletcher, 1976). The usual precipitating event was either pneumonia or a cyanotic attack brought about by the severe disturbance to normal breathing. The cerebral anoxia so induced, perhaps augmented by hypoglycemia, may lead to convulsions, brain damage, mental retardation and death. These and other complications that may arise during the paroxysmal stage of pertussis are listed in Table 13.

In summary, there is good evidence for pertussigen being responsible for some of the clinical signs in whooping cough (leukocytosis and metabolic disturbances) but it is a matter of speculation whether it plays a crucial role in the induction of the paroxysmal cough. Figure 12 presents a diagrammatic scheme (based on an original scheme of Olson, 1975) for the possible roles of the toxins and other biologically-active factors of *B. pertussis* in the overall disease process.

TABLE 13. *Complication Which May Arise During the Paroxysmal Coughing Stage of Pertussis*

A. Hemorrhagic events
    epistaxis
    melena
    subconjunctival hemorrhages
    petechiae
    subdural hematoma
    spinal epidural hematoma

B. Secondary to increased intrathoracic and intra abdominal pressure
    umbilical hernia
    inguinal hernia
    rectal prolapse
    pneumothorax
    mediastinal ephysema
    subcutaneous emphysema

C. Respiratory tract
    bronchopneumonia—primary
    bronchopneumonia—secondary
    atelectasis
    otitis media

D. Encephalopathy

(From Olson, 1975, *Medicine* **521**: 427–458; reproduced with the permission of the author and of Williams & Wilkins, Baltimore.)

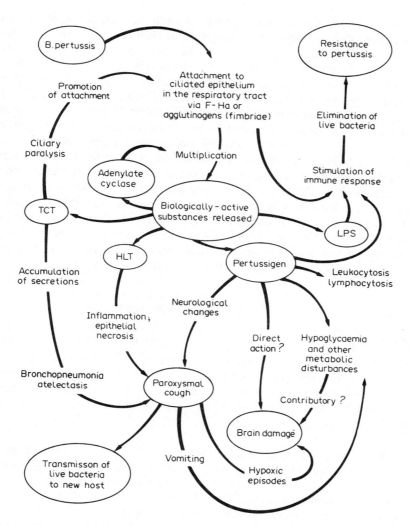

FIG. 12. Scheme showing a network of possible pathophysiological and immunological pathways in human pertussis. TCT is tracheal cytotoxin (section 1.4).

6. ROLE OF THE TOXINS IN THE TOXICITY OF *PERTUSSIS* VACCINE

6.1. NATURE OF PERTUSSIS VACCINE

Despite recent progress in the purification of some of the individual antigens of *B. pertussis*, most of the pertussis vaccines in current use consist of suspensions of whole bacterial cells that have been killed by treatment with formaldehyde or thiomersal or by heating at 56°C, or by a combination of heat, chemicals and storage. The HLT should also be destroyed during these treatments, but the endotoxin and pertussigen are retained. Thus an important corollary to Pittman's (1979) Pertussis Toxin Hypothesis is that immunization against pertussis is currently being done with active toxin as antigen, rather than with toxoid. If the active toxin, as indicated above, produces neurological changes during the disease, it is perhaps not surprizing that pertussis vaccine may on occasion cause neurological changes in the child. Indeed the dose of vaccine used for immunization has to occupy a narrow range bounded as its upper limit by a zone of unacceptable reactivity, and at its lower limit by a zone of inadequate immune stimulation. Much of the recent controversy about the efficacy and safety of pertussis vaccine is due to these opposing requirements. A comprehensive review on pertussis vaccine has been prepared by Wardlaw and Parton (1983).

Although circumstantial evidence points strongly to pertussigen being the major protective antigen for man, the heat-labile agglutinogens on the surface of the organism may also be important (Preston, 1963) although they do not seem to be important in the IC-MPT. While this matter is still unresolved, current formulations of vaccine contain a mixture of representative serotypes of *B. pertussis*, with particular care being taken to include those that are prevalent in the community.

Pertussis vaccine is not a chemically defined product. Not only do different manufacturers use different combinations of strains, media and technical methods, but even from a given laboratory there may be considerable variation in the immunizing potency and toxicity of consecutive batches. Immunizing potency is assayed by the intracerebral mouse protection test, using a standard pertussis vaccine as a reference. For further information, the reader is referred to the World Health Organization report (1979) on the manufacture and testing of pertussis vaccine. Information on fractionation of *B. pertussis* and field trials on partially-purified protective antigens may be found in Pittman (1970) and Manclark and Hill (1979). According to Gonzalez (1982), over one million children in Japan have been immunized with a new partially-purified and detoxified acellular pertussis vaccine containing F-HA and pertussigen; clinical data are not yet available.

6.2. VACCINE TOXICITY IN LABORATORY ANIMALS

6.2.1. *Mouse Weight-Gain Test*

The mouse weight-gain test has been subject to much investigation and some modification since 1949 when it was first prescribed for United States-licenced pertussis vaccines. The work of Pittman (1952) and Pittman and Cox (1965) provided the cornerstones for the universal acceptance and application of this test. Its primary purpose at the time of introduction was to ensure absence of HLT (Pittman, 1970) but it also detects the other toxins.

The test is performed by injecting a weighed group of usually ten 14–16 g mice i.p. with one-half of a single human immunizing dose of pertussis vaccine, and reweighing the animals at 72 hr and 7 days. Normally the animals lose weight within the first 24 hr, but thereafter they should resume normal growth. The pattern of weight change in mice injected with various doses of pertussis vaccine is shown in Fig. 13. For the vaccine under test to be judged satisfactory, the animals should regain their initial group-weight at 72 hr and should show a further average gain in weight of at least 3 g at 7 days.

Unlike the mouse protection test where use of a standard vaccine is mandatory, there is no such standard for the weight-gain test. This is unfortunate because of the many variables that influence the test such as strain of mouse, size of cage, diet, lighting in the animal house and whether the animals are conventionally reared or are germ-free (Pittman, 1967, 1980; Gardner *et al.*, 1969; Cameron, 1976). However, it may be impractical to devise a suitable reference preparation because of the difficulty in deciding how much of each of the *B. pertussis* toxins it should contain. Kurokawa *et al.* (1968) have proposed that each of the three toxins that may be present in vaccine should be assayed separately against reference preparations of the individual purified toxins.

According to Ishida (1968), all three of the *B. pertussis* toxins can be detected, and to some extent differentiated, in the mouse weight-gain test, for each produces a characteristic pattern of either death or change in body weight with time. Unless improperly prepared, the vaccine is unlikely to contain HLT, but the LPS endotoxin and pertussigen will be fully active. The initial 24 hr weight-loss is probably due to LPS, since cholera and typhoid vaccines produced a similar result (Fig. 14), and heating pertussis vaccine at 100°C caused scarcely any loss of the activity (Cameron, 1977). The toxicity of pertussigen may reveal itself in the mouse by late deaths (i.e. after 3 days) and by a failure to resume the preinjection rate of weight-gain (Pittman, 1970).

Several reports (Cohen, 1963, 1968; Muggleton, 1967; Burland *et al.*, 1968; Perkins *et al.*, 1970) suggest that the mouse weight-gain test correlates with reactivity of vaccines in

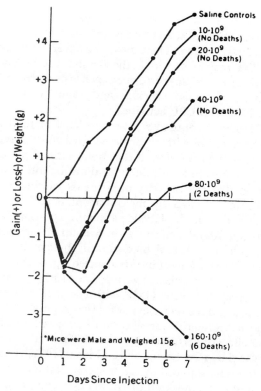

FIG. 13. Effect, on mouse weight and mouse survival, of the i.p. injection of various doses of pertussis vaccine or saline. (From Cameron (1977), In: International Symposium on pyrogenicity, innocuity and toxicity test systems for Biological Products, Budapest 1976; reproduced with the permission of the author and of S. Karger, Basel.)

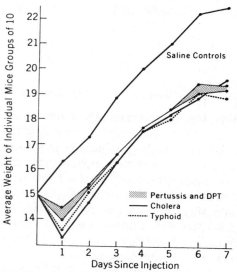

FIG. 14. Pattern of weight loss and gain of mice injected i.p. with cholera, typhoid and pertussis vaccines and with DPT triple vaccine or saline (From Cameron (1976) *Advances in Applied Microbiology* **20**: 57–79; reproduced with the permission of the author and of Academic Press.

children, although there are inherent difficulties in investigating this, notably the ethical barrier to injecting children with a batch of vaccine that has already been found unduly reactive in mice. However, it is generally agreed that the mouse weight-gain tests serves a useful purpose in controlling and minimizing the toxicity of pertussis vaccine, although clearly it has not prevented the rare cases of severe reactions in children.

6.2.2. *Other Tests*

There is no serious competitor of the mouse weight-gain test for controlling the general level of toxicity of pertussis vaccine. There have, however, been proposals to assay the individual toxic factors that may be present in the vaccine, notably endotoxin and HSF and LPF activities. Kurokawa *et al.* (1978b) performed such tests on recently-produced Japanese DPT and DP (diphtheria-pertussis) vaccines and found considerable batch-to-batch variation in endotoxic, HSF and LPF activities.

Manclark *et al.* (1977) have proposed a rat-paw-edema method for assaying pertussis vaccine toxicity but its correlation with other procedures was not reported. Subsequently, however, Munoz *et al.* (1980) have reported that both purified pertussigen and endotoxin cause foot-pad swelling in mice but with different duration and histology.

Amiel (1976) suggested that the capacity of pertussis vaccine to produce neurological complications might be investigated by measurement of changes in cerebral vascular permeability in mice injected with ^{131}I-labelled albumin. He showed that pertussis vaccine indeed had such activity and that the effect was maximum in mice with preexisting cerebral lesion produced by cryo-injury. Actual biochemical changes in brain tissue itself were reported by Askelöf and Bartfai (1979) in rats injected i.p. with pertussis vaccine and by Askelöf and Gillenius (1982) in rats injected with purified LPF. These authors demonstrated a significant elevation in cerebellar cyclic-GMP, with a peak at 2–4 days after injection. Since some convulsive agents also induce such elevations, they suggested that this effect of vaccine may be related to the neurological complications observed in children after pertussis immunization. Another effect of pertussis vaccine and of partially purified HSF on brains of rats, mice and gerbils was shown by Levine and Sowinski (1972). They noted impairment of macrophage response to injury induced by thermal coagulation necrosis and regarded it as analogous to the LPF-induced inhibition of lymphocyte emigration from the blood.

A further rodent model of the brain-damaging potential of pertussis vaccine was proposed by Steinman *et al.* (1982) who showed that a lethal, shock-like syndrome developed in certain strains of mice subjected to a course of injections of vaccine and bovine serum albumin (but not other antigens). Mice of haplotype H-2^d were particularly susceptible. The relationship of this phenomenon to the anaphylactic sensitization (4.6.4) described by Malkiel and Hargis (1952) is unclear.

6.3. VACCINE TOXICITY IN THE HUMAN INFANT

There is an extensive literature on the reactions of the human infant to the injection of pertussis vaccine (Pittman, 1970). However, the reactions have not so far been well correlated with any of the individual toxins produced by *B. pertussis*. Of greatest interest at present are the tragic and unpredictable encephalopathies, and even deaths, which on rare occasions have followed the administration of pertussis vaccine. The very rarity of these severe reactions has made them virtually impossible to investigate experimentally. This issue is also confused by such opposing factors as mistakenly incriminating the vaccine in brain damage from other causes, and underreporting of reactions. The recently published Reports (1981) of the National Childhood Encephalopathy Study in Britain attempt to obtain an objective estimate of the incidence of brain damage that is genuinely attributable to pertussis vaccine and separate it from the background incidence of brain damage from other causes during infancy.

However, before dwelling on the rare, severe reactions, it must be emphasized that the overwhelming majority of children who are given pertussis vaccine show only a mild or moderate reaction, insufficient to cause alarm, or no reaction at all. Indeed if this were not so, pertussis vaccine could scarcely have been used worldwide on such a massive scale over the past 30–40 years. For purposes of discussion, it is convenient to divide pertussis vaccine reactions into mild (i.e. non-alarm causing) and severe, although this should not be taken to imply that there is any natural discontinuity in the spectrum of responses.

6.3.1. *Mild Reactions*

Pertussis vaccine, is common with other injected vaccines, frequently causes both local and systemic reactions, which in the overwhelming majority of recipients are transient and of no persistent concern. Thus, there may be temporary redness, swelling and pain at the site of injection, while the most frequently systemic reactions are fever and irritability. Aspirin is commonly prescribed as a control measure. In a recent study of reactions to DPT vaccine in the United States, only 7% of infants were recorded as exhibiting absolutely no reaction, while 27% and 59% were reported as showing mild and moderate reactions respectively (Barkin and Pichichero, 1979). In another study, Baraff and Cherry (1979) compared DPT vaccine with DT vaccine (i.e. no pertussis) and were able to show that pertussis was the major, but not the sole, contributor of reactogenic material. For example, the incidence of local redness was 51% with DPT and 17% with DT. The role of the individual *B. pertussis* toxins in these 'normal' reactions to pertussis vaccine is not known, but it would seem reasonable to believe that both the LPS and pertussigen may contribute. Thus unless these components can be eliminated or detoxified, pertussis vaccine will probably continue to cause reactions of the type described.

6.3.2. *Severe Reactions*

Ever since Madsen (1933) described the first fatal case of encephalopathy after pertussis vaccine, there have been sporadic reports of this severe, but fortunately rare, occurrence. Still rare, but scarcely less disquieting, are the prolonged shock-like reactions which are not fatal, but which may leave the child with permanent neurological defects, notably mental retardation. Less severe, but still a major cause for concern, are the occasional convulsive episodes, shock syndromes, and prolonged screaming attacks which may follow within 24 hr of the administration of pertussis vaccine. For access to representative literature describing these more or less severe reactions, see Wilson (1967), Hannik (1970), Dick (1974), Kulenkampff *et al.* (1974), Baraff and Cherry (1979), Stewart (1979), Hennessen and Quast (1979), Miller *et al.* (1981; 1982) and Reports (1981).

Recent discussions of this emotive subject have focussed on two particular aspects. Firstly, are all or most of the neurological disturbances truly to be attributed to pertussis vaccine, or in some cases has another disorder coincidently manifested itself shortly after vaccine administration? Secondly, even admitting a certain incidence of wrong attribution, is the continued widespread use of pertussis vaccine still justified as a preventive against the disease, i.e. is the benefit-to-risk ratio still favorable? Although highly important, these questions fall outside the scope of the present review and the reader is referred to other sources for discussion, e.g. Griffith (1979), Koplan *et al.* (1979), Mortimer and Jones (1979), Stewart (1979), Stuart-Harris (1979), Grob *et al.* (1981) and Miller *et al.* (1982). However the following extract from the conclusions of The National Childhood Encephalopathy Study is pertinent (Reports, 1981, p. 149).

(a) Most cases of acute and potentially damaging neurological illness in early childhood are attributable to causes other than immunization.
(b) Such illnesses occur more frequently within 7 days, and particularly within 72 hr, after DPT vaccine and within 7–14 days after measles vaccine than would be expected by chance. Most affected children make a complete recovery.
(c) Taking account of possible alternative explanations of the clinical findings in cases associated with DPT, and of the fact that similar cases occur after DT vaccine, it seems likely that permanent damage as a result of pertussis immunization is a very rare event, and attribution of a cause in individual cases is precarious.

In this report, the estimated rarity of neurological illness attributable to DPT vaccine was 1 in 110,000 immunizations, while 1 in 330,000 showed evidence of permanent neurological damage.

Unfortunately it has not so far been possible to attribute the severe reactions to any of the identified toxins of *B. pertussis*. The very fact that a particular batch of vaccine can be injected into thousands, or tens of thousands, of children without serious result makes it very difficult to explain the tragic response of the individual child who develops a severe reaction leading to permanent brain damage. On the other it must be recognized that if vaccines, such as the several lots of DPT studied by Barkin and Pichichero (1979), produce what looks like an approximately log–normal distribution of responses in a population of children, and with a peak reaction-score in the 'moderate' range (Fig. 15), then it would be expected from the shape of the distribution that a few unfortunate individuals might well register severe or even fatal reactions if the population exposed to risk is sufficiently large. There were in fact no encephalitis cases, seizures or hospitalizations in the 1232 patients in this survey—but perhaps there might have been if the number of children had been 100 or 1000 times larger.

The possibility that *B. pertussis* may possess a neurotoxin, distinct from the three main toxins has been proposed Kuwajima (1978) but awaits confirmation. Indeed it is difficult to explain the rarity of the neurological disturbances in children if vaccine contains neurotoxin. Moreover the association of encephalopathy with convulsions and a shock-like syndrome is more in keeping with the known properties of pertussigen and endotoxin. In addition, Hannik and Cohen (1979) showed that plasma insulin concentrations in children were elevated transiently after administration of the normal dose of pertussis-containing quadruple vaccine. They suggested that the serious reactions shown by some children may be due to inadequate maintenance of glucose homeostasis. In support of this are two early reports (Globus and Kohn, 1949; Anderson and Morris, 1950) that low-blood glucose in one case and extremely low CSF-glucose in another were found in children who developed convulsions 18 and 36 hr respectively after receiving pertussis vaccine.

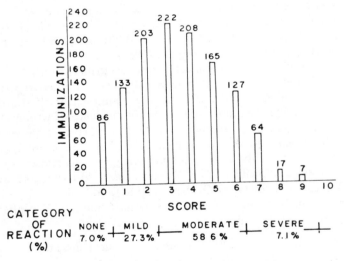

FIG. 15. Distribution of reaction scores to DPT vaccine in children.

Scoring system: Category	Reaction	Points
Systemic febrile response	<100°F	0
	100–102°F	1
	>102°F	3
Acute behavior change	Normal	0
	Irritable	1
	Crying	2
	Screaming	3
Significant local reaction (additive points)	Red	1
	Swollen	1
	Tender	1

(From Barkin and Pichichero (1979) *Pediatrics* **63**: 256–260; reproduced with the permission of the authors; copyright American Academy of Pediatrics, 1979.)

7. *B. PERTUSSIS* TOXINS: HIGHLIGHTS AND PERSPECTIVES

It seems appropriate to end this review with a brief survey of the highlights and desirable growth points in *B. pertussis* toxinology. First, HLT is a neglected toxin—unjustly so, in view of its overwhelming contribution to the toxicity of laboratory-grown *B. pertussis*. Yet there is still no good evidence for HLT having a pathogenic role in whooping cough. Nor do we know whether an antigenically potent HLT-toxoid might function as a protective vaccine. The fact that pertussis convalescent sera lack anti-HLT may be similar to what is said to occur in tetanus where the dose of toxin delivered in a sublethal infection is supposed to be insufficient to stimulate circulating antitoxin. Aside from these clinical considerations are such fundamental and totally unanswered questions as the structure of the HLT molecule, its biochemical mode of action on susceptible cells and the possible analogies with other bacterial toxins. Then there is the intriguing evolutionary implication that HLT from the two other species of *Bordetella* may be identical with, or very similar to, that of *B. pertussis*. Indeed from basic evolutionary theory it would seem to follow automatically that HLT must be essential to the lifestyle of these obligate respiratory tract pathogens or it would not have been so consistently conserved. These and other areas will continue unilluminated so long as HLT research remains in its present state of limbo.

Knowledge of *B. pertussis* LPS, on the other hand, will inevitably benefit from studies on LPS from the more commonly investigated bacterial species. It may be noted, as an aside, that despite immense effort, the biochemical basis of endotoxin action is still unknown. Present information indicates that although *B. pertussis* LPS has many typical endotoxin features there are some novelties of structure—particularly Lipid X—that are worthy of detailed study. Also the serology of the LPS and the nature of its epitopes should be much better defined. Perhaps the most intriguing aspect of *B. pertussis* is the support it provides for the generalization that although lipopolysaccharides are universally present in Gram-negative bacteria and are potent antigens, there are few if any infectious diseases for which LPS makes a useful vaccine or where anti-LPS is protective. One of us has suggested that a general function of LPS in pathogenic Gram-negative bacteria is to act as a 'diversionary antigen', protecting vulnerable target sites on the bacterial cell surface from immune attack and perhaps preempting the possibility of cell-mediated immunity (Wardlaw, 1972).

Undoubtedly the most difficult topic in this review is the third toxin to be discussed, 'pertussigen' or 'pertussis toxin', which until recently has presented problems of un-coordinated research, uncertain composition, diverse activities and confusing nomenclature. An important consequence of Pittman's Pertussis Toxin hypothesis is the unpalatable admission that present-day pertussis vaccines contain an untoxoided toxin as the immu-nogen – a situation which surely would not be tolerated with other infectious diseases where antitoxic immunity is regarded as important. It is therefore encouraging to note the recent success in producing a pertussigen toxoid by treatment with glutaraldehyde (Munoz *et al*, 1981a, b). However, other evidence indicates that protection against whooping cough may not be a simple matter of stimulating the production of circulating antibodies to pertussis toxin. Thus the studies of Robinson and Irons (1983) show that, at least in the mouse intracerebral protection test, pertussigen is not the protective antigen *per se* but functions as a kind of adjuvant towards certain surface components of the bacterium which themselves constitute the immunogen. To go from the mouse intracerebral test to whooping cough in man is a considerable extrapolation. If pertussis toxin indeed causes whooping cough, then should one expect the child to cough, or develop a sensitivity to cough-inducing stimuli, after the first injection of vaccine? Perhaps this is an unreasonable test of the Pittman hypothesis since the vaccine is not delivered by aerosol to the respiratory tract. Nevertheless the problem remains that we do not know whether, or in what way, pertussigen contributes to the paroxysmal coughing syndrome. Likewise its role in induction of whooping cough immunity, whether as primary antigen or as adjuvant, is equally obscure. In a recent article we suggested that immunization and challenge experiments with purified antigens and live *B. pertussis* in adult human volunteers might provide direct answers (Wardlaw and Parton, 1983).

When purified pertussigen becomes more freely available there should also be a useful impact in several biomedical areas unrelated to whooping cough. These include insulin secretion and diabetes, adrenoceptor function, lymphocyte traffic and mitosis, regulation of the immune response, particularly in IgE production and tumor immunology. Research on both pertussigen and HLT should benefit from the reawakening interest in the genetics of *B. pertussis* and from the developments in protein purification methods, particularly for membrane-associated proteins. The continuing demand for a better pertussis vaccine will be a useful stimulus to research on the toxins and other components of *B. pertussis*.

REFERENCES

ADAMS, G. J. and HOPEWELL, J. W. (1970) Enhancement of intracerebral infection of mice with *Bordetella pertussis*. *J. Med. Microbiol.* **3**: 15–27.

ADLAM, C. (1973) Studies on the histamine sensitisation produced in mice by *Corynebacterium parvum*. *J. Med. Microbiol.* **6**: 527–538.

AMIEL, S. A. (1976) The effects of *Bordetella pertussis* vaccine on cerebral vascular permeability. *Br. J. Exp. Path.* **57**: 653–662.

ANDERSON, I. M. and MORRIS, D. (1950) Encephalopathy after combined diphtheria-pertussis inoculation. *Lancet* **1**: 537–539.

ANGELA, G. C., ROSSO, C. and GIULIANI, G. (1962) Effetto della tossina pertossica sulle cellule coltivate in vitro. *Minerva. Med., Roma* **53**: 778–784.

APRILE, M. A. (1972) A reexamination of phase IV *Bordetella pertussis*. *Can. J. Microbiol.* **18**: 1793–1801.

APRILE, M. A. and WARDLAW, A. C. (1973) Immunochemical studies on the lipopolysaccharides of *Bordetella pertussis*. *Can. J. Microbiol.* **19**: 231–239.

ARAI, H. and MUNOZ, J. J. (1981) Crystallization of pertussigen from *Bordetella pertussis*. *Infect. Immun.* **31**: 495–499.

ARAI, H. and SATO, Y. (1976) Separation and characterization of two distinct hemagglutinins contained in purified leukocytosis-promoting factor from *Bordetella pertussis*. *Biochim. Biophys. acta* **444**: 765–782.

ASAKAWA, S. (1969) Effects of the lymphocytosis-promoting factor of *Bordetella pertussis* on antibody production in mice. *Jap. J. Med. Sci. Biol.* **22**: 23–42.

ASHWORTH, L. A. E., IRONS, L. I. and DOWSETT, A. B. (1982) Antigenic relationship between serotype-specific agglutinogen and fimbriae of *Bordetella pertussis*. *Infect. Immun.* **37**: 1278–1281.

ASKELÖF, P. and BARTFAI, T. (1979) Effect of whooping-cough vaccine on cyclic-GMP levels in the brain. *FEMS Microbiol. Lett.* **6**: 223–225.

ASKELÖF, P. and GILLENIUS, P. (1982) Effect of lymphocytosis-promoting factor from *Bordetella pertussis* on cerebellar cyclic GMP levels. *Infect. Immun.* **36**: 958–961.

ASKELÖF, P., GRANSTRÖM, M., GILLENIUS, P. and LINDBERG, A. A. (1982) Purification and characterisation of a fimbrial haemagglutinin from *Bordetella pertussis* for use in an enzyme-linked immunosorbent assay. *J. Med. Microbiol.* **15**: 73–83.

ATHANASSIADES, T. J. (1977) Adjuvant effect of *Bordetella pertussis* vaccine to sheep erythrocytes in mice: Enhancement of cell-mediated immunity by subcutaneous administration of adjuvant and antigen. *Infect. Immun.* **18**: 416–423.

AYME, G., CAROFF, M., CHABY, R., HAEFFNER-CAVAILLON, N., LE DUR, A., MOREAU, M., MUSET, M., MYNARD, M. C., ROUMIANTZEFF, M., SCHULZ, D. and SZABÓ, L. (1980) Biological activities of fragments derived from *Bordetella* pertussis endotoxin: isolation of a nontoxic. Shwartzman-negative Lipid A possessing high adjuvant properties. *Infect. Immun.* **27**: 739–745.

BADR-EL-DIN, M. K., AREF, G. H., KASSEM, A. S., ABDEL-MONEIM, M. A. and AMR ABBASSY, A. (1976a) A beta-adrenergic stimulant, salbutamol, in the treatment of pertussis. *J. Trop. Med. Hyg.* **79**: 218–219.

BADR-EL-DIN, M. K., AREF, G. H., MAZLOUM, H., EL-TOWESY, Y. A., KASSEM, A. S., ABDEL-MONEIM, M. A. and AMR ABBASSY, A. (1967b) The beta-adrenergic receptors in pertussis. *J. Trop. Med. Hyg.* **79**: 213–217.

BARAFF, L. J. and CHERRY, J. D. (1979) Reactogenicity of DTP and DT vaccines. *Pediat. Res.* **13**: 458.

BARKIN, R. M. and PICHICHERO, M. E. (1979) Diphtheria-pertussis-tetanus vaccine: Reactogenicity of commercial products. *Pediatrics* **63**: 256–260.

BARRIE, H. (1982) Treatment of whooping cough. *Lancet.* **2**: 830–831.

BENJAMIN, W. R., KLEIN, T. W., PROSS, S. H. and FRIEDMAN, H. (1980) Inhibition of mononuclear phagocyte elongation, migration, and cellular exudate formation following *Bordetella pertussis* vaccine administration. *Proc. Soc. Exp. Biol. Med.* **166**: 249–256.

BERENBAUM, M. C., UNGAR, J. and STEVENS, W. K. (1960) Intracranial infection of mice with *Bordetella pertussis*. *J. Gen. Microbiol.* **22**: 313–322.

BERGMAN, R. K. and MUNOZ, J. J. (1968) Efficacy of β-adrenergic blocking agents in inducing histamine sensitivity in mice. *Nature, Lond.* **217**: 1173–1174.

BERGMAN, R. K. and MUNOZ, J. J. (1969) Hypoproteinemia in mice after treatment with histamine-sensitizing factor from *Bordetella pertussis*. *Proc. Soc. Exp. Biol. Med.* **131**: 964–969.

BERGMAN, R. K. and MUNOZ, J. J. (1975) Effect of *Bordetella pertussis* extract and vasoactive amines on vascular permeability. *J. Allergy Clin. Immunol.* **55**: 378–385.

BERGMAN, R. K. and MUNOZ, J. J. (1977) Increased histamine sensitivity in mice after administration of endotoxins. *Infect. Immun.* **15**: 72–77.

BERGMAN, R. K., MUNOZ, J. J. and PORTIS, J. L. (1978) Vascular permeability changes in the central nervous system of rats with hyperacute experimental allergic encephalomyelitis induced with the aid of a substance from *Bordetella pertussis*. *Infect. Immun.* **21**: 627–637.

BORDET, J. and GENGOU, O. (1909) L'endotoxine coquelucheuse. *Annls. Inst. Pasteur, Paris* **23**: 415–419.

BURLAND, W. L., SUTCLIFFE, W. M., VOYCE, M. A., HILTON, M. L. and MUGGLETON, P. W. (1968) Reactions to combined diphtheria, tetanus and pertussis vaccine: A comparison between plain vaccine and vaccine adsorbed on aluminium hydroxide. *Med. Offr.* **119**: 17–19.

CAMERON, J. (1967) Variation in *Bordetella pertussis. J. Path. Bact.* **94**: 367–374.

CAMERON, J. (1976) Problems associated with the control testing of pertussis vaccine. *Adv. Appl. Microbiol.* **20**: 57–80.

CAMERON, J. (1977) Pertussis vaccine: mouse-weight-gain (toxicity) test In: *International Symposium on pyrogenecity, innocuity and toxicity test systems for biological products, Budapest, 1976. Dev. Biol. Stand.* **34**: 213–215, S. Karger, Basel.

CHABY, R., MOREAU, M. and SZABÓ, L. (1977) 2-*O*-(β-D-Glucuronyl)-7-*O*-(2-amino-2-Deoxy-α-D-glucopyrano-syl)-L-*glycero*-D-manno-heptose: a constituent of *Bordetella pertussis* endotoxin. *Eur. J. Biochem.* **76**: 453–460.

COHEN, H. H. (1963) Development of pertussis vaccine production and control in the National Institute of Public Health in the Netherlands during the years 1950–1962. *Antonie van Leeuwenhoek* **29**: 183–201.

COHEN, H. H. (1968) Pertussis vaccine research in the Rijks Instituut voor de Volksgezondheid (The Netherlands). *Archs roum. Path. Exp. Microbiol.* **27**: 33–50.

COLLIER, A. M., PETERSON, L. P. and BASEMAN, J. B. (1977) Pathogenesis of infection with *Bordetella pertussis* in hamster tracheal organ culture. *J. Infect. Dis.* **136**: S196–S203.

CONFER, D. L. and EATON, J. W. (1982) Phagocyte impotence caused by an invasive bacterial adenylate cyclase. *Science* **217**: 948–950.

COOK, R. (1979) Pertussis in developing countries: possibilities and problems of control through immunization. In *International Symposium on Pertussis,* 1978, pp. 283–290, MANCLARK, C. R. and HILL, J. C. (eds.) U.S. DHEW Publication no. (NIH) 79–1830, Washington, D. C.

COWELL, J. L., HEWLETT, E. L. and MANCLARK, C. R. (1979) Intracellular localization of the dermonecrotic toxin of *Bordetella pertussis. Infect. Immun.* **25**: 896–901.

COWELL, J. L., SATO, Y., SATO, H., AN DER LAN, B. and MANCLARK, C. R. (1982) Separation, purification, and properties of the filamentous haemagglutinin and the leukocytosis promoting factor—haemagglutinin from *Bordetella pertussis. In: Seminars in Infectious Disease* Vol. IV: *Bacterial Vaccines,* pp. 371–379, ROBBINS J. B., HILL, J. C. and SADOFF, J. C. (eds.). Thieme- Stratton Inc. New York.

CRAVITZ, L. and WILLIAMS, J. W. (1946) Comparative study of "immune response" to various pertussis antigens and the disease. *J. Pediat.* **28**: 172–186.

DHAR, H. L., DHIRWANI, M. K. and SHETH, U. K. (1975) Pertussis vaccine in diabetics requiring high dosage insulin. *Br. J. Clin. Pract.* **29**: 119–120.

DICK, G. (1974) Convulsive disorders in young children. *Proc. R. Soc. Med.* **67**: 371–372.

DOLBY, J. M. (1958) The separation of the histamine-sensitizing factor from the protective antigens of *Bordetella pertussis. Immunology,* **1**: 328–337.

DOLBY, J. M., THOW, D. C. W. and STANDFAST, A. F. B. (1961) The intranasal infection of mice with *Bordetella pertussis. J. Hyg. Camb.* **59**: 191–204.

ENDOH, M. and NAKASE, Y. (1982) Glycerol-releasing activity of histamine-sensitizing factor of *Bordetella pertussis* for rat adipocytes *in vitro. Microbiol. Immunol.* **26**: 689–703.

ENDOH, M., SOGA, M. and NAKASE, Y. (1980) *In vitro* assay for histamine-sensitizing factor of *Bordetella pertussis. Microbiol. Immunol.* **24**: 887–890.

EVANS, D. G. (1940) The production of pertussis antitoxin in rabbits and the neutralization of *pertussis. parapertussis* and *bronchiseptica* toxins. *J. Path. Bact.* **51**: 49–58.

EVANS, D. G. and MAITLAND, H. B. (1939) The failure of whooping cough sera to neutralise pertussis toxin. *J. Path. Bact.* **48**: 465–467.

FARTHING, J. H. (1961) The role of *Bordetella pertussis* as an adjuvant to antibody production. *Br. J. Exp. Path.* **42**: 614–622.

FELTON, H. M., GAGGERO, A. and POMERAT, C. M. (1954) Reaction of cells in tissue culture to *Hemophilus pertussis* I. Effect of whole organisms or brain tissue and results of treatment with specific and normal serum. *Tex. Rep. Biol. Med.* **12**: 960–971.

FINGER, H. (1975) *Bordetella pertussis* as adjuvant. In: *The Immune System and Infectious Diseases,* pp. 132–166, NETER, E. and MILGROM, F. (eds.). 4th Int. Convac. Immunol. Buffalo, N. Y. 1974. Karger, Basel.

FINGER, H., HEYMER, B., HOF, H., RIETSCHEL, E. and SCHLEIFER, K. H. (1976) Über struktur und biologische Aktivität von Bordetella pertussis-Endotoxin. *Zentbl. Bakt. Hyg., I. Abt. Orig. A.* **235**: 56–64.

FISHEL, C. W., SZENTIVANYI, A. and TALMAGE, D. W. (1962) Sensitization and desensitization of mice to histamine and serotonin by neurohumours. *J. Immun.* **89**: 8–18.

FRÖLICH, J. (1897) Beitrag zur Pathologie des Keuchustens. *J. Kinderkrankh.* **44**: 53–58.

FURMAN, B. L., WARDLAW, A. C. and STEVENSON, L. Q. (1981) *Bordetella pertussis*-induced hyperinsulinaemia without marked hypoglycaemia: A paradox explained. *Br. J. Exp. Path.* **62**: 504–511.

GALLAVAN, M. and GOODPASTURE, E. W. (1937) Infection of chick embryos with *H. pertussis* reproducing pulmonary lesions of whooping cough. *Am. J. Path.* **13**: 927–938.

GARDNER, R., BOHNER, H. and PITTMAN, M. (1969) Reactivity of germ-free and conventional mice to pertussis vaccine. *Prog. Immunobiol. Stand.* **3**: 315–318.

GIRARD, R., CHABY, R. and BORDENAVE, G. (1981) Mitogenic responses of C3H/HeJ mouse lymphocytes to polyanionic polysaccharides obtained from *Bordetella pertussis* endotoxin and from other bacterial species. *Infect. Immun.* **31**: 122–128.

GLOBUS, J. H. and KOHN, J. L. (1949) Encephalopathy following pertussis vaccine prophylaxis. *J. Am. Med. Ass.* **141**: 507–509.

GOLDMAN, W. E., KLAPPER, D. G. and BASEMAN, J. B. (1982) Detection, isolation, and analysis of a released *Bordetella pertussis* product toxic to cultured tracheal cells. *Infect. Immun.* **36**: 782–794.

GONZALEZ, E. R. (1982) Newer pertussis vaccines on horizon. *J. Am. Med. Ass.* **248**: 22–23.

Goodnow, R. A. (1980) Biology of *Bordetella bronchiseptica. Microbiol. Rev.* **44:** 722–738.

Griffith, A. H. (1979) The case for immunization. *Scott. Med. J.* **24:** 42–46.

Grob, P. R., Crowder, M. J. and Robbins, J. F. (1981) Effect of vaccination on severity and dissemination of whooping cough. *Br. Med. J.* **282:** 1925–1928.

Gulbenkian, A., Schobert, L., Nixon, C. and Tabachnick, I. I. A. (1968) Metabolic effects of pertussis sensitization in mice and rats. *Endocrinology* **83:** 885–892.

Haeffner, N., Chaby, R. and Szabó, L. (1977) Identification of 2-methly-3-hydroxydecanoic and 2-methly-3-hydroxytetradecanoic acids in the 'Lipid X' fraction of the *Bordetella pertussis* endotoxin. *Eur. J. Biochem.* **77:** 535–544.

Hannik, C. A. (1970) Major reactions after DPT-polio vaccination in the Netherlands. In: *International Symposium on Pertussis,* pp. 161–170, van Hemert, P. A., van Ramshorst, J. D. and Regamey, R. H. (eds). (Symposia Series in Immunobiological Standardization Vol. 13). Karger, Basel.

Hannik, C. A. and Cohen, H. (1979) Changes in plasma insulin concentration and temperature of infants after pertussis vaccination. In: *International Symposium on Pertussis, 1978,* pp. 297–299 Manclark, C. R. and Hill, J. C. (eds). U.S. DHEW Publication no. (NIH) 79–1830, Washington D.C.

Hazeki, O. and Ui, M. (1981) Modification by islet-activating protein of receptor-mediated regulation of cyclic AMP accumulation in isolated rat heart cells. *J. Biol. Chem.* **256:** 2856–2862.

Hennessen, W. and Quast, U. (1979) Adverse reactions after pertussis vaccination. In: *International Symposium on Immunization: Benefit versus Risk Factors,* Brussels, 1978. *Dev. Biol. Stand.* **43:** 95–100 (S. Karger. Basel).

Hewlett, E. L., Myers, G. A., Sauer, K. T., Long, S. A. and Guerrant, R. L. (1982) Alteration of chinese hamster ovary (CHO) cell growth and cyclic AMP metabolism by pertussis toxin (PT). *Clin. Res.* **30:** 368A.

Hewlett, E., Spiegel, A., Wolff, J., Aurbach, G. and Manclark, C. R. (1978) *Bordetella pertussis* does not induce β-adrenergic blockade, *Infect. Immun.* **22:** 430–434.

Hewlett, E. and Wolff, J. (1976) Soluble adenylate cyclase from the culture medium of *Bordetella pertussis:* purification and characterization. *J. Bact.* **127:** 890–898.

Hirano, M., Sinkovics, J. G., Shullenberger, C. C. and Hower, C. D. (1967) Murine lymphoma: Augmented growth in mice with pertussis vaccine-induced lymphocytosis. *Science* **158:** 1061–1064.

Hirashima, M., Yodoi, J. and Ishizaka, K. (1981) Formation of IgE-binding factors by rat T lymphocytes II. Mechanisms of selective formation of IgE-potentiating factors by treatment with *Bordetella pertussis* vaccine. *J. Immun.* **127:** 1804–1810.

Ho, M. K., Kong, A. S. and Morse, S. I. (1979) The *in vitro* effects of *Bordetella pertussis* lymphocytosis-promoting factor on murine lymphocytes III. B-cell dependence for T-cell proliferation. *J. Exp. Med.* **149:** 1001–1017.

Ho, M. K., Morse, S. I. and Kong, A. S. (1981) Studies on a new lymphocyte mitogen from *Bordetella pertussis* I. Induction of proliferation and polyclonal antibody formation. *J. Exp. Med.* **153:** 75–88.

Holt, L. B. (1972) The pathology and immunology of *Bordetella pertussis* infection. *J. Med. Microbiol.* **5:** 407–424.

Huang, C. C., Chen, P. M., Kuo, J. K., Chiu, W. H., Lin, S. T., Lin, H. S. and Lin, Y. C. (1962) Experimental whooping cough. *N. Eng. J. Med.* **266:** 105–111.

Idigbe, E. O., Parton, R. and Wardlaw, A. C. (1981) Rapidity of antigenic modulation of *Bordetella pertussis* in modified Hornibrook medium. *J. Med. Microbiol.,* **14:** 409–418.

Iida, T. and Ajiki, Y. (1974) Growth characteristics of *Bordetella pertussis* in the chick tracheal organ culture. *Jap. J. Microbiol.* **18:** 119–126.

Iida, T. and Ajiki, Y. (1975) The effect of 2,4-dinitrophenol on the growth of *Bordetella pertussis* in chick tracheal organ culture. *Jap. J. Microbiol.* **9:** 381–386.

Iida, T. and Okonogi, T. (1971) Lienotoxicity of *Bordetella pertussis* in mice. *J. Med. Microbiol.* **4:** 51–61.

Imagawa, T., Kanoh, M., Sonoda, S. and Utsumi, S. (1980) Polymorphonuclear leukocyte-inhibitory factor of *Bordetella pertussis* III Inhibition of Arthus reaction and peritoneal infiltration of PMN. *Microbiol. Immunol.* **24:** 895–905.

Irons, L. I. and MacLennan, A. P. (1979a) Substrate specificity and the purification by affinity combination methods of the two *Bordetella pertussis* hemagglutinins. In: *International Symposium on Pertussis, 1978,* pp. 338–349, Manclark, C. R. and Hill, J. C. (eds). US DHEW Publication no. (NIH) 79–1830, Washington, D.C.

Irons, L. I. and MacLennan, A. P. (1979b) Isolation of the lymphocytosis promoting factor–haemagglutinin of *Bordetella pertussis* by affinity chromatography. *Biochim. Biophys. Acta* **580:** 175–185.

Ishida, S. (1968) Characterization of the body weight-decreasing toxicities in mice by the lymphocytosis-promoting factor and the heat-labile toxin of *B. pertussis* and endotoxin. *Jap. J. Med. Sci. Biol.* **21:** 115–135.

Ishida, S., Iwasa, S., Asakawa, S. and Kurokawa, M. (1978) Body temperature reduction of pertussis vaccine-sensitized mice following histamine challenge and a new sensitive assay method for HSF. *Jap. J. Med. Sci. Biol.* **31:** 172–174.

Ishida, S., Kurokawa, M., Asakawa, S., Iwsasa, S., Sato, Y., Arai, H. and Kondo, S. (1979) Multicorrelation analyses of toxic and antigenic components of DPT and DP vaccines produced in Japan. *Jap. J. Med. Sci. Biol.* **32:** 295–304.

Jakus, C. M., McClure, L. and Wardlaw, A. C. (1968) The stability of the protective antigen and histamine-sensitizing factor of *Bordetella pertussis* to acid and alkali. *Can. J. Microbiol.* **14:** 147–151.

Jenkison, D. and Pepper, J. D. (1982) Whooping cough. *Practitioner* **226:** 1479–1487.

Kasai, N. (1966) Chemical studies on the lipid component of endotoxin with special emphasis on its relation to biological activities. *Ann. N.Y. Acad. Sci.* **133:** 486–507.

Kasuga, T., Nakase, Y., Ukishima, K. and Takatsu, K. (1953) Studies on *Haemophilus pertusis* Part I. Antigen structure of *H. pertussis* and its phases. *Kitasato Arch. Exp. Med.* **26:** 121–134.

Kasuga, T., Nakase, Y., Ukishima, K. and Takatsu, K. (1954) Studies on *Haemophilus pertussis* Part III. Some properties of each phase of *H. pertussis. Kitasato Arch. Exp. Med.* **27:** 37–48.

Katada, T., Amano, T. and Ui, M. (1982) Modulation by islet-activating protein of adenylate cyclase activity in C6 glioma cells. *J. Biol. Chem.* **257:** 3739–3746.

Katada, T., Tamura, M. and Ui, M. (1983) The A protomer of islet-activating protein, pertussis toxin, as an active peptide catalyzing ADP-ribosylation of a membrane protein. *Archs. Biochem. Biophys.* **224:** 290–299.

KATADA, T. and UI, M. (1977a) Perfusion of the pancreas isolated from pertussis-sensitized rats: potentiation of insulin secretory responses due to β-adrenergic stimulation. *Endocrinology* **101**: 1247–1255.

KATADA, T. and UI, M. (1977b) Spontaneous recovery from streptozotocin-induced diabetes in rats pretreated with pertussis vaccine or hydrocortisone. *Diabetologia* **13**: 521–525.

KATADA, T. and UI, M. (1979) Islet-activating protein. Enhanced insulin secretion and cyclic AMP accumulation in pancreatic islets due to activation of native calcium ionophores. *J. Biol. Chem.* **254**: 469–479.

KATADA, T. and UI, M. (1980a) Slow interaction of islet-activating protein with pancreatic islets during primary culture to cause reversal of α-adrenergic inhibition of insulin secretion. *J. Biol. Chem.* **255**: 9580–9588.

KATADA, T. and UI, M. (1980b) Potentiation of insulin secretion by islet-activating protein (IAP) in intraportal-islet-transplanted rats. *Biomed. Res.* **1**: 495–501.

KATADA, T. and UI, M. (1981a) Islet-activating protein; a modifier of receptor-mediated regulation of rat islet adenylate cyclase. *J. Biol. Chem.* **256**: 8310–8317.

KATADA, T. and UI, M. (1981b) *In vitro* effects of islet-activating protein on cultured rat pancreatic islets. Enhancement of insulin secretion, adenosine 3′:5′-monophosphate accumulation and ^{45}Ca flux. *J. Biochem.* **89**: 979–990.

KATADA, T. and UI, M. (1982a) ADP ribosylation of the specific membrane protein of C6 cells by islet-activating protein associated with modification of adenylate cyclase activity. *J. Biol. Chem.* **257**: 7210–7216.

KATADA, T. and UI, M. (1982b) Direct modification of the membrane adenylate cyclase system by islet-activating protein due to ADP-ribosylation of a membrane protein. *Proc. Natn. Acad. Sci. U.S.A.* **79**: 3129–3133.

KATORI, A. and YAMASHITA, K. (1982) Stimulatory effect of pertussis toxin on tissue cyclic AMP levels in canine thyroid slices. *Endocrinol. Japan.* **29**: 261–263.

KATSAMPES, C. P., BROOKS, A. M. and BRADFORD, W. L. (1942) Toxicity of washings from *H. pertussis* for mice. *Proc. Soc. Exp. Biol. Med.* **49**: 615–618.

KAWAI, Y. and MORIBAYASHI, A. (1982) Characteristic lipids of *Bordetella pertussis*: simple fatty acid composition, hydroxy fatty acids, and an ornithine–containing lipid. *J. Bact.* **151**: 996–1005.

KENDRICK, P. L., ELDERING, G., DIXON, M. K. and MISNER, J. (1947) Mouse protection tests in the study of pertussis vaccine: a comparative series using the intracerebral route for challenge. *Am. J. Publ. Hlth.* **37**: 803–810.

KIND, L. S. (1953) The altered reactivity of mice after immunization with *Haemophilus pertussis* vaccine. *J. Immunol.* **70**: 411–420.

KONG, A. S. and MORSE, S. I. (1977a) The *in vitro* effects of *Bordetella pertussis* lymphocytosis-promoting factor on murine lymphocytes. I. Proliferative response. *J. Exp. Med.* **145**: 151–162.

KONG, A. S. and MORSE, S. I. (1977b) The *in vitro* effects of *Bordetella pertussis* lymphocytosis-promoting factor on murine lymphocytes. II. Nature of the responding cells. *J. Exp. Med.* **145**: 163–174.

KOPLAN, J. P., SCHOENBAUM, S. C., WEINSTEIN, M. C. And FRASER, D. W. (1979) Pertussis vaccine—an analysis of benefits, risks and costs. *New Engl. J. Med.* **301**: 906–911.

KRZANOWSKI, J. J., POLSON, J. B. and SZENTIVANYI, A. (1976) Pulmonary patterns of adenosine-3′,5′-cyclic monophosphate accumulations in response to adrenergic or histamine stimulation in *Bordetella pertussis*-sensitized mice. *Biochem. Pharmac.* **25**: 1631–1637.

KULENKAMPFF, M., SCHWARTZMAN, J. S. and WILSON, J. (1974) Neurological complications of pertussis inoculation. *Archs Dis. Childh.* **49**: 46–49.

KUROKAWA, M., ISHIDA, S. and ASAKAWA, S. (1969) Attempts at analysis of toxicity of pertussis vaccine II. Quantitative determination of the heat-labile toxin by skin reaction. *Jap. J. Med. Sci. Biol.* **22**: 293–307.

KUROKAWA, M., ISHIDA, S., ASAKAWA, S. and IWASA, S. (1978a) Attempts at analysis of toxicity of pertussis vaccine III. Effects of endotoxin on leukocytosis in mice due to lymphocytosis-promoting factor and reference preparations for determination of lymphocytosis-promoting factor. *Jap. J. Med. Sci. Biol.* **31**: 91–103.

KUROKAWA, M., ISHIDA, S., ASAKAWA, S. and IWASA, S. (1978b) Endotoxin, histamine-sensitizing factor and lymphocytosis-promoting factor contents of pertussis vaccines produced in Japan. *Jap. J. Med. Sci. Biol.* **31**: 377–391.

KUROKAWA, M., ISHIDA, S., IWASA, S., ASAKAWA, S. and KURATSUKA, K.(1968) Attempts at analysis of toxicity of pertussis vaccine I. Bodyweight-decreasing toxicity in mice. *Jap. J. Med. Sci. Biol.* **21**: 137–153.

KUROSE, H., KATADA, T., AMANO, T. and UI, M. (1983) Specific uncoupling by islet-activating protein, pertussis toxin, of negative signal transduction via α-adrenergic, cholinergic, and opiate receptors in neuroblastoma X glioma hybrid cells. *J. Biol. Chem.* **258**: 4870–4875.

KUWAJIMA, Y. (1978) The presence of the heat-stable neurotoxin in the pertussis cells. *Osaka Cy. Med. J.* **24**: 165–174.

LACEY, B. W. (1960) Antigenic modulation of *Bordetella pertussis*. *J. Hyg., Camb.* **58**: 57–93.

LANE, A. G. (1968) Detoxification of liquid cultures of *Bordetella pertussis* by forced aeration at high pH. *Appl. Microbiol.* **16**: 1211–1214.

LANE, A. G. (1969) Effect of pertussis vaccination on the sensitivity of mice to insulin, bicarbonate, and CO_2. *Appl. Microbiol.* **17**: 938–939.

LAUTROP, H. (1960) Laboratory diagnosis of whooping-cough or *Bordetella* infections. *Bull. W.H.O.* **23**: 15–35.

LE DUR, A., CAROFF, M., CHABY, R. and SZABÓ, L. (1978) A novel type of endotoxin structure present in *Bordetella pertussis*. *Eur. J. Biochem.* **84**: 579–589.

LE DUR, A., CHABY, R. and SZABÓ, L. (1980) Isolation of two protein-free and chemically different lipopolysaccharides from *Bordetella pertussis* phenol-extracted endotoxin. *J. Bact.* **143**: 78–88.

LEE, T. P. (1977) Effects of histamine-sensitizing factor and cortisol on lymphocyte adenyl cyclase responses. *J. Allergy clin. Immunol.* **59**: 79–82.

LEHRER, S. B. (1979) Investigation of the biological activities of the histamine sensitizing factor of *Bordetella pertussis*. In: *International Symposium on Pertussis, 1978*, pp. 160–165. MANCLARK, C. R. and HILL, J. C. (eds). US DHEW Publication no. (NIH) 79–1830, Washington, D.C.

LEHRER, S. B., TAN, E. M. and VAUGHAN, J. H. (1974) Extraction and partial purification of the histamine-sensitizing factor of *Bordetella pertussis*. *J. Immunol.* **113**: 18–26.

LEHRER, S. B., VAUGHAN, J. H. and TAN, E. M. (1975a) Immunologic and biochemical properties of the histamine-sensitizing factor from *Bordetella pertussis*. *J. Immunol.* **114**: 34–39.

LEHRER, S. B., VAUGHAN, J. H. and TAN, E. M. (1975b) Adjuvant activity of the histamine-sensitizing factor of *Bordetella pertussis* in different strains of mice. *Int. Archs Allergy Appl. Immunol.* **49**: 796–813.

LEHRER, S. B., VAUGHAN, J. H. and TAN, E. M. (1976) Enhancement of reaginic and hemagglutinating antibody production by an extract of *Bordetella pertussis* containing histamine sensitizing factor. *J. Immunol.* **116**: 178–183.

LESLIE, P. H. and GARDNER, A. D. (1931) The phases of *Haemophilus pertussis. J. Hyg., Camb.* **31**: 423–434.

LEVINE, L. and PIERONI, R. E. (1966) A unitarian hypothesis of altered reactivity to stress mediated by *Bordetella pertussis. Experientia* **22**: 797–800.

LEVINE, S. and SOWINSKI, R. (1972) Inhibition of macrophage response to brain injury. A new effect of pertussis vaccine possibly related to histamine-sensitizing factor. *Am. J. Path.* **67**: 349–357.

LEVINE, S., WENK, E. J., DEVLIN, H. B., PIERONI, R. E. and LEVINE, L. (1966) Hyperacute allergic encephalomyelitis: Adjuvant effect of pertussis vaccines and extracts. *J. Immun.* **97**: 363–368.

LIKHITE, V. V. (1974) The delayed and lasting rejection of mammary adenocarcinoma cell tumours in DBA/2 mice with use of Bordetella pertussis. *Cancer Res.* **34**: 1027–1030.

LINNEMANN, C. C. (1979) Host-parasite interactions in pertussis. In: *International Symposium on Pertussis, 1978*, pp. 3–18, MANCLARK, C. R. and HILL, J. C. (eds). US DHEW Publication no. (NIH) 79–1830, Washington, D.C.

LIVEY, I., PARTON, R. and WARDLAW, A. C. (1978) Loss of heat-labile toxin from *Bordetella pertussis* grown in modified Hornibrook medium. *FEMS Microbiol. Lett.* **3**: 203–205.

LIVEY, I. and WARDLAW, A. C. (1984) Production and properties of *Bordetella pertussis* heat-labile toxin. *J. Med. Microbiol.* **17**: 91–103.

LÜDERITZ, O., GALANOS, C. and RIETSCHEL, E. TH. (1981) Endotoxins of Gram-negative bacteria. *Pharmac. Ther.* **15**(3): 383–402.

MacDONALD, H. and MacDONALD, E. J. (1933) Experimental pertussis. *J. Infect. Dis.* **53**: 328–330.

MacLENNAN, A. P. (1960) Specific lipopolysaccharides of *Bordetella. Biochem. J.* **74**: 398–409.

MADSEN, T. (1933) Vaccination against whooping cough. *J. Am. Med. Ass.* **101**: 187–188.

MAHIEU, J. M., MULLER, R. S., VOORHOEVE, A. M. and DIKKEN, H. (1978) Pertussis in a rural area of Kenya: epidemiology and a preliminary report on a vaccine trial. *Bull. W.H.O.* **56**: 733–780.

MAITLAND, H. B., KOHN, R. and MACDONALD, A. D. (1955) The histamine-sensitizing property of *Haemophilus pertussis. J. Hyg., Camb.* **53**: 196–211.

MALKIEL, S. and HARGIS, B. J. (1952) Anaphylactic shock in the pertussis-vaccinated mouse. *J. Allergy* **23**: 352–358.

MANCLARK, C. R., HANSEN, C. T., TREADWELL, P. E. and PITTMAN, M. (1975) Selective breeding to establish a standard mouse for pertussis vaccine bioassay. II. Bioresponses of mice susceptible and resistant to sensitization by pertussis vaccine HSF. *J. Biol. Stand.* **3**: 353–363.

MANCLARK, C. R. and HILL, J. C. (eds). (1979) *International Symposium on pertussis*, 1978, US DHEW Publication no. (NIH) 79–1830, Washington D.C.

MANCLARK, C. R., URBAN, M. A., SUMMERS, E. P. and VICKERS, J. H. (1977) Assay of pertussis vaccine toxicity by a rat-paw-oedema method. *J. Med. Microbiol.* **10**: 115–120.

MATSUI, T. and KUWAJIMA, Y. (1959) Formation of the toxoid of histamine sensitizing factor in *Bordetella pertussis. Nature, Lond.* **184**: 199–200.

MATSUYAMA, T. (1977) Resistance of *Bordetella pertussis* phase I to mucociliary clearance by rabbit tracheal mucous membrane. *J. Infect. Dis.* **136**: 609–616.

MEDICAL RESEARCH COUNCIL (1951) The prevention of whooping cough by vaccination. *Br. Med. J.* **1**: 1463–1471.

MEDICAL RESEARCH COUNCIL (1956) Vaccination against whooping cough: Relation between protection in children and results of laboratory tests. *Br. Med. J.* **2**: 454–462.

MEDICAL RESEARCH COUNCIL (1959) Vaccination against whooping cough: Final report. *Br. Med. J.* **1**: 944–1000.

MILLER, D. L., ALDERSLADE, R. and ROSS, E. M. (1982) Whooping cough and whooping cough vaccine: the risks and benefits debate. *Epidemiol. Rev.* **4**: 1–24.

MILLER, C. L. and FLETCHER, W. B. (1976) Severity of notified whooping cough *Br. Med. J.* **1**: 117–119.

MILLER, D. L., ROSS, E. M., ALDERSLADE, R., BELLMAN, M. H. and RAWSON, N. S. B. (1981) Pertussis immunization and serious acute neurological illness in children. *Br. Med. J.* **282**: 1595–1599.

MIZUSHIMA, Y., MORI, M., OGITA, T. and NAKAMURA, T. (1979) Adjuvant for IgE antibody islet-activating protein in *Bordetella pertussis. Int. Archs. Allergy Appl. Immunol.* **58**: 426–429.

MOREAU, M., CHABY, R. and SZABO, L. (1982) Isolation of a trisaccharide containing 2-amino-2-deoxy-D-galacturonic acid from the *Bordetella pertussis* endotoxin. *J. Bact.* **150**: 27–35.

MORSE, S. I. (1965) Studies on the lymphocytosis induced in mice by *Bordetella pertussis. J. Exp. Med.* **121**: 49–68.

MORSE, S. I. (1976) Biological active components and properties of *Bordetella pertussis. Adv. Appl. Microbiol.* **20**: 9–26.

MORSE, S. I. (1977a) Lymphocytosis-promoting factor of *Bordetella pertussis:* Isolation, characterisation, and biological activity, *J. Infect. Dis.* **136** (Suppl): S234–S238.

MORSE, S. I. (1977b) Components of *Bordetella pertussis* that modulate the immune response. In: *Microbiology 1977*, pp. 374–379, SCHLESSINGER, D. (ed). American Society for Microbiology, Washington D.C.

MORSE, S. I. and BARRON, B. A. (1970) Studies on the leukocytosis and lymphocytosis induced by *Bordetella pertussis* III. The distribution of transfused lymphocytes in pertussis-treated and normal mice. *J. Exp. Med.* **132**: 663–672.

MORSE, S. I. and BRAY, K. K. (1969) The occurrence and properties of leukocytosis and lymphocytosis-stimulating material in the supernatant fluids of *Bordetella pertussis* cultures. *J. Exp. Med.* **129**: 523–550.

MORSE, S. I., KONG, A. S. and HO, M. K. (1979) *In vitro* effects of lymphocytosis-promoting factor on murine lymphocytes. In: *International Symposium on Pertussis*, 1978, pp. 151–155, MANCLARK, C. R. and HILL, J. C. (eds). US DHEW Publication no. (NIH) 79–1830, Washington, D.C.

MORSE, S. I. and MORSE, J. H. (1976) Isolation and properties of the leukocytosis and lymphocytosis-promoting factor of *Bordetella pertussis. J. Exp. Med.* **143**: 1483–1502.

MORSE, S. I. and RIESTER, S. K. (1967a) Studies on the leukocytosis and lymphocytosis induced by *Bordetella pertussis*. I. Radioautographic analysis of the circulating cells in mice undergoing pertussis-induced hyperleukocytosis. *J. Exp. Med.* **125**: 401–408.

MORSE, S. I. and RIESTER, S. K. (1967b) Studies on the leukocytosis and lymphocytosis induced by *Bordetella pertussis*. II. The effects of pertussis vaccine on the thoracic duct lymph and lymphocytes of mice. *J. Exp. Med.* **125**: 619–629.

MORTIMER, E. A. and JONES, P. K. (1979) An evaluation of pertussis vaccine. *Rev. Infect. Dis.* **1**: 927–932.

MUGGLETON, P. W. (1967) Vaccines against pertussis. *Publ. Hlth, Lond.* **81**: 252–264.

MUNOZ, J. J. (1963a) Immunological and other biological activities of *Bordetella pertussis* antigens. *Bact. Rev.* **27**: 325–340.

MUNOZ, J. J. (1963b) Comparison of *Bordetella pertussis* cells and Freund's adjuvant with respect to their antibody inducing and anaphylactogenic properties. *J. Immun.* **90**: 132–139.

MUNOZ, J. J. (1976) Pertussigen: A substance from *Bordetella pertussis* with many biological activities. *Fedn Proc.* **35**: 813.

MUNOZ, J. J. (1971) Protein toxins from *Bordetella pertussis*. In: *Microbial Toxins*, Vol. **IIa**, *Bacterial Protein Toxins*, pp. 271–300, KADIS, S., MONTIE, T. C. and AJL, S. J. (eds). Academic Press, New York.

MUNOZ, J. J. and ARAI, H. (1982) Studies on crystalline pertussigen. In: *Seminars in Infectious Disease* Vol. **IV**: *Bacterial Vaccines*, pp. 395–400, ROBBINS, J. B., HILL, J. C. and SADOFF, J. C. (eds). Thieme-Stratton Inc. New York.

MUNOZ, J. J., ARAI, H., BERGMAN, R. K. and SADOWSKI, P. L. (1981a) Biological activities of crystalline pertussigen from *Bordetella pertussis*. *Infect. Immun.* **33**: 820–826.

MUNOZ, J. J., ARAI, H. and COLE, R. L. (1981b) Mouse-protecting and histamine-sensitizing activities of pertussigen and fimbrial hemagglutinin from *Bordetella pertussis*. *Infect. Immun.* **32**: 243–250.

MUNOZ, J. J. and BERGMAN, R. K. (1968) Histamine-sensitizing factors from microbial agents, with special reference to *Bordetella pertussis*. *Bact. Rev.* **32**: 103–126.

MUNOZ, J. J. and BERGMAN, R. K. (1977) *Bordetella pertussis*: In: *Immunology Series* vol. 4, ROSE, N. (ed). Marcel Dekker, New York, Basel.

MUNOZ, J. J. and BERGMAN, R. K. (1979a) Biological activities of *Bordetella pertussis*. In: *International Symposium on Pertussis, 1978*, pp. 143–150, MANCLARK, C. R. and HILL, J. C. (eds). US DHEW Publication no. (NIH) 79–1830, Washington, D.C.

MUNOZ, J. J. and BERGMAN, R. K. (1979b) Mechanism of action of pertussigen, a substance from *Bordetella pertussis*. In: *Microbiology, 1979*, pp. 193–197, SCHLESSINGER, D. (ed). American Society for Microbiology, Washington, D.C.

MUNOZ, J. J., BERGMAN, R. K., COLE, R. L. and AYERS, J. C. (1978) Purification and activities of pertussigen, a substance from *Bordetella pertussis*. In: *Toxins: Animal, Plant and Microbial*, pp. 1015–1029, ROSENBERG, P. (ed). Proceedings of the Fifth International Symposium, Pergamon Press, Oxford.

MUNOZ, J. J. and HESTEKIN, B. M. (1966) Antigens of *Bordetella pertussis*. IV. Effect of heat, merthiolate, and formaldehyde on histamine-sensitizing factor and protective activity of soluble extracts from *Bordetella pertussis*. *J. Bact.* **91**: 2175–2179.

MUNOZ, J. J., ROBBINS, K. E. and COLE, R. L. (1980) Reactions in the foot pads of mice induced by pertussigen and endotoxin from *Bordetella pertussis*. *J. Reticuloendothel. Soc.* **27**: 259–268.

MURAYAMA, T., KATADA, T. and UI, M. (1983) Guanine nucleotide activation and inhibition of adenylate cyclase as modified by islet-activating protein, pertussis toxin, in mouse 3T3 fibroblasts. *Archs Biochem. Biophys.* **221**: 381–390.

MURAYAMA, T. and UI, M. (1983) Loss of the inhibitory function of the guanine nucleotide regulatory component of adenylate cyclase due to its ADP ribosylation by islet-activating protein, pertussis toxin, in adipocyte membranes. *J. Biol. Chem.* **258**: 3319–3326.

MUSE, K. E., COLLIER, A. M. and BASEMAN, J. B. (1977) Scanning electron microscopic study of hamster tracheal organ cultures infected with *Bordetella pertussis*. *J. Infect. Dis.* **136**: 768–777.

MUSE, K. E., FINDLEY, D., ALLEN, L. and COLLIER, A. M. (1979) In vitro model of *Bordetella pertussis* infection: pathogenic and microbicidal interactions. In: *International Symposium on Pertussis, 1978*, pp. 41–50, MANCLARK, C. R. and HILL, J. C. (eds). US DHEW Publication no. (NIH) 79–1830, Washington, D.C.

NAGEL, J. (1970) Investigations into the preparation of a non-toxic whole-cell pertussis vaccine. In: *International Symposium on Pertussis*, pp. 234–238, VAN HEMERT, P. A., VAN RAMSHORST, J. D. and REGAMEY, R. H. (eds). Symposia Series in Immunobiological Standardization, vol. **13**, Karger, Basel.

NAKASE, Y. and DOI, M. (1979) Toxicity and potency of a purified pertussis vaccine. In: *International Symposium on Pertussis, 1978*, pp. 350–356, MANCLARK, C. R. and HILL, J. C. (eds). U.S. DHEW Publication no. (NIH) 79–1830, Washington, D.C.

NAKASE, Y., TAKATSU, K., TATEISHI, M., SEKIYA, K. and KASUGA, T. (1969) Heat-labile toxin of *Bordetella pertussis* purified by preparative acrylamide gel electrophoresis. *Jap. J. Microbiol.* **13**: 359–366.

NAKASE, Y., TATEISI, M., SEKIYA, K. and KASUGA, T. (1970) Chemical and biological properties of the purified O antigen of *Bordetella pertussis Jap. J. Microbiol.* **14**: 1–8.

NARIMIYA, M., YAMADA, H., MATSUBA, I., IKEDA, Y., TANESE, T. and ABE, M. (1980) The effect of islet-activating protein on glucagon and insulin secretion. *Jikeikai Med. J.* **27**: 263–273.

NIELSEN, J. H., HANSEN, G. A. and WELINDER, B. S. (1980) Pertussis toxin (Islet Activating Protein) stimulates insulin and glucagon secretion from islets in culture. *Diabetologia* **19**: 283.

ODDY, J. G. and EVANS, D. G. (1940) The effects produced by toxic and non-toxic extracts of *H. pertussis* and *Br. bronchiseptica* on the blood sugar of rabbits. *J. Path. Bact.* **50**: 11–16.

OKAMOTO, T., ITOH, A., YAJIMA, M. and UI, M. (1980) Improvement of diabetic symptoms of hereditary diabetic (KK) mice by a single injection with islet-activating protein (IAP). *J. Pharmacobio-Dyn.* **3**: 470–477.

OLSON, L. C. (1975) Pertussis. *Medicine* **54**: 427–469.

ORTEZ, R. A. (1977) Pharmacologic blockade of the effect of histamine on lung cyclic AMP levels in normal and pertussis-vaccinated mice. *Biochem. Pharmac.* **26**: 529–533.

ORTEZ, R. A., SESHACHALAM, D. and SZENTIVANYI, A. (1975) Alterations in adenyl cyclase activity and glucose utilization of *Bordetella pertussis*-sensitized mouse spleen. *Biochem. Pharmac.* **24**: 1297–1302.

ONOUE, K., KITAGAWA, M. and YAMAMURA, Y. (1963) Chemical studies on cellular components of *Bordetella pertussis* III. Isolation of highly potent toxin from *Bordetella pertussis*. *J. Bact.* **86**: 648–655.

OVARY, Z. and CAIAZZA, S. S. (1975) Further studies on the inheritance of responsiveness to pertussis HSF in mice. *Int. Archs Allergy Appl. Immunol.* **48**: 11–15.

PARFENTJEV, I. A. and GOODLINE, M. A. (1948) Histamine shock in mice sensitized with *Hemophilus pertussis* vaccine. *J. Pharmac. Exp. Ther.* **92**: 411–413.

PARKER, C. D. (1976) Role of the genetics and physiology of *Bordetella pertussis* in the production of vaccine and the study of host–parasite relationships in pertussis. *Adv. Appl. Microbiol.* **20**: 27–42.

PARKER, C. W. and MORSE, S. I. (1973) The effect of *Bordetella pertussis* on lymphocyte cyclic AMP metabolism. *J. Exp. Med.* **137**: 1078–1090.

PARTON, R. and WARDLAW, A. C. (1975) Cell-envelope proteins of *Bordetella pertussis*. *J. Med. Microbiol.* **8**: 47–57.

PELTOLA, H. and MICHELSSON, K. (1982) Efficacy of salbutamol in treatment of infant pertussis demonstrated by sound spectrum analysis. *Lancet* **1**: 310–312.

PERKINS, F. T., SHEFFIELD, F., MILLER, C. L. and SKEGG, J. L. (1970) The comparison of toxicity of pertussis vaccines in children and mice. In: *International Symposium on Pertussis*, pp. 141–149, VAN HEMERT, P. A. VAN RAMSHORST, J. D. and REGAMEY, R. H. (eds). Symposia Series in Immunobiological Standardization. Vol. 13, Karger, Basel.

PIERONI, R. E. and LEVINE, L. (1966) Adjuvant principle of pertussis vaccine in the mouse. *Nature, Lond.* **211**: 1419–1420.

PITTMAN, M. (1951a) Sensitivity of mice to histamine during respiratory infection by *Hemophilus pertussis*. *Proc. Soc. Exp. Biol. Med.* **77**: 70–74.

PITTMAN, M. (1951b) Comparison of the histamine-sensitizing property with the protective activity of pertussis vaccines for mice. *J. Infect. Dis.* **89**: 300–304.

PITTMAN, M. (1952) Influence of preservatives, of heat, and of irradiation on mouse protective activity and detoxification of pertussis vaccine, *J. Immunol.* **69**: 201–216.

PITTMAN, M. (1957) Effect of *Hemophilus pertussis* on immunological and physiological reactions. *Fedn. Proc.* **16**: 867–872.

PITTMAN, M. (1967) Mouse strain variation in response to pertussis vaccine and tetanus toxoid. In: *International Symposium on Laboratory Animals*, pp. 161–166, Symposia Series in Immunolobiological Standardization, Vol. 5, Karger, Basel.

PITTMAN, M. (1970) *Bordetella pertussis*—bacterial and host factors in the pathogenesis and prevention of whooping cough. In: *Infectious Agents and Host Reactions*, pp. 239–270, MUDD, S. (ed). Saunders, Philadelphia.

PITTMAN, M. (1975) Determination of the histamine sensitizing unitage of pertussis vaccine. *J. Biol. Stand.* **3**: 185–191.

PITTMAN, M. (1979) Pertussis toxin: the cause of the harmful effects and prolonged immunity of whooping cough. A hypothesis. *Rev. Infect. Dis.* **1**: 401–412.

PITTMAN, M. (1980) Mouse breeds and the toxicity test for pertussis vaccine. *16th IABS Congress: The standardization of animals to improve biomedical research, production and control*, San Antonio, 1979. *Dev. Biol. Stand.* **45**, 129–135. S. Karger, Basel.

PITTMAN, M. and COX, C. B. (1965) Pertussis vaccine testing for freedom-from-toxicity. *Appl. Microbiol.* **13**: 447–456.

PITTMAN, M., FURMAN, B. L. and WARDLAW, A. C. (1980) *Bordetella pertussis* respiratory tract infection in the mouse: pathophysiological responses. *J. Infect. Dis.* **142**: 56–65.

PRASHKER, D. and WARDLAW, A. C. (1971) Temperature responses of mice to *Escherichia coli* endotoxin. *Br. J. Exp. Path.* **52**: 36–46.

PRESTON, N. W. (1963) Type-specific immunity against whooping-cough. *Br. Med. J.* **2**: 724–726.

PRESTON, N. W. and GARRITY, P. (1967) Histamine-sensitizing factor of *Bordetella pertussis* differentiated from immunogens by neutralisation and passive protection tests. *J. Path. Bact.* **93**: 483–492.

PRESTON, N. W., TIMEWELL, R. M. and CARTER, E. J. (1980) Experimental pertussis infection in the rabbit: similarities with infection in primates. *J. Infect.* **2**: 227–235.

PUSZTAI, Z. and JOÓ, I. (1967) Influence of nicotinic acid on the antigenic structure of *Bordetella pertussis*. *Ann. Immunol. Hung.* **10**: 63–67.

REGAN, J. C. and TOLSTROOUHOV, A. (1936) Relations of acid base equilibrium to the pathogenesis and treatment of whooping cough. *N.Y. St. J. Med.* **36**: 1075–1086.

REPORTS FROM THE COMMITTEE ON SAFETY OF MEDICINES AND THE JOINT COMMITTEE ON VACCINATION AND IMMUNISATION (1981) Whooping Cough. HMSO, London.

ROBINSON, A. and IRONS, L. I. (1983) Synergistic effect of *Bordetella pertussis* lymphocytosis–promoting factor on protective activities of isolated *Bordetella* antigens in mice. *Infect. Immun.* **40**: 523–528.

ROSS, R., MUNOZ, J. J. and CAMERON, C. (1969) Histamine-sensitizing factor, mouse-protective antigens, and other antigens of some members of the genus *Bordetella*. *J. Bact.* **99**: 57–64.

ROWATT, E. (1957) The growth of *Bordetella pertussis*: A review. *J. Gen. Microbiol.* **17**: 297–326.

SANYAL, R. K. (1960) Histamine sensitivity in children after pertussis infection *Nature, Lond.* **185**: 537–538.

SATO, Y., ARAI, H. and SUZUKI, K. (1974) Leukocytosis-promoting factor of *Bordetella pertussis* III. Its identity with protective antigen. *Infect. Immun.* **9**: 801–810.

SATO, Y., IZUMIYA, K., ODA, M. A. and SATO, H. (1979) Biological significance of *Bordetella pertussis* fimbriae or hemagglutinin: A possible role of the fimbriae or hemagglutinin for pathogenesis and antibacterial immunity. In: *International Symposium on Pertussis, 1978*, pp. 51–57, MANCLARK, C. R. and HILL, J. C. (eds). US DHEW Publication no. (NIH) 79–1830, Washington, D.C.

SATO, Y., IZUMIYA, K., SATO, H., COWELL, J. L. and MANCLARK, C. R. (1980) Aerosol infection of mice with *Bordetella pertussis*. *Infect. Immun.* **29**: 261–266.

SATO, Y., IZUMIYA, K., SATO, H., COWELL, J. L. and MANCLARK, C. R. (1981) Role of antibody to leukocytosis-promoting factor hemagglutinin and to filamentous hemagglutinin in immunity to pertussis. *Infect. Immun.* **31**: 1223–1231.

SATO, Y., SATO, H., IZUMIYA, K., COWELL, J. L. and MANCLARK, C. R. (1982) Role of antibody to filamentous hemagglutinin and to leukocytosis promoting factor–hemagglutinin in immunity to pertussis. In: *Seminars in Infectious Disease Vol. IV: Bacterial Vaccines* pp. 380–385, ROBBINS, J. B., HILL, J. C. and SADOFF, J. C. (eds). Thieme-Stratton Inc. New York.

SAUER, L. W. (1933) Whooping cough, a study in immunization. *J. Am. Med. Ass.* **100:** 239–241.

SPASOJEVIĆ, V. (1977) Study on toxicity of *Bordetella pertussis* cultures and antigens. In: *International Symposium on pyrogenicity, innocuity and toxicity test systems for biological products*, Budapest 1976. *Dev. Biol. Stand.* **34:** 197–205, S. Karger, Basel.

STAINER, D. W. (1979) Untitled discussion contribution In: *International Symposium on Pertussis, 1978*, pp. 137–138, MANCLARK, C. R. and HILL, J. C. (eds). US DHEW Publication no. (NIH) 79–1830, Washington, D.C.

STAINER, D. W. and SCHOLTE, M. J. (1971) A simple chemically defined medium for the production of Phase I. *Bordetella pertussis*. *J. Gen. Microbiol.* **63:** 211–220.

STANBRIDGE, T. N. and PRESTON, N. W. (1974) Experimental pertussis infection in the marmoset: Type specificity of active immunity. *J. Hyg., Camb.* **72:** 213–228.

STANDFAST, A. F. B. (1958a) Some factors influencing the virulence for mice of *Bordetella pertussis* by the intracerebral route. *Immunology* **1:** 123–134.

STANDFAST, A. F. B. (1958b) The comparison between field trials and mouse protection tests against intranasal and intracerebral challenges with *Bordetella pertussis*. *Immunology*. **2:** 135–143.

STANDFAST, A. F. B. and DOLBY, J. M. (1961) A comparison between the intranasal and intracerebral infection of mice with *Bordetella pertussis*. *J. Hyg., Camb.*, **59:** 217–229.

STEINMAN, L., SRIRAM, S., ADELMAN, N. E., ZAMVIL, S., McDEVITT, H. O. and URICH, H. (1982) Murine model for pertussis vaccine encephalopathy: linkage to H-2. *Nature, Lond.* **299:** 738–740.

STEWART, G. T. (1979) Toxicity of pertussis vaccine: frequency and probability of reactions. *J. Epidemiol. Community Hlth.* **33:** 150–156.

STŘIŽOVÁ, V. and TRLIFAJOVÁ, J. (1964) The neutralization of *B. pertussis* toxin in a tissue culture. *J. Hyg. Epidemiol. Microbiol. Immunol.* **8:** 428–432.

STRONK, M. G. and PITTMAN, M. (1955) The influence of pertussis vaccine on histamine sensitivity of rabbits and guinea-pigs and on the blood sugar in rabbit and mice. *J. Infect. Dis.* **96:** 152–161.

STUART-HARRIS, C. (1979) Benefits and risks of immunization against pertussis In: *Int. Symp. on Immunization: Benefit Versus Risk Factors*, Brussels. 1978. *Dev. Biol. Stand.* **43:** 75–83, S. Karger, Basel.

SUMI, T. and UI, M. (1975) Potentiation of the adrenergic beta-receptor-mediated insulin secretion in pertussis-sensitized rats. *Endocrinology* **97:** 352–358.

SUZUKI, I., KUMAZAWA, Y., MIYAZAKI, T. and MIZUNOE, K. (1978) Modulation of the antibody response to sheep erythrocytes in murine spleen cell cultures by a T cell mitogen extracted from *Bordetella pertussis*. *Microbiol. Immunol.* **22:** 47–51.

SZENTIVANYI, A., FISHEL, C. W. and TALMAGE, D. W. (1963) Adrenaline mediation of histamine and serotonin hyperglycemia in normal mice and the absence of adrenaline-induced hyperglycemia in pertussis-sensitized mice. *J. Infect. Dis.* **113:** 86–98.

TABACHNICK, I. I. A. and GULBENKIAN, A. (1969) Adrenergic changes due to pertussis: Insulin, glucose and free fatty acids. *Eur. J. Pharmac.* **7:** 186–195.

TAMURA, M., NOGIMORI, K., MURAI, S., YAJIMA, M., ITO, K., KATADA, T., UI, M. and ISHII, S. (1982) Subunit structure of islet-activating protein, pertussis toxin, in conformity with the A-B model. *Biochemistry* **21:** 5516–5522.

TAMURA, M., NOGIMORI, K., YAJIMA, M., ASE, K. and UI, M. (1983) A role of the B-oligomer moiety of islet-activating protein, pertussis toxin, in development of the biological effects on intact cells. *J. Biol. Chem.* **258:** 6756–6761.

TERPSTRA, G. K., RAAIJMAKERS, J. A. M. and KREUKNIET, J. (1979) Comparison of vaccination of mice and rats with *Haemophilus influenzae* and *Bordetella pertussis* as models of atopy. *Clin. Exp. Pharmac. Physiol.* **6:** 139–149.

TOWNLEY, R. G., TRAPANI, I. L. and SZENTIVANYI, A. (1967) Sensitization to anaphylaxis and to some of its pharmacological mediators by blockade of the beta adrenergic receptors. *J. Allergy* **39:** 177–197.

TOYOTA, T., KAI, Y., KAKIZAKI, M., SAKAI, A., GOTO, Y., YAJIMA, M. and UI, M. (1980) Effects of islet-activating protein (IAP) on blood glucose and plasma insulin in healthy volunteers (phase 1 studies). *Tohoku J. Exp. Med.* **130:** 105–116.

TOYOTA, T., KAKIZAKI, M., KIMURA, K., YAJIMA, M., OKAMOTO, T. and UI, M. (1978) Islet activating protein (IAP) derived from the culture supernatant fluid of *Bordetella pertussis*: Effect on spontaneous diabetic rats. *Diabetologia* **14:** 319–323.

TUTA, J. A. (1937) A study of the lymphocytosis following intravenous injections into rabbits of suspensions and extracts of *Hemophilus pertussis*. *Folia haemat. Lpz.* **57:** 122–128.

UI, M. and KATADA, T. (1978) A novel action of the 'islet-activating protein (IAP)' to modify adrenergic regulation of insulin secretions. In: *Proceedings of the Symposium on Proinsulin, Insulin and C-Peptide*, pp. 124–131, BABA, S., KANEKO, T. and YANAIHARA, N. (eds). Elsevier, Amsterdam.

UI, M., KATADA, T. and YAJIMA, M. (1979) Islet-activating protein in *Bordetella pertussis*: Purification and mechanism of action. In: *International Symposium on Pertussis, 1978*, pp. 166–173, MANCLARK, C. R. and HILL, J. C. (eds). US DHEW Publication no. (NIH) 79–1830, Washington, D.C.

UTSUMI, S., SONODA, S., IMAGAWA, T. and KANOH, M. (1978) Polymorphonuclear leukocyte-inhibitory factor of *Bordetella pertussis*. I. Extraction and partial purification of phagocytosis- and chemotaxis-inhibitory activities. *Biken J.* **21:** 121–135.

VAZ, N. M., DE SOUZA, C. M., MAIA, L. C. S. and HANSON, D. G. (1977) Effects of *Bordetella pertussis* on the sensitivity of inbred mice to vasoactive amines. *Int. Archs Allergy Appl. Immunol.* **53:** 560–568.

WALKER, E., PINKERTON, I. W., LOVE, W. C., CHAUDHURI, A. K. R. and DATTA, J. B. (1981) Whooping cough in Glasgow 1969–1980. *J. Infect.* **3:** 150–158.

WARDLAW, A. C. (1970) Inheritance of responsiveness to pertussis HSF in mice. *Int. Archs Allergy Appl. Immunol.* **38:** 573–589.

WARDLAW, A. C. (1972) Possible reasons for the inefficiency of Gram-negative bacterial vaccines. *Prog. Immunobiol. Stand.* **5:** 508–512.

WARDLAW, A. C. and JAKUS, C. M. (1966) The inactivation of pertussis protective antigen, histamine sensitizing factor, and lipopolysaccharide by sodium metaperiodate. *Can. J. Microbiol.* **12:** 1105–1114.

WARDLAW, A. C. and PARTON, R. (1979) Changes in envelope proteins and correlation with biological activities in *B. pertussis*. In: *International Symposium on Pertussis 1978*, pp. 94–98, MANCLARK, C. R. and HILL, J. C. (eds). US DHEW Publication no. (NIH) 79–1830 Washington, D.C.

WARDLAW, A. C. and PARTON, R. (1983) Pertussis vaccine. pp. 207–253 In: *Medical Microbiology Vol. II*, JELJASZEWICZ, J. and EASMON, C. S. F. (eds). Academic Press, London and New York.

WARDLAW, A. C., PARTON, R., BERGMAN, R. K. and MUNOZ, J. J. (1979) Loss of adjuvanticity in rats for the hyperacute form of allergic encephalomyelitis and for reaginic antibody production in mice of a phenotypic variant of *Bordetella pertussis*. *Immunology* **37:** 539–545.

WARDLAW, A. C., PARTON, R. and HOOKER, M. J. (1976) Loss of protective antigen, histamine-sensitizing factor and envelope polypeptides in cultural variants of *Bordetella pertussis*. *J. Med. Microbiol.* **9:** 89–100.

WESTPHAL, O., LÜDERITZ, O. and BISTER, F. (1952) Über die Extraktion von Bakterien mit Phenol/Wasser. *Z. Natur. Teil B.* **7:** 148–155.

WILLIAMS, J. F., LOWITT, S. and SZENTIVANYI, A. (1980) Involvement of a heat-stable and heat-labile component of *Bordetella pertussis* in the depression of the murine hepatic mixed-function oxidase system. *Biochem. Pharmac.* **29:** 1483–1490.

WILSON, G. S. (1967) *The Hazards of Immunization*, Athlone Press, London.

WOOD, M. L. (1940) A filtrable toxic substance in broth-cultures of *B. pertussis J. Immunol.* **39:** 25–42.

WORLD HEALTH ORGANIZATION (1979) Requirements for pertussis vaccine. *W.H.O. Tech. Rep. Ser.* No. **638:** 60–80.

YAJIMA, M., HOSODA, K., KANBAYASHI, Y., NAKAMURA, T., NOGIMORI, K., MIZUSHIMA, Y., NAKASE, Y. and UI, M. (1978a) Islets-activating protein (IAP) in *Bordetella pertussis* that potentiates insulin secretory responses of rats. *J. Biochem., Tokyo*, **83:** 295–303.

YAJIMA, M., HOSODA, K., KANBAYASHI, Y., NAKAMURA, T., TAKAHASHI, I. and UI, M. (1978b) Biological properties of islets-activating protein (IAP) purified from the culture medium of *Bordetella pertussis*. *J. Biochem., Tokyo* **83:** 305–312.

ZOUMBOULAKIS, D., ANAGNOSTAKIS, D., ALBANIS, V. and MATSANIOTIS, N. (1973) Steroids in treatment of pertussis: A controlled clinical trial. *Archs Dis. Childh.* **48:** 51–54.

CHAPTER 19

ANTHRAX TOXIN

JOHN STEPHEN

Department of Microbiology, University of Birmingham, P. O. Box 363, Birmingham B15 2TT, U.K.

1. INTRODUCTION

This topic was actively researched from the early 1950s to the late 1960s in the United States of America and Britain at which point the work came to a halt. During the 1970s a trickle of publications from the Soviet Union continued to appear on the production of toxin (Lesnyak and Saltykov, 1974; Vylchev *et al.*, 1976; Derbin *et al.*, 1977), immunizing antigen preparations (Fedotova, 1974; Kuzmich *et al.*, 1976) biological testing for toxicity (Lesnyak, 1975) and the effect of anthrax toxin on cultured cells (Fedotova, 1970). Very recently, new studies have appeared from American workers on the genetics of anthrax toxin (Mikesell *et al.*, 1983) and on the mode of action of one of its three components in chinese hamster ovary (CHO) and other cells (Leppla, 1982). The bulk of this review will concentrate on the earlier work. The fact that the author was not personally involved in research carried out during the halcyon period from the early 1950s to the late 1960s might enhance rather than detract from this article which is mainly one of retrospective appraisal, since this era closed on a note of as yet unresolved controversy. No attempt will be made to exude a pseudo-scholarship by remarshalling the many primary papers which emanated mainly from the American group at Fort Detrick, the British group at the Microbiological Research Establishment (Porton) and others, since these have been collated and reviewed on several occasions (Smith, 1958; Lincoln *et al.*, 1964; Nungester, 1967; Lincoln and Fish, 1970). My aims are to present, to a later generation, a concise outline of the discovery of this complex toxin, describe its nature and role in the pathogenesis of disease, discuss the controversy that developed as to the pathophysiological changes induced by anthrax toxin and finally to comment on the recent developments which if pursued could, and probably will, lead to a resolution of the extant problems.

The remainder of this introductory section sets out the context in which the work was conceived and developed.

The disease anthrax occurs in two forms. Localized cutaneous infections occur in man, swine, rabbits and horses (Lincoln *et al.*, 1964; Lamb, 1973) in which the most characteristic superficial feature is the black eschar which gives its name to the disease and the causative organisms (Gr. anthrakos = coal). The incidence in humans is low, occurring mainly among veterinarians, meat workers and workers in woollen mills, hence the name wool sorter's disease. This form is readily treatable by antibiotics. The septicaemic form may develop from untreated cutaneous infections, or by primary infection via the respiratory or gastrointestinal routes or by infection of wounds and it is nearly always fatal. In animals, a peracute form of the disease occurs in which the first sign of the disease is often death itself; a less acute form occurs in which signs may be evident over a period of 2–10 days before the, nearly always, fatal outcome (Lincoln *et al.*, 1964). Herbivores are the most usual victims: cattle, sheep, horses and goats, in that order, being most susceptible. The organism is highly invasive, spreading throughout the body from the initial portal of entry and producing a characteristic massive terminal bacteraemia. In certain parts of the world it is of sufficient economic importance to warrant vaccination of animals at risk with attenuated vaccines (Sterne, 1967).

The study of anthrax and its causative organism *B. anthracis* has attracted the attention of microbiologists from Davaine, Pasteur and Koch onward. In the immediate post World-

War II period it was the possible military potential of this aerobic spore-former that stimulated the last major upsurge of interest in the pathogenesis of the disease and led to the discovery of the toxin. However, should reports (Rich, 1980) be confirmed by independent observers, it would appear that the lure of this toxigenic aerobic spore-former for military strategies (Coggins, 1963) may not have completely waned. From the early 1900s to the late 1940s observations had accumulated on the aggressin activities of this organism (i.e. its ability to interfere with or counteract host defence mechanisms), in particular interference with phagocytic activity and anthracidal activity of tissue fluids (summarized by Smith *et al.*, 1953*b*). Before the 1950s several suggestions had been made as to the cause of death but no toxin had ever been implicated. The recognition of the latter arose from studies designed to elucidate the biochemical determinants responsible for this desease, the key work being done by the Porton and Fort Detrick groups. The discovery of the toxin was a modern classic in that the principal determinant of lethal anthrax was detected, having eluded many investigators for many years. The work also gave the kiss of life to bacterial toxinology which at that time was almost moribund. The other equally important discovery of this period was cholera toxin (De and Chatterjee, 1953; De, 1959), but the development of the enterotoxin industry started years later when Field and coworkers (Field *et al.*, 1968; Field *et al.*, 1969) showed that cholera toxin caused the movement of ions across the membranes of epithelial cells *in vitro*.

2. DISCOVERY OF THE TOXIN

2.1. IN VIVO APPROACH: EXPERIMENTAL ANTHRAX IN THE GUINEA-PIG

The fresh thrust of the work at Porton was to examine organisms and their products, derived from *in vivo* sources, in suitably designed biological tests. Anthrax bacilli were injected into the thoracic and peritoneal cavities of guinea-pigs (Smith *et al.*, 1953*a*). From these two anatomical sites large quantities of organisms were readily recovered; exudates from both cavities were also obtained and combined with plasma from infected animals to provide a source of presumptive extracellular factors secreted by organisms *in vivo* (Keppie *et al.*, 1953). It is worthy of note that the strain of organism used was a non-proteolytic (NP) mutant of the Vollum strain, selected from a group of 10 strains examined in preliminary experiments for their ability to produce large volumes of thoracic and peritoneal exudate.

Some of the differing properties of the *in vivo* derived organisms are summarized in Table. 1. Plasma and exudates from both cavities (PE), the product obtained by dissolving

TABLE 1. *Some Properties of* Bacillus anthracis *grown* In vitro *and* In vivo

	Organisms[1]				
	in vitro				in vivo
	TMB	BM	SS	GP	
Possession of capsules[2]	−	+	+	+	+ +
Susceptibility to phagocytosis[3]	+ +	−	−	−	−
Solubility in (NH$_4$)$_2$ CO$_3$[4]	+ +	+	+	+	+ + +

(1) Organisms were grown in four media: tryptic meat broth (TMB), Brewer's media (BM), sheep serum (SS), and guinea-pig plasma (GP) and were compared by three criteria with those obtained from infected guinea-pigs as described by Smith *et al.*, 1953b). For clarity, the relative values are shown as + or − with the significance ascribed to each horizontal row defined in footnotes. Data derived from Smith *et al.* (1953b).

(2) − = no visible capsule. + = visible capsule. + + = visible capsule of significantly greater width than +. It is noteworthy that BM, SS, and GP contained plasma constituents, whereas TMB did not.

(3) + + =highly susceptible to phagocytosis by guinea-pig polymorphonuclear phagocytes. − = resistant to phagocytosis, presumably because of capsules.

(4) + = only a small percentage of organisms dissolved after 24 hr. + + = most of the organisms dissolved after 24 hr. + + + = most of the organisms dissolved after 5 hr. This *rapid* solubility of organisms grown *in vivo* was a highly characteristic property distinguishing them from all *in vitro* grown organisms; the extract was designated ACE (see text).

organisms in ammonium carbonate (ACE), and extracts of organisms obtained by ballotini glass beads (BE) were all tested in the following way. First, direct toxicity tests were performed using guinea-pigs: these were injected intraperitoneally with PE, ACE and BE all of which proved to be non-toxic. Skin tests revealed that PE produced a significant but transient oedema; ACE and BE were inactive. Second, aggressin tests showed that all three types of preparations enhanced the virulence of anthrax spores in that the lethal dose for guinea-pigs was reduced from 1×10^4 to 50, inhibited phagocytosis of organisms by polymorphonuclear cells, and also inhibited the bactericidal effects of fresh defibrinated blood towards vegetative bacilli. Both cellular and extracellular products were therefore active as aggressins. Third, immunity tests showed that only PE would protect guinea-pigs against 1000 lethal doses of organisms, i.e. apparently only the extracellular materials were immunogenic.

2.2. ROLE OF TERMINAL BACTERAEMIA: DISCOVERY OF TOXIN

The results just described yielded no evidence for a lethal anthrax toxin, hence the experimental regimen was changed. Prompted by earlier reports that fatal anthrax was, in a very small number of cases, unaccompanied by the characteristic bacteraemia, Keppie et al. (1955) infected guinea-pigs by injecting anthrax spores intradermally. Quantitative estimates of the time-dependent distribution of organisms throughout the tissues of infected guinea-pigs showed that during the 12 hr period preceding death the number of bacteria in the blood rose from 3×10^5 to 1×10^9 chains/ml. If streptomycin were administered at or before the time that the bacterial burden reached 1/300 that of the terminal level, infected guinea-pigs could be saved; if given after this point, guinea-pigs died even though a massive reduction in bacterial numbers was achieved. Other antibiotics, chlortetracyline, oxytetracyline, and chloramphenicol failed to stop the bacteraemia; penicillin was too toxic for the guinea-pig at bacteriostatic concentrations. Hyperimmune horse anthrax antiserum did not terminate the bacteraemia; further reference is made below to the therapeutic efficiency of antisera. The 'point of no return' type of experiment *proves* the non-essentiality of a bacteraemia and *suggests* a toxic factor as the cause of death; in the case of anthrax the latter was duly found (Smith et al., 1955a). (It is interesting to recall that conceptually similar experiments led Kitasato in 1889 to suspect that experimental tetanus in mice was caused by a toxin; he surgically removed the tissues at the site of injection and, with these, the localized toxin-producing organisms. The work of McCrumb et al. (1953) on human patients infected with *Yersinia pestis* and treated with antibiotics, allowed similar conclusions about the involvement of toxins in human plague.)

At this crucial stage, most organisms were found in the spleen of infected guinea-pigs, but later the majority were found in the blood. Quantitative analyses of blood of infected animals revealed composite physiological disturbances which suggested that guinea-pigs were dying of secondary oligaemic shock. For example, there was a loss of blood (up to 25 % at $1\frac{1}{2}$ hr before death), a dramatic drop in blood pressure from 8 hr before death, and a rise in haematocrit values. There was macroscopic evidence for fluid leakage to the site of infection in the flank and, later, haemorrhage. During the final 6 hr the body temperature dropped from 37 to 31°C. Carbohydrate metabolism was affected—an initial pathological rise in glucose followed by a terminal hypoglycaemia presumed due to bacterial metabolism. Electrolytic imbalances in plasma were observed: pH, Na^+, HCO_3^- fell; K^+, Mg^{2+} rose; there was also histopathological and biochemical evidence of renal failure (Smith et al., 1955a; Smith et al., 1955b).

These features are characteristic of secondary shock which we distinguish from primary or neurogenic shock. The onset of the latter is rapid due to damage to the neurological system with resultant loss of vital motor function. Secondary shock is a term used to describe effects which are secondary to some other primary injury or trauma, which may be of an accidental or surgical nature or induced by pathogenic organisms (Smith 1960). We will return to this question of shock when discussing the pathophysiology of anthrax toxin. The Porton group demonstrated that sterile blood from doomed guinea-pigs reproduced the same syndrome in, and killed, normal guinea-pigs (Smith *et al.*, 1955a). The toxic effects were specifically neutralizable by antisera raised to the Sterne strain, which though attenuated by virtue of having lost its outer capsule, was later shown to produce toxin (Harris-Smith *et al.*, 1958) or by antisera raised in rabbits, monkeys, or humans to an immunizing antigen produced *in vitro* (Smith *et al.*, 1955a). Presumably the failure to find the toxin in PE initially was due to its dilution or inactivation by the exudates which together with plasma constituted PE.

2.3. ISOLATION AND CHARACTERIZATION OF A COMPLEX TOXIN

In its own temporal context, the discovery of this toxin illustrated some fundamental principles in approaching studies in microbial pathogenicity, in particular the search for ecologically significant toxins (Miles, 1955) responsible for disease. In contrast, protein separation technology was only just beginning to develop around this time and as a consequence the early attempts to isolate and purify the lethal toxin highlighted by the experimental pathology were hampered by the lack of good physicochemical separation techniques. For example, initial experiments involving heavy metal salts for differential precipitation of proteins inactivated the toxin. However, the loss of toxic activity by simple preparative ultracentrifugation was more difficult to explain until the pellet and supernatant fractions generated by this mildest of physicochemical procedures were recombined, with concomitant restoration of toxicity. Thus the existence of at least two individually non-toxic factors (pellet, 1; supernatant, 2) comprising a synergistic toxic mixture was revealed. Confirmation of the main findings relating to the composition of the toxin obtained from infected guinea-pigs came from studies on materials derived from *in vitro* culture filtrates. Strange and Thorne (1958) had previously purified an immunizing non-toxic antigen which was later shown to be factor 2. Active toxin was produced by growing the Sterne strain in complex (Harris-Smith *et al.*, 1958) and in defined (Thorne *et al.*, 1960) media. In the latter case, sterilization of the culture filtrates was carried out using fritted-glass filters of appropriate porosity. The filtrate contained a non-toxic product, factor 2, but factor 1 adsorbed to the filter from which it was recovered on washing with alkaline buffers; adsorption could be prevented by addition of horse serum before filtration. The Fort Dietrick group isolated the anthrax toxin from the blood of rhesus monkeys dying of experimental anthrax (Klein *et al.*, 1962) thereby enhancing the relevance of the work done on small animals as a model of the human situation.

It is not possible to predict *a priori* the maximum number of components constituting a synergistic toxic mixture. The number of factors revealed will clearly be a function of the efficiency of the fractionation procedures used together with the number and nature of biological tests used to monitor the process. By monitoring the ratio of LD_{50} in mice to oedema in guinea-pig skin, it was evident that a third factor had been lost in the purification of factors 1 and 2. This was duly found (Stanley and Smith, 1961; Beall *et al.*, 1962); addition of factor 3 to preparations of $1+2$ restored the lethality/oedema ratio to that associated with crude toxin. The most definitive published study on the purification and properties of anthrax toxin components is that of Fish *et al.* (1968b), who used molecular exclusion and adsorption chromatographic techniques to generate preparations of the 3 components, each demonstrably free from the other as judged by serological criteria. Their purified preparations were most stable in the pH range 7.4–7.8, heat labile (as far as biological but not serological activities were concerned), susceptible in differing degrees to inactivation during storage and purification, and apparently capable of existing as different conformers or as aggregates depending on their state of purity or the nature of the environment.

Since the discovery of the synergistic anthrax toxin complex, other toxins have been shown to be synergistic mixtures: these include staphylococcal leucocidin (Woodin, 1970), *Y. pestis* guinea-pig toxin (Smith, 1964), staphylococcal γ-toxin (see McCartney and Arbuthnott, 1978).

3. ROLE IN PATHOGENESIS

If intelligently modified, there are no difficulties in applying the idealized criteria outlined by van Heyningen (1955) to show that anthrax toxin is involved in the pathogenesis of disease. Unlike many bacterial toxins there is unequivocal evidence that it is produced *in vivo* and is therefore of immediate potential relevance. The correlation of toxigenicity and virulence is not so easy since virulence in *B. anthracis* is multifactorial. Fully virulent strains are both capsulated and toxigenic (Smith, 1958, Keppie *et al.*, 1963). The capsule is a highly complex structure (Avakyan *et al.*, 1965) which includes as one of its major constituents poly-D-glutamic acid which acts as an aggressin by inhibiting phagocytosis (Keppie *et al.*, 1963). Loss of capsule produces avirulent strains like the powerfully immunogenic Sterne strain, which will produce toxin *in vitro* (Harris-Smith *et al.*, 1958) but is capable of only limited growth *in vivo* during which sufficient toxin must be produced to evoke an antitoxic immunity. Loss of toxigenic potency produces strains such as the HM strain (Harris-Smith *et al.*, 1958), which though not sufficiently attenuated to be used as a vaccine strain is measurably less virulent than wild type strains. Thus full virulence of *B. anthracis* is associated with at least the possession of both capsule and toxigenicity. Ivanovics *et al.* (1968), on the basis of studies with purine auxotrophic mutants of *B. anthracis*, have suggested the possibility of another factor, distinct from capsule or toxin production, which is necessary for full virulence in mice. To this reviewer's knowledge this has never been pursued or confirmed.

The toxin is not only lethal but also interferes with phagocytic activity (Keppie *et al.*, 1963), macrophage morphology, and retards HeLa and F1 cell growth (Fedotova, 1970). The question as to whether one can demonstrate sterile lesions at sites removed from the initial foci of bacterial multiplication is not relevant, because *B. anthracis* is a highly invasive organism. (This fact has important repercussions as discussed below when dealing with the question of mimicry of the disease).

Can the course of the disease be altered by therapeutic administration of antitoxin or can the initiation of disease be prevented by prophylactic use of antitoxin passively administered or actively induced? As in all bacterial toxaemias, successful antitoxic therapy depends on the timing of the administration of antitoxin; given early enough it is effective. The work of Boyd *et al.* (1972) on the prevention of experimental gas gangrene in sheep is an excellent example of this. Smith *et al.* (1955a) demonstrated that lethality and oedema-production in the guinea-pig were readily neutralizable by specific anthrax antiserum in experiments involving direct injection of performed toxin. Vick *et al.* (1968) showed that primates could also be protected from the lethal effects of toxin if antitoxin were administered before, or not later than 8 hr after, injection of toxin. However, when guinea-pigs, infected with *B. anthracis* and allowed to progress beyond the critical point and treated with streptomycin (under which conditions all animals would normally die), were given antitoxin or antitoxin plus supportive treatment for shock, only a few survived. From such studies it is obvious that therapeutic administration of antitoxin was only partially successful. In general it is necessary not only to neutralize toxin activity but also to reverse the effects already induced by the toxin; this may be difficult or impossible if the toxin induces shock and this has progressed to the terminal stages. In sharp contrast, there is a wealth of evidence to show that active immunity to the toxin and infection can be elicited by toxin or incomplete combinations of its factors, or factor 2 on its own (Stanley and Smith, 1963; see Lincoln and Fish, 1970, for review). However, the definition of the optimal combination of the three factors, the choice of test animals or the criteria for assessing protective levels of immunity without direct challenge are among the points of controversy which have not been completely resolved (see next section). Lincoln and Fish (1970) and Ward *et al.* (1965) described experiments on immunized guinea-pigs which died having demonstrable circulating toxin and antitoxin in their blood. Whether this constitutes sufficient evidence to question the role of anthrax toxin in disease (Ward *et al.*, 1965) or merely emphasizes the difficulty of making an exact analysis of such a highly complex situation (Smith, 1964) is open to question. The weight of evidence in favour of implicating anthrax toxin in disease would seem to this reviewer to be so overwhelming as to constitute sufficient grounds for reexamination of the atypical situations which might arise from using different strains of organisms and animals, and the peculiar patterns of distribution of antibody levels to the three factors which might arise from differing immunization schedules. In the work of Ward *et al.* (1965) only factor 2 was used to immunize guinea-pigs. It is clear from other work (Stanley and Smith, 1963) that combining factor 1 with 2 significantly enhanced the immunogenicity of factor 2; however, addition of factor 3 to factors 2 or 1 + 2 diminished immunogenicity.

Finally, and perhaps most importantly, does injection of the toxin reproduce the major symptomatology of the disease? It is clear from the literature that both the British and American groups claimed to have demonstrated a parallelism between experimental infection and intoxication, thereby ascribing to anthrax toxin a central role in the pathogenesis of the disease. However, the nature of the intoxication process is a highly contentious issue. Clearly, as Lincoln and Fish (1970) rightly point out, there are problems in attempting this type of experiment. For example, in the infected animal, toxin is produced in parallel with the increase in the number of organisms, and therefore the terminal effects of toxin are produced in an already much weakened animal. In sharp contrast, experimental intoxication involves the injection of a preformed lethal dose of toxin consisting of arbitrary combinations of factors 1, 2 and 3 into a healthy animal. The detailed kinetics of production *in vivo* of individual factors, or indeed the order in which they individually interact with, or potentiate, the susceptible tissues for the concerted action of the synergistic complex, have never been firmly established; there is some evidence that factor 2 may be 'fixed' first as judged by studies on the rates of disappearance from the blood (Lincoln and Fish, 1970). No such problems complicated the earlier analyses of the classical bacterial toxaemias such as diphtheria and tetanus since these diseases are caused by organisms which remain highly localized at the primary sites of lodgement and secrete monomolecular toxins. But what is the primary mode of action of anthrax toxin which results in the eventual death of experimental animals? It is at this point that even a superficial reading of the literature reveals disagreements between the British and American groups on a number of points ranging from nomenclatural semantics to the pathophysiology of anthrax.

4. CONTROVERSIAL ASPECTS OF ANTHRAX TOXIN

4.1. PATHOPHYSIOLOGY OF ANTHRAX; WORK ON GUINEA-PIGS

Only two major comparative studies have been published in which host response to toxin *and* infection were correlated: the work of the British group (Smith *et al.*, 1955a, b; Smith, 1960) on guinea-pigs and that of the American group on primates (Klein *et al.*, 1962, 1966, 1968; Vick *et al.*, 1968; Remmele *et al.*, 1968). In the course of very extensive studies on anthrax intoxications, the Americans also used several additional species but concentrated mainly on the rat, in particular the Fischer 344 strain (Fish *et al.*, 1968a). We shall consider each of these three studies.

Smith and coworkers reproduced with toxin the majority of the quantitative and clinical changes observed in infection (Smith *et al.*, 1955a, b; Smith 1960): one notable exception was the lack of change in Na$^+$ levels in intoxicated plasma, although this was variable in plasma from infected guinea-pigs. There was no overt histopathological change observed until late in infection when changes in kidney tubules were observed; kidney dysfunction was correlated with a rise in levels of non-protein nitrogen and alkaline phosphatase in plasma. It was argued (see Smith 1960) that these were not necessarily primary changes caused by anthrax toxin, but secondary effects; this view was based on the fact that other forms of stress or trauma (e.g. crush syndrome or ischaemic shock) would induce similar changes in the kidney. No histopathology was observed in any other tissues—including the CNS (a conclusion based on unpublished work by Ross, quoted by Smith *et al.* (1955a,b), criticized by Lincoln *et al.* (1964) as unevaluable, but later conclusively substantiated by Bonventre *et al.* (1967), in the rhesus monkey and the rat)—and hence the effect of anthrax toxin was described in pathophysiological rather than tissue damaging terms. The syndrome was identified as secondary shock (Smith *et al.*, 1955b) and later more specifically as secondary oligaemic shock (Smith 1960). Now since much of the ensuing controversy between the two rival camps revolved around this point perhaps it would serve some useful purpose to remind ourselves of textbook definitions of relevant terms and concepts. There are four recognizable states in the development of this clinical condition—secondary shock. The *initial* stage is when the volume of circulating blood decreases but is not sufficient to cause serious symptoms. This is followed by a *compensatory* stage when blood volume is further reduced and the body begins to compensate. Blood pressure is maintained by vasoconstriction which selectively diverts blood from skin (hence the blanched appearance) and kidney and depletes main reservoirs like the spleen; blood supply to the central nervous system and mycocardium is maintained. The third or *progressive* stage is one in which the unfavourable changes (falling blood pressure, increasing vasoconstriction, accelerated heart rate, decreased pulse pressure, and oligouria) increase, and the compensatory mechanisms fail to compensate. This leads to the fourth or *irreversible* stage when treatment is hopeless, including transfusing blood which at this stage fails to raise blood pressure; the blood remains pooled in peripheral beds with no significant flow rate and hence poor perfusion of tissues. Now, this clinical state is often seen in infectious disease (Smith 1960), and it is generally agreed that there are many routes to this common clinical terminus. The specificity of disease lies in the inductive mechanism responsible for decreased blood flow and pressure. Clearly this could arise from any direct cardiotoxic action which would affect cardiac output. Alternatively, there are various indirect means whereby the haemodynamic situation could be deleteriously affected. Clearly, any mechanism which affects the venous return to the 'right heart' will affect the ability of the 'left heart' to pump sufficient arterial blood to the tissues. This could happen, for example, by alteration in permeability of capillaries, causing leakage of blood into extravascular spaces. Blocking mechanisms could also operate: release of vasoconstrictors could affect blood flow; physical blockage could also occur in the peripheral circulation. One must also consider effects on the autonomic nervous system, which plays an important role in controlling circulation: toxins may act directly or indirectly on key centres of the central nervous system—here arguments tend to become somewhat circular. Does such neurotoxic activity initiate some of the kinds of responses already described or merely augment or exacerbate them?

It is quite clear that Smith and coworkers established a conclusive case, based on quantitative and clinical data, that anthrax toxin induces a state of secondary oligaemic shock, at least in guinea-pigs; Lamb (1973), also describes the syndrome of patients who were acutely ill or who died from anthrax (or suspected anthrax) in terms of deep shock and cardiovascular failure. However, Lincoln and Fish (1970) claim that 'Smith and Stoner (1967), influenced by the work of Beall and Dalldorf (1966)' (on rats, referred to below), 'amended the secondary shock hypothesis to state that the primary cause of death is fluid loss due to increased permeability of blood vessels'. This is a strange comment since within the text-book definitions outlined above, such a mechanism is, if unchecked, an inducer of shock. Moreover, to claim that 'massive oedema and increased hematocrit changes are found only in the rat' (Lincoln and Fish, 1970) is simply not correct. One might cavil at the use of 'massive' and query the degrees of increase, but Smith and co-workers established that oedema formation and an increase in haematocrit values did take place in both infected and intoxicated guinea-pigs (Smith 1960).

4.2. Pathophysiology of Anthrax; Work on Primates

Let us now consider the work of the Americans on primates. This excellent series of extensive studies was designed to elucidate the cause of 'sudden', 'unexpected', or 'apoplectic' death in man which also occurs in herbivores and is so often preceded by no recognizable signs or symptoms; rhesus monkeys and chimpanzees (and also rabbits) were used in these studies. Changes in the blood cellular, chemical, and, in particular, gaseous elements were observed to occur mainly during the terminal stages of septicaemia or, much more rapidly, upon injection of sterile toxin. Where the measurements were common there was marked agreement between the general picture of anthrax infection and intoxication in primates (and rabbits) and that described by Smith and coworkers in guinea-pigs. The new features of the work included infection of primates by the aerosol as well as the intradermal route and quantitative studies on oxygen levels in the blood of infected or intoxicated animals; the terminal phase of the disease was associated with severe anoxia. This feature of the disease had been reported by Nordberg *et al.*, (1961, 1964) as occurring in rabbits after spore challenge.

Smith and Keppie (1962) dismissed measurements of anoxia as having little relevance in the elucidation of the anthrax syndrome: they claimed that, for a variety of reasons, meaningful measurements could not be carried out in the terminal stages of anthrax in guinea-pigs and that most of the drop in blood oxygen content could be accounted for by a rapidly increasing population of organisms. However, Remmele *et al.* (1968) showed that hypoxia is not only a terminal feature of infections with *B. anthracis* but is also induced by sterile anthrax toxin preparations, thus enhancing the possibility that this is a potentially relevant effect and diminishing the weight of Smith and Keppie's (1962) criticisms.

In addition, hyperesthesia was frequently observed in primates dying of anthrax before this was overshadowed by anoxic muscle fatigue; this 'tended to indicate involvement of the central nervous system' (Klein *et al.*, 1966), as postulated earlier by Lincoln *et al.* (1964). The interpretation of these findings was that anthrax toxin was acting on the central nervous control of the respiratory system and, by implication, all the other effects observed in the cardiovascular system were consequent upon the ensuing anoxia. This idea was supported by direct measurements of cortical electrical activity which was depressed in rhesus monkeys infected with *B. anthracis* (Klein *et al.*, 1968) or rhesus monkeys and chimpanzees intoxicated with whole anthrax toxin or factors 2 + 3 (Vick *et al.*, 1968). These changes were either paralleled by or preceded the onset of respiratory distress. Convincing evidence also came from experiments in which anthrax toxin was injected subdurally. The dose of toxin and the time required for the induction of complex major neuromuscular changes which led ultimately to anoxia and death were considerably reduced from 10,000 to 1000 rat units and 31 hr to 6–10 min respectively (Remmele *et al.*, 1968). Forced ventilation for only 10 min or two injections of isoproterenol (a β-adrenergic stimulant which would promote survival by dilating the pulmonary vasculature or increasing cardiac output) at 7 and 11 min post challenge saved otherwise doomed animals.

The unequivocal demonstration of the involvement of the central nervous system could thus provide the basis of an explanation of the sudden death alluded to above. However, Remmele *et al.* (1968) cautiously admit that the dramatic effects seen on subdural injection could be caused by a component which does not normally penetrate the blood–brain barrier. They regarded the latter possibility as improbable, believing that this route merely accelerates the effects of the toxin. This is a rather dangerous assumption until it is formally proven that there are no intermediates involved in bringing about the action of anthrax toxin (see Stephen and Pietrowski (1981) where a similar situation regarding the dynamics of endotoxin-induced febrile responses after either peripheral or intracerebral injection is summarized in respect of the role of possible intermediate mediators). In their work on primates, the American group observed no kidney dysfunction (Klein *et al.*, 1968) and hence dismissed the idea of slowly developing complications leading to secondary shock and death as proposed by Smith *et al.* (1955b) for guinea-pigs.

Smith and Stoner (1967) criticized the American postulate of a direct effect of anthrax toxin on the central nervous system since there 'does not seem to be any evidence for this and no definite lesions could be found in the central nervous system of infected animals by Ross (quoted by Keppie *et al.*, 1955)'. However, while American workers have also shown in published data that there is no overt histopathological change in the nervous system, they did produce positive evidence (alluded to above) for a functional derangement of the central nervous system: it became more than a postulate. Smith and Stoner (1967) however, cautioned against dismissing the notion that neurological changes of the kind postulated in the pre-1967 literature (and subsequently *shown* to exist in the post 1967 literature) could be caused by fluid loss consequent upon changes in vascular permeability induced by anthrax toxin. For example they quoted the earlier work of Green and Stoner which asserts that rapid death can occur after a period of apparent well-being in oligaemic states at high environmental temperatures.

4.3. PATHOPHYSIOLOGY OF ANTHRAX; WORK ON RATS

In the previous section we considered the two most complete and hence potentially the most relevant of the extant comparative studies on anthrax infection and intoxication. One must also, however, consider the work carried out by the American workers on rats; in particular, the Fischer 344 strain. This is noteworthy for at least two reasons. First, the rat is highly susceptible to anthrax toxin but relatively very resistant to infection by anthrax spores; there is in general a peculiar inverse relationship between susceptibilities of different species to infection and intoxication (Lincoln and Fish 1970). Second, arising from their studies on the effects of anthrax toxin on the rat, the American workers developed a system of nomenclature and a variable concept of anthrax toxin which were quite different from those of the British group.

In general the rat showed responses to toxin that were similar to those of other species examined but with some differences. First, gross pulmonary oedema occurred following injection of toxin; after spore challenge, fluid was observed only in the peritoneum *post mortem*. Both whole toxin (or factors 2 + 3) and live organisms induced highly significant and comparable rises in haematocrit value. Fish *et al.* (1968a) stated that the increase in haematocrit value induced by toxin was caused by the massive pulmonary oedema: electrophoretic analysis of nasal fluid yielded a protein profile indistinguishable from serum. The magnitude and timing of changes in electroencephalograms and the absence of comparable changes in electrocardiograms led these workers to postulate that death was due, as was claimed for primates (Remmele *et al.*, 1968) to the neurotoxic activities of anthrax toxin, causing acute respiratory embarrassment. However, Fish *et al.* (1968a) offered no explanations for haemotocrit increases caused by spore challenge. They asserted that death from anthrax was not attributable to shock even in the Fischer rat. These authors did confirm the work of Ross reported by Smith *et al.* (1955a, b) in guinea-pigs on the elevation of serum- and the depression of kidney-alkaline phosphatase. But, unlike Smith *et al.* (1955a,b), who interpreted their findings as confirmatory evidence supporting the identification of the shock syndrome in guinea-pigs infected with anthrax, Fish *et al.* (1968a) claimed that, because this effect was not specific to anthrax toxin, it must therefore be of doubtful significance. However, as stated above, there are many different routes to common pathological termini; it is the nature and specificity of the determinants that trigger these processes which is important in analyses of pathogenicity.

The validity of the rat model for studies in the pathogenesis of anthrax can be questioned. There are differences between the effects of intoxication and infection. Moreover, it is only in the rat that any histopathological changes are observed: hyperaemic areas, elevation of the thin endothelial cell membranes lining the pulmonary capillaries as a result of oedema, and the presence of granular thrombi were observed in the lung (Lincoln and Fish, 1970). Also, the Fisher strain 344 rat seems to be highly sensitive to factor 3 of the toxin complex, and this leads us to consider the last point of controversy.

Beall *et al.* (1962) independently discovered factor 3 of the anthrax toxin complex. For this and much subsequent work, Fischer 344 rats were used which proved to be highly sensitive to anthrax toxin or certain combinations of its components, i.e. factors 2 + 3. Arising from this study an alternative descriptive nomenclature emerged in which factor 1 became oedema factor (EF), 2 protective antigen (PA) and 3 lethal factor (LF). Bonventre (1970), in an eloquent essay on the nomenclature of microbial toxins, suggested that on semantic grounds the term factor should be dropped and substituted by component and that the terms oedema component, protective antigen component and lethal component should be adopted to describe factors 1, 2 and 3 respectively. Bonventre's argument is based on the fact that in the dictionary definition of factor is implied the dependence of one factor on another in order for the result to manifest itself. As far as lethality is concerned, this is precisely the case with anthrax toxin; there is no argument about the non-lethality of each individual purified component (Lincoln and Fish 1970). The concept of a plurality of toxins was once used explicitly (Lincoln *et al.*, 1964). Although this was later happily dropped it is still implicit in a descriptive nomenclature in which factor 1 is designated EF and factor 3, LF; however, both EF and LF require the presence of PA for oedema and lethality to be expressed. In fact the only component for which there has been demonstrated potentially relevant biological activity on its own is factor 2 (PA). It is immunogenic (Stanley and Smith, 1963), and induces an initial but transient electrical response in primates when injected intravenously (Vick *et al.*, 1968). The properties of the toxin are summarized in Table 2. Some of the apparent discrepancies between the American and British results can be explained on the basis of trace contamination in preparations of certain factors; the preparations obtained by the American workers were almost certainly more pure than those obtained by their British counterparts. Thus it is possible that the 1 + 3 combination which was weakly protective was contaminated with immunogenic traces of 2. The basis of the American nomenclature can be readily appreciated from Table 2. Factor 1 became oedema factor (EF) since in combination with 2 it produced oedema in guinea-pigs; this combination was not lethal to rats. Factor 3 became lethal factor (LF) since in combination with 2 it was highly lethal for rats; the low lethality of 1 + 2 for mice could be explained by trace contamination with 3 or inherent differences between rats and mice. However, some differences are not so easy to explain. For example, PA (Factor 2) protected guinea-pigs against spore challenge but not rats against either spores or toxin; in contrast, LF (Factor 3) protected both guinea-pigs and rats against spore challenge and rats against toxin challenge. This immunogenic role of Factor 3 *per se* disagrees with the British findings for guinea-pigs and would also make the description of Factor 2 as protective antigen somewhat untenable. Smith and coworkers showed that in the guinea-pig, factor 3 tended to depress the immunogenicity of factors 2 or 1 + 2. The question of the immunogenicity of the three factors is obviously a complex and contentious subject.

5. NEW DEVELOPMENTS

5.1. IN VITRO TOXIN PRODUCTION IN DEFINED MEDIUM

Ristroph and Ivins (1983) have produced a new fully synthetic medium which gives up to five-fold (strain-dependent) greater yields of toxin than media previously described; the practical implications of this work, are obvious. Results presented to validate the toxigenic potential of the new 'R' medium against other media are also worthy of comment additional to that made by the authors themselves. The data, recorded in the text as well as in Table 1 (Ristroph and Ivins, 1983) highlight the contribution of EF (factor I) to lethality of anthrax toxin, a fact which (as referred to earlier in this article) tends to become obscured by use of the 'descriptive' nomenclature for the components of this toxin.

5.2. GENETICS OF ANTHRAX TOXIN

Mikesell *et al.* (1983) have shown that the ability to make anthrax toxin in quantity is mediated by a plasmid whose molecular weight ranged from $60-130 \times 10^6$ depending on which of the 3 strains used in their study it was isolated from. The plasmid was heat labile and strains could be cured of the plasmid by multiple passage at $42.5°C$-a regime remarkably close to that used by Pasteur to produce his famous immunizing strains. Two such nontoxigenic vaccine strains were examined by Mikesell *et al.* (1983) and were shown not to possess the plasmid present in two nonencapsulated toxigenic strains (Sterne and V770-NPl-R) and a virulent capsulated toxigenic strain (Vollum 1B). The authors suggest, not unreasonably, that their findings provide an explanation for Pasteur's empirical observations. The converse was also true. Heat-treated non-toxigenic strains were successfully transformed by plasmid DNA from parent strain V770-NPl-R as judged by gel-diffusion and the production of both lethal and oedema producing activities.

TABLE 2. *Properties of Anthrax Toxin*

Factor(s)	Biological											
	oedema[1]			neurotoxicity[2]		lethality[3]			immunogenicity[4]			
									rat		guinea-pig	
											Challenged by	
											Spores	
	guinea pig skin	rabbit skin	rat lung	primate	rat	mouse	rat	primate	Toxin A[5]	Spores A[6]	A[6]	B[5]
1 (EF)	—	—		—	—	—	—		0	−1.9	−1.5	0
2 (PA)	—	—		±	—	—	—		0	−1.8	2.3	38
3 (LF)	—	—		—	—	—	—		100	1.2	2.5	0
1 + 2	100+	4+				+			36	3.3	4.3	70
1 + 3	—	—				+			100	4.0	1.5	14
2 + 3	—	—	+	+	+	2+	+	+	100	2.7[7]	3.0[7]	35
1 + 2 + 3	+	2+	+	+	+	4+	+	+	100	2.0	4.0	58

In this table an attempt has been made to summarize some of the properties of anthrax toxin to give a broad superficial view. In striving for concision some of the complexities inherent in the analysis of an interacting system have been unavoidably obscured: in particular the analysis of immunogenicity and the recognition of the unique or partial (be it additive or synergistic) contribution of each factor is impossible to convey in a simplified manner. It is hoped that this has been sufficiently compensated for by citing in footnotes the primary papers which ought to be consulted. Abbreviations I, EF etc., are as in the text, A and B identify data from the American and British groups respectively.

Physical and chemical

Stability: most stable at pH 7.4–7.8: susceptible to inactivation during storage and purification; may exist as conformers or aggregates; in general, stability high and dependent on environmental conditions and state of purity.

Heat lability: biological but not serological properties are heat labile.

Chemical: toxin components are proteins; factor I is an adenylate cyclase activated by calmodulin.

(1) Data derived from Fish et al. (1968b) (guinea-pig), Stanley and Smith (1961) (rabbit), Fish et al. (1968a) (rat). In the rat column, + indicates 'massive'; for the other two species n+ indicates the relative diameter and thickness of skin lesion (rabbit) or oedema-inducing titre (guinea-pig).

(2) Data derived or inferred from Fish et al. (1968a) (rat), Vick et al. (1968) (primate). + indicates ability of 10,000 rat units to cause changes in EEG patterns, when unprotected animals died; ± = transient effect on EEG.

(3) Data derived from Stanley and Smith (1961) (mouse, n+ indicates relative lethal potencies, statistical analysis showed synergy rather than additivity in combinations), Fish et al. (1968b) (rat, + indicates lethal effect which varied considerably with differing ratios of PA and LF), Vick et al. (1968) (primate, same animals and treatments as in neurotoxic tests).

(4) Data derived from Mahlandt et al. (1966) and Stanley and Smith (1963). It is impossible to convey in a simplified form the data from either group A or B or to readily compare the results between groups A and B. Mahlandt et al. (1966) in a comprehensive study used 5 criteria to assess immunity; only those results obtained by injecting the various factors singly or in combination at a level of 1.0 mg/factor and then challenging animals with live spores or toxin are cited here. Their data are expressed as % animals surviving or as immunity index defined as the log difference in challenge dose of organisms required to cause the same time to death in immunized group as controls. Stanley and Smith (1963) used only guinea-pigs, a smaller number of combinations of factors, and resistance to spore challenge as criterion for immunity.

(5) % of animals surviving challenge after immunization.

(6) Immunity index.

(7) 100 μg LF + 1000 μg PA.

The question as to whether the plasmid codes for structural or regulatory proteins was raised but is as yet not fully answered, but, heat-treated strains did show faint precipitin lines against anti-lethal factor (III) and anti-protective antigen (factor II); no results were given for anti-oedema factor (I).

5.3. MODE OF ACTION

In the last twelve months a new breakthrough has been achieved by Leppla (1982) shedding light on some aspects of the mode of action of this complex toxin. Three cells lines—a variant of Chinese hamster ovary (CHO) cells, baby hamster kidney (BHK) cells and fetal rhesus lung (FRL) cells-were exposed to toxin. EF was shown to be an inactive form of adenylate cyclase which was activated by some heat-stable factor present in CHO-cell lysates which could be replaced by calmodulin; PA and LF were not active. Exposure of the three cell lines to individual factors on their own caused no elevation of cAMP. However, combinations of PA and EF (but not PA and LF) caused large increases in cAMP levels in the three cell lines. The response observed is more rapid and greater than that induced by cholera toxin (CT). The latter is an ADP-ribosylating enzyme which modulates endogenous adenylate cyclase activity. In contrast to CT the anthrax complex is the cyclase and showed no lag phase; its effects were also instantly reversible upon washing the cells. This suggests that the enzyme is either rapidly degraded after internalization or, that it is not completely internalized but associated with the cell membrane in a manner allowing it to be readily removed. These facts together with the observations that LF would block the activity of EF can be summarized as in Fig. 1. This explains how LF blocks the effects of EF. They either compete for the same sites on PA, in which case the explanation is self-evident, or they bind to separate sites on PA which are situated such that occupancy of one occludes access to the other.

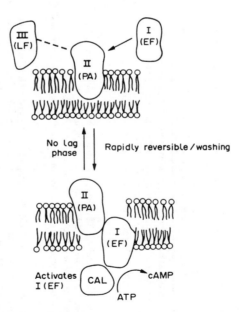

FIG. 1. *Mode of action of anthrax toxin.* This simplified schematic representation of the recent results obtained by Leppla (1982) helps explain some, but not all, of the known effects of anthrax toxin. First, factor II (PA) binds to the cell membrane. Second, factor I (EF) binds to factor II (PA). Third, bound factor I, or its biologically active site, is rapidly exposed to the cytosol when after interactions with calmodulin (CAL) it exhibits adenylate cyclase activity; the level of cAMP, a potent secretagogue, is thus elevated. Factor III (LF) can compete (– – – –►) with factor I (EF) for sites on bound factor II (PA). This picture helps explain the following. Factor II (PA) is a protective antigen, because it induces an antibody which blocks either the binding of factor I (EF) or attachment of itself to cell membrane, or both. Factor I (EF) is an edema factor by virtue of its adenylate cyclase activity (after activation by calmodulin). The ratio oedema/lethality for I + II is > than that for I + II + III: factor III competes with factor I for bound factor II. The model does not explain why I + II + III is more lethal than I + II.

One can extend these observations made *in vitro* to the *in vivo* situation. The model provides a basis for understanding the protective function of PA. Antibodies to PA could either block the initial attachment to the cell membrane of target organs *in vivo* or, prevent the binding of EF to PA, or both. The fact that cAMP is known to be a potent secretagogue could explain how the oedematous reaction occurs when PA and EF are injected into test animals, i.e. EF is, after activation, an oedema factor. Moreover, addition of LF (factor III) depressed oedema production as would be predicted by this model. The observations alluded to earlier that PA was probably fixed first may now be placed on a firmer basis since binding of PA is the apparent *sine qua non* for the expression of EF (and by implication) LF activities.

In my final comments on the significance of this new work and its bearing on the cause of death in animals I wish to draw attention to the third last paragraph in Leppla's important paper (1982). The first sentence is 'Previous work has not demonstrated that EF contributes to the virulence of *B. anthracis*' and the last, 'In the only studies directly implicating EF as a virulence factor, mice were found to be killed by lower doses of the lethal toxins (PA and LF) when EF was administered simultaneously'. This is unfortunate in that it perpetuates the whole controversy discussed above without any attempt to resolve it: the new American impetus could do just that. Insistence on the primacy of LF (with PA) as the cause of death (the Fort Detrick view) is to negate the significance of the new work. In contrast the case for the Smith Keppie view that, in experimental anthrax in guinea pigs animals died (as do humans (Lamb, 1973)) of secondary shock, is placed on a firmer basis with one (perhaps important) reservation. Smith and co-workers claimed that factor III (LF) decreased oedema but increased lethality (Stanley and Smith, 1961). The former but not the latter observation is explicable by the model which is therefore too simplistic to explain the effects of the holotoxin or there are other cell types where LF exerts its activity (with PA) in a manner as yet to be discovered.

6. IN CONCLUSION

It is fascinating that this problem has been reopened in the present climate of enquiry. If highly purified factors, obtained by appropriate combinations of newer techniques, derived from a range of strains of *B. anthracis* were used in the same biological tests in the same test animals, it would be only a matter of time before the phenomenological descrepancies were ironed out. It is highly probable that inherent differences would be observed between different species of experimental animals, leaving the perennial problem of deciding whether a man was a mouse, rat, guinea-pig or monkey when confronted with *B. anthracis*! The question of biochemical modes of action *in vivo* will only be solved if the primary target sites can be identified in individual species. This might be done by following the anatomical fate of appropriately labelled factors of the complex toxin administered by meaningful routes. The examination of effects of mutant strains deficient or excessively proficient in their abilities to produce one or more of the three factors might also be useful in this context. Attempts to identify and clone the genes responsible for the three factors would, if successful, open up new vistas of enquiry.

REFERENCES

AVAKYAN, A. A., KATZ, L. N., LEVINA, K. N. and PAVLOVA, I. B. (1965) Structure and composition of the *Bacillus anthracis* capsule. *J. Bacteriol.* **90**: 1082–1095.

BEALL, F. A. and DALLDORF, F. G. (1966) The pathogenesis of the lethal effect of anthrax toxin in the rat. *J. Infec. Dis.* **116**: 377–389.

BEALL, F. A., TAYLOR, M. J. and THORNE, C. B. (1962) Rapid lethal effects in rats of a third component found upon fractionating the toxin of *Bacillus anthracis*. *J. Bacteriol.* **83**: 1274–1280.

BONVENTRE, P. F. (1970) The nomenclature of microbial toxins: problems and recommendations. In: *Microbial Toxins Vol. I* p. 29–66, AJL. S. J., KADIS, S., and MONTIE, T. C. (Eds). Academic Press, New York.

BONVENTRE, P. F., SUEOKA, L. W., TRUE, C. W., KLEIN, F. and LINCOLN, R. (1967) Attempts to implicate the central nervous system as a primary site of action for *Bacillus anthracis* lethal toxin. *Fed. Proc.* **26**: 1549–1553.

BOYD, N. A., WALKER, P. D. and THOMSON, R. O. (1972) The prevention of experimental *Clostridium novyi* gas gangrene in high-velocity missile wounds by passive immunization. *J. Med. Microbiol.* **5**: 459–465.

COGGINS, C. H. (1963) Weapons of mass destruction. *Military Review.* **42**: 43–50.

DE, S. N. (1959) Enterotoxicity of bacteria-free culture filtrate of *Vibrio cholerae. Nature, London.* **183**: 1533–1534.

DE, S. N. and CHATTERJE, D. N. (1953) An experimental study of the mechanism of action of *Vibrio cholerae* on the intestinal mucous membrane. *J. Path. and Bact.* **66**: 559–562.

DERBIN, M. I., GARIN, N. S., TARUMOV, V. S., MIKHAILOV, V. V., SADOVOY, N. V., KUZMICH, M. K., FEDOROVA, N. V., SHEN, I. V., MUNTYANOV, P. V., KRAVETS, I. D., FOFANOV, P. E., ILYUKLIN, V. P. and SHUMILOV, G. P. (1977) Preparation and study of anthrax protective antigen. Report IV. Harmlessness, reactogenic properties, and efficacy of concentrated purified sorbed chemical anthrax vaccine. *Zh. Microbiol. Epidemiol. Immunobiol.* issue **8**: 115–120.

FEDOTOVA, I. M. (1970) Effect of anthrax toxin on cells in culture *in vitro. Arkh. Patol.* **32**: 30–33.

FEDOTOVA, I. M. (1974) The role of antitoxin in immunity to anthrax. *Zh. Microbiol. Epidemiol. Immunobiol.* issue **8**: 56–59.

FIELD, M., FROMM, D., WALLACE, C. K. and GREENOUGH, W. B. III. (1969) Stimulation of active chloride secretion in small intestine by cholera exotoxin. *J. Clin. Inv.* **48**: 24a.

FIELD, M., PLOTKIN, G. R. and SILEN, W. (1968) Effects of vasopressin, theophylline and cyclic adenosine monophosphate on short-circuit current across isolated rabbit ileal mucosa. *Nature, London*, **217**: 469–471.

FISH, D. C., KLEIN, F., LINCOLN, R. E., WALKER, J. S. and DOBBS, J. P. (1968a) Pathophysiological changes in the rat associated with anthrax toxin. *J. Inf. Dis.* **118**: 114–124.

FISH, D. C., MAHLANDT, B. G., DOBBS, J. P. and LINCOLN, R. E. (1968b) Purification and properties of *in vitro*-produced anthrax toxin components. *J. Bact.* **95**: 907–918.

HARRIS-SMITH, P. W., SMITH H. and KEPPIE, J. (1958) Production *in vitro* of the toxin of *Bacillus anthracis* previously recognized *in vivo. J. Gen. Microbiol.* **19**: 91–103.

IVÁNOVICS, G., MARJAI, E. and DOBOZY, A. (1968) The growth of purine mutants of *Bacillus anthracis* in the body of the mouse. *J. Gen. Microbiol.* **53**: 147–162.

KEPPIE, J., HARRIS-SMITH, P. W. and SMITH, H. (1963) The chemical basis of the virulence of *Bacillus anthracis* IX. Its aggressins and their mode of action. *Brit. J. Exp. Path.* **44**: 446–453.

KEPPIE, J., SMITH, H. and HARRIS-SMITH, P. W. (1953) The chemical basis of the virulence of *Bacillus anthracis*. II: some biological properties of bacterial products. *Brit. J. Exp. Path.* **34**: 486–496.

KEPPIE, J., SMITH, H. and HARRIS-SMITH, P. W. (1955) The chemical basis of the virulence of *Bacillus anthracis*. III: The role of the terminal bacteraemia in death of guinea pigs from anthrax. *Brit. J. Exp. Path.* **36**: 315–322.

KITASATO, S. (1889) On the tetanus bacillus. *Z. Hyg. Infektionskrank.* 7: 225–233. English translation. In: *Three centuries of microbiology.* LECHEVALIER, H. A. and SOLOTOROVSKY, M. pp. 158–160. McGraw-Hill Inc., 1965.

KLEIN, F., HODGES, D. R., MAHLANDT, G. G., JONES, W. I., HAINES, B. W. and LINCOLN, R. E. (1962) Anthrax toxin: causative agent in the death of rhesus monkeys. *Science*, **138**: 1331–1333.

KLEIN, F., LINCOLN, R. E., DOBBS, J. P., MAHLANDT, B. G., REMMELE, N. S. and WALKER, J. S. (1968) Neurological and physiological responses of the primate to anthrax infection. *J. Inf. Dis.* **118**: 97–103.

KLEIN, F., WALKER, J. S., FITZPATRICK, D. F., LINCOLN, R. E., MAHLANDT, B. G., JONES, W. I., DOBBS, J. P. and HENDRIX, K. J. (1966) Pathophysiology of anthrax. *J. Inf. Dis.* **116**: 123–138.

KUZMICH, M. K., DERBIN, M. I., GARIN, N. S., KRAVETS, I. D., SHENTSEV, I. V., TARUMOV, V. S., GORLANOV, A. A., SADOVOY, N. V. and FEDOROVA, N. V. (1976) Preparation and study of the anthrax protective antigen. Report II. Development of test-preparations for the assessment of the quality of anthrax chemical vaccines and of the antigens obtained at various stages of its preparation. *Zh. Microbiol. Epidemiol. Immunobiol.* issue **10**: 94–98.

LAMB, R. (1973) Anthrax. *Brit. Med. J.* **1**: 157–159.

LEPPLA, S. H. (1982) Anthrax toxin edema factor: A bacterial adenylate cyclase that increases cyclic AMP concentrations in eukaryotic cells. *Proc. Natl. Acad. Sci. U.S.A.* **79**: 3162–3166.

LESNYAK, O. T. (1975) Toxic properties of the exotoxin of the anthrax vaccine strain CT-1 in experiments on animals. *Zh. Microbiol. Epidemiol. Immunobiol.* issue **9**: 97–99.

LESNYAK, O. T. and SALTYKOV, R. A. (1974) Preparation of exotoxin of anthrax vaccine strain ST-1. *Zh. Microbiol. Epidemiol. Immunobiol.* issue **2**: 110–113.

LINCOLN, R. E. and FISH, D. C. (1970) Anthrax toxin. In: *Microbial Toxins* Vol. III p. 361–414, MONTIE, T. C., KADIS, S. and AJL, S. J. (Eds). Academic Press, New York.

LINCOLN, R. E., WALKER, J. S., KLEIN, F. and HAINES, B. W. (1964) Anthrax. *Adv. in Vet. Sci.* **9**: 327–368.

MAHLANDT, B. G., KLEIN, F., LINCOLN, R. E., HAINES, B. W., JONES, W. I. and FRIEDMAN, R. H. (1966) Immunologic studies of anthrax. IV. Evaluation of the immunogenicity of three components of anthrax toxin. *J. Immunol.* **96**: 727–733.

MCCARTNEY, A. C. and ARBUTHNOTT, J. P. (1978) Mode of action of membrane-damaging toxins produced by staphylococci. In: *Bacterial toxins and cell membranes* p. 89–127. JELJASZEWICZ, J. and WADSTRÖM, T. (Eds).

MCCRUMB, F. R., MERCIER, S., ROBIC, J., BOUILLAT, M., SMADEL, J. E., WOODWARD, T. E. and GOODNER, K. (1953) Chloramphenicol and terramycin in the treatment of pneumonic plague. *Am. J. Med.* **14**: 284–293.

MIKESELL, P., IVINS, B. E., RISTROPH, J. D. and DREIER, T. M. (1983) Evidence for plasmid-mediated toxin production in *Bacillus anthracis.* **39**: 371–376.

MILES, A. A. (1955) The meaning of pathogenicity. In: *Mechanisms of microbial pathogenicity.* Symp. Soc. Gen. Microbiol. **5**: 1–16.

NORDBERG, B. K., SCHMITERLOW, G. G. and HANSEN, H. J. (1961) Pathophysiological investigations into the terminal course of experimental anthrax in the rabbit. *Acta. Path. Microbiol. Scand.* **53**: 295–318.

NORDBERG, B. K., SCHMITERLOW, G. G. and HANSEN, H. J. (1964) Further pathophysiological investigations into the terminal course of experimental anthrax in the rabbit. *Acta. Path. Microbiol. Scand.* **60**: 108–116.

NUNGESTER, W. J. (1967) Proceedings of the conference on the progress in the understanding of anthrax. *Fed. Proc.* **26**: 1482–1571.

REMMELE, N. S., KLEIN, F., VICK, J. A., WALKER, J. S., MAHLANDT, B. G. and LINCOLN, R. E. (1968) Anthrax toxin: primary site of action. *J. Inf. Dis.* **118**: 104–113.

RICH, V. (1980) Incident at military village no. 19. *Nature*, **284**: 294.

RISTROPH, J. D. and IVINS, B. E. (1983) Elaboration of *Bacillus anthracis* antigens in a new, defined culture medium. *Infect. Immun.* **39**, 483–486.

SMITH, H. (1958) The use of bacteria grown *in vivo* for studies on the basis of their pathogenicity. *Ann. Rev. Microbiol.* **12:** 77–102.

SMITH, H. (1960) The biochemical response to bacterial injury. In: *The biochemical response to injury: a symposium organized by the council for international organizations of medical sciences, established under the joint auspices of UNESCO and WHO*, p. 341–359, STONER, H. B. and THREFALL, C. J. (Eds). Blackwell Scientific Oxford.

SMITH, H. (1964) Microbial behaviour in natural and artificial environments. In: *Microbial behaviour*, in vivo *and* in vitro. Symp. Soc. Gen. Microbiol. **14:** 1–29.

SMITH, H. and KEPPIE, J. (1962) The terminal phase of anthrax. *Brit. J. Exp. Path.* **43:** 684–686.

SMITH, H., KEPPIE, J. and STANLEY, J. L. (1953a) A method for collecting bacteria and their products from infections in experimental animals, with special reference to *Bacillus anthracis*. *Brit. J. Exp. Path.* **34:** 471–476.

SMITH, H., KEPPIE, J. and STANLEY, J. L. (1953b) The chemical basis of the virulence of *Bacillus anthracis*. I: Properties of bacteria grown *in vivo* and preparation of extracts. *Brit. J. Exp.* 447–485.

SMITH, H., KEPPIE, J. and STANLEY, J. L. (1955a) The chemical basis of the virulence of *Bacillus anthracis*. V. The specific toxin produced by *B. anthracis in vivo*. *Brit. J. Exp. Path.* **36:** 460–472.

SMITH, H., KEPPIE, J., STANLEY, J. L. and HARRIS-SMITH, P. W. (1955b) The chemical basis of the virulence of *Bacillus anthracis*. IV: Secondary shock as the major factor in death of guinea pigs from anthrax. *Brit. J. Exp. Path.* **36:** 323–335.

SMITH, H. and STONER, H. B. (1967) Anthrax toxic complex. *Fed. Proc.* **26:** 1554–1557.

STANLEY, J. L. and SMITH, H. (1961) Purification of factor I and recognition of a third factor of the anthrax toxin. *J. Gen. Microbiol.* **26:** 49–66.

STANLEY, J. L. and SMITH, H. (1963) The three factors of anthrax toxin: their immunogenicity and lack of demonstrable enzymic activity. *J. Gen. Microbiol.* **31:** 329–337.

STEPHEN, J. and PIETROWSKI, R. A. (1981) *Bacterial Toxins*. Thomas Nelson.

STERNE, M. (1967) Distribution and economic importance of anthrax. *Fed. Proc.* **26:** 1493–1495.

STRANGE, R. E. and THORNE, C. B. (1958) Further purification studies on the protective antigen of *Bacillus anthracis* produced *in vitro*. *J. Bacteriol.* **76:** 192–202.

THORNE, C. B., MOLNAR, D. M. and STRANGE, R. E. (1960) Production of toxin *in vitro* by *B. anthracis* and its separation into two components. *J. Bact.* **79:** 450–455.

VICK, J. A., LINCOLN, R. E., KLEIN, F., MAHLANDT, B. G., WALKER, J. S. and FISH, D. C. (1968) Neurological and physiological responses of the primate to anthrax toxin. *J. Inf. Dis.* **118:** 85–96.

VAN HEYNINGEN, W. E. (1955) The role of toxins in pathology. In: *Mechanisms of microbial pathogenicity*. Symp. Soc. Gen. Microbiol. **5:** 17–39.

VYLCHEV, V., SIROMASHKOVA, M. and MIRCHEVA, I. (1976) Standardization of a protective anthrax preparation. *Zh. Microbiol. Epidemiol. Immunobiol.* issue **3:** 53–56.

WARD, M. K., McGANN, V. G., HOGGE, A. L., HUFF, M. L., KANODE, R. G. and ROBERTS, E. O. (1965) Studies on anthrax infections in immunized guinea pigs. *J. Inf. Dis.* **115:** 59–67.

WOODIN, A. M. (1970) Staphylococcal leucocidin. In: *Microbial toxins* Vol. III. p. 327–355. MONTIE, T. C., KADIS, S. and AJL, S. J. (Eds). Academic Press.

CHAPTER 20

BACILLUS CEREUS TOXINS

P. C. B. TURNBULL

*Food Hygiene Laboratory, Central Public Health Laboratory,
Colindale Avenue, London, NW9 5HT, England**

1. GENERAL INTRODUCTION

1.1. PATHOGENICITY OF BACILLUS CEREUS

Wide recognition of the pathogenicity of *Bacillus cereus* has been slow to develop; for years, workers encountering *B. cereus* were only concerned with ensuring that it was not the closely related *B. anthracis*. Also contributing to this slow recognition was the state of confusion of the taxonomy within the genus *Bacillus* before Smith *et al.* (1952) brought some order to this.

However, there is ample evidence (Goepfert *et al.* 1972; Gilbert 1979; Tuazon *et al.* 1979; Turnbull *et al.* 1979a; O'Day *et al.* 1981a,b; Anon, 1983; Turnbull and Kramer, 1983) that, under the guise of a variety of names up to 1952 and, since then, as *B. cereus*, this organism has been associated from as early as 1898 with abscess formation, bacteremia and septicemia, cellulitis, ear and eye infections, endocarditis, gastroenteritis, meningitis, kidney and urinary tract infections, osteomyelitis, puerperal sepsis, pulmonary infections and wound infections sometimes gangrenous. Frequently these infections have been severe, occasionally fatal. The organism is also known in veterinary circles particularly in relation to bovine mastitis (Jones and Turnbull, 1981; Francis, 1984).

B. cereus has also been brought into particular focus in approximately the last 20 years in the context of food poisoning. Initially, interest was in what is now described for convenience as the 'diarrheal-type' syndrome characterized by symptoms predominantly or diarrhea and abdominal cramps 8–16 hr after eating the incriminated food; the types of foods involved have ranged widely from meats and vegetable dishes to pastas, desserts, cakes, sauces and milk (Gilbert, 1979). More recently, it has become accepted that *B. cereus* is the etiological agent of a second distinct type of food poisoning referred to as the 'emetic-type' syndrome notably characterized by vomiting after a short incubation period of < 1–5 hr. All but a small number of recorded incidents have been associated with rice dishes. It is becoming apparent from studies on the factors of *B. cereus* thought responsible for these two forms of food poisoning that the types of food involved are relevant from the standpoint of the growth conditions they provide.

Reports of the diarrheal-type of food poisoning were quite numerous between 1950 and 1976, particularly during the 1960's (Gilbert, 1979) and, indeed, *B. cereus* was recorded as the third most common cause of food poisoning in Hungary between 1960 and 1968 (Ormay and Novotny, 1970). Interestingly, these reports have become steadily less numerous in the last decade. Virtually all of them, however, suffered from the common epidemiological defect that the *B. cereus* was not isolated from patient specimens but only from the suspect food. This defect and its interpretation in the light of human volunteer and monkey feeding test results is expanded at the beginning of section 6.1 p 424 on 'Loop fluid-inducing/skin test/necrotic toxin'. One almost classic. *B. cereus* diarrheal-type outbreak was eventually described by Giannella and Brasile (1979); *B. cereus* was isolated from both the implicated

* Present Address: Vaccine Research and Production Laboratory, Public Health Laboratory Service Centre for Applied Microbiology and Research, Porton Down, Salisbury, Witshire SP4 0JG, England.

397

TABLE 1. *The toxins of* Bacillus cereus—*present status*

Toxin	Characteristics

(1) 'Diarrheagenic' toxin
    Fluid accumulation factor
    Vascular permeability factor
    Dermonecrotic toxin
    Intestino-necrotic toxin
    Mouse lethal factor 1
	Two proteinous moieties, precise interrelationships undetermined. MW *ca.* 50,000, pI 5.1 and 5.6 respectively.
	Susceptible to trypsin and pronase digestion. Antigenic. May have role in non-gastrointestinal infections

(2) Cereolysin
    Hemolysin I (H-I)
    Mouse lethal factor 2
	Thiol-activated cytolysin.
	Thermolabile antigenic protein MW 49–59,000, pI 6.3–6.7. Inactivated by cholesterol and antistreptolysin 0 in horse serum. Lethal to mice.

(3) Secondary hemolysin Hemolysin II (H-II)	Thermolabile antigenic protein, MW 29–34,000, pI 4.92. Susceptible to pronase, pepsin and trypsin. *In vitro* activity unaffected by thiols, cholesterol and antistreptolysin 0. *In vivo* toxicity not yet established.

(4) Phospholipases C
    Lecithinase
    Egg yolk turbidity factor
	Relatively stable metallo-enzymes.
	    (a) Phosphatidylcholine hydrolase, MW 23,000, pI disputed 6.5–8.5.
	    (b) Phosphatidylinositol hydrolase, MW 29,000 (Phosphatasemic factor), pI 5.4.
	    (c) Sphingomyelinase, MW 24,000, pI 5.6. Hemolytic depending on sphingomyelin content of erythrocyte.

(5) Emetic	Highly stable compound(s), not formed above 40°C. Survive(s) conditions of 126°C × 1.5 hr, pH extremes and exposure to trypsin and pepsin. May be associated with sporulation or rice breakdown products?
(6a) Toxin of Ezepchuk & Fluer (1973)	Thermolabile antigenic protein MW 57,000. Inactivated by 60°C × 20 min. Lethal to mice and rabbits. I.v. injection induces emesis in cats. Possibly related to (1).
(b) Toxin of Ezepchuk *et al.* (1979)	MW 100,000. 'Previously unknown protein'. Not sensitive to trypsin. Lethal to mice; injection in cats produced mild fever but no emesis. Rabbit loop negative but alters skin permeability. Not compared by the authors with 6(a).

turkey loaf and fecal specimens of 14 symptomatic patients. Subsequent examinations not included in that report showed that the food isolate and isolates from all the patients were serotype 19 (Gilbert and Parry, 1977). However, the numbers of *B. cereus* in the food (1.2×10^3/g) were lower than might have been anticipated and the isolates were not found to be especially good producers of the toxin purported to be the diarrheal factor.

The emetic-type episodes in general have not suffered from the same epidemiological anomalies as the diarrheal-type—the median *B. cereus* count in the foods from 53 episodes where this was assessed was 2×10^7/g while numbers in patients' feces have been as high as 3×10^9/g (Gilbert, 1979). Serotyping has frequently provided supportive evidence of identity between the food and fecal isolates.

The symptoms of the emetic-type syndrome closely resemble those of *Staphylococcus aureus* food poisoning and it was some years before it became accepted that it was *B. cereus* and not *S. aureus* that was causing this food poisoning.

An attempt has been made in Tables 3–5 to pinpoint the current status of *B. cereus* as a pathogen in food poisoning and other clinical conditions as based on published reports. There is reason to believe that its pathogenicity in these conditions is attributable to its production of certain toxic metabolites. This chapter reviews what is known about these

TABLE 2. *Histories of Bacillus cereus strains referred to in the text*

Strain	Serotype	Isolated from	Country of Origin	Reference in relation to original isolation	VPR Category	VPR Necrosis	Incident designation
4433/73 (NCTC 11145)	2	Meat loaf	USA	Midura et al. (1970)	5	3+	Diarrheal
B-4ac(4430/73)	NT	Pea soup		Spira & Goepfert (1975)	2	0	Diarrheal
B-4acL	n	Derivative of B-4ac		Parker & Goepfert (1978)	n	—	—
B-5ac	n		Netherlands (Dr. D. Mossel)		n	—	—
667/78							
668/78							
669/78							
671/78	2	Postoperative Wound Infection	Ireland	Fitzpatrick et al. (1979)	4/5	3+	Clinical
4810/72 (NCTC 11143)	1	Vomitus	UK	PHLS CDR 1972 No. 32	2	0	Emetic
B-48	n	NK	USA	Bonventre & Eckert (1963b)	—	—	?
C9b	n	Derivative of B-48	USA	Coolbaugh & Williams (1978)	—	—	?
No. 96	NT	NK	USSR	Ezepchuk & Fluer (1973)	5	3+	?
4096/73	4	Rice	UK	PHLS CDR 1973 No. 41	3	±	Emetic
2141/74	11	Wound infection	UK	Turnbull et al. (1977a)	3/4	2+	Clinical
243/80(IP 5832)	NSA	?	France	Schaeffer (1950)	2/3	±	?
2532/74	NT	Raw rice	UK	Turnbull (1976)	5	3+	Routine
4370/75	6	Barbecued chicken	Canada	Todd et al. (1974)	5	3+	Diarrheal
837/76	17	Postoperative wound Infection	UK	Turnbull et al. (1977b)	5	3+	Clinical
2769/77	NT	Lobster pate	UK	PHLS CDR 1978 No. 28	3	0	Diarrheal
ATCC 14579 NCTC 2599	n	Baltimore milk	USA	Lawrence & Ford (1916)			?
ATCC 7004	n	Pasteurized milk	USA	USDA Agr. Monogr. 16:58 (1952)	—	—	?
NVH 322	n	Food poisoning	Norway	Fossum (1963)	n	—	Diarrheal
171	1	Vegetable stew	Denmark	Jorgensen (1976)	n	—	Diarrheal
175	NT	Unrecorded food	Denmark	Jorgensen (1976)	n	—	Diarrheal

n = not done; NT = not typable; NSA = non-specific agglutination; PHLS CDR = Public Health Laboratory Service Weekly Communicable Disease Report.

TABLE 3   Bacillus cereus *infections excluding food poisoning* (1898–1984)

Infection	Number of published reports (number of cases involved if different)	
	1898–1949	1950–1984
Abscesses	5	3(9)
Bacteremia/Septicemia	—	12(± 20)
Cellulitis	—	1
Cerebral and respiratory tract necrosis	—	1
Conjunctivitis and panophthalmitis	6 (many)	7* (>10)
Endocarditis	—	4(8)
Meningitis	3	9
Middle ear infection	—	1
Neonatal infection	—	3(>10)
Osteomyelitis	—	2
Puerperal sepsis	2	—
Pulmonary infections including pneumonia	4	9
Pyelonephritis and urinary tract infection	1	1
Vaginitis	—	1
Wounds; postoperative and other; several 'gangrenous'	2	8(>10)
Bovine mastitis; several gangrenous and lethal	—	20 (many)
Bovine abortion	—	4
Caprine mastitis	—	1

* Including one report of a corneal ulcer caused by *B. thuringiensis*

TABLE 4. *The reported incidence of* Bacillus cereus *as a food poisoning agent relative to other bacterial food poisoning agents**

Reporting Centre	Approximate percentages of all outbreaks and cases in which the etiology was established									
	Salmonella		*Staph. aureus*		*C. perfringens*		*B. cereus*		*Other*	
	Outbreaks	Cases	Outbreaks	Cases	Outbreaks	Cases	Outbreaks	Cases	Outbreaks	Cases
England and Wales 1969–79	88	77	2.5	3	8	19	1.3	0.5	0.2	0.4
Scotland 1973–79	61	56	4	2.5	30	39	4	1	1	1
USA 1972–78	36	43	30	28	10	14	2	1	25	14
Canada 1973–76	31	40	41	30	15	27	6**	2**	6	1
Hungary 1960–68	24	25	56	34	n	n	8	15	12	16

* Modified and updated from Turnbull (1979a) with acknowledgements to the authors cited there.
** 'Bacillus species'.
n = not listed.

TABLE 5. *World Reports on* Bacillus cereus *Food Poisoning* (to 1980)

Diarrheal type *(since 1950)*		Vomiting type *(since 1971)*	
Country	*Approx. No. of incidents	Country	*Approx. No. of incidents
Hungary 1960–68	117	UK	120
Finland	50	Canada	10
Netherlands	11	Netherlands	10
Canada	9	Japan	10
USA	9	Australia	7
USSR 1967–70	6 outbreaks 29 isolated cases	USA	6
		India	3
Norway 1950–58	4	Finland	1
Australia, Rumania Sweden, UK	2 each		
Denmark, Germany, India, Italy, Japan, Poland.	1 each		

* Figures and type designations collated within acknowledged limitations in the extent or type of information available to the author.

metabolites. A summary of their characteristics is given in Table 1. A list of the histories of the principal strains used in studies referred to in the text is given in Table 2.

2. METABOLITES OF BACILLUS CEREUS CONTENDING FOR TOXIN STATUS

An enormous range of extracellular metabolites are known to be elaborated by *B. cereus* and the closely related *B. thuringiensis*. Table 6 lists many of these but does not claim to be exhaustive.

In the case of the majority of the well-described metabolites of *B. cereus*, there is little reason to believe they are involved in the pathogenic activities of the organism and that, therefore, they should be considered 'toxins'. Some, such as cereolysin and phospholipase-C, are fairly well characterized, but their role, if any, in the pathogenesis of *B. cereus* infections remains unclear. A third group consists of factors, poorly defined in chemical terms, but which on the basis of experimental evidence, are thought to be likely agents of *B. cereus* virulence. The earliest recognized of these was 'lethal toxin', the precise nature of which still remains unclear. More recently, the existence of two distinct enterotoxins has been proposed in relation to the two types of food poisoning that have been described, the diarrheal-type and the emetic-type. There is now some reason to believe the toxin originally studied in relation to the diarrheal-type syndrome is also of consequence in non-gastrointestinal *B. cereus* infections.

3. LETHAL TOXIN

3.1. INTRODUCTION, HISTORY AND EARLY PATHOGENICITY STUDIES

Given the likelihood already stated that the anthrax-like bacilli recorded before 1952 under various names, such as *B. anthracoides*, *B. anthracis similis*, *B. pseudoanthracis* (reviewed by Grierson, 1928) were frequently, if not invariably what are now classified as *B. cereus*, then the pathogenic activity of this organism as based on mouse lethality has been known since the first decade of this century.

The report of Bainbridge (1903) appears to provide the first demonstration of the lethal effect in mice of a strain of *B. anthracoides* isolated from a bundle of Chinese horse-hairs being examined for anthrax spores. The mice were inoculated s.c. with 0.25–1 ml of 24 hr broth cultures and death was observed over 24–48 hr. Since guinea-pigs survived similar infections, the author concluded that the pathogenic powers of the organism were limited. It is less easy to be certain that at least some of the 25 soil isolates described by Stregulina (1906) as '*B. subtilis*' were probably *B. cereus*, but 16 of these were lethal to guinea-pigs.

Thereafter, there were a significant number of reports of pathogenicity tests of this type on isolates from clinical problems as reviewed by Grierson (1928) whose own pathogenic *B. anthracoides* isolates were, in the opinion of McGaughey and Chu (1948), mostly *B. cereus*.

Interest seems to have waned in the 20 years between these two reports and only two publications were found (Clark, 1937; Burdon, 1947) referring to *B. cereus* pathogenicity. Clark (1937) compared the virulence of a blood culture isolate on i.p. injection of whole-cell cultures in guinea pigs with soil isolates and noted (1) variations in virulence among different strains; (2) that virulence varied with the culture medium employed and (3) that virulence decreased with continuous subculture. Burdon (1947) noted, in common with some of the earlier workers, that virulence could be enhanced by animal passage. He also related the virulence to hemolytic activity.

3.2. DEMONSTRATION OF TOXICITY AND STUDIES TO DETERMINE ITS NATURE

Chu (1949) appears to be the first to have demonstrated the lethal activity in cell-free filtrates (the type of filter is not given). He considered that the metabolite involved might be analogous to *Clostridium perfringens* α-toxin having both lecithinase and hemolytic as well as lethal activities; his ammonium sulfate precipitation method of purification failed to separate these three activities but he was cautious enough to admit that his preparation was too crude to be certain that a single entity was responsible for all three activities. This appears also to be the first reference to i.v. injection in mice (as opposed to other routes) as a measure of lethal activity presumably following procedures already in use for the study of *C. perfringens* α-toxin.

The 1960's saw a resurgence of interest in the lethal activity of *B. cereus* as related both to differentiation of *B. anthracis* from *B. cereus* and to clinical *B. cereus* infections in themselves, and it had become fully accepted that the activity was due to a filterable toxin or toxins. This was well reviewed by Bonventre and Johnson (1970) and Goepfert *et al.* (1972). There was support for the idea that the lethal activity was related to phospholipase and hemolysin (Chu, 1949; Bonventre and Eckert, 1963a,b; Bonventre, 1965) in the fact that *B. anthracis*, which is non-hemolytic and only produces a weak lecithovitellin reaction, did not elaborate a lethal factor resembling that of *B. cereus*.

Molnar (1962), however, using differential ammonium sulphate precipitation, ethanol treatment and calcium phosphate gel chromatography of fritted-glass culture filtrates supplied evidence that the lethal activity was separable from the phospholipase. Slein and Logan (1963) found that fractionation of a culture filtrate (type of filter not given) of two ATCC strains of *B. cereus* resulted in the separation of two fractions with phospholipolytic activity. One of these factors had no hemolytic or lethal powers; while it was less clear for the second fraction, they felt the evidence indicated that the same was true for this also.

That *C. perfringens* α-toxin is a single entity possessing all three activities was subsequently re-examined and confirmed (Park *et al.* 1977). Johnson (1966), Johnson and Bonventre (1966, 1967) and Bonventre and Johnson (1970) finally showed that the analogy between the *B. cereus* toxin and *C. perfringens* α-toxin did not hold. By the use of (1) 2–4 per cent methanol in the growth medium which specifically inhibited phospholipase synthesis, (2) trypsin which destroyed hemolytic and lethal activities, (3) exposure for 24 hr to pH 2.2, which eliminated hemolysin while reducing phospholipase to 19 per cent and lethal activity to only 70 per cent of their zero time levels, and (4) growth in dialyzed and undialyzed beef infusion broth, which resulted in different lethality titers but identical hemolysin titers, they obtained evidence of non-identity between the three activities. They demonstrated that, while all three appeared simultaneously in a complex growth medium, the kinetics of synthesis of each was different. Furthermore, although they were unable to obtain the lethal factor free of either phospholipase or hemolysin, chromatography on Sephadex G-200 and G-75 provided yet more evidence of non-identity between the three activities. Finally, they showed that the *B. cereus* products were antigenically unrelated to *C. perfringens* α-toxin and that, while *C. perfringens* lethality was susceptible to chelating agents, that of *B. cereus* was not (implying that the *B. cereus* factor does not require free divalent cations for activity).

3.3. PROGRESS IN PURIFICATION AND CHARACTERIZATION OF LETHAL FACTOR

In their 1970 review, Bonventre and Johnson pointed out that the relative contributions to toxicity of individual products in *B. cereus* culture filtrates could not be deduced because investigations up to that time had been largely carried out using crude culture filtrates. Although, in the decade since then, some progress has been made, two problems have contributed to it being less than might have been anticipated. The first is the general problem shared by all studying bacterial metabolites—that the criteria for defining purity became ever harder with the rapid appearance of increasingly sophisticated purification methods; secondly, the products of *B. cereus* considered most likely to be at the basis of its pathogenic actions (namely a lethal toxin, hemolysin, phospholipase-C and a so-called enterotoxin) have proved especially hard to separate.

The first report of successful purification of a lethal toxin free of both hemolysin and lecithinase was that of Ezepchuk and Fluer (1973) using Biogel (P-150, according to Spira, 1974) column chromatography following ammonium sulfate precipitation of the culture filtrate of strain No. 96. Unfortunately the materials and methods used were not documented in sufficient detail to allow confirmatory work but evidence of purity as based on sedimentation analysis during ultracentrifuge precipitation, electrophoresis, gel diffusion and immunoelectrophoresis was supplied. Analysis of the purified toxin showed it be a protein free of nucleic acids with a sedimentation coefficient of 4.65 corresponding to the MW of 55,000–60,000. Amino acid analysis revealed that it consisted of 18 amino acids; cystine, cysteine and oxyproline were not found. The toxin was inactivated by 6M urea, hydrogen cyanide and 0.8 per cent formalin, its properties 'modified' by ferrous sulphate and other unspecified salts of heavy metals and toxicity reduced by treatment with 0.01 M and 0.05 M EDTA. The last finding is in conflict with that of Johnson and Bonventre (above) and in part with those of Turnbull *et al.* (1979b—see section 6.4, p 435–436). Ezepchuk and Fleur (1973) interpreted their results as indicating firstly the importance to active toxicity of hydrogen bonding in the spatial configuration and in the attachment of carboxyl groups, and secondly the presence of metal ions within the molecule.

The toxin was fatal to rabbits as well as mice but apparently not to guinea pigs; 7–13 mg/kg body weight injected into cats (presumably i.v.) led to violent vomiting, retching, choking and weakness with onset at 50–60 min. In subsequent reports (Gorina *et al.*, 1975, 1976) the minimum i.v. dose provoking emesis in cats was given as 70–80 μg/kg body weight and the minimum lethal dose for mice was 15 mg/kg (or about 300 μg/mouse). Other reports (in Russian) relating to the isolation, purification and characterization of this toxin by these workers are cited in these papers.

Spira and Goepfert (1972b), Glatz and Goepfert (1973), Glatz *et al.* (1974), Spira (1974) and Spira and Goepfert (1975) observed a close correspondence between the lethal activity and the rabbit loop fluid-inducing and guinea-pig and rabbit skin test activities discussed later in detail under 'Loop fluid-inducing/skin test/necrotic toxin'. Spira and Goepfert (1972a) noted that, in initial rabbit ligated ileal loop tests, most of the rabbits in which one or more of the loops were strongly positive died within 10 hr. Fractions obtained from Sephadex G-75 chromatography of ammonium sulphate precipitated concentrated cell-free filtrates of strain B-4ac which possessed loop-active factor essentially free of hemolysin and phospholipase also possessed the abilities to kill mice and alter the permeability of blood vessels in rabbit skin (Spira and Goepfert, 1975). As a group, however, they remained cautious and felt that, while their evidence strongly supported the possibility that a single protein was responsible for loop, skin and lethal activities, this remained unproven (Spira and Goepfert, 1975).

Turnbull *et al.* (1979b), in examining cell-free culture filtrates of 88 isolates of *B. cereus* from a wide variety of sources, found that, while loop fluid accumulation and vascular permeability alterations correlated almost ideally, their relationship to mouse lethality remained anomalous. Flat bed electrofocusing of culture filtrates of 4433/73, however, yielded fractions in which the loop and skin active factor was well separated from cereolysin and phospholipase-C (see p 431) which focussed coincidentally. Interestingly, both the loop/skin active and the cereolysin/phospholipase fractions were lethal to mice. Using EDTA to neutralize phospholipase-C and heating to destroy hemolysin in the cereolysin/ phospholipase fractions, supported by tests on phospholipase separated from the other activities by Sephadex G-100 chromatography, J. M. Kramer and P. C. B. Turnbull (unpublished results) have determined that lethality in the cereolysin/phospholipase eluate was attributable to the cereolysin.

Thus it became apparent that the lethal activity of a culture filtrate of a strain of *B. cereus* is the result of the combined activities of at least two separate toxins, and since these appear to be elaborated independently, this may go far to explain the anomalies found for so long by those attempting to understand the lethal activity of *B. cereus*.

Further evidence was obtained using antisera to the skin-active fraction of strain 4433/73. Table 7 shows the experimental design and results. It is seen that protection against lethality was given by antiserum to the fraction possessing both skin and lethal activities (Lethal Factor I) but not by pre-inoculation serum from the same rabbit. In contrast, in keeping with the known ability (Bernheimer and Grushoff, 1967a) of normal serum to inactivate the

TABLE 6. *Some extracellular metabolites reported to be produced*
by Bacillus cereus

Antibiotics (peptide)	Hydrolases
biocerin	20β-ketoreductase
cerein	*Lethal toxin
cerexins A & B	*Loop fluid-inducing factor
thiocillins, I, II, III	Milk clotting enzymes
Beta-amylase	(neutral proteases)
Beta-glucanase	Nucleases
Beta-lactamases	DNase/RNase
I penicillinases	Pectinases
II cephalosporinases	*Phospholipases
III	3 C-types
*Cereolysin (hemolysin I)	Phosphatidase
Collagenase	Proteases—neutral
*Exo-enterotoxins	(including caseolytic &
Gelatinase	milk clotting enzymes)
*Hemolysins	Pulcherriminic acid
cereolysin	Thromboplastinase
hemolysin II	Tyramine
Histamine	Urease

* Covered in detail in this review.

TABLE 7. *Protection against the lethal properties of the skin* (*VPR**) *active and*
cereolysin fractions from flat bed electrofocusing of culture filtrates of 4433/73

Fraction	Containing	Incubated before injection with	Intravenous in mice
X	VPR activity (Lethal factor I)	**Pre-inoculation serum	4/4 died
X	VPR activity (Lethal factor I)	Anti-X serum	0/4 died
Y	Cereolysin (Lethal factor II)	**Pre-inoculation serum ⎫ Normal rabbit serum ⎭	0/5 died
Y	Cereolysin (Lethal factor II)	Saline	4/4 died

* VPR = vascular permeability reaction.
** Serum from rabbit before inoculations to raise antibodies were commenced.

hemolytic activity of cereolysin (discussed further under 'Hemolysins'), it was found that pre-inoculation or normal rabbit serum neutralized the lethal activities of the cereolysin fraction (Lethal Factor II). As discussed in section 4.4, p 412, the matter is complicated by a second hemolysin formed in culture filtrates and by the recent finding (Kramer, 1984) that the skin active (VPR) factor can be resolved into two distinct moieties by electrofocusing.

The antisera raised to the skin active fractions of 4433/73 and 671/78 neutralized the lethal activities of crude culture filtrates of both the homologous strains and a number of heterologous strains including strain No. 96 from which Ezepchuk and Fluer (1973) purified their toxin (see below). One must presume that in these tests, the contribution of the cereolysin to the lethal activities of the strains was neutralized non-specifically during pre-incubation with the antiserum.

This evidence suggests that loop fluid induction, vascular permeability alteration (both with accompanying necrosis if occurring in sufficient strength) and lethality are three manifestations of one, possibly two, metabolites—although lethality tests have not been carried out yet on the two newly separated VPR moieties. The proteinaceous material in the VPR/lethal/necrotic factor as described by Turnbull *et al.* (1979b) gave rise to three bands on polyacrylamide gel electrophoresis (J. M. Kramer, personal communication) and was thus already suspected of not being a single protein or pure at that stage.

Bernheimer and Grushoff (1967a) established that their purified cereolysin (see section 4.2, p 411) possessed a minimum lethal dose for mice of $1\mu g$ of protein.

Finally, Ezepchuk *et al.* (1979) have reported purification of lethal toxin using methodology somewhat different from their earlier work (Ezepchuk and Fluer, 1973). In this case, purification was achieved using ion-exchange chromatography on DE-32-cellulose (Whatman) of a modified casein hydrolysate broth culture and the homogeneity of the protein component was checked by SDS-disc electrophoresis and gel diffusion.

As estimated by SDS-disc electrophoresis, the MW of the toxin was 100,000; the MLD_{50} was 4–50 μg/mouse. Perhaps a little strangely, the relation of this metabolite and that reported in 1973 (MW 55,000–60,000 by sedimentation coefficient and MLD 300 μg/mouse) was not specifically discussed and no immunological cross-reactivity tests were apparently done. In fact, they describe this later one as 'a previously unknown protein not identical to any of the known biologically active polymers of *B. cereus*'. It was shown to alter vascular permeability both in rabbit skin after intracutaneous injection and in mouse lungs after intranasal application but it failed to stimulate fluid accumulation in ligated rabbit loops. Two particular differences from the previously described toxin are the sensitivity to trypsin (see below) and the negative results on injection of 300 μg/kg into cats. In this instance, the only response was a weak feverish one. Thus they concluded this lethal toxin had vascular permeability activity but was not an enterotoxin.

Probably because the precise nature of the lethal activity of *B. cereus* culture filtrates is unknown, only rather primitive data is available on its physical and chemical characteristics. Johnson (1966), Johnson and Bonventre (1967) and Bonventre and Johnson (1970) found that, while stable to 45°C for 2 hr, the activity was abolished by 56°C for 30 min. Trypsin at a final concentration of 0.01 per cent reduced the activity to zero within 4 min, at 37°C. Exposure for 24 hr at 4°C of cell-free filtrates to pH's of 2.2, 7.0 and 11.1 reduced lethal activities by 70 per cent, 0 per cent and 50 per cent respectively.

Ezepchuk and Fluer (1973) found that the toxic activity in ammonium sulphate precipitates of their casein hydrolysate cultures was susceptible to pH's outside the range 5.0–10.0 with a minimum stability at pH 4. It was also destroyed by exposure to 60°C for 20 min and by trypsin. Figures for their Biogel-purified preparations (Ezepchuk *et al.*, 1979) were not given but, although they do not give details, they imply that this large MW lethal toxin was unaffected by trypsin and also by thiol-reducing agents.

Balacescu (1975) reported similar heat and pH stability findings to those of Bonventre and Johnson (1970) and Ezepchuk and Fluer (1973).

The toxin in crude culture filtrates appears to tolerate repeated freeze–thawing well (P. C. B. Turnbull, unpublished observations).

3.4. Production and Persistence Kinetics of *B. cereus* Lethal Activity

Johnson (1966), Johnson and Bonventre (1967) and Bonventre and Johnson (1970) noted that production of lethal activity by their strain B-48 in fresh beef infusion broth at 37°C occurred primarily during the transitional phase of growth—that is, the time lapse between termination of vegetative growth (as marked by the point at which the pH ceases to fall and signalling the induction of the tricarboxylic acid cycle [Glatz *et al.*, 1974]) and the initiation of sporulation (Hanson *et al.*, 1963). This finding was supported by Ezepchuk and Fluer (1973) with their strain No. 96 in a casein hydrolysate broth (temperature not given) and by K. Jørgensen (personal communication) with strains B-4ac and 171 in brain-heart infusion broth (Difco) at 30°C. Presumably because of the complex physico-chemical form of the growth media, Ivers and Potter (1977), using strains ATCC 14579 and 7004 found that production of this toxin at 30°C in commercial strained beef and beef broth and blended ripe bananas more-or-less parallelled the growth curve from commencement of measurements.

The persistence at 37°C of lethal activity in beef infusion broth was found by Bonventre and Eckert (1963b) to be very short and its activity had declined from a 9 hr peak to undetectable at 21 hr. Johnson and Bonventre (1967) recorded that the titer of lethal activity of strain B-48 in a fresh beef infusion broth remained stable for 48 hr at this temperature. Ezepchuk and Fluer (1973) recorded a peak in the titer at 12–14 hr after which it dropped to a lower level at which it held steady for the remainder of the 24 hr test period. The titrations of

Balacescu (1975) with a meat extract broth culture showed a peak between 12 and 18 hr falling to undetectable by 36 hr and K. Jørgensen (personal communication) found that, while the activity with B-4ac had dropped from a peak at 12 hr to undetectable by 22 hr, that of strain 171 was still detectable at 22 hr. In the two foods in which the two strains of Ivers and Potter (1977) gave rise to lethal toxin, the titer was at a peak at the end of the 24 hr test period.

It is difficult to say whether the differences in the persistences recorded for the different strains under the different circumstances are significant and, if they are, whether they reflect variable production of other proteolytic enzymes within the culture media which may destroy the toxin. Further related discussion is found under 'Hemolysins' and 'Loop fluid-inducing/skin test/necrotic toxin'.

As inferred, the toxin may be elaborated at 30°C (Ivers and Potter, 1977), 32°C (Glatz and Goepfert, 1973; Spira and Goepfert, 1975; Glatz and Goepfert, 1976; K. Jørgensen, personal communication) and 37°C (Molnar, 1962; Johnson and Bonventre, 1967; Bonventre and Johnson, 1970; Turnbull et al., 1979a,b). Bonventre and Johnson (1970) recorded that the titer of lethality after incubation at 37°C was twice that found after incubation at 30°C when the same growth had been attained. The toxin can also be produced at 25°C (P. C. B. Turnbull, unpublished results).

According to Balacescu (1975), the presence of oxygen in the culture medium is essential and gasification with pure oxygen significantly enhances production of lethal toxin. This contrasts with the findings that, as discussed later, cereolysin (Lethal Factor II) is inactivated by oxygen and the vascular permeability reaction toxin (Lethal Factor I) is produced optimally under limited oxygenation.

3.5. Growth Media

Bonventre and Johnson in their various papers and personal communication noted that, while excellent growth was supported by a variety of complex, semi-synthetic and synthetic media, only their own freshly prepared beef infusion broth could be relied on for consistent production of the lethal factor at significant levels. It was either not detectable or detectable only at very low levels or for only a very brief period during culture growth in commercial beef infusion broth (Difco), trypticase soya broth (BBL), nutrient broth (Difco), casamino acids or acid hydrolysed casamino acids media (Difco and Sheffield Chemical Co.). Using a synthetic amino acids basal salt medium containing 16 amino acids, they established that proline and cystine were not essential to toxin synthesis and that supplementation of the synthetic medium with glucose, peptones, peptides or B vitamins, alone or in combination, did not lead to enhanced synthesis.

The indications from these results, supported further by the finding that Seitz-filtered beef-infusion broth failed to support production of the toxin, was that (an) essential factor(s) is/are required for its elaboration. This, to date, has not been defined.

Since the papers of Bonventre and Johnson, observations made on the lethal activities of *B. cereus* cultures or culture filtrates have been reported as part of studies primarily concerned with other toxins. Goepfert and his colleagues found the medium of choice to be brain–heart infusion broth (Difco) with an extra 0.1 per cent glucose (BHIG) and this continues to be the most satisfactory for routine testing for lethal activity.

3.6. Differences in Lethal Activity among Different Strains

That not all *B. cereus* strains necessarily produced lethal toxin was apparently first indicated by Spira and Goepfert (1975) and Katsaras and Zeller (1977) showed varying titers amongst 9 strains tested, although all did kill mice. Turnbull et al. (1979b) analysed 88 unrelated strains isolated from a wide range of clinical and routine sources; 12 (13.7 per cent) were recorded as producing undetectable levels of the toxin. Exhaustive repeat tests, different growth conditions and the effect of concentration were not carried out, but the results indicated marked differences in the readiness and extent to which different strains will produce lethal activity under standard conditions (BHIG, 9 hr at 37°C on a rotatory shaker at approximately 200 r.p.m.).

3.7. MODE OF ACTION OF THE LETHAL FACTORS

In general, and unless doses are borderline, 0.5 ml of a *B. cereus* culture filtrate possessing lethal potential when injected i.v. into mice or rats acts extremely rapidly and death can result within 30 sec, and usually within 2 min. When very rapid, there is an initial appearance of apprehension followed immediately by a brief period of mild to violent convulsive movements terminating in death, resembling symptoms following i.v. injection of an insupportable volume of air. When less rapid, a period of quiescence with hunching, indrawn waist and panting occurs before the terminal convulsions; the convulsions characteristically involve violent kicking of the rear legs. Other authors have interpreted the indrawn waist and panting as 'respiratory difficult' and Torres–Anjel *et al.* (1979) interpreted the convulsive movements as 'paralysis', but this author does not subscribe to either of these views.

Bonventre and Eckert (1963b) noted that, on necropsy, the only pathological changes were massive congestion with thrombi in the vessels and capillaries of the lungs; no other organs were affected. The finding is corroborated by Balacescu (1975) and Ezepchuk *et al.* (1979) who also recorded large hemorrhagic areas in the lungs. This author has re-examined this carefully and found that, while there is congestion in the lungs, reflected mildly in the liver, he could find no evidence of tissue damage or hemorrhage. He observed that, in contrast to cervically dislocated control mice, the intoxicated mice appeared to have suffered immediate cardiac arrest and it seems likely that congestion seen in the lungs results from this. Death, therefore, appears to result primarily from cardiotoxicity rather than, as previously inferred, from action on the lungs. No obvious histological changes are apparent in the heart muscle.

Intranasal administration results in consistent lethality with 5- to 10-fold lower doses than that generally used in i.v. tests (Stamatin and Anghelesco, 1969; Balacescu, 1975; Ezepchuk *et al.*, 1979) and apparently may be as instantaneous as i.v. inoculation (Ezepchuk *et al.*, 1979). Stamatin and Anghelesco (1969) even claimed that the toxin inoculated by the respiratory route seemed to be the most potent bacterial toxin so far known. Presumably the toxin is very rapidly absorbed into the blood in the alveolar capillaries producing death in the same manner as with the i.v. route.

The toxin is also lethal when administered i.p. or s.c. (Bonventre and Eckert, 1963b; Bonventre and Johnson, 1970; Balacescu, 1975; P. C. B. Turnbull, unpublished observations), but the response is not as consistent and the time to death is much longer (1 to 24 hr— Bonventre and Johnson, 1970). The animals become increasingly comatose up to the point of death which is usually preceded by a brief period of deep breathing and one or two mild convulsive movements. Again (P. C. B. Turnbull, unpublished observations), there is no evidence of respiratory difficulties, paralysis or other signs of neurotoxicity, and histological findings are identical to those following i.v. injection of toxin preparations. Tinted serum emboli were very rarely apparent and there were no significant abnormalities in the heart muscle, liver or intestine. (Bonventre and Eckert, 1963b; Bonventre and Johnson, 1970).

The toxin does not kill mice when administered orally (Balacescu, 1975; P. C. B. Turnbull, unpublished observations) or intra-rectally (Balacescu, 1975). Very strong fermenter-grown preparations of 4433/73 and 668/78 introduced by stomach gavage did not kill adult mice even when stomach contents were pre-neutralized with sodium bicarbonate (P. C. B. Turnbull, unpublished results). Toxin introduced into the stomachs of infant mice according to the test for *Escherichia coli* heat stable toxin, did however, result in death within 1 hr and gross stomach necrosis. Symptoms of gastroenteritis were not noted following any of these enteric route tests.

It is logical to believe that the necrotic nature of either or both lethal factor I (the vascular permeability reaction toxin) and lethal factor II (cereolysin), may play a role in death even if not histologically obvious. As discussed in the relevent sections, they may apply more to the former since cereolysin is inhibited by serum; that no evidence can be seen in histological sections indicating that hemolysis has occurred appears to support this.

3.8. OTHER *BACILLUS* SPECIES AND LETHAL TOXIN

More by inference from the absence of reports of lethal activities in the culture filtrates of other *Bacillus* species than from reports of negative results, it appears that lethal activity is peculiar to *B. cereus* and the closely related *B. thuringiensis*. A wound swab isolate and an unrelated blood culture isolate identified as *B. mycoides* in this laboratory were both positive in mouse lethal tests, although a strain tested by Gorina *et al.* (1975, 1976) was negative. *B. mycoides*, like *B. thuringiensis* is closely related to *B. cereus* and thus it might be anticipated that it would produce similar metabolites. As mentioned earlier, however, culture filtrates of *B. anthracis*, which is also closely related to *B. cereus* (Kaneko *et al.*, 1978) do not exhibit this activity. (P. C. B. Turnbull, unpublished results).

Kreig (1971a,b) reported that lethal toxin was also produced by a strain of *B. subtilis*, but this has not been substantiated for *B. subtilis* in general. Nine representative strains of *B. subtilis* and seven of *B. licheniformis* isolated from patients' (diarrheal) feces in separate food poisoning investigations and eight further strains of *B. licheniformis* thought to be isolates of significance in a variety of non-gastrointestinal human and animal infections (Maddocks and Turnbull, 1978; Turnbull, 1978, 1979b) were all negative when culture filtrates were prepared and injected into mice according to the test used for *B. cereus* toxicity. The culture filtrate of *B. licheniformis* strain 3223/77 originally incriminated in morbidity, mortality and reduced parity in a laboratory colony of CBA/Ca mice (Wright *et al.*, 1979) caused an unusual febrile reaction in the conventional mice used for the lethal test; the culture was also unusually difficult to filter.

Gorina *et al.* (1975, 1976) reported that the toxicity was not produced by a strain each of *B. mesentericus* and *B. megaterium*.

To entomological toxicologists, the lethal toxin as produced by *B. thuringiensis* is known as α-toxin and has been produced by all serotypes for which it has been tested (Krieg, 1970, 1971a,b, 1975; Forsberg *et al.*, 1976; Turnbull—Table 8). In the literature review of Forsberg *et al.* (1976) an interesting parallel can be seen between the entirely independent studies that have been done on *B. thuringiensis* α-toxin and the *B. cereus* lethal activity even to the extent of similar proposals as to their possible identities with hemolysin and phospholipase.

TABLE 8. *Mouse lethal test (MLT) and rabbit vascular permeability reaction (VPR) test results on cell-free BHIG* culture filtrates of* B. thuringiensis

Food Hygiene No.	Milstead Culture No. (where known)	Serotype	MLT** duplicate mice, minutes to death	VPR Category†	VPR Necrosis	Identity in Fig. 2b
2100/78		I	7/6	4	1.1	7T
—	21	II	<2/<2	4	3.1	—
2103/78		IIIA	<1/<1	4	2.5	8T
2105/78		IIIAB	1/<1	4	2.4	9T
2107/78		IVAB (sotte)	<2/<2	4	3.0	—
	23	IVB	<1/<1	4	2.9	—
2110/78		IVAC (kenyae)	2/<2	4	3.4	—
2111/78		VAB	3/4	4	1.2	10T
	72	VI	2/2	2	0	—
2113/78		VI (entomocidus)	2/2	3	1.4	—
	57	VII	10/14	2	0	—
2115/78		VII	7/5	3	0	11T
2116/78		VII	6/5	3	0	12T
	75	VIII	<1/2	3	0	—
	117	IX	4/3	3	0.9	—
2117/78		IX	5/5	3	0.2	—

* Brain–heart infusion broth with extra 0.1 per cent glucose; 37°C for 6 hr with shaking and pH adjustment at 3.5 and 4.5 hr. Inoculated at zero time with a 5 per cent overnight nutrient broth culture. **0.5 ml i.v. †Based on mean radii of perpendicular readings of zones of light blue, dark blue and necrosis in at least duplicate tests.

Heimpel (1955) postulated that 'lecithinase-C' was responsible for the lethality but Krieg (1971a) found that it was not limited to lecithinase-producing strains.

3.9. Lethal Toxin and Public and Animal Health

In contrast to *B. anthracis*, in all probability due to their lack of an equivalent capsule, *B. cereus* and *B. thuringiensis* appear generally to be unable to proliferate systemically or within the bowel of otherwise healthy mammals, although clearly *B. cereus* can multiply in wounds, abscesses, and when able to penetrate into the lens and vitreous chambers of the eye (Turnbull *et al.*, 1977a; Fitzpatrick *et al.*, 1979; Young *et al.*, 1980; O'Day *et al.*, 1981a; b). *B. thuringiensis* has now also been recorded in relation to human infection (Samples and Buettner, 1983; Warren *et al.*, 1984). On occasion, the infections in which the *B. cereus* has multiplied are fatal or the patients or animals are reported to be toxemic before therapy brings the infection under control. One of the more exotic fatalities on record due to *B. cereus* was that of a tiger (Bonventre and Johnson, 1970). The role of the lethal factors of the organism in these infections can, of course, only be guessed at or inferred indirectly from the types of tests carried out by Turnbull *et al.* (1979a).

It is well-known that *B. thuringiensis* viable spores mixed with parasporal crystals are used in various countries of the world in commercial insecticides, including sprays; at least 7000 tons of this type of preparation had been used worldwide by 1979, a significant proportion on food crops (Burges, 1981). There is also a commercial preparation consisting of saline spore suspensions of a strain of *B. cereus* (243/80—see Table 2) which is marketed and prescribed in certain countries for human oral consumption as an antidote to diarrhea. Washed spore preparations of these organisms do not possess lethal activity and, as administered, these preparations appear to have no hazardous potential. However, Forsberg *et al.* (1976) draws attention to the type of environmental concern that might arise from a secondary stage where vegetative growth may occur; their example was development of *B. thuringiensis* septicemia in infected insect larvae.

Any hazard that might arise from secondary situations would presumably occur in a wound-type infection or inhalation since the toxin is apparently ineffective by oral routes (see sections 3.7, p 407 and 6.1, p 424, 425). However, it must be stressed that extensive and exhaustive safety tests have been carried out on the strength of which *B. thuringiensis* has been declared to be non-infective in vertebrates including mammals and man by any route (Fisher and Rosner, 1959; WHO, 1979; Burges, 1981). Similarly, the commercial *B. cereus* preparation has been tested and deemed safe for human use (Pillen, 1971; Vandekerkove, 1979). Balacescu (1974) consumed seven increasing doses (10–70 ml) of mouse lethal test-active *B. cereus* filtrates over seven days without ill effects of any sort.

The single differential test by which *B. cereus* and *B. thuringiensis* can be morphologically distinguished, is the presence in *B. thuringiensis* of parasporal crystal bodies. Apparently plasmid encoded, it seems that the ability of a strain of *B. thuringiensis* to form these crystals is a property that can be lost (reviewed by Warren *et al.*, 1984). Examination for the crystal bodies is not routinely done to ensure that cultures isolated in clinical laboratories and recorded as *B. cereus* are not, in fact, *B. thuringiensis*. For these reasons, it is not known how often, if ever, *B. thuringiensis* may be involved in human or animal infections. During the early years of investigations into *B. cereus* food poisoning in Britain, however, isolates were submitted to a *B. thuringiensis* expert but *B. thuringiensis* was not found (Burges, 1981).

3.10. Summary of Lethal Activities of *B. cereus*

Although the lethal activity of *B. cereus* cultures for laboratory animals has been known for many years, its precise nature still remains unclear. Initially, like *C. perfringens* α-toxin, it was thought to be one of three manifestations of a single toxin—namely lethality, hemolysis and lecithinase activity. Subsequently evidence was provided which suggested that for *B. cereus*, these activities represented differentiable metabolites. The non-identity with phospholipase-C was fully established but differentiation of lethality from hemolysin was not so clear-cut. A toxin which produced fluid accumulation in ligated rabbit loops and altered permeability in skin capillaries with necrosis in both situations if present in sufficient strength was then discovered; this also killed mice on i.v. injection. This fluid accumulation/skin test factor and the cereolysin component of culture filtrates of 4433/73 and 671/78 were successfully separated by an electrofocusing technique (Kramer *et al.*, 1978; Turnbull *et al.*, 1979b) and both were found to kill mice with identical symptoms on i.v. injection. Thus these authors proposed that the lethal activity of culture filtrates of *B. cereus* represent the combined lethal effects of the fluid accumulation/skin test factor (Lethal Factor I) and cereolysin (Lethal Factor II). Further details on these factors are given in sections following.

A group of Russian workers have made two claims to have purified lethal toxin, both from strain No. 96. Two different purification methods were used and the resulting toxins appear to have some markedly different characteristics. One (Ezepchuk and Fluer, 1973) was a compound of MW 55,000–60,000, trypsin sensitive, killed mice at a MLD of 300 μg/mouse and at 300 μg/kg caused severe vomiting in cats. The second (Ezepchuk *et al.*, 1979), referred to as a previously unknown protein, had a MW of 100,000, was apparently insensitive to trypsin, had a MLD_{50} of 40–50 μg/mouse but only produced a mild febrile reaction in cats at a dose of 300 μg/kg. The authors did not report that they had done tests for possible hemolytic activity with either of the toxins. The later one altered vascular permeability in rabbit skin but it did not induce fluid accumulation in rabbit loops. In the 1979 paper, no reference was made to the earlier toxin and the possible identities of these toxins with each other or with cereolysin and the fluid accumulation/skin test factor of Western workers remain unknown. One finding of possible relevance is that strain No. 96 tested in this laboratory elaborated the skin test toxin very strongly although its hemolytic titre of 40 was relatively weak in relation to numerous other *B. cereus* strains tested.

The possible relevance of the lethal properties of cultures of *B. cereus* and the closely related *B. thuringiensis* to human and animal infection has been discussed.

4. HEMOLYSINS

4.1. INTRODUCTION—OBSERVATIONS 1930–1965

One of the primary identification features of *B. cereus*, and a fundamental test for distinguishing it from *B. anthracis* is hemolysis on blood agar. This appears to have been well-known by 1930 (St. John–Brooks, 1930) in relation to the differentiation of 'anthrax and pseudoanthrax bacilli' and was stated specifically for *B. cereus* by Clark (1937). Burdon (1947) considered virulence of strains of *B. cereus* in mice to be directly related to hemolytic activity.

The early idea that the hemolytic activity of *B. cereus* might be one of a number of manifestations of a single metabolite analagous to *C. perfringens* α-toxin was discussed early in section 3.2, p 401, 402. On the basis of differential sensitivities to 50°C for 20 min at pH 8.2, differential absorption by platelets, differential production in nitrogen-deficient media and differences exhibited among variant strains, Ottolenghi *et al.* (1961) proposed that hemolysin and phospholipase activities were different. The separation of hemolysin from egg-yolk turbidity factor in cell-free extracts of *B. cereus* and from one of two phospholipases in culture filtrates was reported independently and respectively by Fossum (1963) and Slein and Logan (1963). Both separations were achieved by DEAE-cellulose chromatography of ammonium sulphate precipitates. Slein and Logan (1965) produced further data supporting the non-identity of hemolysin and phospholipase; their findings are covered in more detail in the section on phospholipases. Fossum (1963) observed two peaks of hemolytic activity in his fractions; the significance of this is discussed below.

4.2. PURIFICATION AND CHARACTERIZATION OF CEREOLYSIN

In the previous section it was discussed how Johnson (1966) and Johnson and Bonventre (1966) provided evidence that the hemolytic, phospholipolytic and lethal activities of *B. cereus* were closely associated but not identical having different kinetics of synthesis and being partially resolved by Sephadex chromatography. Bernheimer and Grushoff (1967a) appear to be the first to have studied *B. cereus* hemolysin in detail. Ammonium sulphate-precipitated cell-free filtrate of a secondary culture in semi-minimal broth was fractionated by electrophoresis and the pooled fraction re-precipitated with ammonium sulphate. The redissolved deposit was further purified by Sephadex G-100 chromatography and, on the basis of acrylamide gel electrophoresis and the schlieren pattern in an analytical ultra-centrifuge, they judged that they had obtained the hemolytic agent, a protein which they named cereolysin, in a 'substantially pure' form. It was entirely free of phospholipolytic activity and, capable of red cell lysis at a concentration of 1 $\mu\mu$g/ml, they rated it as one of the most potent *in vitro* hemolytic agents known. The characteristics of this protein are summarized in Table 9.

They found the molecule to be unstable under most conditions and that it could not be freeze-dried without loss of activity; their storage method of choice was solution in 5 per cent (v/v) glycerol phosphate buffer (pH 6.0) slow-frozen to $-20°C$. The cereolysin was highly lethal to mice; the later support for this given by Kramer *et al.* (1978) and Turnbull *et al.* (1979b) was discussed under 'Lethal Toxin', p 403. The hemolytic activity was (in contrast to that of *C. perfringens* α-toxin) inhibited by human serum and also by cholesterol at 10 μg/ml; 10–50 times this concentration was found to be necessary in the case of five other lipids that were tested to obtain an equivalent inhibition.

The authors, Bernheimer and Grushoff (1967a), were interested in the possible relationship between cereolysin and streptolysin-O and initially concluded that they were unrelated. However, they later found (Bernheimer and Grushoff, 1967b) that while, when human serum was used no antigenic relationship was apparent, anti-streptolysin-O globulins in hyperimmune horse serum did indeed neutralize cereolysin. This was important in establishing that cereolysin was closely related to the oxygen-labile thiol-activated cytolysins. A year later they (Bernheimer *et al.*, 1968) concluded from the results obtained with isoelectric focusing that cereolysin was a homogeneous protein with pI 6.5.

Bernheimer's group published again in 1976 (Cowell *et al.*, 1976) on improved purification of cereolysin using, in addition to their previously described procedure (Bernheimer and Grushoff, 1967a), AH-sepharose chromatography and isoelectric focusing. They confirmed its antigenic relationship with streptolysin-O and found that, in common with the members

TABLE 9. *Properties and Composition of Cereolysin**

Condition	Hemolysin activity Activity remaining	Amino acid analysis (estimated residues/molecule)			
half life at 50°C	1–3 min	alanine	33	proline	29
40°C	45 min	arginine	16	serine	41
5°C	1–3 days	aspartic acid	67	threonine	42
presence at 20°C × 30 mins of:		half cystine	2	tryptophan	2
EDTA	NA	glutamic acid	47	tyrosine	19
cysteine	NA	glycine	56	valine	39
mercaptoethanol	NA	histidine	11		
trypsin (10 μg)	NA	isoleucine	24		
chymotrypsin (100 μg)	NA	leucine	29		
papain (100 μg)	NA	lysine	40	Total 518 residues	
pronase (100 μg)	Lost	methionine	6		
serum	Inhibited	phenylalanine	15		
cholesterol	Inhibited				

MW = approx. 55,500   pH range for optimum stability 5.0–7.0

NA = not affected.
*Bernheimer and Grushoff (1967a) & Cowell *et al.* (1976).

of the thiol-activated cytolysins (and, indeed, many other bacterial toxins), it exhibited microheterogeneity on isoelectric focusing. The cause of this heterogeneity had hitherto been unclear, but, investigating the possibility that thiol-activated toxins exist in at least two forms—an active reduced form requiring free sulfydryl groups for activity and a reversibly inactive oxidised form with the sulfydryl groups in disulfide bonds—they were able to provide the first demonstration that this was true with cereolysin. Discontinuous acrylamide electrophoresis of toxin that had been purified in the presence or absence of the reducing agent dithiothreitol, the two forms, identical in size but separable by charge differences (pI of oxidised form $= 6.3$–6.4; pI of reduced form $= 6.5$–6.6) were observed. The reduced active form with MW of approximately 55,500 as determined by sodium dodecylsulfate (SDS) gel electrophoresis, gel filtration and acrylamide gel electrophoresis with a minimum of 55,636 as calculated from amino acid analysis, was inhibited by sulphydryl reagents; the inhibition could be reversed by dithiothreitol.

Cowell et al. (1976) considered they had successfully purified cereolysin and determined it to be a single polypeptide chain of 518 amino acids.

4.3. HEMOLYSIN VERSUS OTHER TOXIC ACTIVITIES

Other publications featuring hemolysin and appearing during the period spanned by the papers of Bernheimer and colleagues just reviewed, have been concerned with the possible role of hemolysin in animal tests, such as rabbit and guinea-pig skin tests, being used to elucidate the toxicological basis of B. cereus food poisoning. Thus Glatz and Goepfert (1973) and Glatz et al. (1974), found that exposure of cell-free culture filtrates to 45°C for 30 min resulted in a 90–97 per cent reduction in hemolytic activity without a significant alteration either in skin test results or in phospholipase activities. Spira and Goepfert (1975), using Sephadex G-75 chromatography, although unable to obtain vascular permeability factor entirely free of hemolysin felt that the elution profiles were sufficiently different to indicate separate entities.

Ezepchuk and Fluer (1973), as noted under 'Lethal toxin', claimed to have successfully separated hemolysin from lethal toxin.

The reports of Kramer et al. (1978) and Turnbull et al. (1979b), in which they conclude that cereolysin is one of two lethal and skin test activities in culture filtrates of B. cereus, are discussed in the section on purification and characterization of lethal toxin (p 403).

4.4. TWO OR MORE HEMOLYSINS—STABILITY TO HEAT

In 1963, Fossum, examining the culture filtrate of strain NVH 322 (which appears to be the isolate from the first recorded incident incriminating B. cereus as a food poisoning agent—Hauge 1950, 1955), observed two hemolytic peaks, designated H^I and H^{II}, on DEAE-cellulose chromatography of ammonium sulphate precipitated culture supernatants. H^I was readily separable from both of two egg-yolk turbidity peaks E^I and E^{II} but H^{II} could not be separated from E^{II}. A second strain, isolated from a case of bovine mastitis appeared only to produce H^I.

In a paper a year later (Fossum, 1964), he observed the Arrhenius effect in the hemolytic activities of his two strains and noted that the activity of strain NVH 322 was significantly higher at 90°C–100°C than that of the mastitis strain. From this it might be deduced that H^{II} was the component responsible for the Arrhenius effect.

Parker and Goepfert (1978) indicated an awareness of the existence of two hemolysins in that they assayed for both a heat-stable (45°C × 30 min) and a heat-labile hemolysin in culture filtrates of a strain B-4ac-L derived from B-4ac. Kramer et al. (1978) referred to two hemolysin peaks obtained from flat-bed electrofocusing; both were separable from phospholipase. One, referred to as relatively heat-labile, was considered to be cereolysin.

Later in the same year, Coolbaugh and Williams (1978) published detailed studies on two hemolysins from strain B-48. These were partially separable by and distinguishable as two peaks on Sephadex G-100 chromatography and were both distinct from phospholipase. The authors labelled the two hemolysins H-I and H-II and showed that a mutant strain of B-48 (designated C9b) selected for low hemolysin production had mostly lost its ability to produce H-I. B-48 grown in a semi-minimal broth failed to produce H-II. Ammonium sulfate at 40 per cent saturation precipitated only H-I; as the ammonium sulphate concentration was increased, precipitation of H-II was also increased. Taking advantage of these properties, they were able to characterize H-I as a protein of 50,000–52,000 MW which showed signs of loss of activity after 5 min at 40°C, 2 min at 50°C and complete inactivation after 2 min at 60°C. It was inhibited in its hemolytic activity by cholesterol and the authors concluded that it was probably cereolysin.

H-II had a MW of 29,000–31,000, exhibited the Arrhenius effect in showing increased sensitivity to temperatures raised to 60°C but decreased sensitivity again as temperatures increased from 70°C to 100°C. This hemolysin was not inhibited by cholesterol and exhibited a different pattern and rate of hemolysis on rabbit red cells at 37°C from H-I.

The two hemolysins were equally sensitive to chloroform, ether, pH extremes, trypsin and pronase. At least on the basis of the relative temperature sensitivities, it would seem possible that the H^I and H^{II} of Fossum (1963, 1964) corresponded to H-I and H-II as described by Coolbaugh and Williams (1978).

The results reported by Kramer *et al.* (1978) were presented in more detail in the paper of Turnbull *et al.* (1979b) where the flat-bed electrofocusing profiles of strains 4433/73 and 671/78 are shown. The differential heat sensitivities were based on 50°C for 30 min; the stable hemolysin had a pI of 5.0 and the labile hemolysin had a pI of 6.6–the same as that reported by Cowell *et al.* (1976) for cereolysin. Improved equipment and methodologies have subsequently shown the secondary hemolysin to have a pI of 5.3 (Kramer, 1984).

Although the reports of Bernheimer's, Bonventre's, Goepfert's and Turnbull's groups and of Fossum (1963, 1964) and Coolbaugh and Williams (1978) reviewed here have implied that the factors responsible for hemolysis are distinguishable from those responsible for lecithovitellin/lecithinase/phospholipase activity, phospholipase-C (Bowman *et al.*, 1971) and more specifically, the sphingomyelinase form of phospholipase-C (Ikezawa *et al.*, 1976, 1980) has been reported to be hemolytic. It is possible that the method of purification of the phospholipase-C used by Bowman *et al.* (1971) left a hemolysin contaminant in the final product. Sphingomyelinase as a hemolysin is covered in greater detail under 'Phospholipases'. The possibility that phospholipase may render a red cell more fragile and predispose it to hemolysis was proposed by Rawley and Hunter (1951—see p 416 below).

Similarly, the intensely necrotic nature of the loop fluid-inducing/skin test/necrotic toxin is discussed under 'Mode of action' of that toxin and the point is made there that it is hard to understand how this toxin, apparently able to destroy tissue cells, can be non-hemolytic.

4.5. Production of Hemolysins

Hemolysin production by *B. cereus* is a vegetative growth phenomenon and, generally, in the papers reviewed concerned with hemolysin in either a primary or secondary manner, production has been achieved in well-aerated cultures. The sac-culture method of Donnelly *et al.* (1967), found useful for enhanced production of skin test toxin (Parker and Goepfert, 1978), did not enhance hemolysin production.

Clear production kinetics have not been given in any of the papers reviewed concerned with hemolysins apart from that of Ivers and Potter (1977) studying hemolysin production in certain foodstuffs. In the absence of growth and production curves from other authors, Tables 10, 11 and 12 are offered here (A. Wayne, J. M. Kramer and P. C. B. Turnbull, unpublished results). Total and heat stable (50°C for 30 min) hemolysin readings for strain 4433/73 under various conditions and of 671/78 and B-4ac under just two conditions are given. All three strains are strong producers of hemolysin; readings for heat-labile hemolysin (cereolysin) can be assessed by subtracting the heat-stable titers from the total hemolysin titers.

At 36°C in BHIG, measurable hemolysin appears in late exponential phase of growth with peak readings apparent at or near to the point of pH minimum (Tables 10, 11). Within the

TABLE 10. *Growth of* B. cereus *4433/73 and production of hemolysin (HL), phospholipase (PL) and vascular permeability reaction (VPR) factor under varied conditions*

Time (hr)	0	1	2	3	4	5	6	7	8	9	10	24
4433/73 BHIG 36°C Shaker												
Log colony count	4.6	4.8	5.2	6.7	8.2	8.7	8.7	8.8	8.9	8.6	8.8	8.8
pH	7.1	7.0	7.0	7.1	6.7	5.9	5.8	6.4	6.6	6.3	6.5	8.1
Total HL	<5	<5	<5	5	640	640	640	640	640	640	640	320
Heat stable HL	<5	<5	<5	<5	40	40	160	160	320	160	40	80
PL	0	0	0	0	6.2	8.2	8.5	9.0	8.5	8.4	8.0	8.5
VPR	0	0	0	0	2.8	2.8	6.5	6.0	4.8	9.5	10.7	9.5
4433/73 BHIG + 5% FCS 36°C Shaker												
Log colony count	5	5.5	6.7	7.5	8.2	8.3	8.8	8.9	9.3	9.0	8.8	8.8
pH	7.0	7.0	7.0	6.9	6.0	5.8	6.1	6.6	6.4	6.7	6.9	8.0
Total HL	<5	<5	<5	5	640	640	640	640	640	640	640	160
Heat stable HL	<5	<5	<5	<5	160	320	320	320	320	320	320	80
PL	0	0	0	0	10.4	10.2	10.4	10.7	10.1	10.2	10.2	9.0
VPR	0	0	0	0	2.8	4.8	2.8	7.0	2.5	11.2	10.8	4.0
4433/73 BHIG 36°C Stationary												
Log colony count	4.6	4.7	5.2	6.0	7.3	7.5	8.3	7.9	8.6	8.5	8.5	8.3
pH	7.1	7.1	7.1	7.1	7.0	6.9	6.5	6.4	5.9	5.8	6.8	7.7
Total HL	<5	<5	<5	<5	10	80	160	160	320	160	640	80
Heat stable HL	Not done											
PL	0	0	0	0	0	0	7.0	5.5	8.1	7.5	8.0	7.5
VPR	0	0	0	0	0	2.8	3.3	3.5	8.8	6.8	8.5	9.8
4433/73 BHIG 22°C Stationary												
Log colony count	4.2	4.2	4.3	4.1	5.2	5.3	5.8	5.4	6.7	6.7	6.9	8.5
pH	Dropped from 7.0 at zero time to 6.0 at 14 hr											6.3
Total HL	<5	<5	<5	<5	<5	<5	<5	<5	10	10	20	640
Heat stable HL	Not done											
PL	First appeared at 14 hr with reading 7.5											8.5
VPR	First appeared at 14 hr with reading 14.0											14.5
4433/73 BHIG 40°C Stationary												
Log colony count	4.4	4.8	5.6	5.4	7.5	6.7	7.7	7.8	7.5	7.7	7.5	8.5
pH	7.0	7.1	7.1	7.1	7.0	7.0	6.5	6.2	5.6	5.6	5.7	7.6
Total HL	<5	<5	<5	<5	10	40	80	160	160	160	640	40
Heat stable HL	—	—	—	—	—	—	—	—	—	—	—	—
PL	—	—	—	—	—	—	—	1.8	4.5	4.9	10.0	8.6
VPR	—	—	—	—	—	—	—	—	4.2	4.2	6.2	3.5

BHIG = brain–heart infusion broth + 0.1% added glucose; FCS = fetal calf serum.

TABLE 11. *Growth of* B. cereus *strains 671/78 and B-4ac and production of hemolysin (HL), phospholipase (PL) and vascular permeability reaction (VPR) factor*

671/78 BHIG 36°C Shaker

Time (hr)	0	1	2	3	4	5	6	7	8	9	10	24
Log colony count	3.6	—	6.3	6.6	6.2	7.2	9.1	9.0	9.0	9.1	9.1	9.1
pH	7.1	—	7.1	7.0	7.0	6.9	5.9	6.1	6.4	6.4	6.8	8.0
Total HL	<5	—	<5	<5	10	40	>640	>640	>640	>640	>640	160
Heat stable HL	<5	—	<5	<5	<5	<5	20	640	320	320	160	80
PL	0	—	0	0	0	0	9.2	9.6	10.2	9.1	9.7	0
VPR	0	—	0	0	0	6.2	8.5	—	13.2	—	11.2	0

671/78 BHIG + 5% FCS 36°C Shaker

Time (hr)	0	1	2	3	4	5	6	7	8	9	10	24
Log colony count	5.0	5.2	6.4	7.9	8.2	8.8	9.0	9.1	8.9	9.2	9.1	8.9
pH	7.1	7.0	7.1	6.9	6.0	5.8	6.0	6.1	6.0	6.3	6.9	8.0
Total HL	<5	<5	5	320	640	640	>640	640	320	320	640	160
Heat stable HL	<5	<5	<5	10	640	320	320	640	320	160	320	80
PL	0	0	0	0	7.5	7.5	8.0	8.1	7.5	7.2	8.0	6.4
VPR	0	0	0	0	3.2	8.0	13.0	13.0	15.0	15.5	14.8	0

B-4ac BHIG 36°C Shaker

Time (hr)	0	1	2	3	4	5	6	7	8	9	10	24
Log colony count	4.4	5.0	5.6	6.5	7.5	8.5	8.7	8.8	8.8	8.8	8.8	8.6
pH	7.1	7.1	7.1	7.0	6.9	5.9	5.8	6.1	6.3	6.2	6.2	6.5
Total HL	<5	<5	<5	<5	20	640	640	640	>640	320	320	20
Heat stable HL	<5	<5	<5	0	<5	40	—	40	40	20	20	<5
PL	0	0	0	0	0	3.8	3.3	5.0	4.3	3.5	3.3	2.0
VPR	0	0	0	8.5	7.5	11.0	11.3	11.7	11.8	11.0	12.0	8.2

B-4ac BHIG + 5% FCS 36°C Shaker

Time (hr)	0	1	2	3	4	5	6	7	8	9	10	24
Log colony count	4.5	5.2	6.3	7.5	—	8.3	8.7	8.7	9.0	9.8	8.9	8.9
pH	7.1	7.2	7.2	7.0	6.0	6.0	6.2	6.3	6.3	6.3	6.5	7.4
Total HL	<5	<5	<5	40	640	640	320	320	320	320	320	20
Heat stable HL	<5	<5	<5	<5	80	80	160	320	320	160	160	20
PL	0	0	0	0	8.0	8.0	7.1	7.5	7.5	7.3	7.3	6.5
VPR	0	0	0	8.5	15.7	14.5	12.2	13.8	14.3	13.5	15.5	9.2

BHIG = brain–heart infusion broth with 0.1% added glucose; FCS = fetal calf serum.

limits of the experiments, this was coincident with or marginally in advance of the phospholipase and vascular permeability reaction (skin test) peaks. The rise in heat stable hemolysin titer appeared to lag a little behind that of cereolysin. Enrichment with 5 per cent fetal calf serum may have slightly accelerated the cycles of multiplication and production of metabolites and raised them to marginally higher peak values but probably not to a statistically significant extent.

The cycles in stationary cultures were retarded by several hours as compared with shaken cultures although the peak value of total hemolysin finally reached was unchanged. Differences in the results obtained with the different strains were not marked and their significance would require further tests for verification.

Bacterial growth in nutrient broth, milk, oxtail soup and blended peas (Table 12) was good but not accompanied by the pH trough observed in BHIG cultures and around which the kinetics of lethal toxin and the loop fluid-inducing/skin test/necrotic toxin appear to orientate. This probably results from a lack of readily available glucose and, in the foodstuffs, from some natural buffering. Hemolysin production in nutrient broth and soup was poor and better in milk and peas; the results with peas compare favorably with those reported by Ivers and Potter (1977—see below).

A notable fall in titer in both types of hemolysin is noted between 10 and 24 hr readings in the 36° and 40°C cultures with the apparent exception of sterilized milk (Table 12).

Variations among strains in their ability to elaborate hemolysin must have been known since the earliest use of blood agar for isolation and studies of *B. cereus*; formal evidence of widely differing strain variability in this respect is found in the papers of Fossum (1963), Bernheimer and Grushoff (1967b), Katsaras and Zeller (1977) Turnbull *et al.* (1979a, b) and Turnbull and Kramer (1983). In titrations of total hemolysin in cell-free filtrates of 155 strains (mostly isolates from human and animal infections), using 0.5 per cent human blood, 10 (6.5 per cent) were recorded as having titers of less than 1:5, the lowest dilution tested (P. C. B. Turnbull, unpublished results), but it is doubtful that truly hemolysin negative strains exist.

It was interesting to note in those titrations some parallelism between the hemolysin titers and phospholipase activities of the strains determined by the methods of Turnbull *et al.* (1979a). A high proportion of strains exhibiting high hemolysin titers also produced large egg yolk turbidity zones and vice versa with lower hemolysin and phospholipase activities. The relationship was not, however, exclusive (Turnbull and Kramer, 1983).

Blood from a variety of mammals and birds have been used by the various authors and none have been reported as having notable resistance to *B. cereus* hemolysin. In tests done preliminary to the titrations referred to in the preceding paragraph, no significant differences in susceptibilities were noted between human and rabbit blood. The only other reference found to a comparative study was that of Rawley and Hunter (1951) who found that rabbit erythrocytes were considerably less sensitive to *B. cereus* hemolysin than chick red cells. Taking the data of Pendleton (in Smyth and Duncan, 1978) on thuringiolysin for the purposes of analogy, it would be reasonable to expect cereolysin to exhibit similar differences in the sensitivities listed.

Ivers and Potter (1977) studied production *B. cereus* hemolysin in commercially strained beef and peas and in blanched ripe bananas. They reported that hemolysin production at 30°C was supported by the beef and pea preparations but not by the banana which they proposed must be deficient in some essential nutrient or at too low a pH (5.0). J. M. Kramer (personal communication), interested in this from the stand-point of obtaining hemolysin-free skin test toxin, found that hemolysin could be readily detected in similar banana purée cultures of 4433/73 and B-4ac even with maximum colony counts of 5×10^5 to 5×10^6/g. The production of hemolysin in beef and pea (Ivers and Potter, 1977) followed an eccentric pattern over the 24 hr period studied. At 4°C, approximately 55 per cent and 80 per cent of its activity had been lost after 48 hr in the beef and pea preparations respectively and somewhat similar losses were recorded after freezing to -37°C and rethawing at 48 hr. In the beef, only 50 per cent of hemolytic activity was lost on exposure to 65°C for 30 min and 77 per cent after 120 min. This is rather greater stability than recorded by other authors.

TABLE 12. *Growth of B. cereus 4433/73 and production of hemolysin (HL) phospholipase (PL) and vascular permeability reaction (VPR) factor in nutrient broth and three foods*

Time (hr)	0	1	2	3	4	5	6	7	8	9	10	24
4433/73 Nutrient Broth 36°C Shaker												
Log colony count	4.1	4.3	5.1	6.5	7.5	—	7.9	8.6	—	8.8	8.9	8.5
pH	7.1	7.1	7.2	7.2	7.2	—	7.9	7.8	—	7.8	8.0	8.4
Total HL	<5	<5	<5	<5	40	—	20	40	—	20	20	10
Heat stable HL	<5	<5	<5	<5	<5	—	5	10	—	10	10	10
PL	0	0	0	0	0	—	0	6.2	—	6.0	5.0	0
VPR	0	0	0	0	6.0	—	9.2	8.0	—	9.2	6.0	0
4433/73 Sterilized milk—36°C Shaker												
Log colony count	4.2	4.5	5.3	7.0	7.2	7.9	8.0	8.2	8.3	8.4	8.2	8.1
pH	—	6.3	6.4	6.4	6.5	—	6.4	6.4	6.5	6.4	6.5	6.7
Total HL	<5	<5	<5	5	20	640	320	320	320	320	320	320
Heat stable HL	<5	<5	<5	5	5	160	80	80	80	80	160	320
PL	0	0	0	0	0	0	6.0	6.5	8.1	8.4	8.0	7.5
VPR	0	0	0	0	0	6.0	0	0	0	5.8	0	0
4433/73 Commercial oxtail soup—36°C Shaker												
Log colony count	—	3.4	3.7	3.8	4.7	5.8	7.7	7.5	8.0	8.1	8.5	8.9
pH	5.1	5.3	5.1	5.4	5.2	5.4	5.3	5.3	5.5	—	5.2	5.3
Total HL	<5	<5	<5	<5	<5	<5	<5	<5	<5	40	40	<5
Heat stable HL	Not done											
PL	0	0	0	0	0	0	0	0	0	12.0	12.5	0
VPR	0	0	0	0	0	0	0	0	0	5.8	5.0	0
4433/73 Canned mushy peas 1:1 with distilled water and blended 36°C shaker												
Log colony count	4.2	4.8	4.7	6.5	7.5	7.5	7.6	8.8	8.7	8.2	7.8	8.5
pH	6.1	6.1	6.2	6.1	5.8	5.8	6.0	6.1	—	6.2	—	5.8
Total HL	<5	<5	<5	<5	20	40	80	80	160	160	80	5
Heat stable HL	<5	<5	<5	<5	<5	5	20	40	40	40	40	10
PL	0	0	0	0	0	0	6.3	6.5	8.3	7.9	8.9	8.5
VPR	0	0	0	0	7.5	7.8	7.5	8.5	8.5	7.5	7.0	0

10–20 ml vols inoculated with 5 per cent overnight nutrient broth cultures.

4.6. MODE OF ACTION OF *B. CEREUS* HEMOLYSINS

Hunter *et al.* (1949) found that Seitz or Berkefeld filtrates of *B. cereus* cultures in Bacto proteose peptone No. 3 broth had only a little effect on the respiration rate of chicken erythrocytes. Hemolysis as such was not recorded and one cannot be certain in retrospect to what extent hemolysins would pass through those types of filters unadsorbed. However, using a system which observed changes in light transmission through red cell suspensions by which altered red cell volume could be assessed reflecting, in turn, changes in permeability and osmotic effect, Hunter *et al.* (1950) noted that the *B. cereus* filtrates had a 'marked effect' on the osmotic status of chicken and dogfish erythrocytes. Rawley and Hunter (1951) tested fragilities of red cells exposed to '*B. cereus* toxins' by observing subsequent hemolysis during swelling in 0.3 M and 0.6 M Ringer–Locke solution and shrinking in 1.25x and 2x normal strength Ringer–Locke solution and comparing the results with unexposed controls. A $2\frac{1}{2}$ hr exposure rendered chicken red cells significantly fragile while rabbit erythrocytes required $4\frac{1}{2}$ to 7 hr and dogfish cells even longer (not specified).

They concluded that exposure to *B. cereus* toxins weakened the cell surface eventually leading to hemolysis but did not affect the channels through which small lipid-insoluble non-electrolytes (glycerol, ethylene glycol, urea, thiourea and erythritol) penetrate. They evidently thought phospholipase might be the principal factor in causing this weakening.

Pendleton *et al.* (1972) examined the effects of cereolysin on rabbit erythrocyte membranes by electronmicroscopy and found that, although they were smaller in diameter or less frequent, characteristic pits and arc or ring-shaped structures similar to those produced by streptolysin O were also produced by cereolysin. Binding of both lysins was shown to occur in cholesterol-containing cells but not to bacterial membranes in which cholesterol is absent. That membrane cholesterol was the common binding site of cereolysin and streptolysin O was confirmed by Shany *et al.* (1974).

Cowell *et al.* (1976), by placing cereolysin akin to the oxygen-labile (later known as 'thiol-activated') cytolysins defined some of its probable properties and modes of action. These are reviewed for thiol-activated cytolysins in general by Alouf (1977) and Smyth and Duncan (1978) who accepted the position of cereolysin within this classification. The binding site for these toxins on the red cell membrane is cholesterol; pre-incubation of the toxin with cholesterol inhibits hemolysis but cholesterol does not affect the reaction once binding has occurred. Hemolysis is a multi-hit phenomenon; several hundred molecules are required to lyse a single red blood cell. The rate of hemolysis is proportional to the toxin concentration and is a function of temperature although the initial binding of the toxin to the red cell is not temperature-dependent. The hemolysis occurs by a colloidosmotic mechanism in which small holes are produced in the red cell membrane and the ability to prevent free exchange of ions across the membrane is lost. Intracellular K^+ escapes but the net flow of ions and water is into the cell ultimately resulting in rupture.

There is no evidence that these toxins alter membrane components enzymatically; the reviewers proposed that it is just a direct sequestration and depletion of cholesterol which leads to the 'holes' and these toxins can cause permeability changes in a broad spectrum of cell types which contain cholesterol in their membranes. Of the two forms of cereolysin, oxidized and reduced (Cowell *et al.*, 1976), it is apparently the reduced form that is hemolytically active; the oxidised form is either unable to bind to or has decreased affinity for erythrocyte membranes. The mode of interaction of cereolysin with its cholesterol receptor has yet to be elucidated.

Coolbaugh and Williams (1978) found that hemolysis by both of their hemolysins involved two stages: a stage of attachment and a stage of lysis. The rate of hemolysis in the second stage was progressively reduced by cooling to 0°C but attachment still occurred rapidly at 0°C; the required number of red cells removed all hemolysin from a standard suspension in < 1 min. In fact, the ability of erythrocytes to absorb hemolysin at 0°C without lysis was used by Glatz and Goepfert (1973) to remove hemolysin from culture filtrates of B-4ac and to demonstrate that hemolysin and skin activities were differentiable.

In measurements of hemolytic reaction rates at 37°C (Coolbaugh and Williams, 1978) the maximum rate of hemolysis by H-I (cereolysin) was reached in < 1 min at all concentrations tested while that of H-II reached a peak after a lag of 2–7 min. The authors thus proposed that an intermediate step might be involved in hemolysis by H-II and they further showed this to be a temperature-dependent step. Support for their belief that H-I was cereolysin was gained in that it was inhibited by cholesterol; this was not the case for H-II.

The mode of action of sphingomyelinase as a hemolysin and the factors involved are discussed under 'Phospholipases' (p 422).

4.7. HEMOLYSINS AS *IN VIVO* TOXINS

The rapid lethal effect of purified cereolysin on i.v. injection in mice (Bernheimer and Grushoff, 1967a; Turnbull *et al.*, 1979b) allows the hemolysin to be regarded as a toxin and the gross and histological observations (see 'Mode of action of the lethal factors') support the concept that, in keeping with the thiol-activated cytolysins as a whole, it is a cardiotoxin. However, despite the claim by Bernheimer and Grushoff (1967a) that it is one of the most potent *in vitro* hemolytic agents known, it remains uncertain what role it has, if any, in *B. cereus* infections.

The early idea of Burdon (1947) that the pathogenicity of a strain of *B. cereus* is related to its hemolytic activity is clearly over-simplistic. It did appear though from the analysis of exotoxin production by isolates from 120 human infections and 27 environmental strains that cereolysin may play a positive part in production of the clinical manifestations of infections. The manner and extent of this involvement could not however be defined at all precisely (Turnbull and Kramer, 1983).

Johnson and Bonventre (1967) and Bonventre and Johnson (1970) felt that, since normal serum inactivates the hemolytic activity rapidly, it is quite likely that *B. cereus* hemolysin has little if any *in vivo* significance. Neither is hemolysis apparent in histological sections of mice which succumb to the lethal activity of cereolysin (see section 3.7, p 407). Nonetheless, the consistent strength of altered vascular permeability reactions and necrosis produced by cereolysin-containing electrofocusing fractions found by Turnbull *et al.* (1979b) and J. M. Kramer and P. C. B. Turnbull (unpublished results) suggests that cereolysin is a strongly active metabolite and may play a role either in wound and other infections where the opportunity for serum inhibition is limited or before the neutralizing action of serum has completely taken effect.

It is not possible yet to say whether the second hemolysin of Fossum (1963, 1964), Coolbaugh and Williams (1978), Kramer *et al.* (1978), Parker and Goepfert (1978) and Turnbull *et al.* (1979b) can reasonably be called a toxin. To use the terminology of Bonventre and Johnson (1970), it may be an 'auxiliary virulence factor' but this remains to be established.

Coolbaugh and Williams (1978) argue that the ubiquity of hemolysins in bacteriology and the metabolism expended in their production suggests that they must have a (teleological) function, but with *B. cereus* hemolysins as with those of other organisms, their function in the life of the bacteria themselves remains a mystery for the present.

4.8. SUMMARY OF HEMOLYSINS

In summary it appears that *B. cereus* is, in general, capable of producing two hemolysins; the well defined cereolysin of approximate MW 55,500 and now numbered among the thiol-activated cytolysins (Alouf, 1977; Smyth and Duncan, 1978) and a second less well-defined hemolysin of MW in the order of 30,000.

Cereolysin has been isolated to a high degree of purity and found to be a single polypeptide chain of 518 amino acids (Cowell *et al.*, 1976). It exists in two separable species: a reduced active form (pI 6.5–6.6) and an oxidized inactive form (pI 6.3–6.4). It shares the properties of thiol-activated cytolysins in having cholesterol as its receptor on the host cell membrane, in being inhibited by anti-streptolysin O, at least in hyperimmune horse serum, in being lethal on i.v. injection in mice and probably cardiotoxic.

The second hemolysin is relatively more stable to heat than cereolysin, exhibits the Arrhenius effect, and a different pattern and rate of lysis and is not inhibited by cholesterol—therefore presumably having a different receptor site from cereolysin.

Both hemolysins are exponential phase metabolites and are equally sensitive to chloroform, ether, pH extremes, trypsin and pronase (Coolbaugh and Williams, 1978). Their role as *in vivo* toxins have not been established.

The roles of phospholipase-C, especially sphingomyelinase, and the necrotic skin test/loop fluid inducing toxin in hemolysis are considered also.

4.9. PRODUCTION OF HEMOLYSINS BY OTHER *BACILLUS* SPECIES

The inability of *B. anthracis* to elaborate hemolysin has long been a useful criterion for distinguishing it from the otherwise closely related *B. cereus*. The other close relative to *B. cereus, B. thuringiensis* (Kaneko *et al.*, 1978), on the other hand does also produce two hemolysins: thuringiolysin with MW 47,000 and a secondary hemolysin of MW 29,000 (Pendleton *et al.*, 1973). The MWs were estimated by Sephadex G-100 chromatography. These two hemolysins appear to be analagous to those of *B. cereus* and thuringiolysin is also classed as a thiol-activated cytolysin (Alouf, 1977).

Among the other *Bacillus* species reported to produce detectable hemolytic activities are *B. alvei, B. laterosporus, B. licheniformis* (Bernheimer and Grushoff, 1967b) and *B. subtilis* (Büsing, 1950; Williams, 1957). *B. alvei* and *B. laterosporus* were found to produce hemolysins which, like cereolysin, closely resembled streptolysin O while *B. subtilis* gave rise to a relatively weak lysin, not cysteine-activable.

5. PHOSPHOLIPASES-C

The topic of bacterial phospholipases has been thoroughly reviewed most recently by Möllby (1978). It is not within this author's capacity to improve this; to a considerable extent, citation from it is adequate to place phospholipases-C in context among the other metabolites of *B. cereus* variously thought of as toxins and covered by this chapter.

5.1. INTRODUCTION

Phospholipases are a group of enzymes whose substrates are phospholipids found almost exclusively in biological membranes. There are two classes of these: glycerophospholipids and sphingolipids.

Among the most important phospholipids in mammalian membranes are phosphatidyl-choline (= lecithin), a glycerophospholipid, and sphingomyelin, a sphingolipid. In addition, cholesterol in cytoplasmic membranes is associated with the phospholipids in the membrane bilayer and hydrolysis of phospholipids by phospholipases is cholesterol-affected.

Möllby (1978) has reviewed the official classification of the phospholipases A–D according to the International Union of Biochemists (Enzyme Nomenclature, 1973) on the basis of their specific substrates and concluded there is a great need for improved designations. Officially, phospholipase-C is phosphatidylcholine (lecithin) cholinephos-phohydrolase, but it appears that it comprises a group of enzymes which hydrolyze several types of glycerophospholipids and sphingomyelin.

The phospholipases-C are the most thoroughly studied of the phospholipases and are produced by a variety of bacteria, both gram negative and gram positive. Little, other than their existence, is known about many of these. The most thoroughly studied is *C. perfringens* α-toxin and, as has been mentioned in the sections on lethal toxin and hemolysins, this is believed to be a single molecule possessing phospholipase-C, hemolytic and lethal activities. It has long been thought to be a major virulence factor and the most important toxin of *C. perfringens* in gas gangrene. However, as again reviewed by Möllby (1978), the preparations used in studies on which this conclusion has been reached were frequently of inadequate purity and full understanding of *C. perfringens* virulence is far from complete (see section 3.2, p 401 under 'Lethal toxin').

A comparison between *C. perfringens* α-toxin and the *B. cereus* phospholipase-C which hydrolyzes phosphatidylcholine serves to exemplify the variations which may be anticipated when more is known about phospholipases-C from different bacterial species. The *B. cereus* phospholipase-C does not possess either hemolytic or lethal activity, is less active on human fibroblasts, does not affect bacterial protoplasts as does α-toxin, is not affected by chelating agents as is α-toxin, has a pI of 8.1 as compared with that of α-toxin which lies in the vicinity of 4.6–5.7, has a MW of 23,000 compared with 30,000 for α-toxin and is antigenically unrelated (Chu, 1949; Johnson and Bonventre, 1967; Bonventre and Johnson, 1970; Möllby, 1978).

5.2. The Phospholipases-C of *B. cereus*

References to production of phospholipase-A (phosphatidate acylhydrolase) by *B. cereus*, at least under certain circumstances, have been found (Gaäl and Ivánovics, 1972, 1976; Ivánovics *et al.*, 1974, 1976) but equally frequently, searches for phospholipase-A (Slein and Logan, 1965; Johnson, 1966) and phospholipase-D (Johnson, 1966; Cole and Proulx, 1975) in cultures of *B. cereus* have failed to reveal the presence of these enzymes. Early confusion in the nomenclature of the phospholipases (Slein and Logan, 1963) may have given rise to misunderstandings, but it appears to be the general concensus of opinion that the phospholipases of *B. cereus* are exclusively of the C-type.

Although the precise relationship between production of phospholipase and egg yolk turbidity tests has yet to be clarified, the production of phospholipase has long been utilised in the routine identification of *B. cereus* in lecithovitellin or lecithinase tests. In this, the phosphatid lecithin of egg yolk is hydrolyzed (Colmer, 1947). Titration in some manner of the end-products resulting from the hydrolysis of egg-yolk lecithin has long been and remains a basic test for the assay of phospholipase-C activity (Zwaal *et al.*, 1971). In the experience of this laboratory, virtually all strains of *B. cereus* are lecithinase positive although both observations at the routine bench and specific attempts at measurement (Katsaras and Zeller, 1977; Turnbull *et al.*, 1979a, b; Turnbull and Kramer, 1983) show considerable variations in strengths of reaction among different strains under fixed conditions. Lecithinase negative strains have, however, been reported (Kreig, 1969; Lemille *et al.*, 1969; Spira and Goepfert, 1972a; Glatz *et al.*, 1974).

Three different enzymes produced by *B. cereus* were found by Slein and Logan (1963, 1965) to have phospholipase-C activity. All are vegetative growth metabolites, conventionally produced by well-aerated culture at 37°C. The most widely studied is that which hydrolyzes phosphatidylcholine and other natural phospholipids and is the enzyme commonly being referred to when discussing phospholipase-C from *B. cereus* (Möllby, 1978). The second and third enzymes have specificities for phosphatidylinositol and sphingomyelin and these have been characterized by Ikezawa *et al.* (1976, 1977, 1978, 1980).

Phosphatidylcholine cholinephosphohydrolase, the first of the enzymes, has been extensively purified and analyzed and the literature has been fully cited by Möllby (1978) and Little and Johansen (1979). It is a monomeric metalloenzyme of MW 23,000 with maximal activity at pH 7.2–7.5, containing two zinc atoms essential to its conformational stability and no disulphide bonds. Its activity is not influenced by Ca^{2+} ions. The importance of several amino residues and a carboxyl group to the binding and catalytic activities of the enzyme has been revealed. There seems to be some dispute as to its pI; Zwaal and Roelofsen (1974) place it between 7.2 and 8.5, Otnaess *et al.* (1972) at 6.5 while Ikezawa *et al.* (1978) found that isoelectric focusing yielded two species with pI's 6.8 and 7.5 respectively.

It remains accepted that this enzyme is not hemolytic to intact red cells although Möllby (1978) cites two reports attesting to hemolysis of guinea-pig and cod erythrocytes by it; further reports were cited on the susceptibility of human red blood cells after subjection to detergents or hypotoxicity and of chicken and toad red cells after ATP depletion. It is also generally regarded as not being lethal although Otnaess *et al.* (1976) is cited as determining that it had an i.v. LD_{50} of 1.6–1.7 mg/kg which is apparently on the limit for what is generally considered toxic in a protein ($LD_{50} = 1$ ppm). The enzyme is not dermonecrotic in rabbits and does not cause increased permeability in human fibroblast or rat muscle fibre plasma membranes (Möllby, 1978).

Phosphatidylinositol hydrolysing phospholipase-C, the second phospholipase-C of *B. cereus* detected by Slein and Logan (1965) and purified and characterized by Ikezawa *et al.* (1976, 1977) was found to have a MW of 29,000, a pI of 5.4 (Ikezawa *et al.*, 1978) and was not dependent on intact sulphhydryl groups or divalent cations. The enzyme specifically releases membrane-bound alkaline phosphatase from cellular membranes. Slein and Logan (1960, 1962) had noted that crude filtrates of *B. anthracis*, *B. cereus* and *B. thuringiensis* injected i.v. into rabbits produced hyperphosphatasemia. Since antisera to crude *B. anthracis* lecithinase inhibited phosphatasemia but not lecithinase activity in *B. cereus* filtrates and since aged filtrates were also phosphatasemia negative but lecithinase positive, they initially felt that the phosphatasemic factor was not phospholipase-C. However, by the following year (Slein and Logan, 1963) they had been able to demonstrate that *B. cereus* produced a second phospholipase which could be associated with the phenomenon and which they thus named the 'phosphatasemia factor'). Subsequently (Slein and Logan, 1965) they showed this to be the phosphatidylinositol hydrolysing phospholipase-C.

The third phospholipase-C of *B. cereus* is sphingomyelinase, detected by Slein and Logan (1963) and purified by Ikezawa *et al.* (1978). Slein and Logan did not feel this enzyme had hemolytic activity but according to Ikezawa *et al.* (1978), it is a protein of MW 24,000 and pI 5.6 and is apparently capable of breaking down sphingomyelin in the outer leaf of the membrane lipid bilayer of sheep red blood cells ultimately leading to hemolysis.

Ikezawa *et al.* (1980) investigated this hemolytic action in more detail and found that there was a strong correlation between the sphingomyelin content of the red cell and sensitivity to the enzyme. Sheep cells with 51.0 per cent sphingomyelin content were the most sensitive among erythrocytes tested (human 26.9 per cent, rabbit 19.0 per cent, horse 13.8 per cent and rat 12.8 per cent sphingomyelin content respectively). Hot hemolysis was preceded by sphingomyelin breakdown and 10 mM Ca^{2+} inhibited the latter with complete suppression of the former. Hot-cold hemolysis started immediately after contact with the enzyme before appreciable loss of sphingomyelin and occurred to a significant extent in the presence of 10 mM Ca^{2+}. Thus, they concluded that, while hot hemolysis did depend on enzymatic sphingomyelin degradation, hot-cold hemolysis did not. Both types of hemolysis were stimulated by the presence of Mg^{2+}, especially with Ca^{2+} also present. At 37°C in the presence of 10 mM $MgCl_2$ and 10 mM $CaCl_2$, 40 per cent and 85 per cent of sphingomyelin were lost respectively at 15 and 30 min and the red cells had become spherical (spherocytes) at 30 min with approximately 60 per cent lysis. In action, the sphingomyelinase resembled *C. perfringens* α-toxin although, in contrast to this, it was extensively adsorbed onto red cell surfaces during incubation; furthermore, Ca^{2+} ions stimulate rather than inhibit the hydrolytic action of phospholipase-C.

The adsorption phase was not influenced by cations and the receptor sites for adsorption have not been determined. It was not clear whether the pits and vesicles reported in several papers reviewed by the authors examining the action of hemolytic *Staphylococcus aureus* sphingomyelinase (β-toxin) on red blood cells was a feature similarly found with *B. cereus* sphingomyelinase. However, with a MW of 38,000 (Doery *et al.*, 1965; Wiseman, 1965) and pI of 9.4 (Wadström and Möllby, 1971), *S. aureus* sphingomyelinase was clearly a rather different molecule anyway.

5.3. PHOSPHOLIPASES-C AS TOXINS

Early workers influenced by the possible analogy between *B. cereus* toxins and *C. perfringens* α-toxin (Chu, 1949; Bonventre and Eckert, 1963b) thought the toxic activity of *B. cereus* filtrates in mice to be closely associated with the organism's phospholipase. Molnar (1962) presented evidence that toxicity as based on lethality in mice was distinct from phospholipase activity and by 1966 Johnson and Bonventre had established that partially purified preparations of *B. cereus* phospholipase were neither lethal nor hemolytic.

The reasons why it is arguable whether the first of the phospholipases-C, phosphatidylcholine cholinesterese, can legitimately be rated a toxin were discussed six paragraphs earlier.

Slein and Logan (1963) were unclear as to the possible relationship between the second (phosphatasemic) phospholipase-C, phosphatidylinositol hydrolysate, and hemolytic and lethal activities but Ikezawa *et al.* (1976, 1980) did not mention examining this with their purified preparations of this phospholipase-C. By inference it appears that the enzyme was not hemolytic; other bioassays were confined to phosphatasemic activities. Since stability characteristics were not given either (Ikezawa *et al.*, 1976, 1980), it is not possible to draw conclusions on these relationships on the basis of simple factors such as relative heat stabilities.

By means of a series of surgical and immunological tests, Slein and Logan (1962) determined that bone appeared to be the source of the excess serum alkaline phosphatase produced in response to this phospholipase-C. In the sense that elevated serum alkaline phosphatase is used as an indicator of liver or bone disease, this activity of the phosphatidylinositol hydrolysing phospholipase-C might legitimately be regarded as toxic.

There appears to be nothing yet on which to judge whether sphingomyelinase, the third phospholipase-C of *B. cereus*, may or may not be toxic *in vivo*.

Möllby (1978) felt it to be unlikely that the phospholipases-C from *B. cereus* would prove to be of pathological significance *per se*. However, where accessibility to their phospholipid substrates in the host-cell membrane may be prevented under normal *in vivo* circumstances, there may be occasions where they can act secondarily after exposure of the phospholipids by some other factor. An example of this might be the alleged synergistic effect (Gazitt *et al.*, 1975, 1976) between *S. aureus* sphingomyelinase-C and *B. cereus* phospholipase in hemolysing red blood cells. Bonventre and Johnson (1970) similarly proposed they might, like hemolysins, be auxiliary virulence factors.

Glatz *et al.* (1974) noted that injection of commercially purified *B. cereus* phospholipase-C into the skin of rabbits did produce a prominent, though transient alteration in vascular permeability. No relationship could be found (Turnbull *et al.*, 1979a; Turnbull and Kramer, 1983) between phospholipase activities in culture filtrates as measured by a very simple egg-yolk agar/well technique and the recorded severities of the 144 cases of human or animal infections, judged bona fide *B. cereus* infections, from which the strains under test had been isolated.

As far as precise mechanisms of action at cellular and membrane level are concerned in any pathogenic action these enzymes might have, very little is known at present. Analogy with the action of phospholipases-C from other bacteria such as *C. perfringens* and *S. aureus* must be made only with caution since it is clear that there are many properties *B. cereus* phospholipases-C fail to share with these (Möllby, 1978).

5.4. Summary of *B. cereus* Phospholipases-C

Three distinct types of phospholipase-C have been demonstrated in culture filtrates of *B. cereus*: (1) a phosphatidylcholine hydrolase, MW 23,000 (which also hydrolyses phosphatidylethanolamine); (2) phosphatidylinositol hydrolase, MW 29,000—the phosphatasemia factor, and (3) sphingomyelinase, MW 24,000.

Little information appears to be available on the differential kinetics of production of these, but findings such as those of Slein and Logan (1963) that shaking of cultures favors production of (1) while static incubation favors that of (2), indicate that such differences exist. Nor is it entirely apparent whether any one of these is produced in greater abundance by a given strain of *B. cereus* than the others. Phosphatidylcholine hydrolase, the enzyme usually being referred to in discussion on *B. cereus* phospholipase, is the best known and most studied and, indeed, the existence of sphingomyelinase was in doubt until very recently (Möllby, 1978). However, this may reflect problems in separation and identification rather than levels of production.

Phosphatidylcholine hydrolase appears to be, at most, only marginally 'toxic' and is not hemolytic. Whether phosphatidylinositol hydrolase can be regarded as toxic depends on the manner, as yet unidentified, by which it acts on bone tissue and causes raised serum alkaline phosphatase. Sphingomyelinase appears to have hemolytic activity, but its potential *in vivo* toxicity is not yet known.

For all three phospholipases-C, it would seem that any inherent toxic activity they may have probably depends on some other initiating factor which can give them access to their phospholipid substrates in the host cell membranes by removing protective covering proteins. There is little obvious evidence though that the phospholipases-C of *B. cereus* are involved in the clinical manifestations of *B. cereus* infections (Turnbull and Kramer, 1983).

6. LOOP FLUID-INDUCING/SKIN TEST/NECROTIC TOXIN

6.1. DIARRHEA AND *B. CEREUS*

Goepfert *et al.* (1972) traced a number of early publications reporting that *B. cereus* or *B. cereus*-like sporeformers, either as whole-cell or cell-free preparations could cause gastroenteritis or altered intestinal function in animal models. The earliest of these was that of Seitz (1913). However, interest in the idea that *B. cereus* might produce an enterotoxin arose as a logical consequence of increasing numbers of reports in the 1950's and 1960's, starting with that of Hauge (1950), that this organism was being implicated in a type of food poisoning characterized by abdominal pain and diarrhea 8–16 hr after ingestion of a wide range of foods which, on subsequent examination, were found to be heavily contaminated with *B. cereus*.

The general epidemiological history of this type of food poisoning was given in the opening paragraphs of this paper. As reviewed by Goepfert *et al.* (1972) and Gilbert (1979), early human feeding tests following Hauge's report gave some support to the concept of *B. cereus*-induced diarrhea and Nikodemusz (1965–1977, cited by Goepfert *et al.*, 1972 and Gilbert, 1979) found that cats and dogs fed food containing > 10^5 *B. cereus*/g could develop severe diarrhea and dehydration. Since then, feedings of whole cell cultures of strains isolated from food poisoning incidents to monkeys (Melling *et al.*, 1976; Goepfert, 1978; Logan *et al.*, 1979) and of sterile culture filtrates and ammonium sulfate precipitated preparations of strain B-4ac (Goepfert, 1973, 1978) have been reported to have induced diarrhea in these animals. In all the published papers and in our own unpublished results of feeding tests (J. Melling, personal communication) it was only possible to feed a small number of monkeys (2–6) with any one strain or preparation and invariably only a proportion of the animals showed recordable stool looseness. 'Profuse watery diarrhea' was encountered in Goepfert's feeding trials, but the results are not presented in detail and, in the manner recorded (Goepfert, 1978), the impression is gained that this was exceptional.

Melling, in numerous feeding trials with *B. cereus* strains (Melling *et al.*, 1976; Cayton *et al.*, 1978; Logan *et al.*, 1979; J. Melling, personal communication), has rarely noted more than transient looseness. An interesting example resulted from the feeding of strain 2769/77, isolated in heavy growth (2.4×10^8/g) from lobster paté and incriminated in a case of severe diarrhea and dehydration. In monkeys, the strain caused diarrhea in one, loose stools in a second, and no gastroenteritis in two more, but all animals were seriously unwell for 48 hr (Cayton *et al.*, 1978).

Melling's feeding preparations have consisted of rice culture slurries as designed for the search for an emetic toxin (see section 7.1, p 440) and it may be that these do not provide optimal culture conditions in tests for a diarrheal response. However, it is this author's opinion that, despite the number of reports over the years of diarrheal-type food poisoning associated with *B. cereus*, the epidemiological and experimental evidence that the organism is a significant agent of diarrheal disease remains inadequate. Findings during investigations of emetic-type *B. cereus* food poisoning and the results of a human volunteer feeding test in this laboratory using 243/80 (in the form of a proprietary pharmaceutical product [Vandekerkove, 1979] dispensed in various countries of Europe for treatment of antibiotic-induced or other enteritis) indicates that *B. cereus* survives sufficiently well in the gastrointestinal tract to allow ready detection 2–3 days after consumption of a significant dose (Table 13). Despite

TABLE 13. *Survival of* B. cereus *243/80 in human gastrointestinal tract following ingestion of 8 × 10⁹ spores in the form of a proprietary pharmaceutical product and taken as prescribed for therapy in humans against digestive disorders*

Day	Fecal colony counts/g			
	Total aerobic	Coliforms	*E. coli*	*B. cereus*
−1	6.2×10^6	$> 10^6$	$> 10^6$	NF
0 (pre-dose) }	5.0×10^7	$> 10^7$	$> 10^6$	NF
1	6.5×10^6	$> 10^6$	$> 10^6$	4.5×10^6
2	5.2×10^6	$> 10^6$	$> 10^6$	4.5×10^6
3	1.4×10^7	$> 10^7$	$> 10^7$	5.3×10^5
4	1.6×10^7	$> 10^7$	$> 10^7$	8×10^4
7	*B. cereus* present on enrichment*			
8,9	*B. cereus* not found			

*Feces in nutrient broth heated 20 min at 60°C incubated 7 hr at 37°C and subcultured to blood agar.

this, of the well-documented diarrheal-type incidents, the only outbreaks in which it was recorded that the organism was looked for and isolated from the feces of the sufferers as well as from the implicated food were those of Hauge (1950, 1955) and Giannella and Brasile (1979—see section 1.1, p 397).

Numerous tests have been carried out with conventional laboratory animals in an attempt to assess the diarrhea-producing potential of *B. cereus*. Goepfert *et al.* (1972) reviews a number of reports of such tests dating back to 1894; responses to feeding cultures of *B. cereus* or probable *B. cereus* varied from nil to production of enteritis. Papers are cited reporting development of diarrhea in guinea pigs injected i. p. or s.c., rabbits given whole cultures intra-rectally and mice injected i.p. with sterile culture filtrates. However, by today's stringent standards of experimentation and interpretation of results, these reports are less convincing in the demonstration of *B. cereus* as an agent of diarrhea than the summary suggests.

Spira and Goepfert (1972a) found that rabbit loop fluid-inducing cultures of strain B-4ac, when introduced directly into unligated ilea or by stomach catheter, failed to elicit diarrhea in rabbits. Using a stomach gavage this author has administered to mice 0.5 ml volumes of whole cell cultures ($> 10^9$ cells) and cell-free filtrates of highly skin test active (see below) preparations of 4433/73 and 668/78 and of relatively less skin active preparations of 4810/72 and 243/80. Whole cell cultures of 668/78 grown at 37°C, but not those grown at 25°C, killed the mice within 15 hr; the abdomens were recorded as swollen but no evidence of enteritis was seen among these or any others of the mice which remained well. Pre-feeding with 10 per cent $NaHCO_3$ 15–30 min before administration of the test preparations did not alter these results. Good histological sections of the stomach were not obtained but apparently damage was minimal if present at all; intestinal sections were entirely normal.

As covered on p 407, trials with *B. cereus* preparations in the infant mouse test, as used for *E. coli* heat stable toxin detection, simply resulted in the death of a proportion of the animals within 1–2 hr but there were no signs of intestinal fluid accumulation, looseness or dehydration in the remainder which were held for $7\frac{1}{2}$ hr before euthanasia. Madge (1978) demonstrated impaired absorption of D-glucose, D-galactose and four amino acids with slightly lowered fluid transfer in $2–3\frac{1}{2}$-month old mice following a single oral dose of 2×10^8 *B. cereus* cells. However, changes in intestinal histology and differences in the feces of reactors and controls were minimal. The toxigenicity of the strain used as measured by other tests is not known.

6.2. PROPOSED ACTIVE PRINCIPLE OF *B. CEREUS*-INDUCED DIARRHEA

Concern in the 1950's and 1960's was with establishing *B. cereus* as a food poisoning agent capable of causing diarrhea rather than with its possible mechanism of pathogenesis. The earliest suggestion concerning its mode of action was that of Nygren (1962) who postulated that phosphorylcholine, produced by the hydrolysis of lecithin by *B. cereus* phospholipase, might be the toxin of *B. cereus* food poisoning, but this view never gained further support. Even in 1970, Bonventre and Johnson were only able to state that it was not possible to identify the toxic product(s) responsible for *B. cereus* (diarrheal-type) food poisoning and that it could be the lethal toxin or the phospholipase, combination of the two or still another bacterial product.

The first clear indication of the possible existence of an enterotoxin is found in the mention by Goepfert *et al.* (1972) of preliminary success in their laboratory in eliciting fluid accumulation following injection of whole-cell *B. cereus* cultures into ligated rabbit intestinal loops. Later that year, Spira and Goepfert (1972a) gave more details on this. Positive fluid accumulation responses had been obtained with 19 of 22 *B. cereus* and also 4 of 6 *B. thuringiensis* cultures.

They made a number of important observations in this paper: (1) that, under the optimal growth and test conditions they had worked out (12 hr cultures in brain-heart infusion [BHI] broth tested in approximately 1 kg rabbits held 7 hr), different strains produced different degrees of fluid accumulation with fluid volume: loop length ratios varying from nil to 1.39; (2) that although several types of media were tested, while equally effective from the standpoint of bacterial growth, BHI consistently engendered the greatest loop response; nutrient broth cultures were consistently loop negative; (3) the loop response did not differentiate *B. cereus* strains isolated from food poisoning episodes from those of other origins; (4) response was poor and inconsistent in adult rabbits but consistent in young rabbits (< 1200 g) held 7 hr; (5) the response was not significantly affected by the position of the loop along the intestine; (6) when one or more of the loops was strongly positive, the animals were liable to die within 10 hr. Over a period of time using many strains from food poisoning, other clinical, veterinary, routine food and environmental sources, this author has substantiated these observations (Turnbull, 1976; Turnbull *et al.*, 1977b).

Using the loop-positive strain B-4ac, they (Spira and Goepfert, 1972a) made a number of other valuable observations; (7) cultures introduced directly into unligated ilea or by stomach catheter failed to elicit diarrhea; (8) fluid accumulation was significantly associated with approximately 2- to 3-fold increases in bacterial numbers within the ligated loops; in the case of negative accumulation, both with *B. cereus* and other *Bacillus* species tested, a fall in numbers was found. On the other hand, (9) *in situ* growth of the organisms by resuspension in fresh nutrient broth or BHI prior to injection failed to elicit a response. Also (10) large numbers (8×10^9/ml) of washed B-4ac vegetative cells (but not spores) provoked fluid accumulation. Finally, (11) cell-free supernates of 12 hr BHI cultures elicited strong positive responses. From these results (8–11), the authors concluded that increases in cell numbers were a consequence of, rather than a cause of fluid accumulation, that intraluminal multiplication was not involved in fluid accumulation and that, therefore, *B. cereus*-induced diarrhea was likely to be the result of intoxication rather than infection.

This important paper was the first of a series by Goepfert and his colleagues which revealed and delineated a hitherto undefined activity of *B. cereus*. On the basis of its loop fluid-inducing ability, they termed it an 'enterotoxin' but with circumspect caution based on their inability to actually induce diarrhea experimentally, they called it 'diarrheagenic factor' rather than 'diarrheal toxin'. They (Spira and Goepfert, 1972b) presented evidence of non-identity between this loop fluid-inducing factor and both hemolysin and egg-yolk turbidity factor.

Correlations had already been established for a number of enteric pathogens between fluid accumulation in ligated rabbit ileal loops and responses to intradermal injection of culture filtrates in guinea-pigs and rabbits. Glatz and Goepfert (1973) and Glatz *et al.* (1974), examining this for *B. cereus* and a few representative strains of other *Bacillus* species confirmed the correlation between the fluid-inducing abilities reported by Spira and Goepfert (1972a) and the extent of reactions in guinea-pig skin (Glatz and Goepfert, 1973) and vascular permeability reaction (VPR) in rabbit skin (Glatz *et al.*, 1974).

The guinea-pig skin reaction characterized by darkening at the site of inoculation within

5 min developing over a few hours into a necrotic ulcer of size and severity dependent on the toxigenicity of the strain (Figure 1) had previously been noted by Chu (1949), who attributed it to lecithinase, Burdon and Wende (1960) using log phase whole cell cultures and Molnar (1962) who associated it with a toxin she considered was distinct from phospholipase (see page 402).

The rabbit VPR test based on the cholera toxin model of Craig (1965), differed from the guinea-pig skin test in that, at the requisite time interval after intradermal injection of culture filtrates, Evans blue dye (1 ml of a 10 per cent solution/kg body weight) was injected i.v. In addition to the necrotic zone produced by sufficiently potent preparations, larger zones of blueing appear within 1 hr representing release of the dye into the dermal tissue resulting from altered vascular permeability (Fig. 2).

In applying these tests to culture filtrates of *B. cereus*, Glatz and Goepfert (1973) and Glatz *et al.* (1974) again noted that BHI, now supplemented with extra 0.1 per cent glucose (BHIG), gave consistently higher readings than trypticase soya broth and that without prior concentration, nutrient broth cultures gave barely or not detectable readings. On the basis of differential heat-stabilities, immunological tests using antisera to culture filtrates and to purified phospholipase-C, results with four phospholipase-negative strains and a permeability factor negative strain, and selective adsorption with rabbit erythrocytes at 0°C, they demonstrated the non-identity of this toxin with hemolysin and phospholipase-C.

They noted that commercially purified phospholipase-C could also cause a blueing response but that it did so with a different time course, giving prominent blueing at 2 hr post intradermal injection but no blueing at 3 hr. Consequently for testing the new permeability factor, they chose an interval of 3 hr between injection of test preparations and dye to preclude interference by phospholipase-induced reactions.

As judged by (1) the correlation between the extents of loop fluid accumulation and guinea pig skin test reactions associated with different strains of *B. cereus*, (2) their simultaneous

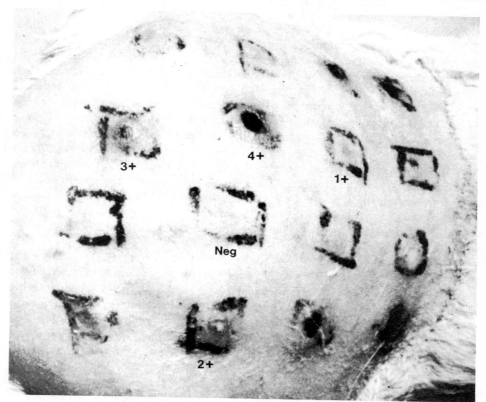

FIG. 1. Guinea-pig skin test. 0.05 ml cell-free culture filtrates injected intradermally. Necrotic reaction read at 18–20 hr; numbers indicate strength of reaction. (Turnbull *et al.*, 1977b). Reproduced by kind permission of the editor of the British Journal of Experimental Pathology.

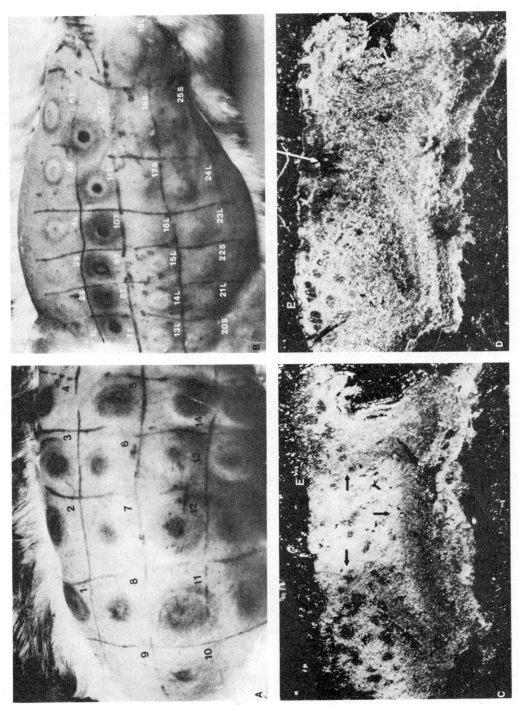

FIG. 2. Vascular permeability reaction (VPR) tests in rabbit skin. 0.05 ml of appropriate cell-free BHIG culture filtrate is injected intradermally at zero time; at 3 hr, 4 ml of 2 per cent Evans blue dye is injected i.v. Readings are taken at 4 hr and zones of necrosis checked at 24 hr. (A) *B. cereus.* Nos. 1,11 = fermenter-grown cultures of (1) 4433/73, (11) 668/78; VPR categories >5. Nos. 5,14 = Conventional shake flask cultures of (5) 4433/73, (14) 668/78; VPR categories 5. Nos. 6 to 9—all strain 243/80 (Vandekerkove, 1979); (6–8) whole spore suspensions, (9) spore filtrate; VPR categories 0–1. No. 10 = 3965/79, ex-aborted calf (Jones and Turnbull, 1981); VPR category 3. No. 12 = 169/80 ex-abscess; VPR category 3. No. 13 = 101/80 ex-drain site swab; VPR category 1. (B) L = *B. licheniformis*; S = *B. subtilis*; T = *B. thuringiensis.* All *B. licheniformis* and *B. subtilis* isolates were from food or feces related to food poisoning incidents (Turnbull, 1978, 1979b) except Nos. 16 (L), 19 (L) and 23 (L) isolated in relation to other infections. For the identities of the *B. thuringiensis* cultures (Nos. 7–12), see Table 8. (C,D) Cross-section (8 × 4 mm) of skin from a VPR category 4 reaction site; (C) unstained: note zone of blue around necrotic center (arrows); (D) stained with hematoxylin-and-eosin showing the necrotic central zone (arrow). E = epidermal surface.

appearance in cultures, (3) the parallel results obtained with different growth media, (4) similar heat-sensitivities and stabilities on storage, and (5) similarities in being precipitated by 60 per cent ammonium sulfate, non-dialyzable and unaffected by EDTA, Glatz and Goepfert (1973) concluded that the loop fluid accumulation factor and the skin test factor were probably one and the same. Antisera to crude filtrates of B-4ac neutralized the lethal and guinea pig skin activities of 5 of 6 other *B. cereus* strains (and a strain of *B. thuringiensis*). They felt this indicated that there was probably more than one antigenically distinct form of the loop fluid-inducing/skin test factor but they were unable to conclude for or against the possible identity between this toxin and lethal activity.

Starting with concentrated cell-free filtrates, the likely identity of the loop-fluid inducing and the VPR factors was established by the highly significant linear regressions found for the two activities (Glatz *et al.*, 1974). The necrotic aspect of the reaction did not fit this regression, but this was not elaborated upon further.

Spira (1974) and Spira and Goepfert (1975) now classifying the diarrheagenic factor as an enterotoxin studied it in 'culture fluids' (CF) which were membrane filtrates of 8 hr (32°C) cultures concentrated, where necessary, by ammonium sulfate precipitation or polyethylene glycol and 'culture extracts' (CE) consisting of buffered saline suspensions of sonically disrupted cells, mostly strain B-4ac. Defining a 'diarrheagenic unit' as that amount of toxin eliciting a volume: length ratio of 0.2 in ligated rabbit loops and a permeability factor unit as the amount eliciting a 7 mm^2 area of blueing (Glatz *et al.*, 1974) they found (1) the toxin was present in CE only in trace amounts, and no more than with unsonicated cells, while being readily demonstrable in CF; this and (2) the results obtained using levels of extracellular DNA as an indicator of cell lysis in CF, showed that cell lysis was not associated with production of the toxin; (3) diarrheagenic and lethal activities showed the same strain-specific neutralization by anti-CF—that is, the activities of B-4ac and two other strains were neutralized but those of B-6ac were not; (4) flushing of loops up to 30 min after initial injection prevented fluid accumulation; interpretation of events after this was not possible since significant fluid increase had begun by 30 min in response to the toxin. This indicated a transient effect on intestinal permeability and an inability to bind tightly to a receptor site; (5) fluid accumulation could, in marked contrast to cholera and *C. perfringens* enterotoxin, be inhibited by injection of antiserum (but not normal serum) 10 min after injection of CF; (6) fluid accumulation was not affected by antisera produced against choleragen, partially purified *C. perfringens* enterotoxin or the lethal toxin of Johnson and Bonventre (1967).

On Sephadex G-75 chromatography, loop fluid-inducing, VPR and lethal activities were recovered coincidentally in a major and a trailing minor peak. Egg yolk turbidity factor was evidently well separated from these activities but hemolysin only poorly; however, the authors felt the elution profiles were sufficiently different to indicate significant differences in MW and that the toxin was not identical to either phospholipase-C or hemolysin. The appearance of an extra erythemal factor eluting just after the void volume and unrelated to any of the other activities increased the complexity of the picture.

Numerical relationships between lethality, loop fluid inducing and VPR activities were established such that 1 MLD = approximately 100 VPR units/ml (1 VPR unit = the quantity producing a 7 mm^2 area of blueing) and 1 diarrheagenic unit (fluid accumulation volume: loop length = 0.2) = approximately 50 VPR units/ml. The authors concluded that this was an exotoxin only synthesized and released by actively growing cells, that there was no appreciable increase during stationary phase and that intracellular concentrations (as measured in CE) was negligible in any moment of bacterial growth.

The findings of Spira and Goepfert (1972a), Glatz and Goepfert (1973), Glatz *et al.* (1974) and Spira and Goepfert (1975) have been confirmed and elaborated upon by other workers. In particular (1) P. C. B. Turnbull and R. J. Gilbert (unpublished findings, 1975) agreed that adult rabbits held for 18 hr as appropriate for cholera and *E. coli* heat labile toxins were not suitable for *B. cereus* toxin tests. Weanling rabbits (about 1 kg) held 5–7 hr gave the most consistent reliability if not more than 6 loops per rabbit were used; (2) the response was not affected by the position of the loop although reversal of the order of a set of injected preparations in duplicate rabbits is routine practice (Turnbull *et al.* 1977b); (3) it was similarly found that the presence of one or more very strong loops frequently led to shock which could not be reversed with adrenalin; (4) a given strain was found to exhibit a characteristic toxigenicity (Turnbull, 1976; Turnbull *et al.*, 1977b; Turnbull *et al.*, 1979a,b Turnbull and Kramer, 1983); (5) excellent correlation was confirmed between loop fluid accumulation and results in the guinea pig skin test (Turnbull *et al.*, 1977b) and VPR tests (Turnbull *et al.*, 1979a,b); (6) food poisoning isolates were no different from isolates of other origins in terms of the spectrum of toxigenicity encountered.

In addition, it was noted that severe mucosal necrosis (Fig. 3A, B) frequently accompanied fluid accumulation caused by strongly toxigenic strains; at first (Turnbull, 1976), this was thought to have been an unusual property of an isolate from a brain abscess (2141/74)

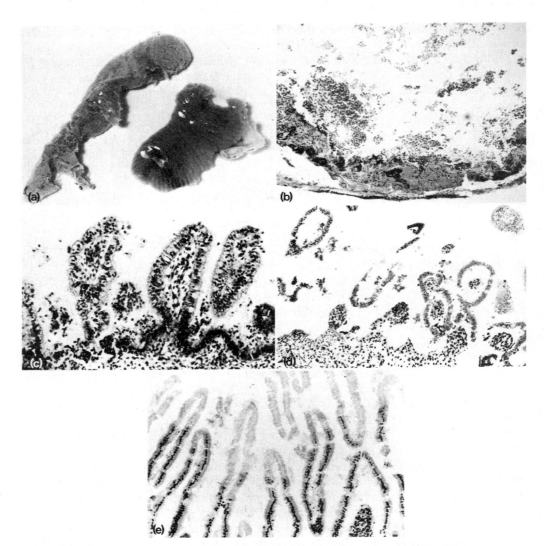

FIG. 3. The necrotic action of strongly toxigenic *Bacillus cereus* cell-free. BHIG culture filtrates (CFCF) on intestinal tissue. a,b. Ligated rabbit ilea after injection of 10-fold concentrated CFCF of (a) 2141/74 (left); sloughing mucosa at 4 hr with control at right (Turnbull, 1976) and (b) 837/76 at 7 hr; severe necrosis of mucosa and submucosa; Hematoxylin– and –Eosin × 30 (Turnbull *et al.*, 1977b). c,d. Human fetal intestine exposed 75 min *in vitro* to (c) BHIG (control) and (d) unconcentrated CFCF of 4433/73. All that remain of the villi in d are the outlines made up of disrupted, presumably dead, epithelial cells. e. Young adult mouse intestine exposed 75 min *in vitro* to unconcentrated CFCF of 4433/73; note the progressive loss of epithelial cell nuclei towards the lumen; c,d,e. Hematoxylin– and –Eosin, 10x objective. (Turnbull *et al.*, 1979b). Permission for reproduction of the figures was received with thanks from the editors of (a) the Journal of Clinical Pathology, (b) the British Journal of Experimental Pathology and (c,d,e) the American Journal of Clinical Nutrition.

but subsequently was found simply to relate to the toxigenicity of the strain (Turnbull *et al.*, 1977b).

In further confirmation of the findings of Goepfert's group, while fully grown whole cell cultures of strongly toxigenic strains in BHIG produced fluid accumulation, when 0.2–0.5 ml of culture was made up to 2 ml with fresh BHIG just before injection into the loop, no fluid accumulation or histological damage resulted from the growth that took place. With an interest in rice-associated food poisoning, rice cultures prepared and dialysed according to the method of Melling *et al.* (1976) were tested; some fluid accumulation and mucosal necrosis was obtained on occasion (Turnbull *et al.*, 1977b) but less than the BHIG equivalents. The casamino acids medium of Evans *et al.* (1973)—found to be good for *Escherichia coli* enterotoxin production—gave negative results with *B. cereus* (P.C.B. Turnbull, unpublished results). BHIG (Gibco) was equally effective as BHIG (Difco— P.C.B. Turnbull and J. Melling, unpublished results). Spore suspensions of strains 4810/72, 4096/73, 4433/73, 2141/74, 2532/74, containing 95 per cent –98 per cent spores, prepared on Tarr's sporulation agar slopes at 30°C for 5 days, were consistently loop negative. The lack of value for *B. cereus* preparations of the infant mouse *E. coli* heat stable toxin test has been covered under 'Lethal toxin' and earlier in this section; the necrotic effect was readily apparent in the stomachs but death intervened before lower intestinal changes occurred and the test was abandoned as of no value.

Satisfied that the correlation between the VPR and loop fluid induction tests was excellent (Turnbull *et al.*, 1979a, b), all further work on this *B. cereus* toxin was based on VPR as the simpler and more sensitive assay. It was found (Turnbull *et al.*, 1979b) that when 116 strains from a wide variety of sources were examined, *B. cereus* could be conveniently placed within 5 categories according to the strength of toxin production under standard test conditions. The total number of strains now examined has been increased to 221 and Fig. 4 and Table 14 show the essentially normal distribution found with these strains. Hemolysin and phospholipase titers obtained on representative strains from all categories revealed no correlation between hemolysin, phospholipase and VPR toxin production although the subsequent findings of some degree of correlation between hemolysin and phospholipase titers in culture filtrates from strains has been noted earlier (see section 4.5, p 413).

Pàrticular care, however, has to be taken when attempting to associate production of this toxin with the isolation histories of the strains as in Table 14. Strains submitted as having been implicated in diarrhea or an extraintestinal infection in fact may not always have been the causative agents. However, insofar as it has been possible to assess the probable involvement of a *B. cereus* strain in an infection from which it was isolated, in human cases at least (Turnbull and Kramer, 1983), a significant relationship was noted between the virulence of the isolate as reflected in the degree to which it appeared responsible for the signs and symptoms of an infection and its VPR toxigenicity. In contrast, the veterinary isolates (Table 14) are of particular interest in that, despite their reported association with gangrenous, sometimes lethal, mastitis, none have been higher than category 3 VPR toxin producers.

Similar gel chromatography profiles to those of Spira and Goepfert (1975) were obtained by Kramer *et al.* (1978), Katsaras and Hartwigk (1979) and Turnbull *et al.* (1979b). Failure to completely separate VPR toxin from hemolysin and phospholipase activities by Sephadex G-75 or G-100 chromatography following the method of Spira and Goepfert (1975) led these groups to trials with electrofocusing. Using strains 4433/73 and 671/78, Kramer *et al.* (1978) and Turnbull *et al.* (1979b) found this method to be highly effective in separating the loop fluid-inducing/VPR factor from cereolysin and phospholipase but, in the case of 4433/73, the fluid-inducing/VPR toxin remained slightly contaminated with the second hemolysin (see 'Two or more hemolysins' section 4.4, p 412) whose peak lay two fractions away; with 671/78, the peaks of this toxin and the second hemolysin were coincident.

Two additional important findings emerged from tests on these electrofocusing fractions—(1) immunologically different mouse lethal activities were separately associated with the fluid-inducing/VPR/necrotic toxin and the cereolysin/phospholipase peaks (see p 403–404, and Table 7); (2) the eluate containing cereolysin and phospholipase (which

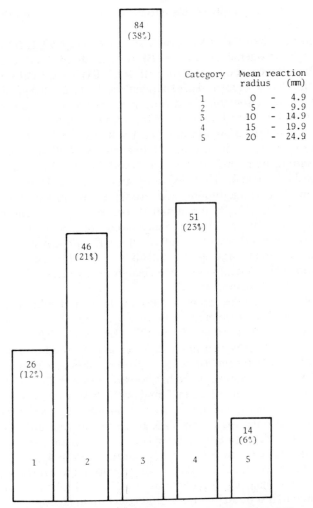

Category	Mean reaction radius	(mm)
1	0 –	4.9
2	5 –	9.9
3	10 –	14.9
4	15 –	19.9
5	20 –	24.9

FIG. 4. Vascular permeability reaction (VPR) toxin production by 221 (100 per cent) broadly selected strains of *Bacillus cereus* (see Table 14).

TABLE 14. *Distribution of* Bacillus cereus *isolates from various sources within five categories based on total vascular permeability reactions (VPR) in rabbit skin*

Type of strain by history	Total number of isolates	Number of isolates in VPR Category				
		1	2	3	4	5
Emetic	30	3	9	17	1	0
Diarrheal	12	1	4	2	3	2
Clinical (human)	109	11	20	35	35	8
Clinical (veterinary)	14	6	3	5	0	0
Routine*	56	5	10	25	12	4
All strains	221 (100%)	26 (11.8%)	46 (20.8%)	84 (38.0%)	51 (23.1%)	14 (6.3%)

*Milk & cream (14), meat & poultry (22), hospital environment (10), miscellaneous (10).

were not separated under the conditions used—i.e. those designed for isolation of the fluid-inducing/VPR/necrotic toxin) produced secondary vascular permeability reactions under the same conditions as used for assaying the fluid-inducing/VPR/necrotic toxin. This is in conflict with the finding of Glatz *et al.* (1974) that other blueing responses are insignificant at

3 hr. The full implications of these observations on the use and interpretation of VPR tests for measurement of the toxin under discussion have yet to be elucidated.

As based on Sephadex chromatography and electrofocusing supported by tests on temperature, enzyme and pH stabilities in crude filtrates or purified fractions, Turnbull *et al.* (1979b) concluded that the toxin was a protein of MW approximately 50,000 and pI in the order of 4.9. Immunological cross-reaction tests in VPR and gel diffusion tests using antisera raised to the purified fractions and to purified choleragen and *C. perfringens* enterotoxin confirmed the findings of Spira and Goepfert (1975) and Katsaras and Hartwigk (1979) that no immunological relationship existed between these three. Three bands resulted from polyacrylamide gel electrophoresis of the fluid-inducing/VPR/necrotic toxin as obtained from isoelectric focusing raising suspicions as to the purity of the electrofocused material (J. M. Kramer, personal communication). Finer resolution isoelectric focusing has indeed now revealed two distinct moieties of pI 5.1 and 5.6, both possessing VPR, necrotic and cytotoxic activities (Kramer, 1984). Analysis and chracterization of these and attempts at determining their interrelationships are underway.

With reference to the toxin of Ezepchuk and Fluer (1973) and Gorina *et al.* (1975, 1976—see section 3.3, p 402, 405), purification was based on mouse lethality and emesis in cats; however, as judged by the molecular size they report it is possible their toxin was the same one as has been described by Goepfert and co-workers and Turnbull and colleagues. Strain No. 96 from which this toxin was isolated and purified produced a very strong VPR in our hands; both its skin test and lethal activities were neutralized with antiserum to the VPR-active electrofocusing fraction of 4433/73. Its hemolysin titer measured according to the method given by Turnbull *et al.* (1979a, b) was 1:40 (relatively low). The relationship between the 100,000 MW permeability-factor-positive/loop-fluid-negative/lethal toxin of Ezepchuk *et al.* (1979), also originating from strain No. 96 (see p 405), and the toxin of Goepfert and colleagues, Turnbull and colleagues and Kramer is not clear at this point.

6.3. Production of Loop-fluid Inducing/VPR/Necrotic Toxin

The toxin is a vegetative growth metabolite. Spira and Goepfert (1972a) found that loop fluid-inducing activity could first be demonstrated about half-way through the exponential phase of growth (i.e. 2–3 hr at 32°C after inoculation with a 0.05 to 1.5 per cent level of a fresh stationary phase culture) with a maximum at about the time growth ceased to be exponential and shortly before the pH reached its minimum at 4–6 hr. Guinea pig skin test (Glatz and Goepfert, 1973) and VPR (Glatz *et al.*, 1974; Spira and Goepfert, 1975) appeared and reached their peaks in parallel with the loop fluid induction. In this respect, the kinetics of these activities closely resemble those of lethal toxin.

Data from other workers on careful studies of these kinetics have been hard to find. Jørgensen (1976) following the method of Glatz *et al.* (1974) but incubating at 30°C instead of 32°C, and using strain B-5ac obtained comparable results; in addition she carried out spore counts. The fairly sudden appearance of the VPR factor after a 2-log increase in vegetative counts and its persistence till the final reading at 12 hr did not relate in any clear manner to the spore counts which showed a small but fluctuating increase from 2×10^2 at 2 hr to 1×10^3 at 12 hr. At 20°C with strains B-4ac, B-5ac and 175, appearance of VPR activity slightly preceded or coincided with appearance of countable levels of spores, although after initial appearance at about 12 hr, spore counts remained fairly steady at levels of about 5×10^2 to 5×10^3 for each culture. Comparable VPR values were found at 20°C and 30°C although at 20°C, maximum values were reached at about 28 hr compared with 7 hr at 30°C and approximately 4.5 hr at 37°C.

It was the experience of Carpenter *et al.* (1975) with B-4ac in a fermenter, K. Jørgensen with B-4ac and 171 (personal communication) and Wayne, Kramer and Turnbull with strains 4433/73, 671/78 and B-4ac (Tables 10, 11) that maximum VPR occurred 1–4 hr after pH had reached its minimum level. Holding cultures of 4433/73 stationary or at 22°C delayed events (Table 10) while enriching the medium with fetal calf serum accelerated them for 4433/73, 671/78 and B-4ac without altering the kinetic pattern. At 40°C, growth of a stationary culture of 4433/73 was marginally poorer than at 36°C and the VPR which was significantly weaker than at 36°C, only appeared at the point of pH minimum. In slight contrast to the findings of Glatz *et al.* (1974) for B-4ac at 32°C, measurable VPR toxin was found in nutrient broth cultures of 4433/73 at 36°C (Table 12); there was no pH fall in this culture, probably because of the absence of glucose from the medium.

Somewhat transient and feeble VPR toxin production by 4433/73 was observed in sterilized milk and commercial oxtail soup (Table 12) but slightly better support for its production was found in blended commercial peas; again no pH fall was observed with these food materials.

In an attempt to determine the conditions for optimal production of the VPR toxin with a view to ultimate purification, Carpenter *et al.* (1975), Glatz and Goepfert (1976, 1977) and Spira and Silverman (1979) studied its production in fermenter-grown cultures of B-4ac in a semi-defined casamino acids based broth. The following findings taken from the three papers together were salient; (1) a 14 hr stationary phase and a 3 hr exponential phase inoculum gave equally good final yields; (2) 0.1 per cent and 1 per cent inocula gave good yields, but a 10 per cent inoculum resulted in a lower toxin yield; (3) optimal yields were achieved when an extra 0.5 per cent to 1 per cent glucose was incorporated into the medium; (4) pH control at 7.0–8.0 had a dramatic effect on yield increase over no pH control or control at other pH's; (5) production occurred at all temperatures between 20° and 40°C, but a marked maximum was found at 32°C; (6) the maximum agitation rate possible without foam being generated gave the highest yields; (7) yields under the optimal conditions given were up to 50-fold greater than by the conventional shake flask method of production and (8) harvest time was at 5 hr.

There was some disagreement as to the dissolved oxygen (DO) levels; Carpenter *et al.* (1975) gave the optimal level as 0–1 per cent, finding that at 10 per cent or greater, toxin yield progressively decreased, even though final cell population increased. Spira and Silverman (1979) expressed DO values in atmospheres but showed the same preference for lower values (0.002 atm) even though greater cell numbers were obtained at a DO of 0.1 atm. Glatz and Goepfert (1976, 1977) in contrast, claimed their maximum yields were obtained with DO levels of >80 per cent saturation. The authors were agreed, however, that significant toxin production was obtained anaerobically. Carpenter *et al.* (1975) felt that their observation of increased enterotoxin production at low DO levels reflected attempts by the organism to overcome oxygen restriction and to dispose of electrons under oxygen-limitation and energy balance regulation.

In relation to pH effect, Glatz and Goepfert (1976, 1977) felt that synthesis rather than toxin stability was pH sensitive since Spira and Goepfert (1975) had found the preformed toxin to be equally stable to pH's in the range 5–10.

The culture volumes involved in the fermenter studies just described were 300–500 ml; Turnbull and Melling (unpublished results) have obtained highly VPR active preparations (Figure 2a) of strains 4433/73 and 668/78 in 20 liter fermenters with the following conditions: a 1 per cent inoculum, pH maintained at 7.5, aeration of 10 l/min, and an agitation rate of 500 r.p.m. at which foaming was minimal. Closedown chillers were attached at $5\frac{1}{2}$–6 hr.

Again with subsequent toxin purification in mind, Parker and Goepfert (1978) tried the sac culture method as one permitting, on the one hand, the use of optimal growth broth (BHI) while, on the other hand, allowing production of enterotoxin in the absence of large MW media components undesirable in subsequent purification attempts. They found a 10-fold increase in yield of VPR toxin by B-4ac over conventional shake flasks and proposed that the method offered a simpler and cheaper alternative to fermenters for preparations destined for purification attempts. They found that phospholipase was enhanced similarly but not hemolysin. K. Jørgensen (personal communication) also tested the sac method using 4433/73, 2532/74 and 667/78 and confirmed the higher VPR toxin yield which could be elevated even further if the sac culture flasks were shaken. Phospholipase and hemolysin levels were not significantly altered from those obtained in conventional shake flasks in her results.

The cellophane-over-agar method as used for *S. aureus* enterotoxin did yield the toxin on BHI agar but at lower levels than the shake flask (K. Jørgensen, personal communication). This author found that rabbit loop fluid could not be induced by cellophane-over-blood agar preparations of 4433/73 and 837/76.

The kinetics of production of the 100,000 MW VPR-positive/lethal toxin of Ezepchuk *et al.* (1979) are not given. Initial culture consisted of 2 liters of an inoculated enzymatic casein hydrolysate-based broth shaken 110 r.p.m. in 5 liter flasks for 16–18 hr at 37°C.

6.4. STABILITY OF THE TOXIN

At 32°C, the loop fluid-inducing factor of B-4ac (Spira and Goepfert, 1972a) retained its maximum activity from 4–15 hr postinoculation, had weakened significantly by 24 hr and was not detectable at 48 hr. It was inactivated in 30 min at 56°C but not at 45°C (Spira and Goepfert, 1972a; Goepfert *et al.* 1973). In further studies, Glatz *et al.* (1974) reported that loop fluid-inducing and VPR factors had, by 21 hr, fallen to undetectable from a peak at 4–6 hr, and they suggested that either surface denaturation of the protein or action of other proteins in the medium might be responsible for this. A similar reduction in activities can be seen in the results of Wayne, Kramer and Turnbull (Tables 10, 11, 12).

Spira and Goepfert (1975) found this factor to be unstable at 25°C and 4°C. Studying the stability at 4°C more thoroughly, they noted that (1) ionic environment, with a minimum ionic strength of 0.3, was critical to maximal stability. Using NaCl, $CaCl_2$, NH_4HCO_3 or sodium or potassium phosphate buffers at pH 7.2 to 7.9 to provide the appropriate ionic environment, they demonstrated that the particular ions involved were irrelevant; (2) untreated toxigenic BHIG culture filtrates lost significant activity over 7 days at 4°C and several weeks at −20°C; (3) alkylation with mercaptoethanol plus iodoacetamide or acrylonitrile partially protected against loss of activity upon dialysis against 0.1 M phosphate buffer; they interpreted this as implying that natural loss of activity was partially attributable to the formation of disulphide bonds leading to molecular aggregation; (4) the stability of the toxin was maximal between pH's 5.0 and 10.0, sharply decreasing outside this range.

The stability of the B-4ac toxin in cultures not harvested at peak activity appears to be dramatically shorter in fermenter cultures with very rapid falls in activity within 2–4 hr (Carpenter *et al.*, 1975; Glatz and Goepfert, 1976; Spira and Silverman, 1979). Spira and Silverman (1979) found that limitation of oxygen reduced this instability somewhat. They also noted that the appearance of proteases was late in stationary phase—i.e. after much of the toxin loss had occurred. They thus concluded that instability was not attributable to protease but rather that the toxin-degrading factor was either an inducible enzyme related transiently to sporulation although insensitive to inhibitors of sporulation or, alternatively, the instability was related to a very early event in sporulation.

During the tests reported by Turnbull *et al.* (1977b), it was found that strongly toxigenic preparations of strains 4096/73, 2141/74 and 837/76 held at −10°C were exhibiting marked reduction in loop fluid-inducing ability within 3 weeks. Within this limitation, the toxin appears unaffected by freezing and thawing (Spira and Goepfert, 1975; P. C. B. Turnbull, routine observations). It is stable to lyophilization (Spira and Goepfert, 1975) and a freeze-dried preparation of ammonium sulphate precipitated B-4ac culture filtrate received from Dr. Goepfert by this author was highly active when tested two years later.

Turnbull *et al.* (1979b) determined that the activity remaining in a cell-free filtrate of 4433/73 was 100 per cent after 14 days at 4°C and 1 hr at 36°C, 53 per cent and 21 per cent after 1 hr at 50°C and 55°C respectively, 26 per cent and 10 per cent after 10 min at 55°C and 60°C respectively, 6 per cent after 5 min at 80°C and 0 per cent after 20 min at 55°C or 10 min at 80°C. Stability tests on purified (electrofocused) preparations have not been carried out yet.

The nature of the natural instability of the toxin at ambient and even refrigerator temperatures is not known, but the data appears to point to greater stability in cell-free filtrates harvested at the point of peak activity than if the culture is allowed to continue in its growth cycle.

The toxin was found by Spira and Goepfert (1972a), Goepfert *et al.* (1973) and Turnbull *et al.* (1979b) to be sensitive to trypsin and pronase but unaffected (Turnbull *et al.*, 1979b) by EDTA and glucuronidase. Both Spira and Goepfert (1975) and Turnbull *et al.* (1979b) found a minimum stability at pH 4 which is in the vicinity of the toxin's pI. This was also the case with the lethal toxin of Ezepchuk and Fluer (1973—see p 405).

The possible relevance of these characteristics to food poisoning is covered below.

6.5. STABILITY OF TOXIN PRODUCTION BY STRAINS

Reports on detailed studies on the ability of a strain to retain its toxigenicity are not available but it is the common experience of those who have studied the loop fluid-inducing/skin test/necrotic factor that frequent subculturing from an agar slant stock culture of a strongly toxigenic strain leads to partial (but not complete) loss of toxigenicity. It is, for example, increasingly difficult to obtain good yields from strains B-4ac (M. Bergdoll, personal communication) and 4433/73 (J. M. Kramer and P. C. B. Turnbull, routine observations).

That the phenomenon is associated with actual subculture rather than storage *per se* has been observed on occasions such as when more than one isolate has been submitted from a single event. Strains 667/78, 668/78, 669/78 and 671/78 were isolated on four separate occasions over four days from a gangrenous postoperative wound (Fitzpatrick *et al.*, 1979). All were serotype 2, morphologically and biochemically similar and strong VPR toxin producers. 671/78, on repeated subculture for further studies on the toxin became progressively weaker; the others, which had not been used, had retained their high toxigenicity on re-testing.

The nature of such loss in activity is not known. Experts on plasmids have asked for and received several strains from this laboratory, including 4810/72, 4433/73 and B-4ac, but in subsequent verbal discussions it appeared, that, while plasmids had been detected, it had not been immediately possible to relate their behavior to strain toxigenicity.

Reports are to be found, especially in the earlier literature of increased virulence of *B. cereus* on animal passage. Cenci (1971) and Candeli *et al.* (1975) associated this with rough/smooth variations; we have no experience to date of retrieved or increased toxigenicity by animal passage.

6.6. NON-ANIMAL DETECTION AND ASSAY

Until very recently no satisfactory alternative to animal tests for detection and assay of loop fluid-inducing/VPR/necrotic toxin had been reported. Crude cell-free culture filtrates were found to non-specifically strip conventional tissue cultures (Bonventre, 1965; Turnbull, 1976). The effect in the case of HeLa cells could not be neutralized by anti-Shiga toxin (A. D. O'Brien, personal communication). Giugliano (1983) and Kramer (1984) now report that human foreskin (HFS) and rabbit kidney (RK-13) cell lines show great promise as both sensitive and specific detectors of loop fluid-inducing/VPR/necrotic activities, capable of distinguishing them from hemolysins and other metabolites which may also be present.

In vitro cultured sections of intestine were found to be sensitive to the necrotic action of toxigenic crude BHIG culture filtrates (Turnbull *et al.*, 1979b; see figures 3C, D, E) but no practical advantages resulted from these findings.

Antisera raised in rabbits to the purified active electrofocusing fractions of 4433/73 and 671/78 were found in preliminary tests to neutralize the VPR activities of 10 other *B. cereus* strains and a *B. thuringiensis* strain; they also gave monospecific precipitin lines against the cell-free filtrates of the homologous cultures and a major with, at most, two minor lines against heterologous strains (Kramer and Turnbull, 1979). On occasion, neutralization was not complete but in-depth tests to determine whether this represented heterogeneous activities or merely that optimal antibody–antigen combination and incubation had not been achieved have not yet been carried out.

Attempts are being made to develop other methods for detection and assay of the toxin in foods or other clinical specimens utilizing these antisera. So far, gel diffusion remains the only technique in which limited success has been achieved. Soups, for instance, artificially contaminated with 4433/73, which grew to a viable count of 10^5-10^6 cfu/ml produced a level of toxin just detectable by this method (Kramer and Turnbull, 1979).

Gorina *et al.* (1975, 1976) report that passive haemagglutination ('aggregation haemagglutination') using antiserum to the purified 'exo-enterotoxin' of Ezepchuk and Fluer (1973) proved to be 1000-fold more sensitive than gel diffusion and was applicable to the detection of the toxin of strain No. 96 in a variety of foodstuffs.

6.7. MODE OF ACTION OF THE TOXIN

Most work to-date on the loop fluid-inducing/VPR/necrotic toxin has been aimed at (1) determining its relationship to diarrheal-type food poisoning, (2) demonstrating its non-identity with hemolysin and phospholipases-C and (3) purification. Only its most basic characteristics have been determined, so a full understanding of its mode of action is still distant.

The reasons for the slow progress in this understanding are (1) that it is produced among a profusion of other metabolites from which it is not readily separated, (2) its lability and (3) the difficulties of finding reliable conditions for large scale production and purification.

Turnbull (1976) attempted to determine whether fluid accumulation in the ileal loop was a cAMP-mediated event. Adenylate cyclase activities (ACA) of homogenized mucosal epithelial cells from ileal loops extracted after exposure *in vivo* for $3-4\frac{1}{2}$ hr to concentrated cell-free culture filtrates of 4810/72, 4433/73, 2141/74, 2532/74 and *V. cholerae* NCTC 7254 were measured. Within the limits of the relatively large probable error inherent in the method used, the results of multiple tests indicated that fluid accumulation might be associated with raised ACA. Fumarola *et al.* (1976) using a platelet aggregation method which they claimed could differentiate enterotoxins affecting ACA, found that, while lyophilized concentrated cell-free filtrate of 4433/73 sent to them failed to pass the test (Fumarola *et al.*, 1976), freshly prepared concentrated cell-free filtrates did subsequently give positive results (D. Fumarola, personal communication). The recent finding by Leppla (1982) that the edema factor component of the toxin of *B. cereus* is an adenylate cyclase may or may not be relevant. *B. anthracis* is a very close relative of *B. cereus* but, on the other hand, there have been no suggestions to-date that *B. cereus* can produce any of the components of anthrax toxin.

Attempts to confirm or negate the findings on ACA in this laboratory using *in vitro* systems have been unproductive. Avian red cells which have proved ideally suitable for such tests with choleragen and *E. coli* heat labile enterotoxin are rapidly lysed by *B. cereus* preparations—even the purified ones. We have been unable to prepare homogeneous preparations of other cell types with sufficient cell density to use as alternatives to red cells. If it is subsequently confirmed that the toxin does alter ACA in a manner analogous to choleragen, it and *Staphylococcus aureus* delta-toxin (O'Brien and Kapral, 1976) would be the first toxins from gram positive bacteria to have been shown to do so. Interestingly, *S. aureus* delta-toxin was also found to be cytotoxic.

Madge (1978), as detailed earlier in this section, showed that the mechanisms typical of malabsorption may be involved.

The importance of the potent necrotizing abilities of this toxin when produced strongly (Turnbull, 1976; Turnbull *et al.*, 1977a, b; Turnbull, 1979a, b—see Figs 1, 2, 3) to its mode of action either in diarrhea or clinical infections is only understood rudimentarily as yet. Necessarily subjective analysis of a large number of *B. cereus*-associated infections (Turnbull and Kramer, 1983) resulted in evidence that it does play a major part in producing the tissue destruction in conditions such as gangrenous wound infections, abscessation, cellulitis and panophthalmitis (Turnbull *et al.*, 1977a; Fitzpatrick *et al.*, 1979; Young *et al.*, 1980; O'Day *et al.*, 1981a; O'Day *et al.*, 1981b; Turnbull and Kramer, 1983). It seemed probable from that analysis that cereolysin also played a role in these manifestations, but not phospholipase. The involvement of other aggressins such as listed in Table 6 remains undetermined. An explanation is needed for the finding that in 24 cases of bovine mastitis, many of which were fatal, gangrenous, peracute or severe (Jones and Turnbull, 1981), the *B. cereus* isolates were all category 3 or less.

The manner in which the organism kills tissue is unknown and it remains a conundrum that, while apparently able to destroy cells (Fig. 3C, D, E)—and this presumably includes blood cells—it is supposedly separable from hemolytic activities.

6.8. CLINICAL IMPORTANCE OF THE TOXIN

The rarity of well-documented *B. cereus* diarrheal-type food poisoning and the evidence for the existence of the syndrome have been discussed at the beginning of the chapter and of this section. Some epidemiological explanations for the rarity were given there. In addition, physiologically, the requirement for an apparently ideal nutrient and the lability to even moderate temperatures and to a digestive enzyme such as trypsin may explain why *B. cereus* is not more frequently involved in food poisoning. Glatz and Goepfert (1976) raise the question as to whether *B. cereus* food poisoning is due to intake of preformed toxin in the food; with the observations of increased cell numbers in ileal loops (Spira and Goepfert, 1972a) in mind, they postulate that, if large numbers of organisms are consumed in mishandled food, they may have just enough time to multiply and produce toxin *in situ* before competitive inhibition of the intestinal microflora brings this to a halt. Spira and Silverman (1979) considered their finding that toxin production is enhanced by low DO levels supported this possibility. A great deal remains to be learnt about the relationship between *B. cereus* and diarrhea.

The association of high category production of this toxin with reportedly severe non-gastrointestinal infections of a wide variety has continued since the paper of Turnbull *et al.* (1979a). Further support for this is given by Andrews and Evans (1979), Barnham *et al.* (1980) Anon (1983) and Turnbull and Kramer (1983). To this author, the evidence is that, in everyday human health, the toxin is of more importance in relation to these infections than to diarrheal disease. However the anomaly provided by the findings in relation to veterinary mastitis and the unknown roles of other *B. cereus* metabolites alone or in combination with this toxin underscore the fact that there is a great deal yet to learn about the clinical importance of this toxin.

6.9. PRODUCTION BY OTHER *BACILLUS* SPECIES

Spira and Goepfert (1972a), when first reporting the existence of loop-fluid accumulation factor in *B. cereus* cultures, noted that the strain of *B. thuringiensis* (ATCC 10792) they included in their tests was similarly capable of producing this factor. Some miscellanies are apparent in references to three other *B. thuringiensis* strains but strains of *B. megaterium, B. subtilis, B. licheniformis* and other incompletely identified aerobic spore formers were negative. Goepfert (1973) noted that fluid accumulation caused by *B. thuringiensis* culture filtrate was neutralized by antiserum to culture filtrate of *B. cereus*.

Glatz and Goepfert (1973), using the guinea-pig skin test, found that 11/11 *B. thuringiensis* strains comprising 9 varieties were positive but that the culture filtrates of four *B. subtilis* strains and single strains of *B. licheniformis* and *B. megaterium* were negative. Similarly Glatz (1973) and Glatz *et al.* (1974) found that 5/5 *B. thuringiensis* and 2/4 *B. mycoides* strains were positive in the rabbit vascular permeability assay while, once again, two strains of *B. licheniformis* and one each of *B. megaterium* and *B. subtilis* were negative.

Production of the skin test toxin by *B. thuringiensis* has been confirmed by Jørgensen (1976, 1977) and Turnbull (Table 8). Skin test toxin production by a strain of *B. thuringiensis* involved in a mixed, laboratory-acquired human infection has been reported by Warren *et al.* (1984) who also underscore the extremely close, plasmid-involved relationship between *B. thuringiensis* and *B. cereus*. Jørgensen (1976) reported significant production of VPR factor in two strains of *B. mycoides*, 4/7 *B. licheniformis* strains, 1/4 *B. subtilis* strains, a single strain of *B. subtilis var niger* and no production from a single strain each of *B. polymyxa*, *B. circulans* and *B. sphaericus*.

Turnbull and Kramer (unpublished results) found that the antiserum to the purified electrofocusing fraction of *B. cereus* 4433/73 neutralized the VPR of a serotype V (variety Shvetsova) strain of *B. thuringiensis*. In addition, eight of the *B. licheniformis* isolates from diarrheal-type food poisoning incidents (Maddocks and Turnbull, 1978; Turnbull, 1978), two isolated in association with pyrexia in humans (Turnbull, 1978), one associated with morbidity and mortality in a colony of laboratory mice (Turnbull, 1978, Wright *et al.*, 1979) and five associated with bovine mastitis (Jones and Turnbull, 1981) were found to be negative or to produce just a faint blue ring of unknown significance in the rabbit VPR (Fig. 2B). Similarly, nine of the *B. subtilis* strains associated with food poisoning (Turnbull, 1979b) and two isolated in pure growth from mastitic milk were either negative or extremely weak or exhibited unusual reactions (Fig. 2B). J. M. Kramer (personal communication), however, found that concentration of the culture filtrates from some of these *B. subtilis* strains resulted in proportionately increased reaction size.

Strains of *B. pumilus* isolated in pure growth from a case of bovine mastitis and from pustules on the leg of a human patient, a strain of *B. alvei* isolated together with *C. perfringens* in a case of gas gangrene, a second unrelated postoperative isolate of *B. alvei* and an unassigned aerobic spore former from bovine mastitis were all negative in the VPR test; culture growth in all cases was excellent (P. C. B. Turnbull, unpublished data). In contrast, a strain of *B. mycoides* isolated as the predominant organism from the discharge in an infected knee was a category 4 producer with necrosis while a second strain from an unrelated blood culture fell into category 3.

The general conclusion is that *B. thuringiensis* and *B. mycoides* which stand very closely related to *B. cereus* (Kaneko *et al.*, 1978; Warren *et al.*, 1984) produce this loop fluid-inducing/skin test/necrotic toxin with similar strain variations to those found with *B. cereus* and that other *Bacillus* species either do not do so or do so only to a very limited extent.

It would appear, then, that if the *B. licheniformis* and *B. subtilis* strains were responsible for the diarrheal-type incidents from which they were isolated (Maddocks and Turnbull, 1978; Turnbull, 1978, 1979b), the diarrhea was not produced by the *B. cereus*-type fluid-inducing/skin test/necrotic toxin. The corollary is, of course, that there may be another undiscovered mechanism common to *Bacillus* species and perhaps including *B. cereus* which is the root cause of the periodic diarrheal-type incident that is encountered.

With regard to the public health importance of the ability of *B. thuringiensis* to produce this toxin, the comments made in relation to lethal (α) toxin and public and animal health are pertinent here also. Given the probability that *B. thuringiensis* α-toxin and its thuringiolysin and VPR activities are related in the same manner as the lethal toxin of *B. cereus* is related to its cereolysin and VPR toxin, it may be a relevant finding (Krieg, 1971b) that intracoelomic injection of the α-toxin in ammonium sulphate-precipitated preparations into larvae of the Greater Wax Moth, *Galleria mellonella*, resulted in *in vivo* degeneration and lysis of the hemocytes.

6.10. SUMMARY OF THE LOOP FLUID-INDUCING/SKIN TEST/NECROTIC TOXIN

The nature of a toxic activity characterized by the ability to induce fluid accumulation in ligated rabbit ileal loops and to cause characteristic reactions and alterations in capillary permeability and tissue in guinea pig and rabbit skin have been discussed. It appears that the activity can be detected to one extent or another in appropriate culture filtrates of virtually all strains of *B. cereus* and the closely related species, *B. thuringiensis* and *B. mycoides* but not, at least to any significant extent, by other *Bacillus* species. Partial loss of toxigenicity appears to occur with repeated subculture of a strain.

The activity is associated with late exponential phase of growth, is unstable in unfrozen crude culture filtrates, heat labile, susceptible to trypsin and pronase and antigenic. It has been shown (Kramer, 1984) to be separable into two components of pI 5.1 and 5.6 respectively and MW in the order of 50,000. Both moieties produce vascular permeability, necrotic and cytotoxic reactions, but the precise interrelationships between the two have not been established yet. Their collective activity is distinct from phospholipases C and the two hemolysins of *B. cereus*, but it appears to constitute one of two lethal factors making up the total lethal activity of these organisms (the other being cereolysin).

The loop fluid-inducing/skin test/necrotic activity is suspected of being the underlying cause of the so-called diarrheal-type of *B. cereus* food poisoning; but the latter is itself, in epidemiological terms, a rather elusive syndrome. Evidence is supplied to support this author's opinion that a great deal more information is needed before the metabolites can be legitimately labelled diarrheal enterotoxins. Their mode of action in causing tissue damage, alteration of the fluid balance in the intestine and other clinical effects is not yet understood either.

The instability of the toxic activity, its sensitivity to various enzymes, the ability of strongly toxigenic strains to partially lose toxigenicity and the problems that have been encountered in differentiating it from other metabolites of *B. cereus* with similar size or charge properties have all contributed to inhibiting progress in defining its nature and what it does. It continues to offer considerable research challenges.

7. EMETIC TOXIN

7.1. NATURE OF THE TOXIN

The characteristics and epidemiological background of the so-called 'emetic-type' of food poisoning caused by *B. cereus* were given at the outset of this chapter (p 397). Since, with just a relatively small number of exceptions, all incidents have been associated with rice dishes, the starting point for studies on the pathogenic mechanisms involved was the feeding of rice cultures of isolates incriminated in such incidents. Autoclaved soaked rice (1 part rice: 4 [w/v] saline) was found to be a good growth medium (Melling *et al.*, 1976). Liquefaction of an overnight culture (30°C) with diastase produces a liquor which, after dialysis for 24 hr at 4°C against 10 per cent polyethylene glycol, is readily fed by intragastric tube to monkeys.

Of three strains chosen in the initial tests (Melling *et al.*, 1976) rice culture slurries of 4810/72 isolated from vomitus in an emetic incident (Table 2) produced emesis in almost half the feedings with diarrhea recorded in one occasion. Strain 4433/73 from a diarrheal-type incident and 2532b/74 from routine raw rice failed to induce emesis but 4433/73 did cause diarrhea in more than half the feedings. Fecal counts before and after feeding (with appropriate serological confirmation of the re-isolates) showed that the differences could not be attributed to differences in the numbers of *B. cereus* in the intestine. The specificity of the rice was demonstrated by the fact that cultures of 4810/72 in a protein hydrolysate and amine broth with or without starch (to observe any obvious relation to sporulation) failed to produce emesis although cultures of 4433/73 in this medium did produce diarrhea in 3/8 feedings. Failure of BHIG cultures of isolates from emetic-type incidents to induce emesis in monkeys had already been noted by Goepfert (1978).

Subsequent feeding trials showed that approximately 50 per cent of monkeys did not respond to the toxin. Melling and Capel (1978) used monkeys selected for their susceptibility to study the toxin further and, using 4810/72, established a number of important findings: (1) $0.45\,\mu$ membrane filtered rice culture supernatants possessed emetic activity which, although only one-tenth the strength (in ED_{50}) of the whole culture, provided the first definite evidence of involvement of a toxin in the syndrome; (2) tryptone soya broth (TSB) cultures and both washings and total agar homogenates of TSB agar slope cultures [in 500 ml flats inoculated with a 1 per cent TSB culture incubated at 30°C for 72 hr] produced emesis in about half the feedings carried out; (3) attempts to concentrate the factor revealed that it passed through a 10,000 MW cut-off Amicon filter and was not retained by dialysis tubing; (4) the factor was highly stable and survived autoclaving, pH extremes and exposure to trypsin and pronase; (5) no apparent resistance developed in four monkeys fed 16 times over an 8-month period indicating poor antigenicity.

From these observations they concluded that, in contrast to the proteinous loop fluid-inducing/skin test/necrotic toxin with its large MW and general lability, the emetic toxin was an entirely distinct stable small MW compound.

In further feeding tests, A. J. Crooks (personal communication) found that certain fractions from gel permeation chromatography of chloroform and methanol extracts of rice and TSB (in which *B. cereus* had not been grown) also induced emesis in monkeys. One possibility, though just speculation at this stage, is that the emetic activity of *B. cereus* may be related to release or elaboration of one or more of these compounds through metabolic action of the organism on rice, TSB or other suitable substrates.

7.2. PRODUCTION OF EMETIC FACTOR

In the absence of any other test than monkey feeding for detection of emetic toxin, and on account of the practical problems involved in carrying out large numbers of feedings, growth and toxin production studies are, in practice, not easy to perform. In view of the fairly exclusive relationship between the emetic type of *B. cereus* food poisoning and cooked rice dishes, it seemed reasonable to suspect that toxin production might be related to sporulation. Melling and Capel (in Turnbull *et al.*, 1979b, and personal communication) carried out two growth and production studies (Table 15) with the inclusion of spore counts and using strain 4810/72. It is seen that in the first trial, emesis appeared in late exponential phase of vegetative growth and before spore levels had become detectable; in the second trial, emetic activity was not apparent until several hours after stationary phase had been reached and the spore count had also reached its approximate maximum.

A relationship between sporulation and emetic toxin production has thus not been confirmed or refuted; if such a relationship exists, it is not a simple one since cultures of 4810/72 in artificial sporulation media containing from 40–98 per cent spores have failed to produce emesis in monkeys (Melling *et al.*, 1976; J. Melling and B. J. Capel, personal communication). As discussed above the possibility cannot be ruled out at this point that the toxic factor may, in fact, be a breakdown product or products resulting from an undefined bacterial action by *B. cereus* on rice and occasionally other foods. The food poisoning incidents not involving rice (vanilla slices, Chinese pancake, omelette, dried milk, pasteurised cream, pasta, and vegetable dishes have been implicated), though small in number, serve to indicate that production of the toxin is not necessarily exclusive to rice; however, it is assumed that obvious signs of spoilage and unpalatability become apparent in most foods when the organism has multiplied sufficiently to produce significant levels of the toxin.

Melling *et al.* (1978) determined that the optimal temperature for production of the toxin in 24 hr rice cultures is 30°C (Table 16). At 35–45°C, even though equivalent or higher vegetative and spore counts were obtained, the emetic response was less than that at 30°C.

TABLE 15. *Production of* Bacillus cereus *(4810/72) emetic toxin in relation to vegetative cell and spore counts in rice cultures*

Time (hr)	Study 1*			Study 2**		
	LVC	LSC	ER	LVC	LSC	ER
0	6.3	<1	0/3	1.8	<1	n
6	8.2	<1	3/3	6.4	3.3	n
14	8.5	7.8	2/2	7.8	4.5	n
18	8.4	8.2	2/2	7.9	6.6	0/4
24	8.6	8.4	3/3	8.1	7.2	0/4
30	n			8.0	7.1	1/4
36	n			8.3	7.4	3/4
42	n			8.5	7.8	3/4

*Turnbull *et al.* (1979b).
**Melling *et al.* (1978).
LVC = log vegetative cell count/ml; LSC = log spore count/ml; ER = emetic response (no. monkeys vomiting/no. fed); n = not done.

TABLE 16. *Effect of growth temperature on the emetic activity of 24 hr rice cultures of* Bacillus cereus *4810/72**

Temp. °C	Vegetative cell count/ml	Spore count/ml	Emetic response**
22	9×10^7	1×10^5	2/4
25	5.5×10^7	2×10^5	3/4
30	3×10^8	1×10^6	4/4
35	9×10^8	8×10^7	1/4
40	3×10^8	5×10^7	1/4
45	3×10^8	1.5×10^7	0/4
50	3×10^4	8×10^1	0/4

*Melling *et al.* (1978).
**No. monkeys which vomited/no. fed.

Due, once again, to the practical difficulties in relying on monkey feeding for assay of this toxin, it is not yet known whether production of the emetic toxin is an all-or-none event or whether different strains produce it to different extents. Sixteen strains of *B. cereus* are now on record (Melling *et al.*, 1976; Logan *et al.*, 1979; Turnbull *et al.*, 1979b) as having been tested by monkey feeding of rice cultures. Although differences in the number of positive responses are recorded for the different strains, the feeding trials were carried out over a period of several years making precise duplication of conditions difficult. Also the number of feedings for each strain was rarely > 4, and other factors which may have accounted for the differences, including animal-to-animal variation, could not be readily assessed.

Two other features of interest about emetic-type *B. cereus* food poisoning incidents are that (1) a very high proportion (over 70 per cent) of incriminated isolates from these incidents are serotype 1; this high frequency is not reflected in isolation rates of serotype 1 from routine raw rice or other food samples or from other environmental or clinical sources (Gilbert, 1979); (2) Parry and Gilbert (1980) have shown that spores of serotype 1 isolates from emetic-type food poisoning frequently exhibit a markedly higher decimal reduction time at 95°C than those of other serotypes.

While the most obvious significance of the second feature lies in the relative abilities of the organisms to survive boiling, these points serve to demonstrate that strains which cause emetic-type food poisoning may possess characteristics not shared by all *B. cereus*. Whether emetic toxin production is a further characteristic peculiar to some strains remains to be conclusively demonstrated. That it may be is suggested by the results from feedings of four strains not isolated from emetic-type incidents (Logan *et al.*, 1979). Only one of these (2769/77) induced emesis and this only once in eight feedings.

7.3. EMETIC TOXIN AND OTHER *BACILLUS* SPECIES

It is not known whether other *Bacillus* species can produce the emetic toxin. *B. subtilis* is periodically isolated in high numbers and occasionally in pure growth during investigations of food poisoning; in some of these incidents, histories similar to those of *B. cereus* emetic type food poisoning are recorded (Mortimer and Meers, 1975; Winton and Sayers, 1975; Turnbull, 1979b), but no feeding tests have been done with such isolates. Although these types of reports are, as yet, rare, the preliminary epidemiological evidence they supply suggests that production of an emetic toxin may not be restricted to *B. cereus* among the *Bacillus* species.

7.4. EMETIC TOXIN VERSUS LOOP FLUID-INDUCING/SKIN TEST/NECROTIC TOXIN

On the evidence available to date, there appears to be no consistent relationship between production of emetic toxin and that of the loop fluid-inducing/skin test/necrotic toxin by a given strain of *B. cereus*. In skin tests on isolates from emetic type incidents which have been shown capable of inducing emesis in monkeys, categories 1–4 have all been represented (Turnbull *et al.*, 1979b). This has the important implication that, if it is finally proven that the fluid-inducing/skin test/necrotic factor is a diarrheal toxin, it would then become clear that some strains could cause either type of food poisoning depending on the conditions of mishandling under which they have been allowed to grow. Diarrhea is sometimes recorded in addition to vomiting in emetic-type incidents and it may be speculated that, when this occurs, it represents the actions of the two separate toxins.

Of four strains isolated from diarrheal-type incidents fed to monkeys in rice cultures, only one (2769/77—skin test category 3) induced emesis in just one of eight feedings; the remainder (4430/73—category 4, 4433/73—category 5 and 4370/75—category 5) failed to induce vomiting. This indicates that not all *B. cereus* strains produce both toxins. However, until our knowledge of these toxins and their production has progressed considerably beyond the present limited state, it should be regarded as being erroneous to designate strains as 'diarrheal strains' or 'emetic strains' as has been observed on occasion (Logan *et al.*, 1979).

ACKNOWLEDGEMENTS

The author wishes to express sincere thanks to colleagues and co-workers in the field of *Bacillus cereus*—Dr. Richard J. Gilbert, Mr. John M. Kramer, Dr. Jack Melling and Ms. Jennifer M. Parry—for their help and encouragement with this review. Warm thanks are also expressed to Mrs. Phyllis Rose for secretarial assistance, Mr. John R. Gibson for assistance with illustrations and Mr. E. A. Leeson for help with miscellaneous items.

REFERENCES

ALOUF, J. E. (1977) Cell membranes and cytolytic bacterial toxins. In: *The Specificity and Action of Animal, Bacterial and Plant toxins.* (*Receptors and Recognition*, series B, Volume 1) pp. 219–270, CUATRECASAS, P. (Ed), Chapman & Hall, London.

ANDREWS, H. J. and EVANS, D. M. (1979) *Bacillus cereus* wound infections. (letter) *J. Clin. Path.* **32:** 1305.

ANON (1983) *Bacillus cereus* as a systemic pathogen. *Lancet* **ii:** 1469.

BAINBRIDGE, F. A. (1903) Some observations on the *Bacillus anthracoides. J. Path. Bact.* **8:** 117–120.

BALACESCU, C. (1974) Über einen Selbstversuch mit *Bacillus cereus.* (Report of autointoxication experiment with *Bacillus cereus.*) *Zbl. Bakt. Hyg., I Abt. Orig. B* **159:** 196–199. English summary.

BALACESCU, C. (1975) Über einen von *Bacillus cereus* synthetitisierten 'lethal factor'. (Report of 'lethal factor' synthesized by *Bacillus cereus.*) *Zbl. Bakt. Hyg., I Abt. Orig. B* **161:** 178–187. English summary.

BARNHAM, M., WHITE, D., MELLING, J. and GILBERT, R. J. (1980) *Bacillus cereus* infections. (letters) *J. Clin. Path.* **33:** 314–315.

BERGDOLL, M., personal communication. Food Research Institute, Madison, Wisconsin, USA.

BERNHEIMER, A. W. and GRUSHOFF, P. (1967a) Cereolysin: production, purification and partial characterization. *J. Gen. Microbiol.* **46:** 143–150.

BERNHEIMER, A. W. and GRUSHOFF, P. (1967b) Extracellular hemolysins of aerobic sporogenic bacilli. *J. Bact.* **93:** 1541–1543.

BERNHEIMER, A. W., GRUSHOFF, P. and AVIGAD, L. S. (1968) Isoelectric analysis of cytolytic bacterial proteins. *J. Bact.* **95:** 2439–2441.

BONVENTRE, P. F. (1965) Differential cytotoxicity of *Bacillus anthracis* and *Bacillus cereus* culture filtrates. *J. Bact.* **90:** 284–285.

BONVENTRE, P. F. and ECKERT, N. J. (1963a) Toxin production as a criterion for differentiating *Bacillus cereus* and *Bacillus anthracis. J. Bact.* **85:** 490–491.

BONVENTRE, P. F. and ECKERT, N. J. (1963b) The biologic activities of *Bacillus anthracis* and *Bacillus cereus* culture filtrates. *Amer. J. Path.* **43:** 201–212.

BONVENTRE, P. F. and JOHNSON, C. E. (1970) *Bacillus cereus* toxin. In: *Microbial toxins, 3, Bacterial Protein Toxins,* pp. 415–435, MONTIE, T. C., KADIS, S., AJL, S. J., (Eds), Academic Press, London.

BOWMAN, M. H., OTTOLENGHI, A. C. and MENGEL, C. E. (1971) Effects of phospholipase C on human erythroctyes. *J. Membrane Biol.* **4:** 156–164.

BRILL, B. M., WASILAUSKAS, B. L. and RICHARDSON, S. H. (1979) Adaptation of the staphylococcal coagglutination technique for detection of heat-labile enterotoxin of *Escherichia coli. J. Clin. Microbiol.* **9:** 49–55.

BURDON, K. L. (1947) The potential pathogenicity of *Bacillus cereus* and its relationship to *Bacillus anthracis. J. Bact.* **54:** 58.

BURDON, K. L. and WENDE, R. D. (1960) On the differentiation of anthrax bacilli from *B. cereus. J. Infect. Dis.* **107:** 224–234.

BURGES, H. D. (1981) Safety, safety testing and quality control of microbial pesticides. In: *Microbial control of pests and plant diseases, 1970–1980,* pp. 738–767, BURGES, H. D. (Ed), Academic Press, New York.

BÜSING, K-H. (1950) Notizen über das subtilis-haemolysin. *Arch. Hyg.* **133:** 63–68.

CANDELI, A., MASTRANDREA, V., CENCI, G. and BARTOLOMEO DE, A. (1975) Fasi dissociative e pathogenicita' di specie diverse del genere *Bacillus. Annali Sclavo* **17:** 102–114.

CARPENTER, D. F., SPIRA, W. M. and SILVERMAN, G. J. (1975) Effects of dissolved oxygen tension on bacterial enterotoxin production. In: *Developments in Industrial Microbiology* (a publication of the Society for Industrial Microbiology) **17:** 363–374.

CAYTON, H. R., TURNBULL, P. C. B. and GILBERT, R. J. (1978) Severe food poisoning associated with *Bacillus cereus*. Public Health Laboratory Service (England & Wales), *Communicable Disease Report* 1978; No. 28.

CENCI, G. (1971) Richerche sull' attività dissociante di alcuni contituenti dell'umor vitreo. *Annali Sclavo* 13: 49–58.

CHU, H. P. (1949) The lecithinase of *Bacillus cereus* and its comparison with *Clostridium welchii* α-toxin. *J. Gen. Microbiol.* 3: 255–273.

CLARK, F. E. (1937) The relation of *Bacillus siamensis* and similar pathogenic spore-forming bacteria to *Bacillus cereus*. *J. Bact.* 33: 435–443.

COLE, R. and PROULX, P. (1975) Phospholipase D activity of gram-negative bacteria. *J. Bact.* 124: 1148–1152.

COLMER, A. R. (1947) The use of the enzyme lecithinase in grouping some members of the genus *Bacillus. J. Bact.* 54: 11–12.

COOLBAUGH, J. C. and WILLIAMS, R. P. (1978) Production and characterization of two hemolysins of *Bacillus cereus. Canad. J. Microbiol.* 24: 1289–1295.

COWELL, J. L., GRUSHOFF-KOSYK, P. S. and BERNHEIMER, A. W. (1976) Purification of cereolysin and the electrophoretic separation of the active (reduced) and inactive (oxidized) forms of the purified toxin. *Infect. & Immun.* 14: 144–154.

CRAIG, J. P. (1965) A permeability factor (toxin) found in cholera stools and culture filtrates and its neutralization by convalescent cholera sera. *Nature, Lond.* 207: 614–616.

DOERY, H. M., MAGNUSSON, B. J., GULASEKHARAM, J. and PEARSON, J. (1965) The properties of phospholipase enzymes in staphylococcal toxins. *J. Gen. Microbiol.* 40: 283–296.

DONNELLY, C. B., LESLIE, J. E., BLACK, L. A. and LEWIS, K. H. (1967) Serological identification of enterotoxigenic staphylococci from cheese. *Appl. Microbiol.* 15: 1382–1387.

EVANS, D. J. JR., EVANS, D. G. and GORBACH, S. L. (1973) Production of vascular permeability factor by enterotoxigenic *Escherichia coli* isolated from man. *Infect. & Immun.* 8: 725–735.

EZEPCHUK, YU. V. and FLUER, F. S. (1973)—authors may be found quoted as JESEPTCUK, J. and FLUER, F.—The enterotoxic effect. *Moderne Medizin,* 3: 20–25.

EZEPCHUK, YU. V., BONDARENKO, V. M., YAKOVLEVA, E. A. and KORYAGINA, I. P. (1979) The *Bacillus cereus* toxin: isolation of permeability factor. *Zbl. Bakt. Hyg., I. Abt. Orig. A* 244: 275–284.

FISHER, R. A. and ROSNER, L. (1959) Toxicology of the microbial insecticide, Thuricide, *J. Agric. Fd. Chem.* 7: 686–688.

FITZPATRICK, D. J., TURNBULL, P. C. B., KEANE, C. T. and ENGLISH, L. F. (1979) Two gas-gangrene-like infections due to *Bacillus cereus. Brit. J. Surg.* 66: 577–579.

FORSBERG, C. W., HENDERSON, M., HENRY, E. and ROBERTS, J. R. (1976) *Bacillus thuringiensis: Its Effects on Environmental Quality*, National Research Council of Canada, NRC Associate Committee on Scientific Criteria for Environmental Quality, Publication No. NRCC 15385, Ottowa K1A 0R6.

FOSSUM, K. (1963) Separation of hemolysin and egg yolk turbidity factor in cell-free extracts of *Bacillus cereus. Acta. Path. Microbiol. Scand.* 59: 400–406.

FOSSUM, K. (1964) The heat sensitivity of *Bacillus cereus* hemolysin. *Acta. Path. Microbiol. Scand.* 60: 523–527.

FRANCIS, P. G. (1984) An approach to the herd mastitis problem. *Br. Vet. J.* 140: 22–26.

FUMAROLA, D., PASQUETTO, N., BRANDONISIO, O., MONNO, R. and MIRAGLIOTTA, G. (1976) L'inibizione dell' aggregazione piastrinica da ADP come possibile test di valutazione dell' enterotossigenicita di alcuni enterobatteri, Studio preliminare, *Giorn. Batt. Virol. Immun.* 69: 234–243.

GAÁL, V. and IVÁNOVICS, G. (1972) Synthesis of inducible phospholipase A with antibacterial activity by *Bacillus cereus. Z. Allg. Mikrobiol.* 12: 393–402.

GAÁL, V. and IVÁNOVICS, G. (1976) Studies on megacinogeny in *Bacillus cereus* I. Multiplication of phage wx causing lysogenic conversion to megacin A (phospholipase A) production. *Acta Microbiol. Hung.* 23: 277–282.

GAZITT, Y. OHAD, I. and LOYTER, A. (1975) Changes in phospholipid susceptibility towards phospholipases induced by ATP depletion in avian and amphibian erythrocyte membranes. *Biochim. Biophys. Acta.* 382: 65–72.

GAZITT, Y., OHAD, I. and LOYTER, A. (1976) Increase in the phospholipid phase extractable by dry ether following ATP-depletion of erythrocytes. *Biochim. Biophys. Res. Commun.* 72: 1359–1366.

GIANNELLA, R. A. and BRASILE, L. (1979) A hospital food-borne outbreak of diarrhea caused by *Bacillus cereus*: clinical, epidemiological and microbiologic studies. *J. Infect. Dis.* 139: 366–370.

GILBERT, R. J. (1979) *Bacillus cereus* gastroenteritis. In: *Foodborne Infections and Intoxications*; 2nd edn, pp. 495–518, RIEMANN, H. and BRYAN, F. L. (Eds), Academic Press, New York.

GILBERT, R. J. and PARRY, J. M. (1977) Serotypes of *Bacillus cereus* from outbreaks of food poisoning and from routine foods. *J. Hyg. (Camb)*, 78: 69–74.

GIUGLIANO, L. G. (1983) Bacterial toxin and tissue culture. Ph.D. Thesis. University of London, London.

GLATZ, B. A. (1973) Alternative dermal assays of enteropathogenicity of *Bacillus cereus* and *Bacillus thuringiensis*. Master's Thesis, University of Wisconsin, Madison, Wisconsin.

GLATZ, B. A. and GOEPFERT, J. M. (1973) Extracellular factor synthesized by *Bacillus cereus* which evokes a dermal reaction in guinea-pigs. *Infect. Immun.* 8: 25–29.

GLATZ, B. A. and GOEPFERT, J. M. (1976) Defined conditions for synthesis of *Bacillus cereus* enterotoxin by fermenter-grown cultures. *Appl. Environ. Microbiol.* 32: 400–404.

GLATZ, B. A. and GOEPFERT, J. M. (1977) Production of *Bacillus cereus* enterotoxin in defined media in fermenter-grown cultures. *J. Fd. Protect.* 40: 472–474.

GLATZ, B. A., SPIRA, W. M. and GOEPFERT, J. M. (1974) Alteration of vascular permeability in rabbits by culture filtrates of *Bacillus cereus* and related species. *Infect. Immun.* 10: 299–303.

GOEPFERT, J. M. (1973) Pathogenicity patterns in *Bacillus cereus* foodborne disease. Abstracts of the 1st International Congress for Bacteriology, International Association of Microbiological Societies, Jerusalem, September 1973, 1: 140–141.

GOEPFERT, J. M. (1978) Monkey feeding trials in the investigation of the nature of *Bacillus cereus* food poisoning. Proceedings of the Fourth International Congress of Food Science and Technology, Spain, 1974, Volume 3, pp. 178–181.

GOEPFERT, J. M., SPIRA, W. M., GLATZ, B. A. and KIM, H. U. (1973) Pathogenicity of *Bacillus cereus*. In: *The Microbiological Safety of Foods*, pp. 69–75, HOBBS, B. C. and CHRISTIAN, J. H. B., (Eds), Proceedings of the Eighth International Symposium on Food Microbiology held in Reading, England, 1972, Academic Press, London.

GOEPFERT, J. M., SPIRA, W. M. and KIM, H. U. (1972) *Bacillus cereus*: Food poisoning organism. A review. *J. Milk Fd Tech.* **35:** 213–227.

GORINA, L. G., FLUER, F. S., OLOVNIKOV, A. M. and EZEPCHUK, YU. V. (1975) Use of the aggregate-hemagglutination technique for determining exo-enterotoxin of *Bacillus cereus*. *Appl. Microbiol.* **29:** 201–204.

GORINA, L. G., FLUER, F. S., OLOVNIKOV, A. M. and EZEPCHUK, YU. V. (1976) Highly sensitive determination of *Bacillus cereus* exo-enterotoxin using the method of aggregate haemagglutination. *J. Hyg. Epidem. Microbiol. Immunol.* **20:** 361–367.

GRIERSON, A. M. M. (1928) '*Bacillus anthracoides*'. A study of its biological characters and relationships and its pathogenic properties under experimental conditions. *J. Hyg. Camb.* **27:** 306–320.

HANSON, R. S., SRINIVASAN, V. R. and HALVORSON, H. O. (1963) Biochemistry of sporulation. 1. Metabolism of acetate by vegetative and sporulating cells. *J. Bact.* **85:** 451–460.

HAUGE, S. (1950) Matforgiftninger fremkalt av *Bacillus cereus*. *Nord. Hyg. T.* **31:** 189–206 (*Biol. Abstr.* **25:** 1063, 1951).

HAUGE, S. (1955) Food poisoning caused by aerobic spore-forming bacilli. *J. Appl. Bact.* **18:** 591–595.

HEIMPEL, A. M. (1955) The pH in the gut and blood of the larch sawfly *Pristiphora erichsonii* (Htg) and other insects with reference to the pathogenicity of *Bacillus cereus* Fr. and Fr. Canad. *J. Zool.* **33:** 99–106.

HUNTER, F. R., MARKER, M. J., BULLOCK, J. A., RAWLEY, J. and LARSH, H. W. (1949) Action of bacterial toxins on respiration of chicken erythrocytes. *Proc. Soc. Exp. Biol. and Med.* **72:** 606–608.

HUNTER, F. R., RAWLEY, J., BULLOCK, J. A. and LARSH, H. (1950) Action of bacterial toxins on the 'fragility' of chicken erythrocytes. *Science* **112:** 206–207.

IKEZAWA, H., MORI, M., OHYABU, T. and TAGUCHI, R. (1978) Studies on sphingomyelinase of *Bacillus cereus*. I. Purification and properties. *Biochim. Biophys. Acta.* **528:** 247–256.

IKEZAWA, H., MORI, M. and TAGUCHI, R. (1980) Studies on sphingomyelinase of *Bacillus cereus*; hydrolytic and hemolytic actions on erythrocyte membranes *Arch. Biochem. Biophys.* **199:** 572–578.

IKEZAWA, H., YAMANEGI, M., TAGUCHI, R., MIYASHITA, T. and OHYABU, T. (1976) Studies on phosphatidylinositol phosphodiesterase (phospholipase C type) of *Bacillus cereus*. I. Purification, properties and phosphatase-releasing activity. *Biochim. Biophys. Acta.* **450:** 154–164.

IKEZAWA, H., YAMANEGI, M., TAGUCHI, R., MIYASHITA, T. and OHYABU, T. (1977) A phosphatidylinositol phospholipase C (phosphatasemia factor) of *Bacillus cereus*. *Jap. J. Med. Sci. Biol.* **30:** 81–82.

IVANOVICS, G., GAÁL, V., NAGY, E., PRÁGAI, B. and SIMON, M. JR. (1976) Studies on megacinogeny in *Bacillus cereus*. II. *Bacillus cereus* isolates characterized by prophage-controlled production of megacin A (phospholipase A). *Acta Microbiol. Hung.* **23:** 283–291.

IVÁNOVICS, G., GAÁL, V. and PRÁGAI, B. (1974) Lysogenic conversion to phospholipase A production in *Bacillus cereus*. *J. Gen. Virol.* **24:** 349–358.

IVERS, J. T. and POTTER, N. N. (1977) Production and stability of hemolysin, phospholipase C, and lethal toxin of *Bacillus cereus* in foods. *J. Food Protec.* **40:** 17–22.

JOHNSON, C. E. (1966) Studies on the lethal toxin of *Bacillus cereus*. Ph. D. Thesis, University of Cincinnati, Cincinnati, Ohio.

JOHNSON, C. E. and BONVENTRE, P. F. (1966) Studies on the lethal toxin of *Bacillus cereus*. *Bact. Proc.* p. 41, M19.

JOHNSON, C. E. and BONVENTRE, P. F. (1967) Lethal toxin of *Bacillus cereus*. I. Relationships and nature of toxin, hemolysin and phospholipase. *J. Bact.* **94:** 306–316.

JONES, T. O. and TURNBULL, P. C. B. (1981) Bovine mastitis caused by *Bacillus cereus*. *Vet. Rec.* **108:** 272–274.

JØRGENSEN, K. (1976) Belysning af enterotoksin produktionen has slaegten *Bacillus* ved anvendelse af cutantest samt taksonomisk bestemmelse af mesofile arter af denne slaegt. (Demonstration of enterotoxin production within the genus *Bacillus* by use of the cutan test and a taxonomic determination of mesophilic species of the genus). *Licentiatafhandling* (Thesis) Institute of Hygiene and Microbiology, the Royal Veterinary and Agricultural University, Copenhagen, Denmark.

JØRGENSEN, K. (1977) Enterotoxin producing abilities among strains of *Bacillus*. pp. 25–35, Proceedings of the World Association of Veterinary Food Hygienists 7th International Symposium held in Garmisch-Partenkirchen, Germany, 1977, Deutscher Veterinärmedizinischer Gesellschaft, Frankfurter Str. 87, D-6300 Giessen/Lahn.

KANEKO, T., NOZAKI, R. and AIZAWA, K. (1978) Deoxyribonucleic acid retatedness between *Bacillus anthracis*, *Bacillus cereus* and *Bacillus thuringiensis*. *Microbiol. Immunol.* **22:** 639–641.

KATSARAS, K. and HARTWIGK, H. (1979) Versuche zur Reinigung der Ektotoxine des *Bacillus cereus*. (Studies of the purification of the exotoxin of *Bacillus cereus*). *Zbl. Bakt. Hyg., I. Abt. Orig.* A **245:** 332–344. English summary.

KATSARAS, K. and ZELLER, U. P. (1977) Nachweis von *Bacillus cereus*-toxinen. *Zbl. Bakt. Hyg., I. Abt. Orig.* A **238:** 255–262. English summary.

KRAMER, J. M. (1984) *Bacillus cereus* exotoxins: production, isolation, detection and properties. In: *Bacterial Protein Toxins*, ALOUF, J. E., FREER, J. H., FEHRENBACH, F. J. and JELJASZEWICZ, J., (Eds) Academic Press, London, pp. 385–386.

KRAMER, J. M. and TURNBULL, P. C. B. (1979) Serological studies on the vascular permeability reaction and haemolytic factors elaborated by *Bacillus cereus*. Proceedings of the FEMS-NWEMG-SGM Joint Symposium on Extracellular Products of Microorganisms—Bacterial Toxins, September 1979, Dublin, Eire.

KRAMER, J. M., TURNBULL, P. C. B., JORGENSEN, K., PARRY, J. and GILBERT, R. J. (1978) Separation of exponential growth exotoxins of *Bacillus cereus* and their preliminary characterization. *J. Appl. Bact.* **45:** xix.

KREIG, A. (1969) *In vitro* determination of *Bacillus thuringiensis*, *Bacillus cereus*, and related bacilli. *J. Invertebr. Pathol.* **15:** 313–320.

KREIG, A. (1970) Über die Differenzierung der Mäuse-Toxizität des *Bacillus cereus* und des *Bacillus thuringiensis* von der Mäuse-Pathogenität des *Bacillus anthracis*. (Differentiation of the toxicity for mice of *Bacillus cereus* and *Bacillus thuringiensis* from the pathogenicity of *Bacillus anthracis* for mice). *Zbl. Bakt. Hyg., I. Abt. Orig.* **215**: 523–529. English summary.

KREIG, A. (1971a) Concerning α-exotoxin produced by vegetative cells of *Bacillus thuringiensis* and *Bacillus cereus*. *J. Invertebr. Pathol.* **17**: 134–135.

KREIG, A. (1971b) Is the potential pathogenicity of bacilli for insects related to production of α-exotoxin? *J. Invertebr. Pathol.* **18**: 425–426.

KREIG, A. (1975) Photoprotection against inactivation of *Bacillus thuringiensis* spores by ultraviolet rays. *J. Invertebr. Pathol.* **25**: 267–268.

LAWRENCE, J. S. and FORD, W. W. (1916) Aerobic spore-bearing non-pathogenic bacteria. *J. Bact.* **1**: 273–320. (*Bacillus cereus* Frankland 1887—pp. 284–287).

LEMILLE, F., DE BARJAC, H. and BONNEFOI, A. (1969) Essai sur la classification biochimique de 97 bacillus du groupe I. Appartenant à 9 espèces différentes. *Ann. Inst. Pasteur.* **116**: 808–819.

LEPPLA, S. H. (1982) Anthrax toxin edema factor: a bacterial adenylate cyclase that increases cyclic AMP concentrations in eukaryotic cells. *Biochemistry,* **79**: 3162–3166.

LITTLE, C. and JOHANSEN, S. (1979) Unfolding and refolding of phospholipase C from *Bacillus cereus* in solutions of guanidinium chloride. *Biochem. J.* **179**: 509–514.

LOGAN, N. A., CAPEL, B. J., MELLING, J. and BERKELEY, R. C. W. (1979) Distinction between emetic and other strains of *Bacillus cereus* using the API system and numerical methods. *FEMS Microbiol. Lett.* **5**: 373–375.

MADDOCKS, A. C. and TURNBULL, P. C. B. (1978) Diarrhoea associated with *Bacillus licheniformis*. Public Health Laboratory Service (England & Wales) *Communicable Disease Report* 1978, No. **48**.

MADGE, D. S. (1978) *Bacillus cereus*—induced malabsorption in young mice. *Digestion* **17**: 332–345.

McGAUGHEY, C. A. and CHU, H. P. (1948) The egg-yolk reaction of aerobic sporing bacilli. *J. Gen. Microbiol.* **2**: 334–340.

MELLING, J. and CAPEL, B. J. (1978) Characteristics of *Bacillus cereus* emetic toxin. *FEMS Microbiol. Lett.* **4**: 133–135.

MELLING, J., CAPEL, B. J., TURNBULL, P. C. B. and GILBERT, R. J. (1976) Identification of a novel enterotoxigenic activity associated with *Bacillus cereus. J. Clin. Path.* **29**: 938–940.

MELLING, J., CAPEL, B. J., WITHAM, M. D. and GILBERT, R. J. (1978) Identification and characterization of *Bacillus cereus* emetic toxin. Proceedings of the 47th Annual Meeting of the Society for Applied Bacteriology, July 1978. University of Birmingham. *J. Appl. Bact.* **45**: xxv.

MIDURA, T., GERBER, M., WOOD, R. and LEONARD, A. R. (1970) Outbreak of food poisoning caused by *Bacillus cereus*. Pub. Hlth. Rpt. (Washington) **85**: 45–48.

MÖLLBY, R. (1978) Bacterial phospholipases. In: *Bacterial toxins and cell membranes,* pp. 367–424, JELJASZEWICZ, J. and WADSTROM, T. (Eds), Academic Press, London.

MOLNAR, D. M. (1962) Separation of the toxin of *Bacillus cereus* into two components and non identity of the toxin with phospholipase. *J. Bact.* **84**: 147–153.

MORTIMER, P. R. and MEERS, P. D. (1975) Two food poisoning incidents possibly associated with a *Bacillus* species. Public Health Laboratory Service (England & Wales) *Communicable Disease Report* 1975, No. 30.

NYGREN, B. (1962) Phospholipase C-producing bacteria and food poisoning. *Acta. Pathol. Microbiol. Scand. Suppl.* **160**: 1–89.

O'BRIEN, A. D. and KAPRAL, F. A. (1976) Increased cyclic adenosine 3′,5′-monophosphate content in guinea pig ileum after exposure to *Staphylococcus aureus* delta-toxin. *Infect. Immun.* **13**: 152–162.

O'DAY, D. M., HO, P. C., ANDREWS, J. S., HEAD, W. S., IVES, J. and TURNBULL, P. C. B. (1981a) Mechanism of tissue destruction in ocular *Bacillus cereus* infections. In: *The cornea in health and disease,* pp. 403–407, TREVOR-ROPER, P. (Ed), (VIth Congress of the European Society of Ophthalmology) Academic Press, London.

O'DAY, D. M., SMITH, R. S., GREGG, C. R., TURNBULL, P. C. B., HEAD, W. S., IVES, J. A. and HO, P. C. (1981b) The problem of bacillus species infection with special emphasis on the virulence of *Bacillus cereus. Ophthalmology* (*Rochester*) **88**: 833–838.

ORMAY, L. and NOVOTNY, T. (1970) Über sogenannte unspezifische Lebensmittelvergiftungen in Ungarn. *Zbl. Bakt. Hyg., I. Abt. Orig.* **215**: 84–89. English Summary.

OTNAESS, A.-B., GIERCKSKY, K. E. and PRYDZ, H. (1976) Parenteral administration of phospholipase C in the rat. Distribution, elimination and lethal doses. *Scand. J. Clin. Lab. Invest.* **36**: 553–559.

OTNAESS, A.-B., PRYDZ, H. BJORKLID, E. and BERRE, A. (1972) Phospholipase C from *Bacillus cereus* and its use in studies of tissue thromboplastin. *Europ. J. Biochem.* **27**: 238–243.

OTTOLENGHI, A., GOLLUB, S. and ULIN, A. (1961) Studies on phospholipase from *Bacillus cereus*. I. Separation of phospholipolytic and hemolytic activities *Bact. Proc.* **171**: 20.

PARK, Y., BABAJIMOPOULUS, M. and MIKOLAJCIK, E. M. (1977) Purification and activity of *Clostridium perfringens* alpha toxin. *J. Fd. Protect.* **40**: 831–834.

PARKER, D. A. and GOEPFERT, J. M. (1978) Enhancement of synthesis of *Bacillus cereus* enterotoxin using a sac-culture technique. *J. Fd. Protect.* **41**: 116–117.

PARRY, J. M. and GILBERT, R. J. (1980) Studies on the heat resistance of *Bacillus cereus* spores and growth of the organism in boiled rice. *J. Hyg., Camb.* **84**: 77–82.

PENDLETON, I. R., BERNHEIMER, A. W. and GRUSHOFF, P. (1973) Purification and partial characterization of hemolysins from *Bacillus thuringiensis. J. Invertebr. Pathol.* **21**: 131–135.

PENDLETON, I. R., KIM, K. S. and BERNHEIMER, A. W. (1972) Detection of cholesterol in cell membranes by use of bacterial toxins. *J. Bact.* **110**: 722–730.

PILLEN, D. (1971) Behandlung von Darmerkrankungen im Doppelblindversuch mit *Bacillus* Stamm 5832 (Pasteur Institut). *Med. Welt.* **22**: 266–268.

RAWLEY, J. and HUNTER, F. R. (1951) Action of *Bacillus cereus* toxins on chicken erythrocytes. *Proc. Soc. Exp. Biol. Med.* (New York) **77**: 99–104.

SAMPLES, J. R. and BUETTNER, H. (1983) Corneal ulcer caused by a biologic insecticide (*Bacillus thuringiensis*). *Am. J. Ophthalmol.* **95**: 258–260.

SCHAEFFER, P. (1950) Croissance et respiration d'une souche streptomycino-exigeante de *Bacillus cereus* privée de l'antibiotique-facteur de croissance. *Ann. Inst. Pasteur* **78**: 624–637.

SEITZ, M. (1913) Pathogener *Bacillus subtilis*. *Zbl. Bakt. Hyg., I. Abt. Orig.* **70**: 113–114.

SHANY, S., BERNHEIMER, A. W., GRUSHOFF, P. S. and KIM, K. W. (1974) Evidence for membrane cholesterol as the common binding site for cereolysin, streptolysin O and saponin. *Molec. Cellul. Biochem.* **3**: 179–186.

SLEIN, M. W. and LOGAN, G. F. JR. (1960) Mechanism of action of the toxin of *Bacillus anthracis*. I. Effect in vivo on some blood serum components. *J. Bact.* **80**: 77–85.

SLEIN, M. W. and LOGAN, G. F. JR. (1962) Mechanism of action of the toxin of *Bacillus anthracis*. II. Alkaline phosphatasemia produced by culture filtrates of various bacilli. *J. Bact.* **83**: 359–369.

SLEIN, M. W. and LOGAN, G. F., JR. (1963) Partial purification and properties of two phospholipases of *Bacillus cereus*. *J. Bact.* **85**: 369–381.

SLEIN, M. W. and LOGAN, G. F., JR. (1965) Characterization of the phospholipases of *Bacillus cereus* and their effects on erythrocytes, bone, and kidney cells. *J. Bact.* **90**: 69–81.

SMITH, N. R., GORDON, R. E. and CLARK, F. E. (1952) *Aerobic Sporeforming Bacteria* pp. 56–64. United States Department of Agriculture Monograph No. 16 Washington, D. C.

SMYTH, C. J. and DUNCAN, J. L. (1978) Thiol-activated cytolysins. In *Bacterial toxins and Cell membranes*. pp. 130–183, JELJASZEWICZ, J. and WADSTRÖM, T. (Eds), Academic Press, London.

SPIRA, W. M. (1974) Animal assay systems for the qualitative and quantitative determination of *Bacillus cereus* enterotoxin. Ph.D. Thesis. University of Wisconsin, Madison, Wisconsin.

SPIRA, W. M. and GOEPFERT, J. M. (1972a) *Bacillus cereus*-induced fluid accumulation in rabbit ileal loops. *Appl. Microbiol.* **24**: 341–348.

SPIRA, W. M. and GOEPFERT, J. M. (1972b) An enterotoxic factor produced by *Bacillus cereus* and assayed in the ligated ileal loop of rabbits. *Abstr. Annu. Meet. Amer. Soc. Microbiol*, p. 23 E133.

SPIRA, W. M. and GOEPFERT, J. M. (1975) Biological characteristics of an enterotoxin produced by *Bacillus cereus*. *Canad. J. Microbiol.* **21**: 1236–1246.

SPIRA, W. M. and SILVERMAN, G. J. (1979) Effects of glucose, pH and dissolved-oxygen tension on *Bacillus cereus* growth and permeability factor production in batch culture. *Appl. Environm. Microbiol.* **37**: 109–116.

STAMATIN, N. and ANGHELESCO, S. (1969) Pouvoir pathogène et toxicité de *Bacillus cereus*. *Ann. Inst. Pasteur* **116**: 210–217.

ST. JOHN-BROOKS, R. (1930) The non-pathogenic spore-bearing aerobic bacteria. In: *A System of Bacteriology in Relation to Medicine*, Volume 5, MRC, Her Majesty's Stationery Office: London.

STREGULINA, A. (1906) Ueber die im Züricher Boden vorkommenden Heubacillen und über deren Beziehungen zu den Erregern der Panophthalmie nach Hackensplitterverletzung. *Zbl. Bact. Hyg., I. Abt. Orig.* **38**: 352–353.

TODD, E., PARK, C., CLEANER, B., FABRICIUS, A., EDWARDS, D. and EWAN, P. (1974) Two outbreaks of *Bacillus cereus* food poisoning in Canada. *Canad. J. Publ. Hlth.* **65**: 109–113.

TORRES-ANJEL, M. J., GONZÁLEZ, G. H., GIRALDO, M. E., ANGEL, M. O., CAMACHO, A. and SEGURA, C. (1979) Enterotoxigenicidad de *Bacillus cereus*. *Rev. lat-amer. Microbiol.* **21**: 5–10.

TUAZON, C. U., MURRAY, H. W., LEVY, C., SOLNY, M. N., CURTIN, J. A. and SHEAGREN, J. N. (1979) Serious infections from *Bacillus* sp. *J. Amer. Med. Ass.* **241**: 1137–1140.

TURNBULL, P. C. B. (1976) Studies on the production of enterotoxins by *Bacillus cereus*. *J. Clin. Path.* **29**: 941–948.

TURNBULL, P. C. B. (1978) *Bacillus licheniformis*: a possible food poisoning agent and clinical pathogen. Public Health Laboratory Service (England & Wales) *Communicable Disease Report* 1978, No. 18.

TURNBULL, P. C. B. (1979a) Food poisoning with special reference to *Salmonella*—its epidemiology, pathogenesis and control. *Clinics in Gastroenterology* **8**: 663–714.

TURNBULL, P. C. B. (1979b) *Bacillus subtilis*. Public Health Laboratory Service (England & Wales) *Communicable Disease Report*, 1979, No. 31.

TURNBULL, P. C. B., FRENCH, T. A. and DOWSETT, E. G. (1977a) Severe systemic and pyogenic infections with *Bacillus cereus*. *Brit. Med. J.* **1**: 1628–1629.

TURNBULL, P. C. B., JØRGENSEN, K., KRAMER, J. M., GILBERT, R. J. and PARRY, J. M. (1979a) Severe clinical conditions associated with *Bacillus cereus* and the apparent involvement of exotoxins. *J. Clin. Path.* **32**: 289–293.

TURNBULL, P. C. B. and KRAMER, J. M. (1983) Non-gastrointestinal *Bacillus cereus* infections: an analysis of exotoxin production by strains isolated over a two-year period. *J. Clin. Path.* **36**: 1091–1096.

TURNBULL, P. C. B., KRAMER, J. M., JØRGENSEN, K., GILBERT, R. J. and MELLING, J. (1979b) Properties and production characteristics of vomiting, diarrheal, and necrotizing toxins of *Bacillus cereus*. *Amer. J. Clin. Nutr.* **32**: 219–228.

TURNBULL, P. C. B., NOTTINGHAM, J. F. and GHOSH, A. C. (1977b) A severe necrotic enterotoxin produced by certain food, food poisoning and other clinical isolates of *Bacillus cereus*. *Brit. J. Exp. Path.* **58**: 273–280.

VANDEKERKOVE, M. (1979) Etude des effets de l'administration du *Bacillus* souche IP 5832 sur la flore intestinale des nourrissons soumis aux traitements antibiotiques. *Annales de Pédiatrie* **26**: 503–506.

WADSTRÖM, T. and MÖLLBY, R. (1971) Studies on extracellular proteins from *Staphylococcus aureus*. VI Production and purification of β-haemolysin in large scale. *Biochim. Biophys. Acta.* **242**: 288–307.

WARREN, R. E., RUBENSTEIN, D., ELLAR, D. J., KRAMER, J. M. and GILBERT, R. J. (1984) *Bacillus thuringiensis* var *israelensis*: protoxin activation and safety. *Lancet* **i**: 678–679.

WHO. (1979) World Health Organization, Biological Control Agent data sheet, No. VBC/BCDS/79.01. *Bacillus thuringiensis israelensis*, de Barjac, H. 1978.

WILLIAMS, G. R. (1957) Haemolytic material from aerobic sporing bacteria. *J. Gen. Microbiol.* **16**: 16–21.

WINTON, F. W. and SAYERS, J. O. (1975) An outbreak of food poisoning caused by *Bacillus subtilis*? *Communicable Disease Scotland*, Weekly Report, No. 46: iii.

WISEMAN, G. M. (1965) Some characteristics of the beta haemolysin of *Staphylococcus aureus*. *J. Path. Bact.* **89**: 187–207.

WRIGHT, D. J. M., FROST, D. J., EATON, P. and TURNBULL, P. C. B. (1979) Waterborne *Bacillus licheniformis* infection in mice. *J. Med. Microbiol.* **12**: p ix.

YOUNG, E. J., WALLACE, R. J., JR. ERICSSON, C. D., HARRIS, R. A. and CLARRIDGE, J. (1980) Panophthalmitis due to *Bacillus cereus. Arch. Int. Med.* **140:** 559–560.

ZWAAL, R. F. A. and ROELOFSEN, B. (1974) Phospholipase C (phosphatidylcholine cholinephosphohydrolase, EC 3.1.4.3) from *Bacillus cereus.* In: *Methods in Enzymology* **32:** 154–161, FLEISCHER, S and PACKER, L. (Eds), Academic Press, New York.

ZWAAL, R. F. A., ROELOFSEN, B., COMFURIUS, P. and VAN DEENEN, L. L. M. (1971) Complete purification and some properties of phospholipase C from *Bacillus cereus. Biochim. Biophys. Acta.* **233:** 474–479.

CHAPTER 21

THE ENTOMOCIDAL TOXINS OF
BACILLUS THURINGIENSIS

PETER LÜTHY and HANS RUDOLF EBERSOLD

Institute of Microbiology, Swiss Federal Institute of Technology, 8092 Zürich, Switzerland

1. INTRODUCTION TO *BACILLUS THURINGIENSIS*

1.1. ENTOMOPATHOGENIC MICROORGANISMS

Invertebrates are affected by pathogenic microorganisms much in the same way as vertebrates. Infectious diseases are caused by viruses, rickettsiae, bacteria, fungi and protozoa. Under natural conditions pathogenic microorganisms are the main control mechanisms which limit the development of insect populations. The microbial reduction of insect populations is as a rule very effective and occurs within short periods of time.

The first observations of invertebrate diseases were made with our two domesticated insects, the silkworm (*Bombyx mori*) and the honey bee (*Apis mellifera*). Aristotle (384–322 B.C.) mentioned outbreaks of diseases among honey bees in his history of animals (Historia animalum).

It is probably not generally known that medically important discoveries were based on observations made with insects. Agostino Bassi, for example, used for the first experimental transmission of a disease from one individual to the other silkworm larvae and the fungus, *Beauveria bassiana*. This important experiment was published in 1835. Also Pasteur was involved in insect pathology. He isolated *Nosema bombycis*, a protozoan pathogen causing the pebrine disease in silkworms. *N. bombycis* represented a severe threat to the French silkworm industry. Pasteur (1870) summarized his investigations in an important publication entitled "Etudes sur la maladie des vers à soie". With his recommendations he helped to reduce the losses in the sericultures.

In 1885 Chesire and Cheyne described the causative agent of the European foulbrood of honey bees, *Bacillus alvei*. The bacterium responsible for the American foulbrood, *Bacillus larvae*, was discovered by White at the beginning of our century.

The first reports of *Bacillus thuringiensis*, the most important pathogen used today for insect control, can be dated back to the first years of the twentieth century. Ishiwata (1902), a Japanese scientist, isolated a bacterium from diseased silkworm larvae which he named *Bacillus sotto*. The isolate of Ishiwata represents today the variety (*var.*) *sotto* (serotype 4a4b) within the species *B. thuringiensis*. Between 1909 and 1912 Berliner working at a research station for grain processing in Berlin investigated an infectious disease of the Mediterranean flour moth (*Anagasta kuehniella*). The infected insects were originally obtained from a mill in the district of Thueringen. In a detailed report (Berliner, 1915) he described a spore former as the causative agent and he designated it as *Bacillus thuringiensis*.

Since the original isolation of *B. thuringiensis* nearly 50 years passed before the potential of this microorganism was recognized. Especially the newly developed organic insecticides which were for some time extremely effective and apparently bare of side effects prevented the interest for biological alternatives. The search for microbial insecticides started only when more and more insects acquired resistance against chemical pesticides and when their impacts on the environment became evident.

But in order to remain realistic, it has to be mentioned that only a few microorganisms will finally reach the insecticide market. Among the successful bacteria we can cite

Bacillus popilliae, a pathogen of the Japanese beetle (*Popillia japonica*) which is a severe pest in grasslands of the Eastern United States. *B. popilliae* was discovered by Dutky in 1940. It is a so-called obligate pathogen which grows only in a limited number of host species which all belong to the scarabaeids (order: *Coleoptera*). Despite great efforts, the production of infectious *B. popilliae* spores on artificial media was not successful. Therefore millions of host larvae had to be used for the production of the pathogen. Treatment of grassland with spores led in many places to reduction of the Japanese beetle populations below economic levels. The mode of action of *B. popilliae* is not yet understood, especially since no toxin seems to be involved in the pathogenesis. Other bacteria with some potential for pest control are strains of *Bacillus sphaericus* and *Bacillus moritai*. *B. sphaericus* is active against mosquito larvae while *B. moritai* can be used for the control of the house fly (*Musca domestica*). *B. sphaericus* seems to produce a toxin which is deposited in the cell wall (Davidson *et al.*, 1975; Myers and Yousten, 1980). Studies are under way in several laboratories to identify this toxin. It has to be added that only a few specific strains within the species of *B. sphaericus* are pathogenic. *B. moritai* preparations were marketed in Japan but for the moment production has been stopped.

Several viruses have been registered for the control of agricultural and forest insect pests. They belong to the group of the nuclear polyhedrosis viruses. Granulosis viruses and cytoplasmic polyhedrosis viruses represent two other groups with the potential to be developed to insecticides. The production of viruses represents a major problem since they multiply only within their hosts. *In vitro* production in cell cultures has in some cases been successful but the yields per cell are too low so that mass rearing of insects for virus production is still the only feasible method.

Although fungi belong to the main microbial insect control agents under natural conditions, the artificial introduction into host populations remains difficult. Problems are encountered with the production of virulent material and with inconsistent infectivity rates, probably due to micro-climate conditions such as relative humidity. While bacteria, viruses as well as protozoa have to be ingested by the hosts, fungal spores germinate on the surface of the insect and the hyphae penetrate through the epidermis supported by exoenzymes like chitinases, lipases and proteases. Numerous fungi produce toxins during their proliferation within the hemocoel of the host.

Protozoa are not suitable for quick and efficient reduction of insect populations. They are known to exist in many insect species in an endemic state. They are capable of limiting insect populations by reducing fecundity and by weakening the natural resistance against adverse environmental influences. Furthermore, protozoa can only be propagated in their hosts or in elaborated tissue culture systems. A similar situation exists for insect pathogenic rickettsiae. In addition, a clear-cut separation between rickettsiae pathogenic for invertebrates and vertebrates is difficult to make since invertebrates serve also as vectors for human pathogenic rickettsiae. The reader interested in basic and applied aspects of microbial insect control is referred to books edited by Burges (1981), by Davidson (1981) and by Kurstak (1981).

The emphasis in this chapter will be on the biologically active metabolites produced by *B. thuringiensis*. But in order to put these metabolites into a frame and in order to understand the importance and potential of *B. thuringiensis* some basic information might be useful.

1.2. THE ACTUAL STAGE OF DEVELOPMENT OF *Bacillus thuringiensis*

It has already been mentioned that *B. thuringiensis* is presently the most widely used microorganism to control insect pests. It possesses all the attributes which are required for an ideal insecticide. The host spectrum is limited to species within one order, *Lepidoptera* or *Diptera*. Predators and parasites belong as a rule to other orders and therefore do not respond to *B. thuringiensis*. They can continue to play their important role in maintaining the balance among insect populations. Up to date no resistance has developed against *B. thuringiensis* which means that the life span of this insecticide has at present no predictable limitation. The production of *B. thuringiensis* does not imply major problems. In contrast to organic pesticides which are based on petro-chemicals the raw materials for *B. thuringiensis* production are waste products of the agriculture or of the food industry. No toxic effects of *B. thuringiensis* against vertebrates could be found so far. Therefore, these products may be applied up to the date of harvest which is especially important in vegetable crops. In 1980 *B. thuringiensis* producers obtained the label by the US authorities (Environmental Protection Agency, EPA) to use *B. thuringiensis* for the protection of stored grain and for the control of dipterous larvae.

It is however wrong to assume that chemical pesticides will be replaced in the near future by biological preparations. If we want to provide enough food for the still increasing human population, we cannot do it without chemical pesticides. However, instead of applying pesticides on a prophylactic basis they should be used only when necessary, preferably within so-called pest management programs where at the same time biological means of pest control are integrated.

It has been mentioned that *B. thuringiensis* can also be used for the control of mosquito and blackfly larvae. This goes back to an important discovery made in 1977 by Goldberg and Margalit. A new *B. thuringiensis* serotype was isolated from a diseased mosquito population encountered in a waterhole in Israel. The new variety, named *israelensis*, has an activity spectrum which is limited to some families within the suborder *Nematocera*. The emphasis lies on the *Culicidae* and *Simulidae* where we find most important vectors of human diseases such as *Aedes aegypti* (yellow fever) and *Anopheles stephensi* (malaria). Efficient mosquito control in tropical countries is badly needed in order to limit especially the spread of malaria. Field tests have been very successful and without measurable side effects on the balance of the other water inhabiting fauna. If no severe drawbacks occur world wide production of *B. thuringiensis* var. *israelensis* will be started.

B. thuringiensis production in the US was estimated for 1980 at 1.5 million pounds. Most of the preparations are used in vegetable crops for the control of the cabbage looper (*Trichoplusia ni*) which is a polyphageous leaf feeder. A list of pest insects which can be controlled by *B. thuringiensis* is found in Table 1. *B. thuringiensis* is also produced on a large scale in the USSR and in France. According to a report by Franz and Krieg (1980) the People's Republic of China is putting much effort in the development of *B. thuringiensis* products. Table 2 shows the countries and the companies involved in the production of *B. thuringiensis*. The companies offer different preparations either in the form of wettable powders or flowables, based on several *B. thuringiensis* strains with typical host ranges.

TABLE 1. *Important Insects Susceptible to* Bacillus thuringiensis, *together with some Host Crops*

Insect species	Crops	
Trichoplusia ni (Cabbage looper)	vegetables, soybean, tobacco	
Plutella maculipennis (Diamond black moth)	vegetables	
Pieris brassicae (Large white butterfly)	vegetables	
Pieris rapae (Imported cabbage looper)	vegetables	
Heliothis zea (Bollworm)	soybean, tobacco	(Heliothis spp. in cotton are difficult to control with *B. thuringiensis*)
Heliothis virescens (Tobacco budworm)	soybean, tobacco	
Ostrinia nubilalis (European corn borer)	corn	
Manduca sexta (Tobacco hornworm)	tobacco	
Lymantria dispar (Gypsy moth)	forest	
Choristoneura fumiferana (Spruce budworm)	forest	
Malacosoma disstria (tent caterpillar)	forest	
Dendrolimus sibiricus (Siberian silkworm)	forest	
Plodia interpunctella (Indian meal moth)	stored grain	
Ephestia cautella (Almond moth)	stored grain	
Anagasta kuehniella (Mediterranean flour moth)	stored flour	
Ades aegypti	vector of the yellow fever	
Anopheles stephensi	vector of malaria	

TABLE 2. *The Producers of* Bacillus thuringiensis *Preparations*

Country	Company	Trade names
USA	Sandoz Inc., Homestead, Florida	Thuricide
USA	Abbott Laboratories, North Chicago, Illinois	Dipel
France	Biochem Products S.A.	Bactospéine, Leptox, Bug Time
USSR	Several plants	Entobacterine-3 Dendrobacilline Toxobacterine Insectine BIP Bitoxibacilline

1.3. THE BIOLOGICALLY ACTIVE METABOLITES OF *Bacillus thuringiensis*

Several toxic metabolites belonging to quite different classes are produced by *B. thuringiensis* during its growth cycle. They are summarized in Table 3. The most important is the delta-endotoxin, an attribute by which *B. thuringiensis* is differentiated from the related species *Bacillus cereus*. The delta-endotoxin is practically alone responsible for the importance as insecticide. The other metabolites, the alpha-exotoxin, the beta-exotoxin and the exoenzymes are not uniformly produced by all *B. thuringiensis* varieties. They are either not wanted in commercial preparations or so labile that activity is lost rapidly.

The delta-endotoxin is a protein, formed early in the sporulation phase. It is crystallized within the sporangium, usually assuming the shape of bipyramid. The weight of these crystals reach about one third of the whole cell. When sporulation is completed, the sporangium is lysed and the heat resistant spore and the crystal are set free separately.

The alpha-exotoxin seems to be a very labile protein excreted during the logarithmic growth phase by strains of *B. thuringiensis* and *B. cereus*, but only under certain culture conditions (Krieg and Lysenko, 1979). The toxicity seems to be very unspecific. The nature of that protein as well as the mode of action are not known.

The beta-exotoxin is a nucleotide excreted into the medium during vegetative growth. About half of the identified *B. thuringiensis* varieties produce the beta-exotoxin. The spectrum of activity is rather broad covering not only insects but also other organisms. The *B. thuringiensis* preparations marketed in the US and Western Europe are based on strains which are free of beta-exotoxin while some of the products in the USSR contain beta-exotoxin because of its synergistic effect in combination with the delta-endotoxin.

Vegetative and sporulating cells excrete enzymes such as lecithinases, chitinases and proteases which especially support the proliferation of *B. thuringiensis* within the hosts.

TABLE 3. *The Biologically Active Metabolites of* Bacillus thuringiensis

Metabolite	Nature	Host spectrum	Significance
Alpha-exotoxin	Protein (not identified)	Insects, and vertebrates at high concentrations	None, not present in commercial preparations
Beta-exotoxin	Nucleotide	Invertebrates and vertebrates	High mosquito and fly activity, not present in preparations of US and Western Europe
Delta-endotoxin	Protein crystal	Lepidoptera and in one case Diptera	Basis for all *B. thuringiensis* preparations
Enzymes	Lecithinases chitinases proteases	Ability of causing damage to cells and organs in the presence of an appropriate substrate	Not reported in commercial preparations

1.4. Microbial Characterization of *Bacillus thuringiensis*

Bacillus thuringiensis, a member of the genus *Bacillus*, forms at the end of the vegetative growth a so-called spore which is able to survive for long periods of time, even under most unfavorable environmental conditions. Morphology and metabolism show a close relationship to *B. cereus*. As already mentioned, the formation of the crystalline proteinaceous inclusion during the sporulation is the only constant distinction between the two species. The crystalline inclusion is also called parasporal body, delta-endotoxin or just crystal.

B. thuringiensis is not frequently encountered in nature. With the exception of the two recently discovered varieties *dakota* and *indiana* (De Lucca *et al.*, 1979) all isolates originate from diseased insects. *B. cereus* has a prevalence to grow on decaying organic material. The same must be true for *B. thuringiensis* since it has identical saprophytic growth requirements. *B. thuringiensis* has acquired an additional niche because of its insecticidal metabolites. Diseased insect populations attract the attention of curious pathologists, and this may be the reason that practically all varieties of *B. thuringiensis* were isolated from insects. Interestingly, the pathogenicity of a given variety is much higher against the original host than against other target insects. This may indicate that long term mutual association between insect and pathogen has existed in such cases. On the other hand the pathogenicity does not decrease when the strains are maintained on laboratory media, even after many transfers.

It may also be surprising that epizootics caused by *B. thuringiensis* occur rarely. Spreading within host populations have been reported from sericultures or from insects colonies in stored products such as flour. This may be because the bacterium does not find ideal conditions within the insect to sporulate and to form concomitantly the parasporal body since oxygen supply which is essential for fast sporulation is poor.

Spore germination and the metabolism of vegetative cells of *B. thuringiensis* have been reviewed by Lüthy *et al.* (1981). Like other bacterial spores, *B. thuringiensis* needs activation in order to germinate. Activation is a process which takes place during the ageing of the spores. It can be accelerated by heat, calcium dipicolinate, low pH values or reducing agents. The germination process then gives rise to a vegetative cell, flagellated peritrichously with average dimensions of $3-5 \times 1.2-1.5 \ \mu m$. Numerous media have been developed either more defined, serving for basic investigations or complex in their composition, aimed at high yields. A suitable medium with only water soluble ingredients has the following composition (Yousten and Rogoff, 1969): (g/l) glucose, 3.0 (originally only 1.0); $(NH_4)_2SO_4$, 2.0; yeast extract, 2.0; $MgSO_4$, 0.2; $CaCl_2 \cdot 2H_2O$, 0.08; $MnSO_4 \cdot H_2O$, 0.05; K_2HPO_4, 0.5. The pH is adjusted with KOH to 7.3. Cultivation is best achieved on agar or in liquid medium under aeration at temperatures between 30–32°C. Sporulation is completed between 24 to 36 hr. The yield of spores lies between $2-5 \times 10^8$/ml. A complex medium developed in our laboratory based on cheap ingredients has the following composition: (g/l) soya bean meal (fatty), 35; corn starch, 12.15; malt extract, 2.0; $K_2HPO_4 \cdot 2H_2O$, 1.3; $MgSO_4 \cdot 7H_2O$, 0.2; $CaCl_2 \cdot 2H_2O$, 0.08; $MnSO_4 \cdot 7H_2O$, 0.08. The pH is adjusted to 7.2. At least 48 hr of incubation time are required in order to achieve total sporulation. The fermented broth contains still a large amount of solid ingredients. An elegant method for the optimization of a medium for *B. thuringiensis* with a continuous chemostat culture has been reported by Goldberg *et al.* (1980). Maximum yields obtained with complex media are 5×10^9 spores/ml.

Serotyping is used for the taxonomic classification of *B. thuringiensis* strains. This is a method which was applied originally for the identification of medically important human pathogens, such as *Salmonella* strains. The H-serotyping for *B. thuringiensis* was elaborated by de Barjac and Bonnefoi (1962, 1973). By the end of 1980 a total of 16 serotypes had been described. Subdivision of the serotypes into varieties is based on serological subfactors and biochemical properties. A list of the *B. thuringiensis* varieties has been prepared in Table 4. The use of the antigenic properties of the flagella is the best available system for the classification of *B. thuringiensis* strains.

TABLE 4. *Varieties of* Bacillus thuringiensis

Serotype (H-antigens)	Name of variety (biotype)	Serotype (H-antigens)	Name of variety (biotype)
1	Thuringiensis	7	Aizawai
2	Finitimus	8	Morrisoni
3a	Alesti	9	Tolworthi
3a–3b	Kurstaki	10	Darmstadtiensis
4a–4b	Sotto	11a–11b	Toumanoffi
4a–4b	Dendrolimus	11a–11c	Kyushuensis
4a–4c	Kenyae	12	Tompsoni
5a–5b	Galleriae	13	Pakistani
5a–5c	Canadensis	14	Israelensis
6	Entomocidus	15	Dakota
6	Subtoxicus	16	Indiana

Serology is also used for the investigation and classification of the delta-endotoxin. In an extended study of the crystal antigens of more than 300 strains Krywienczyk (1977) found that in about 85 per cent of the cases the strains with identical crystal antigens belonged to a given H-serotype. Crystal serology can be very useful at the level of strain classification. For example, Krywienczyk detected that within the variety *kurstaki* strains with two distinct antigenic crystal protein patterns are present. The groups were designated as K-1 and K-73. As a rule crystals of different serotypes share antigens. The variety *israelensis* is an exception in that the crystal possesses no antigenic relationship with any of the other varieties (Krywienczyk and Fast, 1980). Although classification by crystal antigens might correlate better with the toxicity spectra, comparison of data obtained by different laboratories are difficult to compare since the the antigens which are expressed depend on the preparation. Whole crystals, chemically dissolved protein or gut juice incubated material yield distinct antigen patterns. Modification causes loss of existing and appearance of new antigenic determinants.

2. THE DELTA-ENDOTOXIN

2.1. Biosynthesis

Vegetative cells multiply in a medium as long as nutrients (carbon, nitrogen, phosphorous sources) are available in balanced proportions. The nutritional depletion stops proliferation and induces the sporulation process. At this point the tricarbonic cycle is derepressed and the organic acids, acetate and pyruvate which have been accumulated during vegetative growth are metabolized supplying the cell with energy and carbon for the spore and crystal synthesis.

The sporulation process is divided into seven different stages. Stage I cells contain an axial chromatin filament. During stage II the chromatin separates into two chromosomes and the forespore septum is formed separating the sporulation region from the rest of the cell. The following phase comprises the engulfment of the septum and the formation of a forespore. The forespore covers only about one third of the whole cell and it is situated in one of the polar regions. The primordial cell wall and the cortex appear between the inner and outer membrane in stage IV. Subsequently the spore becomes refractile in the phase contrast microscope and gradual resistance against organic solvents is acquired. Spore coat development and completion of the exosporium belong to stage V. The maturation of the spore is concluded in Stage VI and the sporulation process ends with the release of the spore (stage VII) by the lysis of the former vegetative cell wall.

Sporulation and delta-endotoxin formation are closely linked and synchronyzed processes. Up to date no mutants blocked at the entrance of sporulation have been found to produce crystal protein. Microscopic evidence for the presence of delta-endotoxin is obtained in sporulation stage II, concomitant with the septum formation. The biosynthesis proceeds at a fast rate and the crystal reaches its final size at the end of stage IV or at the beginning of stage V. The sporulation and crystal formation have been described in detail by Lüthy *et al.* (1981). Fig. 1a and 1b show a cell of *B. thuringiensis* var. *kurstaki* in sporulation stage III and V, respectively.

Little is known about the regulation of the crystal protein synthesis. Monro (1961 a,b) demonstrated that crystal protein was synthesized *de novo* out of breakdown products from the vegetative cell and that there were no detectable amounts of proteins in the vegetative cells which were antigenically related to the crystal. It seems that surplus protein is degraded and resynthesized to the delta-endotoxin.

The size of the crystals can be influenced for example by the amount of glucose added to the growth medium (Scherrer *et al.*, 1973).

If there is a specific site provided for the synthesis of the crystal in the area outside the spore, it has not yet been located. Somerville (1971) found that the biosynthesis of the crystalline inclusion occurred in close contact with the exosporium. Other authors were not able to confirm this, especially since the delta-endotoxin is visible before structures of the exosporium can be recognized. Ribier (1971) observed that the crystal originated in close association with the cell membrane and that it was surrounded by ribosomes.

A stable mRNA seems to be responsible for the crystal protein synthesis. It has a half-life of about 10 min (Glatron and Rapoport, 1972). Klier *et al.* (1973) described a RNA-polymerase (designated as $\beta'\beta\alpha_2$) from sporulating cells which synthesized the stable mRNA (Klier *et al.*, 1978). The crystal-specific RNA was transcribed principally from the L-strand of the DNA. *In vitro* synthesis of crystal protein was achieved by Petit-Glatron and Rapoport (1975). Polypeptides with molecular weights of up to 40,000 were obtained and the identity of the product was proved by immunoprecipitation.

One would expect that crystal protein synthesis is controlled by plasmids. Final proof is however still missing. *B. thuringiensis* carries numerous plasmids whose number seems to coincide with the serotype. Debabov *et al.* (1977) obtained acrystalliferous strains after curing with ethidiumbromide or after growth at elevated temperatures. The acrystalliferous strains had lost their plasmids. Stahly *et al.* (1978) found that all his strains without crystals were bare of extrachromosomal elements. Miteva (1978) however was not able to establish a relationship between plasmids of wild types and acrystalliferous mutants. A final answer can be expected as soon as reliable transformation systems for *B. thuringiensis* are available.

2.2. COMPOSITION OF THE PROTEIN CRYSTAL

The parasporal inclusions produced by *B. thuringiensis* are as a rule bipyramidal. We find variety specific differences in the shape. For example, the crystals of the variety *thuringiensis* are rather long with pointed ends whereas *sotto* crystals are somewhat thicker with rounded tips. As a rule, a single crystal is produced per cell, but there are exceptions where two or even three inclusions occur. It has to be mentioned that strains of the variety *kurstaki* form a so-called ovoid inclusion (Bechtel and Bulla, 1976) whose composition and function is unknown.

The crystals of the variety *israelensis* represent an exception with their irregular and heterogeneous structure. They represent a complex consisting of at least three fragments. The parasporal inclusion is surrounded by an envelope and it seems that a wrapping exists even around the single fragments (Lüthy *et al.*, 1981).

Micrographs of the crystals, freeze-fractures or thin sections reveal a fine structure. No difference can be recognized among crystals of the lepidopterous active varieties. Holmes and Monro (1965) investigated the crystalline structure by X-ray analysis and they calculated a molecular weight (MW) of 230,000 for the subunit. The inclusion of the dipterous active *israelensis* variety is only partially present in a crystalline form. Amorphous material seems to dominate here. Where a crystalline arrangement is found, it is much finer and differently structured compared to the other varieties. Fig. 2a and 2b exhibit a parasporal body of the variety *thuringiensis* and Fig. 2c and 2d an *israelensis* crystal.

Fermented cultures contain a mixture of spores and crystals. For any analytical study purified crystal suspensions are required. Several methods are available for the separation of the crystals from the spores. Good results are obtained with separation techniques proposed by Ang and Nickerson (1978) and Delafield et al. (1968). The purity of the crystal suspensions should be higher than 99 per cent compared to the number of contaminating spores.

Analytical studies of the crystal have proved very difficult because of extreme insolubility. Taking into account the low half-cystine content between 1.3 and 1.99 per cent (Nickerson, 1980) it should be expected that the crystals are readily soluble in standard protein solvents, but they behave like the highly insoluble wool keratin which has a half-cystine content of 10 per cent. Once dissolved the crystal protein shows a great tendency to reagglomerate. It is therefore not surprising that there was considerable controversy between different working groups concerning the composition of the crystals. Difficulties were also experienced in our laboratory and we had to revise our own ideas and to adjust them to new facts found here or elsewhere.

It is known today that the high stability of the crystals is due to disulfide bonds and to non-covalent interactions. They can be readily solubilized with 10 mM dithiothreitol in 0.05 M carbonate buffer of pH 9.5. Following an incubation time of 30 min undissolved contaminating material is eliminated by centrifugation and the supernatant is dialysed against the carbonate buffer. In order to prevent reaggregation the dissolved proteins should be alkylated. Molecular weight determination by polyacrylamide gel electrophoresis resulted in a homogeneous fraction of 230,000 daltons (Nagamatsu et al., 1978; Huber et al., 1981). This is in good agreement with the X-ray diffraction data of Holmes and Monro (1965). The size of the subunit seems to be identical or at least very similar for all the lepidopterous active varieties. Huber et al. (1981) compared the subunits of 10 varieties and they found no differences. DTT dissolved parasporal bodies of the variety *israelensis* yielded a subunit weight of 25,000.

The MW of the subunit seems to depend on the method used. When the determination was carried out by ultracentrifugation a MW of only 177,000 was calculated (Huber et al., 1981). The discrepancy cannot be explained at the moment. Since most of the MW determinations are made with PAGE, these values should be used in order to have reliable comparisons.

A large number of cysteine residues is located at the surface of the subunit where they are able to form intra- and intermolecular disulfide bonds (Huber and Lüthy, 1981). For the crystal subunit of the variety *thuringiensis* about 20 sulfhydryl groups were readily accessable when titrated with 5,5'-dithiobis (2-nitrobenzoate) or p-chloromercuribenzoate. Fifteen out of the 20 SH-groups exposed on the surface of the molecule formed intramolecular disulfides, indicating that they are available for intermolecular S–S linking, a process which must occur during biosynthesis of the crystal. The number of intermolecular S–S bonds was estimated by sulfitolysis with ^{35}S-labeled sulfite, based on the intact crystal. An average of 6.1 intermolecular disulfides could be determined (Huber and Lüthy, 1981), a number which is by far sufficient for cross linking the subunits. The number of crosslinks is probably not constant and may augment with the age of the crystal. This would lead to an increase in stability. Young and Fitz-James (1959) already found an increasing insolubility for crystals which were stored for some weeks.

The subunit (MW 230,000) of the lepidopterous active crystals represents a dimer. Incubation of DTT dissolved crystal protein with a denaturing agent, e.g. 1 per cent SDS yields the monomer with a MW of 130,000 (determined with PAGE). Again a much lower MW of only 84,000 was calculated when ultracentrifugation was used. Molecular weights for the monomer in the above ranges were reported by Bulla et al. (1977), Chestukhina et al. (1978), Huber et al. (1981), Nagamatsu et al. (1978) and Zalunin et al. (1979) using PAGE and by Bulla et al. (1977), Glatron et al. (1972) and Huber et al. (1981) using ultracentrifugation. Variety specific differences in the size of the monomer might exist but exact determinations are missing. It has to be added that the DTT and SDS incubated *israelensis* protein has a molecular weight of 25,000. This suggests that the subunit is already a monomer.

Crystals of many varieties have been subjected to amino acid analysis. No significant

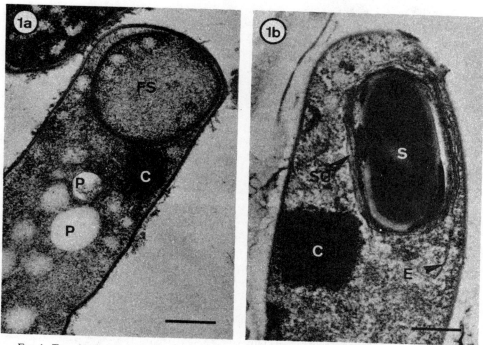

Fig. 1. Two development stages of the crystal of *B. thuringiensis* var. *kurstaki*. The cell in Fig. 1a is in an early sporulation stage III, at the beginning of the forespore (FS) synthesis (C = crystal, P = polybetahydroxybutyric acid inclusions, bar = 380 nm). The synthesis of the crystal is finished in stage V (Fig. 1b), with the ripening of the spore (S). (SC = spore coat, E = exosporium, bar = 340 nm).

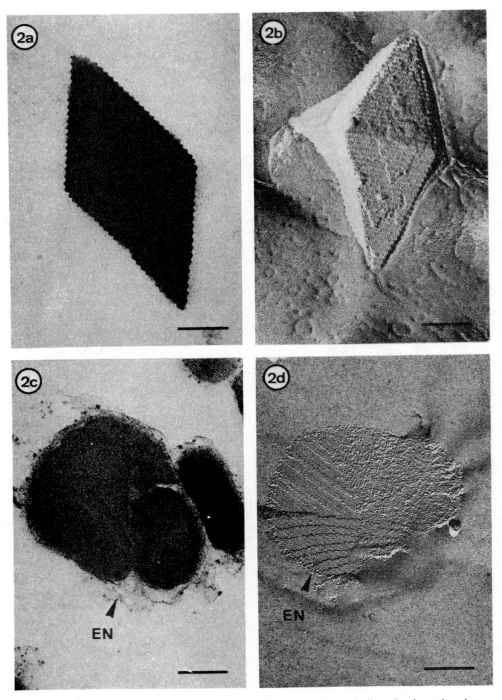

FIG. 2. Crystals of *Bacillus thuringiensis*. The regular composition is indicated only at the edges without a special processing for electron microscopy (Fig. 2a, bar = 230 nm). The crystalline structure is revealed in a freeze-fractured preparation in Fig. 2b (bar = 230 nm). The crystals in Fig. 2a and 2b are derived from the variety *thuringiensis*. Fig. 2c represents an *israelensis* crystal, composed of different particles and surrounded by an envelope (EN), bar = 230 nm). The fine structure of an *israelensis* crystal is shown in a freeze-fracture in Fig. 2d (bar = 170 nm).

variety specific differences could be detected. Results published for the same strain by various laboratories differ often more than the amino acid proportions between varieties. With the exception of ornithin (Aronson and Tillinghast, 1976) no unusual amino acids have been found. Cooksey (1971) has compiled some data of amino acid analyses. Aspartic acid and glutamic acid account for more than 20 per cent of the amino acids. This results in a rather low isoelectric point of about 4.4.

In addition to amino acids the crystals contain carbohydrates. The proportions fluctuate enormously so that a function within the crystal structure and a possible participation in the mode of action appears unlikely (Nickerson, 1980). Bateson and Stainsby (1970) found 12 per cent carbohydrate associated with crystals of the variety *thuringiensis* and Bulla *et al.* (1977) reported 5.6 per cent for the variety *kurstaki*. Variations from 1–5 per cent were determined by Nickerson (1980) examining 12 strains. It can still not yet been excluded that the carbohydrates are a contaminant incorporated together with the protein into the crystal structure.

Several authors have obtained low molecular weight compounds following solubilization. The latest report is by Fast and Martin (1980) who were able to dissociate DTT dissolved crystal protein into low molecular weight fragments which retained toxic activity. KSCN (2–4 M) was used and the peptides possessed MW below 5,000. It remains to be seen if the peptides can be characterized and if one or more can be related to the toxic activity.

2.3. ACTIVATION

The crystal and its subunits are protoxins and they do not exhibit biological activity. Under natural conditions the crystals are ingested with the food whereby the protoxin is transformed by gut juice proteases into the actual delta-endotoxin. Dissolution and activation occur rapidly and the first symptoms are manifested within a few minutes.

An exact measurement of the delta-endotoxin is difficult since no biochemical method is available. Host insects or tissue cultures developed from them are the only means for the determination of the toxic activity. Suitable insects are for example larvae of *Bombyx mori*, *Pieris brassicae* (large white butterfly), or *Trichoplusia ni*. The material to be tested is applied onto leaves, incorporated into synthetic medium or force fed. The activity is determined in terms of paralysis (*B. mori*), of feeding inhibition or of mortality. A force-feeding method with *P. brassicae* larvae permitting an exact measurement of delta-endotoxin has been described by Lüthy (1975). If the state of activation has to be checked, contact with the gut juice must be prevented, and the test solutions are best injected into the hemolymph or assayed in tissue cultures. Suitable tissue culture systems are derived from *Choristoneura fumiferana* (spruce budworm) (Fast *et al.*, 1978; Geiser, 1979) and from *T. ni* (Nishiitsutsuji-Uwo *et al.*, 1979). Figure 3 shows dose-response lines of the delta-endotoxin with *P. brassicae* and with a *C. fumiferana* tissue culture. It should be noted that the sensitivity of the test is in the range of ng per larva while for tissue cultures μg/ml of medium of delta-endotoxin are needed.

The activation process has been intensively studied in our laboratory. We were primarily interested in the activated toxic moieties which were formed by the proteolytic enzymes. The newer investigations were carried out with enzymes bound to activated Sepharose while in the earlier work the proteases were not yet immobilized.

Purified gut juice proteases (e.g. of *P. brassicae* larvae) are able to degrade intact *B. thuringiensis* crystals, a property which trypsin does not possess (Trümpi, 1976). This shows the low specificity of the insect proteases. Lecadet and Dedonder (1966) have investigated the *P. brassicae* proteases. They described two serine proteases both of which were able to cleave disulfide bonds. It is not clear how much other factors of the gut juice, such as the pH (7.5–10 depending on the insect species) contribute to the rapid solubilization. Gut juice of *P. brassicae* whose proteases have been heat inactivated can however no longer dissolve crystals.

The starting material of our investigations was as a rule NaOH dissolved crystal protein. This protoxin was prepared by incubation of crystals in 0.1 N NaOH for 30 min

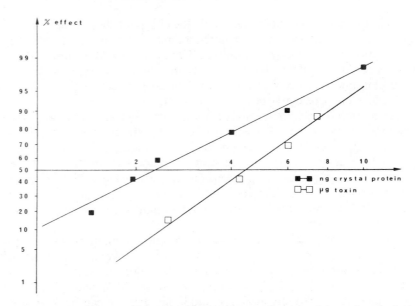

FIG. 3. Dose–response lines (probit) obtained with the crystal protein of the variety *thuringiensis*. The crystal protein was tested against larvae of *P. brassicae* (■———■) and against a cell culture of *Choristoneura fumiferana* (□———□). The per cent feeding inhibition is measured with *P. brassicae* larvae whereas the reaction of the cell culture to the *in vitro* activated toxin is evaluated according to the loss of cellular ATP. The larvae react already to a few ng of crystal protein. For the cell culture several μg/ml are needed to obtain a response.

at 37°C and subsequently dialysed against Na_2CO_3 buffer of pH 9.5. It has to be mentioned that NaOH dissolved crystal material does not yield a clearly defined fraction as in the case of DTT, but a rather wide spread band in the MW range of 320,000. This is because NaOH solubilization is accompanied by a partial denaturation of the protoxin, facilitating the further proteolysis especially by trypsin. Lukač (1980) assumed that partial denaturation of the protoxin occurs also in the gut juice environment during the natural activation process. She found that DTT dissolved protein where subunits are intact, is proteolytically degraded at a much slower pace.

   The degradation speed of crystal protein of the variety *kurstaki* is presented in Fig. 4 (Huber, 1977). It is complete within 20 sec. Crystal protein incubated with trypsin or gut juice proteases becomes toxic upon injection into the hemolymph or in tissue cultures. Proteolytic degradation with immobilized trypsin or gut juice gave a first intermediate compound of MW 80,000. Further active compounds in the range of 60,000 and 40,000 appear as the time of proteolysis proceeds. The gradual transformation to lower MW fractions is shown in Fig. 5 for crystal protein of the variety *thuringiensis* incubated for 1, 3 and 6 hr in diluted gut juice (1:500) of *P. brassicae*. The above described steps in the activation process cannot be generalized for all *B. thuringiensis* varieties. It seems that at this stage variety specific differences of the crystal protein appear. For example we never were able to isolate the fractions MW 80,000 or 60,000 from the variety *kurstaki*. All the activity was found in the region of MW 40,000 (Fig. 6).

   The role of the specificity of the proteases is difficulte to evaluate. Huber (1977) compared the degradation products obtained with gut juice of *P. brassicae* and *Spodoptera littoralis* (cotton leafworm). He was not able to detect significant differences (Fig. 7). Protoxin activated with *S. littoralis* gut juice was fully active when forcefed to *P. brassicae* larvae. *S. littoralis* is one of the lepidopterous insects which exhibits very low susceptibility against the known *B. thuringiensis* varieties. If protoxin is activated with trypsin, the active fractions have MW of 80,000 and 60,000. The obtained results indicate that the choice of the serine protease 'for the activation is not critical for formation of active fragments.

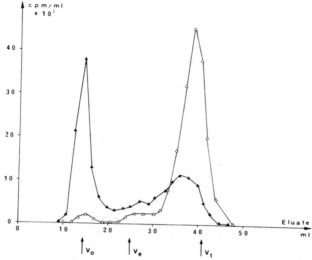

FIG. 4. Demonstration of the degradation speed of the crystal protein of the variety *kurstaki* in undiluted gut juice of *P. brassicae*. Elution profiles on Sephadex G-200 obtained after 1 sec (▲——▲) and after 20 sec (△——△) of incubation are shown. Ve = MW 80,000. Note that the activation of the *kurstaki* protein does not yield a peak at 80,000. The biological activity is found in the region of MW 40,000, corresponding to 30 ml elution volume.

The proteases generate along with the active fractions low molecular weight peptides which are without biological activity and which decrease in size with increasing incubation time (Fig. 6). Upon prolonged exposure of the toxic fractions to proteases they are slowly degraded to inactive low molecular weight compounds. It can be concluded that the stability of the activated compounds is only relative and not absolute.

A wide range of divergent results are found in the literature about the toxic moieties. Toxicity has been attributed to large molecules (MW 80,000–30,000) as well as to small polypeptides (MW down to 500). More recent investigations favor an active delta-endotoxin limited to a large molecule (Geiser, 1979; Lilley and Somerville, 1975; Somerville, 1978; Travers *et al.*, 1976). These authors have determined active compounds ranging from MW 80,000–30,000. Small peptides with biological activity were described by Fast

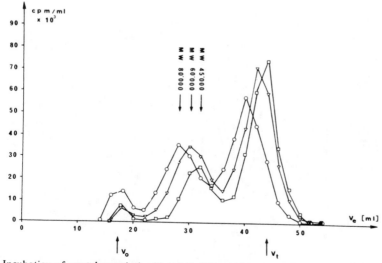

FIG. 5. Incubation of crystal protein in diluted (1:500) gut juice of *P. brassicae*. Incubation was carried out for 1 hr (O——O), 3 hr (▽——▽), and 6 hr (□——□). The toxic peak is gradually translocated from MW 80,000, to 60,000, and to 45,000. Elution profiles obtained with Sephadex G-200; crystal protein: variety *thuringiensis*.

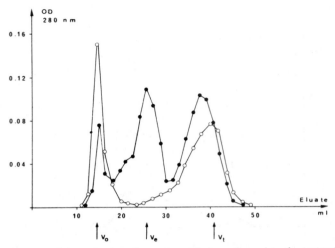

FIG. 6. Comparison of the activation of crystal protein from the variety *thuringiensis* and *kurstaki*. Incubation was carried out in diluted (1:500) gut juice of *P. brassicae*. The elution profiles on Sephadex G-200 shows a peak for the *thuringiensis* digest at MW 80,000 (●———●). Maximum toxicity for the *kurstaki* digest was determined at MW 45,000 (○———○). Ve = MW 80,000.

and Martin (1980) and by Fast and Angus (1970). If the active principle is based on a small molecule it should have been possible to purify this fraction and to analyse it.

Alkaline covalent modification of the protoxin is another possible mode of activation which has been outlined by Nickerson (1980). Dastidar and Nickerson (1978) detected the formation of lysinoalanine during NaOH solubilization of crystals. If the two amino acids are located on the same molecule a cyclic toxic moiety could be produced.

The presence of proteases associated with crystals has been reported by Bulla *et al.* (1977) and by Chestukhina *et al.* (1978, 1979). While the latter are convinced that the proteases are contaminants from the bacteria cell adhering to the crystal surface, Bulla and coworkers suggested that the proteolytic enzymes were prepacked within the crystal and that they had a specific function in the degradation and activation process. In his comprehensive review Nickerson (1980) believes that the proteolytic enzymes are actually contaminants. This would be not the only case where proteases represent an annoyance since they interfere with a protein, induce loss of activity and cause the formation of artifacts.

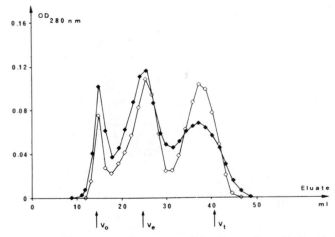

FIG. 7. Comparison of gut juice of *P. brassicae* and *Spodoptera littoralis*. Practically identical elution profiles were obtained when crystal protein of the variety *thuringiensis* was incubated in diluted (1:500) gut juice of *P. brassicae* (□———□) and *S. littoralis* (■———■). Incubation time was 4 hr. Filtration medium was Sephadex G-200. Ve = MW 80,000.

Nothing is known yet about the activation process of the *israelensis* protein. All our attempts to preserve the biological activity of DTT dissolved *israelensis* crystals were in vain. There is little doubt that the principle of activation is similar to that of the lepidopterous active crystal protein. The gut of mosquito larvae has also an alkaline environment (Stiles and Paschke, 1980).

To summarize, the crystal of *B. thuringiensis* which is a protoxin bare of activity, is solubilized by the gut juice proteases. The actual toxin is formed by further proteolytic modification of the crystal subunits. The toxic moieties have molecular weights from 80,000 to around 30,000. The size of the toxic molecule depends on the *B. thuringiensis* variety and on the exposure time to the proteolytic enzymes. The polypeptide is thus toxic over quite a wide range. Below 30,000 the activity is decreasing rapidly because the active center of the molecule is probably exposed to the attack of the proteases. The activation and the appearance of symptoms occur rapidly so that we may assume that under natural circumstances the first toxic product generated by the proteases plays the key role.

2.4. Mode of Action

The gut epithelium is the primary target tissue for the delta-endotoxin. The first symptom, a few minutes following ingestion of crystals is the blockage of further uptake of food. Other microbial toxins, for example the diphteria or the cholera toxins, possess a pronounced latent period, a so-called eclipse, between the first contact and the appearance of symptoms. In the case of the cholera toxin the eclipse lasts 10 hr (Murphy, 1976). The two toxins need this time to interfere with the metabolism of the host cell. During the latent period the action of the toxins cannot be blocked.

Most of the mode of action studies with the *B. thuringiensis* delta-endotoxin were made with larvae of *P. brassicae* and *B. mori*. Both insects are highly susceptible to the delta-endotoxin, they are easy to rear and ideal for histopathological studies because of their respectable size. The pioneering histopathological investigations were made at the Insect Pest Management Institute in Sault Ste. Marie (Canada) by Heimpel and Angus. They have summarized their findings in a review (Heimpel and Angus, 1960).

The cells of the gut epithelium which get in contact with delta-endotoxin increase in volume. Soon the epithelium is covered by bubble-like protrusions (Angus, 1970). The bubbles are formed by columnar cells whereby the foldings of the microvilli are transformed into a single large protrusion. The morphological changes at the gut epithelium occur within 10–30 min depending on the delta-endotoxin concentration. The swollen cells often burst or whole agglomerates are detached from the epithelium. Scanning electron microscopy used by Griego *et al.* (1980) gave an instructive picture about the disruption, viewed from the top part of the gut epithelium of *Manduca sexta* (Tobacco hornworm) larvae.

Electron microscopy was used to demonstrate the histopathological changes on the level of the cell organelles (Lüthy and Ebersold, 1981; Ebersold *et al.*, 1977). The most distinct sign of a delta-endotoxin poisoning is the general intracellular vacuolization. The microvilli, the endoplasmatic reticulum and the mitochondria are the organelles which undergo significant alterations. The microvilli swell and their internal structure disappears. Vacuoles appear within the membraneous network of the rough endoplasmatic reticulum. Mitochondria swell also, are distorted or changed into condensed forms (Endo and Nishiitsutsuji-Uwo, 1980). The changes in goblet cells are relatively minor. Goblet cells are the other cell type of the gut epithelium beside the columnar cells. Figure 8a shows a thin section of an untreated gut epithelium while Fig. 8b summarizes the main histopathological alterations caused by the delta-endotoxin. Vacuolization occurs also between membranes of adjacent cells but the intercellular connections such as the gap junctions remain morphologically intact. Furthermore, a considerable increase of lytic vacuoles (lysosomes, cytosomes and cytosegrosomes) is triggered by the delta-endotoxin. The state of poisoned cells resembles very much that of autolysis i.e. of cells which are normally disposed of and replaced by young ones, generated in the nidi.

The above described histopathological reaction can also be shown with tissue cultures derived from *C. fumiferana* (Fig. 9a, 9c) (Ebersold *et al.*, 1979) and from *T. ni* (Nishiitsut-suji-Uwo *et al.*, 1979). Vacuolization along the nuclear membrane and translocation of the chromatin to peripheral regions of the nucleus are two additional reactions which are not clearly seen in gut epithelial cells. Symptoms develop of course only if proteolytically activated delta-endotoxin is used.

The cell membrane of the gut epithelium is the first site with which the delta-endotoxin gets into contact. It would be one of the rare exceptions if the toxic moiety which is according to the activation studies not smaller than 30,000 daltons, would be able to pass the cell membrane. Therefore, emphasis of our own investigations was put on a toxin–membrane interaction. We were able to demonstrate with the freeze fracture technique that cell membranes were severely affected by delta-endotoxin. The regular membrane pattern (Fig. 9b) had disappeared and the proteins had formed agglomerates which led to large areas where lipids were predominant (Fig. 9d). These changes in the membrane structure were shown with tissue culture cells of *C. fumiferana*.

The next step was aimed at the investigation of the permeability properties of cell membranes under the influence of delta-endotoxin. First, ruthenium red was used, an inorganic stain (MW 852) and also a contrasting agent especially for carbohydrates. Ruthenium red does not pass normally functioning gut epithelial membranes. But after exposure to delta-endotoxin permeability was established within a few minutes. In another experiment the permeability changes were studied with lactate dehydrogenase (LDH), an intracellular enzyme (MW 140,000) which is present in an unbound state. *C. fumiferana* cells released LDH as soon as 10 min following exposure to activated delta-endotoxin. After 60 min about 80 per cent of the total LDH had leaked out of the cells. The action of the delta-endotoxin could be blocked by specific antibodies (Fig. 10). Additional evidence that the delta-endotoxin interferes with the cell membrane was presented by Fast *et al.* (1978). They coupled activated toxin to Sephadex G-25 beads and obtained the typical symptoms. The Sephadex beads had to prevent the entrance of the toxin into the fumiferana cells. The delta-endotoxin caused a rapid loss of cellular ATP. This fact was used by Geiser (1979) to establish a quantitative *in vitro* assay (Fig. 3).

Although the histopathological studies clearly demonstrate that the cell membrane is the target of the delta-endotoxin it cannot be excluded that first of all a selective per-meability change for ions or small molecules takes place. Angus (1968) found that the delta-endotoxin could be mimiced by valinomycin, a peptide antibiotic which acts as ionophore, especially for K^+. Valinomycin induced an influx of K^+ from the gut into the hemolymph of *B. mori* larvae, leading to rapid paralysis. There are however major differences between valinomycin and delta-endotoxin. While the delta-endotoxin is highly specific, valinomycin is generally membrane active. According to own unpublished data, a combination of delta-endotoxin and valinomycin had no additive effect. Geiser (1979) working with black lipid membranes was not able to attribute ionophoric properties to the delta-endotoxin. Further experiments based on the K^+-flux were made by Griego *et al.* (1979). The potassium transport through the gut epithelium was inhibited by delta-endotoxin. The tests were made with *M. sexta* larvae. Unfortunately the first measure-ment of the transepithelial membrane potential was done as late as one hour after delta-endotoxin application. Fast and Donaghue (1971) recorded an increase in the uptake of glucose by the gut epithelium already within 1 min after administration of toxin. After 10 min the transport of glucose came to a halt.

Travers *et al.* (1976) have suggested that the mitochondria represent the primary site of action. Their assay preparation were mitochondria isolated out of the midgut epithelium of *B. mori*. The delta-endotoxin uncoupled the oxidative phosphorylation. An activated toxin fraction of MW 33,000 was used. Molecules of this size are however not known to interfere directly with the oxidative phosphorylation. Classical uncoupling agents are lipophilic with an acid group bound to an aromatic ring as for example 2,4-dinitrophe-nol, carbonyl cyanide or phenylhydrazones. Another type of uncoupling compounds are the already discussed ionophores (e.g. valinomycin). A third group affecting the oxidative

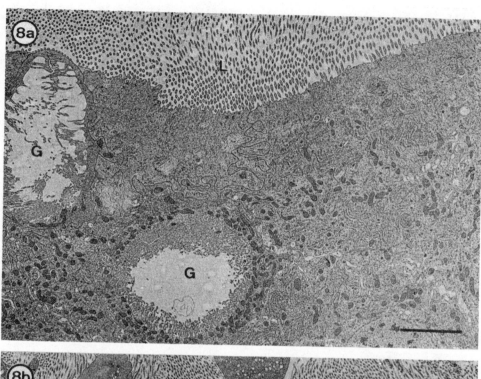

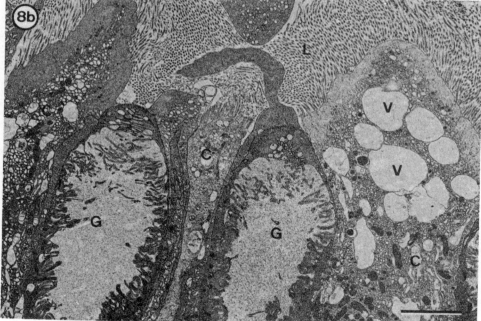

FIG. 8. Thin sections out of the gut epithelium of *P. brassicae*. Figure 8a represents an untreated control (G = goblet cell, L = gut lumen, bar = 3.9 μm. Figure 8b is part of an epithelium of a larva which had obtained a sublethal dose of crystals 20 min before fixation of the tissue. Swelling and vacuole formation (V) are at this rather low magnification the main histopathological alterations. C = columnar cell, bar = 3.9 μm.

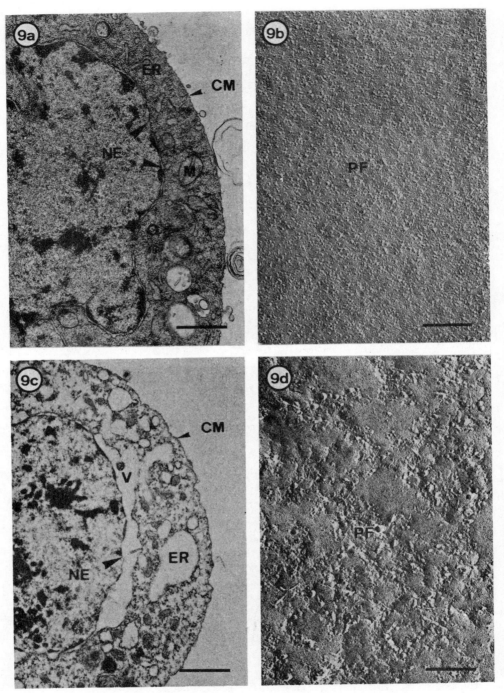

FIG. 9. The effect of the delta-endotoxin shown with tissue culture cells of *Choristoneura fumiferana*. Figure 9a represents a thin section of an untreated cell (NE = nuclear envelope, G = Golgi complex,   M = mitochondria,   ER = endoplasmatic   reticulum,   CM = cell   membrane, bar = 790 nm). In Fig. 9b a freeze-fracture of a cell membrane from a control is shown (PF = plasmatic fracture face). The proteins are regularly distributed (bar = 190 nm). The cell in Fig. 9c is derived from a toxin treated culture (15 µg/ml). General vacuolization (V) is the main feature of the action of the delta-endotoxin (bar = 1.7 µm). In Fig. 9d we find a freeze-fractured cell membrane of a toxin treated culture. The regular appearance has disappeared. The proteins have formed agglomerates. There is no clear-cut fracture plain (bar = 190 nm).

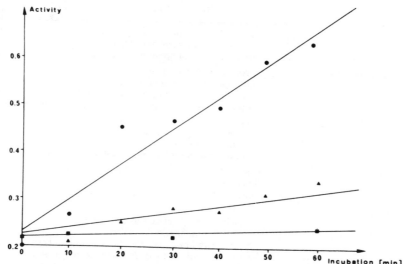

Fig. 10. Gradual loss of lactate dehydrogenase (LDH) of delta-endotoxin treated cells of *C. fumiferana*. LDH can be measured after 10 min in the supernatant. After 60 min the cells have lost about 80 per cent of their LDH. The action of the delta-endotoxin can be blocked by specific antibodies. Extracellular LDH activity of a delta-endotoxin treated culture (●——●), delta-endotoxin + specific antiserum (▲——▲), control (■——■).

phosphorylation are inhibitors of ATP formation such as oligomycin. Ebersold (unpublished) failed to reproduce the results of Travers *et al.* (1976). It has to be mentioned that rat liver mitochondria were used, and this might be the reason why an uncoupling reaction was not observed. An indirect effect on the respiration cannot be excluded since breakdown of the permeability control of the gut epithelium leads to an influx of potassium which may then interfere with the respiration.

We have already seen that the activity of the delta-endotoxin is not limited to the gut epithelium. Activated toxin reacts upon injection into the hemocoel and also with some insect tissue cultures. It is surprising that only few reports about assays with mammalian cell systems have been published. Geiser (1979) showed that chicken fibroblasts did not respond to the presence of delta-endotoxin. Growth and appearance of the cultures remained unaltered. Activity of delta-endotoxin against tumor cells was found by Prasad and Shetna (1974) and by Seki *et al.* (1978). Prasad and Shetna were able to block growth of Yoshida ascites sarcoma cells in mice after injection of delta-endotoxin. Exposure of short time *in vitro* cultures of such tumor cells to the toxin resulted in a general breakdown of the metabolism (Prasad and Shetna, 1976). Since low and high molecular weight compounds leaked out into the medium it was suggested that the delta-endotoxin affected primarily the cell membrane. The results of Seki *et al.* (1978) who were also able to demonstrate activity against mouse sarcoma 180 ascites cells were questioned by Nishiitsutsuji-Uwo *et al.* (1980). The latter found that four types of mammalian cultures including mouse sarcoma 180 ascites cells remained indifferent to delta-endotoxin while an equal number of insect cell cultures showed a reaction. It was concluded that the *in vitro* activity of the delta-endotoxin was limited to some types of insect cells.

The above publications must have prompted similar studies in numerous laboratories because compounds with antitumor activity are highly interesting. But so far there is little evidence for the confirmation of antitumor activity and we have to wait for more informations before any conclusions can be drawn. In this context the publication of negative results would be of great value.

Little is known about the mode of action of the delta-endotoxin of the variety *israelensis*. De Barjac (1978) examined sections of mosquito larvae which had been exposed to the toxin. She was able to confirm that the same histopathological alterations occurred in the gut epithelium.

TABLE 5. *The Properties of the Delta-endotoxin of* B. thuringiensis

1. Biosynthesis	—coupled to the sporulation process —involvement of a stable mRNA —no definite proof about plasmid control
2. Composition of crystal	—protein or glycoprotein —no unusual amino acids detected —subunits (MW 320,000) linked by disulfides —subunit consists of 2 polypeptides (except variety *israelensis*)
3. Activation	—crystal and subunits are protoxins —activation by gut juice proteases of certain insects —products of proteolysis MW 80,000–30,000 —no low MW peptides defined yet as carrier of activity
4. Mode of action	—rapid damage to gut epithelia of target insects —membrane toxin or —uncoupler of oxidative phosphorylation
5. Multifactoral specificity	—variety of toxin —intestine of some insects as site of activation —probably specific membrane receptors necessary —other invertebrate tissues and cell culture only susceptible if *in vitro* activated toxin is used. No definite proof about activity against vertebrate cells

The histopathological part of the mode of action studies can be regarded as concluded. Future research has to emphasize the molecular mode of action. Present knowledge suggests an assignment to the membrane active cytolytic toxins. Since molecular mode of action studies are still missing, it is difficult to judge in which category of the membrane active bacterial metabolites our delta-endotoxin fits. The membrane active bacterial toxins have been reviewed by Freer and Arbuthnott (1976). The high specificity presumes a specific interaction with a cell membrane component, for example with a sterol. On the other hand the rapid action and histopathology resemble very much that of the delta-toxin of *Staphyloccocus aureus* which attacks however a wide range of cell membranes. The *S. aureus* delta-toxin has a detergent like effect with the exception that the pores in the membranes increase step by step while Triton X-100 treated cells are immediately permeable for high molecular weight compounds (Thelestam and Möllby, 1975). Also, we cannot rule out that the delta-endotoxin of *B. thuringiensis* is an enzyme. Metabolites of *S. aureus* (beta-toxin) or *Clostridium perfringens* (alpha-toxin) are membrane active enzymes that degrade the phospholipids.

There is no histopathological evidence that the delta-endotoxin dissolves target membranes. The membrane components seem to be rearranged either permanently or transiently. The histopathological effects caused by the breakdown of the permeability control depend on the environment of the cells. Gut juice is extreme whereas other tissues have a surrounding (pH, osmolarity, enzymes) which diverge much less from the intracellular conditions. There, morphological alterations like swelling and vacuolization are probably less pronounced. The complex but fascinating properties of the delta-endotoxin of *B. thuringiensis* are outlined in a condensed form in Table 5.

3. THE BETA-EXOTOXIN OF *BACILLUS THURINGIENSIS*

3.1. GENERAL CHARACTERIZATION

Some years following the discovery by Angus (1954) that the crystals were responsible for the insecticidal activity against lepidopterous larvae, it was noticed that a second biologically active metabolite had to be present in some varieties of *B. thuringiensis*. McConnell and Richards (1959) gave a first general characterization of this substance which was later called beta-exotoxin. It appeared in the supernatants during vegetative growth and it showed high stability withstanding even autoclaving. Additional basic information was then published by Burgerjon and de Barjac (1960), Briggs (1960) and

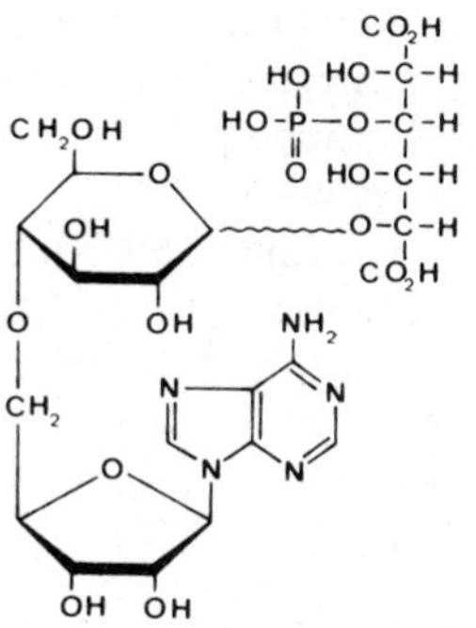

FIG. 11. Structure of the beta-exotoxin of *Bacillus thuringiensis*.

Krieg and Herfs (1963). The host spectrum was not limited to lepidopterous larvae but included *Diptera, Coleptera, Hymenoptera* and other orders. This heat stable compound was found in the supernatants of the varieties *thuringiensis, sotto, kenyae, aizawai, morrisoni, tolworthi, galleriae* and *darmstadtiensis*.

3.2. CHEMISTRY

Purification and analysis of the beta-exotoxin proved to be quite easy compared with the delta-endotoxin. The first steps in the purification were achieved by de Barjac and Dedonder (1965) and by Benz (1966) using adsorption and precipitation techniques. Exotoxin preparations of increasing purity facilitated the study of the chemical structure. Farkaš *et al.* (1969) presented the final chemical structure of the beta-exotoxin. Substantial contributions to the chemistry were also made by de Barjac and Dedonder (1968), Bond *et al.* (1969) and Kim and Huang (1970). The beta-exotoxin is a nucleotide composed of adenin, ribose, glucose and phosphorylated allomucic acid. The structure which is shown in Fig. 11 has been confirmed by chemical synthesis (Prystaš *et al.*, 1976).

3.3. MODE OF ACTION

The wide spectrum of activity indicated interference of the beta-exotoxin with a key function of the cellular metabolism. Šebesta and Horská (1968) showed that the beta-exotoxin inhibited RNA synthesis by blocking the polymerization which is catalized by the DNA-dependent RNA polymerase. It is assumed that the exotoxin enters into direct competition with ATP (Šebesta and Sternbach, 1970). The effects of the beta-exotoxin can be demonstrated also *in vitro* with RNA polymerases from bacteria, invertebrates and vertebrates. Šebesta *et al.* (1969) found that only *de novo* RNA synthesis was blocked and that protein and DNA formation proceeded normally and were only inhibited at extremely high exotoxin concentrations. On the other hand Kim *et al.* (1972) working with cabbage loopers (*Trichoplusia ni*) observed in addition inhibition of DNA and protein synthesis. For more details on the molecular mode of action the reader is referred to a review by Vaňková (1978).

Diptera such as mosquitoes and flies are the most susceptible insects and suitable for bioassays. Death occurs not only during the larval stages but primarily during the transition from one instar to the other, from the larval to the pupal and from the pupal to the adult stage. While the bioassay with Diptera is based on the addition of a certain amount of exotoxin to the corresponding medium, more quantitative results are obtained by injecting lepidopterous larvae such as *Galleria mellonella* (greater wax moth) or *Mamestra brassicae* (cabbage moth). The sensitivity of the larvae is about 250 times higher by intralymphal injection compared to application per os. Intralymphally applied exotoxin gives a LD_{50} of 0.5 µg/g for *G. mellonella*.

Some controversy exists concerning the activity of the beta-exotoxin against mammals, a point which is of course closely connected with safety aspects. Studying the effect of exotoxin injected peritoneally and subcutaneously into mice, de Barjac and Riou (1969) obtained a LD_{50} of about 15 μg/g, results which are also in agreement with Šebesta et al. (1969). On the other hand Krieg and Lysenko (1979) did not observe pathological signs following intraperitoneal injection of concentrated and autoclaved supernatant into mice. Although the amount of beta-exotoxin injected is difficult to estimate. In this case the concentrations must have been high enough to give a representative result. The fate of the beta-exotoxin was investigated by Šebesta and Horská (1973) with a ^{32}P-labeled preparation injected into mice. 20 per cent of the exotoxin was excreted in an unchanged form within half an hour. In the selected organs the exotoxin was present in measurable amounts only for the first five minutes. The ^{32}P appeared soon in other compounds which indicated rapid enzymatic degradation.

There exists general agreement that even high doses of exotoxin applied per os are not toxic for mammals (de Barjac and Riou, 1969; Krieg and Lysenko, 1979). This can be explained by the rapid dephosphorylation which takes place in the intestine by alkaline phosphatases. The activity is lost as soon as the phosphate group is cleaved off.

3.4. THE USE OF BETA-EXOTOXIN AS AN INSECTICIDE

The early B. thuringiensis preparations which were based on the variety thuringiensis contained the beta-exotoxin in quantities which were high enough to kill insects and to increase the potency of the products. Benz (1975) measured a pronounced synergism between the delta- and beta-exotoxin in assays with Zeiraphera diniana (larch bud moth). When it became known that beta-exotoxin interfered with an omnipresent enzyme it was banned from B. thuringiensis preparations in the US and in Western Europe. Eastern European countries continued to use it in some of their products, apparently without undesirable side effects. Even pure exotoxin preparations were applied for the control of Diptera at rates between 50 and 150 g/acre. Some caution is however justified, especially since Meretoja et al. (1977) and Linnainmaa et al. (1977) found some cytogenetic effects caused by the beta-exotoxin, such as an increase in the incidence of chromosomal aberrations in human blood cultures. In a third paper (Kahkonen et al., 1979), the same group of authors considered the risk of cytogenetic damage to humans as negligible if the exotoxin is used in amounts necessary for pest control. It is our personal opinion that the beta-exotoxin will disappear as an insecticide, since the delta-endotoxin of the variety israelensis offers an effective and highly selective alternative for the control of Culicidae and Simulidae.

3.5. MICROBIOLOGY

The biosynthetic pathways of the beta-exotoxin have not been thoroughly investigated since commercial interest in this compound does not exist any longer. It is known that the beta-exotoxin producers are not auxotroph for purine bases which is usually typical for sporeformers which accumulate extracellularly purine bases, nucleosides and nucleotides. Accumulation does not result from RNA degradation but the purine moiety is synthesized de novo. Addition of purine derivates inhibits partially the production of beta-exotoxin. Furthermore there is evidence that the beta-exotoxin is resistant to nucleases, and it may even act as an inhibitor of such enzymes. The only rudimentary knowledge of the exotoxin metabolism is presented in more detail by Bond et al. (1971).

The yield of beta-exotoxin depends on the strain and on the culture medium. Vaňková (1978) showed yields ranging between 100 and 150 mg/l. Fermentation studies for optimum beta-exotoxin yields were carried out by Holmberg et al. (1980). Commercial production can be achieved with cheap complex media without major technological problems.

The degradability of beta-exotoxin has not yet been investigated. But we can assume that the activity disappears readily in the environment since dephosphorylation is all what is needed. Another interesting point is the development of resistance against hosts.

Structure and mode of action let expect a rather fast development of resistant populations.

4. THE ALPHA-EXOTOXIN

A third toxic metabolite but without any practical importance was first reported by Heimpel (1955) and later (1967) designated by the same author as alpha-exotoxin. It is produced by strains of *B. thuringiensis* and *Bacillus cereus* only under certain culture conditions, for example if meat extract is present in the medium (Krieg and Lysenko, 1979). Its activity spectrum is not well defined. While various insect species are susceptible upon peroral application others react only after injection into the hemocoel. High doses of alpha-exotoxin injected by the intraperitoneal or intravenous route can kill mice. It is without effect if applied to mammals per os.

Krieg (1971) and Krieg and Lysenko (1979) characterized the alpha-exotoxin as heat labile protein. It is inactivated at a temperature of 56°C. It is readily degraded by trypsin. The molecular weight can be estimated at 50,000 from a Sephadex G-75 elution-activity diagram. Krieg (1971) was able to exclude identity with one of the known extracellular enzymes of *B. thuringiensis* and *B. cereus*.

The alpha-exotoxin does not interfere with safety aspects since it cannot be traced in commercial preparations. The media which are used do not induce alpha-exotoxin production. Furthermore this metabolite is very unstable and disappears during sporulation.

5. EXOENZYMES

Cells of *B. thuringiensis* and *B. cereus* which gain access to the hemolymph of an insect proliferate apparently without interference by the host. This is a general phenomenon, not limited to certain insect species and not in correlation to the host range of the above described toxins. Other microorganisms, for example *B. subtilis* are readily controlled and eliminated by host defence mechanisms.

Exoenzymes such as phospholipase C, chitinases, proteases and hemolysin are known to be produced by *B. thuringiensis* and *B. cereus* and they must contribute to the pathogenicity as soon as the organisms have penetrated the natural barriers of the insect body. Phospholipase C is probably the most potent enzyme being able to destroy membranes. Lysenko (1974) has shown the toxicity of phospholipase C and of proteases for *Galleria mellonella* upon injection into the hemocoel. Many parts of the insect body contain chitin and it has been suggested that chitinases enhance the activity of *B. thuringiensis* (Smirnoff, 1974). In fact it has been demonstrated that chitinases destroy the peritrophic membrane and this might facilitate the contact of the delta-endotoxin with the gut epithelium. It has to be added that chitinase production of *B. thuringiensis* is very low. In order to work with chitinases they have to be isolated from another source. Since *B. thuringiensis* spores are as a rule not able to germinate in the intestine of a healthy insect exoenzymes play no role during the first stages of pathogenesis or in the absence of delta-endotoxin. Proliferation of vegetative cells in the gut epithelium may start following interruption of the transport mechanisms through the epithelium and uncontrolled exchange of body fluid and gut juice. In this case the lytic exoenzymes support the penetration of the bacteria into the hemocoel and the lethal septicemia.

It is a question of definition which enzymes are called toxins. As a typical example we can mention the phosphodiesterase present in snake venom. From the practical aspect the *B. thuringiensis* exoenzymes play only a minor and secondary role since they are not present in a preformed state in the preparations. They only appear with the development and proliferation of vegetative cells.

Acknowledgements—The authors thank Françoise Jaquet, J. L. Cordier, H. M. Fischer and H. E. Huber for their excellent collaboration. The *Bacillus thuringiensis* project is supported by the Swiss National Science Foundation, project Nr. 3.357–0.78.

REFERENCES

Ang, B. J. and Nickerson, K. W. (1978) Purification of the protein crystal from *Bacillus thuringiensis* by zonal gradient centrifugation. *Env. Microbiol.* **36**: 625–626.

Angus, T. A. (1954) A bacterial toxin paralyzing silkworm larvae. *Nature* **173**: 545.

Angus, T. A. (1968) Similarity of effect of valinomycin and *Bacillus thuringiensis* parasporal protein in larvae of *Bombyx mori*. *J. Invertebr. Pathol.* **11**: 145–146.

Angus, T. A. (1970) Implications of some recent studies of *Bacillus thuringiensis*—a personal purview. *Proc. IV Int. Coll. Insect Pathol., College Park, Maryland, USA.* p. 183–189.

Aronson, J. N. and Tillinghast, J. (1976) A chemical study of the parasporal crystal of *Bacillus thuringiensis*. In: *Spore Research* p. 351–357, Barker, A. N., Wolf, J., Ellar, D. J., Dring, G. J. and Gould, G. W. (Eds). Academic Press, London.

de Barjac, H. (1978) Etude cytologique de l'action de *Bacillus thuringiensis* var. *israelensis* sur larves de Moustiques. *C.R. Acad. Sc. Paris* **286**: 1629–1632, série D.

de Barjac, H. and Bonnefoi, A. (1962) Essai de classification biochimique et sérologique de 24 souches de Bacillus du type *B. thuringiensis*. *Entomophaga* **7**: 5–31.

de Barjac, H. and Bonnefoi, A. (1973) Mise au point sur la classification des *Bacillus thuringiensis*. *Entomophaga* **18**: 5–17.

de Barjac, H. and Dedonder, R. (1965) Isolement d'un nucléotide identifiable à la 'toxine thermostable' de *Bacillus thuringiensis* var. Berliner. *C.R. Acad. Sc. Paris* **260**: 7050, série D.

de Barjac, H. and Dedonder, R. (1968) Purification de la toxine thermostable de *Bacillus thuringiensis* et analyses complémentaires. *Bull. Soc. Chim. Biol.* **50**: 941–944.

de Barjac, H. and Riou, J. Y. (1969) Action de la toxine thermostable de *Bacillus thuringiensis* var. *thuringiensis* administrée à des souris. *Revue Path. Comp. Méd. Exp.* **6**: 367–374.

Bassi, A. (1835) Del mal del segno, calcinaccio o moscardino, malattia che affligge i bachi da seta e sul modo di liberarne le bigattaje anche le più infestate. Parte prima, teoria. *Orcesi Lodi*, 77 pp.

Bateson, J. B. and Stainsby, G. (1970) Analysis of the active principle in the biological insecticide *Bacillus thuringiensis* Berliner. *J. Fd. Technol.* **5**: 403–415.

Bechtel, D. B. and Bulla, L. A. (1976) Electron microscope study of sporulation and parasporal crystal formation in *Bacillus thuringiensis*. *J. Bacteriol.* **127**: 1472–1481.

Benz, G. (1966) On the chemical nature of the heat-stable exotoxin of *Bacillus thuringiensis*. *Experientia* **22**: 81–82.

Benz, G. (1975) Action of *Bacillus thuringiensis* preparation against larch bud moth, *Zeiraphera diniana* (Gn.), enhanced by beta-exotoxin and DDT. *Experientia* **31**: 1288–1290.

Berliner, E. (1915) Ueber die Schlaffsucht der Mehlmottenraupe (*Ephestia kühniella*, Zell.) und ihren Erreger *Bacillus thuringiensis*. *Z. Angew. Entomol.* **2**: 29–56.

Bond, R. P. M., Boyce, C. B. C. and French, S. J. (1969) A purification and some properties of an insecticidal exotoxin from *Bacillus thuringiensis* Berliner. *Biochem. J.* **114**: 477–488.

Bond, R. P. M., Boyce, C. B. C., Rogoff, M. H. and Shieh, T. R. (1971) The thermostable exotoxin of *Bacillus thuringiensis*. In: *Microbial Control of Insects and Mites* p. 275–303, Burges, H. D. and Hussey, N. W. (Eds). Academic Press, London.

Briggs, J. D. (1960) Reduction of adult house-fly emergence by the effect of Bacillus spp. on the development of immature forms. *J. Insect Pathol.* **2**: 418–432.

Bulla, L. A., Kramer, K. J. and Davidson, L. I. (1977) Characterization of the entomocidal parasporal crystal of *Bacillus thuringiensis*. *J. Bacteriol.* **130**: 375–383.

Burges, H. D. (1981) *Microbial Control of Pest and Plant Diseases 1970–1980*. Academic Press, London.

Burgerjon, A. and de Barjac, H. (1960) Nouvelle données sur le rôle de la toxine thermostable produite par *Bacillus thuringiensis* Berliner. *C.R. Acad. Sc. Paris* **251**: 911, série D.

Chestukhina, G. G., Kostina, L. I., Zalunin, I. A., Kotova, T. S., Katrukha, S. P., Kutnetsov, Y. S. and Stepanov, V. M. (1978) Proteinase bound to crystals of *Bacillus thuringiensis*. *Biokhimiya*, **43**: 857–864.

Chestukhina, G. G., Kotova, T. S., Zalunin, I. A. and Stepanov, V. M. (1979) Proteinases during growth and spore formation of *Bacillus thuringiensis*. *Biokhimiya* **44**: 796–802.

Cooksey, K. E. (1971) The protein crystal toxin of *Bacillus thuringiensis*: Biochemistry and mode of action. In: Microbial Control of Insects and Mites p. 247–274, Burges, H. D. and Hussey, N. W. (Eds). Academic Press, London.

Cheshire, F. R. and Cheyne, W. W. (1885) The pathogenic history and the history under cultivation of a new bacillus (*B. alvei*), the cause of a disease of the hive bee hitherto known as foul brood. *J. Roy. Microscop. Soc.*, Ser. 2, pt II, **5**: 581–601.

Dastidar, P. G. and Nickerson, K. W. (1978) Lysinoalanine in alkali-solubilized protein crystal toxin from *Bacillus thuringiensis*. *FEMS Microbiol. Letters* **4**: 331–333.

Davidson, E. W. (1981) Pathogenesis of Invertebrate Microbial Diseases. Allanheld Osmun, New York.

Davidson, E. W., Singer, S. and Briggs, J. D. (1975) Pathogenesis of *Bacillus sphaericus* strain SSII-1 infection in *Culex pipiens quinquefasciatus* (= *C. pipiens fatigans*) larvae. *J. Invertebr. Pathol.* **25**: 179–184.

Debabov, V. G., Azizbekyan, R. R., Khlebalina, O. I., D'yachenko, V. V., Galushka, F. P. and Belykh, R. A. (1977) Isolation and preliminary characterization of extrachromosomal elements of *Bacillus thuringiensis* DNA. *Genetika* **13**: 496–501.

Delafield, F. P., Somerville, H. J. and Rittenberg, S. C. (1968) Immunological homology between crystal and spore protein of *Bacillus thuringiensis*. *J. Bacteriol.* **96**: 713–720.

De Lucca II, A. J., Simonson, J. and Larson, A. (1979) Two new serovars of *Bacillus thuringiensis*: Serovars *dakota* and *indiana* (Serovars 15 and 16). *J. Invertebr. Pathol.* **34**: 323–324.

Dutky, S. R. (1940) Two new spore-forming bacteria causing milky disease of Japanese beetle larvae. *J. Agr. Res.* **61**: 57–68.

EBERSOLD, H. R., LÜTHY, P. and MÜLLER, M. (1977) Changes in the fine structure of the gut epithelium of *Pieris brassicae* induced by the delta-endotoxin of *Bacillus thuringiensis*. *Bull. Soc. Ent. Suisse* **50**: 269–276.

EBERSOLD, H. R., LÜTHY, P. and HUBER, H. E. (1979) Membrane damaging effect of the delta-endotoxin of *Bacillus thuringiensis*. *Experientia* **36**: 495.

ENDO, Y. and NISHIITSUTSUJI-UWO, J. (1980) Mode of action of *Bacillus thuringiensis* delta-endotoxin: Histopathological changes in the silkworm midgut. *J. Invertebr. Pathol.* **36**: 90–103.

FARKAŠ, J., SEBESTA, K., HORSKÁ, K., SAMEK, Z., DOLEJŠ, L. and SORM, F. (1969) The structure of exotoxin of *Bacillus thuringiensis* var. *gelechiae*. *Coll. Czech. Chem. Commun.* **34**: 1118–1119.

FAST, P. G., MURPHY, D. W. and SOHI, S. S. (1978) *Bacillus thuringiensis* delta-endotoxin: Evidence that toxin acts at the surface of susceptible cells. *Experientia* **34**: 762–763.

FAST, P. G. and ANGUS, T. A. (1970) The delta-endotoxin of *Bacillus thuringiensis* var. *sotto*: A toxic low molecular weight fragment. *J. Invertebr. Pathol.* **16**: 465.

FAST, P. G. and DONAGHUE, I. P. (1971) The delta-endotoxin of *Bacillus thuringiensis*. II. On the mode of action. *J. Invertebr. Pathol.* **18**: 135–138.

FAST, P. G. and MARTIN, W. G. (1980) *Bacillus thuringiensis* parasporal crystal toxin: Dissociation into toxic low molecular weight peptides. *Biochem. Biophys. Res. Comm.* **95**: 1314–1320.

FRANZ, J. M. and KRIEG, A. (1980) Mikrobiologische Schädlingsbekämpfung in China. Ein Reisebericht. *Forum microbiol.* **3**: 173–176.

FREER, J. H. and ARBUTHNOTT, J. P. (1976) Biochemical and Morphologic Alterations of Membranes by Bacterial Toxins. In: *Mechanisms in Bacterial Toxinology* p. 170–193, BERNHEIMER, A. W. (Ed). John Wiley, New York.

GEISER, P. (1979) Versuche *in vitro* zum Nachweis einer Wirkung des delta-Endotoxins von *Bacillus thuringiensis*. Diss. ETH Zürich, Switzerland, Nr. 6411.

GLATRON, M. F. and RAPOPORT, G. (1972) Biosynthesis of the parasporal inclusion of *Bacillus thuringiensis*: half-life of its corresponding messenger RNA. *Biochimie* **54**: 1291–1301.

GLATRON, M. F., LECADET, M. M. and DEDONDER, R. (1972) Structure of the parasporal inclusion of *Bacillus thuringiensis* Berliner; Characterization of a repetitive subunit. *Eur. J. Biochem.* **30**: 330–338.

GOLDBERG, I., SNEH, B., BATTAT, E. and KLEIN, D. (1980) Optimization of a medium for a high yield production of spore-crystal preparation of *Bacillus thuringiensis* effective against the Egyptian cotton leaf worm *Spodoptera littoralis* Boisd. *Biotechnol. Letters* **2**: 419–426.

GOLDBERG, L. J. and MARGALIT, J. (1977) Bacterial spore demonstrating rapid larvicidal activity against *Anopheles sergenti*, *Uranotaenia unguiculata*, *Culex univittatus*, *Aedes aegypti* and *Culex pipiens*. *Mosquito News* **37**: 355–358.

GRIEGO, V. M., MOFFETT, D. and SPENCE, K. D. (1979) Inhibition of active K^+ transport in the tobacco hornworm (*Manduca sexta*) midgut after ingestion of *Bacillus thuringiensis* endotoxin. *J. Insect Physiol.* **25**: 283–288.

GRIEGO, V. M., FANCHER, L. J. and SPENCE, K. D. (1980) Scanning electron microscopy of the disruption of tobacco hornworm, *Manduca sexta*, midgut by *Bacillus thuringiensis* endotoxin. *J. Invertebr. Pathol.* **35**: 186–189.

HEIMPEL, A. M. (1955) Investigations of the mode of action of strains of *Bacillus cereus* Fr. and Fr. pathogenic for the larch sawfly, *Pristiphora erichsonii*. *Can. J. Zool.* **33**: 311–326.

HEIMPEL, A. M. (1967) A critical review of *Bacillus thuringiensis* var. *thuringiensis* Berliner and other crystalliferous bacteria. *Ann. Rev. Entomol.* **12**: 287–322.

HEIMPEL, A. M. and ANGUS, T. A. (1960) Bacterial insecticides. *Bacteriol. Rev.* **24**: 266–288.

HOLMBERG, A., SIEVÄNEN, R. and CARLBERG, G. (1980) Fermentation of *Bacillus thuringiensis* for exotoxin production: Process analysis study. *Biotechnol. Bioeng.* **22**: 1707–1724.

HOLMES, K. C. and MONRO, R. E. (1965) Studies on the structure of parasporal inclusions from *Bacillus thuringiensis*. *J. Mol. Biol.* **14**: 572–581.

HUBER, H. E. (1977) Zur Spezifität des delta-Endotoxins von *Bacillus thuringiensis*. Diploma thesis, Faculty Nat. Sci., ETH Zürich, Switzerland.

HUBER, H. E. and LÜTHY, P. (1981) *Bacillus thuringiensis* delta-endotoxin: Composition and activation. In: *Pathogenesis of Invertebrate Microbial Diseases*, DAVIDSON, E. W. (Ed). Allenheld Osmun, New York. In press.

HUBER, H. E., LÜTHY, P., EBERSOLD, H. R. and CORDIER, J. L. (1981) The subunits of the parasporal crystal of *Bacillus thuringiensis*: Size, linkage and toxicity. *Arch. Microbiol.* **129**: 14–18.

ISHIWATA, S. (1902) Koyoto Sanyo Koshujo Sanji Hokoku **2**: 346–347.

KAHKONEN, M., GRIPPENBERG, U., CARLBERG, G., MERETOJA, T. and SORSA, M. (1979) Mutagenicity of *Bacillus thuringiensis* exotoxin: 3. Sister chromatid exchange in rats *in vivo*. *Hereditas* **91**: 1–4.

KIM, Y. T. and HUANG, H. T. (1970) The beta-exotoxin of *Bacillus thuringiensis*. I. Isolation and characterization. *J. Invertebr. Pathol.* **15**: 100–108.

KIM, Y. T., GREGORY, B. G. and IGNOFFO, C. M. (1972) The beta-exotoxins of *Bacillus thuringiensis*. III. Effects on *in vivo* synthesis of macromolecules in an insect system. *J. Invertebr. Pathol.* **20**: 46–50.

KLIER, A. F., LECADET, M. M. and DEDONDER, R. (1973) Sequential modification of DNA-dependent RNA-polymerase during sporogenesis in *Bacillus thuringiensis*. *Eur. J. Biochem.* **36**: 317–327.

KLIER, A. F., LECADET, M. M. and RAPOPORT, G. (1978) Transcription *in vitro* of sporulation specific mRNA's by RNA-polymerase from *Bacillus thuringiensis*. In: *Spores VII* p. 205–212, CHAMBLISS, G. and VARY, J. C. (Eds). American Society for Microbiology.

KRIEG, A. (1971) Concerning alpha-exotoxin produced by vegetative cells of *Bacillus thuringiensis* and *Bacillus cereus*. *J. Invertebr. Pathol.* **17**: 134–135.

KRIEG, A. and HERFS, W. (1963) Empfindlichkeit verschiedener Insektenarten gegenüber dem "Exotoxin" von *Bacillus thuringiensis* Berliner. *Z. Pfl. Krankh. Pflschutz.* **70**: 11–21.

KRIEG, A. and LYSENKO, O. (1979) Toxine und Enzyme bei einigen *Bacillus*-Arten unter besonderer Berücksichtigung der *B. cereus-thuringiensis* Gruppe. *Zbl. Bakt. II. Abt.* **134**: 70–88.

KRYWIENCZYK, J. (1977) Antigenic composition of delta-endotoxin as an aid in identification of *Bacillus thuringiensis* varieties. *Technical Report, Canadian Forestry Service IP-X-12.*

KRYWIENCZYK, J. and FAST, P. G. (1980) Serological relationship of the crystals of *Bacillus thuringiensis* var. *israelensis. J. Invertebr. Pathol.* **36**: 139–140.

KURSTAK, E. (1981) *Microbial Pesticides.* Marcel Dekker, Inc., New York.

LECADET, M. M. and DEDONDER, R. (1966) Les protéases de *Pieris brassicae.* II. Spécificité. *Bull. Soc. Chim. Biol.* **48**: 661–691.

LILLEY, M. and SOMERVILLE, H. J. (1975) The action of proteolytic enzymes on the crystalline insect toxin of *Bacillus thuringiensis. Proc. Soc. Gen. Microbiol.* **3**: 62.

LINNAINMAA, K., SORSA, M., CARLBERG, G., GRIPPENBERG, U. and MERETOJA, T. (1977) Mutagenicity of *Bacillus thuringiensis* exotoxin: II. Submammalian tests. *Hereditas* **85**: 113–122.

LUKAČ, M. (1980) Ueber das delta-Endotoxin von *Bacillus thuringiensis*: Vom Protoxin zur toxischen Einheit und die Herstellung monoklonaler Antikörper. Diploma thesis, Faculty Nat. Sci., ETH Zürich, Switzerland.

LÜTHY, P. (1975) Zur bakteriologischen Schädlingsbekämpfung: Die entomopathogenen Bacillus-Arten, *Bacillus thuringiensis* und *Bacillus popilliae. Vjschr. naturf. Ges. Zürich* **120**: 81–163.

LÜTHY, P. and EBERSOLD, H. R. (1981) *Bacillus thuringiensis* delta-endotoxin: Histopathology and molecular mode of action. In: *Pathogenesis of Invertebrate Microbial Diseases*, DAVIDSON, E. W. (Ed). Allenheld Osmun, New York.

LÜTHY, P., CORDIER, J. L. and FISCHER, H. M. (1981) *Bacillus thuringiensis* as bacterial insecticide: Basic considerations and application. In: *Microbial Pesticides*, KURSTAK, E. (Ed). Marcel Dekker, Inc. New York.

LYSENKO, O. (1974) Bacterial exoenzymes toxic for insects; proteinase and lecithinase. *J. Hyg. Epidemiol. Immunol.* **18**: 347–352.

McCONNELL, E. and RICHARDS, A. G. (1959) The production by *Bacillus thuringiensis* Berliner of a heat-stable substance toxic for insects. *Canad. J. Microbiol.* **6**: 161–168.

MERETOJA, T., CARLBERG, G., GRIPENBERG, U., LINNAINMAA, K. and SORSA, M. (1977) Mutagenicity of *Bacillus thuringiensis* exotoxin: I. Mammalian tests. *Hereditas* **85**: 105–112.

MITEVA, V. J. (1978) Isolation of plasmid DNA from various strains of *Bacillus thuringiensis* and *Bacillus cereus. Dokl. Bulg. Acad. Nauk* **31**: 913–916.

MONRO, R. E. (1961a) Protein turnover and the formation of protein inclusion during sporulation of *Bacillus thuringiensis. Biochem. J.* **81**: 225–232.

MONRO, R. E. (1961b) Serological studies on the formation of protein parasporal inclusions of *Bacillus thuringiensis. J. Biophys. Biochem. Cytol.* **11**: 321–331.

MURPHY, J. R. (1976) Structure activity relationship of diphteria toxin. In: *Mechanisms in Bacterial Toxinology* p. 31–51, BERNHEIMER, A. W. (Ed). J. Wiley, New York.

MYERS, P. S. and YOUSTEN, A. A. (1980) Localization of a mosquito-larval toxin of *Bacillus sphaericus* 1593. *Appl. Environ. Microbiol.* **39**: 1205–1211.

NAGAMATSU, Y. R., TSUTSUI, R., ICHIMARU, T., NAGAMATSU, T., KOGA, M. and HAYASHI, K. (1978) Subunit structure and toxic component of delta-endotoxin from *Bacillus thuringiensis. J. Invertebr. Pathol.* **32**: 103–109.

NICKERSON, K. W. (1980) Structure and function of the *Bacillus thuringiensis* protein crystal. *Biotechnol. Bioeng.* **22**: 1305–1333.

NISHIITSUTSUJI-UWO, J, ENDO, Y. and HIMENO, M. (1979) Mode of action of *Bacillus thuringiensis* delta-endotoxin: Effect on TN-368 cells. *J. Invertebr. Pathol.* **34**: 267–275.

NISHIITSUTSUJI-UWO, J., ENDO, Y. and HIMENO, M. (1980) Effects of *Bacillus thuringiensis* delta-endotoxin on insect and mammalian cells *in vitro. Appl. Ent. Zool.* **15**: 133–139.

PASTEUR, L. (1870) Etudes sur la maladie des vers à soie. Vol. I 322 pp., Vol. II 327 pp. Gauthier-Villars, Paris.

PETIT-GLATRON, M. F. and RAPOPORT, G. (1975) *In vivo* and *in vitro* evidence for the existence of stable messenger ribonucleic acids in sporulating cells of *Bacillus thuringiensis.* In: *Spores VI*, GERHARDT, P., COSTILOW, R. N. and SADOFF, H. L. (Eds). American Society for Microbiology, Washington, D.C.

PRASAD, S. S. S. V. and SHETNA, Y. I. (1974) Purification, crystallization and partial characterization of the antitumor and insecticidal protein subunit from the delta-endotoxin of *Bacillus thuringiensis* var. *thuringiensis. Biochim. Biophys. Acta* **363**: 558–566.

PRASAD, S. S. S. V. and SHETNA, Y. I. (1976) Mode of action of a purified antitumor protein from the proteinaceous crystal of *Bacillus thuringiensis* subsp. *thuringiensis* on Yoshida ascites sarcoma cells. *Antimicrobiol. Agents Chemother.* **10**: 293–298.

PRYSTAŠ, M., KALDOVA, L. and ŠORM, F. (1976) Alternative synthesis of exotoxin from *Bacillus thuringiensis. Coll. Czech. Chem. Commun.* **41**: 1426–1447.

RIBIER, J. (1971) L'inclusion parasporale de *Bacillus thuringiensis* var. Berliner 1715: moment et site de son initiation, rapport avec l'ADN sporangial. *C.R. Acad. Sc. Paris* **273**: 1444–1447 (série D).

SCHERRER, P., LÜTHY, P. and TRÜMPI, B. (1973) Production of delta-endotoxin by *Bacillus thuringiensis* as a function of glucose concentrations. *Appl. Microbiol.* **25**: 644–646.

ŠEBESTA, K., HORSKÁ, K. and VAŇKOVÁ, J. (1969) Inhibition of *de novo* RNA-synthesis by the insecticidal exotoxin of *Bacillus thuringiensis* var. *gelechiae. Coll. Czech. Chem. Commun.* **34**: 1786–1791.

ŠEBESTA, K. and HORSKÁ, K. (1968) Inhibition of DNA-dependent RNA polymerase by the exotoxin of *Bacillus thuringiensis* var. *gelechiae. Biochim. Biophys. Acta* **169**: 281–282.

ŠEBESTA, K. and HORSKÁ, K. (1973) The fate of exotoxin from *Bacillus thuringiensis* in mice. *Coll. Czech. Chem. Commun.* **38**: 2533.

SEBESTA, K. and STERNBACH, H. (1970) The specificity of inhibition of DNA-dependent RNA polymerase by *Bacillus thuringiensis. FEBS Letters* **8**: 233–235.

SEKI, T., NAGAMATSU, M., NAGAMATSU, Y., TSUTSUI, R., ICHIMARU, T., WATANABE, T., KOGA, K. and HAYASHI, K. (1978) Injuring reaction of delta-endotoxin upon sarcoma 180 ascites cells and silkworm midgut cells *in vitro. Sci. Bull. Fac. Agr., Kyushu Univ.* **33**: 19–24.

SMIRNOFF, W. A. (1974) Sensibilité de *Lambdina fiscellaria fiscellaria* (*Lepidoptera, Geometridae*) à l'infection par *Bacillus thuringiensis* Berliner seul ou en presence de chitinase. *Can. Entomol.* **106**: 429–432.

SOMERVILLE, H. J. (1971) Formation of the parasporal inclusion of *Bacillus thuringiensis*. *Eur. J. Biochem.* **18**: 226–237.

SOMERVILLE, H. J. (1978) Insect toxin in spores and protein crystals of *Bacillus thuringiensis*. TIBS, May 1978.

STAHLY, D. P., DINGMAN, D. W., IRGENS, R. L., FIELD, C. C., FEISS, M. G. and SMITH, G. L. (1978) Multiple extrachromosomal deoxyribonucleic acid molecules in *Bacillus thuringiensis*. *FEMS Microbiol. Letters* **3**: 139–141.

STILES, B. and PASCHKE, J. D. (1980) Midgut pH in different instars of three *Aedes* mosquito species and the relation between pH and susceptibility of larvae to a nuclear polyhydrosis virus. *J. Invertebr. Pathol.* **35**: 58–64.

THELESTAM, M. and MÖLLBY, R. (1975) Determination of toxin induced leakage at different size nucleotides through the plasma membrane of human diploid fibroblasts. *Infect. Immun.* **11**: 640–648.

TRAVERS, R. S., FAUST, R. M. and REICHELDERFER, C. F. (1976) Effects of *Bacillus thuringiensis* var. *kurstaki* delta-endotoxin on isolated Lepidopteran mitochondria. *J. Invertebr. Pathol.* **28**: 351–356.

TRÜMPI, B. (1976) Analytische Untersuchungen am delta-Endotoxin von *Bacillus thuringiensis*. *Zbl. Bakt. Abt. II* **131**: 305–360.

VAŇKOVÁ, J. (1978) The heat-stable exotoxin of *Bacillus thuringiensis*. *Folia Microbiol.* **23**: 162–174.

YOUNG, E. I. and FITZ-JAMES, P. (1959) Chemical and morphological studies of bacterial spore formation. II. Spore and parasporal protein formation in *Bacillus cereus* var. *alesti. J. Biophys. Biochem. Cytol.* **6**: 483–489.

YOUSTEN, A. A. and ROGOFF, M. H. (1969) Metabolism of *Bacillus thuringiensis* in relation to spore and crystal formation. *J. Bacteriol.* **100**: 1229–1236.

ZALUNIN, I. A., CHESTUKHINA, G. G. and STEPANOV, V. M. (1979) Protein composition of delta-endotoxin crystals in various serotypes of *Bacillus thuringiensis*. *Biokhimiya* **44**: 693–698.

CHAPTER 22

TOXINS OF *CLOSTRIDIUM PERFRINGENS*
TYPES A, B, C, D AND E

JAMES L. McDONEL, Ph.D.

Immuno AG. Donau Austria

ABSTRACT

Clostridium perfringens types A, B, C, D, and E produce at least 12 different antigens, referred to as *toxins*, that may be involved in *pathogenesis*. These antigens have been given the names *alpha, beta, epsilon,* and *iota* toxin ('major' toxins), and *delta, theta, kappa* (collagenase), *lambda* (protease), *mu* (hyaluronidase), *nu* (deoxyribonuclease), *gamma* and *eta* toxin ('minor' toxins). An *enterotoxin* and *neuraminidase* are also produced by certain strains. Significant progress has been made in characterizing alpha and theta toxin, and the enterotoxin, but relatively little is known about the other toxins. A variety of disease syndromes are believed to be caused by one or more of each of these toxins though their exact role in disease is not clear in most cases.

1. INTRODUCTION

Clostridium perfringens produces at least 12 different soluble antigens, referred to as toxins, that may be involved in pathogenesis. Whether or not all of these antigens are directly involved in production of lesions or contribute to pathogenesis in animals or man is unclear. However, the term 'toxin' is commonly used to describe these antigens. The activities of the different toxins are given in Table 1. At least eight of the toxins are believed to be lethal. The role in pathogenesis of eta and gamma toxins, and the enzymatic kappa, lambda, mu and nu toxins is uncertain. It is not even certain that eta and gamma toxins exist. Four of the lethal toxins, alpha, beta, epsilon, and iota, are considered to be the 'major' toxins and are used to group the species into five toxigenic types of A, B, C, D, and E. Type A strains produce predominantly alpha toxin, type B, beta and epsilon toxins, type C, beta and delta toxins, type D, epsilon toxin, and type E, iota toxin. A strain once classed as type F (Zeissler and Rassfeld–Sternberg, 1949) which has different colony appearance, elongated cell forms, heat resistant spores, and minor antigens, has since been more accurately classified as a subtype of

TABLE 1. *General Description of* Clostridium perfringens *Toxins and Their Activities*

Toxin	Activity
Alpha (lecithinase)	lethal; necrotizing; hemolytic
Beta	lethal; necrotizing
Epsilon	lethal; necrotizing
Iota	lethal; necrotizing
Delta	lethal, hemolytic
Theta	lethal, hemolytic
Kappa (collagenase)	lethal; necrotizing; gelatinase
Lambda (protease)	disintegrates azocoll and hide powder, gelatinase
Mu (hyaluronidase)	release glucosamine from hyaluronic acid
Nu (deoxyribonuclease)	may be leucocidic in gas gangrene and post-uterine infection
Gamma	existence doubtful; may be lethal
Eta	existence doubtful; may be lethal
Enterotoxin	diarrheagenic; cytotoxic, causes gut damage; lethal
Neuraminidase	inhibits cell receptor function

C (Stern and Warrack, 1964). Typing of the organism is accomplished with type-specific antisera. The type neutralized by each specific antisera is given in Table 2. It is important to note that a clear-cut distinction does not always exist between different types of *C. perfringens*, and erroneous typing results can cause problems (Serrano and Schneider, 1978). Nontoxigenic variants are found within the types and 'degraded' types (Dalling and Ross, 1938; Buddle, 1954) are those which have lost their ability to produce a certain toxin. The toxins produced by the different types are given in Table 3. There is not total agreement in the literature about which strains produce which toxins. It should also be noted that a wide variety exists in amounts of toxins produced by different strains. Excellent reviews already have been written that include this kind of information about *C. perfringens* toxins (Willis, 1969; Ispolatovskaya, 1971; Hauschild, 1971; Smith, 1975a).

C. perfringens is widely distributed in nature and normally is present in large numbers in soil, sewage, and the intestinal tract of animals and man (Willis, 1969). However, the organism also is found in air, dust, water, and numerous foods. In fact, *C. perfringens* can be considered to be ubiquitous due to its distribution throughout the ecosystems of the world.

Type A strains are by far the most commonly encountered under non-infectious conditions (Colee, 1974), and they are the only ones associated with the microflora of both soil and the intestinal tract. The 'classical' (hemolytic type A) strains are more numerous in the intestinal tract than are nonhemolytic strains. Except under disease conditions, *C. perfringens* is not usually found in the stomach or upper and middle small intestine, while it may be isolated from the terminal ileum (Vince, *et al.*, 1972). Distribution in the large intestine is believed to be the most widespread. Types B, C, D, and E are invariably restricted to the intestinal tract, primarily of animals, and occasionally of man. Types B, C, and D have been isolated from soil but in areas where enteritis was affecting significant numbers of animals or humans. Even when inoculated directly into soil, strains of *C. perfringens* of intestinal origin die out within a few months at the most. It appears that they are unable to compete with the better adapted normal soil inhabitants (Smith, 1975a).

Table 4 gives the general disease conditions in man and animals known to be caused by the different types of *C. perfringens*. It is not certain which toxins produced by each strain are directly or indirectly responsible for each of these conditions. A detailed description of each toxin's known activity under experimental conditions is given below.

2. ALPHA TOXIN (LECITHINASE, PHOSPHOLIPASE C)

While strains of all five types of *C. perfringens* produce this toxin, type A strains usually produce the greatest quantities. On occasion a strain is isolated that is typical type A except that it does not produce detectable amounts of alpha toxin. Alpha toxin production also varies considerably with growth medium and amount of growth is not necessarily correlated with toxin production (Smith, 1975a). According to a study by Möllby, *et al.* (1976) the yields of alpha toxin produced by type A strains isolated from cases of gas gangrene and abdominal wounds were indistinguishable from those isolated from fecal samples from healthy persons. Not much is known about genetic control of alpha toxin production but one reported attempt to link its production to a plasmid was unsuccessful (Krämer and

TABLE 2. *Types of C. perfringens Neutralized by Various Type-Specific Antisera*

Type-Specific Antiserum	Type Neutralized
A	A
B	A, B, C, D
C	A, C
D	A, D
E	A, E

TABLE 3. *Toxins Produced by the Five Different Types of* C. perfringens

TYPE	Major Toxins				Minor Toxins								Other Toxins	
	alpha	beta	epsilon	iota	delta	theta	kappa	lambda	mu	nu	eta	gamma	enterotoxin	neuraminidase
A	+	−	−	−	−	+	+	−	+	+	⊕	−	+	+
B	+	+	(+)	−	+	+	+	+	+	+	−	⊕	O	+
C	+	+	−	−	+	+	+	−	+	+	−	⊕	+	+
D	+	−	(+)	−	−	+	+	+	+	+	−	−	+	+
E	+	−	−	(+)	−	+	+	+	−	+	−	−	O	+

+ = produced by some strains of the type given. Quantities of toxin produced by different strains can vary.
− = not known to be produced by any strains of the type given.
(+) = prototoxin, activation requires enzymes.
⊕ = existence doubtful
O = not studied.

TABLE 4. *Disease Conditions Caused by Different Types of* C. perfringens

Type	Disease
A	gas gangrene of man and animals; food poisoning; equine grass sickness; necrotizing colitis and enterotoxemia of horses
B	lamb dysentery; enterotoxemia of foals, sheep, goats
C	enterotoxemia of sheep (struck), calves, lambs, piglets, necrotic enteritis of man (pig-bel, Darmbrand), fowl
D	enterotoxemia of sheep, lambs (pulpy kidney or overeating disease), goats, cattle, possibly man
E	role in pathogenicity unclear; found in sheep, cattle; possibly responsible for colitis in rabbits

Schallehn, 1978). Suitable media and conditions for alpha toxin production have been reviewed by Ispolatovskaya (1971) and Smith (1975a).

Alpha toxin, by far the most widely studied of the perfringens toxins, has been demonstrated to have phospholipase C, lethal, necrotizing, hemolytic, and cytolytic activities (Willis, 1977). It was the first bacterial toxin to be identified as an enzyme (a phospholipase C that catalyzes the hydrolysis of the phosphodiester bond in position 3 of the lecithin molecule to produce phosphorylcholine and water-insoluble 1,2-diacylglyceride). It has been realized since the end of the 19th century that *C. perfringens* (then referred to as *Bacillus aerogenes capsulatus* and later as Fraenkel's gas bacillus and *C. welchii*) is the etiological agent for several disease conditions. During World War I *C. perfringens* came into great prominence as the most important causal organism of gas gangrene in man (Willis, 1969). Alpha toxin's enzymatic nature was first observed by Nagler (1939) and Seiffert (1939). Its mode of action as a specific phospholipase C (phosphatidylcholine: cholinephosphohydrolase E.C. 3.1.4.3) was first defined by MacFarlane and Knight (1941). Since then, much work has been done to elucidate the action of this toxin at various levels. There also is considerable interest today in using the toxin as a tool for studying biological membranes and lipids in relation to structure and function of the membranes. Extensive reviews of alpha toxin (Willis, 1969; Ispolatovskaya, 1971; Hauschild, 1971) and its application to the study of cell membranes (Avigad, 1976; Freer and Arbuthnott, 1976; Rosenberg, 1976; Möllby, 1978; Alouf, 1977; Zwaal, *et al.*, 1973), have been written.

Physical Properties. As shown in Table 5, numerous authors have reported molecular weights for alpha toxin, determined by different methods, ranging from 30,000 to 106,000. The most reproducible value appears to be about 30,000 obtained by gel filtration chromatography, while SDS-polyacrylamide gel electrophoresis has yielded higher values (Möllby, 1978). It is interesting to note that alpha toxin has been reported to move with beta toxin in G-100 columns and therefore it has been suggested (Akama, *et al*, 1968; Sakurai and Duncan, 1977) that the molecular weights of both toxins are similar (beta toxin molecular weight, 30,000). Less variation has been reported for the isoelectric point of alpha toxin, with a value of about 5.6 for the main component. The higher molecular weight values obtained with SDS gel electrophoresis may represent a polymer. The data from isoelectric focusing generally reveal two forms of the toxin of which the true enzyme is probably represented by the material with a pI of 5.5 (Smith, 1975a). Some reports suggest the existence of 2–4 isozymes (Sugahara, *et al.*, 1976; Litvinko, *et al.*, 1977). Studies done with SDS gels (Park, *et al.*, 1977) showed two bands for phospholipase C but only one of the bands had enzymatic activity. Both hemolytic and phospholipolytic activity were found to reside with the same (one protein) band. This is unlike *Bacillus cereus* toxin for which hemolytic, phospholipolytic, and lethal activities are each believed to be catalyzed by separate proteins (Ivers, *et al.*, 1977). The physical properties of *C. perfringens* phospholipase C have been reviewed by Smyth and Arbuthnott (1974).

TABLE 5. *Molecular Weights and Isolectric Points Reported for Phospholipase C of* Clostridium perfringens[a]

Authors	Year	Gel Filtration	SDS Acrylamide	Other Methods	Isoelectric Point[b]
Meduski and Volkova	1958			106,000[c]	
Bangham and Dawson	1961				
Bernheimer and Grushoff	1967	31,000			5.0, 5.8
Shemonova, *et al.*	1968			51,000[d]	
Bernheimer, *et al.*	1968				5.2, 5.5
Glushkova, *et al.*	1969	35,000–42,000			
Teodorescu, *et al.*	1970	35,000			
Sugahara and Ohsaka	1970				5.3, 5.6
Casu, *et al.*	1971		90,000		
Isopolatovskaya	1971				5.2, 5.5
Mitsui, *et al.*	1973	49,000			
Möllby, *et al.*	1973				4.6, 5.7
Möllby and Wadström	1973	30,000	55,000		5.7
Stahl	1973		46,500		
Bird, *et al.*	1974		48,000		4.75, 5.5
Smyth and Arbuthnott	1974		53,000		5.2, 5.5
Takahashi, *et al.*	1974		43,000		5.2, 5.3, 5.5
Smyth and Wadström	1975				5.3, 5.3, 5.5
Yamakawa and Ohsaka	1977	31,000	43,000		

[a] Modified from Möllby (1978), Alouf (1977), and Smith (1975a).
[b] Determined by isoelectric focusing.
[c] Gamma irradiation inactivation.
[d] Ultracentrifugation.

Phospholipase C is capable of hydrolyzing both choline—containing phospholipids and glycerophosphatides. The substrate range of the enzyme among the phospholipids commonly occurring in membranes is given in Table 6. There is some uncertainty about hydrolysis of some of these phospholipids due to their reported differences in susceptibility to the enzyme. This depends upon whether they are studied as components of intact membranes, or in their purified form. Möllby (1978) has reviewed some of the problems in relation to water soluble enzymes acting upon water insoluble or partially soluble substrates. Another problem in interpreting published data on this enzyme is the fact that many authors have used preparations of the enzyme from commercial or other sources with insufficient or no regard for the fact that these preparations, unless produced under very rigorous purification standards, may contain as many as 10 contaminating active substances, including theta hemolysin, mu and nu toxins, protease, α-glucosidase, N-acetyl-glucosamine, sulphatase, and β-glucuronidase (Möllby, *et al.*, 1973). Several of these contaminating substances have marked activity with respect to biological membranes (Smyth, *et al.*, 1975; Freer and Arbuthnott, 1976). Phospholipase C is a comparatively thermostable enzyme which can retain 45 % of its activity when heated in a sealed ampule for 10 to 15 minutes at 100°C (Smith and Gardner, 1950). It is also believed to be a zinc metalloenzyme (Ispolatovskaya, 1971) even though the presence of zinc ions has not been demonstrated in purified preparations of the enzyme (Smyth and Arbuthnott, 1974).

TABLE 6. *Substrate Specificity of* C. perfringens *Phospholipase C*[a]

Hydrolyzed	Not Hydrolyzed
Sphingomyelin	Phosphatidylinositol
Phosphatidylcholine (lecithin)	Phosphatidylglycerol
Phosphatidylethanolamine	Diphosphatidylglycerol (cardiolipin)
Phosphatidylserine	*O*-lysylphosphatidylglycerol
Lysophosphatidylcholine	
Lysophosphatidylethanolamine	

[a] See van Deenen (1964), Hill and Lands (1970), Dawson (1973), Freer and Arbuthnott (1976), and Möllby (1978).

However, zinc appears to be important to the stability of the enzyme and its resistance to proteases (Sato, et al., 1978). The enzyme's activity is calcium-dependent (Bangham and Dawson, 1961; Kurioka and Matsuda, 1976), though the role of calcium appears to be limited to its effect on the substrate, not the enzyme (Kurioka and Matsuda, 1976; Avigad, 1976; Dawson, et al., 1976). Divalent cations and positively charged detergents are believed to activate the phospholipase action by giving the substrate a positive charge which optimizes attachment of the negatively charged enzyme. But, trace amounts of calcium ions have been found to be an absolute requirement besides the optimizing effects created just by charge differences (Klein, 1975; Dawson, et al., 1976) because hydrolysis may occur without the positive charges when rotational freedom of individual phospholipid molecules is increased or when a monolayer of the substrate is expanded (Dawson et al., 1976). However, under normal conditions, the phospholipase C activity in vitro is inhibited by phosphate, citrate, fluoride, and other substances that tightly bind calcium (Smith, 1975a). It can also be inhibited by phosphonate and phosphinate analogues of lecithin [i.e., phosphatidylcholine with one or two direct carbon-phosphorus bonds, (Rosenthal and Pousada, 1968; Rosenthal, et al., 1969; Möllby, 1978)], chelating agents (in vitro and in vivo) such as diethylene triamine pentacetate (Senff and Moskowitz, 1969), and specific antitoxin.

   Biological Activity. Hemolysis due to alpha toxin occurs in most erythrocytes except those of horses and goats. Erythrocytes of cattle and mice seem most susceptible while those of rabbits, sheep, and humans are moderate in susceptibility (Smith, 1975a). The hydrolysis of phospholipid in the cell membrane precedes hemolysis, as can be seen by the increasing concentration of acid-soluble phosphate in the suspending medium when red cells are exposed to low concentrations of alpha toxin (Smith, 1975a). This damage to the cell membrane may result directly in hemoglobin release but other factors may be involved. An example of this is the 'hot-cold' lysis phenomenon. Erythrocytes of many species do not lyse when exposed to toxin at 37°C. However, when cooled to 4°C, rapid lysis occurs. At the same time, Möllby (1978) reports that only a comparatively slight hot-cold hemolytic phenomenon is detectable using highly purified phospholipase C from C. perfringens. The hemolytic activity of phospholipase C has been directly correlated with sphingomyelinase C activity. With Sphingomyelinase C the hot-cold phenomenon is striking because when used in its purified form lysis does not occur at all at 37°C. But, lysis of sphingomyelin-depleted red cells can be induced by several things including decreasing the temperature below the lipid phase transition temperature, or synergistic lysis with very small quantities of alpha toxin (Möllby, 1978; Möllby, 1976). Ethylenediamine tetraacetic acid (EDTA) also causes lysis of sphingomyelin-depleted cells in a manner that compares to hot-cold lysis (Smyth, et al., 1975). It has been postulated that the divalent cation (mainly magnesium)-lipid interactions which stabilize the sphingomyelin-depleted membrane may be weakened by lowered temperature or addition of chelating agents (Smyth, et al., 1975; Möllby, 1976). The lowered temperature may weaken hydrophobic forces (Low, et al., 1974; Low and Freer, 1977) and EDTA leads to removal of ionic and hydrogen bonds between the cholesterol molecules and the polar groups of the sphingomyelin, either of which increases permeability and results in eventual lysis (Möllby, 1978). Avigad and Bernheimer (1976) showed that zinc ions (150 μM) conferred resistance to hemolysis of sheep erythrocytes by alpha toxin. They concluded that the zinc does not protect by preventing binding of the alpha toxin to the membrane. This phenomenon may support the idea that cations stabilize the membrane. However, the exact mechanism by which zinc ions protect the red cells is not known.

   Other studies have indicated that alpha toxin is able only to degrade membrane phospholipids and cause hemolysis of ATP-depleted erythrocytes (Frish, et al., 1973; Möllby, et al., 1973; Möllby, et al., 1974). Taguchi and Ikezawa (1976a; 1976b) concluded that the hemolytic activity of phospholipase C depends upon asymmetric distribution of phospholipids in the erythrocyte membrane and accessibility of the enzyme to the phospholipids on the membrane surface (Möllby, 1978). And, several workers have postulated that accessibility of the enzyme to substrate is related to lateral pressure due to lipid packing in the outer leaflet of the phospholipid bilayer found in erythrocytes (Zwaal, et al., 1975; Demel, et al., 1975; van Deenen, et al., 1976). Another example of the importance of accessibility is a phenomenon noted in aged red cells (Shukla, *et al.*, 1978). Aged red cells undergo microvessiculation and eventually become spherocytes which alters the accessibility of membrane phosphatidylethanolamine. This causes the older cells to become more resistant to alpha toxin activity. Further question of the direct involvement of alpha toxin phospholipase activity in hemolysis has arisen from the work of Sabban, *et al.* (1972). They found that chicken erythrocytes are lysed by alpha toxin unable to hydrolyze phospholipids because of treatment with EDTA which binds calcium ions necessary for phospholipase C activity (Bangham and Dawson, 1961; Kurioka and Matsuda, 1976). At the same time, alpha toxin, unable to hemolyse red cells due to heating at 56°C in the presence of calcium, is capable of hydrolyzing membrane phospholipids.

As mentioned before, caution must be exercised in interpreting data generated from membrane studies using alpha toxin preparations of unknown or unproven purity. Möllby, *et al.* (1974) showed that the major portion of membrane damage in mammalian cells treated with phospholipase C was due to a contamination with theta toxin. Membrane damage could be induced by highly purified alpha toxin but lysis of cells was not noted. Further effects of phospholipase upon red cell membranes and the use of phospholipase to study lipids in relation to structure and function of membranes has been reviewed by Möllby (1978). Systems utilizing synergistic lysis of human, guinea pig and sheep erythrocytes with alpha toxin and streptococcal CAMP (Christie Atkins Munch Peterson) factor (Gubash, 1978) or other organisms (Choudhury, 1978) have recently been developed that may generate data that will aid in understanding toxin-induced hemolysis as well as membrane structure and function.

Aside from its effects upon red cells, alpha toxin also lyses platelets and leucocytes (Mihancea *et al.*, 1970), stimulates histamine release from cells *in vivo* (Habermann, 1960) and *in vitro* (Strandberg *et al.*, 1974), and damages membranes in fibroblasts (Möllby *et al.*, 1974; Möllby, 1973) and intact muscle cells (Boethius *et al.*, 1973). Furthermore, it causes aggregation of platelets *in vitro* (Sugahara *et al.*, 1976) and *in vivo* (Ohsaka *et al.*, 1978a,b). Ohsaka *et al.* (1978b) demonstrated that within 1–1.5 minutes of topical application of alpha toxin to rat mesentery, rolling leucocytes along vessel walls occurred in venules but not arterioles. Thrombi then formed in venules, capillaries, and eventually, in arterioles. They have concluded that thrombosis must be involved as an early important step in the pathogenesis of necrosis caused by alpha toxin and that these alpha-toxin induced thrombi (which result in hemostasis) may be one of the factors involved in the causation of toxemia often manifested in the late stage of gas gangrene (Ohsaka *et al.*, 1978b). Otnaess and Holm (1976) showed that just phospholipid degradation in platelet membranes is not sufficient to cause the release reaction or aggregation of platelets. This was concluded because phospholipase C from *Bacillus cereus* (which did not act on sphingomyelin under their reaction conditions) degraded phospholipids but did not cause the aggregation noted to occur in response to *Clostridium perfringens* phospholipase C. This implies that sphingomyelin must be degraded in order for the release reaction or aggregation to occur. It has also been shown (Sugahara *et al.*, 1977) that alpha toxin causes an increase in vascular permeability in guinea pig skin due possibly to release of some mediator(s) from aggregating platelets (Sugahara *et al.*, 1977; Ohsaka *et al.*, 1978a). Wilkinson (1975) has demonstrated that the locomotor response of human monocytes is inhibited by the toxin as well.

Szmigielski *et al.* (1978) showed that five minutes exposure to alpha toxin decreased uptake and increased leakage of ^{86}Rb from a rabbit kidney cell line. At a later time, binding of ouabain, and uptake of ^{3}H-uridine and ^{3}H-glycine were inhibited, apparently due to membrane damage induced by subcytotoxic doses of the toxin. They suggested that the toxin causes disturbances in potassium transport through the cellular membrane with accompanying changes in Na^+-K^+-ATP-ase activity. The phospholipid content of alpha toxin treated versus untreated cultured embryonic chick muscle cells was reported (Kent, 1978) to be similar but cellular degradation and synthesis of phosphatidylcholine and sphingomyelin was reported to be 3–4 times greater in the treated than untreated cells.

There is considerable difficulty in interpreting much of the data published over past years dealing with alpha toxin's role in disease because of lack of purity of the toxin preparations used. With this problem in mind, some attempt will be made to summarize numerous disease syndromes thought to be induced by the toxin. The systemic effects of alpha toxin are affected by the route of administration (Smith, 1975a). When injected intravenously, a 5 to 20 per cent drop in the red cell count occurs within a few hours followed shortly thereafter by death. Other effects are destruction of platelets, a drop in clotting time, and widespread capillary damage. Alpha toxin has been recovered from the serum of a patient suffering from *C. perfringens* septicemia (Moore *et al.*, 1976). Under experimental conditions ninety per cent of the toxin injected disappears from circulating blood within 5 minutes of injection (Ellner, 1961). The toxin that disappears from the blood appears in the following organs: liver, 72%, lungs, 15%, kidneys, 8%, and spleen, 5%. Toxin does not appear to bind to skeletal muscle. In fact, when injected intramuscularly, apparent leakage into blood or lymph, vascular damage, and effects on platelets are absent. The muscle cells' plasma membranes are altered which probably causes the apparent degeneration of mitochondria, sarcoplasmic reticulum, and nuclei (Strunk *et al.*, 1967).

The disease gas gangrene (anaerobic myonecrosis) can be caused by six different species of *Clostridium*, including *perfringens*. Individual lesions often yield more than one species, though *C. perfringens* is recovered from 80% of gas gangrene cases (Weinstein and Barza, 1973). It is believed that between 10,000 and 12,000 cases of this disease occur per year in the United States today (Hitchcock *et al.*, 1975). Mortality varies from 0 to 100%. Once started, the pathological process of gas gangrene can often result in death within 30 to 48 hours. The exact involvement of alpha toxin in the disease is not clear. Kameyama *et al.* (1975) demonstrated that guinea pigs immunized with purified alpha toxin did not develop gas gangrene when challenged simultaneously with the organism, alpha toxin, and kappa toxin. Animals immunized with kappa toxin did develop gas gangrene when challenged with the organism and alpha toxin. It is likely that other toxins of *C. perfringens* type A mentioned in this review play a role in the development of the disease. Theta toxin has lethal, necrotic, and hemolyzing capabilities similar to those of alpha toxin. Kappa toxin is a potent protease, while nu toxin acts as a 'spreading factor'. Mu toxin affects DNA, fibrinolysin is produced, neuraminidase destroys the immunological receptors on erythrocytes, hemagglutinin inactivates the group factor A on erythrocytes, and the 'circulating factor' inhibits phagocytosis (Hitchcock *et al.*, 1975). Intense and 'woody hard' edema develops in the area of the infection which frequently causes occlusion of the microcirculation. This gives rise to hypoxia which enhances growth of the organism. Thrombosis of local vessels occurs followed by production of hydrogen sulfide and carbon dioxide gases. Within as little as 12 to 20 hours the defense mechanisms of the host can be completely overwhelmed. All organs of the body are likely to be involved at this point. The treatment of choice is crystalline sodium penicillin G (recommended doses vary from 10 million to 32 million units per day) given intravenously, and possibly cephalothin (Keflin), coupled with hyperbaric oxygen (3 ATA) for 2 hour periods, and surgical debridement. These procedures, when used in concert, give consistent survival rates of 95% assuming sufficiently early diagnosis and treatment of the disease. None of the treatments alone is nearly as effective. There has been some controversy over the use of hyperbaric oxygen as there has been over the effectiveness of antitoxin in treatment of the disease. Petrov *et al.* (1978) recently reported that polymerization of alpha toxoid can triple the immune response to the monomeric form. The development of highly immunogenic toxoid preparations could give toxoid prophylaxis a more central role in combating this disease. Much work needs yet to be done to distinguish the role played in pathogenesis of each of the toxins (in their highly purified state) produced by *C. perfringens*.

Necrotic enteritis of chickens is thought (Al-Sheikhly and Truscott, 1977a; Al-Sheikhly and Truscott, 1977b; Al-Sheikhly and Truscott, 1977c) to be caused in large part by alpha toxin from *C. perfringens* type A. There is a similar disease, ulcerative enteritis, of quail caused by type C (Bickford, 1975) and, in fact, it has been reported that necrotic enteritis of chickens is due to type C organisms (Smith, 1975b). The disease symptoms described parallel closely those characteristic for type C enteritis in piglets. Typical lesions, which develop as early as 1 hour after infusion of organisms, include edema in the lamina propria, desquamation of epithelial cells, especially at villus tips, coagulation necrosis of villus tips, and eventually (8–12 hours), necrosis of the entire villus structures. Other organs are not overtly affected but abnormal erythrocytes are present in them at 12 hours. The histological damage at villus tips has striking similarities to the histopathology described for *C. perfringens* enterotoxin (see below). Suggestive evidence has been presented (Al-Sheikhly and Truscott, 1977c) that alpha toxin is the primary cause of necrosis in this disease, though more work needs to be done with purified alpha and theta toxins (both potent necrotizing agents) before concrete conclusions can be drawn about their contribution to disease symptoms.

3. BETA TOXIN

Beta toxin, which may be coded for by a plasmid (Duncan *et al.*, 1978), is produced exclusively by *C. perfringens* types B and C. These are the organisms most likely responsible for necrotic enteritis in man and animals. Very little is known about this toxin and interpretation of the few mode-of-action studies that have been done must be made with caution because only recently has the toxin been successfully prepared in a highly purified form. It is particularly likely that toxin preparations used in earlier studies have been contaminated with alpha toxin (and very possibly several other toxins produced by these organisms).

The known physical properties of beta toxin are summarized in Table 7. The earliest report of purification was that of Akama *et al.* (1968). When they performed gel chromatography of crude material it was found that alpha toxin and beta toxin moved together and appeared inseparable by contemporary techniques. To overcome this problem, antiserum to alpha toxin was used to adsorb the toxin component prior to further separation on Sephadex G-100 of the immunoreacted material. The purified beta toxin showed none of the activities associated with toxins produced by type A organisms. It appeared to retain serological activity (guinea pigs were successfully immunized) and biological activity (measured by lethality after IV injection into mice) was retained. Worthington and Mülders (1975b) reported partial purification of beta toxin using chromatography on Sephadex G-50, G-100, and DEAE cellulose. The resultant material was not homogeneous on polyacrylamide gels. The toxin had 800,000 MLD_{50} per mg nitrogen, a typical protein UV absorption spectrum, pI values of 5 and 6, and a molecular weight of $42,000 \pm 2,000$ as determined on SDS gel electrophoresis. Sakurai and Duncan (1977; 1978) reported a 340 fold purification of beta toxin from type C organisms by ammonium sulfate fractionation, gel filtration through Sephadex G-100, isoelectric focusing on a pH 3 to 6 gradient, and immunoaffinity chromatography. The resultant purified toxin gave a single band with polyacrylamide gel electrophoresis. They reported that the toxin appears to be a single polypeptide chain protein with a molecular weight of approximately 30,000 and a major component with a pI value of 5.53 and minor peak with a pI value of 5.06. The toxin was found to be heat labile (75 % loss of biological activity after 5 minutes at 50°C) and destroyed by trypsin after 30 minutes at 37°C. The 50 % lethal dose for a mouse was calculated to be 1.87 μg of the purified beta toxin. Sakurai *et al.* (1980) have demonstrated the existence of thiol groups in the toxin whose reduced state appear to be essential for biological activity. Unpublished data by Al-Saadi and Lauerman (personal communication) indicate that beta toxin has a molecular weight of 20,000, one disulfide bond, and is trypsin sensitive (Table 7). They found that the purified beta toxin has a MLD_{50} of 4 μg.

TABLE 7. *Molecular Weights and Isoelectric Points Reported for Beta Toxin of* C. perfringens

Authors	Year	Gel Filtration	SDS Acrylamide	Isoelectric Point
Worthington and Mülders	1975		$42,000 + 2,000$	5, 6
Sakurai and Duncan	1978	30,000		5.53, 5.06
Al-Saadi and Lauerman	1979[a]		20,000	

[a] Personal communication, unpublished data

In a recent report Sakurai and Duncan (1979) demonstrated that beta toxin production by cultures of type C organisms could be enhanced by pH-controlled medium containing 1 % glucose, starch or sucrose, but that toxin synthesis was not related to growth yield of the organism. They also described a guinea pig skin test that allowed for distinguishing beta and alpha toxin activities, which the mouse lethality test does not necessarily do.

Beta toxin is probably of most widespread concern to veterinary medicine. The most common types of *C. perfringens* to cause problems in animals are B, C, and D. Type B distribution is not thought to be world wide (not found in North America, Australia, or New Zealand) but is found in Europe, South Africa, and the Middle East. Necrotic enteritis from type C is reportedly world wide in distribution affecting calves, lambs, pigs, and possibly feeder cattle (Kennedy *et al.*, 1977). While numerous other toxins are produced by types B and C (see Table 3) it is generally believed that beta toxin is the one primarily responsible for the symptoms noted in necrotic enteritis of the animals listed (Willis, 1969; Hauschild, 1971). Some success has been reported (Hogh, 1976) in immunizing piglets against type C infection using anti-beta toxin serum.

Some slight differences in symptoms between enteritis caused by type B versus type C may be attributed to the production by type B of epsilon toxin which is thought to increase intestinal permeability (Bullen and Batty, 1956), and mu toxin (hyaluronidase) which enable the necrotoxins to spread more widely in the intestinal tissues. This same effect is noted in the development of the characteristic purplish necrotic area produced when beta toxin is injected intradermally in guinea pig skin. Beta reactions produced by type B filtrates are very irregular in shape due to the presence of mu toxin while those produced by type C filtrates (most of which do not contain mu toxin) are smaller and more nearly circular (Willis, 1969).

It is also believed that beta toxin is responsible for necrotizing jejunitis (enteritis necroticans) in man as well. This disease, also known as 'pig bel' (a similar syndrome had the name 'Darmbrand' in Germany and Scandinavia from 1944–1949) is endemic in the highlands of Papua New Guinea and has been reported in Africa, South East Asia, and even America (Lawrence and Walker, 1976). Sporadic cases have been reported in other western countries. Lawrence and Walker (1976) have proposed an interesting hypothesis concerning the development of enteritis necroticans. While the disease is endemic and relatively common in the highlands of New Guinea, it is rare in the lowlands, where poor nutrition and a predominance of type C organisms in the soil are equivalent to the conditions in the highlands. These workers postulated that the sweet potato, a staple food in the highlands, is the indirect cause of the prevalence of the disease. Sweet potatoes have been shown to contain heat-stable inhibitors of trypsin (Sugiura *et al.*, 1973), a protease that readily destroys beta toxin activity. The contributory factors to development of disease are a low protein diet, low pancreatic tryptic activity, plus continuous consumption of trypsin inhibitors which results in inadequate proteolysis of beta toxin. In fact, this proposal has been supported experimentally with guinea pigs. Enteritis developed in guinea pigs given type C toxin filtrates and soybean material (which naturally contains protease inhibitors), while pigs given the same amount of beta toxin preparation but with heat-inactivated soybean material did not develop symptoms. Lawrence and Cooke (1980) have reported that characteristic symptoms developed in the guinea pig model, when injected intragastrically with growing type C cultures, only if protease inhibitors were also given. They reported that an excess of pancreatic enzymes or active or passive immunization against beta toxin protected the animals against intragastric or intrajejunal challenge with cultures or toxic filtrates. The efficacy of vaccination in prevention of pig bel has been described by Knight *et al.* (1979), Lawrence *et al.* (1979) and Walker *et al.* (1979).

Early studies on the pharmacological activity of filtrates from type B and C indicate that it can cause contraction of smooth muscle, liberate pigments from perfused liver, raise pulmonary arterial pressure and venous pressure, and decrease systemic pressure which usually is accompanied by heart block. Type B filtrates can cause liberation of histamine from perfused cat lung, and both types liberate a slowly-acting muscle stimulant (Kellaway and Trethewie, 1941). As mentioned before, however, the presence of unaccounted toxins, and use of 'specific' antiserum prepared against beta toxin that may not have been highly purified necessitates cautious interpretation of these data. More recently Parnas (1976) demonstrated that beta toxin administered into the rabbit jejunum and ileum shows paralysis of the motor activity of the intestine which he believed to be similar to the paralyzing activity in the intestine noted in piglet dysentery. Sakurai *et al.* (1981, 1982) have established a rat model for beta toxin which confirms the dose-related rise in blood pressure (and concomitant decline in heart rate) associated with IV injection of purified toxin. They conclude that the toxin acts on at least preganglionic fiber, and vasomotor centers, and causes increased blood pressure by toxin-induced release of catecholamines such as norepinephrine (see also epsilon toxin).

4. EPSILON TOXIN

C. perfringens type B and D produce an essentially inactive prototoxin that, when digested with trypsin becomes a highly potent toxin called epsilon toxin. This toxin is of particular interest to veterinary medicine in that it causes a rapidly fatal enterotoxemia (also called pulpy kidney disease, and overeating disease) of sheep and other animals (Hauschild, 1971). Some conditions for maximal toxin production in culture have been described by Kulshrestha (1974a, b) and Smith (1975a). Radioimmunoassays for detection of toxin and antibodies (as little as 0.004 IU/ml) have been developed that are useful in laboratory studies and in screening large herds of vaccinated animals (Bernath, 1975; Lieberman, 1975). The purified toxin may also be assayed by a precipitin test, a microcomplement fixation test (Marucci and Fuller, 1971), a single radial diffusion test (Mancini *et al.*, 1965), and reverse phase passive hemagglutination (detects as little as 0.6 ng/ml) (Beh and Buttery, 1978).

Early attempts at purification of the prototoxin by column chromatography were made by Orlans *et al.* (1960) which resulted in a calculated molecular weight of 38,000 ± 5,000 (see Table 8) and a sedimentation coefficient of 2.8 S. Thompson (1962; 1963) reported a molecular weight of 40,500 and a sedimentation coefficient of 2.48 S. Habeeb (1969) reported the presence in purified preparations of multiple electrophoretic forms of the prototoxin that

TABLE 8. *Molecular Weights and Sedimentation Coefficients of Epsilon Prototoxin of* Clostridium perfringens *Type D*

Authors	Year	Molecular Weight	Sedimentation Coefficient
Orlans	1960	38,000 + 5,000	2.8 S
Thompson	1962	40,500	2.48 S
Habeeb	1964	23,000 − 25,000	2.85 S
Habeeb	1972	34,250[a] 33,200[b] + 1,300 24,000[c]	2.15 S
Habeeb	1975	34,250[a] 33,100[b] 25,000[d] 27,500[e]	2.15 S
Worthington and Mülders	1977	32,700[f] 31,200[f, g]	
Al-Saadi and Lauerman	1979	25,000[f, h]	

[a] Determined by ultracentrifugation.
[b] Determined by sedimentation equilibration.
[c] Determined by gel filtration (Sephadex G-100).
[d] Determined by gel filtration (Sephadex G-100 with borate buffer).
[e] Determined by gel filtration (Sephadex G-100 with phosphate buffer).
[f] Activated epsilon toxin.
[g] Determined by SDS gel electrophoresis.
[h] Personal communication, unpublished data.

were immunologically indistinguishable. Habeeb (1964) first reported a molecular weight of 23,500–25,000 and a sedimentation coefficient of 2.85 S then later, values ranging from 24,000–34,250 (Habeeb, 1972) and 25,000–34,250 (Habeeb, 1975) with a stokes radius of 1.96 nm. Worthington and Mülders (1977) reported a molecular weight of 32,700 for the prototoxin and 31,200 for the activated epsilon toxin. The isoelectric point for the major peak of prototoxin was 8.02. The activated toxin had two major peaks with pI values of 5.36 and 5.74. Both peaks contained material toxic for mice though the acidic fraction was more toxic on the average than the basic fraction. The significant change in isoelectric point and the small change in molecular weight that resulted upon activation of the prototoxin suggested that a small highly basic peptide(s) was being removed. This confirmed a similar observation made earlier by Habeeb (1969). Al-Saadi and Lauerman (personal communication, unpublished data) have used SDS gels to estimate a molecular weight of 25,000 for epsilon prototoxin. Epsilon prototoxin consists of one polypeptide chain of 311 amino acids with aspartate, threonine, serine, glutamate, valine, and lysine accounting for over 60 % of the total amino acid residues (Habeeb, 1975). The molecule has no free cysteine but contains one blocked cysteine. The N- and C- terminal residues are lysine.

While activation is usually effected by the enzymatic activity of trypsin, some activation can occur spontaneously in growing cultures, presumably due to the activities of proteolytic enzymes (such as kappa and lambda toxins) produced by the bacteria (Smith, 1975a). It has been shown (Bhown and Habeeb, 1977) that activation is caused by a scission of the peptide bond between lys_{14}-ala_{15} of the prototoxin molecule resulting in a small peptide (14 amino acids) split from the N-terminal to give active epsilon toxin. The epsilon prototoxin and toxin contain a high amount of β-conformation (Habeeb et al., 1973). The activation of prototoxin results in some conformation change. But, there is a tendency of the cleavage product to bind to the remaining active toxin molecule which gives the toxin a conformation and serological identity similar to that of the prototoxin. The rebinding of the cleavage product can be prevented under the proper conditions. It is not clear whether the conformation changes resulting from activation are a necessary prerequisite for toxicity (Bhown and Habeeb, 1977).

While rare or non-existent as a cause for human disease, epsilon toxin is responsible for acute enterotoxemia in animals, most commonly sheep, but found also in goats and cattle. A contributing factor in enterotoxemia is a sudden supply of diet (hence 'overeating disease') which results in passage of undigested food and C. perfringens type D organisms from the rumen to the intestines (Hauschild, 1971). This is followed by multiplication and epsilon prototoxin production by the organism in the intestine where proteolytic enzymes in the intestinal fluid (Niilo, 1965) activate the epsilon toxin. The highly toxic epsilon toxin, which increases intestinal permeability (Bullen and Batty, 1956; Bullen, 1970), then enters the blood (Jansen, 1967a) in substantial doses and causes typically swollen hyperemic kidneys, lung edema, and excess pericardial fluid. The kidneys become pulpy (hence 'pulpy kidney disease') in sheep, but not in cattle, within a few hours of death (Jansen, 1960). Clinical symptoms (prostration and convulsions preceding death) are rarely seen (Hauschild, 1971), though affected sheep do exhibit a typical nervousness (Buxton and Morgan, 1976; Hartley, 1956). Immunity to the disease can be induced by injection of toxin, or toxoid (Jansen, 1967a; Jansen, 1967b; Oxer et al., 1971; Hyder, 1973; Worthington et al., 1973; Kennedy et al., 1977).

A considerable amount of work has been done to study the effects of epsilon toxin on the brains of experimental animals because nervousness is a principal clinical sign in sheep with acute cases of enterotoxemia. Hartley (1956) described a focal symmetrical encephalomalacia (FSE) in brain stems of sheep affected by enterotoxemia caused by C. perfringens type D. Griner (1961) and Griner and Carlson (1961) produced brain lesions in sheep and mice by intravenous injection of epsilon toxin, and Gardner (1974) stated that the primary morphological change in the mouse brain was severe endothelial damage. He reported that the brain edema revealed a quantitative increase in water content of the brain tissue and swelling of protoplasm in astrocyte and astrocyte processes around blood vessels. A more detailed study was reported in 1974 by Morgan and Kelly in which the light and electron microscopes were used to detect morphological changes in periaxonal and intramyelinic edema in the white matter of the cerebellar corpus medulare. There also was noted a swelling of axon terminals and dendrites in the grey matter adjacent to the left ventricles while endothelial degeneration appeared to be a feature of older lesions.

In support of Griner and Carlson (1961) and Gardner (1974), Morgan *et al.* (1975) concluded that the primary lesion of this intoxication in the brain is in the vascular endothelium. They reported the extravasation of horseradish peroxidase (HRP) from the brain vasculature of clinically normal mice given lethal or sublethal doses of epsilon toxin. Within 20 minutes of intravenous administration HRP was found throughout the brain. Since detectable morphological damage usually takes 6 hours to develop (Gardner, 1974; Morgan and Kelly, 1974), vascular leakage occurs several hours before development of observable brain lesions. The minimal dose to produce leakage of HRP in mouse brains was 100 μg. Doses below 50 μg had no effect while 150–200 μg caused extensive leakage. Some differences in description by different investigators in pathology caused by this toxin may be due to the fixation or toxin preparation used.

Worthington and Mülders (1975a) demonstrated vascular leakage in mouse brain using epsilon toxin and ^{125}I-polyvinylpyrrolidone and ^{125}I-human serum albumin. With larger doses (4,000 MLD$_{50}$) death, accompanied by extravassation of the albumin, occurred within 2–3 minutes. With smaller doses the effects took a longer period of time. Buxton and Morgan (1976) further characterized the pathology induced by epsilon toxin in lambs brains (FSE) as severe endothelial damage with swelling of perivascular astrocyte end feet, malacic changes, capillary hemorrhages, and choroidal edema. The extravassation of HRP occurred within 50 minutes of intravenous injection. It is also believed that epsilon toxin acts by binding to receptors in the brain vascular walls because administration of a formalinized toxoid prior to exposure to active toxin prevented extravassation of HRP and other typical vascular alterations (Buxton, 1976). The sequence of events in epsilon toxin intoxication has been described as follows (Buxton and Morgan, 1976). Epsilon toxin reacts with specific receptor sites causing vascular endothelial cells to degenerate. This results in tight junctions becoming patent, which alters fluid dynamics. The effect is that astrocyte end feet begin to swell. As degenerative changes progress, serum proteins, and eventually red cells, leak out, and the end feet rupture which causes edema. The edema then produces the clinical signs of nervousness seen in cases of acute lesions observed in actual cases of enterotoxemia of sheep.

A detailed series of studies have recently been reported by Buxton in which binding and activity of epsilon toxin in mice (1978a), guinea pigs (1978b), and cells from guinea pigs, mice, rabbits, and sheep (1978b) were studied. In the mouse model it was found that epsilon toxin bound to the luminal surface of the endothelial lining of blood vessels in the brain, liver, lungs (sparse), and heart (slight) and to cells lining the loops of Henle, the distal convoluted tubules in kidney, and to the hepatic sinusoids. No binding was detected in the large or small intestines, or smooth (intestinal) and skeletal muscles in the body.

The toxin has also been shown (Buxton, 1978b) to cause an increase in capillary permeability in guinea pig skin, and an elevation of serum levels of cyclic $3'-5'$ adenosine monophosphate (cAMP) in mice. A scheme has been proposed to explain the dramatic increase in blood glucose reported (Gardner, 1973a; Gardner, 1973b) to occur in the pre-clinical phase of type D enterotoxemia whereby hepatocyte-bound epsilon toxin (Buxton, 1978b) stimulates cyclic $3'-5'$ adenosine monophosphate production which in turn causes breakdown of glycogen to glucose. Buxton's use of the term "enterotoxin" for type D epsilon toxin may be premature in that the intestine has not been demonstrated as a target organ. In fact, the evidence available to date suggests that the intestine does not have receptor sites for the toxin (Buxton, 1978a). Utilizing a lamb model, Worthington *et al.* (1979) have proposed that the cAMP-induced glycogenolysis and resultant hyperglycemia occur when epsilon toxin causes rapid brain edema which is the trigger for increased release of catecholamines (which stimulate adenyl cyclase).

Studies done with isolated cells (Buxton, 1978c) showed that guinea pig peritoneal macrophages were altered in morphology and eventually killed. The cells became swollen, the nuclear and cytoplasmic membranes became "blistered" and noncontinuous, and the cytoplasm appeared structureless. It is believed that the outer surface of these cells represents the location of the receptors for epsilon toxin. Other cell types studied did not respond to the toxin (pulmonary alveolar macrophages from guinea pigs and rabbits, lymphocytes from guinea pigs and sheep, and peritoneal marcrophages and Lan Schultz ascites-tumor cells from mice).

5. THETA TOXIN

Theta toxin (also known as perfringolysin 0), which is produced by *C. perfringens* types A-E, is a member of the group of bacterial protein toxins known as 'thiol or SH-activated cytolysins'. These toxins have often been referred to as "oxygen-labile hemolysins" (van Heyningen, 1950; Smith, 1975a) in the past but the variability of oxygen lability and dependence of lability upon degree of purity have caused the nomenclature to be improved (Bernheimer, 1974). The term "cytolysins" more accurately describes their ability to affect many cell types other than erythrocytes (Smyth and Duncan, 1978; Bernheimer, 1976; Alouf, 1977; McCartney and Arbuthnott, 1978). The cytolysins, which are produced by gram positive members of the families Bacillaceae, Streptococcaceae, and Lactobacillaceae, are all related in the following ways: (1) addition of cholesterol causes irreversible loss of biological activity; (2) hyperimmune horse serum causes cross-neutralization; (3) they are lethal and cardiotoxic; (4) they have similar pH and temperature optima for cytolytic activity; (5) they lyse numerous erythrocyte species though mouse erythrocytes are characteristically resistant (Smyth and Duncan, 1978).

Molecular weights and isoelectric points reported for theta toxin are given in Table 9. Smyth *et al.* (1972) reported a molecular weight of 61,500 and Smyth and Arbuthnott (1972) reported a pI value of 6.5. Mitsui *et al.* (1973) reported two species of theta toxin, θ_A and θ_B with molecular weights of 53,000 and 50,000, and pI values of 7.05 and 6.65, respectively. Smyth (1975) reported four electrophoretically distinguishable components of theta toxin which he designated θ_1, θ_2, θ_3, and θ_4. Most recently, Yamakawa *et al.* (1977) reported a molecular weight of 51,000 for theta toxin which was in close agreement with the molecular weight calculated from the amino acid composition. The protein was found to be composed of approximately 465 amino acid residues of which over 51 % were lysine, aspartic acid, serine, glutamic acid, and valine. There was found to be one cysteic acid residue per

TABLE 9. *Physical Characteristics of Theta Toxin from* Clostridium perfringens

Authors	Year	Molecular Weight	Isoelectric Point
Smyth, *et al.*	1972	61,500[b]	
Smyth and Arbuthnott	1972		6.5
Mitsui, *et al.*	1973	θ_A 53,000[a]	7.05
		θ_B 50,000[a]	6.65
Möllby and Wadström	1973	60,000–65,000[a]	6.8
Hauschild, *et al.*	1973	74,000[b]	
Smyth	1975	θ_1 60,800–62,000[b]	6.8–6.9
		θ_2 61,600[b]	6.5–6.6
		θ_3 59,500[b]	6.1–6.3
		θ_4 59,000[b]	5.7–5.9
		θ_1–θ_4 200,000–250,000[c]	
Yamakawa, *et al.*	1977	51,000[b]	
Hauschild, *et al.*	1973	35,000–40,000[a, d]	
Smyth	1974	46,000[a, d]	

[a] Determined by gel filtration.

[b] Determined by SDS gel electrophoresis.

[c] Determined by pore gradient polyacrylamide gel electrophoresis.

[d] These may represent cleavage products of the theta toxin that have reduced or no activity.

molecule. Mitsui *et al.* (1973) also did amino acid analysis of θ_A and θ_B fractions. The molar ratios they reported (converted to number of residues by Smyth and Duncan, 1978) are in agreement with Yamakawa *et al.* (1977) for some amino acids but not others. Lysine was determined to be the N-terminal residue which confirms the earlier observation of Hauschild *et al.* (1973b). The purified theta toxin showed a single band on SDS gel electrophoresis.

Theta toxin is responsible for the zone of clear hemolysis that surrounds colonies on blood agar plates. It is also noted for its lethal and necrotizing activities (Smith, 1975a). A report by Soda *et al.* (1976) suggests that the hemolytic and lethal activities of the toxin may be separate. It is reversibly inactivated by mild exposure to oxygen or oxidizing agents and is reactivated by thiol-reducing agents (but not other reducing agents, Mitsui and Hase, 1979) such as cysteine, 2-mercaptoethanol, dithiothreitol and sodium thioglycolate (Smyth and Duncan, 1978). It seems likely that theta toxin contains SH groups (which are subject to reversible oxidation to S-S linkages) that are essential to its hemolytic activity (Smith, 1975a). Mitsui and Hase (1979) have recently supported this concept with data suggesting that the active form of the toxin has free thiol groups in its active site. These are changed to disulfide bonds with loss of activity by the exchange reaction between disulfide reagents having high E_0' (oxidation-reduction potential) value. In addition, an unknown sulfide bond (possibly extramolecular) in the toxin's inactive form may be reductively cleaved by thiols to form free thiol groups, thereby affecting recovery of the activity. Theta toxin is thermolabile (Duncan, 1975) and markedly temperature-dependent in that its activity rises sharply as temperature increases to 37°C but drops off sharply as the temperature is raised above 37°C. The hemolytic activity also is markedly dependent upon pH with the optimum activity at pH 6.7–6.8. Hydrogen ion concentrations above or below these values cause rapid loss of activity (Smith, 1975a).

It has been known for many years that cholesterol irreversibly inactivates reduced theta toxin (Howard *et al.*, 1953; Smyth and Duncan, 1978). The stereochemical specificity of sterol inhibition of theta toxin has been studied by Howard *et al.* (1953) and Hase *et al.* (1976). Sterols which contain alcohol functional groups, are an important subclass of the compounds called steroids. Steroids are compounds containing the basic perhydrocyclopentanophenanthrene carbon skeleton (see Masoro, 1968, for a lucid description of these substances). The β-OH group on C-3 was found to be essential on cholesterol and related sterol molecules for inhibitory activity. The presence of an α-OH group, an ester bond, or a keto group on C-3 caused the sterols to be incapable of inactivating the toxin. In addition, a hydrophobic group on C-17 (D ring) appears to be a prerequisite for inhibitory activity (Hase *et al.*, 1976). Unpublished data of Watson and Smyth have been reported (1978) to support, for theta toxin, studies done with streptolysin 0 (Watson and Kerr, 1974; Prigent and Alouf, 1976) which showed that various other substitutions on the sterol molecules that interfere with the β-OH of C-3 also alter inactivation potential.

There are numerous problems associated with determining the number of molecules of particular sterol that are necessary to inactivate a molecule of theta toxin (reviewed by Smyth and Duncan, 1978). In view of these problems, Smyth (1975) has reported that 1,500 cholesterol molecules are required per theta toxin molecule to affect inactivation. The exact nature of interaction between cholesterol and theta toxin is not known. Some hypotheses have been presented for other cytolysins that are similar to theta toxin, and more highly studied (Smyth and Duncan, 1978).

Cells that do not contain cholesterol are insensitive to the SH-activated cytolysins which have been studied. The hemolytic activity of theta toxin is abolished if the toxin is preincubated with erythrocyte membranes (Smyth, 1975). It has been shown indirectly that theta toxin appears to bind to erythrocyte membranes and that the inactivating substance in membranes is lipid and must be a fraction containing cholesterol (or ergosterol). Phospholipids do not inactivate the toxin (Hase *et al.*, 1975). Binding of theta toxin to cells appears, unlike hemolysins, to be independent of temperature. Binding occurs at 0°C while lysis does not. But if cells bound with theta toxin are raised in temperature to 37°C they lyse (Hase *et al.*, 1975). It is believed that hemolysis due to cytolysins is a multi-hit phenomenon and theta toxin has been demonstrated to require 2 and sometimes 3 hits for hemolysis to occur (Inoue *et al.*, 1976). Mitsui *et al.* (1979) have suggested that 7 molecules of theta toxin per human erythrocyte are sufficient to cause complete hemolysis. They reported that the toxin causes altered bilayer portions ('cavities') in the membrane structure of the erythrocytes. They also noted a random aggregation of intramembranous particles on the protoplasmic face of membranes treated with low concentrations of theta toxin.

Theta toxin has been shown to have a membrane effect upon several cell types aside from erythrocytes. Wilkinson (1975) demonstrated that the locomotor response of human blood neutrophils is inhibited by theta toxin. Freholm *et al.* (1978) have shown that theta toxin acts quickly, and, prior to development of clear-cut morphological alterations, antagonizes noradrenaline-stimulated cyclic $3'-5'$ adenosine monophosphate (cyclic AMP) accumulation and lipolysis in isolated rat adipocytes. They concluded that the onset of affect is so rapid that an enzymatic mechanism of action is unlikely. They hypothesize that lipolysis inhibition results from a decrease in cellular concentration of cyclic AMP and possibly ions such as calcium. Strandberg *et al.* (1974) demonstrated that theta toxin causes a zinc-inhibitable release of histamine from rat mast cells. Gill and King (1975) reported an interesting phenomenon in that membrane ghosts, prepared by lysing erythrocytes with theta toxin, did not reseal or vessicularize. Thelestam and Möllby (1975a; 1975b) demonstrated that functional pores were formed by theta toxin in human diploid fibroblasts that allowed for passage of nucleotides but not larger molecules. Unlike other membrane-active agents they studied, theta toxin did not cause an increase in the size of the functional pores with time. The size of pores and the functional alterations noted by Thelestam and Möllby led them to support the postulation that theta toxin interacts with membrane cholesterol in these cells. The absence of morphological alterations in fibroblasts may be due to the integrity of the rapid membrane repair mechanisms which are lacking in erythrocyte ghosts. More recently, Thelestam and Möllby (1980), in comparing the activities of theta toxin and streptolysin 0 in human fibroblasts, have called to question the current concept that all thiol-activated cholesterol-inactivated bacterial toxins are similar both structurally and functionally.

The activity of theta toxin is particularly important, aside from pathological considerations, in that many studies on mechanisms of action reported in the past for other substances such as *C. perfringens* alpha toxin (Möllby *et al.*, 1976; Smyth, *et al.*, 1975) and neuraminidase (Chien *et al.*, 1975; Den *et al.*, 1975; Rood and Wilkinson, 1974) have been shown to be contaminated with theta toxin.

Smyth *et al.* (1975) showed that commercial preparations of alpha toxin caused arc-shaped structures to form in the membranes of horse erythrocyte ghosts. These are similar to the 'pits' or 'holes' found during immune lysis of erythrocytes by antibody and complement (Dourmashkin and Rosse, 1966; Iles, *et al.*, 1973). These same structures were found when the ghosts were treated with highly purified theta toxin, while they were absent when treated with highly purified alpha toxin. When large doses of purified theta toxin were used the ghosts were actually fragmented. Similar arc-shaped structures have been shown to be produced by other cytolysins such as cerolysin (Cowell *et al.*, 1978) and tetanolysin (Rottem *et al.*, 1976). By using lipid dispersions and liposomes, Smyth *et al.* (1975) were able to show that cholesterol was the membrane constituent necessary for ring formation.

The relationship of structural alterations to the lytic mechanism is unknown at this time (Smyth and Duncan, 1978). An interesting description of the course of events for hemolysis by a cytolysin such as theta toxin has been postulated by Smyth and Duncan (1978) in which the toxin sequesters cholesterol in the membrane thereby permitting a lipid phase-transition to occur. The result is an increase in membrane fluidity and permeability. Much more work must be done before the exact mechanism whereby the observed structural and functional alterations occur as a result of the action of theta and related thio-activated cytolysins.

The role played by theta toxin in disease is unknown at this time. It has been shown to be lethal upon intravenous injection into mice but its lethal effect is not generally believed to be additive when co-injected with alpha toxin. However, according to Soda *et al.* (1976), theta toxin, when co-injected with alpha toxin into mice, enhances the speed of death even though the dose of toxin necessary to kill the animal is not lowered. Muscle tissue is not thought to adsorb theta toxin and may even suppress its production. For this reason there is question about the toxin's role in clostridial myonecrosis (Duncan, 1975).

6. ENTEROTOXIN

C. perfringens enterotoxin is responsible for one of the most common types of food poisoning in the United States (Genigeorgis, 1975; Duncan, 1970; Chakrabarty *et al.*, 1977; Shandera *et al.*, 1983). It is most often associated with meat, poultry and gravy-containing dishes (Smart *et al.*, 1979; Duncan, 1975; Genigeorgis, 1975; Duncan, 1970) which are served or stored in large quantities. An extensive treatment of all aspects of the disease and the causative organisms has been presented by Walker (1975). While food poisoning due to *C. perfringens* was described as early as 1945 (McClung, 1945) it was not until the classic report by Hobbs *et al.* (1953) that the organism began to acquire its deserved attention as one of major public importance. Most if not all cases of classical *C. perfringens* food poisoning are caused by strains from type A. Strains isolated from human food poisoning cases do not appear to be limited to any particular group of type A, that is to say, they may be (a) beta-hemolytic, heat sensitive, like gas gangrene strains, (b) partially hemolytic, heat-resistant, (c) partially hemolytic, or heat-sensitive (Hauschild, 1973; Hall *et al.*, 1963; Hauschild and Thatcher, 1967; Hauschild and Thatcher, 1968; Sutton and Hobbs, 1968). Pinegar and Stringer recently reported the isolation of lecithinase-negative type A strains believed to be responsible for food poisoning outbreaks (Pinegar and Stringer, 1977). However, caution must be exercised in that many enterotoxin positive strains are very weak producers of alpha toxin, and very sensitive assays are necessary to detect the toxin. The standard egg yolk plate test is likely to be of insufficient sensitivity to detect the small amounts of alpha toxin from a weak producer. And, there are restrictions in the use of this assay to detect alpha toxin (Rigby, 1981). Enterotoxin production appears not to be restricted to any particular agglutinating serotype of type A, though it may be common to the entire group of Hobb's serotypes (Niilo, 1973c; Chakrabarty and Narayan, 1979). Strains of Hobb's serotypes 4, 5, and 7 have not been shown to produce enterotoxin however. It has been proposed that these strains, isolated from food poisoning cases, may have lost their ability to produce enterotoxin. Enterotoxin production by strains of type C (Skjelkvalé and Duncan, 1975a; Skjelkvalé and Duncan, 1975b) and type D (Uemura and Skjelkvalé, 1976) have been described but the role in intestinal disease of enterotoxin produced by these strains is not clear at this time. The disease is thought to be confined to humans though there is a report that may link type A enterotoxin to equine grass sickness (Ochoa and Velandia, 1978).

Onset of primary symptoms of the disease (diarrhea and abdominal cramps) is usually 6–12 hours and duration is usually 12–24 hours. Some cases involve nausea and headache, but emesis and fever are rare (Hobbs, 1969; Yamagishi *et al.*, 1983). Fatal cases are rare but have been associated with elderly or debilitated persons.

Early studies done with whole cells were performed by introduction of viable cultures of *C. perfringens* into the intestinal tracts of lambs (Hauschild *et al.*, 1967), sheep (Niilo *et al.*, 1971) and rabbits (Duncan *et al.*, 1968; Duncan and Strong, 1969b; Duncan and Strong, 1971; Strong *et al.*, 1971). The discovery that an enteropathogenic factor (Duncan and Strong, 1969a; Hauschild *et al*, 1970b; Niilo, 1971; Hauschild *et al.*, 1970a) is produced during sporulation (Duncan and Strong, 1969a; Duncan *et al.*, 1972) led to the isolation and purification (Hauschild and Hilsheimer, 1971; Stark and Duncan, 1972b; Sakaguchi *et al.*, 1973; Hauschild *et al.*, 1973a; Scott and Duncan, 1975; Uemura and Skjelkvalé, 1976; Enders and Duncan, 1977; Granum and Whitaker, 1980a) of a protein toxin. This toxin has been shown to be the factor primarily responsible for experimental disease induced in lambs (Hauschild *et al.*, 1967; Hauschild *et al.*, 1970a; Niilo, 1971), sheep (Niilo, 1971; Niilo, 1972; Niilo *et al.*, 1971), calves (Niilo, 1973a; Niilo, 1973b), chickens (Niilo, 1974; Niilo, 1976), dogs (Bartlett *et al.*, 1972), rats, (McDonel, 1974; McDonel and Asano, 1975; McDonel *et al.*, 1978), rabbits (Duncan and Strong, 1971; Strong *et al.*, 1971; Hauschild *et al.*, 1971a; Niilo, 1971; McDonel *et al.*, 1978; McDonel and Duncan, 1975c; McDonel and Duncan,

1977), guinea pigs (Niilo, 1971), mice (Miwantani *et al.*, 1978; Yamaoto *et al.*, 1979), horses (Ochoa and Kern, 1980), monkeys (Uemura *et al.*, 1975; Duncan and Strong, 1971; Hauschild *et al.*, 1971b) and humans (Strong *et al.*, 1971; Skjelkvalé and Uemura, 1977b).

The physical characteristics of *C. perfringens* enterotoxin are outlined in Table 10. Aside from values obtained with SDS gels, the average molecular weight determined by most workers has been about 35,000. Anomalous aggregation of the enterotoxin into high molecular weight forms when subjected to detergent gel electrophoresis has been reported by Skjelkvalé and Duncan (1975b) and Enders and Duncan (1976). They reported that the high molecular weight values corresponded to multiples of a theoretical subunit of molecular weight of 17,500. However, in our experience, SDS gel electrophoresis of enterotoxin has consistently given a single band with a position equivalent to a molecular weight of about 35,000 (Smith and McDonel, 1980). Yotis and Catsimpoolas (1975) have reported isoelectric focusing and isotachophoretic data that support the concept of the enterotoxin being a two-component entity. However, Enders and Ducan (1976) and Granum and Skjelkvalé (1977) also have demonstrated that the protein is a single polypeptide chain with a molecular weight of about 34,000. Smith and McDonel (1980) recently reported an *in vitro* system to synthesize *C. perfringens* enterotoxin. They found that *in vitro* synthesized material that was precipitated with anti-enterotoxin serum had formed three bands on SDS gels that represented molecular weights of approximately 17,000, 35,000, and 52,000. They have proposed that the enterotoxin may be a precursor (molecular weight > 35,000) of a spore coat component (see below). The spore coat component is envisioned to have a molecular

TABLE 10. *Physical Characteristics of Enterotoxin from* Clostridium perfringens *Type A*

Authors	Year	Molecular Weight	Isoelectric Point	Sedimentation Coefficient
Hauschild and Hilsheimer	1971	36,000[a] ± 4,000	4.3	
Stark and Duncan	1972	34,000[a] ± 3,000 35,000[c]	4.3	3.08
Sakaguchi *et al.*	1973		4.3	
Hauschild *et al.*	1973	40,000[d] 36,000[c] 33,000[e]		2.79
Skjelkvalé and Duncan	1975a	37,000[f]-Type C		
Skjelkvalé and Duncan	1975b	36,000[a] 33,400[c] 68,000[b] 85,000[b] 105,000[b] 140,000[b]	4.3	2.92
Yotis and Catsimpoolas	1975		4.5 major 4.6 minor	
Freiben and Duncan	1975	38,000[f]		4.43
Enders and Duncan	1976	33,500[b] 52,000[b] 69,000[b]-most common 82,000[b] 108,000[b] 140,000[b]	4.38 major 4.50 minor	
Granum and Skjelkvalé	1977	34,000[c]		
McDonel and Smith	1979	17,500[b] 35,000[b] 52,000[b]		

[a]Determined by filtration chromatography.
[b]Determined by SDS gel electrophoresis.
[c]Determined by sedimentation equilibration.
[d]Determined by ultracentrifugation (Archibald method).
[e]Determined by amino acid analysis.
[f]Determined by polyacrylamide gel electrophoresis.

weight of approximately 17,000, while the precursor (enterotoxin) is a single polypeptide chain that has one or more components contained within. This may explain the 'subunits' reported by Enders and Duncan, and Skjelkvalé and Duncan, and the homology between enterotoxin and spore coat components (Freiben and Duncan, 1973, 1975). Freiben and Duncan (1975) reported the existence of enterotoxin-like proteins, that were serologically reactive with anti-enterotoxin serum, which could be extracted from spores of enterotoxin-positive as well as enterotoxin-negative strains. These proteins were labeled Type I (mol. wt. = 36,500; pI = 4.43), Type II (mol. wt. = 23,000; pI = 4.36), and Type III (mol. wt. = 14,500; pI = 4.52). The enterotoxin reported by Skjelkvalé and Duncan (1975a; 1975b) to have a molecular weight of 36,000–37,000 was purified from type C strains and is apparently indistinguishable from enterotoxin produced by type A strains. Sakaguchi *et al.* (1973) reported that the molecular weight of enterotoxin purified by ammonium sulfate and gel filtration through Sephadex G-200 was similar to that reported elsewhere, but they did not report the exact values they obtained.

Amino acid analysis of the enterotoxin has been done which indicates that the enterotoxin molecule, with approximately 300 amino acid residues, is composed predominantly of aspartic acid, serine, leucine, glutamic acid, isoleucine, glycine and threonine (Hauschild *et al.*, 1973a). Granum and Skjelkvalé (1977) reported results that agreed closely with those of Hauschild *et al.* (1973a). However, Hauschild *et al.* reported the presence of 2 cysteic acid residues per molecule of enterotoxin while Granum and Skjelkvalé reported 1 cysteic acid residue. Enders and Duncan (1976) alluded to having found an amino acid composition comparable to that reported by Hauschild *et al.*, but values were not given. Recent studies have reconfirmed that the enterotoxin is a single polypeptide chain. The sequence of the first 20 amino acids of the NH_2-terminal has been determined to be: Met-Leu-Ser-Asn-Asn-Leu-Asn-Pro-Met-Val-Phe-Glu-Asn-Ala-Lys-Glu-Val-Phe-Leu-Ile (Duffy *et al.*, 1982). This sequence has been more recently confirmed by Richardson and Granum (1983) and carried further up to the first 66 amino acids. Granum *et al.* (1981), while not identifying the NH_2-terminal, reported that glycine is the C-terminal residue. Salinovich *et al.* (1982) have reported observations on the molecular conformation of the enterotoxin molecule under various conditions of temperature, pH and detergents and conclude that the conformational properties are very similar to those observed for the lectins. Dasgupta and Pariza (1982) have reported two different forms of the enterotoxin but this could likely be due to improper technique, such as failure to routinely autoclave buffers to destroy contaminating proteases.

Other characteristics of the enterotoxin molecule that have been reported are as follows. It is heat labile, i.e., 60°C for 5 minutes destroys biological activity though serological activity can be retained (10 % of original serological activity) even after 80 minutes at 60°C (Naik and Duncan, 1978a). Loss of serological activity is more rapid at 60°C if the pH is 6.0 or less. If heat-inactivated in food samples, about 12 % of the serological activity destroyed by heating at 60°C can be restored by treatment with urea for 1 hour at room temperature (Naik and Duncan, 1978a). Granum and Skjelkvalé (1977) reported 90 % loss of biological activity at 60°C after 1 minute. They reported that enterotoxin heat-inactivated at 55°C for 1 minute (70 % loss of activity) regained 50 % of the original activity after 4 days. Enterotoxin heated for 15 minutes or more did not regain activity. The enterotoxin loses its activity during pronase and subtilisin treatment, but is insensitive to trypsin, chymotrypsin, bacterial lipase, steapsin, α-amylase, papain, and neuraminidase (Duncan and Strong, 1969a; Hauschild and Hilsheimer, 1971). Loss of activity occurs at pH 1.0, 3.0, 5.0, and 12.0 (Duncan and Strong, 1969a). It is essentially free of nucleic acids, fatty acids, lipid phosphorus, and reducing sugars, and has a UV absorption spectrum with a maximum of 278–280 nm and a minimum of 250 nm. It has a stokes' radius of 2.6 nm (Hauschild and Hilsheimer, 1971; Sakaguchi *et al.*, 1973). Enders and Duncan (1976) have suggested that the acidic protein may have hydrophobic regions created by clustered hydrophobic amino acids which comprise about 40 % of the residues in the molecule. They also were unable to find in the enterotoxin the presence of ligands, free fatty acids, protease activity, or phospholipase activity. They reported the presence of less than 0.1 % lipid, 0.2 % nucleic acid, and no protein-bound carbohydrate.

Whitaker and Granum (1980) have studied the lability of enterotoxin biological and serological activity with modification of amino groups by reductive alkylation, acelylation and succinylation. Granum and Whitaker (1980b) have proposed an amphiphatic model for the enterotoxin based upon protein modification studies using sodium dodecyl sulfate, guanidine hydrochloride, pH, and heat.

As mentioned above, Duncan and Strong (1969a) and Duncan et al. (1972) have demonstrated that enterotoxin is produced only by sporulating cells which distinguishes this toxin from other toxins produced by C. perfringens. Sporulation and enterotoxin production have been shown to be dependent upon pH, temperature, and carbohydrate availability in culture (Labbe and Duncan, 1974; Labbe and Duncan, 1975). Mutants blocked in sporulation earlier than stage III do not produce enterotoxin while ones blocked at stage III produce small amounts, and ones blocked at late stage IV and stage V are able to produce enterotoxin (Duncan et al., 1972). They concluded that the enterotoxin is a sporulation-specific gene product. Duncan (1973) and Labbe and Duncan (1977a; 1977b) have suggested that enterotoxin formation, which may involve a stable messenger RNA, appears to begin approximately 2.5 to 3 hours after inoculation into sporulation medium. This corresponds to late stage II or early stage III of sporulation. Smith and McDonel (1980) have isolated polysomes from cultures 1 hr after inoculation that produce enterotoxin in vitro. Duncan et al. (1973) described a paracrystalline inclusion that is found only in sporulating cells that are enterotoxin producers, which may be an aggregate of enterotoxin or enterotoxin-like spore coat protein material. When sporulation mutants were studied the inclusions appeared only in cells blocked no earlier than stage IV of sporulation. The relationship of enterotoxin to spore coat proteins was further detailed by Frieben and Duncan (1973, 1975). They found that anti-enterotoxin serum precipitated protein material extracted from spores of enterotoxin-positive as well as negative strains. Furthermore, the material was associated with spore 'coat' fractions but not spore 'core' fractions. They concluded that the enterotoxin is a spore coat structural component. Further characterization of this spore coat protein revealed that three distinct enterotoxin-like proteins can be extracted which Frieben and Duncan (1975) named types I, II, and III (mol. wts., 14,500, 23,000 and 36,500, respectively; see Table 10). All three of these proteins retained biological activity characteristic of purified enterotoxin (mol. wt., 35,000). The enterotoxin-like proteins (types I and II) particularly support the concept of a subunit(s) within the enterotoxin molecule that has typical biological and serological activity. Smith and McDonel (1980) have demonstrated that proteins synthesized in vitro by polysomes extracted from vegetative cells do not produce protein(s) precipitable by anti-enterotoxin serum. However, polysomes from cells grown in Duncan–Strong sporulation medium (1968) produced anti-enterotoxin serum precipitable proteins after one hour (early stage of sporulation) of incubation. At six hours, 12% of the total protein produced by the polysomes was precipitable with the anti-enterotoxin serum. The precipitated material (see Table 10) had molecular weights of 17,000, 35,000, and 52,000 as determined by SDS gel electrophoresis. These data support the earlier observation that enterotoxin is a sporulation-specific product (Duncan and Strong, 1969a; Duncan et al., 1972) and has given rise to the suggestion (McDonel, and Smith 1980) that enterotoxin may be precursor molecule for the spore coat component described by Frieben and Duncan (1973, 1975). Only recently has further work been undertaken to elaborate in more detail the physiology of sporulation and enterotoxin production by this organism (Löffler and Labbe, 1983).

The presence of plasmids has been described for C. perfringens (Sebald et al., 1975; Sebald and Bréfort, 1975; Rood et al., 1978a; Rood et al., 1978b) but aside from one identified plasmid that may control beta toxin production (Duncan et al., 1978), plasmid control of other toxins including enterotoxin has not yet been demonstrated.

Several biological and serological assay systems have been developed for the detection and quantitation of enterotoxin. It appears that the biological activity of the enterotoxin is more labile than the serological activity (McDonel and McClane, 1981) and the specific (biological/serological) activity tends to vary considerable from one preparation to another. While biologically active material will always be serologically active, the converse is not necessarily true. Conversion factors (Niilo, 1975) from assays of one activity to the other should be avoided. For mode of action studies, enterotoxin doses that are presented only in terms of mass (i.e., 10 μg/injection) have very limited meaning. It is also important to note that the biological activity of enterotoxin solutions, even when stored frozen at $-20°C$ begin to lose activity within weeks of storage (McDonel and McClane, 1981). While reference will be made in the discussions to follow of quantities of enterotoxin (mass units) it is to be understood that biological activity/unit mass varies considerably from one enterotoxin preparation to another.

The earliest assay of the enterotoxin's biological activity was the rabbit ligated ileal loop test (Duncan and Strong, 1969a). This assay is based upon the response of the intestine to the enterotoxin, which is a net secretion of fluid and electrolytes into the lumen. The result is a noticeable expansion of the loops due to the excess fluid. The assay is inconvenient, relatively insensitive, and expensive. Stark and Duncan (1972a) reported that the minimal dose detectable by this assay is 140–200 EU (erythemal units, see definition below) or 29 μg (Genigeorgis et al., 1973). Hauschild et al. (1971a) described a rapid and more sensitive ligated loop technique in rabbits that could detect as little as 2.5 EU (6.25 μg) within 90 minutes of intraluminal challenge with enterotoxin. Niilo (1974) has described a chicken ligated ileal loop assay system that will detect 20 to 30 μg per loop (biological activity unknown).

Probably the most generally applicable assay of biological activity reported to date is one based on the observations by Hauschild (1970) and Stark and Duncan (1971) that the enterotoxin, when injected intradermally, causes erythema in guinea pig or rabbit skin. The erythemal unit has been defined as that amount of enterotoxin that causes a zone of erythema 0.8 cm in diameter on the skin of a dipilitated guinea pig which has received intradermal injections of the enterotoxin (Stark and Duncan, 1971). Results are usually read at 18–24 hours after injection. This assay is more sensitive, less expensive, and easier than the ileal loop test. It can detect, with reasonable accuracy, quantities of enterotoxin as low as 0.25–0.5 EU. Detection has been reported of quantities as small as 0.06–0.125 μg (Genigeorgis et al., 1973). However, a linear dose-response curve can be seen only over a range of about 0.5 to 2.0 EU, at best. Specific activities of highly purified enterotoxin range from as high as 5,000 to as low as 2,000 EU/mg protein. It is very unusual to encounter specific activities over 3,600 EU/mg and the most commonly encountered activity is around 2,000 to 2,500 EU/mg.

Another assay that has received some use is the mouse lethality assay (Hauschild and Hilsheimer, 1971; Stark and Duncan, 1971; Genigeorgis et al., 1973; Niilo, 1975). It has been proposed that mouse lethality results from the enterotoxin's activity on the portion of the brain controlling respiration (Miwantani et al., 1978). No effect upon the heart, embryonic heart cells grown in culture, or neuromuscular junctions was noted. Niilo (1975) reported that one LD_{50} for the average 18 g mouse was about 5 EU (1.46 μg) when injected intravenously.

The most highly sensitive biological assay has recently been developed by McDonel and McClane (1981) that utilizes inhibition by the enterotoxin of plating efficiency of Vero (African green monkey kidney) cells grown in tissue culture (McClane and McDonel, 1979). This effect has been used to detect as little as 2.5×10^{-4} EU (0.1 ng of protein). This corresponds to a concentration of 2.5×10^{-3} EU/ml (1 ng/ml). A linear dose-response curve is obtained with dilutions containing between 1.25×10^{-3} and 1.25×10^{-2} EU (0.5–5 ng). Doses over 0.25 EU (100 ng) cause inhibition of plating efficiency to approach 100%. They have described a new unit of biological activity, called the plating efficiency unit (PEU), which is defined as that amount of enterotoxin causing inhibition of plating of 25% of 200 cells inoculated into the test wells (100 μl). Enterotoxin with a specific activity of 2,000 EU/mg has 400,000 PEU/mg (1 PEU = 2.5 ng, or 2.5 ng/ml). Erythemal activity and plating efficiency inhibiting activity correlate very closely with one another.

Granum (1982) has adapted into an assay the observation of McClane and McDonel (1981) that protein synthesis by Vero cells is inhibited by the enterotoxin. He reports detection of as little as 30 ng of enterotoxin which is about four times more sensitive than the erythemal skin test but 300 times less sensitive than the Vero cell plating efficiency assay mentioned above. Granum also reports trypsin-induced breakdown of the molecule and enhancement of biological activity which has not been noted by others (Duncan and Strong, 1969a; and personal communications with other laboratories studying this problem currently). More work needs to be done to confirm either the trypsin sensitivity or insensitivity of this enterotoxin molecule (Richardson and Granum, 1983).

Serological assays have been developed with excellent sensitivity and reproducibility. The Ouchterlony double-immunodiffusion method performed on standard microscope slides (Stark and Duncan, 1971) allows identification of enterotoxin (Genigeorgis et al., 1973). However, this method is not nearly as sensitive as electroimmunodiffusion, single gel diffusion tube, or reverse passive hemagglutinin (RPHA) techniques. Duncan and Somers (1972) reported that electroimmunodiffusion could detect as little as 0.01 μg (1 μg/ml) of enterotoxin while single gel diffusion could detect 3 μg/ml. Genigeorgis et al. (1973) reported that microslide diffusion could detect 0.013 μg (0.50 μg/ml) while the single gel diffusion method could detect 0.3 μg (0.9 μg/ml). Counter-immunoelectrophoresis (CIEP), a rapid, sensitive, and specific assay, has been used to detect as little as 0.002 μg (0.2 μg/ml) of enterotoxin (Naik and Duncan, 1977b). RPHA is reported to be sensitive to quantities of enterotoxin as small as 0.05 ng (0.5 ng/ml) (Genigeorgis et al., 1973; Uemura et al., 1973). Olsvik et al. (1982) have reported detection of as little enterotoxin as 0.1 ng/ml in the purified state and 1.0 ng/ml in heterogeneous solutions utilizing a four-layer sandwich ELISA (enzyme-linked immunosorbent assay). Similar values are reported by McClane and Strouse (unpublished observations) in a more rapid indirect ELISA for the enterotoxin. Fluorescent antibody has been used to detect intracellular enterotoxin in small numbers of sporulating cells (Niilo, 1977). The efficacy of numerous of these serological tests for laboratory detection of enterotoxigenic C. perfringens has been reviewed by Niilo (1978, 1979). Skjelkvalé and Uemura (1977a) have utilized RPHA and CIEP to detect enterotoxin in feces of food poisoning victims. Naik and Duncan (1977a, 1978b) have used CIEP to detect enterotoxin in foods and human feces.

At one time it was believed that fluid accumulation in the gut resulting from C. perfringens enteritis was due to alpha toxin (Nygren, 1962), but alpha toxin now is known not to be responsible for the diarrhea in this disease (Hauschild et al., 1967; Hauschild et al., 1971b). The enterotoxin's ability to cause fluid accumulation in intestinal loops was first demonstrated in rabbits (Duncan and Strong, 1969a) and lambs (Hauschild et al., 1970b). The erythemal reaction to the enterotoxin in guinea pig and rabbit skin (Hauschild, 1970) was used by Stark and Duncan (1971) to develop an assay for its biological activity. They also demonstrated that the erythema is associated with an increase in capillary permeability (Stark and Duncan, 1972a). The increase in capillary permeability was reported by Niilo (1971) to occur within 15–20 minutes of intradermal injection. In the same report Niilo described the systemic effects of the enterotoxin when injected intravenously into rabbits, lambs, and guinea pigs. The responses of all three species are outlined in Table 11. The enterotoxin has been shown to be capable of causing depression of blood pressure in sheep as well (Niilo, 1972). Marked differences were noted in a similar study done with calves (Niilo, 1973b) in that they did not develop lacrimation, salivation, nasal discharge, or diarrhea, but intestinal hyperemia and mucosal sloughing did occur. It is believed that the enterotoxin has a strong predilection for the intestinal capillary bed. Niilo also reported that fluid accumulation in bovine thirty fistulas can occur within 30 minutes exposure to the enterotoxin (1973a).

All biological activities of C. perfringens enterotoxin so far described have been found to be neutralizable with specific antiserum prepared against the enterotoxin. Immunization of sheep (Niilo et al., 1971) against the enterotoxin prevented development of characteristic systemic reactions upon intravenous injection of the enterotoxin. However, the immunized sheep were as susceptible as control sheep to intraluminal enterotoxin challenge. At the same time Uemura et al. (1975) showed that intraluminal enterotoxin challenge in monkeys confers no detectable immunity (serum anti-enterotoxin titer) in the animals. It appears that with intraluminal challenge (the challenge route of C. perfringens food poisoning)

TABLE 11. *Systemic Effects of Enterotoxin When Injected Intravenously into Lambs, Rabbits, and Guinea Pigs*[a]

I. Parasympathomimetic Properties
capillary permeability
vasodilation in intestine
increased intestinal motility

II. Other Effects
diarrhea
lacrimation
salivation
nasal discharge
lassitude
dyspnea
hyperemic intestinal mucosa
congestion of:
    liver
    lungs
    spleen
    kidneys

[a] From Niilo (1971).

enterotoxin does not penetrate to the immune system either to induce formation of specific antibodies or to be neutralized by them. But, Uemura *et al.* (1974) found that 85 % Brazilians and 65 % of Americans sampled had substantial antienterotoxin serum titers. Niilo and Bainborough (1980) have reported detectable antienterotoxin titers in the blood of humans, cattle, horse and swine in western Canada. While the results of the study by Niilo *et al.* (1971) would imply that these titers in humans are unable to prevent *C. perfringens* food poisoning, accessibility of the enterotoxin to the blood stream must be possible by a mechanism absent in simple intraluminal challenge with enterotoxin in experimental models. The frequency of detectable titers in humans studied gives good indication of the high exposure and carrier rate of *C. perfringens* type A food poisoning organisms. Skjelkvalé and Uemura (1977a; 1977b) reported an increase in serum antienterotoxin titer over a 60 day period in cases of human food poisoning due to *C. perfringens* but enterotoxin was not detected in the serum.

Progress has been made during the last five years in defining precisely the physiological and pathological changes caused in the gut by *C. perfringens* enterotoxin (McDonel, 1979). It is important to review the literature during these years in considerable detail since current reports and reviews continue to be published that appear to be without awareness of the considerable progress that has been made (Yamamoto *et al.*, 1979; Plotkin *et al.*, 1979). The rat ileum was used as the first model system to describe transport alterations due to the enterotoxin (McDonel, 1974). In the rat ileum, when treated with the enterotoxin, there was a reversal of transport from absorption in controls, to secretion of fluid, sodium, and chloride. Glucose absorption was inhibited while transport of potassium and bicarbonate was unaffected. Fluid secretion was found to increase with enterotoxin dose up to a point beyond which excess enterotoxin had no effect. This saturation phenomenon was confirmed in another report in which rabbit ileal loops were challenged with a range of 50 (minimum dose to cause fluid accumulation) to 1,000 erythemal units (EU) of enterotoxin (McDonel and Duncan, 1977). The amount of fluid accumulation was indistinguishable in loops treated with each dose. Protein levels (an indication of tissue damage) in loop contents increased with dose in loops treated with 50 to 250 EU but did not change with challenges from 250 to 1,000 EU. Desquamation of intestinal epithelial cells was noted to occur at villus tips in enterotoxin-treated loops. Niilo (1971) has reported epithelial desquamation after intravenous injection of enterotoxin. Intestinal epithelial desquamation from intraluminal challenge with the enterotoxin has since been confirmed in rats (McDonel and Asano, 1975; McDonel and Duncan, 1975b) and rabbits (McDonel and Duncan, 1977; Hauschild *et al.*, 1973a; McDonel *et al.*, 1978). The increased intestinal motility that has been observed in these animal models has been quantitated by Justus *et al.* (1980). They conclude that the enterotoxin-induced increase in myoelectric activity could explain the characteristic abdominal cramps and mucosal injury associated with experimental or actual cases of perfringens food poisoning.

When net transport of sodium in the rat ileum was resolved into unidirectional fluxes (McDonel and Asano, 1975) it was found that sodium uptake (influx) was identical in control and enterotoxin-treated animals. Net loss of sodium in enterotoxin-treated animals was shown to be due to nearly a two-fold increase in sodium efflux to the lumen.

Studies done with rat everted ileal sacs (McDonel and Duncan, 1975a) revealed that the enterotoxin causes a significant reduction in oxygen consumption by the sacs. It was concluded that oxidative metabolism is inhibited while glycolysis is unaffected because glucose was absorbed and lactate produced in equivalent quantities by enterotoxin-treated and control sacs. A similar (30%) enterotoxin-induced decrease in oxygen consumption by mitochondria from rat liver and beef heart was reported (McDonel and Duncan, 1976) though the rate of phosphate esterification (ATP production) coupled to substrate oxidation (P:O ratios) was unaffected.

Removal of enterotoxin from the rat gut after as little as 10 minutes exposure will not prevent typical responses from developing at their normal rate, and overt tissue damage can occur within 15 minutes of exposure to the enterotoxin (McDonel and Duncan, 1975a; McDonel, 1974). Yamamoto et al. (1979) reported that removal of enterotoxin from mouse ligated loops caused a reduction in fluid accumulation, even if the loop was exposed to enterotoxin for 30 minutes prior to removal. They concluded that the enterotoxin does not bind freely to the intestinal cells. However, much more sophisticated binding techniques must be used before conclusions can be made about cell membrane-enterotoxin binding interactions (see below). Studies with the rabbit have revealed that the enterotoxin is most active in the ileum, mildly active in the jejunum, and nearly inactive in the duodenum (McDonel and Duncan, 1977). Activities measured included tissue damage and transport of fluid, sodium, chloride, and glucose. Net sodium fluxes in all three sections of the small intestine were resolved into unidirectional fluxes (McDonel, unpublished data). The results in the ileum confirmed those already reported for the rat (McDonel and Asano, 1975), but sodium transport appeared unaffected in the jejunum and duodenum. However, slight tissue damage was evident in jejunal sections so the relationship between tissue damage and electrolyte transport in this model system is not yet clear (McDonel, 1980a). McDonel and Demers (1982) have demonstrated that the colon of rabbits does not respond to the enterotoxin even though binding to the colonic mucosal cells occurs at levels equivalent to binding to ileal cells which are very responsive to the enterotoxin. While binding is essential for biological activity, binding does not necessarily result in biological activity.

It is becoming increasingly evident that C. perfringens enterotoxin acts by direct cell membrane damage (McDonel, 1979). McDonel and Duncan (1975b) have shown that cycloheximide, an inhibitor of protein synthesis, does not prevent tissue damage and fluid and glucose transport alterations induced by the enterotoxin. This evidence indicates that induction of de novo synthesis of protein does not play a role in the mode of action. Furthermore, levels of cyclic 3'−5' adenosine monophosphate are not different in control and enterotoxin-treated intestinal mucosa. It appears that, rather than to activate novel metabolic pathways, synthesis, or existing enzymes, the enterotoxin acts through interference with energy production and cellular maintenance of structure and function.

Support for the concept of direct membrane effect is found in data from an electron microscopic analysis of rat and rabbit intestinal tissue (McDonel et al., 1978). Scanning electron micrographs revealed that the enterotoxin causes the formation of blebs and morphologically altered epithelial cells localized at villus tips. With transmission electron micrographs it could be seen that blebs were forming in the apical membrane of epithelial cells. Brush borders lost their characteristic folded configuration and large quantities of membrane and cytoplasm from the terminal web region and below were being lost to the lumen. A sequential process was described whereby the highly structured brush borders were losing their characteristic folded configuration with the concomitant loss of significant quantities of membrane and cytoplasm to the intestinal lumen. Prior to lysis of these cells, internal organelles and membranes appeared essentially normal. This suggested that later changes in organelles were due to cell destruction rather than cell destruction resulting from organelle deterioration. No effect was noted upon epithelial cell basolateral membranes until cellular lysis caused a general breakdown of the cytoplasmic membrane. The chronology of these events implicates the brush border membrane of villus tip epithelial cells as being the enterotoxin's primary site of action (McDonel, 1980a).

Gyobu and Kodama (1978) have reported that *C. perfringens* enterotoxin is cytotoxic for Vero (African green monkey kidney) cells. An *in vitro* model system for studying the mechanism of action of the enterotoxin has recently been established (McClane and McDonel, 1979) which utilizes Vero cells. The cells have proven to be very sensitive in that enterotoxin alters their morphology, viability, and macromolecular synthesis. Gross morphological damage was observed within 30 minutes exposure of monolayers to enterotoxin, and approximately 75% of the cells had detached within 40 minutes. The affected cells had large blebs on their cytoplasmic membranes that were reminiscent of those described for intestinal cells treated with the enterotoxin (McDonel *et al.*, 1978). Vero cell viability dropped to nearly 50% within 35 to 40 minutes. Doses of enterotoxin as low as 0.1 ng (1 ng/ml) caused small but detectable inhibition of plating efficiency while more than 100 ng (1 μg/ml) caused the inhibition to approach 100%. The enterotoxin-induced formation of blebs in Vero and HeLa cells has been reported to be calcium and temperature-dependent (Matsuda and Sugimoto, 1979).

It has been demonstrated (McClane and McDonel, 1980) that functional 'holes' (Thelestam and Möllby, 1976) are being formed in Vero cell membranes by the enterotoxin. The holes allow nearly 100% of ^{14}C-amino-isobutyric acid (AIB, mol. wt. 103), 50–60% of ^{3}H-uridine (mol. wt. 244), 25–30% of ^{51}Cr (complexed with polypeptides, mol. wt. 3,000–3,500), and 0% of ^{3}H-RNA (mol. wt. > 25,000) to pass out of treated cells within 30 minutes. The size of these holes does not appear to increase with time since length of exposure to enterotoxin does not increase the minimum size for molecules to pass through the membrane. The degree of leakage is, however, dose dependent. They have also noted that growing cells are more sensitive to the enterotoxin than cells in confluent monolayer. More than 50% protection can be conferred on the cells by pretreating them with 0.3 M sucrose, 5% albumin, or 20–40% polyethylene glycol (McClane and McDonel, 1981).

Membrane damage and resulting permeability changes have been used to explain the depression by enterotoxin of glucagon-stimulated AIB transport, enhancement of sodium uptake, and rapid exodus of L-glucose, 3-0-methylglucose, and aminoisobutyric acid from cultured rat hepatocytes (Giger and Pariza, 1978, 1980). Further evidence of a membrane effect comes from binding studies (McDonel and McClane, 1979) in which it has been demonstrated that ^{125}I-enterotoxin binds in a specific (binding inhibitable by pretreatment with native enterotoxin) manner to the Vero cells. After the isolation of a strain of Vero cells resistant to the enterotoxin from the highly sensitive cells, the apparent existence of high and low affinity binding sites was described in both cell types. The difference was that the site density on the resistant cells (1.35×10^5 sites/cell) was ten-fold less than that on the sensitive cells (1.30×10^6 sites/cell). The association constants for high and low affinity sites were similar for both cell types. This indicates that the primary difference between the two cell types is in the density of sites. The biological effect of the enterotoxin in resistant cells (as determined by analysis of DNA synthesis, ^{3}H-uridine release, and plating efficiency inhibition) was found also to be ten-fold less than on sensitive cells. It has been concluded that binding of the membrane is necessary for biological activity. Work is currently in progress to identify and isolate a specific compound (receptor) within the cell membrane with which the enterotoxin interacts. It is believed (McDonel, 1979; McDonel, 1980b) that the enterotoxin is altering the configuration or structure of some component of the membrane which results in structural and functional changes in the membrane.

Other binding studies have been performed with cells isolated from rabbit intestine, liver, kidney, and brain (McDonel, 1980b). The ^{125}I-enterotoxin was found to bind equally to cells from the intestine, liver, and kidney, but not the brain. Detailed studies with the intestinal cells revealed two classes of saturable binding sites. The rate and amount of binding to cells appeared to be temperature dependent in that lesser amounts of enterotoxin bound as the temperature was lowered from 37° C to 4° C. The binding site density on intestinal cells was 1.96×10^6 sites/cell. A problem exists in that spontaneous dissociation was observed to be much slower than expected from calculations based on the rate of association. Either the enterotoxin interacts with a compound in the membrane in such a way as to become trapped, or it is being absorbed into the membrane or the cell in such a way that escape is impossible. Skjelkvalé (1980), Skjelkvalé et al. (1980), and Granum and Skjelkvalé (1982) have radioiodinated the enterotoxin and performed in vivo binding studies in mice and rats. Tolleshaug et al. (1982) have repeated the in vitro work of McDonel (1980b) and McDonel and McClane (1979) using isolated rat liver cells. They reported similar results and confirmed the apparent number of binding sites on cell and reaffirmed the concept that the enterotoxin acts at the cell membrane surface. Petrie et al. (1982) have further reinforced the concept of cell membrane surface localization of enterotoxin activity by demonstrating that Vero cells cannot be protected from enterotoxin by microinjection into the cytoplasm of active, purified anti-enterotoxin IgG. And, Jarmund and Telle (1982) have confirmed the formation of blebs and specific binding of the enterotoxin to Vero cells and intestinal epithelial cells though they report the presence of only one class of binding site as opposed to two reported by McDonel (1980b). Wnek and McClane (1983) have isolated a protein with apparent molecular weight of 50,000 from intestinal epithelial cells that appears to be a specific receptor for the enterotoxin. When enterotoxin is treated with this putative receptor it looses its biological activity in the Vero cell system.

C. perfringens enterotoxin is similar in ways to cholera, Escherichia coli, staphylococcal and shigella enterotoxins in that they all cause fluid and electrolyte accumulation in treated ileal loops. Staphylococcal and shigella enterotoxins have been shown to cause gut tissue damage under the proper conditions although the mechanisms appear dissimilar to that of perfringens (McDonel et al., 1978). However, in contrast to the other enterotoxins, perfringens enterotoxin inhibits glucose uptake, energy production, and macromolecular synthesis. It also causes breakdown of membrane structure and function by an apparently direct interaction with the outer cell membrane. Therefore, perfringens enterotoxin probably falls into a separate category from the other enterotoxins with regard to mechanism of action.

7. IOTA TOXIN

Iota prototoxin, produced only by type E strains, was first described in 1943 (Bosworth, 1943). It is similar to epsilon prototoxin in that it must be activated to a toxic form by proteolytic enzymes. The enzymes can be those produced by the growing organisms such as lambda toxin (proteinase) (Craig and Miles, 1961) or by those added to the prototoxin such as trypsin (Ross et al., 1949).

Very little is known about the iota toxin molecule. Purification has not yet been reported and therefore the few studies that have been done to define its activity must be interpreted with caution. Orcutt et al. (1978) have reported that iota toxin has an estimated molecular weight of about 70,000 and that toxoid (formalinized toxin) can be used to produce antisera which protects against experimental challenge with active iota toxin. The toxin has been shown to be heat labile (it is inactivated with 15 minutes treatment at 53°C) and it is rapidly inactivated by pH values between 5.2 and 4.2 (Craig and Miles, 1961). Craig and Miles (1961) have shown that iota toxin causes an increase in capillary permeability when injected intradermally into a guinea pig. Larger doses injected intradermally cause necrosis. When injected intravenously, the toxin is lethal.

Some controversy has existed over the role of type E strains in disease. Generally speaking, most sources conclude that these strains do not appear to play a role in pathogenicity (Cowie–Whitney, 1970; Flatt et al., 1974; Sterne and Batty, 1975). However, indirect evidence has recently been published by Patton et al. (1978) and Orcutt et al. (1978) that type E strains producing iota toxin may be responsible for enterotoxemia, or 'hemorrhagic typhlitis' in rabbits that have experienced diet-related stress. Patton et al. (1978) described cecal hemorrhage and edema in rabbits with the enterotoxin attributed to type E. However, there were difficulties reported in isolating type E organisms from many of the affected animals, and iota toxin was not detected in the isolated cultures grown on artificial medium. Fernie and Eaton (1980), Eaton and Fernie (1980), Baskerville *et al.* (1980), and Rehg and Pakes (1982) have also implicated the presumptive involvement of iota toxin in recent explosive outbreaks of enteropathic disease in rabbit colonies. Until iota toxin is purified, characterized, and shown to induce characteristic lesions in experimental models, no firm conclusions can be made about the role of iota toxin in disease in animals or man.

A recent report by LaMont *et al.* (1979) has described a toxin from cecal contents of rabbits with clindamycin-associated colitis that is neutralized by *C. perfringens* type E antiserum. The toxin has an apparent molecular weight (as determined by column chromatography) of 45,000, is heat labile (loss of activity with 60°C for 10 minutes), and pronase-sensitive. Its activity includes mouse lethality, HeLa cell toxicity, and severe epithelial cell necrosis in rabbit rectal explants maintained in organ culture. These authors suggest that the toxic material may be iota toxin but an organism was not isolated and the toxic material was not generated in culture. Further work will be necessary before the nature and origin of this toxic material can be identified.

8. DELTA TOXIN

Delta toxin is produced only by young cultures of certain strains of types B and C. There appears not to be any correlation between delta toxin production and isolation of organisms from diseased animals. For example, strains of type B associated with lamb dysentery have been shown to produce delta toxin while strains from enterotoxemia of sheep and goats in Iran reportedly have not (Smith, 1975a). Type C strains which have been isolated from sheep with 'struck' in England, and cattle in Japan are producers of delta toxin (Yamagishi *et al.*, 1971) while type C strains isolated from calves and lambs in the United States, and man in Germany and New Guinea do not appear to be active producers (Smith, 1975a).

Very little is known about delta toxin's role, if any, in disease. It has been shown to be hemolytic only for erythrocytes of sheep, goats, pigs, and cows (Oakley and Warrack, 1953; Brooks *et al.*, 1957), and it is lethal but not necrotizing upon intradermal injection. Tixier and Alouf (1976) have described a purification scheme for delta toxin which involves ammonium sulfate precipitation and gel chromatography with Sephadex G-75. They reported that the purified toxin is a basic protein occurring as two forms with pI values of 8.8 and 9.4, and a molecular weight, as estimated by SDS gel electrophoresis, of about 42,000. More recently, Alouf and Jolivet–Reynaud (1981) have characterized the toxin as being a single polypeptide chain composed of 391 amino acids, a molecular weight of 42,000, an isoelectric point of 9.1, and having 320,000 hemolytic units per mg protein. The toxin's lytic activity, inhibitable by G_{M2} ganglioside, was reported to be restricted to even-toed ungulates (sheep, ox, goats, and pigs). They also have shown (Jolivet–Reynaud *et al.*, 1982) that delta toxin is selectively cytotoxic for various rabbit leukocyte populations and have proposed delta toxin's application to possible identification of leukocyte subpopulations based upon this selective activity. Based upon this report they now conclude that delta toxin is also lytic for human, horse, rabbit, and guinea pig platelets as well. Jolivet–Reynaud and Alouf (1983) have demonstrated that specific binding of the delta toxin to various cell types is directly correlated with the known hemolytic specificity. They also demonstrated that binding and membrane damage are separate sequential events. The binding phenomenon was characterized as rapid (2–5 min), temperature-dependent, saturable, irreversible, and inhibitable by competition with G_{M2} ganglioside or pretreatment of cells with pronase.

9. KAPPA TOXIN

Kappa toxin attacks collagen and gelatin and therefore is categorized as a collagenase (Oakley *et al.*, 1946) and a gelatinase (Oakley *et al.*, 1948). The enzyme catalyzes the hydrolysis of nonpolar regions of the collagen molecule characterized by the sequence (Gly-

Pro-R)$_n$, where R is an amino acid (Duncan, 1975). It is produced primarily by strains of types A, D, and E, though strains of types B and C have been reported to produce the toxin. Testing for kappa toxin should be done with native collagen since other proteolytic enzymes which are unable to act on native collagen will attack gelatin and hide powder (Smith, 1975a). Azocoll (hide powder coupled with an azo dye) can be used as an indicator of kappa toxin with some reliability and specificity if pretreated with papain and polyvinylpyrrolidone (PVP). The resultant azocoll is called azocoll EP (Kameyama and Akama, 1970).

Relatively little is known about the kappa toxin molecule or its role in disease. Kameyama and Akama (1971) have purified the molecule by gel filtration (Sephadex G-100) and DEAE-cellulose. They have concluded from their studies that kappa toxin apparently is protein in nature, free of carbohydrate and phosphorus, heat labile (enzymatic activity destroyed by 60°C for 10 minutes), and sensitive to low pH (activity destroyed by pH 4.5). The molecular weight, as determined by gel filtration (Sephadex G-150 − 200) was estimated to be about 80,000.

Kappa toxin has been shown to be lethal (approximately 30 μg is lethal to a mouse within one hour) and necrotic when injected intravenously into mice and intracutaneously into rabbits, respectively (Kameyama and Akama, 1971). Hemorrhage in the rabbits, appeared as early as 5 minutes after injection of as little as 0.7 μg of the toxin. Necrosis developed within a few days. Extensive destruction of connective tissue in the absence of visible changes in the muscle layer was noted in guinea pigs injected subcutaneously with the toxin. Extensive hemorrhage in lungs but not other organs was noted after subcutaneous and intramuscular injection in guinea pigs. From these observations it is possible to envision kappa toxin playing a role in the development of gas gangrene by softening muscle tissue and contributing to the spread of alpha toxin and the organisms producing these toxins. Some muscle damage has been reported to occur from purified alpha toxin as well (Strunk et al., 1967; Kameyama and Akama, 1971) though the absolute purity question is still a problem in the interpretation of these observations. Kameyama et al. (1975) have reported that guinea pigs immunized with kappa toxin were resistant to challenge with the organisms (type A) and kappa toxin but not the organisms and alpha toxin. On the other hand, guinea pigs immunized against alpha toxin were resistant to challenge with the organisms and either alpha or kappa toxin. They concluded that alpha toxin is the main contributor to development of local infection and gas gangrene. However, gas gangrene is difficult to quantitate in degree as a response, and the purity of their toxin preparations for immunization and challenge is not that well documented. Much further study is needed to ascertain the roles and interdependence of these agents in development of disease (see lambda toxin, also).

10. LAMBDA TOXIN

Lambda toxin is a protease that is produced by strains of types B, E, and some strains of D. Very little is known about this toxin and little if any meaningful work has been done with it in the past 20 years. Lambda toxin degrades numerous proteins such as hide powder, azocoll, gelatin, casein, hemoglobin, and seracin. It can be distinguished from kappa toxin (collagenase) in that it does not degrade native collagen. Early studies indicate that it is inhibited by normal nonimmune serum, is destroyed by pH below 5 or above 9, is heat labile, and is inhibited by lambda 'antitoxin', egg albumin, cysteine, cyanide, and citrate (Smith, 1975a; Willis, 1969). The purity and exact identity of preparations used in these studies are unknown and therefore these observations should not be regarded as firm.

The role of lambda toxin in disease is unclear though its likely contribution to breakdown of muscle and connective tissue is bound to be of some significance (see kappa toxin). Lambda and kappa toxin both would be expected to contribute to spread of infection (supply of amino acids and peptides for organism growth, and breakdown of physical barriers) and other toxins (such as alpha toxin). Some amounts of these toxins are likely absorbed and distributed systemically and therefore able to contribute to generalized toxemia. The possibility has also been suggested that conversion of epsilon prototoxin to active toxin may be enhanced in some instances by lambda toxin (Willis, 1969).

11. MU TOXIN

Mu toxin, which is a hyaluronidase, is produced in largest amounts by strains of type B, but is also produced by strains of types A and D, and, according to some sources, by type C (Smith, 1975a; Willis, 1969). It acts by releasing glucosamine from hyaluronic acid, a polysaccharide universally present in connective tissue that probably binds water to hold cells together in a jellylike matrix. Like most of the other minor toxins, very little of real substance is known about this toxin because it has not been studied in detail in recent years. Studies with material of undefined purity have indicated that mu toxin is heat labile (activity is destroyed rapidly by temperatures above 50°C) (Robertson *et al.*, 1940), is relatively resistant to high and low pH values (activity remains at pH values from 3.9–8.5) (Rogers, 1948) though it is inactivated by pH 9 (Hale, 1944). Mu toxin has been demonstrated to have hemolytic, necrotic, and lethal activities. It has been shown to increase skin permeability (Willis, 1969; Smith, 1975a) and therefore it may contribute to more rapid spread of infection in gas gangrene cases. However, no relationship has been found between mu toxin production and organism virulence. The same problem exists for this toxin as exists for the others that have not been studied in depth in a purified state. The importance of mu toxin in disease is unknown, though certainly it does not appear to be essential for development of gas gangrene. It may contribute to severity or speed of spread of the disease.

12. NU TOXIN

Nu toxin, which is a deoxyribonuclease, is produced by strains from all five types of *C. perfringens*, though most frequently by types A and C. It is believed to have lethal, hemolytic, or necrotic activities. It is, however, a leucocidin in that its ribonuclease activity results in destruction of nuclei or polymorphonuclear leucocytes and muscle cells when injected intramuscularly in rabbits (Robb–Smith, 1945). Nu toxin's involvement in gas gangrene appears to be reflected by the absence of a leucocyte response during the disease.

13. GAMMA AND ETA TOXINS

The existence of gamma toxin (strains of types B and C) and eta toxin (one strain of type A) is doubtful. Suggestive evidence of their existence has arisen from discrepancies in neutralizing values of specific antisera used with these strains of organisms. However, until specific active substances are isolated and purified from suspect cultures, the existence of these toxins must be considered speculative at best.

14. NEURAMINIDASE

Neuraminidase (sialidase) has been shown to be produced by strains of types A, B, C, D, and E (McCrea, 1947; Collee, 1965; Fraser and Collee, 1975; Fraser, 1978). A neuraminidase is an enzyme which cleaves acylneuraminic acid residues from oligosaccharides, glycoproteins, glycolipids or colonimic acid (Cabexas, 1978). Rood and Wilkinson (1976) have described three neuraminidase enzymes produced by *C. perfringens* with molecular weights of 310,000, 105,000 and 64,000. The role of neuraminidase in disease is unclear at this time. Various activities of neuraminidase in numerous systems have been reviewed by Rosenberg and Schengrund (1976). Ogier *et al.* (1979) have reported that neuraminidase concentration is proportional to a decrease in viability of human myeloblasts treated with the enzyme. Neuraminidase may contribute to the virulence and invasiveness of an organism but certain neuraminidase-negative organisms such as *C. novyi* type A are invasive and cause gas gangrene (Fraser, 1978). And there are neuraminidase-positive organisms such as *C. tertium* that are not thought to be pathogenic. At this time it is only possible to suggest that neuraminidase may contribute to a large number of other factors responsible for the development of disease caused by certain organisms that produce the enzyme.

15. OTHER SUBSTANCES

Certain strains of all types of *C. perfringens* produce a hemagglutin. Numerous other factors have been described and referred to as fibrinolysin, thyroid stimulating factor (Macchia *et al.*, 1967), bursting factor, hemolytic (non-alpha, theta, or delta) factor, and circulating factor. The activities (and in some instances the existence) of these factors are either unknown, in question, or in doubt. Generally speaking, the studies that have been done with these substances were carried out many years ago in the absence of sophisticated modern techniques and standards. There may be considerable value to reinvestigation of these components in contemporary laboratories.

Numerous clinical conditions other than those already mentioned, have been attributed to *C. perfringens* though it seems that little attention has been paid by clinicians to identification of the type or strain of the organisms causing diseases. Clostridial septicemia has been described in association with postpartum and postabortal infection (Bornstein *et al.*, 1964; MacLennon, 1962; Mariona and Ismail, 1980), traumatic wound infections (MacLennon, 1962) and neoplastic disease (Wynne and Armstrong, 1972; Burrell *et al.*, 1980). Less common clinical syndromes are septic arthritis (Schiller *et al.*, 1979), pneumonia and empyema (Bayer *et al.*, 1975), meningitis (MacKay *et al.*, 1971), corneal ulcer (Stern *et al.*, 1979), myonecrosis (Mohr *et al.*, 1978; Seradge and Anderson, 1980), necrotizing enterocolitis in infants (Kosloske *et al.*, 1978; Kliegman *et al.*, 1979), and cystitis (Maliwan, 1979). Animal diseases such as focal abscess and intestinal disease in horses (MacKay *et al.*, 1979; Wierup, 1977) and myositis in marine mammals (Greenwood and Taylor, 1978) have been reported as well.

C. perfringens is a ubiquitous organism that emerges from time to time as a confirmed or suspected etiologic agent in a variety of diseases in animals and man. Surprisingly little is known about ecological and physiological factors that cause the organism to move from being a passive resident to an active pathogen. Furthermore, relatively little is known about the numerous toxins produced by the organism and their role in pathogenicity. Clinicians traditionally have paid minimal attention to *C. perfringens* in the stools of patients with intestinal disorders. Reports abound where 'clostridia' have been isolated without regard for identifying the species, and *C. perfringens* has been identified without regard for type, or toxins produced. In the late 1960's and early 1970's the number of reported outbreaks of *C. perfringens* food poisoning rose to unprecedented levels because public health officials spent more time looking for this organism as a cause of disease previously categorized as 'etiology unknown'. It is likely that a similar change in incidence of other intestinal disorders of unconfirmed etiology would occur if *C. perfringens* were given more serious consideration as the responsible agent. Basic science has equally ignored the toxin's physical and chemical properties, and modes of action. Hopefully more attention will be paid in the future to the possible if not probable role of *C. perfringens* toxins in intestinal disease ranging from simple diarrhea to necrotizing enterocolitis.

REFERENCES

AKAMA, K., OTANI, S. and KAMEYAMA, S. (1968) Purification of beta toxin of *Clostridium perfringens* type C. *Jap. J. Med. Sci. Biol.* **21**: 423–426.

ALOUF, J. E. (1977) Cell membranes and cytolytic bacterial toxins. In: *The specificity and action of animal, bacterial and plant toxins. Receptors and Recognition.* p. 219–270. CUATRECASAS, P. (ed.) Series B, Vol. **1**. John Wiley and Sons, N.Y.

ALOUF, J. E. and JOLIVET–REYNAUD, C. (1981) Purification and characterization of *Clostridium perfringens* delta-toxin. *Infect. Immun.* **31**: 536–546.

AL-SHEIKHLY, F. and TRUSCOTT, R. B. (1977a) The pathology of necrotic enteritis of chickens following infusion of both cultures of *Clostridium perfringens* into the duodenum. *Avian Dis.* **21**: 230–240.

AL-SHEIKHLY, F. and TRUSCOTT, R. B. (1977b) The pathology of necrotic enteritis of chickens following infusion of crude toxins of *Clostridium perfringens* into the duodenum. *Avian Dis.* **21**: 241–255.

AL-SHIEKHLY, F. and TRUSCOTT, R. B. (1977c) The interaction of *Clostridium perfringens* and its toxins in the production of necrotic enteritis of chickens. *Avian Dis.* **21**: 256–263.

AVIGAD, G. (1976) Microbial Phospholipases. In: *Mechanisms in bacterial toxinology.* p. 99–167. BERNHEIMER, A. W. (ed.) John Wiley and Sons, N.Y.

AVIGAD, L. S. and BERNHEIMER, A. W. (1976) Inhibition by zinc of hemolysis induced by bacterial and other cytolytic agents. *Infect. Immun.* **13**: 1378–1381.

BANGHAM, A. D. and DAWSON, R. M. C. (1961) Electrokinetic requirements for the reaction between *Cl. perfringens* α-toxin (phospholipase C) and phospholipid substrates. *Biochim. Biophys. Acta* **59**: 103–115.

BARTLETT, M. L., WALKER, H. W. and ZIPRIN, R. (1972) Use of dogs as an assay for *Clostridium perfringens* enterotoxin. *Appl. Microbiol.* **23**: 196–197.

BASKERVILLE, M., WOOD, M. and SEAMER, J. H. (1980) *Clostridium perfringens* type E enterotoxaemia in rabbits. *Vet. Record.* **107**: 18–19.

BAYER, A. S., NELSON, S. C., GALPIN, J. E., CHOW., A. W. and GUZE, L. B. (1975) Necrotizing pneumonia and empyema due to *Clostridium perfringens*. Report and review of the literature. *Am. J. Med.* **59**: 851–856.

BEH, K. J. and BUTTERY, S. H. (1978) Reverse phase passive haemagglutination and single radial immunodiffusion to detect epsilon antigen of *Clostridium perfringens* type D. *Austr. Vet. J.* **54**: 541–544.

BERNATH, S. (1975) Solid phase radioimmunoassays for quantitative antibody determination of *Clostridium perfringens* type D epsilon toxin. *Appl. Microbiol.* **30**: 499–502.

BERNHEIMER, A. W. (1974) Interactions between membranes and cytolytic bacterial toxins. *Biochim. Biophys. Acta* **344**: 27–50.

BERNHEIMER, A. W. (1976) Sulfhydryl activated toxins. In: *Mechanisms in bacterial toxinology.* p. 85–97. BERNHEIMER, A. W. (ed.) John Wiley and Sons, N.Y.

BERNHEIMER, A. W. and GRUSHOFF, P. (1967) Cereolysin: Production, purification and partial characterization. *J. Gen. Microbiol.* **46**: 143–150.

BERNHEIMER, A. W., GRUSHOFF, P. and AVIGAD, L. S. (1968) Isoelectric analysis of cytolytic bacterial proteins. *J. Bacteriol.* **95**: 2439–2441.

BERNHEIMER, A. W. and SCHWARTZ, L. L. (1965) Effect of staphylococcal and other bacterial toxins on platelets in vitro. *J. Pathol. Bacteriol.* **89**: 209–223.

BHOWN, A. S. and HABEEB, A. F. S. A. (1977) Structural studies on epsilon prototoxin of *Clostridium perfringens* type D localization of the site of tryptic scission necessary for activation to epsilon toxin. *Biochem. Biophys. Res. Commun.* **78**: 889–896.

BICKFORD, A. A. (1975) Comments on ulcerative enteritis. *Am. J. Vet. Res.* **36**: 586.

BIRD, R. A., LOW, M. G. and STEPHEN, J. (1974) Immunopurification of phospholipase C (α-toxin) from *Clostridium perfringens*. FEBS Lett. **44**: 279–281.

BOETHIUS, J., RYDQUIST, B., MÖLLBY, R. and WADSTRÖM, T. (1973) Effect of a highly purified phospholipase C on some electrophysiological properties of the frog muscle fiber membrane. *Life Sci.* **13**: 171–176.

BORNSTEIN, D. L., WEINBERG, A. N., SWARTZ, M. N. and KUNZ, L. J. (1964) Anaerobic infections. Review of current experience. *Medicine* **43**: 207–232.

BOSWORTH, T. J. (1943) On a new type of toxin produced by *Clostridium welchii*. *J. Comp. Pathol.* **53**: 245–255.

BROOKS, M. E., STERNE, M. and WARRACK, G. H. (1957) A reassessment of the criteria used for type differentiation of *Clostridium perfringens*. *J. Pathol. Bacteriol.* **74**: 185–195.

BUDDLE, M. B. (1954) "Degraded" strains of *Clostridium welchii* type C isolated from sheep in New Zealand. *J. Comp. Path. Ther.* **64**: 217–224.

BULLEN, J. J. (1970) Role of toxins in host-parasite relationships. In: *Microbial Toxins.* p. 233. SJL, S. J. KADIS, S. and MONTIE, T. C. (eds.) Vol. I Academic Press, N.Y.

BULLEN, J. J. and BATTY, I. (1956) The effect of *Clostridium welchii* type D culture filtrates on the permeability of the mouse intestine. *J. Path. Bact.* **71**: 311–323.

BURRELL, M. I., HYSON, E. A. and WALKER–SMITH, G. J. (1980) Spontaneous clostridial infection and malignancy. *Am. J. Roentgen.* **134**: 1157–1159.

BUXTON, D. (1976) Use of horseradish peroxidase to study the antagonism of *Clostridium welchii* (*Clostridium perfringens*) type D epsilon toxin in mice by the formalinized epsilon prototoxin. *J. Comp. Pathol.* **86**: 67–72.

BUXTON, D. (1978a) The use of an immunoperoxidase technique to investigate by light and electron microscopy the sites of binding *Clostridium welchii* type D epsilon toxin in mice. *J. Med. Microbiol.* **11**: 289–292.

BUXTON, D. (1978b) Further studies on the mode of action of *Clostridium welchii* type D epsilon toxin. *J. Med. Microbiol.* **11**: 293–298.

BUXTON, D. (1978c) In vitro effects of *Clostridium welchii* type D epsilon toxin on guinea pig, mouse, rabbit and sheep cells. *J. Med. Microbiol.* **11**: 299–302.

BUXTON, D. and K. T. MORGAN (1976), Studies of lesions produced in the brains of colostrum deprived lambs by *Clostridium welchii* (*Clostridium perfringens*) type D toxin. *J. Comp. Pathol.* **86**: 435–447.

CABEXAS, M. (1978) Determination of the inhibitory effect of several compounds of neuraminidases from virus influenza, *V. cholerae* and *Cl. perfringens*. *Int. J. Biochem.* **9**: 47–49.

CASU, A., PALA, V. MONACELLI, R. and NANNI, G. (1971) Phospholipase C from *Clostridium perfringens*: purification by electrophoresis on acrylamide-agarose gel. *Ital. J. Biochem.* **20**: 166–178.

CHAKRABARTY, A. K. and NARAYAN, K. G. (1979) Pathogenesis of Hobbs' heat-sensitive spore forming *Clostridium perfringens* type A strain. *Microbiol. Immunol.* **23**: 213–221.

CHAKRABARTY, A. K., NARAYAN, K. G. and CHANDIRAMANI, N. K. (1977) Association of *Clostridium perfringens* type A with human diarrhoeal cases. *Ind. J. Med. Res.* **65**: 495–499.

CHIEN, S.-F., YEVICH, S. J., LI, S.-C. and LI, Y.-T. (1975) Presence of endo β-N-actylglucosaminidase and protease activities in the commercial neuraminidase preparations isolated from *Clostridium perfringens*. *Biochem. Biophys. Res. Commun.* **65**: 683–691.

CHOUDHURY, T. K. (1978) Synergistic lysis of erythrocytes by *Propionibacterium acnes*. *J. Clin. Microbiol.* **8**: 238–241.

COLLEE, J. G. (1965) A myxovirus receptor-inactivating agent occurring in cultures of *Clostridium welchii*. *J. Pathol. Bacteriol.* **90**: 1–11.

COLLEE, J. G. (1974) *Clostridium perfringens* (*Cl. welchii*) in the human gastrointestinal tract. In: *The Normal Microbial Flora of Man.* p. 205–219. SKINNER, F. A. and CARR, J. G. (eds.) Academic Press, N.Y.

COWELL, J. L., KIM, K. S. and BERNHEIMER, A. W. (1978) Alteration by cereolysin of the structure of cholesterol-containing membranes. *Biochim. Biophys. Acta* **507**: 230–241.

COWIE–WHITNEY, J. (1970) Some aspects of the enteritis complex of rabbits. In: *Nutrition and disease in experimental animals.* p. 122–131. TAVERNOR, W. D. (ed.) Williams & Wilkins Co., Baltimore.

CRAIG, J. P. and MILES, A. A. (1961) Some properties of the iota-toxin of *Clostridium welchii*, including its action on capillary permeability, *J. Path. Bact.* **81**: 481–493.

DALLING, T. and ROSS, H. E. (1938) *Clostridium welchii*: Notes on the relationship between the types of cultures and the production of toxin. *J. Comp. Path. Ther.* **51**: 235–249.

DASGUPTA, B. R. and PARIZA, M. W. (1982) Purification of two *Clostridium perfringens* enterotoxin-like proteins and their effects on membrane permeability in primary cultures of adult rate hepatocytes. *Infect. Immun.* **38**: 592–597.

DAWSON, R. M. C. (1973) Specificity of enzymes involved in the metabolism of phospholipids. In: *Form and function of phospholipids.* p. 97–116. ANSELL, G. B., HAWTHORNE, J. N. and DAWSON, R. M. C. (eds.) Elsevier, Amsterdam.

DAWSON, R. M. C., HEMINGTON, N. L., MILLER, N. G. A. and BANGHAM, A. D. (1976) On the question of electrokinetic requirement for phospholipase C action. *J. Membrane Biol.* **29**: 179–184.

DEMEL, R. A., GUERTS van KESSEL, W. S. M., ZWALL, R. F. A., ROELOFSEN, B. and van DEENEN, L. L. M. (1975) Relation between various phospholipase actions on human red cell membranes and the interfacial phospholipid pressure in monolayers. *Biochim. Biophys. Acta.* **406**: 97–107.

DEN, H., MALINZAK, D. A. and ROSENBERG, A. (1975) Cytotoxin contaminants in commercial *Clostridium perfringens* neuraminidase preparations purified by affinity chromatography. *J. Chromat.* **111**: 217–222.

DOURMASHKIN, R. R. and ROSSE, W. F. (1966) Morphologic changes in the membranes of red blood cells undergoing hemolysis. *Am. J. Med.* **41**: 699–709.

DUFFY, L. K., McDONEL, J. L., McCLANE, B. A. and KUROSKY, A. (1982) *Clostridium perfringens* type A enterotoxin: characterization of the aminoterminal region. *Infect. Immun.* **38**: 386–388.

DUNCAN, C. L. (1970) *Clostridium perfringens* food poisoning. *J. Milk Food Technol.* **33**: 35–41.

DUNCAN, C. L. (1973) Time of enterotoxin formation and release during sporulation of *Clostridium perfringens* type A. *J. Bacteriol.* **113**: 932–936.

DUNCAN, C. L. (1975) Role of clostridial toxins in pathogenesis. In: *Microbiology–1975.* p. 283–291. SCHLESSINGER, D. (ed.) American Society for Microbiology, Washington, D.C.

DUNCAN, C. L., KING, G. J. and FRIEBEN, W. R. (1973) A paracrystalline inclusion formed during sporulation of enterotoxin-producing strains of *Clostridium perfringens* type A. *J. Bacteriol.* **114**: 845–859.

DUNCAN, C. L., ROKOS, E. A., CHRISTENSON, C. M. and ROOD, J. I. (1978) Multiple plasmids in different toxigenic types of *Clostridium perfringens* possible control of beta toxin production. In: *Microbiology 1978.* p. 246–248. SCHLESSINGER, D. (ed.) American Society for Microbiology, Washington, D.C.

DUNCAN, C. L. and SOMERS, E. B. (1972) Quantitation of *Clostridium perfringens* type A enterotoxin by electro-immunodiffusion. *Appl. Microbiol.* **24**: 801–804.

DUNCAN, C. L. and STRONG, D. H. (1968) Improved medium for sporulation of *Clostridium perfringens*. *Appl. Microbiol.* **16**: 82–89.

DUNCAN, C. L. and STRONG, D. H. (1969a) Ileal loop fluid accumulation and production of diarrhea in rabbits by cell-free products of *Clostridium perfringens*. *J. Bacteriol.* **100**: 86–94.

DUNCAN, C. L. and STRONG, D. H. (1969b) Experimental production of diarrhea in rabbits with *Clostridium perfringens*. *Can. J. Microbiol.* **15**: 765–770.

DUNCAN, C. L. and STRONG, D. H. (1971) *Clostridium perfringens* type A food poisoning. I. Response of the rabbit ileum as an indication of enteropathogenicity of strains of *Clostridium perfringens* in monkeys. *Infect. Immun.* **3**: 167–170.

DUNCAN, D. L., STRONG, D. H. and SEBALD, M. (1972) Sporulation and enterotoxin production by mutants of *Clostridium perfringens*. *J. Bacteriol.* **110**: 378–391.

DUNCAN, C. L., SUGIYAMA, H. and STRONG, D. H. (1968) Rabbit ileal loop response to strains of *Clostridium perfringens*. *J. Bacteriol.* **95**: 1560–1566.

EATON, P. and FERNIE, D. S. (1980) Enterotoxaemia involving *Clostridium perfringens* iota toxin in a hysterectomy-derived rabbit colony. *Lab. Animals* **14**: 347–351.

ELLNER, P. D. (1961) Fate of partially purified C^{14}-labelled toxin of *Clostridium perfringens*. *J. Bacteriol.* **82**: 275–283.

ENDERS, G. L., JR. and DUNCAN, C. L. (1976) Anomalous aggregation of *Clostridium perfringens* enterotoxin under dissociating conditions. *Can. J. Microbiol.* **22**: 1410–1414.

ENDERS, G. L., JR. and DUNCAN, C. L. (1977) Preparative polyacrylamide gel electrophoresis purification of *Clostridium perfringens* enterotoxin. *Infect. and Immun.* **17**: 425–429.

FERNIE, D. S. and EATON, P. (1980) The demonstration of a toxin resembling *Clostridium perfringens* iota toxin in rabbits with enterotoxaemia. *FEMS Microbiol. Lett.* **8**: 33–35.

FLATT, R. E., WEISBROTH, S. H. and KRAUS, A. L. (1974) Metabolic, traumatic, mycotic, and miscellaneous diseases of rabbits. In: *The biology of the laboratory rabbit.* p. 437–440. WEISBROTH, S. H., FLATT, R. E. and KRAUS, A. L. (eds.) Academic Press, N.Y.

FRASER, A. G. (1978) Neuraminidase production by Clostridia. *J. Med. Microbiol.* **11**: 269–280.

FRASER, A. G. and COLLEE, J. G. (1975) The production of neuraminidase by food-poisoning strains of *Clostridium welchii* (*C. perfringens*). *J. Med. Microbiol.* **8**: 251–263.

FREER, J. H. and ARBUTHNOTT, J. P. (1976) Biochemical and morphologic alterations of membranes by bacterial toxins. In: *Mechanisms of bacterial toxinology.* p. 169–193. BERNHEIMER, A. W. (ed.) John Wiley & Sons, N.Y.

FREHOLM, B. B., MÖLLBY, R., ANDERSON, P., MALMQUIST, T. and SMYTH, C. J. (1978) Inhibition of noradrenaline-stimulated lipolysis and cyclic AMP accumulation in isolated rat adipocytes by purified phospholipase C and theta-toxin from *Clostridium perfringens*. *Acta Pharmacol. Toxicol.* **42**: 23–34.

FRIEBEN, W. R. and DUNCAN, C. L. (1973) Homology between enterotoxin protein and spore structural protein in *Clostridium perfringens* type A. *Eur. J. Biochem.* **39**: 393–401.

FRIEBEN, W. R. and DUNCAN, C. L. (1975) Heterogeneity of enterotoxin-like protein extracted from spores of *Clostridium perfringens* type A. *Eur. J. Biochem.* **55**: 455–463.

FRISH, A., GAZIIT, Y. and LOYTER, A. (1973) Metabolically controlled hemolysis of chicken erythrocytes. *Biochim. Biophys. Acta.* **291**: 690–700.

GARDNER, D. E. (1973a) Pathology of *Clostridium welchii* type D enterotoxaemia. I. Biochemical and haematological alterations in lambs. *J. Comp. Pathol.* **83**: 499–507.

GARDNER, D. E. (1973b) Pathology of *Clostridium welchii* type D enterotoxaemia. III. Basis of the hyperglycaemic response. *J. Comp. Pathol.* **83**: 525–529.

GARDNER, D. E. (1974) Brain oedema: an experimental model. *Br. J. Expt. Pathol.* **55**: 453–457.

GENIGEORGIS, C. (1975) Public health importance of *Clostridium perfringens. J. Am. Vet. Med. Assoc.* **167**: 821–827.

GENIGEORGIS, C., SAKAGUCHI, G. and RIEMANN, H. (1973) Assay methods for *Clostridium perfringens* type A enterotoxin. *Appl. Microbiol.* **26**: 111–115.

GIGER, O. and PARIZA, M. (1978) Depression of amino acid transport in cultured rat hepatocytes by purified enterotoxin from *Clostridium perfringens. Biochem. Biophys. Res. Commun.* **82**: 378–383.

GIGER, O. and PARIZA, M. W. (1980) Mechanism of action of *Clostridium perfringens* enterotoxin. Effects on membrane permeability and amino acid transport in primary cultures of adult rat hepatocytes. *Biochim. Biophys. Acta.* **595**: 264–276.

GILL, D. M. and KING, C. A. (1975) The mechanism of action of cholera toxin in pigeon erythrocyte lysates. *J. Biol. Chem.* **250**: 6424–6432.

GLUSHKOVA, A. I., NENASHEAV, V. P. and GOLDSHMID, V. K. (1969) A study of nutrient medium and the toxin of *Cl. perfringens* type A by means of gel filtration through Sephadex gel. In: *Proceedings of the Inter-Institute Conference,* Stavropol, 1966. In Russian, cited by Smyth and Arbuthnott, 1974.

GRANUM, P. E. (1982) Inhibition of protein synthesis by a tryptic polypeptide of *Clostridium perfringens* type A enterotoxin. *Biochem. Biophys. Acta.* **708**: 6–11.

GRANUM, P. E. and SKJELKVALÉ, R. (1977) Chemical modification and characterization of enterotoxin from *Clostridium perfringens* type A. *Acta Pathol. Microbiol. Scand. Sect. B* **85**: 89–94.

GRANUM, P. E. and SKJELKVALÉ, R. (1981) Endogenous radiolabeling of enterotoxin from *Clostridium perfringens* type A on a defined medium. *Appl. Environ. Microbiol.* **42**: 596–598.

GRANUM, P. E. and WHITAKER, J. R. (1980a) Improved method for purification of enterotoxin from *Clostridium perfringens* type A. *Appl. Environ. Microbiol.* **39**: 1120–1122.

GRANUM, P. E. and WHITAKER, J. R. (1980b) Perturbation of the structure of *Clostridium perfringens* enterotoxin by sodium dodecyl sulfate, gyanidine hydrochloride, pH and temperature. *J. Food Biochem.* **4**: 219–234.

GRANUM, P. E., WHITAKER, J. R. and SKJELKVALÉ, R. (1981) Trypsin activation of enterotoxin from *Clostridium perfringens* type A. Fragmentation and some Physiochemical properties. *Biochim. Biophys. Acta.* **668**: 325–332.

GREENWOOD, A. G. and TAYLOR, D. C. (1978) Clostridial myositis in marine mammals. *Vet. Record.* **103**: 54–55.

GRINER, L. A. (1961) Enterotoxemia of sheep. I. Effect of *Clostridium perfringens* type D toxin on the brains of sheep and mice. *Am. J. Vet. Res.* **22**: 429–442.

GRINER, L. A. and CARLSON, W. D. (1961) Enterotoxemia of sheep. II. Distribution of ^{131}I-radioiodinated serum albumin in brains of *Clostridium perfringens* type D intoxicated lambs. *Am. J. Vet. Res.* **22**: 443–446.

GUBASH, S. M. (1978) Synergistic hemolysis phenomenon shown by an alpha-toxin-producing *Clostridium perfringens* and streptococcal CAMP factor in presumptive streptococcal grouping. *J. Clin. Microbiol.* **8**: 480–488.

GYOBU, Y. and KODAMA, H. (1978) Vero cell microcell culture technique for the detection of neutralization antibody against *Clostridium perfringens* enterotoxin and its application to sero-epidemiology. *J. Food Hyg. Soc. Jap.* **19**: 294–298.

HABEEB, A. F. S. A. (1964) Studies on ε-prototoxin of *Clostridium perfringens* type A. *Can. J. Biochem.* **42**: 545–554.

HABEEB, A. F. S. A. (1969) Studies on ε-prototoxin of *Clostridium perfringens* type D. I. Purification methods: evidence for multiple forms of ε-prototoxin. *Arch. Biochem. Biophys.* **130**: 430–440.

HABEEB, A. F. S. A. (1972) Chemical and physicochemical properties of ε-prototoxin of *Clostridium perfringens* type D. *Fed. Proc.* **31**: 932.

HABEEB, A. F. S. A. (1975) Studies on ε-prototoxin of *Clostridium perfringens* type D physicochemical and chemical properties of ε-prototoxin. *Biochim. Biophys. Acta* **412**: 62–69.

HABEEB, A. F. S. A., LEE, C. L. and ATASSI, M. Z. (1973) Conformatial studies on modified proteins and peptides, Part 7. Conformation of epsilon prototoxin and epsilon toxin from *Clostridium perfringens*, conformational changes associated with toxicity. *Biochim. Biophys. Acta* **322**: 245–250.

HABERMANN, E. (1960) Zur Toxikologie und Pharmakologie des Gasbrandgiftes (*Clostridium welchii* type A) und seiner Komponenten. *Naunyn-Schmiedeberg's Arch. Exp. Path. Pharmak.* **238**: 502–524.

HALE, C. W. (1944) Studies on diffusing factors 5. The influence of some environmental conditions on the activity of hyaluronidase. *Biochem. J.* **38**: 368–370.

HALL, H. E., ANGELOTTI, R., LEWIS, K. H. and FOTER, M. J. (1963) Characteristics of *Clostridium perfringens* strains associated with food and food-borne disease. *J. Bacteriol.* **85**: 1094–1103.

HARTLEY, W. J. (1956) A focal symmetrical encephalomalacia of lambs. *N.Z. Vet. J.* **4**: 129–135.

HASE, J., MITSUI, K. and SHONAKA, E. (1975) *Clostridium perfringens* exotoxins. III. Binding of θ-toxin to erythrocyte membrane. *Japan. J. Exp. Med.* **45**: 433–438.

HASE, J., MITSUI, K. and SHONAKA, E. (1976) *Clostridium perfringens* exotoxins. IV. Inhibition of the θ-toxin induced hemolysis by steroids and related compounds. *Japan. J. Exp. Med.* **46**: 45–50.

HAUSCHILD, A. H. W. (1970) Erythemal activity of the cellular enteropathogenic factor of *Clostridium perfringens* type A. *Can. J. Microbiol.* **16**: 651–654.

HAUSCHILD, A. H. W. (1971) *Clostridium perfringens* toxins types B, C, D, and E. In: *Microbial Toxins.* Vol. IIA. *Bacterial Protein Toxins.* p. 159–188. KADIS, S., MONTIE, T. C. and AJL, S. J. (eds.) Academic Press, N. Y.

HAUSCHILD, A. H. W. (1973) Food poisoning by *Clostridium perfringens. Can. Inst. Food Sci. Technol. J.* **6**: 106–110.

HAUSCHILD, A. H. W. and HILSHEIMER, R. (1971) Purification and characteristics of the enterotoxin of *Clostridium perfringens* type A. *Can. J. Microbiol.* **17**: 1425–1433.

HAUSCHILD, A. H. W., HILSHEIMER, R. and MARTIN, W. G. (1973a) Improved purification and further characterization of *Clostridium perfringens* type A enterotoxin. *Can. J. Microbiol.* **19**: 1379–1382.

HAUSCHILD, A. H. W., HILSHEIMER, R. and ROGERS, C. G. (1971a) Rapid detection of *Clostridium perfringens* enterotoxin in a modified ligated intestinal loop technique in rabbits. *Can. J. Microbiol.* **17**: 1475–1476.

Hauschild, A. H. W., Lecroisey, A. and Alouf, J. E. (1973b) Purification of *Clostridium perfringens* type C theta toxin. *Can. J. Microbiol.* **19**: 881–885.

Hauschild, A. H. W., Niilo, L. and Dorward, W. J. (1967) Experimental enteritis with food poisoning and classical strains of *Clostridium perfringens* type A in lambs. *J. Infect. Dis.* **117**: 379–386.

Hauschild, A. H. W., Niilo, L. and Dorward, W. J. (1970a) Enteropathogenic factors of food-poisoning *Clostridium perfringens* type A. *Can. J. Microbiol.* **16**: 331–338.

Hauschild, A. H. W., Niilo, L. and Dorward, W. J. (1970b) Response of ligated intestinal loops in lambs to an enteropathogenic factor of *Clostridium perfringens* type A. *Can. Microbiol.* **16**: 339–343.

Hauschild, A. H. W. and Thatcher, F. S. (1967) Experimental food poisoning with heat-susceptible *Clostridium perfringens* type A. *J. Food Sci.* **32**: 467–469.

Hauschild, A. H. W. and Thatcher, F. S. (1968) Experimental gas gangrene with food-poisoning heat-susceptible *Clostridium perfringens* type A. *Can. J. Microbiol.* **14**: 705–709.

Hauschild, A. H. W., Walcroft, M. J. and Campbell, W. (1971b) Emesis and diarrhea induced by enterotoxin of *Clostridium perfringens* type A in monkeys. *Can. J. Microbiol.* **17**: 1141–1143.

Hill, E. E. and Lands, W. E. M. (1970) Phospholipid metabolism. In: *Lipid metabolism*. p. 185–277. Wakil, S. J. (ed.) Academic Press, N.Y.

Hitchcock, C. R., Demello, F. J. and Haglin, J. J. (1975) Gangrene infection, new approaches to an old disease. *Surg. Clin. N. Am.* **55**: 1403–1410.

Hobbs, B. C. (1969) *Clostridium perfringens* and *Bacillus cereus* infections. In: *Food-borne infections and intoxications*. p. 131–173. Rieman, H. (ed.) Academic Press, N.Y.

Hobbs, B. C., Smith, S. F., Oakley, C. T., Warrack, G. H. and Cruichshank, J. F. (1953) *Clostridium welchii* food poisoning. *J. Hyg.* **51**: 74–101.

Hogh, P. (1976) Experimental studies on serum treatment and vaccination against *C. perfringens* type C infection in piglets. *Dev. Biol. Stand.* **32**: 69–76.

Howard, J. G., Wallace, K. R. and Wright, G. P. (1953) The inhibitory effects of cholesterol and related sterol on haemolysis by streptolysin O. *Br. J. Exp. Pathol.* **34**: 174–180.

Hyder, G. (1973) Enterotoxemia or pulpy kidney disease vaccine. *Indian Vet. J.* **50**: 972–978.

Iles, G. H., Seeman, P., Naylor, D. and Cinader, B. (1973) Membrane lesions, immune lysis surface rings, globule aggregates and transient openings. *J. Cell. Biol.* **56**: 528–539.

Inoue, K., Akiyama, Y., Kinoshita, T., Higashi, Y. and Amano, T. (1976) Evidence for a one-hit theory in the immune bactericidal reaction and demonstration of a multi-hit response for hemolysis by streptolysin O and *Clostridium perfringens* theta-toxin. *Infect. Immun.* **13**: 337–344.

Ispolatovskaya, M. V. (1971) Type A *Clostridium perfringens* toxin. In: *Microbial Toxins*. Vol. IIA. *Bacterial Protein Toxins*. p. 109–158. Kadis, S., Montie, T. C. and Ajl, S. J. (eds.) Academic Press, N. Y.

Ivers, J. T. and Potter, N. N. (1977) Production and stability of hemolysin, phospholipase C, and lethal toxin of *Bacillus cereus* in food. *J. Food Prot.* **40**: 17–21.

Jansen, B. C. (1960) The diagnosis of pulpy kidney disease. *J. S. African Vet. Med. Assoc.* **31**: 15–20.

Jansen, B. C. (1967a) The production of a basic immunity against pulpy kidney disease. *Onderstepoort. J. Vet. Res.* **34**: 65–80.

Jansen, B. C. (1967b) The duration of immunity to pulpy kidney disease of sheep. *Onderstepoort J. Vet. Res.* **34**: 333–334.

Jarmund, T. and Telle, W. (1982) Binding of *Clostridium perfringens* enterotoxin to hepatocytes, small intestinal epithelial cells and Vero cells. *Acta Path. Microbiol. Immunol. Scand. Sect. B.* **90**: 377–381.

Jolivet-Reynaud, C. and Alouf, J. E. (1983) Binding of *Clostridium perfringens* ^{125}I-labeled Δ-toxin to erythrocytes. *J. Biol. Chem.* **258**: 1871–1877.

Jolivet-Reynaud, C., Cavaillon, J. and Alouf, J. E. (1982) Selective cytotoxicity of *Clostridium perfringens* delat toxin on rabbit leukocytes. *Infect. Immun.* **38**: 860–864.

Justus, P. G., Mathias, J. R., Carlson, G. M., Martin, J. L., Formal, S. and Shields, R. P. (1980) The myoelectric activity of the small intestine in response to *Clostridium perfringens* A enterotoxin and *Clostridium difficile* culture filtrate. In: Gastrointestinal Motility. p. 379–386. Christensen, J. (Ed.) Raven Press, New York.

Kameyama, S. and Akama, K. (1970) Titration of kappa toxin of *Clostridium perfringens* and kappa antitoxin by a modified azocoll method. *Japan. J. Med. Sci. Biol.* **23**: 31–46.

Kameyama, S. and Akama, K. (1971) Purification and some properties of kappa toxin of *Clostridium perfringens*. *Japan. J. Med. Sci. Biol.* **24**: 9–23.

Kameyama, S., Sato, H. and Murata, R. (1975) The role of α-toxin of *Clostridium prefringens* in experimental gas gangrene in guinea pigs. *Japan. J. Med. Sci. Biol.* **25**: 200.

Kellaway, C. H. and Trethewie, E. R. (1941) The injury of tissue cells and the liberation of pharmacologically active substances by the toxins of *Cl. welchii* types B and C. Aust. *J. Exp. Biol. Med. Sci.* **19**: 17–27.

Kennedy, K. K., Norris, S. J., Beckenhauer, W. H. and White, R. G. (1977) *Clostridium perfringens* type C and Type D toxoid. *Am. J. Vet. Res.* **38**: 1515–1518.

Kent, C. (1978) Inhibition of muscle cell fusion by phospholipase C alterations in phospholipid metabolism. *Fed. Proc.* **37**: 1404.

Klein, R. (1975) The action of phospholipase C from *Clostridium welchii* by quinine: an absolute requirement for calcium ions. *Chem. Phys. Lipids* **15**: 15–26.

Kliegman, R. M., Fanaroff, A. A., Izant, R. and Speck, W. T. (1979) Brief clinical and laboratory observations: Clostridia as pathogens in neonatal necrotizing enterocolitis. *J. Pediatr.* **95**: 287–289.

Knight, P. A., Lucken, R., Foster, W. H. and Walker, P. D. (1979) Development, preparation and safety testing of a *Clostridium welchii* type C toxoid. II. Laboratory studies on potency. *J. Biol. Stand.* **7**: 373–381.

Kosloske, A. M., Ulrich, J. A. and Hoffman, H. (1978) Fulminant necrotising enterocolitis associated with clostridia. *Lancet* **ii**. 1014–1016.

Krämer, J. and Schallehn, G. (1978) Characterization of plasmid DNA in a lecithinase-positive and in a lecithinase-negative strain of *Clostridium perfringens*. *Zbl. Bakt. Hyg. I. Abt. Orig. A* **241**: 438–447.

KULSHRESTHA, S. B. (1974a) Effect of carbohydrates on the production of lethal toxin by *Clostridium perfringens* types B and C with particular reference to beta toxin and epsilon toxin. *Indian. J. Anim. Sci.* **43**: 628–631.

KULSHRESTHA, S. B. (1974b) Effect of period of incubation and pH on the production of beta and epsilon toxins by *Clostridium welchii* type B and type C. *Indian. J. Anim. Sci.* **43**: 987–990.

KURIOKA, S. and MATSUDA, M. (1976) Phospholipase C assay using p-nitrophenylphosphorycholine together with sorbital and its application to studying the metal and detergent requirement of the enzyme. *Anal. Biochem.* **75**: 281–289.

LABBE, R. G. and DUNCAN, C. L. (1974) Sporulation and enterotoxin production by *Clostridium perfringens* type A and under conditions of controlled pH and temperature. *Can. J. Microbiol.* **20**: 1493–1501.

LABBE, R. G. and DUNCAN, C. L. (1975) Influence of carbohydrates on growth and sporulation of *Clostridium perfringens* type A. *Appl. Microbiol.* **29**: 345–351.

LABBE, R. G. and DUNCAN, C. L. (1977a) Evidence for stable messenger ribonucleic acid during sporulation and enterotoxin synthesis by *Clostridium perfringens* type A. *J. Bacteriol.* **129**: 843–849.

LABBE, R. G. and DUNCAN, C. L. (1977b) Spore coat protein and enterotoxin synthesis in *Clostridium perfringens. J. Bacteriol.* **131**: 713–715.

LAMONT, J. T., SONNENBLICK, E. B. and ROTHMAN, S. (1979) Role of Clostridial toxin in the pathogenesis of clindamycin colitis in rabbits. *Gastroenterology* **76**: 356–361.

LAWRENCE, G. and COOKE, R. (1980) Experimental pigbel: the production and pathology of necrotizing due to *Clostridium welchii* type C in the guinea pig. *Br. J. Exp. Pathol.* **61**: 261–271.

LAWRENCE, G., SHANN, F., FREESTONE, D. S. and WALKER, P. D. (1979) Prevention of necrotising enteritis in Papua New Guinea by active immunization. *Lancet* **1**: 227–230.

LAWRENCE, G. and WALKER, P. D. (1976) Pathogenesis of enteritis necroticans in Papua New Guinea. *Lancet* **1**: 125–126.

LIEBERMAN, M. (1975) A highly efficient solid phase radio-immunoassay for a clostridial toxin. *Anal. Biochem.* **67**: 115–121.

LITVINKO, N. M., KHURGIN, Y. I. and SHEMANOVA, G. F. (1977) Effect of low molecular weight substrate fragments and their analogs on activity of isoenzymes of phospholipase C E.C.–3.1.4.3. from *Clostridium perfringens* type A. *Biochemistry* (Engl. Transl. Biokhimiya) **42**: 838–842.

LÖFFLER, A. and LABBE, R. G. (1983) Intracellular proteases during sporulation and enterotoxin formation by *Clostridium perfringens* type A. *Current Microbiology* **8**: 187–190.

LOW, D. K. R. and FREER, J. H. (1977) Biological effects of highly purified β-lysin (sphingomyelinase C) from *Staphylococcus aureus. FEMS Microbiol. Lett.* **2**: 133–138.

LOW, D. K. R., FREER, J. H., ARBUTHNOTT, J. P., MÖLLBY, R. and WADSTRÖM, T. (1974) Consequences of sphingomylin degradation in erythrocyte ghost membranes by staphylococcal β-toxin (sphingomyelinase C). *Toxicom.* **12**: 279–285.

MACCHIA, V., BATES, R. W. and PASTAN, I. (1967) The purification and properties of a thyroid-stimulating factor isolated from *Clostridium perfringens. J. Biol. Chem.* **242**: 3726–3730.

MACFARLANE, M. G. and KNIGHT, B. C. J. G. (1941) The biochemistry of bacterial toxins. I. The lecithinase activity of *Cl. welchii* toxins. *Biochem. J.* **35**: 884–902.

MACKAY, N. N. S., GRUNEBERG, R. N., HARRIES, B. J. and THOMAS, P. K. (1971) Primary *Clostridium welchii* meningitis. *Br. Med. J.* **1**: 591–592.

MACKAY, R. J., CARLSON, G. P. and HIRSH, D. C. (1979) *Clostridium perfringens* associated with a focal abscess in a horse. *J. Amer. Vet. Med. Assoc.* **175**: 71–72.

MACLENNON, J. D. (1962) Histotoxic clostridial infections of man. *Bact. Rev.* **26**: 177–276.

MALIWAN, N. (1979) Emphysematous cystitis associated with *Clostridium perfringens* bacteremia. *J. Urol.* **121**: 819–820.

MANCINI, G., CARBONARA, A. O. and HEREMANS, J. F. (1965) Immunochemical quantitation of antigens by single radial immunodiffusion. *Immunochem.* **2**: 235–254.

MARIONA, F. G. and ISMAIL, M. A. (1980) *Clostridium perfringens* septicemia following cesarean section. *Obset Gynecol.* **56**: 518–521.

MARUCCI, A. A. and FULLER, T. C. (1971) Quantitative microcompliment fixation test. *Appl. Microbiol.* **21**: 260–264.

MASORO, E. J. (1968) *Physiological chemistry of lipids in mammals.* Saunders Co., Philadelphia.

MATSUDA, M. and SUGIMOTO, N. (1979) Calcium-independent and dependent steps in action of *Clostridium perfringens* enterotoxin on HeLa and Vero cells. *Biochem. Biophys. Res. Comm.* **91**: 629–636.

McCARTNEY, C. and ARBUTHNOTT, J. P. (1978) Mode of action of membrane-damaging toxins produced by staphylococci. In: *Bacterial toxins and cell membranes.* p. 89–127. JELJASZEWICZ, J. and WADSTRÖM, T. (eds.) Academic Press, N.Y.

McCLANE, B. A. and McDONEL, J. L. (1979) The effects of *Clostridium perfringens* enterotoxin on morphology, viability, and macromolecular synthesis in vero cells. *J. Cell. Physiol.* **99**: 191–200.

McCLANE, B. A. and McDONEL, J. L. (1980) Characterization of membrane permeability alterations induced in Vero cells by *Clostridium perfringens* enterotoxin. *Biochim. Biophys. Acta.* **600**: 974–985.

McCLANE, B. A. and McDONEL, J. L. (1981) Protective effects of osmotic stabilizers on morphological and permeability alterations induced in Vero cells by *Clostridium perfringens* enterotoxin. *Biochim. Biophys. Acta.* **641**: 401–409.

McCLUNG, L. S. (1945) Human food poisoning due to growth of *Clostridium perfringens* (*C. welchii*) in freshly cooked chicken. *J. Bacteriol.* **50**: 229–231.

McCREA, J. F. (1947) Modification of red-cell agglutinability by *Cl. welchii* toxins. *Aust. J. Exp. Biol. Med. Sci.* **25**: 127–136.

McDONEL, J. L. (1974) *In vivo* effects of *Clostridium perfringens* enteropathogenic factors on the rat ileum. *Infect. Immun.* **10**: 1156–1162.

McDONEL, J. L. (1979) The molecular mode of action of *Clostridium perfringens* enterotoxin. *Am. J. Clin. Nutr.* **32**: 210–218.

McDONEL, J. L. (1980a) Mechanism of action of *Clostridium perfringens* enterotoxin. *J. Food Technol.* **34**: 91–95.

McDONEL, J. L. (1980b) Binding of *Clostridium perfringens* ^{125}I-enterotoxin to rabbit intestinal cells. *Biochemistry* **21**: 4801–4807.

McDONEL, J. L. and ASANO, T. (1975) Analysis of unidirectional sodium fluxes during diarrhea induced by *Clostridium perfringens* enterotoxin in the rat terminal ileum. *Infect. Immun.* **11**: 526–529.

McDONEL, J. L., CHANG, L. W., POUNDS, J. G. and DUNCAN, C. L. (1978) The effects of *Clostridium perfringens* enterotoxin on rat and rabbit ileum: an electron microscopic study. *Lab. Invest.* **39**: 210–218.

McDONEL, J. L. and DEMERS, G. W. (1982) *In vivo* effects of enterotoxin from *Clostridium perfringens* type A in rabbit colon: binding vs. biologic activity. *J. Infect. Dis.* **145**: 490–494.

McDONEL, J. L. and DUNCAN, C. L. (1975a) Effects of *Clostridium perfringens* enterotoxin on metabolic indexes of everted rat ileal sacs. *Infect. Immun.* **12**: 274–280.

McDONEL, J. L. and DUNCAN, C. L. (1975b) Mechanism of action of *Clostridium perfringens* enterotoxin in the rat ileum: protein synthesis and cyclic 3′–5′ adenosine monophosphate. Proceeding of the 11th Joint Conference U. S. -Japan Cooperative Medical Science Program, Cholera Panel, p. 297–305.

McDONEL, J. L. and DUNCAN, C. L. (1975c) Histopathological effects of *Clostridium perfringens* enterotoxin in the rabbit ileum. *Infect. Immun.* **12**: 1214–1218.

McDONEL, J. L. and DUNCAN, C. L. (1976) Effect of *Clostridium perfringens* enterotoxin on mitochondrial respiration. *Infect. Immun.* **15**: 999–1001.

McDONEL, J. L. and DUNCAN, C. L. (1977) Regional localization of activity of *Clostridium perfringens* type A enterotoxin in the rabbit ileum. *J. Infect. Dis.* **136**: 661–666.

McDONEL, J. L. and McCLANE, B. A. (1979) Binding versus biological activity of *Clostridium perfringens* enterotoxin in vero cells. *Biochem. Biophys. Res. Commun.* **87**: 497–504.

McDONEL, J. L. and McCLANE, B. A. (1981) Highly sensitive assay for *Clostridium perfringens* enterotoxin that uses inhibition of plating efficiency of Vero cells grown in culture. *J. Clin. Microbiol.* **13**: 940–946.

MEDUSKI, J. W. and VOLKOVA, M. S. (1958) *Clostridium perfringens* (*welchii*) inaktywowaniem promieniami gamma. *Medycyna Dosw. Mikrobiol.* **10**: 247–254. (Biol. Abs. 1960, **35**: 38506).

MIHANCEA, N., BITTNER, J., TOACSEN, E., CEACURUANU, A. and TEODORESCU, G. (1970) Influence de la toxine perfringens sur la phagocytose et la viabilité leucocytaire. *Arch. Roum. Pathol. Exp. Microbiol.* **6**: 159–167.

MITSUI, K., MITSUI, N. and HASE, J. (1973) *Clostridium perfringens* exotoxins. I. Purification and properties of α-toxin. *Japan. J. Exp. Med.* **43**: 65–80.

MITSUI, K., MITSUI, N. and HASE, J. (1973) *Clostridium perfringens* exotoxins. II. Purification and some properties of θ-toxin. *Japan. J. Exp. Med.* **43**: 377–391.

MITSUI, K. and HASE, J. (1979) *Clostridium perfringens* enterotoxins. VI. Reactivity of perfringolysin 0 with thiol and disulfide compounds. *Japan. J. Exp. Med.* **49**: 13–18.

MITSUI, K., SEKIYA, T., NOZAWA, Y. and HASE, J. (1979) Alteration of human erythrocyte plasma membranes by perfringolysin 0 as revealed by freeze-fracture electron microscopy. Studies on *Clostridium perfringens* exotoxins V. *Biochim. Biophys. Acta* **554**: 68–75.

MIWANTANI, T., HONDA, T., ARAI, S. and NAKAYAMA, A. (1978) Mode of lethal activity of *Clostridium perfringens* type A enterotoxin. *Japan. J. Med. Sci. Biol.* **31**: 221–223.

MOHR, J. A., GRIFFITHS, W., HOLM, R., GARCIA-MORAL, C. and FLOURNOY, D. J. (1978) Clostridial myonecrosis ('gas gangrene') during cephalosporin porphylaxis. *J. Am. Med. Assoc.* **239**: 847–849.

MÖLLBY, R. (1973) Purification of two bacterial phospholipases C and some effects on cell membranes. Ph.D. Dissertation, Karolinska Institute, Stockholm.

MÖLLBY, R. (1976) Effect of staphylococcal beta-haemolysin (sphingomyelinase C) on cell membranes. In: *Staphylococci and Staphylococcal diseases.* pp. 665–667. JELJASZEWICZ, J. (ed.) Gustav Fischer Verlag, Stuttgart, N. Y.

MÖLLBY, R. (1978) Bacterial Phospholipases. In: *Bacterial toxins and cell membranes.* p. 367–424. JELIJASZEWICZ, J. and WADSTRÖM, T. (eds.) Academic Press, N. Y.

MÖLLBY, R., HOLME, T., NORD, C. -E., SMYTH, C. J. and WADSTRÖM, T. (1976) Production of phospholipase C (alpha toxin) haemolysis and lethal toxins by *Clostridium perfringens* types A to D. *J. Gen. Microbiol.* **96**: 137–144.

MÖLLBY, R., NORD, C. E. and WADSTRÖM, T. (1973) Biological activities contaminating preparations of phospholipase C (α-toxin) from *Clostridium perfringens.* *Toxicon.* **11**: 139–147.

MÖLLBY, R., THELESTAM, M. and WADSTRÖM, T. (1974) Effect of *Clostridium perfringens* phospholipase C (alpha toxin) on the human diploid fibroblast membrane. *J. Membrane Biol.* **16**: 313–330.

MÖLLBY, R. and WADSTRÖM, T. (1973) Purification of phospholipase C (α-toxin) from *Clostridium perfringens.* *Biochim. Biophys. Acta* **321**: 569–584.

MOORE, A., GOTTFRIED, E. L., STONE, P. H. and COLEMAN, M. (1976) Case report. *Clostridium perfringens* septicemia with detection of phospholipase C activity in the serum. *Am. J. Med. Sci.* **271**: 59–63.

MORGAN, K. T. and KELLY, B. G. (1974) Ultrastructural study of brain lesions produced in mice by the administration of *Clostridium perfringens* type D toxin. *J. Comp. Pathol.* **84**: 181–191.

MORGAN, K. T., KELLY, B. G. and BUXTON, D. (1975) Vascular leakage produced in the brains of mice by *Clostridium welchii* type D toxin. *J. Comp. Pathol.* **85**: 461–466.

NAGLER, F. P. O. (1939) Observations on a reaction between lethal toxins of *Cl. welchii* (Type A) and human serum. *Br. J. Exp. Path.* **20**: 473–485.

NAIK, H. S. and DUNCAN, C. L. (1977a) Enterotoxin formation in foods by *Clostridium perfringens* type A. *J. Food Safety* **1**: 7–18.

NAIK, H. S. and DUNCAN, C. L. (1977b) Rapid detection and quantitation of *Clostridium perfringens* enterotoxin by counterimmunoelectrophoresis. *Appl. Environ. Microbiol.* **34**: 125–128.

NAIK, H.S. and DUNCAN, C. L. (1978a) Thermal inactivation of *Clostridium perfringens* enterotoxin. *J. Food Prot.* **41**: 100–103.

NAIK, H. A. and DUNCAN, C. L. (1978b) Detection of *Clostridium perfringens* enterotoxin in human fecal samples and antienterotoxin in sera. *J. Clin. Microbiol.* **7**: 337–340.

NIILO, L. (1965) Bovine enterotoxemia. III. Factors affecting the stability of the toxins of *Clostridium perfringens* types A, C, and D. *Can. Vet. J.* **6**: 38–42.

NIILO, L. (1971) Mechanism of action of the enteropathogenic factor of *Clostridium perfringens* type. A. *Infect. Immun.* **3**: 100–106.

NIILO, L. (1972) The effect of enterotoxin of *Clostridium welchii* (*perfringens*) on the systemic blood pressure of sheep. *Res. Vet. Sci.* **13**: 503–505.

NIILO, L. (1973a) Fluid secretory response of bovine Thiry jejunal fistula to enterotoxin of *Clostridium perfringens*. *Infect. Immun.* **7**: 1–4.

NIILO, L. (1973b) Effect of calves of the intravenous injection of the enterotoxin of *Clostridium perfringens* type A. *J. Comp. Pathol.* **83**: 265–269.

NIILO, L. (1973c) Antigen homogeneity of enterotoxin from different agglutinating serotypes of *Clostridium perfringens*. *Can. J. Microbiol.* **19**: 521–524.

NIILO, L. (1974) Response of ligated intestinal loops in chickens to the enterotoxin of *Clostridium perfringens*. *Appl. Microbiol.* **28**: 889–891.

NIILO, L. (1975) Measurement of biological activities of purified and crude enterotoxin of *Clostridium perfringens*. *Infect. Immun.* **12**: 440–442.

NIILO, L. (1976) The effect of enterotoxin of *Clostridium welchii* (*perfringens*) type A on fowls. *Res. Vet. Sci.* **20**: 225–226.

NIILO, L. (1977) Enterotoxin formation by *Clostridium perfrigens* type A studied by the use of fluorescent antibody. *Can. J. Microbiol.* **23**: 908–915.

NIILO, L. (1978) Efficacy of laboratory tests for the detection of enterotoxigenic *Clostridium perfringens*. *Can. J. Microbiol.* **24**: 633–635.

NIILO, L. (1979) Identification of enterotoxigenic *Clostridium perfringens* type A in mixed cultures. *Can. J. Comp. Med.* **43**: 98–101.

NIILO, L. and BAINBOROUGH, A. R. (1980) A survey of *Clostridium perfringens* enterotoxin antibody in human and animal sera in western Canada. *Can. J. Microbiol.* **26**: 1162–1164.

NIILO, L., HAUSCHILD, A. H. W. and DORWARD, W. J. (1971) Immunization of sheep against experimental *Clostridium perfringens* type A enteritis. *Can. J. Microbiol.* **17**: 391–395.

NYGREN, B. (1962) Phospholipase C-producing bacteria and food poisoning. *Acta Pathol. Microbiol. Scand.* (Suppl.) **160**: 1–88.

OAKLEY, C. L. (1949) The toxins of *Clostridium welchii* type F. *Br. Med. J.* **1**: 269–270.

OAKLEY, C. L. and WARRACK, G. H. (1953) Routine typing of *Clostridium welchii*. *J. Hyg., Camb.* **51**: 102–107.

OAKLEY, C. L., WARRACK, G. H. and VAN HEYNINGEN, W. E. (1946) The collagenase (κ toxin) of *Cl. welchii* type A. *J. Pathol. Bacteriol.* **58**: 229–235.

OAKLEY, C. L., WARRACK, G. H. and WARREN, M. E. (1948) The kappa and lambda antigens of *Clostridium welchii*. *J. Pathol. Bacteriol.* **60**: 495–503.

OCHOA, R. and KERN, S. R. (1980) The effects of *Clostridium perfringens* type A enterotoxin in Shetland ponies – clinical, morphologic and clinicopathologic changes, *Vet. Pathol.* **17**: 737–747.

OCHOA, R. and VELANDIA, S. (1978) Equine grass sickness: serologic evidence of association with *Clostridium perfringens* type A enterotoxin. *Am. J. Vet. Res.* **39**: 1049–1051.

OGIER, C., SJÖGREN, A. M. and REIZENSTEIN, P. (1979) Effect of *Clostridium perfringens* neuraminidase on viability and antigenicity of human leukemic myeloblasts. *Biomedicine* **31**: 250–252.

OHSAKA, A., SUGAHARA, T., TAKAHASHI, T. and YAMAYA, S. (1978a) Effects of α-toxin (phospholipase C) of *Clostridium perfringens* on micro-circulation. In: *Toxins, animal, plant, and microbial.* p. 1031–1048 ROSENBERG, P. (ed.) (Suppl. No. 1, Toxicon) Pergamon Press, N. Y.

OHSAKA, A., TSUCHIYA, M., OSHIO, C., MIYAIRA, M., SUZUKI, K. and YAMAKAWA, Y. (1978b) Aggregation of platelets in the mesenteric micro-circulation of the rat induced by α-toxin (phospholipase C) of *Clostridium perfringens*. *Toxicon.* **16**: 333–341.

OLSVIK, O., GRANUM, P. E. and BERDAL, B. P. (1982) Detection of *Clostridium perfringens* type A enterotoxin by ELISA. *Acta Path. Microbiol. Immunol. Scand. Sect. B.* **90**: 445–447.

ORCUTT, R. P., FOSTER, H. L. and JONAS, A. M. (1978) *Clostridium perfringens* type E enterotoxemia as the cause of acute diarrheal death or "hemorrhagic typhlitis" in rabbits. Abstract # 100. *Am. Assoc. Lab. Animal Sci. Publ. 78-4.*

ORLANS, E. S., RICHARDS, C. B. and JONES, V. E. (1960) *Clostridium welchii* epsilontoxin and antitoxin. *Immunology* **3**: 28–44.

OTNAESS, A-B. and HOLM, T. (1976) The effect of phospholipase C on human blood platelets. *J. Clin. Invest.* **57**: 1419–1425.

OXER, D. T., MINTY, D. W. and LIEFMAN, C. E. (1971) Vaccination trials in sheep with clostridial vaccines with special reference to passively acquired *Cl. welchii* type D antitoxin in lambs. *Aust. Vet. J.* **47**: 134–140.

PARK, Y., BABAJIMOPOULUS, M. and MIKOLAJCIK, E. M. (1977) Purification and activity of *Clostridium perfringens* alpha toxin. *J. Food Prot.* **40**: 831–834.

PARNAS, J. (1976) About the influence of β toxin of *Clostridium perfringens* type C on the motorics of testine segments *in vitro*. Part 1. Zentralbl. *Bacteriol. Parasitenkd.* **234**: 243–246.

PATTON, N. M., HOLMES, H. T., RIGGS, R. J. and CHEEKE, P. R. (1978) Enterotoxemia in rabbits. *Lab. Anim. Sci.* **28**: 536–540.

PETRIE, H. L., MCDONEL, J. L. and SCHLEGEL, R. A. (1982) Intracellular antibody against *Clostridium perfringens* enterotoxin fails to counteract enterotoxin-induced damage. Cell Biology International Reports **6**: 705–711.

PETROV, R. V., SHEMANOVA, G. F., KAVERZNEVA, E. D., LISSEL, V. L., PANTELEEV, E. I., DMITRIEVA, L. N. and RUDNEVA, T. B. (1978) Immunogenicity and thymus-dependence of polymerized *Clostridium perfringens* α-toxoid. *Bull. Expt. Biol. Med.* **84**: 1743–1737.

PLOTKIN, G. R., KLUGE, R. M. and WALDMAN, R. G. (1979) Gastroenteritis: etiology, pathophysiology and clinical manifestations. *Med.* **58**: 95–114.

PINEGAR, J. A. and STRINGER, M. F. (1977) Outbreaks of food poisoning attributed to lecithinase-negative *Clostridium welchii*. *J. Clin. Pathol.* **30**: 491–492.

PRIGENT, D. and ALOUF, J. E. (1976) Interaction of streptolysin 0 with sterols. *Biochim. Biophys. Acta* **443**: 288–300.

REHG, J. E. and PAKES, S. P. (1982) Implication of *Clostridium difficile* and *Clostridium perfringens* Iota Toxins in Experimental Lincomycin-Associated Colitis of Rabbits[1,2,3] *Lab. Anim. Sci.* **32**: 253–257.

RICHARDSON, M. and GRANUM, P. E. (1983) Sequence of aminoterminal part of enterotoxin from *Clostridium perfringens* type A: identification of points of trypsin activation. *Infect. Immun.* **40**: 943–949.

RIGBY, G. J. (1981) An egg-yolk agar diffusion assay for monitoring phospholipase C in cultures of *Clostridium welchii*. *J. Appl. Bacteriol.* **50**: 11–19.

ROBB-SMITH, A. H. T. (1945) Tissue changes induced by *Cl. welchii* type A filtrates. *Lancet* **2**: 362–368.

ROBERTSON, W. B., ROPES, M. W. and BAUER, W. (1940) Mucinase: a bacterial enzyme which hydrolyzes synovial fluid mucin and other mucins. *J. Biol. Chem.* **133**: 261–276.

ROGERS, H. J. (1948) The complexity of the hyaluronidases produced by microorganisms. *Biochem. J.* **42**: 633–640.

ROOD, J. I., SCOTT, V. N. and DUNCAN, C. L. (1978a) Identification of a transferable tetracycline resistance plasmid (pCW3) from *Clostridium perfringens*. *Plasmid* **1**: 563–570.

ROOD, J. I., MAHER, E. M., SOMERS, E. B., CAMPOS, E. and DUNCAN, C. L. (1978b) Isolation and characterization of multiple antibiotic-resistant *Clostridium perfringens* strains from porcine feces. *Antimicrob. Agents Chemother.* **13**: 871–880.

ROOD, J. I. and WILKINSON, R. G. (1974) Affinity chromatography of *Clostridium perfringens* sialidase non specific adsorption of haemagglutinin, haemolysin and phospholipase C to Sepharosyl-glycyl-tryosyl [N-(p-aminophenyl) oxamic acid]. *Biochim. Biophys. Acta* **334**: 168–178.

ROOD, J. I. and WILKINSON, R. G. (1976) Relationship between haemagglutinin and sialidase from *Clostridium perfringens* CN3870: chromatographic characterization of the biologically active proteins. *J. Bacteriol.* **126**: 841–844.

ROSENBERG, A. and SCHENGRUND, C. L. (1976) Sialidases: In: *Biological roles of sialic acid.* p. 259–359. ROSENBERG, A. and SCHENGRUND, C. L. (eds.) Plenum Press, N. Y.

ROSENBERG, P. (1976) Bacterial and snake venom phospholipases: enzymatic probes in the study of structure and function in bioelectrically excitable tissues. In: *Animal, plant, and microbial toxins,* vol. II. p. 229–262. OHSAKA, A., HAYASHI, K. and SAWAI, Y. (eds.) Plenum Press, N.Y.

ROSENTHAL, A. F., CHODSKY, S. V. and HAN, S. C. H. (1969) Relationship between chemical structure and platelet-aggregation activity of prostagladins. *Biochim. Biophys. Acta* **187**: 385–392.

ROSENTHAL, A. F. and POUSADA, M. (1968) Inhibition of phospholipase C by phosphonate analogs of glycerophosphatides. *Biochim. Biophys. Acta* **164**: 226–237.

ROSS, H. E., WARREN, M. E. and BARNES, J. M. (1949) *Clostridium welchii* iota toxin: its activation by trypsin. *J. Gen. Microbiol.* **3**: 148–152.

ROTTEM, S., HARDEGREE, M. C., GRABOWSKI, M. W., FORNWALD, R. and BARILE, M. F. (1976) Interaction between tetanolysin and mycoplasma cell membrane. *Biochim. Biophys. Acta* **455**: 876–888.

SABBAN, E., LASTER, Y. and LOYTER, A. (1972) Resolution of the hemolytic and the hydrolytic activities of phospholipase-C preparations from *Clostridium perfringens*. *Eur. J. Biochem.* **28**: 373–380.

SAKAGUCHI, G., UEMURA, T. and TIEMANN, H. P. (1973) Simplified method for purification of *Clostridium perfringens* type A enterotoxin. *Appl. Microbiol.* **26**: 762–767.

SAKURAI, J. and DUNCAN, D. L. (1977) Purification of beta toxin from *Clostridium perfringens* type C. *Infect. Immun.* **18**: 741–745.

SAKURAI, J. and DUNCAN, C. L. (1978) Some properties of beta toxin produced by *Clostridium perfringens* type C. *Infect. Immun.* **21**: 678–680.

SAKURAI, J. and DUNCAN, C. L. (1979) Effect of carbohydrates and control of culture pH on beta toxin production by *Clostridium perfringens* type C. *Microbiol. Immunol.* **23**: 313–318.

SAKURAI, J. FUJII, Y. and MATSUURA, M. (1980) Effect of oxidizing agents and sulfhydril group reagents on beta toxin from *Clostridium perfringens* type C. *Microbiol. Immunol.* **24**: 595–601.

SAKURAI, J., FUJII, Y., MATSUURA, M. and ENDO, K. (1981) Pharmacological effect of beta toxin of *Clostridium perfringens* type C on rats. *Microbiol. Immunol* **25**: 423–432.

SAKURAI, J., FUJII, Y., DEZAKI, K. and ENDOH, K. (1982) Study of hypertension caused by beta toxin of *Clostridium perfringens* type C. *Jap. J. Med. Science and Biology.* **35**: 126–127.

SALINOVICH, O., MATTICE, W. L. and BLAKENEY, JR., E. W. (1982) Effects of temperature, pH and detergents on the molecular conformation of the enterotoxin of *Clostridium perfringens*. *Biochim. Biophys. Acta.* **707**: 147–153.

SATO, H., YAMAKAWA, Y., ITO, A. and MURATA, R. (1978) Effect on zinc and calcium ions on the production of alpha-toxin and proteases by *Clostridium perfringens*. *Infect. Immun.* **20**: 325–333.

SCHILLER, M., DONNELLY, P. J., MELO, J. C. and RAFF, M. J. (1979) *Clostridium perfringens* septic arthritis. *Clin. Orthop.* **139**: 92–96.

SCOTT, V. N. and DUNCAN, C. L. (1975) Affinity chromatography purification of *Clostridium perfringens* enterotoxin. *Infect. Immun.* **12**: 536–543.

SEBALD, M., BOUANCHAUD, D. and BIETH, G. (1975) Nature plasmiquide de la resistance a plusieurs antibiotiques chez *C. perfingens* type A, soche 659. *C. R. Acad. Sci.* (Paris) **280**: 2401–2404.

SEBALD, M. and BRÉFORT, G. (1975) Transfer du plasmide tetracycline-chloramphenicol chez *Clostridium perfringens*. *C. R. Acad. Sci.* (Paris) **281**: 317–319.

SEIFFERT, G. (1939) A reaction in human serum with *Cl. perfringens* toxin. *Z. Immun. Forsch.* **96**: 515–520.

SENFF, L. M. M. and MOSKOWITZ, M. (1969) Relation of *in vitro* inhibition by chelates of *Clostridium perfringens* α-toxin to their ability to protect against experimental toxemia. *J. Bacteriol.* **98**: 29–35.

SERADGE, H. and ANDERSON, M. G. (1980) Clostridial myonecrosis following intra-articular steroid injection. *Clin. Orthop.* **147**: 207–209.

SERRANO, A. M. and SCHNEIDER, I. S. (1978) New modification of Willis and Hobb's method for identification of *Clostridium perfringens*. *Appl. Environ. Microbiol.* **35**: 809–810.

SHANDERA, W. X., TACKET, C. O. and BLAKE, P. A. (1983) Food poisoning due to *Clostridium perfringens* in the United States *J. Infect. Dis.* **147**: 167–170.

SHEMANOVA, G. R., VLASOVA, E. G., TSVETKOV, V. S., LOGUNOV, A. I. and LEVIN, F. B. (1968) Extraction and properties of *Clostridium perfringens* lecithinase. *Biochemistry*, N.Y. (Eng. ed) **33**: 110–115.

SHUKLA, S. D., COLEMAN, R., FINEAN, J. B. and MICHELL, R. H. (1978) The use of phospholipase C to detect structural changes in the membranes of human erythrocytes aged by storage. *Biochim. Biophys. Acta* **512**: 341–349.

SKJELKVALÉ, R. (1980) Radioiodination of enterotoxin from *Clostridium perfringens* type A using chloramine T. *J. Appl. Bacteriol.* **48**: 283–295.

SKJELKVALÉ, R. and DUNCAN, C. L. (1975a) Enterotoxin formation by different toxigenic types of *Clostridium perfringens*. *Infect. Immun.* **11**: 563–575.

SKJELKVALÉ, R. and DUNCAN, C. L. (1975b) Characterization of enterotoxin purified from *Clostridium perfringens* type C. *Infect. Immun.* **11**: 1061–1068.

SKJELKVALÉ, R., TOLLESHAUG, H. and JARMUND, T. (1980) Binding of enterotoxin from *Clostridium perfringens* type A to liver cells *in vivo* and *in vitro*. *Acta Path. Microbiol. Scand. Sect. B*. **88**: 95–102.

SKJELKVALÉ, R. and UEMURA, T. (1977a) Detection of enterotoxin in faeces and anti-enterotoxin in serum after *Clostridium perfringens* food-poisoning. *J. Appl. Bacteriol.* **42**: 355–363.

SKJELKVALÉ, R. and UEMURA, T. (1977b) Experimental diarrhoea in human volunteers following oral administration of *Clostridium perfringens* enterotoxin. *J. Appl. Bacteriol.* **43**: 281–286.

SMART, J. L., ROBERTS, T. A., STRINGER, M. F. and SHAH, N. (1979) The incidence and serotypes of *Clostridium perfringens* on beef, pork, and lamb carcasses. *J. Appl. Bacteriol.* **46**: 377–383.

SMITH, L. DS. (1975a) *The pathogenic anaerobic bacteria*. (2nd Ed.) Charles C. Thomas. Springfield. IL.

SMITH, L. DS. (1975b) Clostridial infections. In: *Isolation and identification of Avian Pathogens*. p. 95–96. HITCHNER, S. B., DOMERMUTH, C. H., PURCHASE, H. G. and WILLIAMS, J. E. (eds.) *Am. Assoc. of Avian Pathologists*.

SMITH, L. DS. and GARDNER, V. M. (1950) The anomalous heat inactivation of *Clostridium perfringens* lecithinase *Arch. Biochem.* **25**: 54–60.

SMITH, W. P. and McDONEL, J. L. (1980) *Clostridium perfringens* type A: *In vitro* systems for sporulation and enterotoxin synthesis. *J. Bacteriol.* **144**: 306–311.

SMYTH, C. J. (1974) Multiple forms of *Clostridium perfringens* θ-toxin (θ-haemolysin): physical properties and biological characteristics. *Proc. Soc. Gen. Microbiol.* **1**: 56.

SMYTH, C. J. (1975) The identification and purification of multiple forms of θ-haemolysin (θ-toxin) of *Clostridium perfringens* type A. *J. Gen. Microbiol.* **87**: 219–238.

SMYTH, C. J. and ARBUTHNOTT, J. P. (1972) Characteristics of *Clostridium perfringens* type A θ-toxin purified by isoelectric focusing. *J. Gen. Microbiol.* **71**: ii (abstract).

SMYTH, C. J. and ARBUTHNOTT, J. P. (1974) Properties of *Clostridium perfringens* (*welchii*) type A θ-toxin (Phospholipase C) purified by electrofocusing. *J. Med. Microbiol.* **7**: 41–66.

SMYTH, C. J., ARBUTHNOTT, J. P. and FREER, J. H. (1972) Purification properties and biological characteristics of *Clostridium perfringens* type A θ-toxin. *J. Gen. Microbiol.* **73**: xxvi (abstract).

SMYTH, C. J. and DUNCAN, C. L. (1978) Thiol-activated (oxygen-labile) cytolysins. In: *Bacterial toxins and cell membranes*. p. 129–183. JELJASZEWICZ, J. and WADSTRÖM, T. (eds.) Academic Press. N.Y.

SMYTH, C. J., FREER, J. H. and ARBUTHNOTT, J. P. (1975) Interaction of *Clostridium perfringens* θ-hemolysin, a contaminant of commercial phospholipase C, with erythrocyte membranes and lipid dispersions, a morphological study. *Biochim. Biophys. Acta* **382**: 479–493.

SMYTH, C. J. and WADSTRÖM, T. (1975) Isoelectric focusing in this layer polyacrylamide gel combined with a zymogian method for detecting enzyme microheterogeneity: sample application. *Anal. Biochem.* **65**: 137–152.

SODA, S., ITO, A. and YAMAMOTO, A. (1976) Production and properties of θ-toxin of *Clostridium perfringens* with special reference of lethal activity. *Japan. J. Med. Sci. Biol.* **29**: 335–349.

STAHL, W. L. (1973) Phospholipase C purification and specificity with respect to individual phospholipids and brain microsomal membrane phospholipids. *Arch. Biochem. Biophys.* **154**: 47–55.

STARK, R. L. and DUNCAN, C. L. (1971) Biological characteristics of *Clostridium perfringens* type A enterotoxin. *Infect. Immun.* **4**: 89–96.

STARK, R. L. and DUNCAN, C. L. (1972a) Transient increase in capillary permeability induced by *Clostridium perfringens* type A enterotoxin. *Infect. Immun.* **5**: 147–150.

STARK, R. L. and DUNCAN, C. L. (1972b) Purification and biochemical properties of *Clostridium perfringens* type A enterotoxin. *Infect. Immun.* **6**: 662–673.

STERN, G. A., HODES, B. L. and STOCK, E. L. (1979) *Clostridium perfringens* corneal ulcer. *Arch. Ophthmalmol.* **97**: 661–663.

STERN, M. and WARRACK, G. H. (1964) The types of *Clostridium perfringens*. *J. Pathol. Bacteriol.* **88**: 279–283.

STERNE, M. and BATTY, I. (1975) Criteria for diagnosing clostridial infection. In: *Pathogenic clostridia*. p. 79–84. Butterworth & Co. London.

STRANDBERG, K., MÖLLBY, R. and WADSTRÖM, T. (1974) Histamine release from mast cells by highly purified phospholipase C (α-toxin) and theta from *Clostridium perfringens*. *Toxicon*. **12**: 199–208.

STRONG, D. H., DUNCAN, C. L. and PERNA, G. (1971) *Clostridium perfringens* type A food poisoning. II. Response of the rabbit ileum as an indication of enteropathogenicity of strains of *Clostridium perfringens* in human beings. *Infect. Immun.* **3**: 171–178.

STRUNK, S. W., SMITH, C. W. and BLUMBERG, J. M. (1967) Ultrastructural studies on the lesion produced in skeletal muscle fibers by crude type A *Clostridium perfringens* toxin and its purified alpha fraction. *Amer. J. Pathol.* **50**: 89–107.

SUGAHARA, T. and OHSAKA, S. (1970) Two molecular forms of *Clostridium perfringens* α-toxin associated with lethal, hemolytic and enzymatic activities. *Japan. J. Med. Sci. Biol.* **23**: 61–66.

SUGAHARA, T., TAKAHASHI, T., YAMAYA, S. and OHSAKA, A. (1976) *In vitro* aggregation of platelets induced by alpha-toxin (phospholipase C) of *Clostridium perfringens*. *Japan. J. Med. Sci. Biol.* **29**: 255–263.

SUGAHARA, T., TAKAHASHI, T., YAMAYA, S. and OHSAKA, A. (1977) Vascular permeability increase by α-toxin (phospholipase C) of *Clostridium perfringens*. *Toxicon*. **15**: 81–87.

SUGIURA, M., OGISO, T., TAKEUTI, K., TAMURO, S. and ITO, A. (1973) Studies on trypsin inhibitors in sweet potato. I. Purification and some properties. *Biochim. Biophys. Acta* **328**: 407–417.

SUTTON, R. G. A. and HOBBS, B. C. (1968) Food poisoning caused by heat-sensitive *Clostridium welchii*. A report of five recent outbreaks. *J. Hyg. Camb.* **66**: 135–146.

SZMIGIELSKI, S., JANIAK, M., MÖLLBY, R., WADSTRÖM, T. and JELJASZEWICZ, J. (1978) Metabolism of rabbit kidney cells incubated *in vitro* with phospholipase C from *Staphylococcus aureus* and *Clostridium perfringens*. *Toxicon.* **16:** 567–574.

TAGUCHI, R. and IKEZAWA, H. (1976a) Studies on the hemolytic and hydrolytic actions of phospholipases against mammalian erythrocyte membranes. *Archs. Biochem. Biophys.* **173:** 538–545.

TAGUCHI, R. and IKEZAWA, H. (1976b) Studies on the mode of action of phospholipases on mammalian erythrocytes. In: *Animal, plant, and microbial toxins.* Vol. I. p. 429–436. OHSAKA, A., HAYASHI, K. and SAUAI, Y. (eds.) Plenum Press, N.Y.

TAKAHASHI, T., SUGAHARA, T. and OHSAKA, A. (1974) Purification of *Clostridium perfringens* phospholipase C (α-toxin) by affinity chromatography on agarose-linked egg-yolk lipoprotein. *Biochim. Biophys. Acta* **351:** 155–171.

TEODORESCU, G. H., BITTNER, J. and CERCARCANU, A. (1970) Données preliminaires sur la purification et la structure de l'alphatoxine *Clostridium perfringens. Arch. Roum. Pathol. Exp. Microbiol.* **29:** 541–544.

THELESTAM, M. and MÖLLBY, R. (1975a) Determination of toxin-induced leakage of different size nucleotides through the plasma membrane of human diploid fibroblasts. *Infect. Immun.* **11:** 640–648.

THELESTAM, M. and MÖLLBY, R. (1975b) Sensitive assay for detection of toxin-induced damage to the cytoplasmic membrane of human diploid fibroblasts. *Infect. Immun.* **12:** 225–232.

THELESTAM, M. and MÖLLBY, R. (1976) Cytotoxic effects on the plasma membrane of human diploid fibroblasts, a comparative study of leakage tests. *Med. Biol.* **54:** 39–49.

THELESTAM, M. and MÖLLBY, R. (1980) Interaction of streptolysin O from *Streptococcus pyrogenes* and theta-toxin from *Clostridium perfringens* with human fibroblasts. *Infect. Immun.* **29:** 863–872.

THOMPSON, R. O. (1962) Crystalline ε-prototoxin from *Clostridium welchii. Nature* **193:** 69–70.

THOMPSON, R. O. (1963) The fractionation of *Clostridium welchii* ε-antigen on cellulose ion exchangers. *J. Gen. Microbiol.* **31:** 79–90.

TIXIER, G. and ALOUF, J. E. (1976) Purification and some properties of *Clostridium perfringens* delta toxin. *Ann. Microbiol.* (Paris) **127B:** 509–524.

TOLLESHAUG, H., SKJELKVALE, R. and BERG, T. (1982) Quantitation of binding and subcellular distribution of *Clostridium perfringens* enterotoxin in rat liver cells. *Infect. Immun.* **37:** 486–491.

UEMURA, T., GENIGEORGIS, C., RIEMANN, H. P. and FRANTI, C. E. (1974) Antibody against *Clostridium perfringens* type A enterotoxin in human sera. *Infect. Immun.* **9:** 470–471.

UEMURA, T., SAKAGUCHI, G., ITOH, T., OKAZAWA, K. and SAKAI, S. (1975) Experimental diarrhea in cynomolgus monkeys by oral administration with *Clostridium perfringens* type A viable cells or enterotoxin. *Japan. J. Med. Sci. Biol.* **28:** 165–177.

UEMURA, T., SAKAGUCHI, G. and RIEMANN, H. P. (1973) *In vitro* production of *Clostridium perfringens* enterotoxin and its detection by reversed passive hemagglutination. *Appl. Microbiol.* **26:** 381–385.

UEMURA, T. and SKJELKVALE, R. (1976) An enterotoxin produced by *Clostridium perfringens* type D. Purification by affinity chromatography. *Acta Pathol. Microbiol. Scand. Sect. B* **84:** 414–420.

VAN DEENEN, L. L. M. (1964) The specificity of phospholipases. In: *Metabolism and physiological significance of lipids.* p. 155–178. DAWSON, R. M. C. and RHODES, D. N. (eds.) John Wiley, London.

VAN DEENEN, L. L. M., DEMEL, R. A., GUERTS VAN KESSEL, W. S. M., KAMP, H. H., ROELOFSEN, B., VERKLEIJ, A. J., WIRTZ, K. W. A. and ZWAAL, R. F. A. (1976) Phospholipases and monolayers as tools in studies on membrane structure. In: *The structural basis of membrane function.* p. 21–38. HATEFI, Y. and DJAVADI-OHANIANCE, L. (eds.) Academic Press, N.Y.

VAN HEYNINGEN, W. E. (1950) *Bacterial toxins.* C. J. Thomas, Springfield, Ill.

VINCE, A., DYER, N. H., O'GRADY, F. W. and DAWSON, A. M. (1972) Bacteriological studies in Crohn's disease. *J. Med. Microbiol.* **5:** 219–229.

WALKER, H. W. (1975) Food borne illness from *Clostridium perfringens. Crit. Rev. Food Sci. Nutr.* **7:** 71–104.

WALKER, P. D., FOSTER, W. H., KNIGHT, P. A., FREESTONE, D. S. and LAWRENCE, G. (1979) Development, preparation and safety testing of a *Clostridium welchii* type C Toxoid. I. Preliminary observations in man in Papua New Guinea. *J. Biol. Standard.* **7:** 315–323.

WATSON, K. C. and KERR, E. J. C. (1974) Sterol structural requirements for inhibition of streptolysin O activity. *Biochem. J.* **140:** 95–98.

WEINSTEIN, L. and BARZA, M. A. (1973) Gas gangrene. *N. Engl. J. Med.* **289:** 1129–1131.

WHITAKER, J. R. and GRANUM, P. E. (1980) The role of amino groups in the biological and antigenic activities of *Clostridium perfringens* type A enterotoxin. *J. Food Biochem.* **4:** 201–217.

WIERUP, M. (1977) Equine intestinal clostridiodis. An acute disease in horses associated with high intestinal count of *Clostridium perfringens* type A. *Acta Vet. Scand.* (suppl.) 62–64.

WILLIS, T. A. (1969) *Clostridia of Wound Infection.* Butterworth, London.

WILLIS, A. T. (1977) *Anaerobic Bacteriology: Clinical and Laboratory Practice.* (3rd Edition) Butterworth, London.

WILKINSON, P. C. (1975) Inhibition of leukocyte locomotion and chemotaxis by lipid specific bacterial toxins. *Nature* (Lond.) **255:** 485–487.

WNEK, A. P. and MCCLANE, B. A. (1983) Identification of a 50,000 M_r protein from rabbit brush border membranes that binds *Clostridium perfringens* enterotoxin. *Biochem. Biophys. Res. Commun.* **112:** 1099–1105.

WORTHINGTON, R. W., BERTSCHINGER, H. J. and MULDERS, M. S. G. (1979) Catecholamine and cyclic nucleotide response of sheep to the injection of *Clostridium welchii* type D epsilon toxin. *J. Med. Microbiol.* **12:** 497–501.

WORTHINGTON, R. W. and MÜLDERS, M. S. G. (1975a) Effect of *Clostridium perfringens* epsilon toxin on the blood brain barrier of mice. *Onderstepoort J. Vet. Res.* **42:** 25–28.

WORTHINGTON, R. W. and MÜLDERS, M. S. G. (1975b) The partial purification of *Clostridium perfringens* beta toxin. *Onderstepoort J. Vet. Res.* **42:** 91–98.

WORTHINGTON, R. W. and MÜLDERS, M. S. G. (1977) Physical changes in the epsilon prototoxin molecule of *Clostridium perfringens* during enzymatic activation. *Infect. Immun.* **18:** 549–551.

WORTHINGTON, R. W. and MÜLDERS, M. S. G. and VAN RENSBURG, J. J. (1973) Enzymatic activation of *Clostridium perfringens* epsilon toxin and some biological properties of activated toxin. *Onderstepoort J. Vet. Res.* **40:** 151–154.

WYNNE, J. W. and ARMSTRONG, D. (1972) Clostridial septicemia. *Cancer* **29:** 215–221.

YAMAGISHI, T., YOSHIZAWA, J., KAWAI, M., SEO, N. and NISHIDA, S. (1971) Identification of isolates of *Clostridium perfringens* types C and D by agglutination and fluorescent-antibody methods. *Appl. Microbiol.* **21**: 787–793.

YAMAGISHI, T., SAKAMOTO, K., SAKURAI, S., KONISHI, K., DAIMON, Y., MATSUDA, M., GYOBU, Y., KUBO, Y. and DODAMA, H. (1983) A nosocomial outbreak of food poisoning caused by enterotoxigenic *Clostridium perfringens*. *Microbiol. Immunol.* **27**: 291–296.

YAMAKAWA, Y., ITO, A. and SATO, H. (1977) Theta toxin of *Clostridium perfringens*. I. Purification and some properties. *Biochim. Biophys. Acta* **494**: 301–313.

YAMAKAWA, Y. and OHSAKA, A. (1977) Purification and some properties of phospholipase C (α-toxin) of *Clostridium perfringens*. *J. Biochem.* **81**: 115–126.

YAMAMOTO, K., OHISHI, I. and SAKAGUCHI, G. (1979) Fluid accumulation in mouse ligated intestine inoculated with *Clostridium perfringens* enterotoxin. *Appl. Environ. Microbiol.* **37**: 181–186.

YOTIS, W. W. and CATSIMPOOLAS, N. (1975) Scanning isoelectric focusing and isotachophoresis of *Clostridium perfringens* type A enterotoxin. *J. Appl. Bacteriol.* **39**: 147–156.

ZEISSLER, J. and RASSFELD–STERNBERG, L. (1949) Enteritis necroticans due to *Clostridium welchii* type F. *Br. Med. J.* **1**: 267–269.

ZWAAL, R. F. A., ROELOFSEN, B. and COLLEY, C. M. (1973) Localization of red cell membrane constituents. *Biochim. Biophys. Acta* **300**: 159–182.

ZWAAL, R. F. A., ROELOFSEN, B., COMFURIUS, P. and VAN DEENEN, L. L. M. (1975) Organization of phospholipids in human red cell membranes as detected by the actions of various purified phospholipases. *Biochim. Biophys. Acta* **406**: 83–96.

CHAPTER 23

CLOSTRIDIUM BOTULINUM TOXINS

Genji Sakaguchi

*University of Osaka Prefecture, College of Agriculture, 804 Mozu-ume-machi 4-cho,
Sakai-shi, Osaka 591, Japan*

1. HISTORICAL ASPECTS

1.1. Discovery of Different Types of Botulinum Toxin

Botulinum toxin is a neurotoxin of high molecular weight protein produced by *Clostridium botulinum* and the cause of human and animal botulism with high fatality rates. Botulism, sausage poisoning in Latin, is the term given to designate such an acute food poisoning caused by the ingestion of spoiled sausages that has been known in Europe for more than 2,000 years (Dack, 1956). In 1895, members of a musical party who partook of a festive meal at a wake at Elzele, Belgium, developed the symptoms of botulism and three of them died. Van Ermengem (1897) isolated anaerobic, spore-forming bacilli from the remains of the incriminated raw ham and the livers of the dead. Culture filtrates of the isolates, when administered to various experimental animals through different routes, produced paralytic symptoms resembling those of human botulism and led to death. He ascribed the extracellular toxin produced by the isolate to human botulism.

In 1904, 11 persons died from eating wax-bean salad in Darmstadt, Germany (Landmann, 1904). This episode proved that botulinum toxin is produced not only in meat and meat products but also in boiled vegetables. The antitoxic serum prepared against the toxin of Elzele strain did not neutralize the toxin of Darmstadt strain, nor did the antitoxic serum against the toxin of Darmstadt strain neutralize the toxin of Elzele strain. Thus, the toxins produced by the two strains were immunologically distinct (Leuchs, 1910). Botulinum toxins were later classified into types A and B (Meyer and Gunnison, 1929); the toxin of Darmstadt strain may have corresponded to type A and that of Elzele strain to type B.

Type C toxin was found in the United States in the cultures isolated from fly larvae (Bengtson, 1922) and in Australia in the cultures isolated from carcasses of cattle which died of bulbar paralysis (Seddon, 1922). The antitoxin prepared against the toxin of Bengtson strain neutralized the toxins of both Bengtson and Seddon strains, whereas the antitoxin against the toxin of Seddon strain neutralized the toxin of the homologous strain but did not neutralize that of Bengtson strain. It was proposed, therefore, that Bengtson strain be called *C. botulinum* type Cα and Seddon strain type Cβ (Pfenninger, 1924). Type D toxin was first reported by Theiler (1927).

It was later found that type C toxin cross-reacted with type D toxin (Mason and Robinson, 1935; Bulatova *et al.*, 1967). Mason and Robinson (1935) reported that type C strains produced three immunologically distinct toxin components, C1, C2, and a small amount of D, and that type D strains chiefly produced the D component and also a small quantity of the C component. More recently, Jansen (1971) demonstrated that type Cα strains produced C1, C2 and D factors; type Cβ produced C2 factors only and type D produced C1 and D factors. Except for type C and D strains, it had generally been believed that one strain of *C. botulinum* produces an antigenically single toxin until the isolation of a strain producing both type A and F toxins (Giménez and Ciccarelli, 1970a).

The cultures isolated from the intestines of sturgeons in Russia were identified as type E by Gunnison *et al* (1936). Møller and Scheibel (1960) isolated, from the liver paste that caused human botulism in Denmark, a new type *C. botulinum*, which was then designated as type F by Dolman and Murakami (1961). *C. botulinum* type G was isolated from a soil sample collected in Argentina (Giménez and Ciccarelli, 1970b).

1.2. CHARACTERIZATION OF BOTULINUM TOXINS

Purification of botulinum toxin was attempted and type A toxin was obtained in crystalline form for the first time as a bacterial toxin by Lamanna *et al.* (1946), who proved that botulinum toxin is a simple protein. In the following year, purification of type B toxin was reported (Lamanna and Glassman, 1947).

C. botulinum types A and B produce, in 1 ml of culture medium, a quantity of toxin corresponding to more than one million mouse intraperitoneal (i.p.) lethal doses, whereas type E organisms produce at most several hundred mouse i.p. lethal doses. To explain such a low toxigenicity of *C. botulinum* type E in contrast to such a high morbidity and mortality of human type E botulism comparable to those of type A and B botulism, several hypotheses were presented; e.g. a relatively higher sensitivity of man to type E toxin than to type A or B toxin and/or a higher rate of intestinal absorption of type E toxin than of type A or B toxin (Dolman, 1957). It was found that type E toxin is produced in a virtually nontoxic 'precursor' form. The precursor is 'activated' accompanying a several hundred-fold increase in the parenteral toxicity when treated with a proteolytic enzyme produced by an anaerobic microorganism (Sakaguchi and Tohyama, 1955a,b). In the following year it was found that trypsin activates type E precursor much more efficiently (Duff *et al.*, 1956). Jansen and Knoetze (1971) reported that C2 toxin is also activated upon trypsinization. The optimum reaction for activation of C2 toxin was found to be pH 7.5; in contrast, the optimum pH for activation of type E toxin is 6.0. It was found that the production of botulinum toxin, at least C1 and D toxins, is governed by infection of the bacterial cells with bacteriophages (Inoue and Iida, 1970).

It was demonstrated earlier that crystalline type A toxin, with a molecular weight of about 900,000, is a complex of neurotoxin and hemagglutinin (Lamanna, 1948), and that it dissociates reversibly under slightly alkaline conditions (Lowenthal and Lamanna, 1951, 1953). It has been demonstrated later that botulinum toxins of different types, regardless of the hemagglutinin activity, are commonly composed of a neurotoxin component of a molecular weight of about 150,000 and a nontoxic component of a molecular weight of about 150,000 or higher (Boroff *et al.*, 1966; Kitamura *et al.*, 1967). Some strains produce a toxin of a uniform molecular size, while others of two or three different molecular sizes. Botulinum toxin in the complexed form can be classified into three groups based on their molecular size, namely 12S, 16S, and 19S. All these three forms were shown with type A toxin (Sugii and Sakaguchi, 1977) and two forms, 12S and 16S, were shown with type B (Kozaki *et al.*, 1974), type C (Iwasaki and Sakaguchi, 1978), and type D toxins (Miyazaki *et al.*, 1977); whereas only a single form, 12S, was shown with type E (Kitamura *et al.*, 1968) and type F toxins (Ohishi and Sakaguchi, 1975). Within the same immunological type, the larger the molecular size of the toxin, the higher the oral toxicity but the lower the parenteral toxicity (Sakaguchi and Sakaguchi, 1974; Sugii *et al.*, 1977; Ohishi and Sakaguchi, 1980).

C2 toxin produced by most type C and some type D strains was purified and characterized (Iwasaki *et al.*, 1980; Ohishi *et al.*, 1980a). Its molecular structure is distinct from that of the toxin of types A–F, being constructed with two independent and dissimilar components with molecular weights of approximately 50,000 and 100,000. The toxicity is elicited by cooperation of the two components not held together. In addition to the lethal activity, C2 toxin has a vascular permeability activity (Ohishi *et al.*, 1980b).

1.3. NOMENCLATURE OF BOTULINUM TOXINS

Botulinum toxins produced in food and culture were proved to be 12S or larger (Schantz and Spero, 1967; Sakaguchi *et al.*, 1974; Sugii and Sakaguchi, 1977), being the complexes of a neurotoxic component of 7S and a nontoxic component of 7S or larger. The term 'progenitor toxin' was proposed to designate such a toxin complex appearing first in food or culture (Lamanna and Sakaguchi, 1971). The toxic component is released when the progenitor toxin is exposed to slightly alkaline conditions, pH 7.2 or higher. The term 'derivative toxin' was proposed by the same authors to designate the freed toxic component. Type E progenitor toxin is a nonactivated toxin; the trypsinized toxin is not called derivative toxin but 'activated progenitor toxin', since trypsinization does not accompany the dissociation (Kitamura *et al.*, 1968). 'Type E derivative toxin', therefore, designates the dissociated toxic component, regardless of whether or not it has been activated.

Of the three differently molecular-sized progenitor toxins, the 12S toxin was named 'medium-sized' or 'M toxin'; the 16S toxin 'large-sized' or 'L toxin'; the 19S toxin 'extra large-sized' or 'LL toxin'; and the 7S derivative toxin 'small-sized or 'S toxin' (Kozaki *et al.*, 1974; Sugii and Sakaguchi, 1975).

1.4. PATHOGENESIS OF BOTULISM

Van Ermengem (1897) considered that the characteristic neuroparalytic symptoms of botulism resulted from lesions of the central nervous system. It was soon made clear that the site of action of botulinum toxin is not central but peripheral (Dickson and Shevky, 1923a,b; Edmunds and Long, 1923). It was then made clear that botulinal toxin acts on the peripheral cholinergic nervous system (Ambache, 1948, 1949, 1951, 1952). The toxin, attacking on the presynaptic terminals, causes cholinergic blockade by inhibiting the release of the transmitter substance, acetylcholine (Burgen *et al.*, 1949; Brooks, 1956; Koelle, 1962). The toxin interacts with the peripheral nerve terminal (Simpson, 1973, 1974). The inhibition of neuromuscular transmission may involve at least two steps; the initial binding step, which does not impair transmission, is fast and temperature-independent, and the lytic step, which paralyzes transmission, is slow and is dependent on temperature and neuronal activity (Simpson, 1979). In addition, the necessity of a translocation step was suggested between the binding and the lytic steps (Simpson, 1980).

It is generally regarded that human and animal botulism is caused by ingestion of botulinum toxin preformed in food or feed, although intoxication with the toxin produced in the intestines (Minervin, 1967) or the organs of the host (Boroff and Reilly, 1962) has been suggested. Human wound infection, first reported in 1943, is caused by the toxin produced locally in the wound (Merson and Dowell, 1973). Infant botulism affecting those aged between 3 weeks and 8 months without any toxin source has often been reported since 1976 (Midura and Arnon, 1976). Thus, botulism caused by intravitally produced toxin has recently been given much attention.

2. HUMAN AND ANIMAL BOTULISM

2.1. HUMAN BOTULISM

Human botulism is classified into the following four types based on the mode of intoxication (Center for Disease Control, 1979). There is no transmission from one person to another, although sometimes many people are affected at one time after consumption of a common toxin source (Iida *et al.*, 1964; Rouhbakhsh-Khaleghdoust and Pourtaghva, 1977; Terranova *et al.*, 1978).

2.1.1. *Food-Borne Botulism*

It is the most common type caused by ingestion of the toxin preformed in food. Adult cases are mostly of this type. Usually two or more persons are intoxicated at a time from consumption of a common toxin source. Type A, B and E toxins have often been involved; type F toxin has been involved in two outbreaks. Laboratory diagnosis of food-borne botulism is dependent upon the detection and identification of the toxin in the blood serum of the patient and the incriminated food. Detection of the toxin in the fecal specimen is also useful for diagnosis (Craig *et al.*, 1970; Fukuda *et al.*, 1970; Dowell *et al.*, 1977).

2.1.2. *Wound Botulism*

This was first found in 1943, and 21 cases have been reported in the United States (anonymous, 1980a). A single case has been reported in Australia (Fullerton *et al.*, 1980). If a wound is infected with type A or B spores, they germinate, grow and produce toxin locally. The incubation period has ranged from 4 to 18 days. A single case per outbreak is a characteristic feature, and young boys (the median age for all cases has been 19 yr) have most often been affected.

2.1.3. *Infant Botulism*

This was first recognized in 1975 (Pickett *et al.*, 1976), but may not be a new disease (Arnon *et al.*, 1979). Only infants aged between 3 weeks and 8 months have been affected. At least 188 cases in the United States (anonymous, 1981), three cases in Australia (Douglas *et al.*, 1980) and single cases in the United Kingdom, Czechoslovakia and Canada have been reported (anonymous, 1980b). No toxin source has been found in any case. It is considered that the infant ingests viable spores, which may germinate, proliferate and produce toxin somewhere in the body; probably in the large intestines (Sugiyama, 1979). Honey has been incriminated as a probable vector of the spores (Arnon *et al.*, 1978a), although there are many other potential vectors. A single case per outbreak is also a characteristic feature; no other family members of the infant patient, except a set of twins (anonymous, 1980b), have ever developed the symptoms. Type A and B cases are common; a single type F case has been reported (anonymous, 1980c). The case–fatality rate has been 2.7%; however, it may have actually been higher since at least 5% of cases of sudden infant death syndrome were suspected of infant botulism (Arnon *et al.*, 1978b). No toxin in blood serum has been found in any case except one. Detection and identification of the toxin in the fecal materials are the key diagnosis. Excretion of the toxin and the organisms in the feces continues for a long period, although the cases recover spontaneously.

2.1.4. *Classification Undetermined*

Cases aged over one year where there has been no detection of the toxin source are classified into this category. There have been at least 13 outbreaks of this type involving 18 cases in the United States. It is considered that at least some of them must have been caused by the toxin produced intraintestinally like infant botulism. Recently, type G organisms were detected in necropsy specimens of four adults and an 18-week-old infant died suddenly and unexpectedly in Switzerland. Type G toxin was detected in the serum of two of the adults and the infant. Type D organisms and type A toxin were also detected in necropsy specimens of five other persons who died suddenly and unexpectedly (Sonnabend *et al.*, 1981).

2.2. ANIMAL BOTULISM

In contrast to human botulism, the outbreak of animal botulism sometimes involves thousands or tens of thousands of cases.

In captive minks, the same composite feed (raw animal offal, miscellaneous fish, etc.) is given to all animals on a farm. Therefore, if toxin (type C) is present in the feed, many animals develop symptoms and die at one time. In farmed fish, spores (type E) originally contained in feed would germinate, proliferate and produce the toxin in the bottom sludge of the pond, resulting in contamination of the water with the toxin, causing deaths of all the fish in the pond. In north European countries, particularly in Denmark, such outbreaks of type E botulism ('bankrupt disease') occur occasionally among cultured rainbow trouts in hot summer (Huss and Eskildsen, 1979).

In wild waterbirds, particularly in wild ducks, if an individual, a bird or animal carrying spores of *C. botulinum* (type C) in its intestines dies from any cause, the spores would germinate, proliferate and produce toxin in the carcass as an ideal culture medium. The toxin produced is ingested by the fly larvae that have developed in the rotten carcasses. The flesh protein is liquefied by the proteolytic enzymes excreted by the fly larvae, while the botulinum toxin seems to be resistant to such proteolysis and remains active in the live larvae. If a healthy duck picks up such toxic fly larvae, it would develop botulism from absorption of the toxin released from the larvae in the digestive tract. The spores ingested together with the toxin would again proliferate in the duck carcass. Thus, more and more healthy ducks are affected, resulting in deaths of tens and hundreds of thousands of birds in one outbreak (Kalmbach, 1968). A similar mode of intoxication is the case in reared pheasants (Lee *et al.*, 1962; Fish *et al.*, 1967; Borland, 1976). In such outbreaks among ducks or reared pheasants it appears as if botulism were a highly contagious disease. 'Lamziekte', a cattle botulism which used to prevail in South Africa, also affects one cow after another from ingestion of type D toxin formed in cattle carcasses as a culture medium (Theiler *et al.*, 1927).

Broiler chickens are occasionally affected by botulism (type C) without any toxin source (Roberts *et al.*, 1973). It is considered that there are many chances for broilers to ingest type C spores contained in feed, soil, litter, worms and bugs or other organic matters. The ingested spores germinate, proliferate and produce toxin, most likely in the ceca (Miyazaki and Sakaguchi, 1978), where the conditions are anerobic. Chickens are relatively insusceptible to type C toxin and they are often asymptomatic even if type C toxin is detectable in the circulating blood (Gunnison and Coleman, 1932; Roberts, 1975). Chickens are characteristic for coprophagy, by which they eat cecal droppings containing the toxin, the vegetative cells and the spores. The toxin is absorbed from the upper intestines and the viable organisms again proliferate and produce the toxin in the ceca. Such an intracecal toxin production–coprophagy cycle turns round until the blood toxin level reaches a certain threshold (unpublished data). This type of pathogenesis may be distinguished from feed-borne botulism and toxico-infection.

3. CLASSIFICATION OF BOTULINUM TOXIN AND ASSAY PROCEDURES

3.1. CLASSIFICATION OF BOTULINUM TOXIN

C. botulinum toxin is classified by the toxin–antitoxin neutralization test. It has been classified into types A through G in the chronological order of discovery except for types A and B as described earlier. The susceptibility of animals to botulinum toxin of a certain type differs from one animal species to another and that of animals of a certain species to botulinum toxins differs from one immunological type to another.

C. botulinum type C is classified into two subtypes, Cα and Cβ. It has long been known that the toxins of types Cα, Cβ and D cross-react one to another (Mason and Robinson, 1935; Bulatova *et al.*, 1967). A minor cross-reaction has also been reported between type E and F toxins (Møller and Scheibel, 1960; Dolman and Murakami, 1961). It is generally regarded that one strain of *C. botulinum* produces an immunologically single toxin, but type Cα, D, E, and F strains produce immunologically multiple toxin factors. Type A and F toxins produced by a single strain (strain 84) (Gimenez and Ciccarelli, 1970a) were proved to be borne by separate molecules (Sugiyama *et al.*, 1972); whereas C1 and D toxins produced by type C and D organisms appear to be borne by the same toxin molecule (Oguma *et al.*, 1980, 1981). It has been proved that C2 toxin produced by type C and D organisms is borne by an independent molecule (Ohishi *et al.*, 1980a). It has not been clarified whether type E and F toxins produced by a type E or F strain are borne by a single molecule or separate molecules.

The species of *C. botulinum* is distinguished from other species by the production of specific botulinum toxin, and it includes biologically heterogeneous groups of organisms. It includes both proteolytic and nonproteolytic strains. *C. botulinum* was once used to designate only nonproteolytic strains; proteolytic strains used to be called *C. parabotulinum*. Now all the strains producing the specific neurotoxin are called *C. botulinum*. Therefore, *C. botulinum* strains producing toxin which is immunologically of the same type are not necessarily the same in their cultural or biochemical characteristics. *C. botulinum* now includes at least four biologically different groups, I–IV (Smith, 1977).

Group I strains are strongly proteolytic and include all type A strains and some type B and F strains. The spores of the strains of this group are highly heat resistant.

Group II strains are strongly saccharolytic but nonproteolytic. They are psychrophilic, producing toxin at low temperatures such as 3.3°C (Schmidt *et al.*, 1962; Eklund *et al.*, 1967). The spores of this group are relatively heat labile (Dolman *et al.*, 1960; Eklund and Poysky, 1970; Roberts *et al.*, 1965). Group II includes all type E and some type B and F strains. The toxin produced by the organism of this group requires tryptic activation for its full toxicity.

Group III strains are nonproteolytic but gelatinolytic and saccharolytic. All type C and D strains belong to this group. The heat resistance of the spores of this group is intermediate (Segnar and Schmidt, 1971).

Group IV contains only type G strains, which are proteolytic but nonsaccharolytic. Type G toxin requires tryptic activation for its full toxicity (Smith, 1977; Solomon and Kautter, 1979).

3.2. PROCEDURES FOR ASSAYING BOTULINUM TOXIN

3.2.1. *Bioassay*

The most sensitive and widely used method for assaying botulinum toxin is i.p. injection of material into mice weighing 15–20 g. Cultures and extracts in gelatin phosphate diluent (pH 6.2) of food, feces and other solid materials are clarified by centrifugation. The clarified material is injected i.p. into mice, usually in 0.5 ml doses. Deaths from botulism usually occur within 24 hr but may often be delayed. The toxins of group II organisms are markedly potentiated upon trypsinization, except when in the serum of the patient; mouse tests therefore should be done with trypsinized as well as untrypsinized materials. It is necessary to trypsinize the material at pH 6 or lower; if the reaction of a material is pH 7 or higher, trypsinization decreases the toxicity (Duff *et al.*, 1956). The symptoms of mice often develop within 4 hr after injection and include initial characteristic vibration of the abdominal wall, followed by the wasp-shape abdomen and labored breathing with or without paralysis of the limbs. The lethal i.p. dose does not change depending upon the body weight or age of the mouse (Lamanna *et al.*, 1955).

Since the toxin is specifically neutralized with the antitoxin of a single type, the type of the toxin is indicated by the type of the antitoxin specifically neutralizing the toxicity of the material. Antitoxins are usually used at a concentration of 10 international units (IU)/ml, but to avoid cross-reactions between types C and D as well as types E and F, one IU/ml may be recommended. If the toxicity is too high, the toxin material is diluted appropriately in the gelatin phosphate diluent and neutralization tests are repeated.

For the quantitative determination of the toxin by the mouse i.p. injection method, the material is usually diluted two-fold serially in the gelatin phosphate diluent and each dilution is injected i.p. into four or more mice at 0.5 ml doses. After 4 days, the LD_{50} is calculated, often by the method of Reed and Muench (1938), and the toxicity of botulinum toxin is expressed generally in mouse i.p. LD_{50} per milliliter or per milligram protein nitrogen.

Quantitative determination of toxicity by mouse i.p. injection requires relatively large numbers of animals and a period of four days. If the toxin is injected i.v. into mice, the log dose is linearly proportional to log time-to-death in minutes between about 30 and 180 min (10^6–10^3 i.p. LD_{50}) (Boroff and Fleck, 1966; Sakaguchi *et al.*, 1968). Therefore, the mouse i.v. injection method is rapid, more accurate and simple with less mice to titrate botulinum toxin of any type. The standard curve must be prepared with the toxin of each type. The standard curve for a given type is applicable to the toxin of any molecular size, 19S, 16S, 16S and 7S, although Lamanna *et al.* (1970) claimed that crystalline type A toxin (mainly of 19S) and its dissociated toxic component (7S) gave different curves. This is contradictory to the known fact that the progenitor toxin dissociates into the 7S toxic and the nontoxic components as soon as it is injected i.v. (Hildebrand *et al.*, 1961; Kitamura *et al.*, 1969).

The i.v. injection method, however, should be applied only to the fully activated toxin, because activated and nonactivated type E toxin gave parallel but distinct curves (Sakaguchi *et al.*, 1968). It is also inadequate to apply this method to titrate a crude type C or D toxin, since they are usually mixtures of C1, C2 and D toxins, which give different curves. The time-to-death method can also be applied to titrate C2 toxin (Iwasaki *et al.*, 1980).

Guinea-pigs, gold fish, and other experimental animals have been used for titration of botulinum toxin, but are no longer used.

3.2.2. In vitro *Assay*

Botulinum toxin can be titrated by such *in vitro* methods as agar gel diffusion (Vermilyea *et al.*, 1968), immunoelectrophoresis (Miller and Anderson, 1971), capillary tube immunodiffusion (Mestrandrea, 1974), hemagglutination inhibition (Johnson *et al.*, 1966), reversed passive hemagglutination (Johnson *et al.*, 1966; Sakaguchi *et al.*, 1974), radioimmunoassay (Boroff and Chen, 1973), enzyme-linked immunosorbent assay (ELISA) (Notermans *et al.*, 1978; Kozaki *et al.*, 1979), etc., but the sensitivities of all these *in vitro* immunological methods are lower than that of the mouse i.p. injection method.

The antigenicity of the toxic component of each type is specific, whereas the nontoxic components of type A and B and of type C and D progenitor toxins share common antigenicity (Sakaguchi *et al.*, 1974). Furthermore, anti-crystalline type A toxin serum contains a significantly higher titer against the nontoxic component than against the toxic component (Sugiyama *et al.*, 1974b). Therefore, the titer obtained by any immunological assay method would not directly parallel the toxicity or the quantity of the toxic component (Betly and Sugiyama, 1979; Guilfoyle and Mestrandrea, 1980), unless antibody specific to the toxic component is used (Sugiyama *et al.*, 1974). Antibody specific to the toxic component can be prepared by immunizing animals with the purified toxic component or by affinity chromatography of anti-progenitor toxin on a Sepharose column conjugated with the purified nontoxic component (Sakaguchi *et al.*, 1974). Tryptic activation is not necessary for nonactivated toxins to be titrated by any immunological procedure, as trypsinization does not alter the antigenic specificity (Kondo *et al.*, 1969; Sugiyama *et al.*, 1967).

4. TOXIN PRODUCTION BY *C. BOTULINUM*

4.1. Growth and Toxin Production

C. botulinum is a spore-bearing, anaerobic organism. Germination of the spores, outgrowth and the subsequent anaerobic growth are prerequisites to toxin production. Spores are often in a state of dormancy. Heat treatment for 30–60 min at 80°C for group I and III organisms (Rowley and Feehery, 1970) or for 10 min at 60°C for group II organisms (Ando and Iida, 1970), trypsinization (Treadwell *et al.*, 1958; Kautter and Lilly, 1970), treatment with lysozyme (Alderton *et al.*, 1974), the presence of carbon dioxide gas or bicarbonate ion (Rowley and Feeherry, 1970; Treadwell *et al.*, 1958), etc., accelerate germination of dormant spores. Anaerobic conditions may not be essential for germination of spores (Ando *et al.*, 1975).

C. botulinum grows and produces toxin in such hermetically sealed foods as canned and bottled foods and in sausages, hams and other meat products. The oxygen tolerance, however, differs from one group to another. The group I organisms show the highest oxygen tolerance, tolerating 7–9% O_2; the group II organisms show the lowest tolerance, tolerating only 3.8% O_2 (Meyer, 1929). They can grow and produce toxin in food and culture medium if the oxydation–reduction potential is satisfactorily low. Tissues of animals and plants are aerobic as long as they are alive and, therefore, may not support the growth of *C. botulinum*; however, once they die, the oxygen supply stops, their tissues become anaerobic, and their oxydation–reduction potential drops owing to the reducing substances present in the tissues, allowing *C. botulinum* to grow. Type E organisms grow at an oxydation–reduction potential lower than 0–100 mV (Ando and Iida, 1970). Addition of thioglycolic acid (0.05–0.1% sodium thioglycolate) or cysteine (0.1–0.2%) to a liquid medium allows *C. botulinum* to grow and produce toxin even when incubated in the air. To obtain botulinum toxin in large amounts, complexed media containing combinations of meat hydrolysate, casein hydrolysate, yeast autolysate, yeast extract and glucose supplemented with one or more reducing agents are used.

The organisms of group I can grow and produce toxin in a synthetic culture medium containing inorganic salts, amino acids, vitamins, and glucose (Gullmar and Molin, 1967a,b). Vegetables (boiled string beans, corn, mushrooms, spinach, asparagus, etc.) rather than meat and meat products have more often been implicated in food-borne botulism in the United States. String beans and mushrooms autoclaved in an equal quantity of saline proved to be excellent culture media, supporting toxin production by type A and B organisms to a similar extent (3.5×10^5–1×10^6 mouse i.p. LD_{50}/ml in 7 days at 30°C) as in laboratory media, while addition of glucose was required by type E and F organisms to grow in boiled vegetables (Sugii and Sakaguchi, 1977). What is more, type A and B toxins produced in string beans and mushrooms tended to be larger in the molecular size, 16S and 19S being predominant, than those produced in pork or tuna fish, 12S being predominant. As will be discussed later, the larger the molecular size of the toxin, the higher the oral toxicity in the same immunological type (Ohishi *et al.*, 1977). Iron and/or manganese ions contained in larger quantities in meat may inhibit botulinum 12S progenitor toxin binding to hemagglutinating protein to become 16S and 19S toxins (Sugii and Sakaguchi, 1977).

As seen in cases of infant botulism (types A, B and F) and broiler chicken botulism (type C), *C. botulinum* should grow and produce toxin intraintestinally. The locus of toxin production is the colon in mice (Sugiyama and Mills, 1978) and perhaps in human infants and the ceca in broiler chickens (Miyazaki and Sakaguchi, 1978). Cases of infant botulism have been restricted to infants aged between 3 weeks to 8 months; the intestines of newborn infants may not support the growth of *C. botulinum* and the growth inhibition in those older than 8 months may be due to the antagonism by microflora settled in them (Moberg and Sugiyama, 1979). Certain aerobic microorganisms consume oxygen during respiration resulting in reduction of the oxidation–reduction potential and hence in acceleration of the growth of *C. botulinum* (Baird-Parker, 1971).

The optimum temperatures for growth of *C. botulinum* of groups I, II, and III are 37–39°C, 28–32°C, and 39–43°C, respectively (unpublished data). The optimum temperature for growth may not necessarily be that for toxin production. The optimum temperature for toxin production by *C. botulinum* is generally regarded as 20–35°C. The higher the incubation temperature, the more rapid the toxin production and enzymatic and nonenzymatic destruction of the preformed toxin. The lowest limiting temperatures for toxin production are 10°C for groups I and III (Ohye and Scott, 1953) and 3.3°C for group II (Schmidt *et al.*, 1961; Eklund *et al.*, 1967). Botulinum toxin is not produced at pH 4.6 or lower or pH 8.5 or higher (Townsend *et al.*, 1954; Bonventre and Kempe, 1959). At pH above 7, the progenitor toxin may be dissociated into the toxic and the nontoxic components. The dissociated toxic component is much more labile than is the progenitor toxin and therefore destroyed very rapidly at pH above 7. Toxin production does not occur in an environment with a water activity lower than 0.95 for type A, 0.94 for type B and 0.97 for type E (Ohye and Christian, 1967). The quantity of toxin produced reaches the largest usually in 3–5 days at 30°C, when the growth has reached the stationary phase and sporulation has reached the maximum. Sporulation is not associated with production of the toxin other than C2 toxin. C2 toxin is produced by many type C and D organisms more rapidly than are other botulinum toxins, reaching the highest potential toxicity in 1–2 days at 37°C, and its production is apparently associated with sporulation (Nakamura *et al.*, 1978).

Botulinum toxin is defined as an 'exotoxin,' that is released out of the cells into the medium when the cells lyse. The group II organisms, which are characterized by nonproteolysis and lack of autolysis, do not efficiently release the toxin out of the cells. The author took advantage of such characteristic and established procedures for isolation of type E progenitor toxin from the young-cultured bacterial cells rather than from the culture supernatant (Sakaguchi and Sakaguchi, 1959; Kitamura *et al.*, 1968).

4.2. BACTERIOPHAGES AND TOXIN PRODUCTION

Cultures of *C. botulinum* type C or D, when irradiated with u.v. light to remove extrachromosomal elements or treated with acridine orange to induce lysis of the cells, can be cured of their prophages or extrachromosomal elements and become nontoxigenic and sensitive to the bacteriophage of the parent toxigenic strain. Such nontoxigenic mutants, upon reinfection with the bacteriophage isolated from the toxigenic parent strain restore the toxigenicity (Inoue and Iida, 1970; Eklund *et al.*, 1972). In addition, the immunological type of the toxin produced is dependent upon the origin of the bacteriophage; if it is of type C origin, the toxin produced is type C, irrespective of whether the nontoxigenic mutant is derived from type C or D organisms, and if the phage is type D origin, the toxin produced is type D, irrespective of whether the nontoxigenic mutant is derived from type C or D organisms (Inoue and Iida, 1971; Eklund and Poysky, 1974). The cured nontoxigenic culture can be converted not only to type C or D toxin producer, but also to an entirely different species, *C. novyi* type A, depending upon the specific bacteriophage used (Eklund *et al.*, 1974).

The quantity of the toxin produced by the converted strain depends upon the passage history of the bacteriophage (Oguma and Iida, 1979). The relationship between the bacteriophage and the host cell is considered to be pseudo-lysogeny, since the phage and the toxigenicity are lost simultaneously after successive transfer in the presence of anti-phage serum or after transfer in the spore state (Eklund *et al.*, 1971, 1972; Eklund and Poysky, 1974). The phage-converted type C and D strains lost their toxigenicity more rapidly during serial transfers in a medium containing antiserum against the converting phage than in the same medium containing no antiserum (Oguma, 1976). The phenomenon was interpreted that the converted strains spontaneously lose their phages but in the absence of anti-phage serum reinfection may occur and they are again converted to toxigenic, while the nontoxigenic variants were resistant to lysis and conversion by the original converting phage. In the presence of anti-phage serum, the nontoxigenic variants appeared to remain sensitive to lysis and conversion by the original phage (Oguma, 1976). The nontoxigenic mutant resistant to lysis and conversion by the original phage may have been caused by reinfection of such a nonconverting but lytic mutant with the original phage (Oguma *et al.*, 1975). It has not been proved whether toxin production by *C. botulinum* of other types than types C and D is governed also by infection of bacteriophage.

Unlike production of C1 and D toxin, production of C2 toxin does not seem to be dependent upon phage infection, since some nontoxigenic mutants of type C and D strains, obtained by curing of their prophages, continued to produce C2 toxin which was demonstrated by trypsinization of the culture (Eklund *et al.*, 1972).

5. PURIFICATION OF *C. BOTULINUM* PROGENITOR TOXINS

5.1. HISTORICAL ASPECTS

Many reports have been published on procedures for purification of botulinum toxins since 1946. Some procedures allowed obtaining intact progenitor toxins, while others allowed obtaining dissociated toxic components or derivative toxins.

C. botulinum type A toxin was purified for the first time among bacterial toxins by Lamanna *et al.* (1946) and by Abrams *et al.* (1946), who both obtained it in crystalline form. Purification and crystallization were accomplished by such procedures that were used for purification of various proteins, such as acid precipitation, shaking with chloroform, and salting out with ammonium sulfate. Characterization of type A crystalline toxin definitively ruled out the then prevailing hypothesis of a nonprotein nature of botulinum toxin originating from the apparent indigestibility (Putnum *et al.*, 1947; Buehler *et al.*, 1947). Attempts to purify type B toxin were made by Lamanna and Glassman (1947), who principally applied the acid precipitation method.

Since then, many investigators have attempted purification of botulinum toxins of different immunological types. Until 1960, the purification procedures were based principally upon initial acid precipitation of the toxin from the whole culture at pH 3.5–4.0, followed by extraction of the toxin from the precipitate, and salting out with ammonium sulfate and/or alcohol precipitation. Type A (Duff *et al.*, 1957b), type B (Duff *et al.*, 1957a), and type D toxins (Cardella *et al.*, 1960) were purified to 90% or higher purity by such classical procedures, but type C (Cardella *et al.*, 1958; Vinet and Raynaud, 1963) or type E (Gordon *et al.*, 1957; Fiock *et al.*, 1961) toxin did not seem to have been purified to such a high level.

At the end of 1950's, the techniques of ion exchange chromatography on cellulose or dextran gel and molecular sieving on dextran gel were introduced. Such modern techniques were applied to purification of botulinum toxins. Gerwing and her associates applied DEAE-cellulose chromatography at pH 4.5 or 5.6 to purification of type A (Gerwing *et al.*, 1965a), type B (Gerwing *et al.*, 1966) and type E toxins (Gerwing *et al.*, 1961, 1962, 1964, 1965b). Strangely, the toxins they purified were of low molecular substances, the molecular weight being 12,200 for type A (Gerwing *et al.*, 1965a), 9,000–10,000 for type B (Gerwing *et al.*, 1966), 18,600 for nonactivated type E toxin (Gerwing *et al.*, 1964) and 10,000–12,000 for activated type E toxin (Gerwing *et al.*, 1965b). They claimed that acid precipitation and other harsh methods used by many other workers might have caused aggregation of the toxin (Gerwing *et al.*, 1965a,b). This explanation does not seem valid since Schantz and Spero (1967) determined the sedimentation constants ($S_{20,w}$) of type A through F toxins in spent cultures and obtained 14S for type C, E, and F toxins, 16S for type B and D toxins, and 19S for type A toxin. Type E toxin produced in 'izushi' was proved to be 12S (Sakaguchi *et al.*, 1966). The molecular sizes of type A and B toxins produced in food varied depending upon the constituents, probably depending largely upon the contents of such divalent metal ions as Fe^{2+} and Mn^{2+}, but they were at least in a dimension of 12S; those of type E and F toxins always being 12S (Sugii and Sakaguchi, 1977).

Chromatography on acidified DEAE-cellulose or DEAE-Sephadex was followed to isolate type A (DasGupta *et al.*, 1970) and B toxins (DasGupta *et al.*, 1968; Beers and Reich, 1969). No such small molecular-sized toxins as those reported by Gerwing and her associates were obtained, but the purified type A and B toxins had molecular weights of 150,000 and 167,000, respectively. These toxins were free from hemagglutinin and considered to be the dissociated toxic components of type A and B progenitor toxins.

Purification of botulinum toxins of types A through F in the same molecular form as they are in food and culture has been attempted. It appeared that the initial acid precipitation step would not cause molecular aggregation of the toxin, but chromatography on anion exchangers, even if the matrix is acidified, would cause molecular dissociation. Therefore, chromatography on such cation exchangers as CM- and SP-Sephadex was utilized by the author and his associates to purify *C. botulinum* type A, B, C, D, E and F progenitor toxins. Recently, C2 toxin has also been obtained in pure form (Ohishi *et al.*, 1980a).

The procedures for purification of different progenitor toxins without causing molecular aggregation nor dissociation may be summarized as follows:

5.2. PURIFICATION OF PROGENITOR TOXINS OF GROUP I ORGANISMS

The medium for toxin production by type A, B and F organisms of group I consisted of glucose 0.5%, peptone of meat origin 2.0%, yeast extract 0.5%, and sodium thioglycolate 0.05% (pH 7.0). A spore suspension of each type was inoculated and the culture was incubated for 4 days at 30°C, when the whole culture was adjusted to pH 4.0 by adding 3 N sulfuric acid. The precipitate formed was separated by siphoning the supernatant liquid, then packed by centrifugation, and extracted with 0.2 M phosphate buffer, pH 6.0. The toxin extracted was again precipitated at 50% saturation of ammonium sulfate, and the precipitate was dissolved in a small amount of an appropriate buffer. The extract contained a large quantity of RNA and other acidic substances, which were removed by treating with protamine at pH 4.5. Without removal of such acidic substances, a heavy precipitate coprecipitating the toxin would be formed when the extract was dialyzed against a buffer of pH 4–4.5 with a low ionic strength, e.g. 0.05 M acetate buffer, pH 4.5. The dialyzed material was chromatographed on an SP-Sephadex column equilibrated to pH 4.0–4.5 by elution with linear gradient increase in sodium chloride concentration. The toxin was usually eluted in a single fraction but sometimes in two separate fractions. The toxic fractions were pooled and concentrated by salting out with ammonium sulfate or by ultrafiltration and subjected to gel filtration on a column of Sephadex G-200. Type A (Sugii and Sakaguchi, 1975) and B toxins (Kozaki *et al.*, 1974) were eluted in two separate fractions and type F toxin in a single fraction (Ohishi and Sakaguchi, 1974). Gel filtration on Sephadex G-200 did not allow L and LL toxins to resolve into separate fractions. Type B toxin of a nonproteolytic strain of group II was purified also by the same procedures (Miyazaki *et al.*, 1976).

5.3. PURIFICATION OF TYPE E PROGENITOR TOXIN OF GROUP II ORGANISMS

The ingredients of the medium for toxin production by group II organisms were the same as those used for group I organisms, but the reaction was adjusted to pH 6.2. Such a low pH was chosen so as to minimize the toxin release from the bacterial cells. A spore suspension was inoculated and the culture was incubated for 2–3 days at 30°C, when it was centrifuged to collect the bacterial cells. Prolonged incubation would result in releasing more toxin out of the cells. The precipitated cells contained most toxin, which was extracted with 0.2 M phosphate buffer, pH 6.0. The extract was chromatographed on a CM-Sephadex column equilibrated with 0.01 M phosphate buffer, pH 6.0. No toxin was adsorbed onto the column, since the toxin at this stage was a complex with RNA (Sakaguchi and Sakaguchi, 1959). The pass-through fraction was treated with ribonuclease to remove the RNA associated with the toxin. Type B toxin of Group II organisms, unlike type E toxin, did not seem to be bound to RNA. Type E toxin freed of RNA was chromatographed on CM-Sephadex under the same conditions as the preceding chromatography. The toxin freed of RNA was adsorbed onto the column and eluted with linear gradient increase in sodium chloride concentration in the same buffer. The toxin fraction eluted was concentrated by salting out and subjected to gel filtration on Sephadex G-200 to obtain a single sharp peak at a position near the void volume (Kitamura *et al.*, 1968).

Type E toxin thus obtained was a weakly toxic form, which was activated upon treatment with trypsin at pH 6.0. Re-gel filtration of the trypsinized toxin on Sephadex G-200 under the same conditions as before gave activated progenitor toxin free from trypsin at the same elution position as that of unactivated progenitor toxin (Kitamura *et al.*, 1968).

Type F toxin of group II organisms has not been purified.

5.4. PURIFICATION OF TYPE C AND D PROGENITOR TOXINS (C1 AND D TOXIC FACTORS) OF GROUP III ORGANISMS

The medium of the same ingredients as those for group I and II organisms was used; 0.05% sodium thioglycolate seemed to be inhibitory upon group III organisms and therefore it was replaced with 0.1% cysteine. The spores were inoculated and the cultures were incubated for 3 days at 30°C. The RNA contents of whole culture of group III organisms were usually lower than those of group I or II organisms. Therefore, acid precipitation of C1 and D toxins often required addition of yeast RNA to the whole culture to a concentration of 0.4 mg/ml as a precipitation aid and adjusting the mixture to pH 4.0 with 3 N sulfuric acid (Iwasaki and Sakaguchi, 1978). The acid precipitate was extracted with 0.2 M phosphate buffer, pH 6.0, concentrated by salting out, and treated with protamine sulfate to remove the exogenous as well as endogenous RNA and other acidic substances. The protamine-treated material was dialyzed against 0.05 M acetate buffer, pH 4.0, and subjected to SP-Sephadex chromatography with the same buffer as eluant with linear gradient increase in sodium chloride concentration, followed by concentration and gel filtration on Sephadex G-200. C1 and D toxins were each eluted in two separate fractions (Miyazaki et al., 1977).

5.5. PURIFICATION OF C2 TOXIN OF GROUP III ORGANISMS

One of the strains resembling C. botulinum type C but producing no C1 nor D toxin but C2 toxin only, isolated from soil samples (Serikawa et al., 1977), was grown in a fortified cooked meat medium [Cooked meat medium (Difco) fortified with calcium carbonate 0.5%, ammonium sulfate 1.0%, glucose 0.8%, yeast extract 1.0% (Segnar et al., 1971), and cysteine 0.1%, pH 7.6] for 2 days at 37°C, when the spore population and the potential toxicity of C2 toxin was the highest (Nakamura et al., 1978). The gauze filtrate of the culture was centrifuged to obtain a clear supernatant, to which ammonium sulfate was added to 60% saturation. The formed precipitate was dialyzed against 0.05 M Tris-HCl buffer, pH 7.5, and subjected to chromatography on DEAE-Sephadex equilibrated with the same buffer. The pass-through fraction contained a large quantity of protein but no potential C2 toxicity and the retained fraction eluted with the same buffer containing 0.3 M sodium chloride recovered the potential C2 toxicity. The C2 toxin fraction was dialyzed against 0.01 M acetate buffer, pH 6.0, and applied to CM-Sephadex equilibrated with the same buffer. C2 toxin was resolved into two fractions; component I was recovered in the pass-through fraction and component II was adsorbed onto the column and eluted with the buffer containing 0.3 M sodium chloride. Components I and II were each concentrated by ultrafiltration through Amicon PM30 membrane and subjected to gel filtration on Sephadex G-100. Each component was eluted in a single peak behind the 7S position; component I was eluted further behind component II. Neither component I nor II was toxic, but when they were mixed together at a protein ratio of 1:2.5 (perhaps the equimolar ratio) and the mixture was trypsinized at pH 8.0 for 30 min at 35°C, the highest toxicity, being $1.3-2.5 \times 10^5$ mouse i.p. LD_{50}/mg protein nitrogen, was obtained (Ohishi et al., 1980a).

6. MOLECULAR STRUCTURE OF C. BOTULINUM PROGENITOR TOXINS

Type A crystalline toxin was found to be a simple protein composed of nothing but 19 kinds of amino acids (Buehler et al., 1947). It behaved as a homogeneous protein in ultracentrifugation and electrophoresis, while the presence of more than one component was indicated in solubility and boundary spreading in diffusion tests (Putnam et al., 1948). Its molecular weight was estimated at 900,000 with an $S_{20,w}$ of 17.4 (Putnam et al., 1948). It was found that crystalline type A toxin contained, in addition to its neurotoxic activity, a hemagglutinating activity (Lamanna, 1948). Hemagglutinin-free neurotoxin was obtained by absorption of a solution of the crystalline toxin with chicken erythrocytes at pH 8 (Lowenthal and Lamanna, 1953).

Lamanna and Glassman (1947) reported that the type B toxin they purified had a molecular weight as low as 60,000 determined by diffusion at pH 2. Wagman and Bateman (1951) demonstrated its molecular weight to be 500,000 by ultracentrifugation at pH 3.0.

The progenitor toxins can be classified into three groups according to the molecular size: 19S, 16S, and 12S or extra-large (LL), large (L) and medium (M). Type A progenitor toxin involves all the three forms, 19S, 16S, and 12S (Sugii and Sakaguchi, 1977); type B (Kozaki *et al.*, 1974), type C (Iwasaki and Sakaguchi, 1978) and type D (Miyazaki *et al.*, 1977) involve two forms, 16S and 12S; and type E (Kitamura *et al.*, 1968) and type F (Ohishi and Sakaguchi, 1975) involve a single form, 12S. The exact sedimentation constant ($S_{20,w}$) determined for type F progenitor toxin was 10.3 and the molecular weight was 235,000 (Ohishi and Sakaguchi,, 1975). The figures are significantly smaller than those for the M toxins of the other types. The derivative toxin dissociated from the progenitor toxins of all immunological types and all molecular forms, obtained by DEAE-Sephadex chromatography or sucrose density gradient ultracentrifugation at pH 7.5–8.0, are uniform in the molecular size. According to Ohishi and Sakaguchi (1975), the molecular size of type F derivative toxin was 5.8S, but according to DasGupta and Sugiyama (1977b), it was about 150,000, being the same as the derivative toxins of other types. The molecule of the progenitor toxin, therefore, is a complex of one molecule each of the 7S toxic and the 7S or larger molecular-sized nontoxic components held together with a noncovalent bond(s). It is characteristic that the 12S progenitor or M toxin of all types is a complex of two components, toxic and nontoxic, of the same or nearly the same molecular sizes. Hemagglutinin activity is shown with the nontoxic component of L and LL toxins only.

The molecular structures and the specific mouse i.p. toxicities of *C. botulinum* progenitor toxins of types A through F are shown in Fig. 1.

The mouse i.p. LD_{50}/mg protein nitrogen of the progenitor toxin differs from one immunological type to another and from one molecular form to another. Within the same immunological type, it is apparent that the smaller the molecular size, the smaller the quantity of nontoxic protein and therefore the higher the specific toxicity. The specific toxicities of type A, B and D-M toxins are on the same level. The specific toxicities of type C and F-M toxins, being on the same level, are about 20% and that of type E activated progenitor toxin about 10% those of type A, B and D-M toxins. The M toxin purified from cultures of nonproteolytic type B strain QC possessed a still higher potential toxicity, being $8–9 \times 10^8$ mouse i.p. LD_{50}/mg protein nitrogen (Miyazaki *et al.*, 1976). At any rate, the i.p. toxicity is entirely dependent upon the toxic component, and the nontoxic component seems to play little or no role in the parenteral toxicity, although it plays a critically important role in the oral toxicity as will be discussed later.

The antigenic specificity of the toxic component is the basis for classifying botulinum toxin, although there are some cross-reactions between types C and D and types E and F. The toxic components of M and L (and LL) toxins of the same type proved to be antigenically identical. The antigenic specificities of the nontoxic components of M, L and LL toxins of the same type proved to be only partially identical, suggesting that the nontoxic component of M toxin is a part of that of L and LL toxins. In addition, the nontoxic component of type A-M toxin is antigenetically the same with the corresponding component of type B-M toxin (Sakaguchi *et al.*, 1974). Similar relation is seen with the nontoxic components of type C and D-M toxins (Miyazaki *et al.*, 1977). The interpretation of the antigenicity of the other part of the nontoxic component of L (or LL) toxin is difficult, because isolation of the second part of the nontoxic component of L toxin has been unsuccessful (Sugii and Sakaguchi, 1975; DasGupta and Sugiyama, 1977a). The antigenic relation among hemagglutinins possessed by L and LL toxins of different types has not been clarified.

The molecular dissociation of the progenitor toxin into toxic and nontoxic com-

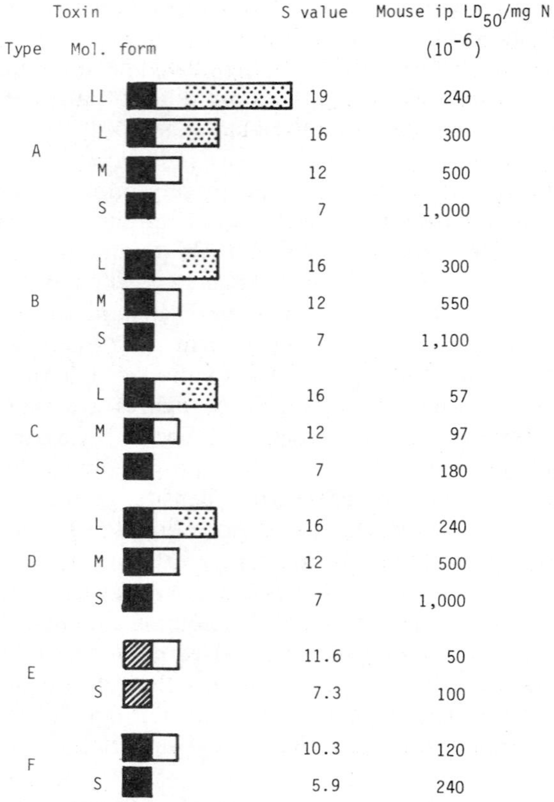

Toxin Type	Mol. form		S value	Mouse ip LD_{50}/mg N (10^{-6})
A	LL		19	240
	L		16	300
	M		12	500
	S		7	1,000
B	L		16	300
	M		12	550
	S		7	1,100
C	L		16	57
	M		12	97
	S		7	180
D	L		16	240
	M		12	500
	S		7	1,000
E			11.6	50
	S		7.3	100
F			10.3	120
	S		5.9	240

FIG. 1. Molecular sizes and structures and toxicities of *C. botulinum* progenitor and derivative toxins. Black area: fully toxic; blank area: nontoxic; diagonally hatched area: nonactivated; dotted area: hemagglutinin active.

ponents is reversible. When type E toxic and nontoxic components at an equimolar ratio are mixed together and the mixture is dialyzed against 0.05 M phosphate buffer, pH 6.0, reassociation occurs forming molecules indistinguishable from the parental progenitor toxin (Kitamura and Sakaguchi, 1969). It is possible to make a hybrid toxin, e.g. between the toxic component of a proteolytic type B strain and the nontoxic component of a nonproteolytic type B strain (Miyazaki *et al.*, 1976).

Type E progenitor toxin sediments in a single boundary to the 12S position when ultracentrifuged at pH 6.0–6.6, and also in a single boundary to the 7S position when ultracentrifuged at pH 7.2–8.0. This indicates that the progenitor toxin molecule dissociates into the components of the same molecular sizes, whereas it sediments in a single boundary to the 10S position when centrifuged at pH 6.8–7.0. This was interpreted as a molecular unfolding taking place (Kitamura *et al.*, 1967; Kitamura and Sakaguchi, 1969). It was also considered that the toxic and the nontoxic components are bound together with at least two qualitatively different bonds; one is susceptible to pH 6.8 or higher, whereas the other is resistant to pH 7.0 but susceptible to pH 7.2 or higher. Electron micrographs showed particulate forms of type E progenitor and derivative toxins and the nontoxic component with diameters of 90–100, 40–50, and 50–60 Å, respectively (Kitamura and Sakaguchi, 1969).

Type E progenitor toxin extracted from young cultured bacterial cells is a complex with two or more molecules of RNA of about 3S forming 15.5–16.5S molecules. It was demonstrated that RNA molecules are bound with only the toxic component (Kitamura and Sakaguchi, 1969). The presence of RNA associated with the toxic component does not disturb the molecular dissociation of RNA–progenitor toxin complex.

The derivative toxin is usually obtained by DEAE-Sephadex chromatography of the progenitor toxin, any one of LL, L, and M toxins, at pH above 7.2 (DasGupta *et al.*, 1977a,b; Kitamura *et al.*, 1969). Type C (C1 toxin) toxic component was purified in the pass-through fraction in affinity chromatography at pH 8.0 on CNBr-activated Sepharose 4B coupled with antihemagglutinin IgG (Syuto and Kubo, 1977). Purification of type A derivative toxin from crystalline toxin by affinity chromatography was reported by Moberg and Sugiyama (1978). The method consisted of irreversible binding of the hemagglutinin to *p*-aminophenyl-β-D-thiogalactopyranoside coupled to CN-Sepharose at pH 6.3 and the subsequent elution of the toxic component with a buffered saline of pH 7.9.

7. MOLECULAR STRUCTURE OF DERIVATIVE TOXIN

When the 7S derivative toxins of types A, B, and F of Group I organisms are analyzed by electrophoresis in polyacrylamide gel in the presence of a reducing agent and sodium dodecyl sulfate, they are each resolved into two bands corresponding to molecular weights of about 100,000 and 50,000 (Beers and Reich, 1969; DasGupta and Sugiyama, 1972c), whereas when those of types B and E of Group II organisms are analyzed under the same conditions, they each migrate in only a single band. When the latter are trypsinized and analyzed by electrophoresis under the same conditions, however, they each migrate in two bands corresponding to molecular weights of 100,000 and 50,000 as do those of group I organisms (DasGupta and Sugiyama, 1972c). These findings show that the toxic component of group II organisms is a single polypeptide chain molecule and that trypsinization at pH 6.0 apparently hydrolyzes one peptide bond in it. The findings show also that the proteolytic enzyme(s) produced by group I organisms hydrolyzes endogenously one peptide bond, perhaps the same one as that cleaved by trypsin, of the toxic component of group II organisms. Although type C and D organisms are both regarded as nonproteolytic, the toxic component of type C toxin is the dichain molecule (Syuto and Kubo, 1977), while that of type D toxin is a single chain molecule (Miyazaki *et al.*, 1977). It is now accepted that the toxic component of any type is produced as a single polypeptide chain. In cultures of Group I organisms, such a single polypeptide chain is transformed into two polypeptide chains that are linked together by at least one disulfide bond, by a certain proteolytic enzyme(s) produced endogenously, while in cultures of Group II organisms, it remains unnicked and treatment with trypsin or other enzymes can bring forth the nicking. Type B toxic component may contain a maximum of three disulfide bonds (Beers and Reich, 1969), while that of type A only one (Knox *et al.*, 1970). The presence of two or more disulfide bonds in type A toxic component was alluded (Sugiyama, 1980).

Sulfhydryl-dependent proteolytic enzymes were isolated from cultures of *C. botulinum* types A, B, and F, and demonstrated to have the same substrate specificity as that of trypsin (DasGupta, 1971; DasGupta and Sugiyama, 1972b; Ohishi *et al.*, 1975; Ohishi and Sakaguchi, 1977b). This enzyme, resembling clostripain produced by *Clostridium histolyticum*, does not nick, though it activates single-chain type E toxic component (Sugiyama, 1980). The enzyme also activates type B toxic component of group I organisms, but to a much lesser extent than does trypsin (Ohishi and Sakaguchi, 1977b).

It is apparent that the toxic component bears the total parenteral toxicity of the progenitor toxin. The reduced nicked derivative toxin was reported to have lost not only its toxicity, but also its antigenicity and immunogenicity (Beers and Reich, 1969; Sugiyama *et al.*, 1973, 1974a). It was confirmed that neither of the two fragments of type B derivative toxin was toxic, but they both possessed distinct antigenic properties (Kozaki and Sakaguchi, 1975) and stimulated animals to produce specific antibodies (Kozaki *et al.*, 1977).

The fragment with the molecular weight of 100,000 was named 'fragment I' or 'H chain' and that with the molecular weight of 50,000 'fragment II' or 'L chain'. Fragment I can be separated from fragment II by gel filtration on Sephadex G-200, superfine, equilibrated with a buffer containing a reducing agent such as dithiothreitol and urea that prevents aggregation of the reduced toxic component (Kozaki and Sakaguchi, 1975; Kozaki *et al.*, 1977). When type A toxic component is reduced with dithiothreitol, it forms an aggregate. Since the aggregate was mostly of L chains, its H chain was isolated by reducing the toxic component in a buffer containing reduced nicotinamide adenine dinucleotide (Krysinski and Sugiyama, 1980). The two fragments of type C toxin (C1 toxin) were separated from each other by reducing the toxic component after adsorption onto a column of QAE-Sephadex with 2-mercaptoethanol (Syuto and Kubo, 1981). When type A toxic component was adsorbed onto QAE-Sephadex and then reduced with dithiothreitol instead of 2-mercaptoethanol, the two fragments were separated from each other by two-step elution (Kozaki *et al.*, 1981).

A mixture of the two fragments at an equimolar ratio restored 30–40% of the original toxicity upon reoxidation by dialysis (Kozaki *et al.*, 1977). The recovery has increased up to 80% (unpublished data).

Various molecular sizes smaller than 7S have been reported for *C. botulinum* toxins in natural or artificially induced state; in the light of the present knowledge, it seems difficult to explain whether there really are small peptides having specific toxicity or if small molecular substances were contaminated with a minute amount of the large molecular toxin or toxic component. Thus, the smallest unit of the toxicity of botulinum toxin may be regarded as the 7S toxic component and a certain tertiary structure of fragments I and II bound together with at least one disulfide bond seems necessary.

Fragment I differs from fragment II in its antigenicity and the antibody to fragment I plays a more important role in neutralization than does fragment II, as a significantly less amount of fragment I than fragment II is required to neutralize the same amount of the derivative toxin (Kozaki *et al.*, 1977).

Antitoxins of type B obtained from each of the type B toxins of group I and II organisms both neutralize reciprocally but there is more efficient neutralization of the homologous toxin than the heterologous one (Shimizu and Kondo, 1973). Kozaki *et al.* (1977) ascribed the different antigenicities to the difference in the antigenicity of fragment I of the two toxins. In agar gel diffusion, fragment II of the two toxins were identical, but fragment I only partially identical.

C2 toxin has a molecular structure entirely different from that of progenitor or derivative toxin of any type. C2 toxicity is elicited by two immunologically distinct, substantive protein components, component I with a molecular weight of 55,000 and component II with a molecular weight of 105,000, that strangely coincide with the molecular weights of fragments I and II of the derivative toxin and are present substantively without binding together (Ohishi *et al.*, 1980a). Mouse lethal and guinea-pig erythemal activities can be shown when the two components are injected simultaneously or one after the other (Ohishi *et al.*, 1980b).

8. ACTIVATION OF BOTULINUM TOXINS

Group I organisms, particularly types A and B, cultured in a laboratory medium usually produce toxin with potencies higher than one million mouse i.p. LD_{50}/ml, whereas type E cultures produce toxin on a magnitude of only 10^2 mouse i.p. LD_{50}/ml. Yet, the morbidity (49% of those at risk) and the case fatality rate (19–33%, including those treated with specific antitoxin) of human type E botulism are compatible to those of type A and B cases (Dolman and Iida, 1963; Center for Disease Control, 1979). A higher rate of absorption of type E toxin than the toxins of other types from the intestinal tract of man or higher susceptibility of man than mice to type E toxin was hypothesized (Dolman, 1957).

The activation phenomenon of type E toxin was found from the observation that the parenteral toxicity of a culture of a type E strain was markedly enhanced upon incubation with a proteolytic strain of genus *Clostridium* originating from 'izushi' incriminated for an outbreak (Sakaguchi and Tohyama, 1955a,b). The phenomenon was interpreted that the virtually nontoxic precursor of type E toxin present in, or on, type E cells was activated by a proteolytic enzyme produced by the contaminating strain. Activation did not occur at either pH 2 or pH 8, but occurred at pH 5–6 (Sakaguchi and Tohyama, 1955a,b). Duff *et al.* (1956) found more marked activation of type E toxin with trypsin at pH 6. Activation of type E toxin occurs not only in test tubes but also in the digestive tract of the mouse and of man.

Activation of type E toxin was once interpreted as the result of fragmentation of 5.6S toxin molecules by trypsin into many small peptide fragments smaller than 1S, releasing more toxic sites (Gerwing *et al.*, 1961). Later, it was ascribed to splitting off a peptide fragment containing at least 18 amino acid residues from the N-terminus, thus reducing the molecular weight from 18,600 or 14,000–16,000 to 10,000–12,000 (Gerwing *et al.*, 1964 and 1965b).

Type E progenitor toxin was extracted from young-cultured bacterial cells in the form of a complex with RNA. Tryptic activation of this precursor accompanied removal of the RNA (Sakaguchi and Sakaguchi, 1959). Removal of the RNA by treatment with ribonuclease did not increase the toxicity at all. Type E progenitor toxin (12S) freed of RNA was purified. It was then activated with trypsin. The progenitor toxin with a toxicity of 1×10^5 mouse i.p. LD_{50}/mg protein nitrogen, and the activated progenitor toxin with a toxicity of 5×10^7 LD_{50}/mg protein nitrogen were compared physicochemically and immunologically. They were not different from each other in the sedimentation constant (12S), electrophoretic mobility, amino acid composition (Sakaguchi and Sakaguchi, 1967), behavior in molecular dissociation and reassociation (Kitamura and Sakaguchi, 1969), or the antigenicity (Kondo *et al.*, 1969; Sugiyama *et al.*, 1967). There was no indication to show that trypsination removed a peptide of a detectable size from the type E progenitor toxin molecule. Activation and molecular dissociation and reassociation of type E toxin are shown schematically in Fig. 2. The highest rate of tryptic activation is attained at pH around 6. At pH 7.5, activation occurs very rapidly but the destruction of the activated toxin is also rapid, resulting in a diminution of the toxicity by 90% or more in 60 min at 37°C (Sakaguchi and Sakaguchi, 1967). It was concluded that tryptic activation does not accompany fragmentation nor release of any peptide chain from type E progenitor or derivative toxin molecule (Kitamura and Sakaguchi, 1969).

DasGupta and Sugiyama (1972c) and Sugiyama *et al.* (1973) found that tryptic activation of type E derivative toxin accompanies cleavage of a certain peptide bond (nicking) in the single polypeptide chain molecule transforming it into a two-polypeptide chain molecule. The two-polypeptide chains had molecular weights of approximately 50,000 and 100,000 and they were held together with at least one disulfide bond. Type A,

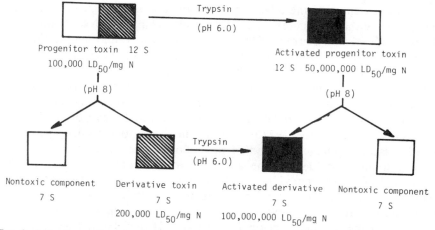

FIG. 2. Activation and molecular structure of *C. botulinum* progenitor and derivative toxins. Black area: activated toxic component or derivative toxin; blank area: nontoxic component; diagonally hatched area: nonactivated toxic component or derivative toxin.

B and F derivative toxins that are regarded to have been activated endogenously were proved to be two-polypeptide chain molecules. It was then considered that the toxic component of *C. botulinum* of any type is synthesized as a single polypeptide chain with a molecular weight of about 150,000 without an apparent toxicity. If the culture does not produce such a proteolytic enzyme that activates the toxin, as is the case with group II organisms, the toxic component remains in an inactive state and in a single polypeptide chain, whereas if the culture produced such a proteolytic enzyme capable of activating the toxin, as is the case with group I organisms, its toxic component recovered is in a fully activated state and is in the nicked form.

It was pointed out that type A, B and F derivative toxins of group I organisms were often only being partially nicked. Trypsinization of such partially nicked derivative toxin brought about complete nicking without any appreciable accompanying increase in the parenteral toxicity (DasGupta and Sugiyama, 1976; Ohishi and Sakaguchi, 1977a; Krysinski and Sugiyama, 1981). The two fragments, with molecular weights of approximately 100,000 and 50,000, formed with trypsin and those formed with endogenous trypsin-like enzyme were not distinguishable from each other.

Sulfhydryl-dependent proteases produced by *C. botulinum* types A, B, and F, *C. histolyticum*, *C. sporogenes* and *C. perfringens*, activate type E progenitor toxin but not type B progenitor toxin, although trypsin activates both much more efficiently (Ohishi *et al.*, 1975). It was interpreted by DasGupta and Sugiyama (1972a,b) that activation in culture may involve two steps; in the first step, the sulfhydryl-dependent protease partially activates the progenitor toxin without nicking, and in the second step, another enzyme completes the activation by nicking the molecule of the toxic component. The enzyme purified from a culture of *C. botulinum* type F of group I was shown to activate type E toxin to the same exent as did trypsin if the concentration of the enzyme was as high as 2.5 mg/ml (equivalent to 10 μg/ml trypsin), whereas under the same conditions it activated type B progenitor toxin to only about 10% that attained with trypsin (Ohishi and Sakaguchi, 1977b). The potentiated toxicity of progenitor toxin persisted, whereas that of derivative toxin was decomposed very rapidly (Ohishi and Sakaguchi, 1977b).

Trypsinization of *C. botulinum* type B derivative toxin at pH 6 results in simultaneous activation and nicking, whereas at pH 4.5 complete activation occurs, though apparently more slowly, but nicking is only partial by the time activation is complete. The observation may indicate that nicking occurs only incidentally and is not directly associated with activation (Ohishi and Sakaguchi, 1977a). Krysinsky and Sugiyama (1981) observed that trypsinization of the single-chain derivative toxin extracted from young cultured type A cells nicked all the molecules not being accompanied by activation and drew the same conclusion.

The fact that trypsinization of the RNA–progenitor toxin complex simultaneously causes increased toxicity and the release of RNA molecules (Sakaguchi and Sakaguchi, 1959) might indicate that the increased toxicity results from hydrolysis of an ester bond formed between the carboxyl group of the C-terminal basic amino acid (perhaps lysine) and a hydroxyl group of ribose in the attached nucleic acid (Sakaguchi and Sakaguchi, 1967). No direct proof of this hypothesis has been obtained.

Trypsin hydrolyzes preferentially *p*-toluene sulfonyl-L-lysine methyl ester (TLME) over *p*-toluene sulfonyl-L-arginine methyl ester (TAME), while the sulfhydryl-dependent trypsin-like enzyme produced by *C. botulinum* type F preferentially hydrolyzes TAME over TLME (Ohishi and Sakaguchi, 1977b). This is the basis to consider that activation involves hydrolysis of lysine–ester bond. It was reported later that when type E derivative toxin was treated with 1,2-cyclohexanedione, which modifies arginine residues, in borate buffer, pH 8.0, it was detoxified and became resistant to nicking with trypsin and that the site of nicking is an arginyl bond, and an arginyl residue is involved in maintaining the toxigenic structure (DasGupta and Sugiyama, 1980). Tryptic activation of type B, E, and F toxins of the organisms belonging to group II may be achieved by the same mechanism (Ohishi and Sakaguchi, 1977a), although little has been studied with activation of type B or F toxin of group II.

Tryptic activation of C2 toxin requires an optimum pH between 7.5 and 8.0 (Iwasaki *et al.*, 1980), which is significantly higher than that required for activation of type E toxin. Trypsinization is necessary for component II only. It is not known whether trypsin causes fragmentation of component II or a modification as minute as just a nicking furnished to type E progenitor toxin.

9. INTESTINAL ABSORPTION OF BOTULINUM TOXIN

Botulinum toxin is an oral toxin. The oral lethal dose of type A crystalline toxin to experimental animals was estimated at 50,000 to 250,000 times that of the i.p. lethal dose (Lamanner and Meyers, 1960). A similar ratio was obtained with type E activated progenitor toxin (Sakaguchi and Sakaguchi, 1974). Various factors such as the nature of the intestinal flora, the nature of the masticated food in the intestines, etc. may affect the oral lethal dose (Lamanna and Carr, 1967). The higher sensitivity of the large, rather than the small mouse, to oral administration of the toxin was explained by a higher rate of absorption of the toxin from the larger surface area of the intestines possessed by the large mouse (Lamanna, 1960).

Attempts were made to correlate the molecular size of botulinum toxin with its oral toxicity to mice. The results obtained are shown in Table 1. The derivative toxin showed an oral LD_{50} of several tens of million the i.p. LD_{50}. It seems impossible for the derivative toxin, if any was ingested, to cause food-borne human botulism (Sakaguchi and Sakaguchi, 1974). The M toxin showed an oral LD_{50} of 95,000–3,600,000 times and L toxin of 1,500–120,000 times the i.p. LD_{50} of the respective toxin. The oral toxicity of the progenitor toxin is much higher than that of the derivative toxin, and that of L toxin is apparently higher than that of M toxin of the same antigenic type.

If the same toxicities in mouse i.p. LD_{50} are ingested, L toxin would be more toxic than M toxin, or if the same levels of toxin are present, such foodstuffs that would support production of L toxin are more fatal than those supporting production of M toxin. Vegetables (string beans and mushrooms) were shown to support production of L and LL toxins and meat (pork and tuna fish) supported production of M toxin by type A and B organisms (Sugii and Sakaguchi, 1977). These findings may explain, at least in part, why boiled vegetables have caused fatal human botulism more often than have meat and meat products (Center for Disease Control, 1979).

Heat stabilities of *C. botulinum* toxins of different types were compared in acid foods

TABLE 1. *Oral LD_{50}:i.p. LD_{50} in mice of Botulinum Toxins of Different Molecular Sizes*

Toxin		Oral LD_{50}:i.p. LD_{50} in mice ($\times 10^{-3}$)
Type	Molecular size	
A	LL	120
	L	2,200
	M	3,600
	S	43,000
B	L	1.5
	M	1,100
	S	24,000
C	L	5.3
	M	160
D	L	62
	M	370
E	M	220
	S	>750
F	M	1,100
	S	>6,000

The data for types A, B, F were from Ohishi *et al.* (1977); those for types C and D from Ohishi and Sakaguchi (1980); those for type E from Sakaguchi and Sakaguchi (1974).

and buffer systems (Woodburn *et al.*, 1979; Bradshaw *et al.*, 1981). In these experiments, the toxins used were crude or purified progenitor toxins. Type A crystalline toxin and type E progenitor toxin are more stable than their derivative toxins and such higher stabilities are more profound at pH lower than 4 and 5, respectively (Kitamura *et al.*, 1969). The stabilities were compared among type A-S, M, and L (a mixture of L and LL) toxins and among type B-S, M and L toxins in buffers at pH 1–6 at 35°C (Sugii *et al.*, 1977). The larger the molecular size of the toxin, the more stable at any pH value.

In vitro destruction curves of type A and B toxins of different molecular sizes upon exposure to pepsin at pH 2.0 were compared; the larger the molecular size of the toxin, the slower in the loss of the lethal activity. Similar results were obtained when type B toxins of different molecular sizes were exposed *in vitro* to rat gastric juice (pH 1.4) at 35°C (Sugii *et al.*, 1977).

Thus, the nontoxic component attached to the toxic component plays an important role as a stabilizer of the rather unstable toxic component in the digestive tract, particularly in the stomach. The larger the molecular size of the nontoxic component attached to the toxic component, the larger the protection afforded from digestion with pepsin and destruction by acidity of the gastric juice.

The toxin is absorbed from all areas of the alimentary tract including the colon (Lamanna and Carr, 1967). The toxin is absorbed mostly from the upper intestines (Dack and Gibbard, 1926a,b). The toxin absorbed from the intestines appears in the lymphatics (May and Whaler, 1958). The toxin in the thoracic lymph duct was demonstrated to be the derivative toxin (Heckley *et al.*, 1960; Kitamura *et al.*, 1969). The lymph fluid collected by cannulation of the thoracic duct of the rat after administration of type B-L, M, or S toxin into the ligated duodenum was titrated for both the toxic and nontoxic components by reversed passive hemagglutination with sheep red blood cells coupled with anti-toxic component immunoglobulin and those coupled with anti-nontoxic component (of B-M toxin) immunoglobulin (Sugii *et al.*, 1977). The toxic activity of the rat lymph was determined by i.p. injection into mice. The rates of absorption of type B toxins of different molecular sizes in terms of antigenicity were nearly the same, however the lymph of the animals given L toxin was highly lethal to mice, that of the animals given M toxin slightly lethal, and that of the animals given S toxin was not lethal at all. The quantities of the toxic and the nontoxic components in terms of the antigenicity appearing in the lymph of the animals given either L or M toxin were nearly the same (Sugii *et al.*, 1977).

Thus, the rate of intestinal absorption of botulinum toxin protein does not change depending upon the molecular size. The whole toxin molecule, no matter whether it is 19S, 16S, or 12S, seems to be absorbed without molecular dissociation in the intestines. In ultracentrifugation of B-L and B-M toxins in sucrose density gradient (5–20%) prepared in rat intestinal juice of pH 7.0, no indication of molecular dissociation was obtained, whereas molecular dissociation of the same toxin preparations was shown in a buffer system of the same pH value. The progenitor toxin, therefore, would not dissociate in the digestive tract, including the lumen of the duodenum. Only the toxicity surviving before, during, and after absorption differs depending upon the molecular size of the toxin. The molecular dissociation occurs immediately after the toxin is absorbed into the lymphatics (Hildebrand *et al.*, 1961; Kitamura *et al.*, 1969).

The mechanism involved in absorption of the toxin from the intestines may be endocytosis as in absorption of nutritional proteins (Bonventre, 1979). The exact mechanism of the subsequent transport of the toxin (derivative toxin) to the target cells is not known. It was estimated that 3.5×10^{11} molecules of type A toxin reaching the peripheral nervous system may be sufficient for an adult to develop clinical botulism (Bonventre, 1979).

10. MODE OF ACTION OF BOTULINUM TOXIN

Botulinum toxin is a potent neurotoxin which is lethal to all vertebrates through paralysis of the skeletal muscles, particularly of the respiratory muscles. It is now known that the toxin interferes with transmission at the peripheral cholinergic motor nerve terminals of the parasympathetic nervous system. The smallest toxic unit of botulinum toxin is regarded as the derivative toxin, which seems to be transported to the nerve terminals. The toxin, due to its large molecular size, does not seem to go through the blood–brain barrier. It is not certain whether the central nervous system is actually affected in botulism, although type A toxin inhibits the release of various centrally acting transmitters (Bigalke and Habermann, 1981). There is no definitive proof to show that the toxin acts on the adrenergic nervous system (Bigalke et al., 1981b).

Most studies on the action of botulinum toxin have been made with type A toxin. Burgen et al. (1949) reported that the isolated rat diaphragm, when treated with a toxin of $1–5 \times 10^3$ LD_{50}/ml, developed paralysis after a lag period of 20–40 min and the paralysis became complete in 70–100 min. Once the diaphragm was exposed to the toxin, washing it did no longer prevent or reduce the paralysis. The temperature-dependency of the toxic action was demonstrated. Simpson (1974) reported that the binding of the toxin to the diaphragm was not influenced by temperature but required an ionic strength of the medium higher than 0.1. The lag period from the exposure of the diaphragm to the toxin to the development of paralysis varied depending upon the toxin concentration; the higher the toxin concentration, the shorter the lag period. It was demonstrated further that the toxin acts at the tip of the nervous cell of the nerve–muscle preparation (Brooks, 1956). The toxin does not inhibit acetylcholinesterase, that decomposes acetylcholine, either *in vitro* or *in vivo* (Simpson and Morimoto, 1969) and the nerve muscle preparation paralyzed with botulinum toxin reacts by contraction upon addition of exogenous acetylcholine (Torda and Wolf, 1947). From these results, it is believed that the site of action of botulinum toxin is located on the presynapse. Simpson (1980) reported that the action of botulinum toxin involves at least three steps: the initial binding step which is not temperature-dependent and by which the toxin rapidly binds to the membrane, the second translocation step, by which the toxin directly moves from the binding site to the lytic site, and the third lytic step, which is temperature-dependent and requires calcium ion and by which acetylcholine release is inhibited.

The toxin has an *in vitro* affinity to the homogenate of the brain matter (Habermann and Heller, 1975), particularly to the synaptosome (Habermann, 1974). Utilizing ^{125}I-labeled toxin, Hirokawa and Kitamura (1979) observed electron microscopically the binding of the toxin to the presynaptic membrane. The toxin inhibits acetylcholine release from the synaptosome induced by K^+ stimulation (Wonnacott and Marchbanks, 1976). It has been demonstrated that, like the findings with the diaphragm and the nerve–muscle preparation, the rate of inhibition of acetylcholine release from synaptosomes is dependent upon the dose of the toxin, there is a lag time before the development of toxic action, and washing the synaptosome after exposure to the toxin does not reduce the toxic action (Wonnacott, 1980).

When the nerve–muscle preparation, paralyzed with botulinum toxin, is treated with black widow spider venom (BWSV), a burst of miniature end plate potentials occurs to the same extent as that in normal nerve–muscle preparations (Kao et al., 1976). This finding attests that intravesicular acetylcholine is not reduced in quantity upon the treatment with the toxin. Similarly, the quantity of acetylcholine synthesized by the synaptosomes is not reduced by the treatment with the toxin. It has been reported that the toxin does not inhibit the activity of choline acetyltransferase, which catalyzes the synthesis of acetylcholine from choline (Tonge et al., 1975). That the toxin inhibits synthesis of acetylcholine has been reported from the experiments using brain slices (Gundersen and Howard, 1978) or primary cell cultures (Bigalke et al., 1978). These results were interpreted as a gradual inhibition of high-affinity uptake of choline (Gundersen and Howard, 1978), or the secondary action of the toxin, resulting from the impaired choline transport system due to the altered compartmentation of acetylcholine at the nerve endings (Bigalke et al., 1978; Gundersen and Howard, 1978).

The toxin inhibits the release of acetylcholine, but not completely. Harris and Miledi (1971) observed abnormal, low amplitude miniature end-plate potentials in the nerve-muscle preparation of the frog teated with the toxin. Kao *et al.* (1976) studied, by electron microscopy, the nerve–muscle preparations treated with BWSV and then with botulinum toxin and demonstrated vesicles at the release site. Gundersen and Howard (1978) reported that it was newly synthesized acetylcholine rather than that stored, the release of which is inhibited with the toxin. From these results, there may be two kinds of synaptic vesicles involved in acetylcholine release. It is the acetylcholine release from the vesicles involved in the normal release–refill cycle that is inhibited with the toxin. The toxin inhibits either the apparatus of acetylcholine release or the interaction of the vesicle and the membrane at the release site (Gundersen and Howard, 1978). Mechanical block-ade of acetylcholine release by the botulinum derivative toxin molecule was proposed by Lamanna (1976) and Hanig and Lamanna (1979).

In exocytotic acetylcholine release from the synaptic vesicles, Ca^{2+} influx may serve as a trigger. Simpson and Tapp (1967) reported that the lag time of the toxic action to the nerve–muscle preparation changed depending upon the ratio between Mg^{2+} and Ca^{2+} concentrations. The higher the Ca^{2+} concentration, the shorter the period from the exposure to the toxin to the development of paralysis. In the presence of Ca^{2+} the toxin inhibits acetylcholine release by BWSV, but no such effect was shown in the absence of Ca^{2+} (Pumplin and Reese, 1977). The rat extensor digitorum longus muscle paralyzed locally showed increased miniature end-plate potentials in the presence of Ca-ionophore A23187 and Ca^{2+} at 4 mM or higher concentration, thus counteracted the paralysis due to the toxin (Cull-Canday *et al.*, 1976). Lundh *et al.* (1977) reported that the inhibition of acetylcholine release from the nerve muscle preparation by the toxin could be counter-acted by such chemicals as tetraethylamine, guanidine and 4-aminopyridine, that enhance Ca^{2+} influx.

These results show that the reactivity of Ca^{2+} inhibited by the toxin was restored by the increased Ca^{2+} influx, resulting in improved acetylcholine release, and also that the acetylcholine release from the synaptosome poisoned with the toxin is increased by the increased concentration of exogenous Ca^{2+} or the addition of Ca-ionophore A23187 and that $^{45}Ca^{2+}$ influx into the synaptosome is not inhibited by the toxin (Wonnacott *et al.*, 1978; Bigalke *et al.*, 1981a). From these results, it seems more reasonable to think that the action of botulinum toxin is to decrease the susceptibility to Ca^{2+} of the Ca^{2+}-dependent release process rather than to inhibit the Ca^{2+} influx associated with depolar-ization (Wonnacott *et al.*, 1978). Recently, however, Hirokawa and Heuser (1981) stated that the blockade of neuromuscle transmission by botulinum toxin is due to the impaired calcium influx.

Most studies on the receptor of the toxin on the membrane of the nerve cells, like those on the action of the toxin, have been made with type A toxin. Habermann (1974) found that type A toxin bound to synaptosome was released partially upon treatment with neuraminidase and concluded that the toxin-binding site on the membrane is sensi-tive to neuraminidase. Simpson and Rapport (1971) reported earlier that type A toxin was inactivated *in vitro* with gangliosides, particularly with a trisialo ganglioside, G_{T1}. Such inactivation of the toxin with G_{T1} was not dependent upon the temperature. Thus, it appeared that G_{T1} is the receptor substance of the toxin on the nerve cell membrane. The pretreatment of synaptosomes with *V. cholera* neuraminidase did not significantly diminish the inhibition of choline uptake (Habermann *et al.*, 1981). To the contrary, van Heyningen and Mellanby (1973) stated that the toxin is not inactivated with G_{T1} in the presence of gelatin. Recently, Kitamura *et al.* (1980) studied the binding of type A toxin to gangliosides and found that it is bound to ganglioside G_{T1b} on a molar ratio of 1:6. They found that the inactivation of the toxin with G_{T1b} was temperature dependent.

It is known that the susceptibility to botulinum toxin of a certain animal species differs from one toxin type to another and that the toxin of a certain type shows toxicities differing from one animal species to another. The interaction between G_{T1} and each of type A, B and E toxins was examined. It was confirmed that type A toxin was inactivated with G_{T1}, whereas type B and E toxins were each only partially inactivated. These results indicate that the concept that G_{T1} is the receptor substance of botulinum toxin may be true with type A toxin, but not with the toxin of other types, and that some other substances may be the receptors for the toxin of other types. In further experiments, the binding of the ^{125}I-labeled toxin to synaptosomes was inhibited only with the unlabeled toxin of the same type; unlabeled toxin of other types only partially inhibited the binding (Kozaki, 1979). The possibility that the receptor substance on the nerve cell membrane may be specific to the toxin type and that the binding of toxin to G_{T1} differs from one type to another, may serve as a clue to explain the different susceptibilities of a certain species of animal to the toxin of different types or different toxicities of the toxin of a certain type to different animal species.

Of the two fragments of the toxic component, fragment I with a molecular weight of 100,000 only inhibits the binding of the toxin to synaptosome (Kozaki, 1979). The quantities of type E unactivated and activated toxins bound to the synaptosome were the same. The results may indicate that the binding site on fragment I is not modified by trypsinization and that the potentiation by trypsinization is caused by the change occurring on the other fragment (fragment II).

These results are of interest if considered in conjunction with the findings that the action of the toxin to the nerve–muscle preparation or synaptosome involves three distinct steps: (1) binding of the toxin to the membrane, (2) translocation of the toxin, and (3) inhibition of acetylcholine release. Simpson (1980) hypothesized that one fragment is concerned with the binding to the membrane while the other with the inhibition of acetylcholine release. If this hypothesis is true, it is fragment I that is concerned with the binding and it may be fragment II that might penetrate into the nerve cell, possibly by endocytosis (Simpson, 1981) and inhibit the Ca^{2+}-sensitive acetylcholine release.

REFERENCES

ABRAMS, A., KEGELES, G. and HOTTLE, G. A. (1946) The purification of toxin from *Clostridium botulinum* type A. *J. biol. Chem.* **164**: 63–79.

ALDERTON, G., CHEN, J. K. and ITO, K. A. (1974) Effect of lysozyme on the recovery of heated *Clostridium botulinum* spores. *Appl. Microbiol.* **27**: 613–615.

AMBACHE, N. (1948) Peripheral action of botulinum toxin. *Nature* **161**: 482–483.

AMBACHE, N. (1949) The peripheral action of *Cl. botulinum* toxin. *J. Physiol.* **108**: 127–141.

AMBACHE, N. (1951) A further survey of the action of *Clostridium botulinum* toxin upon different types of autonomic nerve fibre. *J. Physiol.* **113**: 1–17.

AMBACHE, N. (1952) Effect of botulinum toxin upon the superior cervical ganglion. *J. Physiol.* **116**: 9.

ANDO, Y. and IIDA, H. (1970) Factors affecting the germination of spores of *Clostridium botulinum* type E. *Jap. J. Microbiol.* **14**: 361–370.

ANDO, Y., KAMEYAMA, K. and KARASHIMADA, T. (1975) Studies on germination of spores of clostridial species capable of causing food poisoning (IX) Effect of glycine on the growth from spores of *Clostridium botulinum*. *J. Food Hyg. Soc. Japan* **16**: 258–263.

ANONYMOUS (1980a) Wound botulism—Texas, California, Washington. *Morbid. Mortal. Weekly Rep.* **29**: 34–46.

ANONYMOUS (1980b) Infant botulism—California, Australia, Czechoslovakia. *Calif. Morbid.* **28** (July 18).

ANONYMOUS (1980c) Type F infant botulism—New Mexico. *Morbid. Mortal. Weekly Rep.* **29**: 85–87.

ANONYMOUS (1981) Botulism—United States, 1979–1980. *Morbid. Mortal. Weekly Rep.* **30**: 121–123.

ARNON, S. S. and CHIN, J. (1979) The clinical spectrum of infant botulism. *Rev. infect. Dis.* **1**: 614–621.

ARNON, S. S., MIDURA, T. F., DAMUS, K., THOMPSON, B., WOOD, R. M. and CHIN, J. (1978a) Honey and other environmental risk factors for infant botulism. *J. Pediatr.* **94**: 331–336.

ARNON, S. S., MIDURA, T. F., DAMUS, K., WOOD, R. M. and CHIN, J. (1978b) Intestinal infection and toxin production by *Clostridium botulinum* as one cause of sudden infant death syndrome. *Lancet* i (8077): 1273–1277.

ARNON, S. S., WERNER, S. B., FABER, H. K. and FARR, W. H. (1979) Infant botulism in 1931: Discovery of a misclassified case. *Am. J. Dis. Child.* **133**: 580–582.

BAIRD-PARKER, A. C. (1971) Factors affecting the production of bacterial food poisoning toxins. *J. appl. Bacteriol.* **34**: 181–197.

BEERS, W. H. and REICH, E. (1969) Isolation and characterization of *Clostridium botulinum* type B toxin. *J. biol. Chem.* **244**: 4473–4479.

BENGTSON, I. A. (1922) Preliminary note on a toxin-producing anaerobe isolated from the larvae of *Lucilia caesar*. *Publ. Hlth Rep.* **37**: 164–170.

BETLEY, M. and SUGIYAMA, H. (1979) Noncorrelation between mouse toxicity and serologically assayed toxin in *Clostridium botulinum* type A culture fluids. *Appl. envir. Microbiol.* **38**: 297–300.

BIGALKE, H. and HABERMANN, E. (1981) Botulinum A toxin inhibits the release of noradrenaline, acetylcholine, γ-aminobutyric acid and glycine from particles of rat brain and spinal cord. *IRCS Med. Sci.* **9**: 105–106.

BIGALKE, H., DIMPFEL, W. and HABERMANN, E. (1978) Suppression of ^{3}H-acetylcholine release from primary nerve cell cultures by tetanus and botulinum-A toxin. *Naunyn-Schmiedeberg's Archs Pharmac.* **303**: 133–138.

BIGALKE, H., AHNERT-HILGER, G. and HABERMANN, E. (1981a) Tetanus toxin and botulinum A toxin inhibit acetylcholine release from but not calcium uptake into brain tissue. *Naunyn-Schmiedeberg's Archs Pharmac.* **316**: 143–148.

BIGALKE, H., HELLER, I., BIZZINI, B. and HABERMANN, E. (1981b) Tetanus toxin and botulinum A toxin inhibit release and uptake of various transmitters, as studied with particulate preparations from rat brain and spinal cord. *Naunyn-Schmiedeberg's Archs Pharmac.* **316**: 244–251.

BONVENTRE, P. F. (1979) Absorption of botulinal toxin from the gastrointestinal tract. *Rev. infect. Dis.* **1**: 663–667.

BONVENTRE, P. F. and KEMPE, L. L. (1959) Physiology of toxin production by *Clostridium botulinum* types A and B. III. Effect of pH and temperature during incubation on growth, autolysis, and toxin production. *Appl. Microbiol.* **7**: 374–377.

BORLAND, E. D. (1976) Outbreak of botulism in reared East Anglian pheasants. *Vet. Rec.* **99**: 220–221.

BOROFF, D. A. and FLECK, U. (1966) Statistical analysis of a rapid *in vivo* method for the titration of the toxin of *Clostridium botulinum.* *J. Bacteriol.* **92**: 1580–1581.

BOROFF, D. A. and REILLY, J. R. (1962) Studies of the toxin of *Clostridium botulinum.* VI. Botulism among pheasants and quail, mode of transmission and degree of resistance offered by immunization. *Int. Archs Allergy* **20**: 306–313.

BOROFF, D. A. and SHU-CHEN, G. (1973) Radioimmunoassay for type A toxin of *Clostridium botulinum.* *Appl. Microbiol.* **25**: 545–549.

BOROFF, D. A., TOWNEND, R., FLECK, U. and DASGUPTA, B. R. (1966) Ultracentrifugal analysis of the crystalline toxin and isolated fractions of *Clostridium botulinum* type A. *J. biol. Chem.* **241**: 5165–5167.

BRADSHAW, J. G., PEELER, J. T. and TWEDT, R. M. (1981) Thermal inactivation of *Clostridium botulinum* types F and G in buffer and in beef and mushroom patties. *J. Food Sci.* **46**: 688–690 + 696.

BROOKS, V. B. (1956) An intracellular study of the action of repetitive nerve alloys and of botulinum toxin on miniature end-plate potentials. *J. Physiol.* **134**: 264–277.

BUEHLER, H. J., SCHANTZ, E. J. and LAMANNA, C. (1947) The elemental and amino acid composition of crystalline *Clostridium botulinum* type A toxin. *J. biol. Chem.* **169**: 295–302.

BULATOVA, T. I., MATVEEV, K. I. and SAMSONOVA, V. S. (1967) Biological characteristics of *Cl. botulinum* type C strains isolated from minks in U.S.S.R. In: *Botulism 1966,* pp. 391–399, INGRAM, M. and ROBERTS, T. A. (eds). Chapman & Hall, London.

BURGEN, A. S. V., DICKENS, F. and ZATMAN, L. J. (1949) The action of botulinum toxin on the neuro-muscular junction. *J. Physiol.* **109**: 10–24.

CARDELLA, M. A., DUFF, J. T., GOTTFRIED, C. and BEGEL, J. S. (1958) Studies on immunity to toxins of *Clostridium botulinum.* IV. Production and purification of type C toxin for conversion to toxoid. *J. Bacteriol.* **75**: 360–365.

CARDELLA, M. A., DUFF, J. T., WINGFIELD, B. H. and GOTTFRIED, C. (1960) Studies on immunity to toxins of *Clostridium botulinum.* VI. Purification and detoxification of type D toxin and the immunological response to toxoid. *J. Bacteriol.* **79**: 372–378.

CENTER FOR DISEASE CONTROL (1979) *Botulism in the United States, 1899–1977. Handbook for Epidemiologists, Clinicians, and Laboratory Workers.* Center for Disease Control, Atlanta, Georgia.

CRAIG, J. M., IIDA, H. and INOUE, K. (1970) A recent case of botulism in Hokkaido, Japan. *Jap. J. med. Sci. Biol.* **23**: 193–198.

CULL-CANDY, S. G., LUNDH, H. and THESLEFF, S. (1976) Effects of botulinum toxin on neuromuscular transmission in the rat. *J. Physiol.* **260**: 177–203.

DACK, G. M. (1956) *Food Poisoning* (3rd edn.) Univ. Chicago Press, Chicago, Ill.

DACK, G. M. and GIBBARD, J. (1926a) Studies on botulinum toxin in the alimentary tract of hogs, rabbits, guinea-pigs and mice. *J. infect. Dis.* **39**: 173–180.

DACK, G. M. and GIBBARD, J. (1926b) Permeability of the small intestine of rabbits and hogs to botulinum toxin. *J. infect. Dis.* **39**: 181–185.

DASGUPTA, B. R. (1971) Activation of *Clostridium botulinum* type B toxin by an endogenous enzyme. *J. Bacteriol.* **108**: 1051–1057.

DASGUPTA, B. R. and SUGIYAMA, H. (1972a) Role of a protease in natural activation of *Clostridium botulinum* neurotoxin. *Infec. Immunity* **6**: 587–590.

DASGUPTA, B. R. and SUGIYAMA, H. (1972b) Isolation and characterization of a protease from *Clostridium botulinum* type B. *Biochim. biophys. Acta* **268**: 719–729.

DASGUPTA, B. R. and SUGIYAMA, H. (1972c) A common subunit structure in *Clostridium botulinum* types A, B, and E toxins. *Biochem. biophys. Res. Commun.* **48**: 108–112.

DASGUPTA, B. R. and SUGIYAMA, H. (1976) Molecular forms of neurotoxins in proteolytic *Clostridium botulinum* type B cultures. *Infec. Immunity* **14**: 680–686.

DASGUPTA, B. R. and SUGIYAMA, H. (1977a) Comparative sizes of type A and B botulinum neurotoxins. *Toxicon* **15**: 357–363.

DASGUPTA, B. R. and SUGIYAMA, H. (1977b) Single chain and dichain forms of neurotoxin in type F *Clostridium botulinum* culture. *Toxicon* **15**: 446–471.

DASGUPTA, B. R. and SUGIYAMA, H. (1980) Role of arginine residues in the structure and biological activity of botulinum neurotoxin types A and E. *Biochem. biophys. Res. Commun.* **93**: 369–375.

DASGUPTA, B. R., BERRY, L. J. and BOROFF, D. A. (1970) Purification of *Clostridium botulinum* type A toxin. *Biochim. biophys. Acta* **214**: 343–349.

DASGUPTA, B. R., BOROFF, D. A. and CHEONG, K. (1968) Isolation of chromatographically pure toxin of *Clostridium botulinum* type B. *Biochem. biophys. Res. Commun.* **32**: 1057–1063.

DASGUPTA, B. R., BOROFF, D. A. and ROTHSTEIN, E. (1966) Chromatographic fractionation of the crystalline toxin of *Clostridium botulinum* type A. *Biochem. biophys. Res. Commun.* **22**: 750–756.

DICKSON, E. C. and SHEVKY, R. (1923a) Botulism, studies on the manner in which the toxin of *Clostridium botulinum* acts upon the body. I. The effect upon the autonomic nervous system. *J. exp. Med.* **37**: 711–731.

DICKSON, E. C. and SHEVKY, R. (1923b) Botulism, studies on the manner in which the toxin of *Clostridium botulinum* acts upon the body. II. The effect on the voluntary nervous system. *J. exp. Med.* **38**: 327–346.

DOLMAN, C. E. (1957) Recent observations on type E botulism. *Can. J. Publ. Hlth* **48**: 187–198.

DOLMAN, C. E. and IIDA, H. (1963) Type E botulism: Its epidemiology, prevention and specific treatment. *Can. J. Publ. Hlth* **54**: 293–308.

DOLMAN, C. E. and MURAKAMI, L. (1961) *Clostridium botulinum* type F with recent observations on other types. *J. infect. Dis.* **109**: 107–128.

DOLMAN, C. E., TOMSICH, M., CAMPBELL, C. C. R. and LAING, W. B. (1960) Fish eggs as a cause of human botulism (Two outbreaks in British Columbia due to types E and B botulinus toxins). *J. infect. Dis.* **106**: 5–19.

DOUGLAS, H. M., MANSON, J. I., PATON, J. C., HANSMAN, D. J., MURRELL, W. G. and STEWART, B. J. (1980) Infant botulism. *Med. J. Aust.* Oct. 4, 398.

DOWELL, V. R., McCROSKEY, L. M., HATHEWAY, C. L., LOMBARD, G. L., HUGHES, J. M. and MERSON, M. H. (1977) Coproexamination for botulinal toxin and *Clostridium botulinum*. *J. Am. med. Ass.* **238**: 1829–1832.

DUFF, J. T., KLERER, J., BIBLER, R. H., MOORE, D. E., GOTTFRIED, C. and WRIGHT, G. G. (1957a) Studies on immunity to toxins of *Cl. botulinum*. II. Production and purification of type B toxin for toxoid. *J. Bacteriol.* **73**: 597–601.

DUFF, J. T., WRIGHT, G. G., KLERER, J., MOORE, D. E. and BIBLER, R. H. (1957b) Studies on immunity to toxins of *Clostridium bolutinum*. I. A simplified procedure for isolation of type A toxin. *J. Bacteriol.* **73**: 42–47.

DUFF, J. T., WRIGHT, G. G. and YARINSKY, A. (1956) Activation of *Clostridium botulinum* type E toxin by trypsin. *J. Bacteriol.* **72**: 455–460.

EDMUNDS, C. W. and LONG, P. H. (1923) Contribution to the pathologic physiology of botulism. *J. Am. med. Ass.* **81**: 542–547.

EKLUND, M. W. and POYSKY, F. T. (1970) The significance of non-proteolytic *Clostridium botulinum* types B, E and F in the development of radiation-pasteurized fishery products. In: *Preservation of Fish by Irradiation*. pp. 125–148. International Atomic Energy Agency, Vienna.

EKLUND, M. W. and POYSKY, F. T. (1974) Interconversion of type C and D strains of *Clostridium botulinum* by specific bacteriophages. *Appl. Microbiol.* **27**: 251–258.

EKLUND, M. W., POYSKY, F. T. and REED, S. M. (1972) Bacteriophage and toxigenicity of *Clostridium botulinum* type D. *Nature New Biol.* **235**: 16–18.

EKLUND, M. W., POYSKY, F. T., MEYERS, J. A. and PELROY, G. A. (1974) Interspecies conversion of *Clostridium botulinum* type C to *Clostridium novyi* type A by bacteriophage. *Science* **186**: 456–458.

EKLUND, M. W., POYSKY, F. T., REED, S. M. and SMITH, C. A. (1971) Bacteriophage and the toxigenicity of *Clostridium botulinum* type C. *Science* **172**: 480–482.

EKLUND, M. W., WIELER, D. I. and POYSKY, F. T. (1967) Outgrowth and toxin production of nonproteolytic type B *Clostridium botulinum* at 3.3 to 5.6 C. *J. Bacteriol.* **93**: 1461–1462.

FIOCK, M. A., YARINSKY, A. and DUFF, J. T. (1961) Studies on immunity to toxins of *Clostridium botulinum*. VII. Purification and detoxification of trypsin-activated type E toxin. *J. Bacteriol.* **82**: 66–71.

FISH, N. A., MITCHELL, W. R. and BARNUM, D. A. (1967) A report of a natural outbreak of botulism in pheasants. *Can. Vet. J.* **8**: 10–16.

FUKUDA, T., KITAO, T., TANIKAWA, H. and SAKAGUCHI, G. (1970) An outbreak of type B botulism occurring in Miyazaki prefecture. *Jap. J. med. Sci. Biol.* **23**: 243–248.

FULLERTON, P., GOGNA, N. K. and STODDART, R. (1980) Wound botulism. *Med. J. Aust.* **1**: 662–663.

GERWING, J., DOLMAN, C. E. and ARNOTT, D. (1961) Purification and activation of *Clostridium botulinum* type E toxin. *J. Bacteriol.* **81**: 819–822.

GERWING, J., DOLMAN, C. E. and ARNOTT, D. (1962) Activation phenomenon of *Clostridium botulinum* type E toxin. *J. Bacteriol.* **84**: 302–306.

GERWING, J., DOLMAN, C. E. and BAINS, H. S. (1965a) Isolation and characterization of a toxic moiety of low molecular weight from *Clostridium botulinum* type A. *J. Bacteriol.* **89**: 1383–1386.

GERWING, J., DOLMAN, C. E. and KO, A. (1965b) Mechanism of tryptic activation of *Clostridium botulinum* type E toxin. *J. Bacteriol.* **89**: 1176–1179.

GERWING, J., DOLMAN, C. E., REICHMANN, M. E. and BAINS, H. S. (1964) Purification and molecular weight determination of *Clostridium botulinum* type E toxin. *J. Bacteriol.* **88**: 216–219.

GERWING, J., DOLMAN, C. E., KASON, D. V. and TREMAINE, J. H. (1966) Purification and characterization of *Clostridium botulinum* type B toxin. *J. Bacteriol.* **91**: 484–487.

GIMÉNEZ, D. F. and CICCARELLI, A. S. (1970a) Studies on strain 84 of *Clostridium botulinum*. *Zbl. Bakt., I. Abt. Orig.* **215**: 212–220.

GIMÉNEZ, D. F. and CICCARELLI, A. S. (1970b) Another type of *Clostridium botulinum*. *Zbl. Bakt., I. Abt. Orig.* **215**: 221–224.

GORDON, M., FIOCK, M. A., YARINSKY, A. and DUFF, J. T. (1957) Studies on immunity to toxins of *Clostridium botulinum*. III. Preparation, purification and detoxification of type E toxin. *J. Bacteriol.* **74**: 533–538.

GUILFOYLE, D. E. and MESTRANDREA, L. W. (1980) Problems encountered with the capillary tube immunodiffusion method for detection of botulinal toxin. *Appl. envir. Microbiol.* **40**: 847–848.

GULLMAR, B. and MOLIN, N. (1967a) Effect of choline on cell division of *Clostridium botulinum* type E. *J. Bacteriol.* **93**: 1734–1735.

GULLMAR, B. and MOLIN, N. (1967b) Effect of nutrients on physiological properties of *Clostridium botulinum* type E. *J. Bacteriol.* **94**: 1924–1929.

GUNDERSEN, C. B. JR. and HOWARD, B. D. (1978) The effects of botulinum toxin on acetylcholine metabolism in mouse brain slices and synaptosomes. *J. Neurochem.* **31**: 1005–1013.

GUNNISON, J. B. and COLEMAN, G. E. (1932) *Clostridium botulinum*, type C, associated with western duck sickness. *J. infect. Dis.* **51**: 542–551.

GUNNISON, J. B., CUMMINGS, J. R. and MEYER, K. F. (1936) *Clostridium botulinum* type E. *Proc. Soc. exp. Biol. Med.* **35**: 278–280.

HABERMANN, E. (1974) ^{125}I-Labeled neurotoxin from *Clostridium botulinum* A: Preparation, binding to synaptosomes and ascent to the spinal cord. *Naunyn-Schmiedeberg's Archs Pharmac.* **281**: 47–56.

HABERMANN, E. and HELLER, I. (1975) Direct evidence for the specific fixation of *Cl. botulinum* A neurotoxin to brain matter. *Naunyn Schmiedeberg's Archs Pharmac.* **287**: 97–106.

HABERMANN, E., BIGALKE, H. and HELLER, I. (1981) Inhibition of synaptosomal choline uptake by tetanus and botulinum A toxin. Partial dissociation of fixation and effect of tetanus toxin. *Naunyn Schmiedeberg's Archs Pharmac.* **316**: 135–142.

HANIG, J. P. and LAMANNA, C. (1979) Toxicity of botulinum toxin: a stoichiometric model for the locus of its extraordinary potency and persistence at the neuromuscular junction. *J. theor. Biol.* **77**: 107–113.

HARRIS, A. J. and MILEDI, R. (1971) The effect of type D botulinum toxin on frog neuromuscular junctions. *J. Physiol.* **217**: 497–515.

HECKLY, R. J., HILDEBRAND, G. J. and LAMANNA, C. (1960) On the size of toxic particle passing the intestinal barrier in botulism. *J. exp. Med.* **111**: 745–759.

HILDEBRAND, G. J., LAMANNA, C. and HECKLY, B. J. (1961) Distribution and particle size of type A botulinum toxin in body fluids of intravenously injected rabbits. *Proc. Soc. exp. Biol. Med.* **107**: 284–289.

HIROKAWA, N. and HEUSER, J. E. (1981) Structural evidence that botulinum toxin blocks neuromuscular transmission by impairing the calcium influx that normally accompanies nerve depolarization. *J. Cell Biol.* **88**: 160–171.

HIROKAWA, N. and KITAMURA, M. (1979) Binding of *Clostridium botulinum* neurotoxin to the presynaptic membrane in the central nervous system. *J. Cell Biol.* **81**: 43–49.

HUSS, H. H. and ESKILDSEN, U. (1979) Botulism in farmed trout caused by *Clostridium botulinum* type E. *Nord. Vet. Med.* **26**: 733–738.

IIDA, H., KANZAWA, K., NAKAMURA, Y., KARASHIMADA, T., ONO, T. and SAITO, T. (1964) Botulism outbreaks encountered in Hokkaido in 1962; with special reference to the therapeutic value of specific antitoxin. *Rep. Hokkaido Inst. Publ. Hlth* **14**: 6–18.

INOUE, K. and IIDA, H. (1970) Conversion of toxigenicity in *Clostridium botulinum* type C. *Jap. J. Microbiol.* **14**: 87–89.

INOUE, K. and IIDA, H. (1971) Phage conversion of toxigenicity in *Clostridium botulinum* types C and D. *Jap. J. med. Sci. Biol.* **24**: 53–56.

IWASAKI, M. and SAKAGUCHI, G. (1978) Acid precipitation of *Clostridium botulinum* type C and D toxins from whole culture by addition of ribonucleic acid as a precipitation aid. *Infec. Immunity* **19**: 749–751.

IWASAKI, M., OHISHI, I. and SAKAGUCHI, G. (1980) Evidence that botulinum C2 toxin has two dissimilar components. *Infec. Immunity* **29**: 390–394.

JANSEN, B. C. (1971) The toxic antigenic factors produced by *Clostridium botulinum* types C and D. *Onderstepoort J. vet. Res.* **38**: 93–98.

JANSEN, B. C. and KNOETZE, P. C. (1971) Tryptic activation of *Clostridium botulinum* type Cβ toxin. *Onderstepoort J. vet. Res.* **38**: 237–238.

JOHNSON, H. M., BRENNER, K., ANGELOTTI, R. and HALL, H. E. (1966) Serological studies of types A, B, and E botulinal toxins by passive hemagglutination and bentonite flocculation. *J. Bacteriol.* **91**: 967–974.

KALMBACH, E. R. (1968) Type C botulism among wild birds—A historical sketch. *Bureau of Sport Fisheries and Wildlife Special Scientific Report.* Wildlife, No. 110. Washington, D.C.

KAO, I., DRACHMAN, D. B. and PRICE, D. L. (1976) Botulinum toxin: Mechanism of presynaptic blockade. *Science* **193**: 1256–1258.

KAUTTER, D. A. and LILLY, T. JR. (1970) Detection of *Clostridium botulinum* its toxin in food. I. Detection of *Clostridium botulinum* type E in smoked fish. *J. Ass. off. agric. Chem.* **53**: 710–712.

KITAMURA, M. and SAKAGUCHI, G. (1969) Dissociation and reconstitution of 12S toxin of *Clostridium botulinum* type E. *Biochim. biophys. Acta* **194**: 564–571.

KITAMURA, M., IWAMORI, M. and NAGAI, Y. (1980) Interaction between *Clostridium botulinum* neurotoxin and gangliosides. *Biochim. biophys. Acta* **628**: 328–335.

KITAMURA, M., SAKAGUCHI, S. and SAKAGUCHI, G. (1967) Dissociation of *Clostridium botulinum* type-E toxin. *Biochem. biophys. Res. Commun.* **29**: 892–897.

KITAMURA, M., SAKAGUCHI, S. and SAKAGUCHI, G. (1968) Purification and some properties of *Clostridium botulinum* type-E toxin. *Biochim. biophys. Acta* **168**: 207–217.

KITAMURA, M., SAKAGUCHI, S. and SAKAGUCHI, G. (1969) Significance of 12S toxin of *Clostridium botulinum* type E. *J. Bacteriol.* **98**: 1173–1178.

KNOX, J. N., BROWN, W. P. and SPERO, L. (1970) The role of sulfhydryl groups in the activity of type A botulinum toxin. *Biochim. biophys. Acta* **214**: 350–354.

KOELLE, G. B. (1962) A new general concept of the neurohumoral functions of acetylcholine and acetylcholinesterase. *J. Pharm. Pharmac.* **14**: 65–90.

KONDO, H., KONDO, S., MURATA, R. and SAKAGUCHI, G. (1969) Antigenicity of *Clostridium botulinum* type-E formol toxoid. *Jap. J. med. Sci. Biol.* **22**: 75–85.

KOZAKI, S. (1979) Interaction of botulinum type A, B and E derivative toxins with synaptosomes of rat brain. *Naunyn Schmiedeberg's Archs Pharmac.* **308**: 67–70.

KOZAKI, S. and SAKAGUCHI, G. (1975) Antigenicities of fragments of *Clostridium botulinum* type B derivative toxin. *Infec. Immunity* **11**: 932–936.

KOZAKI, S., DUFRENNE, J., HAGENAARS, A. M. and NOTERMANS, S. (1979) Enzyme linked immunosorbent assay (ELISA) for detection of *Clostridium botulinum* type B toxin. *Jap. J. med. Sci. Biol.* **32**: 199–205.

KOZAKI, S., MIYAZAKI, S. and SAKAGUCHI, G. (1977) Development of antitoxin with each of two complementary fragments of *Clostridium botulinum* type B derivative toxin. *Infec. Immunity* **18**: 761–766.

KOZAKI, S., SAKAGUCHI, S. and SAKAGUCHI, G. (1974) Purification and some properties of progenitor toxins of *Clostridium botulinum* type B. *Infec. Immunity* **10**: 750–756.

KOZAKI, S., TOGASHI, S. and SAKAGUCHI, G. (1981) Separation of *Clostridium botulinum* type A derivative toxin into two fragments. *Jap. J. med. Sci. Biol.* **34**: 61–68.

KRYSINSKI, E. P. and SUGIYAMA, H. (1980) Purification and some properties of H chain subunit of type A botulinum neurotoxin. *Toxicon* **18**: 705–710.

KRYSINSKI, E. P. and SUGIYAMA, H. (1981) Nature of intracellular type A botulinum neurotoxin. *Appl. envir. Microbiol.* **41**: 675–678.

LAMANNA, C. (1948) Haemagglutination by botulinal toxin. *Proc. Soc. exp. Biol. Med.* **69**: 332–336.

LAMANNA, C. (1960) Oral poisoning by bacterial exotoxins exemplified in botulism. *Ann. N.Y. Acad. Sci.* **88**: 1109–1114.

LAMANNA, C. (1976) The pipe and valve hypothesis of the mechanism of action of botulinal toxin. *Spec. Publ. Acad. Sci. Art Bosnia Herzegovina* **29**: 213–221.

LAMANNA, C. and CARR, C. J. (1967) The botulinal, tetanal, and enterostaphylococcal toxins: A review. *Clin. Pharmac. Ther.* **8**: 286–332.

LAMANNA, C. and GLASSMAN, H. N. (1947) The isolation of type B botulinum toxin. *J. Bacteriol.* **54**: 575–584.

LAMANNA, C. and SAKAGUCHI, G. (1971) Botulinal toxins and the problem of nomenclature of simple toxins. *Bacteriol. Rev.* **32**: 242–249.

LAMANNA, C., JENSEN, W. I. and BROSS, D. J. (1955) Body weight as a factor in the response of mice to botulinal toxins. *Am. J. Hyg.* **62**: 21–28.

LAMANNA, C., MACELROY, O. E. and EKLUND, H. W. (1946) The purification and crystallization of *Clostridium botulinum* type A toxin. *Science* **103**: 613–614.

LAMANNA, C. and MEYERS, C. E. (1960) Influence of ingested foods on the oral toxicity in mice of crystalline botulinal type A toxin. *J. Bacteriol.* **79**: 406–410.

LAMANNA, C., SPERO, L. and SCHANTZ, E. J. (1970) Dependence of time to death on molecular size of botulinal toxin. *Infec. Immunity* **1**: 423–424.

LANDMANN, G. (1904) Über die Ursache der Darmstädter Bohnenvergiftung. *Hyg. Rundschau* **14**: 449.

LEE, V. H., VADLAMUDI, S. and HANSON, R. P. (1962) Blow fly larvae as a source of botulinum toxin for game farm pheasants. *J. Wildl. Man.* **26**: 411–413.

LEUCHS, J. (1910) Beiträge zur Kenntnis des Toxins und Antitoxins des *Bacillus botulinus*. *Z. Hyg. Infektionsk.* **65**: 55–84.

LOWENTHAL, J. P. and LAMANNA, C. (1951) Factors affecting the botulinal hemagglutination reaction, and the relationship between hemagglutinating activity and toxicity of toxin preparations. *Am. J. Hyg.* **54**: 342–353.

LOWENTHAL, J. P. and LAMANNA, C. (1953) Characterization of botulinal hemagglutination. *Am. J. Hyg.* **57**: 46–59.

LUNDH, H., LEANDER, S. and THESLEFF, S. (1977) Antagonism of the paralysis produced by botulinum toxin in the rat. The effects of tetraethylammonium, guanidine and 4-aminopyridine. *J. neurol. Sci.* **32**: 29–43.

MASON, J. H. and ROBINSON, E. M. (1935) The antigenic components of the toxins of *Clostridium botulinum* types C and D. *Onderstepoort J. vet. Sci. Anim. Indust.* **5**: 65–75.

MAY, A. J. and WHALER, B. C. (1958) The absorption of *Clostridium botulinum* type A toxin from the alimentary canal. *Br. J. exp. Path.* **39**: 307–316.

MERSON, M. H. and DOWELL, V. R. JR. (1973) Epidemiologic, clinical and laboratory aspects of wound botulism. *New Engl. J. Med.* **289**: 1005–1010.

MESTRANDREA, L. W. (1974) Rapid detection of *Clostridium botulinum* toxin by capillary tube diffusion. *Appl. Microbiol.* **27**: 1017–1022.

MEYER, K. F. (1929) Maximum oxygen tolerance of *Cl. botulinum* A, B and C, of *Cl. sporogens* and *Cl. welchii*. *J. infect. Dis.* **44**: 408–411.

MEYER, K. F. and GUNNISON, J. B. (1929) European strains of *Cl. botulinum* XXXVI. *J. infect. Dis.* **45**: 96–105.

MIDURA, T. F. and ARNON, S. S. (1976) Infant botulism: Identification of *Clostridium botulinum* and its toxins in feces. *Lancet* **ii**: 934–936.

MILLER, C. A. and ANDERSON, A. W. (1971) Rapid detection and quantitative estimation of type A botulinum toxin by electroimmunodiffusion. *Infec. Immunity* **4**: 126–129.

MINERVIN, S. M. (1967) On the parenteral–enteral method of administering serum in cases of botulism. In: *Botulism 1966*, pp. 336–345, INGRAM, M. and ROBERTS, T. A. (eds). Chapman & Hall, London.

MIYAZAKI, S. and SAKAGUCHI, G. (1978) Experimental botulism in chickens: The cecum as the site of production and absorption of botulinum toxin. *Jap. J. med. Sci. Biol.* **31**: 1–15.

MIYAZAKI, S., IWASAKI, M. and SAKAGUCHI, G. (1977) *Clostridium botulinum* type D toxin: Purification, molecular structure, and some immunological properties. *Infec. Immunity* **17**: 395–401.

MIYAZAKI, S., KOZAKI, S., SAKAGUCHI, S. and SAKAGUCHI, G. (1976) Comparison of progenitor toxins of nonproteolytic with those of proteolytic *Clostridium botulinum* type B. *Infec. Immunity* **13**: 987–989.

MOBERG, L. J. and SUGIYAMA, H. (1978) Affinity chromatography purification of type A botulinum neurotoxin from crystalline toxic complex. *Appl. envir. Microbiol.* **35**: 878–880.

MOBERG, L. J. and SUGIYAMA, H. (1979) Microbial ecological basis of infant botulism as studied with germfree mice. *Infec. Immunity* **25**: 653–657.

MØLLER, V. and SCHEIBEL, I. (1960) Preliminary report on the isolation of an apparently new type of *Clostridium botulinum*. *Acta path. microbiol. scand.* **48**: 80.

NAKAMURA, S., SERIKAWA, T., YAMAKAWA, K., NISHIDA, S., KOZAKI, S. and SAKAGUCHI, G. (1978) Sporulation and C2 toxin production by *Clostridium botulinum* type C strains producing no C1 toxin. *Microbiol. Immunol.* **22**: 591–596.

NOTERMANS, S., DUFRENNE, J. and VAN SCHOTHORST, M. (1978) Enzyme-linked immunosorbent assay for detection of *Clostridium botulinum* toxin type A. *Jap. J. med. Sci. Biol.* **31**: 81–85.

OGUMA, K. (1976) The stability of toxigenicity in *Clostridium botulinum* types C and D. *J. gen. Microbiol.* **92**: 67–75.

OGUMA, K. and IIDA, H. (1979) High and low toxin production by a non-toxigenic strain of *Clostridium botulinum* type C following infection with type D phages of different passage history. *J. gen. Microbiol.* **112**: 203–206.

OGUMA, K., IIDA, H. and INOUE, K. (1975) Observations on nonconverting phage, C-n71, obtained from a nontoxigenic strain of *Clostridium botulinum* type C. *Jap. J. Microbiol.* **19**: 167–172.

OGUMA, K., SYUTO, B., IIDA, H. and KUBO, S. (1980) Antigenic similarity of toxins produced by *Clostridium botulinum* type C and D strains. *Infec. Immunity* **30**: 656–660.

OGUMA, K., SYUTO, B., AGUI, T., IIDA, H. and KUBO, S. (1981) Homogeneity of toxins produced by *Clostridium botulinum* type C and D toxins. *Infec. Immunity* **34**: 382–388.

OHISHI, I. and SAKAGUCHI, G. (1974) Purification of *Clostridium botulinum* type F progenitor toxin. *Appl. Microbiol.* **28**: 923–928.

OHISHI, I. and SAKAGUCHI, G. (1975) Molecular construction of *Clostridium botulinum* type F progenitor toxin. *Appl. Microbiol.* **29**: 444–447.

OHISHI, I. and SAKAGUCHI, G. (1977a) Activation of botulinum toxins in the absence of nicking. *Infec. Immunity* **17**: 402–407.

OHISHI, I. and SAKAGUCHI, G. (1977b) Response of type B and E botulinum toxins to purified sulfhydryl-dependent protease produced by *Clostridium botulinum* type F. *Jap. J. med. Sci. Biol.* **30**: 179–190.

OHISHI, I. and SAKAGUCHI, G. (1980) Oral toxicities of *Clostridium botulinum* type C and D toxins of different molecular sizes. *Infec. Immunity* **28**: 303–309.

OHISHI, I., IWASAKI, M. and SAKAGUCHI, G. (1980a) Purification and characterization of two components of botulinum C2 toxin. *Infec. Immunity* **30**: 668–673.

OHISHI, I., IWASAKI, M. and SAKAGUCHI, G. (1980b) Vascular permeability activity of botulinum C2 toxin elicited by cooperation of two dissimilar protein components. *Infec. Immunity* **31**: 890–895.

OHISHI, I., OKADA, T. and SAKAGUCHI, G. (1975) Responses of *Clostridium botulinum* type B and E progenitor toxins to some clostridial sulfhydryl-dependent proteases. *Jap. J. med. Sci. Biol.* **28**: 157–164.

OHISHI, I., SUGII, S. and SAKAGUCHI, G. (1977) Oral toxicities of *Clostridium botulinum* toxins in response to molecular size. *Infec. Immunity* **16**: 107–109.

OHYE, D. F. and CHRISTIAN, J. H. B. (1967) Combined effects of temperature, pH and water activity on growth and toxin production by *Cl. botulinum* types A, B and E. In: *Botulism 1966*, pp. 217–223, INGRAM, M. and ROBERTS, T. A. (eds.). Chapman & Hall, London.

OHYE, D. F. and SCOTT, W. J. (1953) The temperature relations of *Clostridium botulinum*, types A and B. *Aust. J. biol. Sci.* **6**: 178–189.

PFENNINGER, W. (1924) Toxico-immunologic and serologic relationship of *B. botulinus*, type C, and *B. parabotulinus*, "Seddon." XXII. *J. infect. Dis.* **35**: 347–352.

PICKETT, J., BERG, B., CHAPLIN, E. and SHAFER, M. B. (1976) Syndrome of botulism in infancy: Clinical and electrophysiologic study. *New Engl. J. Med.* **295**: 770–772.

PUMPLIN, D. W. and REESE, T. S. (1977) Action of brown widow spider venom and botulinum toxin on the frog neuromuscular junction examined with the freeze-fracture technique. *J. Physiol.* **273**: 443–457.

PUTNAM, F. W., LAMANNA, C. and SHARP, D. G. (1947) Molecular weight and homogeneity of crystalline botulinus A toxin. *J. biol. Chem.* **165**: 735–736.

PUTNAM, F. W., LAMANNA, C. and SHARP, D. G. (1948) Physicochemical properties of crystalline *Clostridium botulinum* type A toxin. *J. biol. Chem.* **176**: 401–412.

REED, L. J. and MUENCH, H. (1938) A simple method of estimating fifty per cent endpoints. *Am. J. Hyg.* **27**: 493–497.

ROBERTS, T. A. (1975) Botulism in poultry. *Vet. Ann. Bristol Engl.* **15**: 144–148.

ROBERTS, T. A., INGRAM, M. and SKULBERG, A. (1965) The resistance of spores of *Clostridium botulinum* type E to heat and radiation, with an addendum on the radiation resistance of *Clostridium botulinum* type E toxin. *J. appl. Bacteriol.* **28**: 125–141.

ROBERTS, T. A., THOMAS, A. I. and GILBERT, R. J. (1973) A third outbreak of type C *Clostridium botulinum* in broiler chickens. *Vet. Rec.* **92**: 107–109.

ROUHBAKHSH-KHALEGHDOUST, A. and POURTAGHVA, M. (1977) A large outbreak of type E botulism in Iran. *Trans. R. Soc. trop. Med. Hyg.* **71**: 444.

ROWLEY, D. B. and FEEHERRY, F. (1970) Conditions affecting germination of *Clostridium botulinum* 62A spores in a chemically defined medium. *J. Bacteriol.* **104**: 1151–1157.

SAKAGUCHI, G. and SAKAGUCHI, S. (1959) Studies on toxin production of *Clostridium botulinum* type E. III. Characterization of toxin precursor. *J. Bacteriol.* **78**: 1–9.

SAKAGUCHI, G. and SAKAGUCHI, S. (1967) Some observations on activation of *Cl. botulinum* type E toxin by trypsin. In: *Botulism 1966*. pp. 266–277, INGRAM, M. and ROBERTS, T. A. (eds.). Chapman & Hall, London.

SAKAGUCHI, G. and SAKAGUCHI, S. (1968) Rapid bioassay for *Clostridium botulinum* type-E toxins by intravenous injection into mice. *Jap. J. med. Sci. Biol.* **21**: 369–378.

SAKAGUCHI, G. and SAKAGUCHI, S. (1974) Oral toxicities of *Clostridium botulinum* type E toxins of different forms. *Jap. J. Med. Sci. Biol.* **27**: 241–244.

SAKAGUCHI, G. and TOHYAMA, Y. (1955a) Studies on the toxin production of *Clostridium botulinum* type E. I. A strain of genus *Clostridium* having the action to promote type E botulinal toxin production in a mixed culture. *Jap. J. med. Sci. Biol.* **8**: 247–253.

SAKAGUCHI, G. and TOHYAMA, Y. (1955b) Studies on the toxin production of *Clostridium botulinum* type E. II. The mode of action of the contaminant organisms to promote toxin production of type E organisms. *Jap. J. med. Sci. Biol.* **8**: 255–262.

SAKAGUCHI, G., SAKAGUCHI, S. and KARASHIMADA, T. (1966) Molecular size of *Clostridium botulinum* type E toxin in "izushi". *Jap. J. med. Sci. Biol.* **19**: 201–207.

SAKAGUCHI, G., SAKAGUCHI, S. and KONDO, H. (1968) Rapid bioassay for *Clostridium botulinum* type-E toxins by intravenous injection into mice. *Jap. J. med. Sci. Biol.* **21**: 369–378.

SAKAGUCHI, G., SAKAGUCHI, S., KOZAKI, S., SUGII, S. and OHISHI, I. (1974) Cross reaction in reversed passive hemagglutination between *Clostridium botulinum* type A and B toxins and its avoidance by the use of anti-toxic component immunoglobulin isolated by affinity chromatography. *Jap. J. med. Sci. Biol.* **27**: 161–172.

SCHANTZ, E. J. and SPERO, L. (1967) Molecular size of *Cl. botulinum* toxins. In: *Botulism 1966*, pp. 296–301, INGRAM, M. and ROBERTS, T. A. (eds.). Chapman & Hall, London.

SCHMIDT, C. F., LECHOWICH, R. V. and FOLINAZZO, J. F. (1961) Growth and toxin production by type E *Clostridium botulinum* below 40°F. *J. Food Sci.* **26**: 626–630.

SCHMIDT, C. F., LECHOWICH, R. V. and NANK, W. K. (1962) Radiation resistance of spores of type E *Clostridium botulinum* as related to extension of the refrigerated storage life of foods. *J. Food Sci.* **27**: 85–89.

SEDDON, H. R. (1922) Bulbar paralysis in cattle due to the action of a toxicogenic bacillus, with a discussion on the relationship of the condition to forage poisoning (Botulism). *J. comp. Path. Ther.* **35**: 147–190.

SEGNER, W. P. and SCHMIDT, C. F. (1971) Heat resistance of spores of marine and terrestrial strains of *Clostridium botulinum* type C. *Appl. Microbiol.* **22**: 1030–1033.

SEGNER, W. P., SCHMIDT, C. F. and BOLTZ, J. K. (1971) Enrichment, isolation, and cultural characteristics of marine strains of *Clostridium botulinum* type C. *Appl. Microbiol.* **22**: 1017–1024.

SERIKAWA, T., NAKAMURA, S. and NISHIDA, S. (1977) Distribution of *Clostridium botulinum* type C in Ishikawa Prefecture, and applicability of agglutination to identification of nontoxigenic isolates of *C. botulinum* type C. *Microbiol. Immunol.* **21**: 127–136.

SHIMIZU, T. and KONDO, H. (1973) Immunological difference between the toxin of a proteolytic strain and that of a nonproteolytic strain of *Clostridium botulinum* type B. *Jap. J. med. Sci. Biol.* **26**: 269–271.

SIMPSON, L. L. (1973) The interaction between divalent cations and botulinum toxin type A in the paralysis of the rat phrenic nerve-hemidiaphragm preparation. *Neuropharmacology* **12**: 165–176.

SIMPSON, L. L. (1974) Studies on the binding of botulinum toxin type A to the rat phrenic nerve-hemidiaphragm preparation. *Neuropharmacology* **13**: 683–691.

SIMPSON, L. L. (1979) Pharmacological studies on the subcellular site of action botulinum toxin type A. *J. Pharmac. exp. Ther.* **206**: 661–669.

SIMPSON, L. L. (1980) Kinetic studies on the interaction between botulinum toxin type A and the cholinergic neuromuscular junction. *J. Pharmac. exp. Ther.* **212**: 16–21.

SIMPSON, L. L. (1981) The origin, structure, and pharmacological activity of botulinum toxin. *Pharmac. Rev.* **33**: 155–188.

SIMPSON, L. L. and MORIMOTO, H. (1969) Failure to inhibit *in vitro* or *in vivo* acetylcholinesterase with botulinum toxin type A. *J. Bacteriol.* **97**: 571–575.

SIMPSON, L. L. and RAPPORT, M. M. (1971) The binding of botulinum toxin to membrane lipids: phospholipids and proteolipid. *J. Neurochem.* **18**: 1761–1767.

SIMPSON, L. L. and TAPP, J. T. (1967) Actions of calcium and magnesium on the rate of onset of botulinum toxin paralysis of the rat diaphragm. *Int. J. Neuropharmac.* **6**: 485–492.

SMITH, L. DS. (1977) *Botulism. The Organism, Its Toxins, the Disease.* C. C. Thomas, Springfield, Ill.

SOLOMON, H. M. and KAUTTER, D. A. (1979) Sporulation and toxin production by *Clostridium botulinum* type G. *J. Food Protec.* **42**: 965–967.

SONNABEND, O., SONNABEND, W., HEINZLE, R. SIGRIST, T., DIRNHOFER, R. and KRECH, U. (1981) Isolation of *Clostridium botulinum* type G and identification of type G botulinal toxin in humans: report of five sudden unexpected deaths. *J. infect. Dis.* **143**: 22–27.

SUGII, S. and SAKAGUCHI, G. (1975) Molecular construction of *Clostridium botulinum* type A toxins. *Infec. Immunity* **12**: 1262–1270.

SUGII, S. and SAKAGUCHI, G. (1977) Botulogenic properties of vegetables with special reference to the molecular size of the toxin in them. *J. Food Safety* **1**: 53–65.

SUGII, S., OHISHI, I. and SAKAGUCHI, G. (1977) Correlation between oral toxicity and *in vitro* stability of *Clostridium botulinum* type A and B toxins of different molecular sizes. *Infec. Immunity* **16**: 910–914.

SUGIYAMA, H. (1979) Animal models for the study of infant botulism. *Rev. infect. Dis.* **1**: 683–687.

SUGIYAMA, H. (1980) *Clostridium botulinum* neurotoxin. *Microbiol. Rev.* **44**: 419–448.

SUGIYAMA, H. and MILLS, D. C. (1978) Intraintestinal toxin in infant mice challenged intragastrically with *Clostridium botulinum* spores. *Infec. Immunity* **21**: 59–63.

SUGIYAMA, H., DASGUPTA, B. R. and OHISHI, I. (1974a) Disulfide-immunogenicity relationship of botulinal toxins. *Proc. Soc. exp. Biol. Med.* **145**: 1306–1309.

SUGIYAMA, H., DASGUPTA, B. R. and YANG, K. H. (1973) Disulfide-toxicity relationship of botulinal toxin types A, E, and F. *Proc. Soc. exp. Biol. Med.* **143**: 589–591.

SUGIYAMA, H., OHISHI, I. and DASGUPTA, B. R. (1974b) Evaluation of type A botulinal toxin assays that use antitoxin to crystalline toxin. *Appl. Microbiol.* **27**: 333–336.

SUGIYAMA, H., VON MYERUSUSER, B., GOGAT, G. and HESMSCH, L. C. (1967) Immunological reactivity of trypsinized *Clostridium botulinum* type E toxin. *Proc. Soc. exp. Biol. Med.* **126**: 690–694.

SUGIYAMA, H., MIZUTANI, K. and YANG, K. W. (1972) Basis of type A and F toxicities of *Clostridium botulinum* strain 84. *Proc. Soc. exp. Biol. Med.* **191**: 1063–1067.

SYUTO, B. and KUBO, S. (1977) Isolation and molecular size of *Clostridium botulinum* type C toxin. *Appl. envir. Microbiol.* **33**: 400–405.

SYUTO, B. and KUBO, S. (1981) Separation and characterization of heavy and light chains from *Clostridium botulinum* type C toxin and their reconstitution. *J. biol. Chem.* **256**: 3712–3717.

TERRANOVA, W., BREMAN, J. G., LOCEY, R. P. and SPECK, S. (1978) Botulism type B: Epidemiologic aspects of an extensive outbreak. *Am. J. Epidemiol.* **108**: 150–156.

THEILER, A., VILJOEN, P. R., GREEN, H. H., DU TOIT, P. J., MEIER, H. and ROBINSON, E. M. (1927) Lamsiekte (parabotulism) in cattle in South Africa. In: *Union of S. Africa, Dept. of Agric., 13th and 14th repts. of the Director of vet. Ed. and Research*, pp. 821–1361.

TONGE, D. A., GARDIDGE, T. J. and MARCHBANKS, R. M. (1975) Effects of botulinum and tetanus toxins on choline acetyltransferase activity in skeletal muscle in the mouse. *J. Neurochem.* **25**: 329–331.

TORDA, C. and WOLFF, H. G. (1947) On the mechanism of paralysis resulting from toxin of *Clostridium botulinum. J. Pharmac. exp. Ther.* **89**: 320–324.

TOWNED, C. T., YEE, L. and MERCER, W. A. (1954) Inhibition of the growth of *Clostridium botulinum* by acidification. *Food Res.* **19**: 1–7.

TREADWELL, P. E., JANN, G. J. and SALLE, A. J. (1958) Studies on factors affecting the rapid germination of spores of *Clostridium botulinum. J. Bacteriol.* **76**: 549–556.

VERMILYEA, B. L., WALKER, H. W. and AYRES, J. C. (1968) Detection of botulinal toxins by immunodiffusion. *Appl. Microbiol.* **16**: 21–24.

VAN ERMENGEM, E. (1897) Über einen neuen anaeroben Bacillus und seine Beziehungen zum Botulismus. *Z. Hyg. Infektkrh.* **26**: 1–56.

VAN HEYNINGEN, W. E. and MELLANBY, J. (1973) A note on the specific fixation, specific deactivation and non-specific inactivation of bacterial toxins by gangliosides. *Naunyn-Schmiedeberg's Archs. Pharmac.* **276**: 297–302.

VINET, C. and RAYNAUD, M. (1963) Preliminary note on production and purification of botulinal toxin type C. *Rev. Can. Biol.* **22**: 119–120.

WAGMAN, J. and BATTEMAN, J. B. (1951) The behavior of the botulinus toxins in the ultracentrifuge. *Archs Biochem. Biophys.* **31**: 424–430.

WONNACOTT, S. (1980) Inhibition by botulinum toxin of acetylcholine release from synaptosomes: latency of action and the role of gangliosides. *J. Neurochem.* **34**: 1567–1573.

WONNACOTT, S. and MARCHBANKS, R. M. (1976) Inhibition of botulinum toxin of depolarization-evoked release of [^{14}C]-acetylcholine from synaptosomes. *in vitro. Biochem. J.* **156**: 701–712.

WONNACOTT, S., MARCHBANKS, R. M. and FIOL, C. (1978) Ca^{2+} uptake by synaptosomes and its effect on the inhibition of acetylcholine release by botulinum toxin. *J. Neurochem.* **30**: 1127–1134.

WOODBURN, M. J., SOMERS, E., RODRIGUEZ, J. and SCHANTZ, J. (1979) Heat inactivation rates of botulinum toxins A, B, E and F in some foods and buffers. *J. Food Sci.* **44**: 1658–1661.

CHAPTER 24

TETANUS TOXIN

SIMON VAN HEYNINGEN

*Department of Biochemistry, University of Edinburgh, Hugh Robson Building,
George Square, Edinburgh EH8 9XD, Great Britain*

ABSTRACT

Tetanus toxin (molecular weight about 150,000) is made up of an H-chain (molecular weight about 100,000) and L-chain (50,000) joined by disulphide bonds. The biological activity of the toxin is not well understood. Following uptake at *neuromuscular junctions*, the toxin is transported by retrograde axonal transport in the alpha motoneurones to synapses, where it seems to act by presynaptic blocking of the release of *inhibitory transmitters*, especially gamma-aminobutyric acid. The toxin binds to cells through an interaction between the H-chain and a *ganglioside* in the plasma membrane, and this binding is specific for *neuronal cells* and important in the transport and activity of the toxin. There are similarities in the binding of toxin and of *thyrotropin*, and also in the structure and binding of tetanus and other toxins.

1. INTRODUCTION

The dramatic muscular spasms of tetanus make it one of the world's most feared diseases, and one which has been known since the earliest days of medicine. An understanding of its pathogenesis was approached towards the end of the last century, but it is a rather depressing fact that although some knowledge has been available for so long it remains a poorly understood disease.

It is one of the classical exotoxinoses, clearly caused by a simple protein toxin secreted into the environment by infective *Clostridium tetani* growing anaerobically in a wound. The fact that the tetanic symptoms are not restricted to the site of infection where the bacteria are multiplying was an early clue that the disease was due to some secreted toxin. Tetanus toxin was the second such to be discovered (the first being diphtheria toxin) and has been studied for most of this century. Indeed, the great success of prophylaxis against the disease achieved by immunization with tetanus toxoid (toxin treated with formaldehyde so destroying activity while retaining immunogenicity) has meant that the toxin is produced commercially in large amounts all over the world, and so its production and properties have been investigated for longer and perhaps by more people than the other toxins.

However comparatively little is known about it still, and its action at a molecular level remains essentially unknown. This is in sharp contrast with, for example, diphtheria and cholera toxins which are now quite well understood, and perhaps reflects the fact that tetanus toxin is producing a lesion in an area of physiology (the nervous system) itself less understood at a molecular level than those affected by cholera or diphtheria.

In this review, I want to consider as much as possible what is known about the toxin itself and its direct action on cells, concentrating less on clinical aspects and on the effects of the toxin on the whole body and the nervous system which have been reviewed in detail recently elsewhere (e.g. Haberman, 1978; Bizzini, 1979; Mellanby and Green, 1981).

2. THE TOXIN PROTEIN

2.1. PREPARATION AND TOXICITY

Tetanus toxin is a simple protein (without lipid or carbohydrate) that is secreted into its medium by *Cl. tetani*.

The gene for the toxin is plasmid associated (Laird *et al.*, 1980). The bacteria are normally grown on a synthetic medium supplemented with beef heart infusion (Mueller and Miller, 1954, and for the more usual modern medium see Latham *et al.*, 1962; Mellanby, 1968). It is often prepared from young cultures towards the end of the exponential phase by release of the toxin from inside the washed bacteria following ultrasonication or treatment with hypertonic solutions (Raynaud, 1947). This technique usually produces a slightly different form of the toxin (see below).

Several different estimates of the toxicity of purified toxin have been published; they are difficult to compare because of variations in the assay as well as in the preparation of the toxin, but a typical value seems to be around 2×10^8 mouse MLD (minimum lethal doses) per mg (see for example Dawson and Mauritzen, 1967).

Because of its high toxicity, tetanus toxin can be dangerous to work with. Everybody in the laboratory must be immunized regularly and their levels of serum antitoxin checked every year to make sure they are high enough (0.2–0.5 units/ml; R. O. Thomson, personal communication). All glasswear and surfaces that might be contaminated with toxin must be washed in dilute acid, which destroys the toxin very rapidly.

2.2. PURIFICATION

The toxin is comparatively easy to purify by chromatography on ion-exchange resins, followed by gel-permeation (see Dawson and Mauritzen, 1967). For example, van Heyningen (1976) showed that a single DEAE-cellulose column using a gradient of phosphate buffer concentration at pH 7.2 purified the toxin enough for most purposes, although gel permeation chromatography on a column of Ultrogel AcA 34 was necessary to produce a protein completely homogeneous on polyacrylamide gel electrophoresis.

During purification of the toxin (and of its chains and fragments), a major problem is partial digestion caused by the proteolytic enzymes that seem to be present in the bacterial culture filtrate almost unavoidably. This is particularly troublesome when the protein is unfolded in the presence of chaotropic reagents such as urea and guanidine which make it vulnerable to proteolytic attack. It is very important to have protease inhibitors present in all the solutions: a mixture of 0.1 mM phenylmethylsulphonylfluoride (which is irreversible but must be freshly prepared as it has a short half life in aqueous solution) and 1 mM benzamidine (which is reversible but does not decay) is usually enough to prevent protease activity (P. Britton and S. van Heyningen, unpublished).

Crystals of the pure toxin have recently been prepared, but they are not of the form most suitable for x-ray diffraction studies (Chiu *et al.*, 1982).

2.3. STRUCTURE OF THE PROTEIN

There has been disagreement in the past about the molecular weight of the purified toxin, and the older literature contains many values difficult to reconcile with modern structural ideas. Most recent workers report a value of around 150,000 determined by gel-permeation chromatography or in the ultracentrifuge, although there is usually some aggregation at high protein concentration (Holmes and Ryan, 1971; Bizzini *et al.*, 1973a; Craven and Dawson, 1973; Matsuda and Yoneda, 1974; Robinson *et al.*, 1975).

Modern ideas of its structure have come in the main from experiments using poly-acrylamide gel electrophoresis in the presence of sodium dodecylsulphate (SDS) a technique that has also provided the crucial information about cholera and diphtheria toxins as well as many other proteins (for review, see Robinson and Hash, 1982).

Most recent authors are agreed that the toxin is made up of two polypeptide chains linked by disulphide bonds: the H- or α-chain, molecular weight about 100,000, and the L- or β-chain, molecular weight about 50,000 (Craven and Dawson, 1973; Matsuda and Yoneda, 1974; van Heyningen, 1976; Helting and Zwisler, 1977; Robinson *et al.*, 1982). These chains can be split apart in the presence of denaturing agents such as SDS by any of the usual techniques for breaking disulphide bonds such as reduction with excess thiol in the form of dithiothreitol or mercaptoethanol, or even by the less usual technique of sulphitolysis (Dawson, 1975). The L-chain is readily soluble in aqueous buffers at neutral pH, but the H-chain is soluble only at very low protein concentrations (e.g. 50 μg ml^{-1} or less). It remains in solution in the presence of 1 M urea. This obviously reflects some differences in the amino acid residues on the exterior of the two chains, but as they probably are never separated under physiological conditions, this is probably not significant.

It turns out that the two chains must be tightly associated together by non-covalent forces in the intact molecule, because even under conditions when the covalent disulphide bonds are broken, it is not easy to separate the two chains quantitatively. Several workers have purified them by gel-permeation chromatography in the presence of denaturing agents, most successfully on Ultrogel AcA 44 in 2 M urea, 1 mM dithiothreitol at pH 8.5 (Matsuda and Yoneda, 1975a), but in all cases the purification is incomplete: the H-chain which comes through the column first is contaminated with L-chain, although the L-chain is comparatively pure.

To prepare really pure chains, it is necessary to repeat the chromatography several times, or to use immunoabsorption with insolubilized antibody to the contaminating chain (Bizzini, 1978), or to carry out preparative gel electrophoresis in SDS (P. Britton and S. van Heyningen, unpublished), which can usefully be done in a discontinuous system (DiMari et al., 1982a).

This tightness of binding suggests a complicated three-dimensional structure with the two chains closely inter-woven; which makes it surprising that the two separated and purified chains can be reassembled to form active toxin (Matsuda and Yoneda, 1975b).

Circular dichroism spectra indicated little difference between the three-dimensional conformation of the chains when isolated and when combined, suggesting that they may make up relatively separate domains in the intact toxin (Robinson et al., 1982).

Most modern theories of protein biosynthesis and assembly would predict that almost all multi-chain proteins (except the immunoglobulins) are the products of proteolytic cleavage of a single chain formed on the ribosomes, and this has been shown to be true for diphtheria toxin and for subunit A of cholera toxin (van Heyningen, 1977). Tetanus toxin is no exception. Matsuda and Yoneda (1974) found a single chain form of the toxin (molecular weight about 160,000) present in protein taken from bacterial extracts (i.e. by the method of Reynaud (1947) mentioned above), which they called 'intracellular' toxin. It can be cleaved by trypsin to give the H- and L-chains, no longer joined by a peptide bond, but remaining joined by disulphides just as in the other 'extracellular' form of the protein. It is quite difficult to prepare the 'unnicked' form of the toxin because of the contaminating proteolytic activity usually present in the preparations.

A protease that probably catalyses this 'nicking' in vivo has been purified from culture filtrates of Cl. tetani (Helting et al., 1979).

The cleavage of the intact chain into two smaller chains is a complicated process. There is evidence that the site of 'nicking' can be in at least two different places, probably either side of an intrachain disulphide bond (DiMari et al., 1982a). Analysis of N-terminal residues (see below) shows that even these cleavage points are ragged in the sense that there are perhaps several susceptible peptide bonds rather close together. Gel electrophoresis shows no sign of any 'connecting peptide' joining the two chains that might be released after proteolysis; but Robinson et al. (1982) made careful measurements of molecular weight in the ultra-centrifuge, and found 140,000 $\pm$ 5000 for the intact toxin, and 128,000 for the 'nicked' toxin, suggesting that there is some loss of material on proteolysis.

The individual chains have little or no toxicity; what toxicity is found can be reasonably ascribed to contamination with the other chain (see above), and is said to be removed by careful treatment with antiserum to the other chain (Bizzini, 1978). The reconstituted toxin is toxic. Figure 1 summarizes current ideas on the structure of the toxin.

Comparatively little detailed work on the structure of the toxin has been reported. Amino acid analyses of the intact toxin have come from several different laboratories; they differ slightly from each other, but probably no more than would be expected from normal experimental error (Dawson and Mauritzen, 1967; Bizzini et al., 1970; Holmes and Ryan,

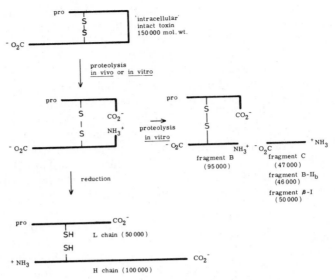

FIG. 1. A summary of the chemistry of tetanus toxin.

1971; Robinson et al., 1975). They are in no way remarkable, and are compatible with the isoelectric point which is 5.1 (Bizzini et al., 1974). The number of sulphydryl groups and disulphide bonds in the protein is not accurately known, but it is large. Craven and Dawson (1973) and Bizzini et al. (1970) found six free SH groups and one disulphide bond, while Murphy et al. (1968) found two disulphide bonds. Britton (1981) found four disulphide bonds and one or two free SH groups. There is no obvious reason for these differences, but DiMari et al. (1982a) found evidence for rearrangement of some of these disulphide bonds when the chains are separately isolated; this may be one reason for the tendency of the chains to precipitate during purification.

Very few sequencing results have been published so far, but Neubauer and Helting (1979) have done some N-terminal studies which may clear up what had been a complicated picture with many authors reporting different results perhaps because of heterogeneous or partially degraded proteins. They found proline to be the N-terminal residue of the intact chain and of the L-chain (thus showing that the L-chain must be N-terminal in the intact toxin), and leucine to be N-terminal in the H-chain. Britton (1981) and DiMari et al. (1982b) also found proline in the whole toxin and in the L-chain, but DiMari et al. (1982b) found chiefly asparagine and serine. Ragged 'nicking' (as described above) is doubtless the main reason for these discrepancies.

Recently, Taylor et al. (1983) have made an observation which may change our view of the structure of the toxin. They noticed remarkable similarity in the amino acid compositions of the H- and L-chains, and applied a published and well-tried mathematical test to judge the significance of these similarities. Their conclusion, which is still tentative but is backed up by some experimental evidence based on similar peptides produced after proteolytic digestion of the two chains, is that the H-chain may contain two domains having partially homologous amino acid sequence, and that the L-chain may also be homologous with those domains. In other words, the whole toxin may be made up of three rather similar regions. This might easily be due to some gene multiplication during the evolution of the toxin.

Many bacterial toxins have some hydrophobic regions, probably involved with their transport across the cell membrane. Charge shift experiments, in which the hydrophobicity of proteins is measured indirectly from their ability to bind various detergents, showed tetanus toxin to be, in general, a hydrophilic protein as would be expected from its solubility and other properties (Ward et al., 1981). However, although the purified L-chain was also hydrophilic, there was good evidence for some hydrophobic arease on the surface of the H-chain. Boquet and Duflot (1982) measured binding of radioactive detergent to the toxin directly, and also found evidence for a hydrophobic regions in the H-chain (see below, section 4.6).

2.4. Proteolytic Fragments

In recent years, several workers have attempted to probe the structure of the molecule further by looking at proteolytic fragments of the toxin. Thus, Helting and Zwisler (1977) digested toxin with papain, and, in a very reproducible manner, obtained two fragments, B and C, both of which reacted with antitoxin although they were not themselves toxic. Analysis showed that fragment C (molecular weight 47,000) was a portion of the heavy chain alone, and so must have come from the C-terminal end of the single-chain form of the toxin; whereas fragment B (95,000) was made up of the rest of the H-chain and all of the L-chain. N-terminal analysis confirmed this idea (Neubauer and Helting, 1981).

The two fragments could not be reconstituted to form active material. Antibodies to fragment C would neutralise toxin action in vivo. Purified fragment B, although not toxic at levels sufficient to promote antibody synthesis, was toxic at high concentration (20 μg per mouse, Helting et al., 1978). However, the symptoms were not the convulsions or paralysis of tetanus, but rather a less dramatic syndrome involving general loss of weight and flaccidity. The authors suggest that the fragment may have retained some of the active parts of the toxin molecule, enough to give it some, but not all, of its characteristic effects (see section 4). Sato et al. (1979) obtained a fragment S by digestion with subtilisin, which may be similar to the B fragment. When guinea-pigs were injected with a mixture of toxin and antibodies to this fragment S, they developed another unusual form of tetanus without local symptoms.

Another fragment B-IIb was obtained by Bizzini et al. (1977) and seems to be spontaneously produced by endogenous proteases: it gives a single band of molecular weight about 46,000 on polyacrylamide gel electrophoresis in the presence or absence of SDS and so seems very similar to the fragment C of Helting and Zwisler (1977). It was not toxic (or at least was 10^5 times less so than native toxin) but did retain some of the properties of native toxin in that it bound ganglioside and was capable of migrating by retrograde axonal transport towards the central nervous system (see below).

Matsuda and Yoneda (1977) also reported similar results. Their fragment β-2 again seemed very like fragment C and had similar antigenic properties. They also studied proteolytic cleavage with trypsin.

Finally, Robinson et al. (1978) obtained a fragment whose molecular weight they put at 59,000 and which seemed (in that it had two chains) to be part of the fragment B of Helting and Zwisler; they found no sign of fragment C. Circular dichroism spectra showed it to have a different conformation from the native toxin, with much less α-helix, (see below). There is no explanation for the discrepancies among different authors.

2.5. Modification of the Protein. Tetanus Toxoid

The chief interest in the protein chemistry of tetanus toxin from a practical point of view has been in the mechanism of production of toxoid, defined as protein so treated that it can elicit the production of antibodies that neutralize the activity of toxin, but is not itself toxic. Of all the infectious diseases, immunization against tetanus has proved one of the most effective (see Habermann, 1978).

Toxoiding is usually done by prolonged incubation of the protein in formaldehyde solution and surprisingly little work has been done on it in recent years although the older literature contains many discussions of the reaction between proteins and formaldehyde (e.g. French and Edsall, 1945). It is unlikely that the formaldehyde leads to the formation of any cross-linking between molecules, but cross-links within individual molecules are certainly formed (see for example Bizzini and Raynaud, 1974). Labeled formaldehyde is gradually incorporated into the protein molecule as toxoiding proceeds and the conversion into toxin is not an all or none process (Habermann, 1976).

Toxoiding does not seem to lead to any very large conformational changes in the structure of the toxin, judging from circular dichroism spectra (Robinson et al., 1975), which are a very sensitive probe for conformational change: they indicated that both toxin and toxoid have roughly 20 per cent of both α-helix and β-sheet, although such quantitative interpretation of

CD spectra is fraught with difficulties. Of course this applies only in cases where the whole molecule is toxoided: the proteolytic fragments described above could be thought of as toxoids since some of them do elicit the production of antibodies that react with toxin.

Chemical modification with reagents other than formaldehyde that might be expected to lead to more specific and easily investigated changes should be a more useful approach. Particularly detailed results have been reported for example for experiments with tetranitromethane, a highly specific nitrating agent for tyrosine residues (Bizzini et al., 1973b). Modification of different numbers of tyrosine residues suggested that there were three different groups of antigenic determinants. Thirty-three nitro groups had to be introduced into the toxin before it lost the ability to elicit neutralising antibodies: a degree of modification that most enzymologists would regard as very large, and which produced material having less than 10^{-8} times the toxicity of native toxin. Reductive methylation has a rather similar effect on lysine residues to that of formaldehyde, but it never completely destroyed toxicity (Robinson et al., 1975).

No doubt many other residues are also essential for activity and in any event modification of more than a few residues often has such a profound effect on the conformation of a protein that it becomes very difficult to assign changes in its properties to any particular residue. Further investigation of the role of particular residues and the mechanism of loss of activity should await a more detailed understanding of the molecular mechanism of that activity.

Many groups (e.g. Mizuguchi et al., 1982) are currently preparing monoclonal antibodies to the toxin and toxoid; these may be helpful in mapping particular antigenic regions.

2.6. BINDING TO GANGLIOSIDE

Almost the only part of the mechanism of the toxin that can be related at all to any of the structure is the binding to ganglioside receptor, discussed below, section 4.

3. BIOLOGICAL ACTION OF THE TOXIN

3.1. TRANSPORT OF TETANUS TOXIN IN THE BODY; ROUTES TO THE TARGET

Tetanus toxin is produced by the invading bacteria at one site of infection, but its effects are widespread throughout the body, although only the nervous system is directly affected. This implies immediately that there must be some transport to the site of action. The mechanism of this transport has been studied in great detail and is one of the few problems concerning the action of tetanus toxin which can perhaps be said to have been solved at least in outline.

For many years there were two basic theories: that the toxin reached the spinal cord via the blood (see for example Abel et al., 1935) or via a neural route of some sort (Meyer and Ransom, 1903). Early work in this area was very difficult to do because the toxin could be detected only by assaying it; this problem has been solved by using toxin labeled with radioactive iodine which is confidently assumed to have the same properties as native toxin (see Habermann 1970; Price et al., 1975).

Iodination of the toxin does seem to produce some changes in structure, although these are not related to changes in activity (An Der Lan et al., 1980).

Most human tetanus falls into one of two categories: 'general' tetanus, which is characterized by generalized convulsions all over the body following on early spasticity, first in the jaw and then moving towards the trunk and outer limbs; and 'local' tetanus in which the muscles of one specific infected limb become spastic. General tetanus can be thought of as multiple local tetanus (Erdmann and Habermann, 1977). Intramuscular injection of toxin into a limb produces local tetanus, but intravenous injection produces general tetanus, showing that there must be at least some transport in the blood (where the half life of toxin is quite high; 10 hr in rats, Habermann, 1970). The toxin cannot however penetrate the blood-brain barrier (Habermann and Dimpfel, 1973). It is now thought that the toxin reaches its site of action by uptake into terminals at the neuromuscular junction followed by retrograde axonal transport in the alpha motoneurones.

Direct evidence for this mode of transport has come from several sources. For example, Price et al. (1975) investigated the fate of iodinated toxin after both intramuscular and intraneural injection. Immediately after the injection the appropriate nerve was crushed proximally and later removed for investigation by autoradiography; using a crush meant that small amounts of activity were localized into a single site and so could be more easily detected. The toxin accumulated within axons on the distal side of the crush, showing direct evidence for retrograde axonal transport of the toxin, which presumably had been initially taken up at nerve terminals. When labelled toxin was injected directly into the nerve there was no axonal transport.

Several other workers have obtained similar results and this transport seems to be common to all (or at least all peripheral) neurones (Erdmann et al., 1975; Stöckel et al., 1975; Price and Griffin, 1977; Habermann and Erdmann, 1978; Wernig et al., 1977). That the route is via the peripheral nerves at least in local tetanus can be shown by looking at the label in the spinal cord using autoradiography. It is present at the highest concentration in just those parts which correspond to the particular limbs affected.

Transport along these nervous paths, which is quite fast (0.5–1 cm per hr in rodents, Habermann, 1972), has been investigated in some detail using different approaches. For example tetanus toxin absorbed to colloidal gold particles makes an excellent tracer for electron microscopy (Schwab and Thoenen, 1978). It was found to be selectively associated with the membranes of nerve terminals and preterminal axons, localized inside them primarily in the smooth endoplasmic reticular membrane apparatus—something not found with the gold complexes of control proteins.

Objections have been raised to much of the work using iodinated toxin on the grounds that what is now being followed is the label rather than the protein, and so may represent nothing but inactive fragments of the toxin formed proteolytically. However an immunological study gave similar results (Carrol et al., 1978). Rats were injected with toxin intramuscularly and both sciatic nerves isolated with double ligatures. Twenty four hours later the nerves were removed, fixed and examined for toxin using the immunoperoxidase technique (i.e. reaction in a sequence: toxin—goat antitoxin—rabbit antigoat—peroxidase, and then staining for peroxidase). This experiment showed toxin antigen within axons on the distal but not on the proximal side of the distal ligature and so demonstrated retrograde axonal transport. There is still no proof (although equally no reason to doubt) that the toxin within the neurones is biologically active.

Tetanus toxin is far from the only protein that is transported by this route; several others can also pass along the neurones, for example cholera toxin, nerve growth factor and several lectins. However it is not a general property of all proteins; most are not transported (Schwab and Thoenen, 1978; and see below, section 4.5).

Once the toxin has reached the cell body after the axonal transport, it is transferred rather selectively from the dendrites into the terminals which form the synapses on the cell (where it is believed to act, see below) (Schwab and Thoenen, 1976, 1977; Schwab et al., 1979).

There has been some controversy about the type of neurone affected. Thus there was a suggestion that at least some of the spasticity of early local tetanus was due to an action of toxin on gamma-motoneurones rather than alpha (Takano and Henatsch, 1973; Benecke et al., 1977). Certainly there is good evidence for hyperactivity of both types of neurone in early local tetanus but it is not clear if this is related to the spasticity. Hyperactivity of gamma motoneurones is not surprising when there has been a profound disturbance of motor mechanisms in general, and the direct evidence is that the toxin is not transported in gamma axons and does not reach the gamma-motoneurones in early local tetanus (Green et al., 1977).

Investigation of the intraspinal distribution of the toxin also lead Erdmann et al. (1981) to deduce that any action of the toxin in alpha-motoneurones is not important in clinical tetanus.

3.2. ACTION OF THE TOXIN AT SYNAPSES

The fundamental electrophysiological consequence of tetanus is the muscular rigidity that is caused by hyperactivity of the spinal cord motoneurones, and which is itself a consequence of the total or partial loss of activity of the inhibitor pathways. The toxin therefore seems to work by inhibiting the release of inhibitory transmitters.

Toxin has been shown directly to block transmission at a number of different types of synapse including, in the central nervous system, pre- and post-synaptic inhibitory synapses where gamma-aminobutyric acid (GABA) is the transmitter (Curtis et al., 1973; Davis and Tongroach, 1979) as well as post-synaptic inhibition using glycine (Curtis and de Groat, 1968). Some cholinergic synapses of the parasympathetic and somatic motor systems are also affected (Ambache et al., 1948; Diamond and Mellanby, 1971; Duchen and Tonge, 1973; Mellanby and Thompson, 1972; Kryzhanovksy, 1973). The block of transmission has always been found to be presynaptic, and it is the release of transmitter rather than its synthesis that is affected. However, as yet, there is no consensus about the mechanism of this blocking (see for example Kryzhanovsky, 1973; Mellanby and Thompson, 1972; King, Fedinec and Latham, 1978). There are some similarities between the effects of tetanus and botulinum toxins at some synapses (Mellanby, Thompson and Hampden, 1973; Matsuda et al., 1982), so a mechanism involving the release mechanism for calcium such as has been suggested for botulinium toxin (Lundh et al., 1977) is a possibility.

Many tetanus patients (especially those treated with curare to control their convulsions and with intermittent positive pressure ventilation) show an instability of the autonomic nervous system (see Hörtnagl et al., 1979). This may be due to some action of the toxin on those parts of the central inhibitor processes which normally modulate sympathetic output (Paar and Wellhöner, 1973).

3.3. IN VITRO STUDIES

In the last few years, there have been several reports of actions of tetanus toxin in vitro on particulate preparations, synaptosomes, and cells in culture. This is very encouraging, as the observation of comparatively simple effects in comparatively simple systems may bring closer the time when the toxin can be studied and even understood in biochemical terms.

In one of the earliest experiments of this sort, a preparation of rat synaptosomes treated with toxin showed a decrease in the release of a wide variety of different things: glycine (the strongest effect), GABA, aspartate, and alanine (Osborne and Bradford, 1973). However it is not easy to be sure of the significance of this result since so many different compounds were affected and toxin in comparatively high concentrations was present throughout the experiment.

More recent experiments have used lower concentrations under what may be more realistic conditions, although it remains impossible to be sure how many of the results, genuine though they undoubtedly are, are relevant to the action of the toxin in vivo. In perhaps one of the most basic of these experiments, tetanus toxin (0.05 to 20 μg/ml) produced paralysis in a mouse phrenic nerve hemidiaphragm preparation (Habermann et al., 1980). The effect was preceded by a latent period in which the toxin became more and more resistant to washing and to antitoxin, perhaps reflecting gradual internalization (as discussed in section 4.5 below) (Habermann et al., 1980; Schmitt et al., 1981).

Other experiments have been concerned principally with the uptake and release of neurotransmitters. For example, tetanus toxin inhibited the uptake of [^{3}H]-choline into synaptosomes from rat brain cortex; the maximum inhibition was about 50 % (Habermann et al., 1981). Again, there was an initial lag phase before inhibition, and the results closely paralleled the paralysis experiments just described. Uptake of glycine and GABA as well as choline are also affected in synaptosomes from different sources (Bigalke et al., 1981a).

The toxin also inhibits the K$^+$-evoked release of acetyl choline both from primary nerve cell cultures derived from the rat CNS (Bigalke et al., 1978) and from brain slices (Bigalke et al., 1981b). There was also inhibition by the toxin of neurotransmitter release from rat spinal cord and (with ten to fifty times less potency) brain particles. Glycine, GABA, and acetylcholine were all affected (in decreasing order of relative sensitivity). The basal and K^+-evoked release of noradrenalin from brain cortex was also inhibited by toxin (Habermann, 1981) and this system seemed a particularly useful one for further study.

In quite separate experiments, Collingridge et al. (1981) and Collingridge and Davies (1982) also found about 30% inhibition of Ca^{2+}-dependent K^+-evoked release of GABA from rat hippocampal slices and substantia nigra. A similar effect on cerebellar cells in culture turned out to be dependent on the age of the culture (Pearce et al., 1983): only 7- to 14-day-old cultures were affected, perhaps because it takes this long for the cells to develop some toxin-sensitive mechanism.

These and other experiments with nerve cells in culture (e.g. Dimpfel, 1979; and references cited in section 4.4) have made it seem possible to begin to investigate the action of the toxin in a comparatively simple system, and one might hope to find some molecular mechanism. So far there has been little success with this. Wendon and Gill (1982) found no evidence for any covalent modification of any protein (e.g. phosphorylation or ADP-ribosylation) by the toxin in cultured cells. Kryzhanovskii et al. (1980) have evidence for a direct action of the toxin on the contractile proteins of nerve endings: a very interesting possibility that deserves to be followed up. They have also suggested that the toxin interferes with the interaction of calcium ions at the nerve endings (Kryzhanovskii et al., 1981).

4. TOXIN BINDING

4.1. BINDING TO GANGLIOSIDE

So far, the mechanism by which tetanus toxin acts on cells is largely unknown, principally because there is as yet no clear biological effect on cells that can be ascribed to it and investigated. Advance in the investigation of other toxins such as cholera and diphtheria came after a clear understanding of what part of metabolism was affected by the toxins. However even in the case of tetanus, some facts are clear.

For a large protein to affect the internal metabolism of a cell, it must either interact in some way with a receptor on the outer membrane or itself be transported to the interior of the cell. Either way, the toxin must first bind to the cell, and it is in the study of the binding that the most progress has been made.

It has been known for a long time (Wassermann and Takaki, 1898) that tetanus toxin is fixed by nervous tissue; that is to say that toxin activity is removed from solution after suspension with such tissue. Tetanus toxoid and other proteins are not fixed, and other tissues are ineffective, so the reaction seems to be a specific one, presumably reflecting the in vivo activity of the toxin.

Further work has shown that it is gangliosides in the nervous tissue that actually bind the toxin. Gangliosides are complex amphiphilic lipids found almost ubiquitously in the plasma membranes of cells (for reviews see Fishman and Brady, 1976; van Heyningen, 1974; and for a typical structure, see Fig. 2). They are very suitable molecules as cell-surface receptors because their hydrophobic portion (a ceramide derivative), which has long-chain fatty acids linked to sphingosine, dissolves in the lipid membrane, leaving the hydrophilic portion (complex sugars, acetylated hexosamines, and N-acetyl neuraminic acid) on the outside of the cell dissolved in the aqueous environment. In aqueous solution, gangliosides form micelles with a hydrophobic interior. The gangliosides have some binding affinity for almost all proteins, but this is weak, non-specific, and easily distinguishable from the specific binding to certain toxins and other proteins (van Heyningen and Mellanby, 1973).

Measuring the binding of gangliosides to proteins is not easy to do quantitatively: equilibrium dialysis experiments are very difficult if not impossible because of the high molecular-weight ganglioside micelles which do not penetrate the membrane. Gangliosides have a very low critical micelle concentration: about 10^{-8} M (Formisano et al., 1979). The earliest method used the ultracentrifuge to observe the separation of toxin and toxin-ganglioside complex by Schlieren optics during a sedimentation-velocity run of a mixture of

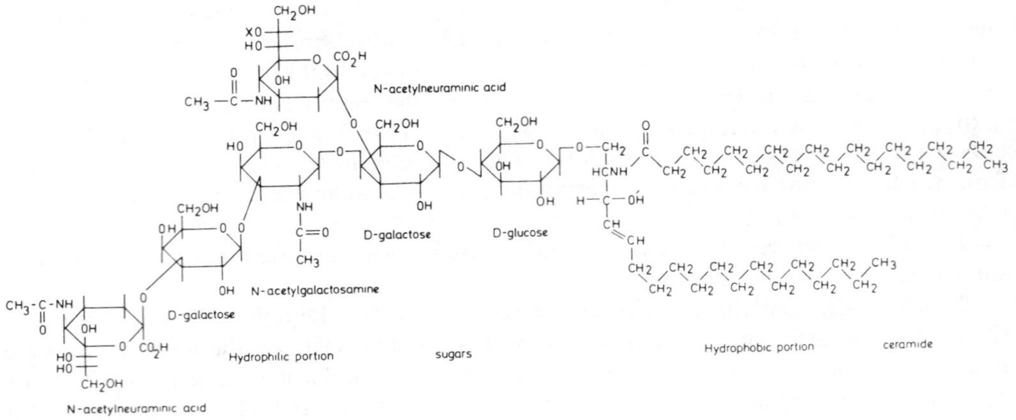

FIG. 2. *The structure of gangliosides.* In gangliosides GT1 and GD1b, X = *N*-acetylneuraminic acid linked to the other *N*-acetylneuraminic acid residue 8 → 2. Ganglioside GD1b lacks the terminal *N*-acetylneuraminic acid residue linked to galactose on the left of the figure.

toxin (5 mg ml^{-1}) and ganglioside (about 0.5 mg ml^{-1}). The two species separate easily in this system (van Heyningen and Miller, 1961).

An alternative approach is to make an insoluble complex with cerebroside (an unreactive insoluble lipid); this will fix toxin. The complex is suspended in a toxin solution, the suspension is incubated and then centrifuged, and the amount of toxin remaining in solution is estimated from its toxicity (van Heyningen and Mellanby, 1968).

A method capable of giving more accurate results and quantitative binding data is that of Helting *et al.* (1977) using tritiated ganglioside (prepared by reduction with sodium borotritiide of ganglioside previously oxidized with galactose oxidase). There are two variants of this method. In the first a small column of Sephadex G-100 is equilibrated with buffer containing radiative ganglioside and a sample of tetanus toxin is then applied to the column. For reasons not entirely clear, the toxin remains stuck to the column, and the radioactivity then eluting from it is decreased by the amount of ganglioside that has bound to the toxin. The amount of radioactivity adsorbed was indeed found to be proportional to the amount of toxin applied, and it could be eluted quantitatively with 0.1 per cent NaOH. Since in this method the toxin is adsorbed to the Sephadex matrix, the experiment can also be carried out the other way round. Tetanus toxin was applied first to a column in the absence of ganglioside, and a charge of ganglioside then put through. The ganglioside not eluting from the column must have been bound to the toxin. These two methods are simple and quantitative and can be used with as little as 10 μg of toxin (although they are expensive in labeled ganglioside). The main objection to them is that the nature of the interaction between the toxin and the gel matrix is not clear; but there is no obvious reason why this should affect the results.

Other methods include a ganglioside enzyme-linked immunosorbent assay in which the binding of toxin to ganglioside absorbed on polystyrene is measured (Holmgren *et al.*, 1980), and measurement of the competition by gangliosides for the binding of ^{125}I-labelled toxin to cell membranes (Rogers and Snyder, 1981, and see section 4.4).

4.2. SPECIFICITY OF BINDING

There are several different kinds of ganglioside that differ from each other in the arrangement of sugar residues, and in particular in the number of N-acetylneuraminic (sialic) acid residues. Tetanus toxin shows an enzyme-like specificity for two particular types of ganglioside, each of which has two such residues linked to the ganglioside by bonds that can be cleaved with neuraminidase (van Heyningen, 1963). In the most common of the many different nomenclatures of gangliosides, these are known as GD1b and GT1 (Svennerholm, 1963); their structure is shown in Fig. 2. These gangliosides will fix up to about twenty times their own weight of toxin: a molar ration of about one to two, toxin to ganglioside. Gangliosides GM1 (which does bind cholera toxin very strongly, see below) and GD1a will also bind tetanus toxin but their binding capacity is about six times less.

In contrast to the ganglioside binding of cholera toxin which has been investigated in great detail in the past few years, little has been published on the nature of this binding. The specificity presumably is in the carbohydrate part of the molecule. There is no evidence that the ganglioside itself is changed in any way by the reaction with toxin. Removal of the ceramide portion of the ganglioside does not affect the binding (Helting et al., 1977). Detailed binding constants have not been measured: they would be very difficult to determine because of the micelle formation. But Helting et al. (1977) found that nanomolar solutions of toxin were half saturated at about 5×10^{-8} M ganglioside suggesting a very tight binding, especially as some of that ganglioside may well have been in micelles and so perhaps not involved directly in the binding. It cannot be clear as yet whether micelles of ganglioside or single molecules only or both can bind. Their results (which were the same for gangliosides GD1b and GT1) suggested a one to one ganglioside to toxin binding ratio.

4.3. GANGLIOSIDE BINDING AND THE STRUCTURE OF THE TOXIN

Further investigation has shown that only one of the two chains of the toxin actually binds the ganglioside.

This has been demonstrated in two different ways. First (van Heyningen, 1976), a solution of toxin was incubated in a suspension with ganglioside insolubilized by complexing with cerebroside as described above. Toxin was quantitatively absorbed to the complex (as judged by electrophoresis of the supernatant); but could be eluted from it with 8 M urea, or solutions of high ionic strength (e.g. 2 M NaCl). Cerebroside alone did not adsorb the toxin. The result with purified heavy chain (in 1 M urea) was very similar; it adsorbed to the complex and could be eluted with 8 M urea. Purified light chain did not adsorb at all.

Helting et al. (1977) used their Sephadex binding assay to obtain similar results. Heavy chain bound ganglioside, but neither light chain nor proteolytic fragment B (light chain and part of the heavy chain, see page 4) bound any significant amount.

These experiments show that the binding site for ganglioside must lie on the heavy chain, and also that its ability to bind ganglioside is retained when the heavy chain is free from the light chain (or at least enough of it is retained for the difference in binding not to be measurable in these assays). This suggests that the conformation of the heavy chain does not change much on binding to the light chain, which is surprising since they are so difficult to separate. Perhaps the binding site is on a section of the chain separate from the rest of the molecule.

There is some evidence from proteolytic digestion for conformational change following ganglioside binding (Britton, 1981).

4.4. BINDING OF THE TOXIN TO CELLS AND ORGANELLES

From the original observation that tetanus toxin bound to nervous tissue, it has now become possible to be rather more specific. Subcellular fractionation of brain showed that synaptosomes bound the most toxin (Mellanby et al., 1964); and that this was a property of the synaptic membranes rather than of the synaptic vesicles (Mellanby and Whittaker, 1967). More direct studies with ^{125}I-labelled toxin have also shown binding to synaptosomes in the spinal cord and elsewhere (Habermann, 1973; Habermann et al., 1973); and this binding can be prevented in vitro by treatment with neuraminidase, presumably because it brings about hydrolysis of the sialic acid residues from the ganglioside molecules so that they can no longer bind the toxin.

Rogers and Snyder (1981) have criticized some of this early work as showing binding of toxin only at concentrations greater than those needed to produce an effect in vivo, or those needed in vitro with gangliosides. Using very low concentrations of brain membranes, they were able to show binding of ^{125}I-labelled toxin particularly to grey matter and at the synapses showing a dissociation constant of about 1.2 nM (comparable to that found with free gangliosides, see section 4.2). This binding was inhibited by gangliosides GD1b and GT1 more than by other gangliosides.

Habermann (1976) was able to show that tetanus toxin could be purified by affinity chromatography on a column of synaptosomes adsorbed to insoluble supports (bromoacetyl cellulose or Kieselgur). Toxin was adsorbed to the column at low ionic strength and could be eluted when the ionic strength was increased. A large excess of unlabelled toxin could not elute labelled toxin from the column, implying that the number of possible receptor sites on the synaptosomes was very large.

Subsequent experiments have confirmed that the toxin can bind to gangliosides in membranes in this way and have raised the suggestion that the toxin makes a good marker of neuronal cells (but not glial cells) in culture. This was first shown by Dimpfel et al. (1975) who used autoradiography to study binding to neurones in culture coming from mouse brain and spinal cord.

In a thorough study of binding by different kinds of cell, Dimpfel et al. (1977) found that only those cell lines which contained gangliosides GD1b and GT1 (and could synthesize them de novo from glutamine) bound the toxin. These were primary cultures derived from embryonic mouse CNS; continuous cultured cells had no ganglioside and would not bind toxin. A hybrid cell of neuroblastoma and glioma normally bound only just detectable amounts of toxin (and did not have the relevant gangliosides). However when these cells were incubated with a solution of the free gangliosides, binding increased very much. Presumably the gangliosides are taken up the hydrophobic membrane and can then act as receptors. This technique has been used very much in cholera toxin research.

Mirsky et al. (1978) extended these results using immunofluorescence (with rabbit antitoxin and goat anti-rabbit gamma globulin conjugated with the fluorescent label). They investigated a number of different cells coming from all parts of the nervous system, and showed that the toxin bound highly specifically to neuronal cells from cortex, cerebellum, spinal cord, and dorsal root ganglia of rats and to spinal cord, optic lobe, retina, and dorsal root and sympathetic ganglia of chicks. In fact, they suggested that toxin binding is a uniquely good marker for neuronal cells in culture (see also Fields et al., 1978). Furthermore, since toxin binds in vitro to cultured cells from all parts of the neuronal system, the more restricted binding found in vivo is probably caused by availability and transport rather than by binding. Chick cells bind toxin avidly although the chick is a highly resistant species to tetanus.

In amphibian cells at least, the toxin does not bind to precursor cells of neurons in embryos: the receptors seem to be acquired only after morphological differentiation is complete (Vulliamy and Messenger, 1981). The binding specificity of the toxin for neurons is marked, but is not absolute: toxin does not bind to some large neurons present in late culture (Raju and Dahl, 1982), and, in the retina, binding to neurons is stronger than to other cells but not exclusive to them (Beale et al., 1982). The toxin will also bind to pancreatic islet cells, which are known to have some cell surface differentiation markers in common with neurons (Eisenbarth et al., 1982).

The ability to bind both to cells and to organelles must clearly be a function of only a small part of the toxin and even of the H-chain, since it is retained by some of the proteolytic fragments described in section 2.4 above. For example, fragment C (part of the H-chain) binds to neural, thyroid (see section 4.7 below) or rat brain membranes in a very similar way to the whole toxin, and the variation with pH, ionic strength and concentration are all the same. The same gangliosides are bound and the fragment can be transported retrogradely in the axons just like toxin (Morris et al., 1980; Goldberg et al., 1981). Fragment B (most of the rest of the molecule) does not bind. Bizzini et al. (1980, 1981) have obtained the same sort of results with their papain fragments, and have shown that it is possible to conjugate other proteins to the binding fragment without losing its ability to bind to ganglioside or to synaptic membranes. This has prompted their suggestion that the fragment might be a useful carrier into the central nervous system for other pharmacologically active agents.

4.5. What is the Role of the Ganglioside Receptors?

Tetanus toxin treated with ganglioside does not lose its toxicity (van Heyningen and Mellanby, 1973). At first sight, this suggests that the ganglioside binding may not after all be obligatorily involved with the activity since molecules already binding ganglioside can presumably no longer bind cells. However the *in vivo* assays are difficult to analyse since one cannot know whether the ganglioside (which is comparatively weakly bound) has remained bound to the toxin when it reaches its site of action. Most other evidence does point clearly to ganglioside binding as a prerequisite for toxin action. The main evidence for this is in the specificity of binding and the observation that modified toxins and partial toxoids that no longer bind to ganglioside always lose toxicity (Habermann, 1976). No derivative of the toxin is known that is toxic but does not bind, although there are some slightly formalinized preparations that bind weakly but are not toxic, perhaps because they have a lower but still measurable affinity for ganglioside. Of course, this kind of evidence can never be definitive, and modification of a ganglioside-binding site might always involve change at some other vital site on the protein particularly if the two were close together. But there is no reason to believe that is what is happening.

Some reports disagree markedly with the idea of ganglioside as a receptor. Zimmerman and Piffaretti (1977) have drawn a distinction between what they see as two different types of binding. 'Non-effective' binding is observed only with non-differentiating mouse neuroblastoma cells in culture, and is due to binding to membrane gangliosides. This binding produced no biological effects on the growth of the cells. However, 'effective' binding, which had nothing to do with gangliosides (and was not affected by pretreatment of the membranes with neuraminidase or with β-galactosidase), was found only with differentiating cells and led to a shortening of the division times and a decrease in adherence to the glass. It is not clear what relationship, if any, these observations have to the *in vivo* activity of the toxin.

Probably more important is the observation of Habermann (1981) who found an inhibitory effect of the toxin on the basal and K^+-evoked release of $[^3H]$-noradrenaline from preloaded particulate rat forebrain cortex (see section 3.3), an effect which may or may not be associated with the pathological action of the toxin, but certainly looks interesting. About 30 % of the total ganglioside in these membranes is ganglioside GD1b. Treatment of the membranes with neuraminidase cleaves off some of the N-acetyl neuraminic acid residues, converting essentially all the ganglioside to ganglioside GM1, which does not bind tetanus toxin. However cells treated in this way still responded to toxin, if anything slightly more than control cells did. Binding to ganglioside GD1b certainly cannot have been a prerequisite for activity here, and there is similar evidence that it is not important from several other experiments *in vitro* (e.g. Habermann *et al.*, 1980, 1981; Bigalke *et al.*, 1981b).

It is always possible that the main role played by ganglioside binding is in the transport process rather than in the activity directly. The retrograde transport of the toxin in all peripheral neurones must be due to some property common to all such neurones, and this could be the ganglioside content (Stöckel *et al.*, 1977). Tetanus toxin and cholera toxin (which binds to a different ganglioside), and wheat-germ agglutinin (which is a lectin binding to certain glycoproteins) were all three transported efficiently in peripheral neurones. Preincubation of cholera toxin with ganglioside GM1 (the one it binds to) abolished its transport, but that of the agglutinin was not affected. Preincubation of tetanus toxin with its ganglioside, GT1, reduces transport only by 50 per cent. Ganglioside GM1 did not affect it at all. The fact that the inhibition was only 50 per cent may have been caused by spontaneous hydrolysis of GT1 to GM1 which is known to occur. But it could also be because, as suggested by Zimmerman and Piffaretti (1977, see last paragraph) there are two different kinds of binding site of which only one involves a ganglioside.

Of one thing there is no doubt: gangliosides could serve as very efficient receptors for tetanus toxin as they certainly do for several other possible ligands, notably cholera toxin (see below, section 5.1). Some physical chemical experiments (Clowes, Cherry and Chapman, 1972) have shown that gangliosides can be absorbed into artificial lipid bilayer membranes and there interact efficiently with the toxin without altering the structure of the toxin or the ganglioside. All the interaction took place exclusively on the membrane surface and there was no appreciable change in the structure of the bilayer. It seems unlikely that binding of toxin to ganglioside would in itself disrupt a biological membrane.

Many other bacterial toxins that have been studied in detail, for example cholera and diphtheria toxins, have been shown to affect intracellular targets, and so to have to cross the cell membrane before they can work. Some recent experiments suggest that tetanus toxin is also taken up into cells (Yavin, E., et al., 1981; Yavin, Z. et al., 1982). Thus a pure culture of rat cerebral neurons took up and internalized [^{125}I]-labelled toxin, and did so rather more at $0°$ than at room temperature. Most of the internalized toxin (which cannot have been degraded during uptake as it retained full activity) seemed to have entered a particular cellular compartment from which it could not be released by treating the cells with detergent, neuraminidase, or trypsin. Internalization must have been dependent on initial binding of toxin or a receptor, presumably ganglioside, since it was inhibited by excess unlabelled toxin, by ganglioside, and by antibodies to the toxin. It seems highly likely that this internalization will turn out to be relevant to the action of the toxin, but this has not been proved.

If any protein is going to cross a cellular membrane, it has to face the difficult problem of getting through a highly hydrophobic lipid bilayer. There is good evidence, from studies in model systems, that a hydrophobic region in fragment B of the toxin (a fragment of the L-chain and part of the H-chain that cannot bind gangliosides, section 2.4) can interact with membranes to form channels at low pH through molecules perhaps such as some other part of the toxin might pass (Boquet and Duflot, 1982). In vivo such channel formation might follow the binding of the toxin to ganglioside through fragment C. Similar experiments with diphtheria toxin have been used to put forward a mechanism for the entry of its active fragment A (section 5.2 below). So little is known about how tetanus toxin works that these experiments cannot be more suggestive at present.

4.6. Relationship between the Receptors for Tetanus Toxin and for Thyrotropin

Mullin et al., (1976a) showed that the receptor for thyrotropin in bovine thyroid plasma membranes among several other types of membrane was related to a ganglioside. Thus gangliosides inhibited the binding of labelled hormone, and some were more efficient at this than others; the best were GD1b and GT1, the ones that bind tetanus toxin. Initially the relationship between cholera toxin and thyrotropin seemed more exciting; this toxin competes for binding sites with the hormone (Mullin et al., 1976b), and is thought to have some amino acid sequence similarities with it. The suggestion is not that the thyrotropin receptor is actually as simple as a ganglioside, but rather that it is more complex than that and has ganglioside-like lipid or carbohydrate components.

The clear follow-up of these results was to investigate the interaction between tetanus toxin and the receptors (Ledley et al., 1977), and these experiments did show clearly that thyroid plasma membranes will bind toxin, and that the variation with time, pH and ionic-strength of this binding are the same as they are with thyrotropin. Further thyrotropin binding can be blocked or chased with tetanus toxin and vice-versa, and cholera toxin inhibits the binding of both. This is yet further evidence that the receptors for the two ligands are similar.

Another approach to this binding is to look at cases of membrane dysfunction. Although normal rat thyroid membranes bind both toxin and hormones, membranes from a rat thyroid tumor having a defect in the thyrotropin receptor do not bind or absorb neurotoxicity, showing some correlation between the two affinities (Habig et al., 1978).

More direct measurement using partially purified thyrotropin receptor gave similar results (Lee et al., 1978). The glycoprotein component of the receptor can be purified to near homogeneity following solubilization of the membrane with lithium iodosalicylate. Its binding characteristics can then be investigated when it is left free in solution or incorporated into liposomes. Binding of tetanus toxin to this receptor was inhibited by unlabelled hormone or toxin but not by several other proteins such as glucagon and growth hormone. It was also inhibited by a purified fragment of the receptor itself. Interestingly, a change in the lipid component of the liposomes increased the binding of hormone without affecting that of the toxin. These and other observations do suggest that the true receptor even for tetanus toxin may be rather more complicated than just the ganglioside.

This work was followed by a study of the binding of both toxin and hormone to membranes from rat thyroid and brain (Lee *et al.*, 1979). Both bound to both membranes, but toxin bound to brain about 20 times better than hormone did, and hormone bound to thyroid about four times better than toxin. The binding of toxin and hormone to neural tissue *in vivo* and *in vitro* showed very similar kinetics except for one awkward fact (which was also true of model systems containing mixed brain gangliosides in liposomes): binding of labelled toxin was enhanced rather than inhibited by excess unlabelled hormone. Furthermore, thyrotropin could undergo retrograde axonal transport *in vivo* just like tetanus toxin, although this is presumably not physiologically significant.

These interesting observations raise several points. Firstly they may possibly be relevant to the progress of the disease of tetanus: could the observed syndrome of sympathetic overactivity be related to some hyperfunction of the thyroid induced directly by the toxin rather than to some indirect effect as has generally been assumed? Secondly, it is suggested that the toxin might have some effect on electrochemical gradient across the membrane similar to that of thyrotropin and that might be an important part of its mechanism of action. There seems no further evidence for this.

However it remains interesting if toxin is using a receptor that has some normal physiological role. The function of membrane gangliosides is on the whole unclear, but they cannot be there solely to bind pathological toxins.

5. COMPARISON OF TETANUS TOXIN WITH OTHER COMPOUNDS

In recent years, there has been vigorous research into the mechanism and structure of several bacterial toxins, and a number of intriguing common features have emerged (for review, see van Heyningen, 1982a). It is clear that tetanus toxin shares at least some of them.

5.1. GANGLIOSIDE BINDING

Tetanus toxin was the first discovered ligand for ganglioside receptors, but since then several others have been found. Of these, the most intensely studied has been cholera toxin, an activator of the adenylate cyclase of almost all eukaryotic cells. Cholera toxin has two different types of subunit: one subunit A which catalyses a reaction leading to the activation of the cyclase, and five subunits B which bind to ganglioside GM1 on the outer cell membrane. This ganglioside has less N-acetylneuraminic acid residues than the ones that bind tetanus toxin. Following the initial binding of the whole toxin molecule to the cell surface through the B subunits, it seems that either the whole or part of subunit A enters the cell and is active internally.

There is also a striking analogy between cholera toxin and some polypeptide hormones that also activate adenylate cyclase. One of these is thyrotropin which, as discussed above, seems to have a binding site rather similar to the binding site for tetanus toxin. Both thyrotropin and cholera toxin have a similar subunit structure, with a binding and active component; and there is some evidence that there are similarities in amino acid sequence, although this is open to some doubt. So in this respect, tetanus and cholera toxins as well as thyrotropin all have some similarities. *Escherichia coli* also secretes a toxin that seems extraordinarily like cholera toxin in structure, binding and activity, although there has been some discussion about whether or not it binds ganglioside. Interferon certainly does bind to ganglioside, and its action can be blocked by preincubation of the cell with cholera or tetanus toxins. For a review of cholera toxin and more detailed discussion of these points, see van Heyningen (1982a, b).

5.2. STRUCTURAL SIMILARITIES

As mentioned above, cholera toxin has two active components, a binding component and an activating component, and the hormones have a similar arrangement. Diphtheria toxin also has a similar strategy. In this case there are two polypeptide fragments, originally part of the same chain but cleavable from each other proteases. Fragment B binds to a receptor in the cell surface (probably a glycoprotein, certainly not a ganglioside); this brings about the passage of fragment A into the cell where it catalyses a reaction bringing protein synthesis to a halt (Collier, 1975; Uchida, 1982).

Tetanus toxin also has a two component structure: the heavy and light chains. And again only one of these can bind the receptor ganglioside. This suggests the possibility that the overall strategy of the toxin may be similar to the others. If it could be established what the molecular activity of the toxin is, this might turn out to be a property of the light chain. The light chain is not itself active against whole cells, but nor are the active components of the other toxins.

All the other toxins have some simple metabolic action that can occur in a wide variety of cells. Tetanus toxin differs from them in being much more organ and cell-type specific. However this may simply reflect the comparatively restricted range of cells which contain the tetanus-binding gangliosides. It does not prove that the metabolic action of the toxin, whatever it is, could not occur in many more different types of cell if they had the receptor. Since these receptors gangliosides can easily be incorporated artificially into cells, this could be a useful further line of investigation.

ACKNOWLEDGEMENTS

I am grateful to the Medical Research Council for grants for my own research, and Dr. J. Mellanby, Dr. J. Green, Dr. P. Britton, and Miss C. Taylor for helpful discussions.

REFERENCES

ABEL, J. J., HAMPIL, B. and JONAS, A. F. (1935) Researches on tetanus. III. Further experiments to prove that tetanus toxin is not carried in peripheral nerves to the central nervous system. *Bull. Johns Hopk. Hosp.* **56**: 317–336.

AMBACHE, N., MORGAN, R. S. and PAYLING WRIGHT, G. (1948) The action of tetanus toxin on the acetylcholine and cholinesterase contents of the rabbit's iris. *Br. J. Exp. Path.* **29**: 408–418.

AN DER LAN, B., HABIG, W. H., HARDEGREE, M. L. and CHRAMBACH, A. (1980) Heterogeneity of ^{125}I-labeled tetanus toxin in isoelectric focusing on polyacrylamide gel and polyacrylamide gel electrophoresis. *Arch. Biochem. Biophys.* **200**: 206–215.

BEALE, R., NICHOLAS, D., NEUHOFF, V. and OSBORNE, N. N. (1982) The binding of tetanus toxin to retinal cells. *Brain Res.* **248**, 141–149.

BENECKE, R., TAKANO, K., SCHMIDT, J. and HENATSCH, H. -D. (1977) Tetanus toxin induced actions on spinal Renshaw cells and Ia-inhibitory interneurons during development of local tetanus in the cat. *Exp. Brain Res.* **27**: 271–286.

BIGALKE, H., DIMPFEL, W. and HABERMANN, E. (1978) Suppression of ^{3}H-acetylcholine release from primary nerve cell cultures by tetanus and botulinum-A toxin. *Naunyn-Schmiedeberg's Arch. Pharmacol.* **303**: 133–138.

BIGALKE, H., HELLER, I., BIZZINI, B. and HABERMANN, E. (1981a) Tetanus toxin and botulinum A toxin inhibit release and uptake of various transmitters as studied with particular preparations from rat brain and spinal cord. *Naunyn-Schmiedeberg's Arch. Pharmacol.* **316**: 244–251.

BIGALKE, H., AHNERT-HILGER, G. and HABERMANN, E. (1981b) Tetanus toxin and botulinum A toxin inhibit acetylcholine release from but not calcium uptake into brain tissue. *Naunyn-Schmiedeberg's Arch. Pharmacol.* **316**: 143–148.

BIZZINI, B. (1978) Chemical studies on a pharmacologically active polypeptide fragment isolated from tetanus toxin. *Toxicon* **16**: 141.

BIZZINI, B. (1979) Tetanus Toxin. *Microbiol. Rev.* **43**, 224–240.

BIZZINI, B. and RAYNAUD, M. (1974) La détoxication des toxines protéiques par le formol: mécanismes supposés et nouveaux développements. *Biochimie* **56**: 297–303.

BIZZINI, R. J., BLASS, J., TURPIN, A. and RAYNAUD, M. (1970) Chemical characterization of tetanus toxin and toxoid. *Eur. J. Biochem.* **17**: 100–105.

BIZZINI, B., TURPIN, A. and RAYNAUD, M. (1973a) On the structure of tetanus toxin. *Naunyn-Schmiedeberg's Arch. Pharmacol.* **276**: 271–288.

BIZZINI, B., TURPIN, A. and RAYNAUD, M. (1973b) Immunochemistry of tetanus toxin. *Eur. J. Biochem.* **39**: 171–181.

BIZZINI, B., TURPIN, A. and RAYNAUD, M. (1974) Immunochimie et méchanisme d'action de la toxine tétanique. *Bull. Inst. Pasteur* **72**: 117–219.

BIZZINI, B., STÖCKEL, K. and SCHWAB, M. (1977) An antigenic polypeptide fragment isolated from tetanus toxin: chemical characterization, binding to gangliosides and retrograde axonal transport in various neuron systems. *J. Neurochem.* **28:** 529–542.

BIZZINI, B., AKERT, K., GLICKSMAN, M. and GROB, P. (1980) Preparation of conjugates using two tetanus toxin derived fragments: their binding to gangliosides and isolated synaptic membranes and their immunological properties. *Toxicon* **18:** 561–572.

BIZZINI, B., GROB, P. and AKERT, K. (1981) Papain-derived fragment IIc of tetanus toxin: its binding to isolated synaptic membranes and retrograde axonal transport. *Brain Res.* **210:** 291–299.

BOQUET, P. and DUFLOT, E. (1982) Tetanus toxin fragment forms channels in lipid vesicles at low pH. *Proc. Natl. Acad. Sci. U.S.A.* **79:** 7614–7618.

BRITTON, P. (1981) Tetanus toxin. Ph.D. thesis, University of Edinburgh.

CARROLL, P. T., PRICE, D. L., GRIFFIN, J. W. and MORRIS, J. (1978) Tetanus toxin: immunocytochemical evidence for retrograde transport. *Neurosci. Lett.* **8:** 335–339.

CHIU, W., RANKERT, D., CUMMING, M. A. and ROBINSON, J. P. (1982) Characterization of crystalline filtrate tetanus toxin. *J. Ultrastruct. Res.* **79:** 285–293.

CLOWES, A. W., CHERRY, R. J. and CHAPMAN, D. (1972) Physical effects of tetanus toxin on model membranes containing ganglioside. *J. Molec. Biol.* **67:** 49–57.

COLLIER, R. J. (1975) Diphtheria toxin: mode of action and structure. *Bacteriol. Rev.* **39:** 54–85.

COLLINGRIDGE, G. L., THOMPSON, P. A., DAVIES, I. and MELLANBY, J. (1981) *In vitro* effect of tetanus toxin on GABA release from rat hippocampal slices. *J. Neurochem.* **37:** 1039–1041.

COLLINGRIDGE, G. L. and DAVIES, J. (1982) The *in vitro* inhibition of GABA release by tetanus toxin. *Neuropharmacol.* **21:** 851–855.

CRAVEN, C. J. and DAWSON, D. J. (1973) The chain composition of tetanus toxin. *Biochim. Biophys. Acta* **317:** 277–285.

CURTIS, D. R. and DE GROAT, W. C. (1968) Tetanus toxin and spinal inhibition. *Brain Res.* **10:** 208–212.

CURTIS, D. R., FELIX, D., GAME, C. J. A. and McCULLOCH, R. M. (1973) Tetanus toxin and the synaptic release of GABA. *Brain Res* **51:** 358–362.

DAVIES, J. and TONGROACH, P. (1979) Tetanus toxin and synaptic inhibition in the substantia nigra and striatum of the rat. *J. Physiol.* **290:** 23–36.

DAWSON, D. J. (1975) The properties of sulfite-treated tetanus toxin. *FEBS Lett.* **56:** 175–178.

DAWSON, D. J. and MAURITZEN, C. M. (1967) Studies on tetanus toxin and toxoid. *Aust. J. Biol. Sci.* **20:** 253–263.

DIAMOND, J. and MELLANBY, J. (1971) The effect of tetanus toxin in the goldfish. *J. Physiol.* **215:** 727–741.

DIMARI, S. J., CUMMING, M. A., HASH, J. H. and ROBINSON, J. P. (1982a) Purification of tetanus toxin and its peptide components by preparative polyacrylamide gel electrophoresis. *Arch. Biochem. Biophys.* **214,** 342–353.

DIMARI, S.J., HASH, J. H. and ROBINSON, J. P. (1982b) Characterization of tetanus toxin and toxin components by amino terminal analyses. *Arch. Biochem. Biophys.* **214:** 354–365.

DIMPFEL, W. (1979) Hyperexcitability of cultured central nervous system neurons caused by tetanus toxin. *Exp. Neurology* **65:** 53–65.

DIMPFEL, W., NEALE, J. H. and HABERMANN, E. (1975) ^{125}I-labelled tetanus toxin as a neuronal marker in tissue cells derived from embryonic CNS. *Naunyn-Schmiedeberg's Arch. Pharmacol.* **290:** 329–333.

DIMPFEL, W., HUANG, R. T. C. and HABERMANN, E. (1977) Gangliosides in nervous tissue cultures and binding of ^{125}-labelled tetanus toxin, a neuronal marker. *J. Neurochem.* **29:** 329–334.

DUCHEN, L. W. and TONGE, D. A. (1973) The effects of tetanus toxin on neuromuscular transmission and on the morphology of motor end-plates in slow and fast skeletal muscle of the mouse, *J. Physiol.* **228:** 157–172.

EISENBARTH, G. S., SHIMIZU, K., BOWRING, M. A. and WELLS, S. (1982) Expression of receptors for tetanus toxin and monoclonal antibody A2B5 by pancreatic islet cells. *Proc. Natl. Acad. Sci. U.S.A.* **79:** 5066–5077.

ERDMANN, G. and HABERMANN, E. (1977) Histoautoradiography of the central nervous system in rats with generalized tetanus due to ^{125}I-labelled toxin. *Naunyn-Schmiedeberg's Arch. Pharmacol.* **301:** 135–138.

ERDMANN, G., WIEGAND, H. and WELLHÖNER, H. H. (1975) Intra-axonal and extraaxonal transport of ^{125}I-tetanus toxin in early local tetanus. *Naunyn-Schmiedeberg's Arch. Pharmacol.* **290:** 357–373.

ERDMANN, G., HANAUSKE, A. and WELLHONER, H. H. (1981) Intraspinal distribution and reaction in the grey matter with tetanus toxin of intracisternally injected anti-tetanus toxoid F(ab')$_2$ fragments. *Brain Res.* **211:** 367–377.

FIELDS, K. L., BROCKES, J. P., MIRSKY, R. and WENDON, L. M. (1978) Cell surface markers for distinguishing different types of rat dorsal ganglion cells in culture. *Cell* **14:** 43–51.

FISHMAN, P. H. and BRADY, R. O. (1976) Biosynthesis and function of gangliosides. *Science* **194:** 906–915.

FORMISANO, S., JOHNSON, M. L., LEE, G., ALOJ, S. M. and EDELHOCH, H. (1979) Critical micelle concentrations of gangliosides. *Biochemistry* **18:** 1119–1124.

FRENCH. D. and EDSALL, J. T. (1945) The reactions of formaldehyde with amino acids and proteins. *Adv. Protein Chem.* **2:** 277–335.

GOLDBERG, R. L., COSTA, T., HABIG, W. H., KOHN, L. D. and HARDEGREE, M. C. (1981) Characterization of fragment C and tetanus toxin binding to rat brain membranes. *Mol. Pharmacol.* **20:** 565–570.

GREEN, J., ERDMANN, G. and WELLHÖNER, H. H. (1977) Is there retrograde axonal transport of tetanus toxin in both alpha and gamma fibres? *Nature* **265:** 370.

HABERMANN, E. (1970) Pharmakokinetische Besonderheiten des Tetanustoxins und ihre Beziehungen zur Pathogenese des lokalen bzw. generalisierten Tetanus. *Naunyn-Schmiedeberg's Arch. Pharmacol.* **267:** 1–19.

HABERMANN, E. (1972) Distribution of ^{125}I-tetanus toxin and ^{125}I-toxoid in rats with local tetanus, as influenced by antitoxin. *Naunyn-Schmiedeberg's Arch. Pharmacol.* **272:** 75–88.

HABERMANN, E. (1973) Interaction of labelled tetanus toxin and toxoid with substructures of rat brain and spinal cord *in vitro*. *Naunyn-Schmiedeberg's Arch. Pharmacol.* **276:** 341–359.

HABERMANN, E. (1976) Affinity chromatography of tetanus toxin, toxoid, and botulinum A toxin on synaptosomes, and differentiation of their acceptors. *Naunyn-Schmiedeberg's Arch. Pharmacol.* **293:** 1–9.

HABERMANN, E. (1978) Tetanus. In: *Handbook of Clinical Neurology* pp. 491–547, VINKEN, P. J. and BRUYN, G. W. (Eds.). North Holland, Amsterdam.

HABERMANN, E. (1981) Tetanus toxin and botulinum A neurotoxin inhibit and at higher concentrations enhance noradrenaline outflow from particulate brain cortex in batch. *Naunyn-Schmiedeberg's Arch. Pharmacol.* **318:** 105–111.

HABERMANN, E. and DIMPFEL, W. (1973) Distribution of ^{125}I-tetanus toxin and ^{125}I-toxoid in rats with generalized tetanus as influenced by antitoxin. *Naunyn-Schmiedeberg's Arch. Pharmacol.* **276:** 327–340.

HABERMANN, E. and ERDMANN, G. (1978) Pharmacokinetic and histoautoradiographic evidence for the intraaxonal movement of toxin in the pathogenesis of tetanus. *Toxicon* **16:** 611–623.

HABERMANN, E., DIMPFEL, W. and RÄKER, K. O. (1973) Interaction of labelled tetanus toxin with substructures of rat spinal chord *in vitro. Naunyn-Schmiedeberg's Arch. Pharmacol.* **276:** 361–373.

HABERMANN, E., DREYER, F. and BIGALKE, H. (1980) Tetanus toxin blocks the neuromuscular transmission *in vitro* like botulinum A toxin. *Naunyn-Schmiedeberg's Arch. Pharmacol.* **311:** 33–40.

HABERMANN, E., BIGALKE, H. and HELLER, I. (1981) Inhibition of synaptosomal choline uptake by tetanus and botulinum A toxin. *Naunyn-Schmiedeberg's Arch. Pharmacol.* **316:** 135–142.

HABIG, W. H., GROLLMAN, E. F., LEDLEY, R. D., MELDOLESI, M. F., ALOJ, S. M., HARDEGREE, M. C. and KOHN, L. D. (1978) Tetanus toxin interactions with the thyroid:decreased toxin binding to membranes from a thyroid tumour with a thyrotropin receptor defect and *in vivo* stimulation of thyroid function. *Endocrinology* **102:** 844–851.

HELTING, T. B. and ZWISLER, O. (1977) Structure of tetanus toxin. I. Breakdown of the toxin molecule and discrimination between polypeptide fragments. *J. Biol. Chem.* **252:** 187–193.

HELTING, T. B., ZWISLER, O. and WIEGANDT, H. (1977) Structure of tetanus toxin. II. Toxin binding to ganglioside. *J. Biol. Chem.* **252:** 194–198.

HELTING, T. B., RONNEBERGER, H.-J., VOLLERTHUN, R. and NEUBAUER, V. (1978) Toxicity of papain-digested tetanus toxin. *J. Biol. Chem.* **253:** 125–129.

HELTING, T. B., PARSCHAT, S. and ENGELHARDT, H. (1979) Structure of tetanus toxin. *J. Biol. Chem.* **254:** 10728–10733.

HOLMES, M. J. and RYAN, W. L. (1971) Amino acid analysis and molecular weight determination of tetanus toxin. *Infect. Immun.* **3:** 133–140.

HOLMGREN, J., ELWING, H., FREDMAN, P. and SVENNERHOLM, L. (1980) Polystyrene-absorbed gangliosides for investigation of the structure of the tetanus toxin receptor. *Europ. J. Biochem.* **106:** 371–379.

HÖRTNAGL, H., BRÜCKE, TH. and HACKL, J. M. (1979) The involvement of the sympathetic nervous system in tetanus. *Klin. Wochenschr.* **57:** 383–389.

KING, L. E., FEDINEC, A. A. and LATHAM, W. C. (1978) Effects of cyclic nucleotides on tetanus toxin paralyzed rabbit sphincter pupillal muscles. *Toxicon* **16:** 625–631.

KRYZHANOVSKY, G. N. (1973) The mechanism of action of tetanus toxin: effect on synaptic processes and some particular features of toxin binding by the nervous tissue. *Naunyn-Schmiedeberg's Arch. Pharmacol.* **276:** 247–270.

KRYZHANOVSKII, G. N., GLEBOV, R. N. and SANDALOV, YU. G. (1980) Contractile proteins of nerve endings as a possible target for the presynaptic action of tetanus toxin. *Bull. Eksp. Biol. Med.* **89:** 664–667.

KRYZHANOVSKII, G. N., POLGAR, A. A., ZINKEVICH, V. A. and SMIRNOVA, V. S. (1981) Effect of tetanus toxin on mechanisms of regulation of transmitter secretion in neuromuscular junctions by calcium ions. *Bull. Eksp. Biol. Med.* **92:** 648–651.

LAIRD, W. J., AARONSON, W., SILVER, R. P., HABIG, W. H. and HARDEGREE, M. C. (1980) Plasmid-associated toxigenicity in *Clostridium tetani. J. Infect. Dis.* **142:** 623.

LATHAM, W. C., BENT, D. F. and LEVINE, L. (1962) Tetanus toxin production in the absence of protein. *Appl. Microbiol.* **10:** 146–152.

LEDLEY, F. D., LEE, G., KOHN, L. D., HABIG, W. H. and HARDEGREE, M. C. (1977) Tetanus toxin interactions with thyroid plasma membranes. *J. Biol. Chem.* **252:** 4049–4055.

LEE, G., CONSIGLIO, E., HABIG, W. H., DYER, S., HARDEGREE, M. C. and KOHN, L. D. (1978) Structure:function studies of receptors for thyrotropin and tetanus toxin:lipid modulation of effector binding to the glycoprotein receptor component. *Biochem. Biophys. Res. Commun.* **83:** 313–320.

LEE, G., GROLLMAN, E. F., DYER, S., BEGHINOT, F., KOHN, L. D., HABIG, W. H. and HARDEGREE, M. C. (1979) Tetanus toxin and thyrotropin interactions with rat membrane preparations. *J. Biol. Chem.* **254:** 3826–3832.

LUNDH, H., LEANDER, S. and THESLEFF, S. (1977) Antagonism of the paralysis produced by botulinum toxin in the rat—the effects of tetraethyl-ammonium, guanidine, and 4-aminopyridine. *J. Neurol. Sci.* **32:** 29–43.

MATSUDA, M. and YONEDA, M. (1974) Dissociation of tetanus neurotoxin into two polypeptide fragments. *Biochem. Biophys. Res. Commun.* **57:** 1257–1262.

MATSUDA, M. and YONEDA, M. (1975a) Isolation and purification of two antigenically active 'complementary' polypeptide fragments of tetanus neurotoxin. *Infect. Immun.* **12:** 1147–1153.

MATSUDA, M. and YONEDA, M. (1975b) Reconstitution of tetanus neurotoxin from two antigenically active polypeptide fragments. *Biochem. Biophys. Res. Commun.* **68:** 668–674.

MATSUDA, M. and YONEDA, M. (1977) Antigenic substructure of tetanus toxin. *Biochem. Biophys. Res. Commun.* **77:** 268–274.

MATSUDA, M., SUGIMOTO, N., OZUTSUMI, K. and HIRAI, T. (1982) Acute botulinum-like intoxication by tetanus neurotoxin in mice. *Biochem. Biophys. Res. Commun.* **104:** 799–805.

MELLANBY, J. (1968) The effect of glutamate on toxin production by *Clostridium tetani. J. Gen. Microbiol.* **54:** 77–82.

MELLANBY, J. and GREEN, J. (1981) How does tetanus toxin act? *Neuroscience,* **6:** 281–300.

MELLANBY, J. and THOMPSON, P. A. (1972) The effect of tetanus toxin at the neuromuscular junction in the goldfish. *J. Physiol.* **224:** 407–419.

MELLANBY, J. and WHITTAKER, V. P. (1967) The fixation of tetanus toxicity synaptic membranes. *J. Neurochem.* **15:** 205–208.

MELLANBY, J., VAN HEYNINGEN, W. E. and WHITTAKER, V. P. (1964) Fixation of tetanus toxin by subcellular fractions of brain. *J. Neurochem.* **12:** 77–79.

MELLANBY, J., THOMPSON, P. A. and HAMPDEN, N. (1973) On the similarity of tetanus and botulinum toxins. *Naunyn-Schmiedeberg's Arch. Pharmacol.* **276:** 303–310.

MEYER, H. and RANSOM, F. (1903) Untersuchungen über den Tetanus. *Arch. Exp. Path u. Pharmakol.* **49:** 369–416.

MIRSKY, R., WENDON, L. M. B., BLACK, P., STOLKIN, C. and BRAY, D. (1978) Tetanus toxin: a cell surface marker for neurones in culture. *Brain research* **148:** 251–259.

MIZUGUSHI, J., YOSHIDA, T., SATO, Y., NAGAOKA, F., KONDO, S. and MATUHASI, T. (1982) Requirement of at least two distinct monoclonal antibodies for efficient neutralization of tetanus toxin *in vitro*. *Naturwiss.* **69:** 597–598.

MORRIS, N. P., LONSIGLIO, E., KOHN, L. D., HABIG, W. H., HARDEGREE, M. C. and HELTING, T. B. (1980) Interaction of fragments B and C of tetanus toxin in the neural and thyroid membranes and with gangliosides. *J. Biol. Chem.* **255:** 6071–6076.

MUELLER, J. H. and MILLER, P. A. (1954) Variable factors influencing the production of tetanus toxin. *J. Bacteriol.* **67:** 271–277.

MULLIN, B. R., FISHMAN, P. H., LEE, G., ALOJ, S. M., LEDLEY, F. D., WINAND, R. J., KOHN, L. D. and BRADY, R. O. (1976a) Thyrotropin-ganglioside interactions and their relationship to the structure and function of thyrotropin receptors. *Proc. Natl. Acad. Sci. U.S.A.* **73:** 842–846.

MULLIN, B. R., ALOJ, S. M., FISHMAN, P. H., LEE, G., KOHN, L. D. and BRADY, R. O. (1976b) Cholera toxin interactions with thyrotropin receptors on thyroid plasma membranes. *Proc. Natl. Acad. Sci. U.S.A.* **73:** 1679–1683.

MURPHY, S. G., PLUMMER, T. H. and MILLER, K. D. (1968) Physical and chemical characterization of tetanus toxin. *Fed. Proc.* **27:** 268.

NEUBAUER, V. and HELTING, T. B. (1979) Structure of tetanus toxin. N-terminal amino acid analysis of the two molecular forms of tetanus toxin and its composite chains. *Biochem. Biophys. Res. Commun.* **86,** 635–642.

NEUBAUER, V. and HELTING, T. B. (1981) Structure of tetanus toxin. *Biochim. Biophys. Acta* **668:** 141–148.

OSBORNE, R. H. and BRADFORD, H. F. (1973) Tetanus toxin inhibits amino acid release from nerve endings *in vitro*. *Nature New Biol.* **244:** 157–158.

PAAR, G. H. and WELLHÖENER, H. H. (1973) The action of tetanus toxin on preganglionic sympathetic reflex discharges. *Naunyn-Schmiedeberg's Arch. Pharmacol.* **276:** 437–445.

PEARCE, B. R., GARD, A. L. and DUTTON, G. R. (1983) Tetanus toxin inhibition of K^+-stimulated [^{3}H]GABA release from developing cell cultures of the rat cerebellum. *J. Neurochem.* **40:** 887–890.

PRICE, D. L. and GRIFFIN, J. W. (1977) Tetanus toxin: retrograde axonal transport of systematically administered toxin. *Neurosci. Lett.* **4:** 61–65.

PRICE, D. L., GRIFFIN, J., YOUNG, A., PECK, K. and STOCKS, A. (1975) Tetanus toxin: direct evidence for retrograde intraaxonal transport. *Science* **188:** 945–947.

RAJU, T. R. and DAHL, D. (1982) Immunofluorescence staining of cultured neurons: a comparative study using tetanus toxin and neurofilament antisera. *Brain Res.* **248:** 196–200.

RAYNAUD, M. (1947) Extraction de la toxine tétanique et de la toxine de *Clostridium sordelli* a partir des corps bactériens. *C. R. Acad Sci. (Paris)* **225:** 543–544.

ROBINSON, J. P. and HASH, J. H. (1982) A review of the molecular structure of tetanus toxin. *Mol. Cell. Biochem.* **48:** 33–44.

ROBINSON, J. P., PICKELSIMER, J. B. and PUETT, D. (1975) Tetanus toxin. *J. Biol. Chem* **250:** 7435–7442.

ROBINSON, J. P., CHEN, H.-C. J., HASH, J. H. and PUETT, D. (1978) Enzymatic fragmentation of tetanus toxin. Identification and characterization of an atoxic immunogenic product. *Mol. Cell. Biochem.* **21:** 23–31.

ROBINSON, J. P., HOLLADAY, L. A., HASH, J. H. and PUETT, D. (1982) Conformational and molecular weight studies of tetanus toxin and its major peptides. *J. Biol. Chem.* **257:** 407–411.

ROGERS, T. B. and SNYDER, S. H. (1981) High affinity binding of tetanus toxin to mammalian brain membranes. *J. Biol. Chem.* **256:** 2402–2407.

SATO, H., ITO, A., YAMAKAWA, Y. and MURATH, R. (1979) Toxin-neutralizing effect of antibody against subtilisin-digested tetanus toxin. *Infect. Immun.* **24:** 958–961.

SCHMITT, A., DREYER, F. and JOHN, C. (1981) At least three sequential steps are involved in the tetanus toxin-induced bluch of neuromuscular transmission. *Naunyn-Schmiedeberg's Arch. Pharmacol.* **317:** 326–330.

SCHWAB, M. and THOENEN, H. (1976) Electron microscopic evidence for a trans-synaptic migration of tetanus toxin in spinal motoneurones: an autoradiographic and morphometric study. *Brain Res.* **105:** 213–224.

SCHWAB, M. and THOENEN, H. (1977) Selective trans-synaptic migration of tetanus toxin after retrograde axonal transport in peripheral sympathic nerves: a comparison with nerve growth factor. *Brain Res.* **122:** 459–474.

SCHWAB, M. E. and THOENEN, H. (1978) Selective binding, uptake, and retrograde transport of tetanus toxin by nerve terminals in the rat iris. *J. Cell Biol.* **77:** 1–13.

SCHWAB, M., SUDA, K. and THOENEN, H. (1979) Selective retrograde trans-synaptic transfer of a protein, tetanus toxin, subsequent to its retrograde axonal transport. *J. Cell Biol.* **83:** 798–810.

STÖCKEL, K., SCHWAB, M. and THOENEN, H. (1975) Comparison between the retrograde axonal transport of nerve growth factor and tetanus toxin in motor, sensory and adrenergic neurons. *Brain Res.* **99:** 1–16.

STÖCKEL, K., SCHWAB, M. and THOENEN, H. (1977) Roll of ganglioside in the uptake and retrograde axonal transport of cholera and tetanus toxin as compared to nerve growth factor and wheat germ agglutinin. *Brain Res.* **132:** 273–285.

SVENNERHOLM, L. (1963) Chromatographic separation of human brain gangliosides. *J. Neurochem.* **10:** 613–623.

SVENNERHOLM, L. (1970) Ganglioside Metabolism. In: *Comprehensive Biochemistry,* vol. 18, pp. 201–227, FLORKIN, M. and STOTZ, E. H. (Eds.). Elsevier, Amsterdam.

TAKANO, K. and HENATSCH, H.-D. (1973) Tension-extension diagram of the tetanus-intoxicated muscle of the cat. *Naunyn-Schmiedeberg's Arch. Pharmacol.* **276:** 421–436.

TAYLOR, C. F., BRITTON, P. and VAN HEYNINGEN, S. (1983) Similarities in the heavy and light chains of tetanus toxin suggested by their amino acid compositions. *Biochem. J.* **209:** 897–899.

UCHIDA, T. (1982) Diphtheria toxin: biological activity. *In Molecular Action of Toxins and Viruses* pp. 1–31 COHEN, P. and VAN HEYNINGEN, S. (Eds.) Elsevier Biomedical, Amsterdam.

VAN HEYNINGEN, S. (1976) Binding of ganglioside by the chains of tetanus toxin. *FEBS Lett.* **68**: 5–7.

VAN HEYNINGEN, S. (1977) Cholera toxin. *Biol. Rev.* **52**: 509–549.

VAN HEYNINGEN, S. (1982a) Similarities in the action of different toxins. In *Molecular Action of Toxins and Viruses* pp. 169–190, COHEN, P. and VAN HEYNINGEN, S. (Eds.) Elsevier Biomedical, Amsterdam.

VAN HEYNINGEN, S. (1982b) Cholera toxin. *Biosci. Rep.* **2**: 135–146.

VAN HEYNINGEN, W. E. (1963) The fixation of tetanus toxin, strychnine, serotonin and other substances by ganglioside. *J. Gen. Microbiol.* **31**: 375–387.

VAN HEYNINGEN, W. E. (1974) Gangliosides as membrane receptors for tetanus toxin, cholera toxin and serotonin. *Nature* **249**: 415–417.

VAN HEYNINGEN, W. E. and MELLANBY, J. (1968) The effect of cerebroside and other lipids on the fixation of tetanus toxin by gangliosides. *J. Gen. Microbiol.* **52**: 447–454.

VAN HEYNINGEN, W. E. and MELLANBY, J. (1975) A note on the specific fixation, specific deactivation and non-specific inactivation of bacterial toxins by gangliosides. *Naunyn-Schmiedeberg's Arch. Pharmacol.* **276**: 297–302.

VAN HEYNINGEN, W. E. and MILLER, P. A. (1961) The fixation of tetanus toxin by ganglioside. *J. Gen. Microbiol.* **24**, 107–119.

VULLIAMY, T. and MESSENGER, E. A. (1981) Tetanus toxin: a marker of amphibian neuronal differentiation *in vitro*. *Neurosci. Lett.* **22**: 87–90.

WARD, W. H. J., BRITTON, P. and VAN HEYNINGEN, S. (1981) The hydrophobicities of cholera toxin, tetanus toxin, and their components. *Biochem. J.* **199**: 457–460.

WASSERMANN, A. and TAKAKI, I. (1898) Über tetanusantitoxische Eigenschaften des normalen Centralnervensystems. *Berl. Klin. Wschr.* **35**: 5–6.

WENDON, L. M. B. and GILL, D. M. (1982) Tetanus toxin action on cultured nerve cells, does it modify a neuronal protein? *Brain Res.* **238**: 292–297.

WERNIG, A., STÖVER, and TONGE, D. (1977) The labelling of motor endplates in skeletal muscle of mice with ^{125}I-tetanus toxin. *Naunyn-Schmiedeberg's Arch. Pharmacol.* **298**: 37–42.

YAVIN, E., YAVIN, Z., HABIG, W. H., HARDEGREE, M. C. and KOHN, C. D. (1981) Tetanus toxin association with developing neuronal cell cultures. *J. Biol. Chem:* **256**: 7014–7022.

YAVIN, Z., YAVIN, E. and KOHN, L. D. (1982) Sequestration of tetanus toxin in developing neuronal cell cultures. *J. Neurosci. Res.* **7**: 267–278.

ZIMMERMAN, J. M. and PIFFARETTI, J.-CL. (1977) Interaction of tetanus toxin and toxoid with cultured neuroblastoma cells. *Naunyn-Schmiedeberg's Arch. Pharmacol.* **296**: 271–277.

NOTE ADDED IN PROOF

Section 2.1 There is new, stronger evidence that the tetanus toxin gene is on a plasmid, of which a partial restriction map has been prepared, (Finn *et al.*, 1984).

Section 2.5 Several new accounts of the production of monoclonal antibodies to tetanus toxin have been published, (Larrick *et al.*, 1983; Ahnert–Hilger *et al.*, 1983; Sheppard *et al.*, 1984; Volk *et al.*, 1984; Goretzki and Habermann, 1985). Some of them show evidence for similar epitopes in the Heavy and Light chains.

Section 4.4 The binding of toxin to cultured cells has been studied in detail, (Yavin and Habig, 1984; Yavin, 1984). Incorporated exogenous gangliosides GD1b and GT1b can bind toxin. Lazarovici and Yavin, (1985, *a,b*) have shown that human erythrocytes can also bind toxin when incubated with gangliosides; they suggest that this may be a useful system for further study. Critchley *et al.* (1985) have shown that toxin initially bound to gangliosides on the surface of primary neurones in culture is rapidly taken up into some subcellular compartment where it escapes degradation. It seems most likely that this internalization is important in the action of the toxin. Isolated fragment C of the toxin (M_r about 50 000, from the carboxyterminus of the heavy chain) binds to cells and is internalized just like intact whole toxin (Simpson, 1985). This portion presumably contains the ganglioside-binding site.

Section 4.5 It is becoming clear that the transport of toxin at least across artificial membranes is very much affected by pH. Thus low pH induces a hydrophobic domain in the toxin which is probably involved with this transport (Boquet *et al.*, 1984). Similarly, at low pH, toxin can enter asolectin vesicles and become protected from external proteolytic action (Roa and Boquet, 1985), and can promote fusion and aggregation of lipid vesicles containing phosphatidylinositol (Cabiaux *et al.*, 1985). Gangliosides can also be involved with channels formed by the toxin in planar lipid bilayers (Borochov–Neori *et al.*, 1984). Hoch *et al.* (1985) have discussed the pH-dependent formation of such channels by botulinum, tetanus, and diphtheria toxins and its possible function *in vivo*.

There is good new evidence that botulinum and tetanus toxins have similar membrane determinants, (Simpson, 1984*a*): fragment C of tetanus toxin antagonizes the neuromuscular blocking properties of intact whole tetanus toxin (Simpson, 1984*b*) and botulinum toxin (Simpson, 1984*c*). Mellanby (1984) has compared the activities of the two toxins, and suggested a possible common mechanism.

REFERENCES

AHNERT–HILGER, G., BIZZINI, B., GORETZKI, K., MULLER, H., VOLCKERS, C. and HABERMANN, E. (1983) Monoclonal antibodies against tetanus toxin. *Med. Microbiol. Immunol.* **172**: 123–135.

BOQUET, P., DUFLOT, E. and HAUTTECOEUR, B. (1984) Low pH induces a hydrophobic domain in the tetanus toxin molecule. *Europ. J. Biochem.* **144:** 339–344.

BOROCHOV–NEORI, H., YAVIN, E. and MONTAL, M. (1984) Tetanus toxin forms channels in planar lipid bilayers containing gangliosides. *Biophys. J.* **45:** 83–85.

CABIAUX, V., LORGE, P., VANDENBRANDEN, M., FALMAGNE, P. and RUYSSCHAERT, J. M. (1985) Tetanus toxin induces fusion and aggregation of lipid vesicles containing phosphatidylinositol at low pH. *Biochem. Biophys. Res. Commun.* **128:** 840–849.

CRITCHLEY, D. R., NELSON, P. G., HABIG, W. H. and FISHMAN, P. H. (1985) Fate of tetanus toxin bound to the surface of primary neurones in culture: evidence for rapid internalization. *J. Cell Biol.* **100:** 1499–1507.

FINN, C. W., SILVER, R. P., HABIG, W. H., HARDEGREE, M. C., ZON, G. and GARON, C. F. (1984) The structural gene for tetanus neurotoxin is on a plasmid. *Science* **224:** 881–884.

GORETZKI, K. and HABERMANN, E. (1985) Enzymatic hydrolysis of tetanus toxin by intrinsic and extrinsic proteases. Characterization of the fragments by monoclonal antibodies. *Med. Microbiol. Immunol.* **174:** 139–150.

HOCH, D. H., ROMERO–MIRA, M., EHRLICH, B. E., FINKELSTEIN, A., DASGUPTA, B. R. and SIMPSON, L. L. (1985) Channels formed by botulinum, tetanus, and diphtheria toxins in planar lipid bilayers: relevance to translocation of proteins across membranes. *Proc. Natl. Acad. Sci. U.S.A.* **82:** 1692–1696.

LARRICK, J. W., TRUITT, K. E., RAUBITSCHEK, A. A., SENYK, G. and WANG, J. C. N. (1983) Characterization of human hybridomas secreting antibody to tetanus toxoid. *Proc. Natl. Acad. Sci. U.S.A.* **80:** 6376–6380.

LAZAROVIC, P. and YAVIN, E. (1985a) Tetanus toxin interaction with human erythrocytes. I. Properties of polysialoganglioside association with the cell surface. *Biochim. Biophys. Acta* **812:** 523–531; (1985b) Tetanus toxin interaction with human erythrocytes. II. Kinetic properties of toxin association and evidence for a ganglioside-toxin macromolecular complex formation. *Biochim. Biophys. Acta* **812:** 532–542.

MELLANBY, J. (1984) Comparative activities of tetanus and botulinum toxins. *Neuroscience* **11:** 29–34.

ROA, M. and BOQUET, P. (1985) Interaction of tetanus toxin with lipid vesicles at low pH. *J. Biol. Chem.* **260:** 6827–6835.

SHEPPARD, A. J., CUSSELL, D. and HUGHES, M. (1984) Production and characterization of monoclonal antibodies to tetanus toxin. *Infect. Immun.* **43:** 710–714.

SIMPSON, L. L. (1984a) Botulinum toxin and tetanus toxin recognize similar membrane determinants. *Brain Research* **305:** 177–180.

SIMPSON, L. L. (1984b) Fragment C of tetanus toxin antagonizes the neuromuscular blocking properties of native tetanus toxin. *J. Pharmacol. Exp. Ther.* **228:** 600–604.

SIMPSON, L. L. (1984c) The binding fragment from tetanus toxin antagonizes the neuromuscular blocking actions of botulinum toxin. *J. Pharmacol. Exp. Ther.* **229:** 182–187.

SIMPSON, L. L. (1985) Pharmacological experiments on the binding and internalization of the 50,000 dalton carboxyterminus of tetanus toxin at the cholinergic neuromuscular junction. *J. Pharmacol. Exp. Ther.* **234:** 100–105.

VOLK, W. A., BIZZINI, B., SNYDER, R. M., BERNHARD, E. and WAGNER, R. R. (1984) Neutralization of tetanus toxin by distinct monoclonal antibodies binding to multiple epitopes on the toxin molecule. *Infect. Immun.* **45:** 604–609.

YAVIN, E. (1984) Gangliosides mediate association of tetanus toxin with neural cells in culture. *Arch. Biochem. Biophys.* **230:** 129–137.

YAVIN, E. and HABIG, W. H. (1984) Binding of tetanus toxin to somatic neural hybrid cells with varying ganglioside composition. *J. Neurochem.* **42:** 1313–1320.

CHAPTER 25

CLOSTRIDIUM DIFFICILE TOXINS

Te-Wen Chang,* John G. Bartlett,[†] Nadine M. Sullivan**
and Tracy D. Wilkins**

*Tufts University School of Medicine, Boston, MA,
[†]Johns Hopkins University School of Medicine, Baltimore, MD, and
** Virginia Polytechnic Institute and the State University, Blacksburg, VA.

1. INTRODUCTION

Acute pseudomembranous colitis (PMC) may occur in association with abdominal surgery, bowel obstruction, vascular insufficiency, uremia and a number of other clinical settings. The vast majority of cases described during the past three decades, however, have occurred in association with antibiotic usage. The precise mechanism was not known until recently, when it became apparent that PMC is associated with toxins produced by *Clostridium difficile*. This organism is not normally present in the colonic flora of adults. When present, the exposure to certain antimicrobials appears to allow this organism to flourish, produce toxins and cause colitis.

There are two distinct toxins, A and B, produced by *C. difficile*. Although there are differences in biological activities, both toxins are pathogenic and probably responsible for diseases caused by *C. difficile* in animals as well as in man.

2. *CLOSTRIDIUM DIFFICILE*

Clostridium difficile was first described by Hall and O'Toole (1935) who studied several strains isolated as normal flora from the feces of healthy infants. Although these infants showed no signs of clinical diseases, all of the strains were lethal when injected into small rodents. The organism was not considered to be a human pathogen until very recently. Indeed, in 1962 Smith and King reported that when *C. difficile* was isolated from human infections it usually was not considered to be the primary pathogen; they concluded that either the organism did not produce the toxin *in vivo* or that humans were not sensitive to the lethal action of the toxin. In latter studies (Gorbach and Thadepalli, 1975), *C. difficile* was not listed as a common isolate from non-intestinal infections.

Similarities between antibiotic-associated cecitis in hamsters and pseudomembranous colitis in human were noted and studied with the hamster as the experimental model. This led to the eventual identification of *C. difficile* as the causative agent. The preliminary studies were complicated by the fact that *C. difficile*, even in seriously ill patients and animals, was a minor component of the intestinal flora and thus was difficult to isolate. Also, the cytopathic activity of fecal extracts from patients and animals with disease was neutralized by *Clostridium sordellii* antiserum which led some researchers to believe the agent was *C. sordellii*. Selective media incorporating either antibiotics (George *et al.*, 1979; Bartlett *et al.*, 1980) or alcohol (Borriello and Honour, 1981) inhibited most of the normal flora, and *C. difficile* was easily isolated from fecal specimens with these techniques. Culture filtrates of this organism were cytopathic and this activity was neutralized by *C. sordellii* antitoxin.

C. difficile is found as normal flora in a high percentage of healthy infants. It is interesting that the presence of the organism or its toxins in the intestine of these infants does not appear to cause any ill effects, whereas, in adults, the presence of the toxin is usually associated with disease. *C. difficile* or its toxin has been found in the feces of 80 to 95% of patients with antibiotic-associated PMC (Bartlett, *et al.*, 1980; Borriello and Larson, 1981; George *et al.*,

1982; Lishman *et al.*, 1981; Viscidi *et al.*, 1981). *C. difficile* is not considered a frequent component of the adult intestinal flora (Bartlett, *et al.*, 1980; Borriello and Larson, 1981; George *et al.*, 1982; Willey and Bartlett, 1979). The carriage rate in healthy adults ranges from 0 to 3 %, except in Japan (Nakamura *et al.*, 1980) where the carriage rate is about 10 %.

Although almost all patients with pseudomembraneous colitis have cytotoxic stools, many patients that do not have such severe symptoms also will excrete the toxin. Occasionally adults who do not have diarrhea or any other symptoms may have *C. difficile* isolated from their feces, but in these instances the cytotoxin cannot be detected (Lishman *et al.*, 1981; Nakamura *et al.*, 1980; Viscidi *et al.*, 1981). The only common exception was in a report by George *et al.* (1982) who observed the cytotoxin in feces of some asymptomatic patients who had been treated with antibiotics.

3. *CLOSTRIDIUM DIFFICILE* TOXINS

3.1. Purification and Characterization of Toxins A and B by *Clostridium difficile*

After the discovery of that *C. difficile* caused PMC, several research groups became involved in the purification and characterization of its toxin. Preliminary studies suggested the presence of a single toxin with reported molecular weights ranging from 107,000 to 600,000 (Taylor and Bartlett, 1979; Humphrey *et al.*, 1979; Rolfe and Finegold, 1979; Aswell *et al.*, 1979). The culture filtrates and partially purified preparations were cytopathic, lethal for animals, inactivated by heat and acid, and caused fluid accumulation in rabbit ileal loops. Taylor *et al.* (1981) and Banno *et al.* (1981) showed that as the cytotoxic activity was purified further the enterotoxic activity was lost. Both groups demonstrated the presence of a separate enterotoxin that had a molecular weight very similar to the cytotoxin. This toxin is now referred to as toxin A, because it elutes first from ion exchange columns, and the cytotoxin is referred to as toxin B. Both Taylor *et al.* (1981) and Banno *et al.* (1981) partially purified both toxins, and Taylor *et al.* were able to cut toxin A from acrylamide gel and used this small amount of toxin to produce antitoxin. This antitoxin was specific for toxin A and did not neutralize the cytotoxicity of toxin B.

Our research has been directed toward the purification and characterization of both toxins (Sullivan *et al.*, 1982; Sullivan N. M. and Wilkins, T. D., unpublished data). We selected a strain of *C. difficile* (VPI 10463) that produced much larger amounts of the toxins than the strains that were being used by other research groups, and we grew this strain in dialysis flask cultures which resulted in about a 100-fold concentration of the toxins. The crude supernatants from the dialysis sacks contained about 1000 fold more of both toxins per ml than had been obtained previously. We then concentrated this supernatant further by ultrafiltration and then put the concentrate on an ion exchange column which separated toxin A from toxin B. Toxin A was dialyzed against low ionic strength acetate buffer at a pH near its isoelectric point (pH 5.5). Under these conditions, the toxin precipitated while the contaminants remained in solution. Contaminants could not be detected in this preparation when it was analyzed by crossed immunoelectrophoresis and PAGE. This toxin preparation was used to immunize goats and the resulting antitoxin specifically neutralized the enterotoxin but had no effect on the cytotoxin. In crossed immunoelectrophoresis, this antitoxin also did not react with toxin B or any other antigens of *C. difficile* other than toxin A (Ehrich *et al.*, 1980). This confirmed the conclusion of Taylor, *et al.* (1981) that the two toxins were immunologically unrelated.

For the purification of toxin B, a better yield was obtained if the concentrated ultrafiltrate on a hydrophobic interaction column was used prior to the ion exchange step. These purification steps removed a large number of contaminants; however, at least two contaminants remained which could not be removed by isoelectric focusing, hydroxylapatite adsorption, cation exchange chromatography, chromatofocusing, or by columns of concanavalin A or glycoboronate. The contaminants were finally removed by an immunoabsorbent column which contained coupled antibodies against the antigens of nontoxigenic strains of *C. difficile*. The toxin B preparation, after this last step, had 4 to 5 protein bands when analyzed by PAGE; but these bands were found to be immunologically related by crossed immunoelectrophoresis. In addition, all the bands were cytopathic and each was neutralized by antiserum that specifically neutralized toxin B activity (Libby and Wilkins, 1982). Thus, toxin B exists in multiple forms, and this explains some of the conflicting reports about the properties of the cytotoxin. These multiple forms of toxin B were not merely artifacts of the purification procedure since they were also detected in the feces from a patient with PMC as well as in the crude culture supernatants before purification (Sullivan, N. M., unpublished observations). The purified cytotoxin has at least four to five forms which have estimated molecular weights of 70,000, 160,000, 250,000/280,000 and 340,000 (determined by gradient PAGE). The smaller forms have much less cytotoxic activity than the large forms.

The high molecular weight values of toxin A and the larger forms of toxin B strongly suggest that the toxins are composed of subunits, but it has been unsuccessful in dissociating either toxin into subunits using several methods for dissociation of proteins (Sullivan *et al.*, 1982; Sullivan, N. M. and Wilkins, T. D., unpublished data). Both toxins are hydrophobic and, therefore tend to aggregate with conventional sodium dodecyl sulfate (SDS) procedures. The smaller forms of toxin B may be subunits, but it is not possible to produce them from the larger forms by the use of normal dissociating conditions. These forms are more likely degradation products caused by the action of a protease on the native toxin B.

The isoelectric point for the cytotoxin is much lower than previously reported; the toxin readily precipitated at pH 3.8 (Sullivan *et al.*, 1982) and is retained on a chromatofocusing column at pH 4.0 (Sullivan, N. M., unpublished data). The isoelectric point of the enterotoxin appears to have a lower isoelectric point, it is more sensitive to the effects of low pH and is inactivated after several minutes at pH 4.0.

Proteolytic enzymes including trypsin, chymotrypsin, and pronase inactivate both toxins (Rolfe and Finegold, 1979; Banno *et al.*, 1981; Sullivan *et al.*, 1982). Rolfe and Finegold (1979) also reported that their cytotoxin preparation was inactivated by high amounts of amylase and suggested that the cytotoxin might be a glycoprotein. It is not possible to inactivate the cytotoxin preparations with amylase, and the cytotoxin does not bind to gels which bind most glycoproteins (Sullivan *et al.*, 1982). Banno *et al.* (1981) also could not inactivate their toxin preparations with amylase. The cytotoxin is not inactivated by RNAase, DNAase, or lipase (Taylor and Bartlett, 1979; Rolfe and Finegold, 1979; Banno *et al.*, 1981). The toxins do not contain detectable amounts of lipid or phosphorous and toxin A contains no detectable carbohydrate (Sullivan *et al.*, 1982).

3.2. Effects of Physical Agents on Toxins

Studies from our laboratory have shown that crude toxins are stable at $-70°C$. They are inactivated at $100°C$ for 1 min. At $60°C$ for 10 min there is a 99.99% reduction in cytotoxicity, and at $37°C$ there is a 90% loss of activity in 24 hr. At pH 3 or 10.4, marked reduction of toxicity occurs. As the purification process progresses, the toxins become less and less stable. However, both toxin A and toxin B can be stabilized by the addition of albumin and remain stable at $4°C$ for months.

3.3. Cytopathic Effects

The discovery of the cytopathic effects in tissue culture is probably the most important finding toward the recognition and characterization of *C. difficile* cytotoxin. Ironically, it was first observed in virus laboratories where tissue cultures were employed for viral cultivation (Larson *et al.*, 1977; Chang *et al.*, 1978a). The appearance of cytopathic effects of cultured cells following inoculation with stool specimens from patients with pseudomembranous colitis was originally thought to be due to enterovirus but it soon became clear that this was not the case, since subsequent passages had resulted in only diminishing cytopathic activity. An alternative explanation for cytotoxicity was that a toxin was responsible for the changes in tissue cultured cells.

The cytopathic effect observed in human lung fibroblast cell (MRC5) culture (Larson *et al.*, 1977) had a characteristic pattern, occurring diffusely and simultaneously throughout the cell sheet, progressing to a maximum at 48 hr. Cells became rounded and refractile, and then came off the glass. Subsequently, a more detailed description was reported (Chang *et al.*, 1979b). It was noted that cytopathic changes varied with cell types. With lung fibroblasts (WI-38) and baby hamster embryo kidney cells the changes were similar to those described by Larson *et al.* (1977). In human amnion cells, however, the affected cells showed actinomorphic changes, i.e. stringing of cell processes with radiation in all directions. The actinomorphic feature remained for 2–3 days before cell rounding and detachment from the glass took place. The time of appearance of cytopathic changes varied inversely with the amount of toxin present in the cell culture. With high concentrations of toxin the changes could be seen as early as 1 hr. With low toxin concentrations, the changes did not appear until 24–48 hr later.

A number of other cell cultures have been tested for their susceptibility to *C. difficile* toxin. All are found to be sensitive but with somewhat variable degrees of sensitivity (Chang *et al.*, 1979a). Those which appeared to be the most susceptible were human amnion cells, WI-38 cells, baby hamster kidney cells, and mouse fibroblasts. Less sensitive cells included Hela, monkey kidney, and rabbit kidney cell cultures. Other susceptible cells to which the degree of susceptibility was not determined are baby mouse kidney, human chorion cells, cells derived from human brain, dagol kidney and lung, and guinea pig kidney. Thus, cytopathic effects produced by toxin have been observed in all types of tissue culture cells tested, including all mammalian cells. The difference in susceptibility between various cell types has been noted, but is not extensive. Both toxins A and B are cytopathic. However, toxin B is at least 1,000 times more potent than toxin A.

3.4. ULTRASTRUCTURAL CHANGES FOLLOWING EXPOSURE TO TOXIN

Surface changes of cells exposed to toxin have been dramatic when examined by scanning electron microscopy (Chang *et al.*, 1979b). Primary human amnion cell culture showed marked changes in the shape and distribution of microvilli. Cells with demarcated borders showed rearrangement of microvilli into globular chains or ridges which lined up with the branching membranes. Cells without demarcated borders exhibited studlike microvilli, all arranged into globular ridges. Typical changes were noted after 1 hr of toxin exposure, and they persisted without further progression, in spite of continued toxin exposure, for periods up to 48 hr. Both toxin A and toxin B are capable of producing similar changes. It is of interest to note that cecal mucosal cells from hamsters with clindamycin-induced cecitis also exhibited surface changes which consisted of numerous globular projections arranged into ridges (Lusk *et al.*, 1978).

In addition to microvilli, other parts of cytoskeletal system are also damaged by toxin B. Microfilaments were disorganized and eventually disappeared (Thelestam and Brönnegard, 1980). There was a loss of surface fibronectin (Ahlgren *et al.*, 1983). While surface fibronectin was not required for the appearance of cytotoxic effects, it is not known if the microvilli are the primary site of toxin activity.

Cytotoxic effects of toxin B were prevented by lowering incubation temperature to 0°C or by treatment with 2,4 nitrophenol, indicating the involvement of oxidative energy in intoxicating process (Florin and Thelestam, 1981). However, these treatments may also influence the integrity of microtubules, which in turn alter or prevent toxin binding to these structures.

3.5. TOXIN NEUTRALIZATION BY ANTITOXINS

Cross neutralization between *C. difficile* toxin and *C. sordellii* antitoxin was one of the first observations that led to the discovery of the etiology of pseudomembranous colitis. In fact, this led some investigators to the belief that pseudomembranous colitis was related to *C. sordellii*. It soon became clear that this was not the case. Toxin produced by *C. sordellii* though lethal to mice did not cause cytopathic changes in tissue culture (Chang *et al.*, 1978a). Stool from patients with pseudomembranous colitis almost invariably yielded *C. difficile* and its toxins, but not *C. sordellii* (Bartlett *et al.*, 1978).

Neutralization between *C. difficile* toxin and *C. sordellii* antitoxin takes place almost instantaneously and with a readily demonstrable zone of equivalence. The speed of neutralization, because of its rapidity, was not significantly affected by the temperature of incubation. Toxin-antitoxin union may be readily dissociated by either simple dilution or by ammonium sulfate precipitation followed by dilution (Chang *et al.*, 1978b). Although these observations may be consistent with antigen-antibody reactions in general, the fact that the union between *C. difficile* toxin and *C. sordellii* antitoxin is easily reversible suggests that this represents a cross-reaction rather than a specific reaction.

Based on these observations a practical diagnostic test for *C. difficile* colitis or diarrhea can be carried out as follows: Equal amounts of stool and antibiotic-containing phosphate buffer (penicillin 1000 units, streptomycin and neomycin 100 g each, bacitracin, 100 g and fungizone 50 g/ml) are mixed and centrifuged at 3000 g for 30 min or at 10,000 g for 10 min. Aliquots (0.1 ml) of the supernatant fluid are then added to WI-38 cell cultures containing 0.9 ml of medium. Serial 10-fold dilutions are made directly in culture tubes. An additional tissue culture tube is inoculated with 0.1 ml of *C. sordellii* antitoxin or gas gangrene antitoxin (which contains *C. sordellii* antitoxin) diluted 1:10 followed by 0.1 ml of stool supernatant fluid. Cytotoxicity is recorded after overnight incubation at 37°C, and again after 48 hr. The toxin titer is reported as the highest dilution showing definite cytopathic effects which are absent in the tube containing antiserum. Occasionally antibiotic-resistant bacteria may grow but they rarely affect the morphological features of the cells. The test can also be carried out in microtiter wells. Our experience with this assay showed that the test was positive in specimens from 136 (96%) of 141 patients with antibiotic-associated pseudomembranous colitis and 9 (2%) of 562 individuals with gastrointestinal complications unrelated to antibiotic usage.

Naturalization of toxins A and B with specific antitoxins can be readily demonstrated. There is no cross neutralization, in contrast to Sordelli antitoxin which neutralizes both toxins A and B, but with different potency. Sordelli antitoxin was at least 25 times more potent against toxin B than against toxin A (Chang, T.-W., unpublished data). The kinetics of neutralization of purified toxins was found to be different from that of crude toxins or stool toxins in two aspects: First, the amount of toxin neutralized increased with the duration of exposure to antitoxin until 45 minutes, when a maximum was reached. Thus, neutralization of purified toxin with specific antitoxin was not instantaneous. Second, toxin-antitoxin union was firm when specific antitoxins were tested. Dissociation occurred only when Sordelli antitoxin was used, especially against toxin A (Chang, T.-W., unpublished data).

3.6. Toxin Induced Biochemical Changes

While cytotoxicity is a distinct feature of *C. difficile* toxins, biochemical changes caused by the toxins are less clear. Adrenal Y1 cells exposed to toxin failed to activate adenylate cyclase or to increase production of steroid (Donta *et al.*, 1980). On the other hand, toxin B treated cells showed increased intracellular levels of cyclic guanine monophospate with concomitant decrease of cyclic AMP, as a result of stimulation of guanylate cyclase and inhibition of adenylate cyclase (Vesely *et al.*, 1981). The significance in these findings, especially in the pathogenesis of diarrhea, however, is not clearly known. More study is needed.

3.7. Animal Pathogenicity

Animal models are frequently used to study human disease and, in the case of PMC, antibiotic treatment of small rodents produced a disease similar to PMC in human (Bartlett *et al.*, 1977; Rifkin *et al.*, 1978a). This was a very useful model system that helped greatly in the study of the human disease. Cecal contents of antibiotic-treated hamsters killed healthy animals when injected intracecally, and the active agent in the disease was neutralized by *C. sordellii* antiserum (Chang *et al.*, 1978b; Rifkin *et al.*, 1978b; Willey and Bartlett, 1979). Although *C. sordellii* was not isolated from the cecal contents of the infected animals, another *Clostridium*, later identified as *C. difficile*, was isolated in high numbers (Bartlett *et al.*, 1978). Culture supernatants of *C. difficile* killed hamsters and produced the same pathology with intracecal challenge as was seen in the antibiotic-associated enterocolitis.

After intracecal injection of culture supernatants or after clindamycin treatment, all animals became lethargic, dehydrated, and developed watery and sometimes hemorrhagic diarrhea, followed by death. Post-mortem examination revealed a dilated and hemorrhagic terminal ileum and cecum, and histologically, the cecum showed diffuse mucosal inflammation and fibrinopurulent exudates which were often adherent to degenerated mucosal epithelium and resembled pseudomembranes. The toxic effects of cecal contents from antibiotic-treated animals and *C. difficile* culture supernatants were neutralized by *C. sordellii* antitoxin, and inactivated by heat. The culture filtrates from *C. difficile* also caused the accumulation of fluid in rabbit ileal loops (Taylor *et al.*, 1981; Humphrey *et al.*, 1979; Rifkin *et al.*, 1978b), increased skin permeability (Taylor and Bartlett, 1979), and killed mice with ip injection (Aswell *et al.*, 1979). The enterotoxic activity of the *C. difficile* toxin was lost during the purification of the major cytotoxic activity, which led investigators to believe there was a second toxin present. Taylor *et al.* (1981) and Banno *et al.* (1981) described the second toxin (toxin A) which causes a fluid accumulation response. Higaki *et al.* (1982) confirmed these results.

The availability of more purified toxin preparations has enabled more definitive studies to be performed on the biological activities of the two toxins. Nanogram amounts of either toxin injected into the skin of rabbits elicit erythematous, hemorrhagic lesions, and increase vascular permeability (Banno *et al.*, 1981; Taylor *et al.*, 1981; Lyerly *et al.*, 1982). Toxin A produces a positive fluid response when *u*g amounts are injected into ligated rabbit intestinal loops, whereas, the cytotoxin is consistently negative (Lyerly *et al.*, 1982; Banno *et al.*, 1981). We have also found that submicrogram amounts of the enterotoxin produces a positive fluid response in infant mice (Lyerly *et al.*, 1982). In addition, toxin B elicits a weak response in infant mice challenged with *u*g amounts, but toxin A is at least 10 times more potent.

Studies by Arnon *et al.*, with monkeys (1982, ASM Meetings, Atlanta, GA) and by Ehrich (1982) with mice showed injection of either toxin caused abnormalities which included hypotonia, hypothermia, and elevated serum concentrations of potassium, magnesium, phosphorous, and intracellular enzymes. Both toxins were equally lethal.

Injection of toxin A into the ceca of untreated hamsters produced mucosal necrosis, primarily affecting the epithelium. Epithelial necrosis was the primary lesion, although there was inflammation of the lamina propria and submucosal congestion, and hemorrhage (Libby *et al.*, 1982). The ceca were dilated and filled with fluid. Intracecal injections of toxin B produced multiple areas of epithelial cell necrosis, polymorphonuclear leukocytic infiltration, congestion, and hemorrhage. The size of the ceca was the same as normal animals but was very hemorrhagic.

When toxin A was first discovered, some investigators thought that toxin B might not be important in pseudomembranous colitis. However, studies by our research group (Libby *et al.*, 1982) have shown that both toxins appear to be involved in the similar disease of hamsters. In this study, hamsters were immunized against either toxin alone or with a mixture of both toxins. After high neutralizing serum titers were present in the blood, the hamsters were challenged with clindamycin. *C. difficile* grew in the ceca of all the animals and produced both toxins; only those animals immunized against both toxins A and B survived and did not have any symptoms nor damage to their cecal mucosa. All those immunized against a single toxin died of the disease.

Based on the current data, we suggest that pseudomembranous colitis in human is caused by both toxins A and B with neither being necessarily more important than the other. Toxin A would increase the permeability of the mucosa and produce excessive fluid exudation into the intestinal lumen. Toxin B would cause localized areas of tissue destruction and hemorrhage. If either toxin gained access to the general circulation, systemic symptoms would occur, and death could result from action of the toxins on other organs. The resistance of younger people and especially infants to the presence of the toxins in their colons could be because the toxins do not gain access to the mucosal cells. Nothing is known about the binding sites for these toxins or their mechanisms of action. Therefore, several important questions remain to be answered in this area as well as the determination of the relationship of the toxins to one another and their actual role in human pathogenesis.

4. ANTIBIOTIC-TREATED COLITIS IN MAN

4.1. CLINICAL FEATURES OF PMC

Nearly all patients with antibiotic-associated colitis have diarrhea as the initial and most prominent symptom. This usually consists of relatively large volumes of mucoid or watery stools (Tedeso *et al.*, 1974; Bartlett and Gorbach, 1977; Keighley *et al.*, 1978). Some patients with antibiotic-associated PMC have few symptoms other than diarrhea. However, most experience some abdominal cramps, abdominal tenderness, fever and leukocytosis. The onset of diarrhea may occur at any time during antimicrobial administration, but at least one-third of patients fail to note any change in bowel habits until antimicrobial agents have been discontinued. Nearly all agents with antibacterial spectrum of activity have been implicated. The most frequent are ampicillin, clindamycin and cephalosporins (Bartlett, 1981; George *et al.*, 1982; Aronsson *et al.*, 1982).

The course of PMC is highly variable. Many patients improve spontaneously without specific forms of therapy, although these individuals often have prolonged bouts of diarrhea which may persist for several weeks or months. Major complications include dehydration, electrolyte imbalance, hypoalbuminemia with anasarca, toxic megacolon, and colonic perforation. The mortality rate in patients who receive no specific forms of therapy varies from none in one series (Tedesco *et al.*, 1974) to 20 percent (Mogg *et al.*, 1979).

4.2. PATHOLOGY

Pathologic changes in the colons of patients with antibiotic-associated diarrhea include an entirely normal mucosa, erythema and edema, colitis which may be histologically indistinguishable from idiopathic ulcerative colitis, and pseudomembranous colitis. *C. difficile* has been implicated in the full spectrum of these pathologic changes. However, the incidence varies with a direct correlation according to the severity of pathologic changes (Table 1). The most characteristic forms of antibiotic-associated colitis is pseudomembranous colitis. This lesion was originally described by Finney in 1893 as a 'pseudodiphtheritic membrane' lining the intestinal mucosa (Finney, 1893). Subsequent work showed that intestinal pseudomembranes may be found in a variety of clinical settings, although the vast majority of cases reported in the past three decades have been ascribed to antimicrobial exposure (Bartlett and Gorbach, 1977). Gross inspection of the pseudomembranes shows raised, punctate, exudative plaques which study the colonic mucosa. Microscopic findings

TABLE 1. *Tissue culture assay for* C. difficile *toxin*

Patient Category	No. Positive/No. Tested
Antibiotic-associated PMC	136/141 (96%)
Antibiotic-associated diarrhea without PMC	193/710 (27%)
Gastrointestinal diseases unrelated to antibiotics	9/562 (02%)
Antibiotic exposure without diarrhea	2/110 (02%)
Healthy adults	0/60
Healthy neonates	12/45 (27%)

may be classified in three categories according to Price and Davies which tend to be uniform in individual patients. The earliest lesion consists of focal necrosis with acute inflammatory cells and an eosinophilic exudate in the lamina propria. There is a collection of fibrin and polymorphonuclear cells splaying out from a necrotic focus in the form of the characteristic 'summit lesion'. A somewhat more advanced lesion shows disrupted glands containing mucin and acute inflammatory cells surmounted by typical pseudomembranes. Both of these lesions show a normal intervening mucosa with the inflammatory changes restricted to the superficial portion of the lamina propria. The third and most advanced form shows complete structural necrosis of the bowel mucosa which is overlaid by a thick, confluent pseudomembrane.

4.3. Incidence of *C. difficile* Toxin

Stool assays of *C. difficile* toxin have been performed in a variety of clinical settings and show several rather striking observations (Table 1) (Bartlett *et al.*, 1980). The vast majority of patients over the age of 1 year with this toxin have diarrhea or colitis which occurs in the presence of antibiotic exposure. As noted above, the frequency of the toxin seems to correlate directly with the severity of the disease. *C. difficile* toxin has also been occasionally noted in adults with 'sporadic diarrhea' (Brettle *et al.*, 1982), patients with PMC which is not associated with antibiotic exposure (Wald *et al.*, 1980) and in patients with relapse of idiopathic inflammatory bowel disease (Trnka and LaMont, 1981). Nevertheless, the association with antibiotic exposure has been a rather consistent observation in the vast majority of cases. A notable exception is the experience in neonates who show a high carriage rate of both *C. difficile* and its toxin, usually without apparent consequences (Sheretz and Sarubbi, 1982). Carriage rates of the toxin decreases substantially as the infant becomes older, reaching baseline levels at 8–12 months of age. The relatively high incidence of *C. difficile* toxin in this group remains enigmatic, but the practical application of the data is that the toxin assay is not considered valid for clinical interpretation except for children over the age of 1–2 years.

4.4. Treatment

The detection of a microbial pathogen led to several available forms of specific therapy. The drug which has been used most extensively is orally administered vancomycin. This drug is active against virtually all strains of *C. difficile* (Dzink and Bartlett, 1980), oral administration results in exceptionally high levels within the colonic lumen, and there is virtually no toxicity with oral administration since the drug is not absorbed (Tedesco *et al.*, 1978). The initial clinical trials showed that virtually all patients respond (Keighley *et al.*, 1978; Tedesco *et al.*, 1978). Our experience with 189 patients showed 183 (97%) had a favorable response (Bartlett, 1983). The major problems encountered with this treatment are that 46 of the 189 (24%) patients had a relapse when vancomycin was discontinued, usually requiring retreatment. These relapses usually occurred 3–20 days after vancomycin was discontinued, stool specimens from these patients showed positive toxin assays and cultures yielded strains of *C. difficile* which were invariably susceptible to vancomycin (Bartlett *et al.*, 1979; Bartlett, 1983). It is of interest to note that hamsters with antibiotic-induced colitis respond well to vancomycin treatment also, but these animals almost invariably relapse when therapy is discontinued (Bartlett *et al.*, 1978). The presumed mechanism of relapse is failure to eradicate *C. difficile* due to sporulation (Onderdonk *et al.*, 1980). Alternative antibiotics which appear promising include metronidazole (Cherry *et al.*, 1982) and bacitracin (Chang *et al.*, 1980). An alternative approach is cholestyramine which binds the toxin of *C. difficile*. The experience with this drug is highly variable with almost universal success in some series (Kreutzer *et al.*, 1978) and nearly 50% failures according to the experience of others (Tedesco *et al.*, 1979).

5. CONCLUDING REMARKS

The evidence of the role of *C. difficile* in antibiotic-associated colitis is convincing. The organism is seldom isolated from the stools of normal healthy persons, but it is commonly present in patients with PMC. Toxin is also present in the stools of patients with PMC: its characteristics are indistinguishable from those produced by broth cultures of the organism. Partially purified toxin causes colitis when introduced intracecally into experimental animals. Finally, the elimination of toxin from the stool is accompanied by the subsidence of symptoms and resolution of lesions. Other factors, however, may be contributory to the development of PMC. For instance, infants may carry *C. difficile* and the toxin in the stool without evidence of disease. The amount of toxin detected in diarrhea stools from patients with PMC does not necessarily correlate with the severity of symptoms or pathological changes.

The mode of action of toxins A and B has not been clearly determined. While cytotoxicity is a distinct feature of both toxins especially B, and is enough to explain many features of colitis, other contributory factors may also be important. One such factor is the stimulation of guanylate cyclase activity which may cause excessive intestinal fluid secretion, much like ST of toxigenic *Escherichia coli*.

REFERENCES

AHLGREN, T., FLORIN, I., JARSTRAND, C. and THELESTAM, M. (1983) Loss of surface fibronectin from human lung fibroblasts exposed to cytotoxin from *Clostridium difficile*. *Infect. Immun.* **39:** 1470–1472.

ARNON, S., MILLS, D., DAY, P., HENRICKSON, R., SULLIVAN, N. and WILKINS, T. (1982) Rapid death of infant rhesus monkeys after I.P. injection of *Clostridium difficile* toxins A and B: Physiological and pathological basis. Abstracts of the Annual Meeting of the Amer. Soc. Microbiol., Atlanta, GA, B121.

ARONSSON, B., MÖLLBY, R. and NORD, C. E., (1982) *Clostridium difficile* and antibiotic associated diarrhoea in Sweden. *Scand. J. Infect. Dis.* (suppl.) **35:** 53–58.

ASWELL, J. E., EHRICH, M., VAN TASSELL, R., TSAI, G. C., HOLDEMAN, L. V. and WILKINS, T. D. (1979) Characterization and comparison of *Clostridium difficile* and other clostridial toxins. In D. SCHLESSINGER (ed.) Microbiology-1979, American Society for Microbiology, p. 272–275. Washington, D. C.

BANNO, Y., TOKYO, K., WATANABE, K., UENO, K. and NAZAWA, Y. (1981) Two toxins (D-1 and D-2) of *Clostridium difficile* causing antibiotic-associated colitis: purification and some characterization. *Biochem. Internat.* **2:** 629–635.

BARTLETT, J. G. (1981) Antimicrobial agents implicated in *Clostridium difficile* toxin associated diarrhea or colitis. *Johns Hopkins Med. J.* **149:** 6–9.

BARTLETT, J. G. (1983) The recognition and treatment of antibiotic-associated colitis. *Survey Dig. Dis.* **1:** 154–163.

BARTLETT, J. G. and GORBACH, S. L. (1977) Pseudomembranous colitis. In: Advances in Internal Medicine. STOLLERMAN, G. H. (ed.). Yearbook Medical Publishers, Chicago, Illinois, pp. 455–476.

BARTLETT, J. G., CHANG, T. W., GURWITH, M., GORBACH, S. L. and ONDERDONK, A. B. (1978) Antibiotic-associated pseudomembranous colitis due to toxin producing clostridia. *New Engl. J. Med.* **298:** 531–534.

BARTLETT, J. G., ONDERDONK, A. B., CISNEROS, R. L. and KASPER, D. L. (1977) Clindamycin-associated colitis due to a toxin-producing species of *Clostridium* in hamsters. *J. Infect. Dis.* **136:** 701–705.

BARTLETT, J. G., TEDESCO, F. J., SCHULL, S. and LOWE, B. (1979) Relapse following oral vancomycin therapy of antibiotic-associated pseudomembranous colitis. *Gastroenterology* **78:** 431–434.

BARTLETT, J. G., TAYLOR, N. S., CHANG, T.-W. and DZINK, J. A. (1980) Clinical and laboratory observations in *Clostridium difficile*-induced colitis. *Amer. J. Clin. Nutr.* **33:** 2521–2527.

BORRIELLO, S. P. and HONOUR, P. (1981) Simplified procedure for the routine isolation of *Clostridium difficile* from faeces. *J. Clin. Pathol.* **34:** 1124–1127.

BORRIELLO, S. P. and LARSON, H. E. (1981) Antibiotics and pseudomembranous colitis. *J. Antimicrob. Chemother.* **7:** A53–A62.

BRETTLE, R. P., POXTON, I. R. and MURDOCK, J. M. (1982) *Clostridium difficile* in association with sporadic diarrhea. *Brit. Med. J.* **284:** 230–233.

CHANG, T.-W., BARTLETT, J. G., GORBACH, S. L. and ONDERDONK, A. B. (1978a) Clinidamycin-induced enterocolitis in hamsters as a model of pseudomembranous colitis. *Infect. Immun.* **20:** 526–529.

CHANG, T.-W., GORBACH, S. L. and BARTLETT, J. G. (1978b) Neutralization of *Clostridium difficile* toxin by *Clostridium sordellii* antitoxins. *Infect. Immun.* **22:** 418–422.

CHANG, T.-W. LAUERMANN, M. and BARTLETT, J. G. (1979a) Cytotoxicity assay in antibiotic-associated colitis. *J. Infect. Dis.* **140:** 765–770.

CHANG, T.-W., LIN, P. S., GORBACH, S. L. and BARTLETT, J. G. (1979b) Ultrastructural changes of cultured human amnion cells by *Clostridium difficile* toxin. *Infect. Immun.* **23:** 795–798.

CHANG, T.-W., GORBACH, S. L., BARTLETT, J. G. and SAGINUR, R. (1980) Bacitracin treatment of antibiotic-associated colitis and diarrhea caused by *Clostridium difficile* toxin. *Gastroenterology* **78:** 1584–1586.

CHERRY, R. D., PORTNOY, D., JABBARI, M., DALY, D. S., KINNEAR, D. G. and GORESKY, C. A. (1982) Metronidazole: An alternative therapy for antibiotic associated colitis. *Gastroenterology* **82:** 849–851.

DONTA, S. J. and SHAFFER, S. J. (1980) Effects of *Clostridium difficile* toxin on tissue cultured cells. *J. Infect. Dis.* **141:** 218–220.

DZINK, J. A. and BARTLETT, J. G. (1980) In vitro susceptibility of *Clostridium difficile* isolates from patients with antibiotic-associated diarrhea or colitis. *Antimicrob. Ag. Chemother.* **17:** 695–698.

EHRICH, M., VAN TASSELL, R., LIBBY, J. M. and WILKINS, T. D. (1980) Production of *Clostridium difficile* antitoxin. *Infect. Immun.* **28:** 1041–1043.

Ehrich, M. (1982) Biochemical and pathological effects of *Clostridium difficile* toxins in mice. *Toxicon.* **20:** 983–989.

Finney, J. M. T. (1893) Gastroenterostomy for cicatrizing ulcer of the pylorus. *Bull. Johns Hopkins Hosp.* **4:** 53–55.

Florin, K. and Thelestam, M. (1981) Intoxication of cultured human lung fibroblasts with *Clostridium difficile* toxin. *Infect. Immun.* **33:** 67–74.

George, W. L., Sutter, V. L., Citron, D. and Finegold, S. M. (1979) Selective and differential medium for isolation of *Clostridium difficile*. *J. Clin. Microbiol.* **9:** 214–219.

George, W. L., Rolfe, R. D. and Finegold, S. M. (1982) *Clostridium difficile* and its cytotoxin in feces of patients with antimicrobial agent-associated diarrhea and miscellaneous conditions. *J. Clin. Microbiol.* **15:** 1049–1053.

Gorbach, S. L. and Thadepalli, H. (1975) Isolation of *Clostridium* in human infections: Evaluation of 114 cases. *J. Infect. Dis.* **131:** 581–585.

Hall, I. C. and O'Toole, E. (1935) Intestinal flora in new-born infants with a description of a new pathogenic anaerobe, *Bacillus difficilis*. *Am. J. Dis. Child.* **49:** 390–402.

Higaki, M., Honda, T., Takeda, Y. and Miwatani, T. (1982) Purification and some properties of an enterotoxin from *Clostridium difficile*. *Jap. J. Med. Sci. Biol.* **35:** 125–126.

Humphrey, C. D., Condon, C. W., Cantey, J. R. and Pittman, F. E. (1979) Partial purification of a toxin found in hamsters with antibiotic-associated colitis. *Gastroenterology* **76:** 468–476.

Keighley, M. R. B., Burdon, D. W., Arabi, Y., Alexander–Williams, J., Thompson, H., Youngs, D., Johnson, M., Bentley, S., George, R. H. and Mogg, G. A. G. (1978) Ramdomized controlled trial of vancomycin for pseudomembranous colitis and postoperative diarrhoea. *Brit. Med. J.* **2:** 1667–1669.

Kreutzer, E. W. and Milligan, F. D. (1978) Treatment of antibiotic-associated pseudomembranous colitis with cholestyramine resin. *Johns Hopkins Med. J.* **143:** 67–72.

Larson, H. E., Parry, J. V., Price, A. B., Davies, D. R., Dolby, J. and Tyrrell, D. A. J. (1977) Undescribed toxin in pseudomembranous colitis. *Brit. Med. J.* **1:** 1246–1248.

Libby, J. M. and Wilkins, T. D. (1982) Production of antitoxins to two toxins of *Clostridium difficile* and immunological comparisons of the toxins by crossed neutralization studies. *Infect. Immun.* **35:** 374–376.

Libby, J. M., Jortner, B. S. and Wilkins, T. D. (1982) Effects of two toxins of *Clostridium difficile* in antibiotic-associated cecitis in hamsters. *Infect. Immun.* **36:** 822–829.

Lishman, A. H., Al-Jumaili, I. J. and Record, C. O. (1981) Spectrum of antibiotic-associated diarrhoea. *Gut.* **22:** 34–37.

Lusk, R. H., Fekety, R., Silva, J., Browne, R. A., Ringler, D. H. and Abrams, G. D. (1978) Clindamycin-induced enterocolitis in hamsters. *J. Infect. Dis.* **137:** 464–475.

Lyerly, D. M., Lockwood, D. E., Richardson, S. J. and Wilkins, T. D. (1982) Biological activities of toxins A and B of *Clostridium difficile*. *Infect. Immun.* **35:** 1147–1150.

Mogg, G. M., Keighley, M., Burdon, D., Alexander-Williams, J., Youngs, D., Johnson, M., Bentley, S. and George, R. (1979) Antibiotic-associated colitis: A review of 66 cases. *Brit. J. Surg.* **66:** 738–743.

Nakamura, S., Mikawa, M., Nakashio, S., Takabake, M., Okado, I., Yamakawa, K., Serikawa, T., Okumura, S. and Nishida, S. (1980) Isolation of *Clostridium difficile* from the feces and the antibody in sera of young and elderly adults. *Microbiol. Immunol.* **25:** 345–351.

Onderdonk, A. B., Cisneros, R. L. and Bartlett, J. G. (1980) *Clostridium difficile* in gnotobiotic mice. *Infec. Immun.* **28:** 277–282.

Rifkin, G. D., Silva, J., Jr. and Fekety, R. (1978a) Gastrointestinal and systemic toxicity of fecal extracts from hamsters with clindamycin-induced colitis. *Gastroenterology* **74:** 52–57.

Rifkin, G. D., Fekety, R. and Silva, J. (1978b) Neutralization by *Clostridium difficile* antitoxin of toxins implicated in clindamycin-induced cecitis in the hamster. *Gastroenterology* **75:** 422–424.

Rolfe, R. D. and Finegold, S. M. (1979) Purification and characterization of *Clostridium difficile* toxin. *Infect. Immun.* **25:** 191–201.

Sheretz, R. J. and Sarubbi, R. A. (1982) The prevalence of *Clostridium difficile* and toxin in a nursery population. *J. Pediat.* **100:** 435–439.

Smith, L. D. S. and King, E. O. (1962) Occurrence of *Clostridium difficile* in infections in man. *J. Bacteriol.* **84:** 65–67.

Sullivan, N. M., Pellet, S. and Wilkins, T. D. (1982) Purification and characterization of toxins A and B of *Clostridium difficile*. *Infect. Immun.* **35:** 1032–1040.

Taylor, N. S. and Bartlett, J. G. (1979) Partial purification and characterization of a cytotoxin from *Clostridium difficile*. *Rev. Infect. Dis.* **1:** 379–385.

Taylor, N. S., Thorne, G. M. and Bartlett, J. G. (1981) Comparisons of two toxins produced by *Clostridium difficile*. *Infect. Immun.* **34:** 1036–1043.

Tedesco, F. J., Markam, R., Gutwith, M., Christie, D. and Bartlett, J. G. (1978) Oral vancomycin therapy of antibiotic-associated pseudomembranous colitis. *Lancet* **ii:** 226–228.

Tedesco, F. J., Napier, J., Gamble, W., Chang, T. W. and Bartlett, J. G. (1979) Cholestyramine therapy of antibiotic-associated pseudomembranous colitis. *Gastroenterology* **1:** 51–54.

Thelestam, M. and Brönnegard, M. (1980) Interaction of cytopathogenic toxin from *Clostridium difficile* with cells in tissue culture. *Scand. J. Infect. Dis. Suppl.* **22:** 16–29.

Trnka, Y. M. and LaMont, J. T. (1981) Association of *Clostridium difficile* toxin with symptomatic relapse of chronic inflammatory bowel disease. *Gastroenterology* **80:** 693–696.

Vesely, D. L., Straub, K. D., Nolan, C. N., Rolfe, R. D., Finegold, S. M. and Monson, T. P. (1981) Purified *Clostridium difficile* cytotoxin stimulates guanylate cyclase activity and inhibits adenylate cyclase activity. *Infect. Immun.* **33:** 285–291.

Viscidi, R., Wiley, S. and Bartlett, J. G. (1981) Isolation rates and toxigenic potential of *Clostridium difficile* isolated from various patient populations. *Gastroenterology* **81:** 5–9.

Wald, A., Mendelow, H. and Bartlett, J. G. (1980) Non-antibiotic associated pseudomembranous colitis due to toxin-producing clostridia. *Ann. Intern. Med.* **92:** 798–799.

Willey, S. and Bartlett, J. G. (1979) Cultures for *Clostridium difficile* in stools containing a cytotoxin neutralized by *Clostridium sordellii* anti-toxin. *J. Clin. Microbiol.* **10:** 880–884.

CHAPTER 26

TOXINS OF *STAPHYLOCOCCUS AUREUS*

J. H. Freer* and J. P. Arbuthnott†

*Department of Microbiology, Anderson College, Glasgow, Scotland
†Department of Microbiology, Trinity College, Dublin, Eire

1. INTRODUCTION

Staphylococcus aureus is capable of producing a formidable array of extracellular proteins, many of which are inimical to the tissues of man and animals. These include enzymes capable of degrading connective tissue (hyaluronidase), membranes and serum components (phospholipases and lipases), nucleic acids (deoxyribonuclease), proteins (proteases) and a variety of esterases (sugar phosphates and cholesteryl esters). In addition the clotting of plasma is induced by staphylococcal coagulase and clot dissolution promoted by staphylokinase.

There is yet another group of extracellular proteins, the exotoxins, also produced by this species. These include the membrane-damaging agents α-, β-, γ- and δ-lysins (also called cytolysins, hemolysins or toxins); Panton–Valentine leucocidin active against human and rabbit leucocytes; epidermolytic toxins A and B (exofoliatins A and B), which induce cell separation in the stratum granulosum of the epidermis resulting in a variety of skin lesions; enterotoxins A, B, C_1, C_2, D and E responsible for the symptoms of staphylococcal food poisoning and the pyrogenic exotoxins A, B and C, implicated in the generation of scarletiniform rash in cases of staphylococcal scarlet fever.

More recently, pyrogenic exotoxin C and enterotoxin F have been implicated in the syndrome known as staphylococcal toxic shock (TSS).

In addition to these activities, the property of lymphocyte mitogenicity is shared by leucocidin, α-, γ- and δ-lysins, enterotoxins A and B and the pyrogenic exotoxins (Petrini and Möllby, 1981; Langford *et al.*, 1978a; Peavy *et al.*, 1970; Schlievert *et al.*, 1979a).

The variety and number of such exoproteins, many of which are produced simultaneously by a single strain, provide the organism with an awesome armory for the pursuance of its pathogenic activities. However, the very diversity of such products has made the task of defining their individual roles in the pathogenesis of staphylococcal disease extremely difficult. This is illustrated by the fact that in spite of a vast amount of literature on properties of individual exoproteins (including the ones recognized as toxins), only in the cases of the enterotoxins and epidermolytic toxins have clear roles been established for these products in the pathogenesis of staphylococcal disease.

In this review, we confine our remarks to the staphylococcal protein exotoxins namely the α-, β-, γ- and δ-lysins, the P–V leucocidin, epidermolytic toxins, the enterotoxins and the erythrogenic toxins. The possible involvement of the latter two toxins in the toxic shock syndrome is discussed briefly.

Inevitably in a review such as this, personal research interests tend to bias the coverage afforded to different topics. While we recognize this, we make no apology, since such differences in emphasis are desirable and informative. We have concentrated on the production, purification, physicochemical properties and mode of action of the staphylococcal toxins. For more background information the reader is referred to the excellent recent review by Rogolsky (1979) and to the earlier informative reviews by McCartney and Arbuthnott (1978), Freer and Arbuthnott (1976) and Wiseman (1975). More detailed coverage of the biological effects of these toxins can be found in the review by Jeljaszewicz *et al.* (1978).

2. STAPHYLOCOCCAL ALPHA-TOXIN

2.1. Description

Staphylococcal α-toxin, produced by most strains of *S. aureus* is a toxic, immunogenic, surface-active extracellular protein with a molecular weight in the region of 33,000 and a pI of approximately 8.5. It is cytolytic and cytotoxic for a wide range of cells by virtue of its membrane-damaging activities and is lethal, dermonecrotizing and neurotoxic for laboratory animals. It is most frequently assayed by its hemolytic activity against rabbit erythrocytes.

2.2. Production of Alpha-Toxin

In spite of the α-toxin being one of the major extracellular proteins of *S. aureus*, there is still a dearth of information on both environmental factors which control its production and the metabolic control of its biosynthesis and release from the cell. Only in relatively recent years have attempts been made to systematically investigate these aspects. Earlier workers were preoccupied with increasing toxin yields by empirical approaches. Studies prior to 1970 showed that factors such as pH value, CO_2 tension, available glucose and amino acid composition of the medium all affected the yield of α-toxin. These earlier studies were comprehensively reviewed by Arbuthnott (1970). The most commonly used strain of *S. aureus* for studies on α-toxin is Wood 46, although there is little doubt that considerable variation in properties occurs even within this so called 'strain'. However, α-toxin produced by different strains is very similar in its biological and physicochemical properties (Goode and Baldwin, 1974).

There is general agreement that α-toxin is produced in a biphasic manner in liquid batch cultures. Low levels of the toxin are produced during exponential growth with a marked increase occurring just prior to the onset of a slower rate of growth prior to stationary phase. By stationary phase, α-toxin can account for up to 2 % of the total dry weight of the culture (Duncan and Cho, 1971).

Uncertainty still exists about whether or not toxin is released from cells due to autolysis (see Bernheimer and Schwartz, 1963; Duncan and Cho, 1971), with conflicting reports of the extent of autolysis during peak toxin appearance in culture supernatant fluids. Both the above mentioned groups used nucleic acid as a marker for autolysis, but this is unsatisfactory as an indication of cell leakiness. Most of the high molecular weight DNA remains associated with the cells or remains intracellular in spite of extensive membrane disruption as seen by electron microscopy and cytoplasmic enzyme release (J. H. Freer, unpublished observations). A more reliable estimate of membrane damage (autolysis) would be gained by measuring the activity of cytoplasmic enzyme markers of molecular weight in the region of 30,000–40,000.

Coleman and Abbas-Ali (1977), confirmed the findings of Duncan and Cho (1971) that the α-toxin is produced in a biphasic manner, most of the toxin appearing in culture supernatant fluids during the post-exponential phase of growth. There is no evidence that toxin accumulates in any appreciable quantities intracellularly prior to its release. This is entirely compatible with current ideas on synthesis and release of exported proteins (Davis and Tai, 1980) which may involve concurrent synthesis on membrane bound polysomes and export through the membrane. It is interesting to note that cerulenin, an antibiotic inhibiting fatty acid synthesis, selectively inhibits exoprotein release in *S. aureus* at concentrations not inhibitory to growth (Saleh and Freer, 1984). This is in keeping with mechanisms which require specific fatty acid synthesis for insertion of proteins into the membrane, be they specific receptor proteins involved in transport/export sites for signalled exoproteins or insertion of the signal sequence of the exported proteins themselves. The exact mechanism involved in export of the protein toxins in *S. aureus* is one area which has received little attention, but has a bearing on the models published on possible control mechanisms for exoprotein production in *S. aureus* (Coleman, 1981).

Circumstantial evidence for the involvement of the plasma membrane as a key control site in the export of exoproteins comes from the work of Yoshikawa *et al.* (1974). They confirm the earlier observations of Voureka (1952) on pleiotropic alterations to hyperproduction of a range of extracellular proteins in nitrosoguanidine (NTG)-induced mutants of *S. aureus*. Revertants were also commonly pleiotropic with respect to hypo-production of extracellular proteins. More interestingly, they noted that pleiotropic effects were associated with loss of yellow pigment which is largely lipid-soluble carotenoid. This suggests that alterations occur in the membrane lipid fraction. Similar loss of pigment also occurs under nongrowth inhibitory concentrations of cerulenin which almost fully inhibit secretion of α-toxin, and reduce markedly the secretion of several other exoproteins (Saleh and Freer, 1984). The effect of cerulenin is to inhibit membrane lipid synthesis (Omura, 1976). Abbas-Ali and Coleman (1977a,b) suggested that increased production of extracellular proteins after exponential growth ceased could be explained by a regulatory mechanism based on 'competition' at the transcriptional level between cell protein and extracellular protein synthesizing machinery. Two separate effects were implicated, namely, an increase in available RNA polymerase after rRNA synthesis is switched off, and an increase in substrate concentrations due to RNA 'turnover'.

Recent results presented by Coleman (1981) showed that the differential rates of total extracellular protein produced by Wood 46 and a low α-toxin producing variant were identical, whereas the contribution of α-toxin to the extracellular proteins was very different in each case. These results are consistent with the pleiotropic alteration of multiple functions reported by Yoshikawa *et al.* (1974) who suggested a common regulatory mechanism for the synthesis and release of exoprotein and the suggestions by Coleman *et al.* (1975) of a competition model for exoprotein formation. It is conceivable however, that there could also be some control exercised at the level of the membrane which may be related to compositional changes in the membrane as a response to growth rate and growth phase. Bjorklind and Arvidson (1980) recently suggested a more detailed model (resembling catabolite repression in some respects) for the regulation of exoprotein synthesis in *S. aureus*. This followed an analysis of the exoprotein patterns found in a series of spontaneous mutants of strain V8 selected during continuous cultivation. Spontaneous protease 1-negative mutants accumulated rapidly during continuous culture and were altered in the formation of most other exoproteins, both those produced during exponential growth (notably protein A and coagulase) and those which appeared primarily in the post-exponential phase of growth.

Different patterns of exoprotein production in the mutants were explained in terms of differing affinities between a putative 'transcription-activating protein' (EX)/'coactivator' (S) complex (EXS) or an EXS–RNA polymerase complex and the individual promotor regions of the structural genes involved in exoprotein production. Both protein A and coagulase are thought to be under positive repressor control in the post-exponential phase of growth, the repressor being transcribed as a response to the presence of the EXS complex, just as structural genes for post-exponential phase exoproteins are transcribed. Coactivator S is thought to be a secondary metabolite associated with amino acid metabolism which accumulates after exponential growth.

In some strains of *S. aureus*, there appears to be a link between production of α-toxin and lysogeny. An early report by Blair and Carr (1961) that toxigenicity could be conferred on nontoxigenic strains by lysogenization with phages from toxigenic strains, conflicts with the failure of Hendricks and Altenbern (1968) to find evidence of lysogenic conversion. In a genetic study of α-toxin mutants of *S. aureus*, strain 233, by transduction (McClatchy and Rosenblum, 1966), results of two-point reciprocal transductions indicated that the mutants fell into two distinct genetic groups, one group showing pleiotropic effects on α-lysin and fibrinolysin production and probably representing a regulatory gene locus for both proteins, and a second group, which included hemolysin-regulatory mutants which produced material cross-reacting with α-lysin, probably representing mutants in the structural gene for α-lysin.

In a more recent report, Brown and Patee (1980) examined mutants of strains NCTC 8325 by transformation techniques and showed that the *hla*⁺ (Hla⁺ phenotype, α-hemolytic) gene resided in the sequence '*pur B 110-bla*⁺ − *hla*⁺ − *ilv-129–pig-131*'. Naturally occurring

(Strain Ps6) or induced mutations (Strains 8325, 233) in the *hla* gene also mapped between *bla*$^+$ and *ilv−129*. Again Hla$^+$ phenotypes in strain 8325 were always fibrinolytic and Hla$^-$ phenotypes always nonfibrinolytic, similar to the findings for group II mutants (regulatory) of McClatchy and Rosenblum (1966). Wheller (1975) also found a close association between u.v.-induced loss of α-hemolysin activity and loss of fibrinolysin.

Witte (1976) after examination of several isolates from human pus concluded that in five out of ten isolates, plasmids were probably involved in control of hemolysin activity. His conclusions were based on SDS-curing and no increased frequency of transduction of Hla$^+$ after u.v. irradiation of the transducing phage. However, the physical loss of plasmid DNA concomitant with loss of Hla$^+$ phenotype was not shown in this study. It would be of interest to follow fibrinolytic activity as well as the α-lysin activity in view of the close association of these two properties reported by other workers, along with DNA profiles after curing. The absence of plasmids in strain 8325 eliminates the possibility of plasmid involvement in Hla activity in this strain and possibly in all strains of lytic group III.

The chromosomal location of the *hla* gene in this group is not in doubt, but it is still not clear what the nature of the *hla* gene product is. As pointed out by Brown and Patee (1980), the close association between α-lysin production and fibrinolysin production in *hla* mutants may indicate an undefined role for the *hla* gene in regulation of several extracellular proteins. Also, the high instability of the Hla$^+$ phenotype, noted repeatedly by workers in the field of α-toxin, is not characteristic of chromosomal genes. Both Rogolsky (1979) and Brown and Patee (1980) suggested that a transposon location for the *hla* gene would go some way towards explaining some of the anomalous properties noted previously in relation to α-toxin activity. Certainly, it is difficult to escape from this possibility when trying to reconcile earlier reports of phage conversion, plasmid control and high-frequency loss of hemolysin activity with no detectable rate of reversion to Hla$^+$.

2.3. Purification of Alpha-Toxin (Lysin)

The number of different published schemes for purification of α-lysin probably matches, if not exceeds the number of laboratories that have at one time or another been involved in α-lysin research. There are several excellent reviews which discuss the development of these earlier purification procedures (Arbuthnott, 1970; Wiseman, 1975; Rogolsky, 1979). In recent years, attention has been concentrated on reducing the complexity of the procedures without sacrificing the yield but improving purity. The importance of rapid purification under carefully controlled conditions from culture supernatants is emphasized by the results of Dalen (1976a), which showed that considerable degradation of α-lysin occurred during isolation procedures, presumably due to endogenous proteases which are readily demonstrable in culture supernatant fluids of strain Wood 46 and many other α-toxin producing strains.

Loss of α-lysin activity during purification probably arises mainly from either proteolysis or denaturation, particularly at low-ionic strengths (Lominski *et al.*, 1963; Coulter, 1966). Also the relatively high surface-activity of this protein (Buckelew and Colacicco, 1971) may lead to loss of hemolytic activity by polymer formation which is enhanced at liquid−air interfaces (Arbuthnott *et al.*, 1967; Colacicco and Buckelew, 1971) and during adsorption to glass surfaces. For these reasons it is advisable to store purified lysin under saturated ammonium sulfate at 4°C.

In recent years several reports have appeared giving details of purification methods of α-toxin along with extensive analyses of purity of the product. Indeed, with a complex procedure involving zinc chloride precipitation, gel filtration, starch zone electrophoresis, ion-exchange chromatography and Pevikon zone electrophoresis followed by dialysis against ammonium sulfate, Watanabe and associates (Watanabe, 1976; Watanabe and Kato, 1974) succeeded in producing crystalline toxin. Concurrently, Harshman and colleagues (Cassidy and Harshman, 1976a) published a much simpler purification procedure involving chromatography on controlled-pore glass followed by ion-exchange chromatography. This procedure resulted in purified α-toxin in high yield. Using the above method in our laboratory, it was necessary to substitute isoelectric-focusing on broad gradients (pH 4–10) for the ion-exchange chromatography step in order to remove all detectable proteolytic activity as well as acidic proteins from the final product. Possible improvements in convenience and yield may be achieved by substituting isoelectric-focusing in thin-layer granulated gels as a final step in purification. Also some improvements in the yield of hemolytic activity can be achieved by incorporating the protease inhibitor phenyl-methyl-sulfonyl fluoride (PMSF) in the buffers during purification procedures (Saleh and Freer, 1984).

2.4. Physicochemical Characteristics of Purified Alpha-Toxin

2.4.1. *Molecular Weight and Isoelectric Point*

The α-toxin is a protein and in all probability a single polypeptide. Earlier claims that it contains a carbohydrate moiety (Goshi *et al.*, 1963) have not been substantiated by later investigations. Some of the characteristics of α-toxin are shown in Table 1. The molecular weight estimations range from 10^4 to 4×10^4 daltons, undoubtedly some of this range reflecting the methods of estimation used by different groups.

However, for a single product assessed by four different methods (SDS-Page, sedimentation equilibrium centrifugation in 8 M urea and in 6 M guanidine HCl, sedimentation velocity centrifugation and amino acid analysis), the molecular weight determinations fell within the range $2.6–3.1 \times 10^4$ daltons (Six and Harshman, 1973b). Sedimentation coefficients for active toxin in the range 2.85–3.15 have been reported frequently although additional minor components in the range 10S–16S have been frequently reported (see Table 1).

The reported values for the isoelectric point of the major α-toxin component in purified preparations fall within the narrow range of 8.4–8.7. (Wadström, 1968; McNiven and Arbuthnott, 1972; Six and Harshman, 1973b; Goode and Baldwin, 1974; Watanabe and Kato, 1974; Fackrell and Wiseman, 1976b; Dalen, 1975, 1976b). Several authors report minor components with different pI values, but these generally amount to a relatively small proportion of the total toxic protein. It is possible that some of the so-called 'multiple forms' of the lysin arise during the purification procedures. Multiple forms of yeast enolase were generated by electrofocusing (Porcelli *et al.*, 1978), possibly as a result of exposure to high pH. Other mechanisms which may induce charge alterations are cation binding and deamidation. Focusing in granular gels should overcome some of these problems. Values for the specific hemolytic activity of purified lysin from different laboratories show a wide range (10^4), no doubt reflecting toxin instability as well as purity. However, most of the more recently reported purification procedures yielded toxin with specific hemolytic activity in the range of $2–5 \times 10^4$ HU mg^{-1}.

2.4.2. *Amino Acid Analyses and End Group Composition*

Results of amino acid analyses from five different laboratories, are shown in Table 2. The first analysis published by Bernheimer and Schwartz (1963) showed a complete absence of half-cystine. Their figures for residues per molecule were calculated assuming a molecular weight of 44,000. Coulter (1966) calculated the number of residues per molecule for a monomer of MW 31,000. Fackrell and Wiseman (1976b) published their analysis in terms of residues per molecule after assigning histidine a value of 4, as were the results of Watanabe and Kato (1974). It is not clear how the figures of Kato and Watanabe (1980) were derived since they do not correspond with their published values for molecular weight. There is overall similarity in the results of analyses from different laboratories, in that half-cystine is absent and there are relatively large amounts of lysine, aspartic and glutamic acids. The high figures for ammonia reported in many of the analyses may indicate that aspartic and glutamic acids were present as corresponding amines, which would also account for the pronounced basicity of the α-toxin molecule. Data from Watanabe and Kato (1974) and

TABLE 1. *Some Characteristics of Purified Staphylococcal Alpha-Lysin*

Reference	Strain of organism	Molecular weight	N-terminal amino acid	Sedimentation coefficient ($S_{20,w}$)	C-terminal amino acid	Isoelectric point (pI)	Specific hemolytic activity (hemolytic units mg^{-1} protein)
Madoff & Weinstein (1962)	Wood 46	—*		—		—	4.2×10^4
Kumar et al. (1962)	Wood 46	$1.0–1.5 \times 10^4$		1.45		—	1.9×10^4
Bernheimer & Schwartz (1963)	Wood 46	4.4×10^4		3.0†; 12.0‡		—	8×10^8
Goshi et al. (1963)	—	—				—	1.2×10^5
Lominski et al. (1963)	Wood 46	—		3.1			
Jackson (1963)	209–60	—				—	
Robinson & Thatcher (1963)	Wood 46	—	Hist. Arg.	2.8		—	1.2×10^6
Cooper et al. (1966)	Wood 46	—		2.8		—	10^4
Coulter (1966)	Wood 46	2.1×10^4		3.0		—	2×10^8
Arbuthnott et al. (1967)	Wood 46	—					
Wadström (1968)	Wood 46, V8, M18	—	Hist.			8.5† (alpha I)	
Wiseman & Caird (1970)	Wood 46	—		2.8		—	
Forlani et al. (1971)	(Wood 46?)	3.3×10^4				8.55† (Alpha A)	
McNiven & Arbuthnott (1972)	Wood 46	3.6×10^4					1.3×10^5
Fackrell (1973)	Wood 46		Ala(A + B)	3.0(A) 3.0(B)	Lys(A + B)	7.2(A); 8.4(B)	1.8×10^4
Six & Harshman (1973a,b)	Wood 46	2.8×10^4		3.0†; 10.5		8.65†; 5.8	
Goode & Baldwin (1973)	Wood 46	—					
Goode & Baldwin (1974)	57, 2079, 3558, 3565	—		3.0†; 10.5		8.65 ± 0.15 7.98 ± 0.05	
Watanabe & Kato (1974)	Wood 46	3.6×10^4					
Dalen (1975a, 1976b)	Wood 46	3.9×10^4				8.6†; 7.4	
Fackrell & Wiseman (1976b)	Wood 46	4.5×10^4	His.	1.4§		8.5	
Cassidy & Harshman (1976a)	Wood 46	—				—	2.8×10^4

*Not reported.
†Major component.
‡Inactive aggregate.
§Changed to 2.8 on standing.

TABLE 2. *Amino Acid Analyses of Staphylococcal Alpha-toxin*

Amino acid	Bernheimer & Schwartz* (1963)	Coulter* (1966)	Fackrell & Wiseman‡ (1974)	Six & Harshman† (1973b)		Watanabe & Kato† (1974)	Kato & Watanabe (1980)
				A	B		
Trp				4	4	4.2	
Asp	44	52	20 (40)	40	43	48	43
Met	10	5	2 (4)	6	6	5.5	8
Thr	23	26	10 (20)	22	23	24.3	24
Ser	22	21	10 (20)	19	19	18	21
Glu	21	23	16 (32)	19	20	20.1	20
Pro	7	10	14 (28)	8	9	5.3	10
Gly	23	25	28 (56)	20	24	22.5	36
Ala	12	14	12 (24)	11	11	12.1	17
Val	12	17	8 (16)	13	14	16.2	19
Lle	13	16	6 (12)	13	14	15	16
Leu	15	15	8 (16)	13	14	14.5	16
Tyr	9	10	6 (12)	9	10	12.5	7
Phala	10	10	4 (8)	8	8	9.3	9
Lys	23	27	12 (24)	21	23	25.5	31
His	4	4	4 (8)	4	4	4	8
Arg	10	8	6 (12)	8	8	9.5	8
No. residues	258	283	166 (332)	239	254	267	297
Calculated MW of single peptide of above composition	28,500*	31,000	17,300 (34,600)	26,500	28,200	30,000	31,000

*Number of residues calculated for a peptide of MW 44,000 (Bernheimer and Schwartz) and 31,000 (Coulter).
†Figures for each residue calculated assuming four residues histidine per molecule.
‡Figures derived from those originally published by assigning 4 or 8 residues to histidine.

Kato and Watanabe (1980) on crystalline toxin, produced by the same procedure in each study, show close similarity in amino acid composition with the exception of histidine which shows four residues per molecule in the earlier preparation and eight in the preparation described in the later publication.

The progress in sequencing the toxin is summarized in Fig. 1. The first 10 residues from the amino terminus are identical in the toxin of Six and Harshman (1973b) and Kato and Watanabe (1980) as is the C-terminal residue (lysine). The amino terminal region of the lethal fragment of the toxin (Kato and Watanabe, 1980) shows a predominance of hydrophobic residues (Fig. 1, heavy chain).

Recently molecular cloning techniques have been used to analyse the α-haemolysin determinant of *S. aureus* strain Wood 46. A 12 kilobase pair DNA sequence encoding the α-haemolysin gene(s) was cloned on a λ bacteriophage vector into *Escherichia coli* K12 (Kehoe *et al.*, 1984). Using detection and transposon mutagenesis the determinant was localized to a 1.65 kilobase pair sequence which was shown to express two polypeptides of molecular weights 34,000 and 33,500 daltons in *E. coli* minicells. The α-haemolysin activity remained cell-associated when the toxin was expressed from *E. coli* plasmid vectors. The determinant was subsequently introduced into *Bacillus subtilis*. Two polypeptides of molecular weight 34,000 daltons and 33,500 daltons were precipitated using anti-α-haemolysin sera from these *B. subtilis* cells. The α-haemolysin could be detected in the supernatant of growing *B. subtilis* cultures. The cloned α-haemolysin determinant was also reintroduced, using plasmid vectors, back into several strains of *S. aureus* where it was expressed in a stable manner. DNA sequencing techniques have been used to determine the amino-acid sequence of the α-haemolysin (Kehoe *et al.*, 1984). The sequence will facilitate the construction of specific mutations in the α-haemolysin gene and may help in elucidating the mode of action of the toxin.

2.5. Biological Activities of Alpha-Toxin

2.5.1. *Lethal and Hemolytic Activity*

Staphylococcal α-toxin is defined as having membrane-damaging activity (encompassing cytolytic and hemolytic activity), it is also cytotoxic and neurotoxic (see reviews by Freer and Arbuthnott, 1976; Rogolsky, 1979). Superficial injection causes dermonecrosis in laboratory animals and intravenous injection is lethal at appropriate doses (LD_{50} mouse = 1 μg; rabbit = 4 μg).

Because of the pronounced sensitivity of rabbit erythrocyte membranes to the action of α-toxin when compared with other mammalian species (rabbit erythrocytes are approximately 100 times more sensitive to lysis by α-toxin than other mammalian erythrocytes), the hemolytic assay with rabbit erythrocytes is the most convenient and sensitive for active toxin. With highly purified preparations of toxin (> 10,000 HU mg^{-1} protein) this assay represents a sensitivity of detection in the region of > 0.1 μg toxic protein.

2.5.2. *Membrane Lesions Induced by Alpha-Toxin*

An indication of the type of membrane damage caused to human embryonic lung diploid fibroblasts was provided by the studies of Thelestam and colleagues (Thelestam and Möllby, 1975a,b; 1979). By following the kinetics of release of three different sized radiolabeled cytoplasmic markers, they concluded that α-toxin caused small (0.6–0.8 nm diameter) 'functional holes' in the cytoplasmic membrane. In a comparative study, similar leakage patterns were observed with the polyene antibiotics Amphotericin B and Nystatin. These patterns of release differed markedly from those induced by such agents as Triton-X100, melittin or staphylococcal δ-lysin. With α-toxin, leakage of the smallest marker (α-[^{14}C]-amino isobutyric acid, MW = 103) was almost complete between 0.01 and 0.1 μg toxin ml^{-1} whereas this concentration range caused no release of the higher molecular weight nucleotide label (MW < 10,000) or RNA label (MW > 200,000). This leakage pattern differed

NH$_2$-Ala-Asp-Ser-Asp-Leu/Ile-Asn-Ile-Lys-Pro-Gly------Gly-Arg----Ile-Leu-His-Val-Arg-Ala-Val-Val---Thr-Tyr-Val-Lys-COOH

1 2 3 4 5   6 7 8 9 10........ 121 122....149 150 151 152 153 154 155 156...291 292 293 294

1..............light chain...............122/ /149.............heavy chain...............294

MW = 14,000 unstable nontoxic   MW = 17,000 Lethal, nonhemolytic
                                                    nondermonecrotic

123 to 148 = 26 residue short chain(s) released in trypsin-cleavage region

FIG. 1. Partial amino acid sequence of staphylococcal alpha-toxin (after Kato and Watanabe, 1980).

in most respects from that caused by the synthetic detergents, where leakage rates of the different sized cell labels were similar indicating 'large functional holes'. An exception to this pattern was found with the cationic detergent, cetyltrimethyl-ammonium bromide (CTAB), where the induced leakage pattern showed a common feature with α-toxin in that RNA label was markedly retained in the detergent-treated cells. In both the case of α-toxin (pI 8.6) and the cationic detergent CTAB, the retention of RNA label, and to some extent the nucleotide label, may be due to an accumulation of positive charges from the lytic agent in the region of the induced membrane 'pore'. Some caution is required in interpretation of these data, since on a weight for weight basis, CTAB is 10–100 fold *more* active in releasing hemoglobin (MW 67,000, pI 6.8) from rabbit erythrocytes than detergents such as Triton-X100 or sodium dodecyl sulfate (J. H. Freer, unpublished observation).

2.5.3. *Interaction of Alpha-Toxin with Isolated Membranes and Liposomes*

There have been numerous reviews published in recent years covering this aspect of α-toxin activity (Harshman, 1979; Rogolsky, 1979). However, a brief summary will be presented here which emphasizes some of the more recent work. An early indication of the importance of membrane lipids in toxin–membrane interactions came from the demonstration of Weissmann *et al.* (1966) that α-toxin (probably contaminated with δ-lysin) disrupted liposomes composed of lecithin: cholesterol and dicetyl phosphate. This observation was confirmed and the work extended by Freer *et al.* (1968) using α-toxin of greater purity than previously used. They showed that disruption of liposomes was accompanied by a loss of hemolytic activity as was the interaction with erythrocyte ghosts. On both toxin-treated liposome and erythrocyte membranes, there appeared a large number of small (10 nm diameter) ring-structures identical in appearance to the inactive polymeric form of the toxin, (α 12S) which is usually present in low concentrations along with active monomeric toxin (α 3S) in purified toxin preparations (Arbuthnott *et al.*, 1967). They concluded that polymer formation was probably promoted by accumulation of toxin in a specific orientation at the membrane surface, a process akin to surface denaturation, and since confirmed by Lo and Fackrell (1979). In the same study it was shown that α-toxin was surface-active and could penetrate mixed lipid films of 17 mN m^{-1} (dynes cm^{-1}) but not 34 mN m^{-1}. The preparation was accompanied by an increase in surface pressure of about 10 mN m^{-1} and an increase in surface potential, suggesting hydrophobic interaction as a mechanism for penetration. Later work by Demel *et al.* (1975) provided circumstantial evidence that the surface pressure in the lipid bilayer regions of intact human erythrocyte membranes may be in the region of 31–34 mN m^{-1}. Taken together with the results of Freer *et al.* (1968), this figure for surface pressure may partly explain why human erythrocytes are relatively low in sensitivity to lysis by α-toxin. Alpha-toxin is surface-active as measured by ability to penetrate mixed lipid films (Freer *et al.*, 1968; Colacicco and Buckelew, 1971), ability to form protein films at an air–water interface in the absence of lipid (Colacicco and Buckelew, 1971) and ability to release marker molecules from liposomes (Freer *et al.*, 1968). At relatively high toxin: membrane ratios, it causes changes in the hydrophobic domain of the erythrocyte membrane (Freer *et al.*, 1973) identical to the changes induced by treatment of erythrocytes ghosts with phospholipase A (Speth *et al.*, 1972). The raised 'plaques' in the fracture plane were thought to arise by deviation of the fracture between closely adherent membranes, induced by the penetration of protein (either α-toxin or phospholipase A) into the hydrophobic domain. Prolonged treatment of erythrocyte membrane with α-toxin resulted in a predominance of cross fractures and destruction of the hydrophobic fracture planes in the membrane. Additional evidence of the high affinity of α-toxin for amphiphilic substrates comes from the data of Bhakdi *et al.* (1981), who demonstrated a deoxycholate-induced transition of the hydrophilic toxin monomer to the amphiphilic hexameric ring form of the toxin. This transition was specific for deoxycholate and did not occur after interaction with either Triton X-100 or with synthetic lysolecithin analogues. Moreover, it occurred only when deoxycholate was present above the critical micellar concentration. In a more comprehensive study (Fussle *et al.*, 1981), this ring form of the toxin (MW = 200,000) was the only one present on toxin-treated erythrocyte membranes and was characterized by electron microscopy as a short cylindrical structure of approximately 10 nm outer diameter, in agreement with the earlier report by Freer *et al.*, (1968). The isolated membrane-derived toxin hexamer consisted of a single protein species of MW = 34,000. The amphiphilic nature of the membrane-derived rings was evident by their ability to bind detergent, to integrate into bilayers of phospholipids, and to release sequestered markers from resealed erythrocyte ghosts in a manner which demonstrated their capacity to discriminate differences in molecular size. From the results of this detailed investigation, it was concluded that the primary membrane lesion was most likely to be a transmembrane pore, formed as a consequence of the integration of the membrane-induced hexameric ring form of the toxin into the lipid bilayer of the membrane.

Although the precise mode of action of staphylococcal α-toxin in cytolysis is still unknown, there are several areas of general agreement regarding its action on natural and artificial membranes which can be summarized as follows:

1. Binding of toxin to membranes is a separate event from the formation of functional lesions (Barei and Fackrell, 1979).
2. Cytolysis can be delayed by hypertonic buffers, by low temperature or by low levels of Zn^{2+} (Avigad and Bernheimer, 1978).
3. The toxin has pronounced surface activity, forms thick solid films at the air–water interface, penetrates mixed lipid monolayers and releases sequestered markers from liposomes.
4. At high concentrations ($10-100 \, \mu g \, ml^{-1}$) the toxin forms hexameric ring structures on erythrocyte ghosts or liposomes.
5. The specificity of the toxin for certain membranes does not solely depend on lipid composition of the membrane.

2.5.4. *Interaction of Alpha-Toxin with Rabbit Erythrocytes*

A question which has preoccupied investigators for some years involves the basis for the relatively high sensitivity of rabbit erythrocytes to lysis by the α-toxin.

Cassidy and Harshman (1976a,b,c) used [^{125}I]-labeled α-toxin in a series of studies investigating the binding characteristics and hemolytic activity of radiolabeled toxin. A fortuitous observation was that monoiodinated α-toxin lost about 90 per cent of its hemolytic activity due to iodination of a single reactive tyrosine but retained its binding activity to rabbit erythrocytes. Iodination with two iodine atoms per molecule (maximum possible) abolished both binding and hemolytic activities, thus confirming earlier suggestions that binding and hemolysis are separate events.

Using monoiodinated toxin, they showed that human erythrocytes bound only 1 per cent of the toxin bound by rabbit erythrocytes. Further, they showed that binding of [^{125}I]-toxin to rabbit erythrocytes could be blocked by native toxin suggesting the presence of high specificity toxin receptors on the rabbit erythrocyte membrane. The rate and extent of binding were temperature dependent. A suggested sequence of events leading to cell damage was:

1. A relatively rapid time dependent binding of free α-toxin;
2. a slower, time dependent induction of foci of membrane damage, leading to K^+ (^{86}Rb) release;
3. eventual osmotic lysis of the cells with hemoglobin release.

Using [^{125}I]-monoiodinated toxin Cassidy and Harshman (1979) also described the isolation by sucrose density gradient centrifugation, of a 12S-Triton extractable toxin–receptor complex, molecular weight 10^6, from toxin-treated rabbit erythrocytes. The high molecular weight component was temperature sensitive and treatment with SDS at 100°C resulted in all the radioactivity comigrating with native toxin. Cassidy and Harshman (1979) suggested that the high MW complex represents a hexameric or dodecameric complex of toxin and receptor molecules.

Triton-X100 extract of α-lysin treated rabbit vagus nerve also yielded a 12S complex on gradient centrifugation. This complex was much less stable than that from the treated rabbit erythrocytes, extraction only being possible if done at $0°C$ (Szmigielski and Harshman, 1978). There is now agreement from several laboratories that the 'specific' receptor of rabbit erythrocytes is sensitive to pronase digestion (Kato et al., 1975b; Cassidy and Harshman, 1976c; Maharaj and Fackrell, 1980), which correlates with the sensitivity of the erythrocyte glycoprotein, band 3, recently suggested as being the specific receptor for α-toxin (Maharaj and Fackrell, 1980). However, the reported sensitivity of the high affinity α-toxin receptor of rabbit erythrocytes to trypsin argues against band 3 as the only receptor molecule involved (Kato et al., 1975b).

A paradoxical finding of Cassidy and Harshman (1979) was that antiserum to whole human erythrocytes precipitated the toxin–receptor complex extracted from rabbit erythrocytes yet human erythrocytes totally lacked the high affinity toxin receptors. The ubiquity of the postulated receptor band 3 minor glycoprotein (Maharaj and Fackrell, 1980), may explain the cross-reaction but necessitates the proviso that either band 3 in the human erythrocyte is not accessible to α-toxin (yet is still effective as a surface antigen) or that human erythrocyte band 3 has lost its toxin-binding site yet retained its immunological cross-reactivity with rabbit erythrocyte band 3. To complicate matters further, Bernheimer and Avigad (1980) recently reported that hemolysis of rabbit erythrocytes by a wide variety of cytolytic agents, including staphylococcal α-toxin, was inhibited strongly by the presence of purified glycophorin from human erythrocytes. They reported that amphiphilic structure, basicity and low molecular weight were the properties, together or singly, which correlated best with sensitivity to inhibition by glycophorin. They postulated that hydrophobic interactions between toxin and glycophorin as well as ionic interactions may account for loss of toxin hemolytic activity. Cassidy and Harshman (1979) also investigated the binding of iodinated lysin to mouse tissue in vivo and in vitro. The 12S toxin–receptor complex was detected only in skeletal muscle when labelled toxin was administered into live mice. However, in vitro the 12S peak material was recovered from toxin treated mouse diaphragm. In this instance, binding was shown to be 'nonspecific' since it was not reduced by the presence of an excess of unlabeled α-toxin. This type of binding was also found by Phimister and Freer (1984) using iodinated α-toxin which retained full hemolytic activity after iodination, in contrast to the iodinated toxin of both Cassidy and Harshman (1976a, b) and Kato et al. (1977). They found binding to be nonspecific to both rabbit and horse erythrocytes and that binding was not affected by the presence of concanavalin A, contrasting with the results of Cassidy and Harshman (1976a, b) and Kato et al. (1977) and more recently, those of Maharaj and Fackrell (1980).

While there is increasing evidence in favor of the presence of high affinity protein or glycoprotein receptors on rabbit erythrocytes, Maharaj and Fackrell (1980) proposed that two different binding mechanisms, specific and nonspecific, were involved in toxin/membrane interactions in order to account for the considerable sensitivity to α-toxin-induced hemolysis of species which apparently lack high affinity receptors on their membranes. Nonspecific 'hydrophobic' binding by toxin was also recognized by Cassidy and Harshman (1976c), who showed that binding of α-toxin to rabbit erythrocytes was reversed by chaotropic salts, the extent of inhibition of binding following the chaotropic series.

Further confusion was added by the results of Kato and Naiki (1976), who showed that binding of radiolabeled α-toxin to rabbit erythrocytes was inhibited by an N-acetyl glucosamine-containing ganglioside isolated from human (sic) erythrocytes. Manifestations of the surface activity of α-toxin are probably reflected in recent reports by Cassidy et al. (1978) of smooth muscle being 'functionally skinned' by α-toxin and also that it acts as a very effective demyelinating agent.

It is clear from the above considerations and contradictions on the binding properties of this toxin that more work is required to resolve the structure–function relationships of this molecule. The way is now open for investigation of specificity of interaction of the toxin with putative receptor molecules such as band 3 glycoprotein, glycophorin or gangliosides incorporated into defined lipid environments in liposomes. Until these definitive experiments are done, it is unlikely that the conflicting reports on the binding properties of this lysin to erythrocytes will be resolved.

2.5.5. α-toxin 'in vivo'

Knowledge of the chemical and biological properties of α-toxin and its effect on mammalian cells provides certain clues as to its involvement in pathogenic mechanisms. Such studies, however, can be criticized on the grounds that *in vitro* effects may bear little relation to the situation that exists within a focus of infection *in vivo*. Using experimental animal model systems, we have attempted to assess the *in vivo* role of α-toxin in pathogenesis.

A direct relationship between virulence and inhibition of weight gain in neonatal mice has been demonstrated (Kinsman and Arbuthnott, 1980). Alpha-toxin deficient mutants of *S. aureus* do not inhibit weight gain to the same extent as the parent strain in the newborn mouse model (Kinsman *et al.*, 1980). This suggests that α-toxin may be an important virulence factor of *S. aureus*.

Convincing evidence for the role of α-toxin also came from the studies of experimental rabbit mastitis by Adlam *et al.* (1977). They showed that the introduction of low numbers of certain strains into mammary tissue caused a spreading lesion in which the mammary tissue became oedematous and haemorrhagic while other strains induced the formation of pus-filled abscesses. In rabbits immunized with highly purified α-toxin the lethal, haemorrhagic, oedematous form of the disease was reduced to a localized abscess form indicating that α-toxin is a prime factor in the initiation and spread of the haemorrhagic type of lesion.

Day *et al.* (1980) have looked at the host response to strain Wood 46, an α-toxinogenic strain, using a chamber system *in vivo*. Chambers, constructed from short lengths of plastic syringe barrels, are filled with suspensions of staphylococci and sealed at both ends with membrane filters; these are implanted intraperitoneally in mice or rabbits. Using this system, it was noted that the chambers became encased with fibrin and granulation tissue between two to six days after implantation. Strain Wood 46 induced the accumulation of more capsulation material than *S. epidermidis* (AW 269) but less than strain SM9, a strain which produces leucocidin but not α- or β-toxins. The production of membrane damaging toxins, chemotactic factors and/or coagulase could therefore influence the amount of granulation tissue formed *in vivo*. That α-toxin is produced in such a system and diffuses from the chamber was shown by following the increase in anti α-toxin titre following implantation of strain Wood 46. In rabbits, serum levels of antitoxin began to rise 10 days after implantation and reached a maximum at 24–28 days. The response was slower in mice, beginning at 18 days and reaching a maximum at about 28 days (Day, 1983). This type of approach which allows both the study of the growth of staphylococci *in vivo* and the response of the host to the production of virulence factors, is likely to play an important part in elucidating the role of membrane-damaging toxins in disease.

3. STAPHYLOCOCCAL BETA-TOXIN (LYSIN)

3.1. Description

Staphylococcal β-lysin (β-toxin) was first described as a toxin serologically distinct from the α-toxin by Glenny and Stevens (1935). They showed that the so-called β-toxin contrasted with the α-toxin in being hemolytic for sheep erythrocytes but not for rabbit erythrocytes, nondermonecrotizing in guinea-pig skin and nonlethal for mice. They also noted that the hemolytic effect of β-toxin was greatly intensified by chilling the toxin-treated erythrocytes below 10°C after incubation at 37°C, a phenomenon reported in earlier studies (the hot–cold effect) on undefined staphylococcal 'hemolysin' by Walbum (1921) and Bigger *et al.* (1927). The undefined hemolysin studied by both these groups was almost certainly a mixture containing both α- and β-toxins and possibly others. Beta-toxin is produced predominantly by bovine strains of *S. aureus* and bovine and ovine erythrocytes are highly susceptible to its hemolytic action, whereas those of rat, guinea-pig, ferret and koala are resistant (Bryce and

Rountree, 1936). Human erythrocytes are sensitive, but less so than those of sheep or cow. A predominance of β-toxin producing strains in animal isolates was also noted by Elek and Levy (1950) and strains isolated from cases of bovine mastitis were predominantly beta producers (Slanetz and Bartley, 1953). The toxin is an immunogenic extracellular protein, with a molecular weight of approximately 30,000 and a pI in the region of 9.0–9.5. It is a phospholipase C with a substrate range restricted to sphingomyelin and lysophosphatidyl choline (EC 3.1.4.12.), requiring Mg^{2+} for activity. Susceptibility of erythrocytes to lysis by β-lysin correlates with membrane sphingomyelin content, those of sheep, ox and goat being highly sensitive. Full manifestation of toxin-induced membrane damage in susceptible erythrocytes is seen only after treated cells are chilled (the 'hot–cold' effect), when lysis follows rapidly. The lethality of the toxin for laboratory animals is equivocal, but it is reported to be cytotoxic for a variety of mammalian cell types *in vitro*.

3.2. Production of Staphylococcal Beta-Lysin

Previous work on the conditions used for production of β-lysin has been comprehensively reviewed by Wiseman (1975) and by Jeljaszewicz (1972). Its production is enhanced by growth of the producer strain in an atmosphere of 10–25% (v/v) CO_2 in air, but this requirement for increased CO_2 tension can be obviated by using a yeast diffusate medium as is the case for optimum production of staphylococcal α-toxin (Wadström and Möllby, 1971a; Bernheimer *et al.*, 1974).

Using the basal salts medium of Gladstone (1938), Wiseman (1970) reported an absolute requirement for proline, arginine and glycine for growth and toxin production. Toxin titers were reduced when either valine or a mixture of cysteine and methionine were omitted from the complete medium. Full growth and toxin production required the presence of both cysteine and methionine; omission of aspartic and glutamic acids had little effect on growth but reduced the level of toxin produced. The growth factors thiamine and nicotinamide were essential for both growth and toxin production, whereas the addition of free fatty acids to the medium increased the rate of growth without increasing levels of toxin (Fritsche and Zitz, 1973). Bernheimer *et al.* (1974), using a yeast diffusate medium and strain G-128, estimated that as much as 8 mg of β-toxin were produced per liter of culture, with possible yields of purified toxin in the region of $1–2\,mg\,l^{-1}$ of culture fluid. Toxin is produced at the maximal rate at neutral pH during early exponential growth (Wiseman, 1970) and reaches maximum concentration at the end of exponential growth (Low and Freer, 1977a).

3.3. Purification of Staphylococcal Beta-Lysin

Table 3 summarizes the strains used and the purification procedures of earlier studies. Those involving an ion-exchange chromatography step usually give rise to a considerable degree of activation of the lysin. This phenomenon was noted by several groups (Haque and Baldwin, 1969; Wadström and Möllby, 1971a; Low and Freer, 1977a); as an example of this phenomenon, Low and Freer reported a 3000 per cent 'recovery' of hemolytic activity and an apparent 23,000-fold purification at the ion-exchange step in their procedure. This activation is thought to result from removal of an inhibitor at this stage in the procedure.

Several groups have reported hemolytic activity against sheep erythrocytes being separable into two main protein peaks, one anionic and one cationic, after ion-exchange fractionation, (Haque and Baldwin, 1969; Wadström and Möllby, 1971a; Maheswaran *et al.*, 1967; Low and Freer, 1977a). The majority of the hemolytic activity against sheep erythrocytes is associated with the cationic peak, the anionic one probably containing β-lysin bound to acidic material as well as other contaminating staphylococcal hemolysins active against sheep erythrocytes at 37°C. This second impure peak may partly explain the origins of the two different antigenic forms of β-toxin found by Chesbro *et al.* (1965), Doery *et al.* (1965) and Wiseman and Caird (1967).

Like the α-toxin of *S. aureus*, β-lysin also gives several different forms, some of which show reduced specific activity after isoelectric focusing in columns. Their significance is unclear,

TABLE 3. *Purification of Staphylococcal Beta-Lysin*

Reference	Strain	Procedures*	Specific activity hemolytic units mg^{-1} protein
Robinson et al. (1958)	L16	A, C, A, D	
Jackson (1963)	J32A	A, A, C	
Chesbro et al. (1965)	UNH-Donita	C	6×10^4
Doery et al. (1965)	1061-17	A, A, C	3.7×10^4
Wiseman (1965)	R-1, 252F	C, A	1.2×10^6
Maheswaran et al. (1967)	J19	A, B, C, C	6.8×10^4
Wiseman & Caird (1967)	R-1, 252F	C, A, C	
Gow & Robinson (1969)	MB534	A, B, C, D†	5.2×10^8
Haque & Baldwin (1969)	681	A, C	6.6×10^6
Wadström & Möllby (1971a)	R-1	C, E, B	$10^7 - 10^8$ (2 IU mg^{-1})‡
Colley et al. (1973)		A, B	(1 IU/20 μl)
Bernheimer et al. (1974)	G-128, R-1, 234	A, B, E	4.7×10^5 (140 IU mg^{-1})
Zwaal et al. (1975)	269HH	A, B, C, C	(1900 IU mg^{-1})
Low & Freer (1977a)	G-128	A, B, C, E	6.3×10^7 (312 IU mg^{-1})

*A, precipitation; B, Gel filtration (molecular sieve); C, ion exchange chromatography; D, electrophoresis (starch block); E, isoelectric focusing.
†Electrophoresis (sucrose gradient).
‡Figures in brackets indicate specific activity of sphingomyelinase in International Units (IU) mg^{-1}.

and a study of the variety of charged forms which result after use of different procedures involving both column and flat bed electrofocusing in toxin purification would help to resolve this question.

3.4. PHYSICOCHEMICAL PROPERTIES OF STAPHYLOCOCCAL BETA-LYSIN

3.4.1. *Molecular Weight and Isoelectric Point*

The relatively low yields after purification and instability of purified β-toxin probably explains the paucity of data on physicochemical properties of this lysin. Table 4 summarizes those properties which have been reported.

Beta-lysin is a protein, but reported values for molecular weight are not consistent, nor do they correlate with reported sedimentation coefficients. More highly purified preparations of toxin, which have resulted from improved purification procedures used in the last decade, in combination with more rigorous definitions of purity, generally have reported molecular weights in the region of 30,000 and pI values for the major components of 9–9.5. The molecular weight of 33,000 reported by Low and Freer (1977a) is in keeping with their value for the sedimentation coefficient of 3.1.

3.4.2. *Amino Acid Composition*

Reports of the amino acid composition of β-lysin from two laboratories show overall similarities but by no means identity (Fackrell and Wiseman, 1976b; Bernheimer et al., 1974). Notable differences are the absence of proline and methionine and the presence of cysteine in Fackrell's toxin compared with that of Bernheimer. The exact significance of these differences is not clear, especially since the lysin preparations from the two different strains used in these studies behave identically on analysis by polyacrylamide gel electrophoresis (Bernheimer et al., 1974).

It is perhaps more than coincidence that the similarity between amino acid composition of β-toxin and that reported for staphylococcal α-toxin (Six and Harshman, 1973b) is closer than the two independent reports for β-lysin (see Table 5). This degree of similarity in composition between two extracellular proteins of the same organism may suggest extensive homology and conservation in certain peptide sequences in the two molecules. Other similar properties are their molecular weights in the region of 30,000 and their pI values of 9.0–9.5.

Table 4. *Properties of Purified Staphylococcal Beta-Lysin*

Reference	Strain of organism	Molecular weight†	Sedimentation coefficient ($S_{20,w}$)	Isoelectric point (pI)	Specific hemolytic activity (hemolytic activity mg⁻¹ protein)‡
Robinson et al. (1958)	L16	—*	—	—	—
Jackson (1963)	J32A	—	—	—	—
Chesbro et al. (1965)	UNH-Donita	59,000[u]	—	8.6–8.9	6×10^4
Doery et al. (1965)	1061–17	—	—	—	3.7×10^4
Wiseman (1965)	R1-252F	—	—	—	1.2×10^4
Maheswaran et al. (1967)	J19	—	—	9.5	6.8×10^4
Wiseman & Caird (1967)	R1-252F	—	—	—	—
Gow & Robinson (1969)	MB534	—	1.7	—	5.2×10^8
Haque & Baldwin (1969)	681	—	—	—	6.6×10^6
Wadström & Möllby (1971a)	R-1	38,000[f]; 33,000[f] 15,500[u,f]	—	9.4	10^7–10^8 (2 IU mg⁻¹)
Chesbro & Kucic (1971)	UNH-15	15,000[u]; 13,800[f]	—	—	—
	243-B1	13,600[u]; 11,000[f]	—	—	—
	243-B2	—	—	—	—
Bernheimer et al. (1974)	G-128; R-1; 234	30,000[e]; 29,000[e] 29,000[e]	—	9.0	4.7×10^5 (140 IU mg⁻¹)
Zwaal et al. (1975)	**269HH**	—	—	—	(1900 IU mg⁻¹)
Fackrell & Wiseman (1976b)		26,000[f]; 16,000[a]	1.8	9.5	—
Low & Freer (1977a)	G-128	33,000[e]; 32,500[f]	3.1	9.3; 9.7	6.2×10^7 (312 IU mg⁻¹)

*Not reported.

†MW determined by: u, ultracentrifugation; f, gel filtration; e, sodium dodecyl sulfate polyacrylamide gel electrophoresis; a, amino acid analysis.

‡Figures in brackets refer to specific activity of sphingomyelinase in International Units mg⁻¹.

TABLE 5. *Comparison of Amino Acid Composition of Beta-Lysin and Alpha-Lysin of* S. aureus.

Amino acid	Number of residues		
	α-Toxin B (Six & Harshman 1973b)*	β-Lysin (Bernheimer *et al.* 1974)†	β-Lysin (Fackrell 1973)‡
Aspartic acid	43	44	44
Threonine	23	14	17
Serine	19	23	33
Glutamic acid	20	25	38
Proline	9	10	0
Glycine	24	21	39
Alanine	11	12	25
Valine	14	12	18
Cystine/Cysteine	0	0	4
Methionine	6	4	0
Isoleucine	14	9	17
Leucine	14	12	20
Tyrosine	10	14	1
Phenylalanine	8	8	13
Lysine	23	28	33
Histidine	4	8	8
Tryptophan	4	6	
Arginine	8	6	13
Ammonia			143

*Histidine set at 4 in original data.
†Methionine set at 4.
‡Histidine set at 8.

3.4.3. *Stability of Staphylococcal Beta-Lysin*

A notable feature of β-lysin is its marked instability which increases as purification proceeds. Wadström and Möllby (1971a) reported that their crude lysin had a half-life of 120 days at $-20°C$, but in the highly purified form the half-life fell to 1–2 days at $-20°C$. Zwaal *et al.* (1975) retained high specific activity in their preparations by storage of the enzyme in 50% (v/v) glycerol.

3.4.4. *Enzyme Activity of Staphylococcal Beta-Lysin*

Following the initial observation of Jackson and Mayman (1958) that β-lysin was activated by divalent metal ions, it was first shown to have phospholipase C activity by Doery *et al.*, (1963), who demonstrated release of water-soluble phosphorus (phosphorylcholine) from both sheep and rabbit red cell stromata. They further showed that the lysin was an enzyme with a substrate range limited to sphingomyelin and lyso-phosphatidylcholine and that its activity was inhibited by commercial antitoxin containing anti β-toxin activity. The suggested degradation sequence is as follows:

$$\text{Sphingomyelin} + \text{water} \xrightarrow[\text{Mg}^{2+}]{\beta\text{-lysin}} N\text{-acyl sphingosine} + \text{phosphorylcholine}$$

Loss of sphingomyelin from phospholipid extracts was shown by thin layer chromatography and the appearance of water soluble phosphorus was demonstrated in the supernatant fluid. These observations have since been confirmed by numerous investigators and the enzyme activity of β-toxin is defined as:

Sphingomyelin cholinephosphohydrolase, EC 3.1.4.12.

The requirement for Mg^{2+} can be replaced by Co^{2+}, but Ca^{2+} acts as an inhibitor of this enzyme. The phospholipase activity and hemolytic spectrum of β-lysin was the subject of detailed investigations by Wiseman and Caird (1967), who confirmed the earlier findings of Doery *et al.* (1963, 1965) that the enzymic activity of the lysin was restricted to sphingomyelin and lysophosphatidylcholine. They reported no hydrolytic activity against aqueous dispersions of phosphatidylethanolamine, phosphatidylcholine or the phosphate esters in RNA, β-glycerophosphate and phenyl phosphate. Differences in susceptibility of erythrocytes from different mammalian species to lysis by β-toxin was explained by showing that there was a close correlation between sphingomyelin content of the membranes and lytic sensitivity. This was later supported by the work of Wadström and Möllby (1971b) and Bernheimer et al. (1974), who showed that sheep, ox and goat erythrocytes, which contained greater than 40% sphingomyelin in the membrane lipids, were more sensitive to lysis by several orders of magnitude than human erythrocytes (see Table 6). Colley et al. (1973) determined the level of sphingomyelin hydrolysis in erythrocytes from different mammalian species (Table 7) and showed that approximately 50 per cent of the sphingomyelin in ovine and bovine erythrocytes was degraded by β-lysin. These cells contain approximately 50 per cent of the membrane lipid as sphingomyelin. In contrast, human erythrocytes which are less sensitive to hemolysis by β-lysin contain approximately 25 per cent of their membrane phospholipid as sphingomyelin. In these cells, β-toxin degraded 77 per cent of the sphingomyelin. Thus, the degradation of a high percentage of the membrane sphingomyelin does not necessarily lead to lysis. Lysis appears to depend on the percentage of *total* membrane phospholipid which is hydrolyzed. In all cases examined there is a fraction of membrane sphingomyelin which is not degradable even when membranes are present as ghosts. This may reflect sphingomyelin being in at least two different modes of association in the membrane, one fraction being tightly bound to other membrane constituents and not available for hydrolysis by exogenous enzyme. A further factor suggested by Low and Freer (1977b) may involve progressive loss of membrane surface charge as sphingomyelin degradation proceeds, which may alter both binding of lysin and also available levels of membrane associated Mg^{2+} ions.

3.4.5. The 'Hot–Cold' Effect in Hemolysis

One of the most unusual features of β-lysin is the phenomenon of 'hot–cold' hemolysis. Incubation at 37°C of sensitive erythrocytes with small quantities of β-lysin in the presence of Mg^{2+} results in little or no lysis, but if the treated erythrocytes are then chilled to below 10°C, rapid lysis follows (Smyth et al., 1975).

A knowledge of the distribution of phospholipid types in the bilayer of the erythrocyte membrane (Bretscher, 1972; Casu et al., 1969; Zwaal et al., 1973) together with information from light microscope and ultrastructural studies of β-toxin-treated erythrocytes and erythrocyte ghosts, permit the formulation of a working hypothesis to account for changes in the membrane resulting in hot–cold hemolysis. There is considerable evidence suggesting that the choline-containing phospholipids are located in the external leaflet of the membrane lipid bilayer. Hydrolysis of sphingomyelin in ghost membranes is accompanied by shrinkage

TABLE 6. *Sensitivity of Erythrocytes from Different Animals to Lysis by Purified Beta-Lysin*

	'Hot–cold' hemolytic titer (HU ml^{-1})*	% Phospholipid as sphingomyelin†
Sheep	10^9	51.0
Ox	10^8	46.2
Goat	10^5	45.9
Rabbit	10^2	19.0
Pig	10	26.5
Cat	10	26.1
Chicken	10	22.7[a]
Fowl	10	21.4[b]
Human	10	20.1
Horse	10	13.5
Guinea-pig	10	11.1

*From Wadström & Möllby (1971b).
†From Rouser et al. (1968), *except* [a]Kleinig et al. (1971) and [b]Kates & James (1961).

TABLE. 7. *Hydrolysis of Sphingomyelin in Different Erythrocytes by Staphylococcal β-Toxin*

Erythrocyte type	Sph. as % membrane phospholipid	Sph:PC ratio in membrane	% Sph. hydrolysis by β-toxin	% Total phospholipid hydrolysed by β-toxin
Man	26	0.8	77	20
Pig	21.4	0.8	75	16
Ox	44.8	15	50	23
Sheep	50	23	48	29

Sph = Sphingomyelin; PC = phosphatidyl choline.

of the membrane and the appearance of phase-dense droplets; numerous internal membrane vesicles are also formed (Low *et al.*, 1974; Bernheimer *et al.*, 1974). In addition Low and Freer (1977b), studying intact β-lysin-treated erythrocytes by phase contrast optics, found that phase dense droplets appeared on cooling. They suggested that at temperatures of about 20°C, the cohesive forces of the intact erythrocyte membrane are sufficient to hold the hydrolysis product of β-toxin, ceramide, in position in the membranes, with Mg^{2+} ions possibly preventing collapse of the weakened bilayer. On cooling, a phase separation occurs with condensation of ceramide into large pools and the collapse of the bilayer follows rapidly.

3.5. Biological Activities of Staphylococcal Beta-Lysin

3.5.1. *Lethality*

In contrast to the relatively well defined activity of β-lysin on membranes and phospholipid dispersions, its toxicity for laboratory animals is still in doubt (for review of earlier work see Wiseman, 1975). Low and Freer (1977b) found that highly purified β-lysin injected intravenously was nontoxic for mice up to the highest dose tested (150 μg, i.e. 7.14 mg kg^{-1} body tissue). Doses up to this level had no detrimental effect on weight gain and intradermal injection did not result in formation of any lesion or evidence of increased vascular permeability. Earlier reports on toxicity for laboratory animals are conflicting. Heydrick and Chesbro (1962) claimed that the toxin was lethal for guinea-pigs by intraperitoneal injection if Mg^{2+} was injected along with the toxin and Gow and Robinson (1969) reported that β-lysin was lethal for rabbits at doses of 40–60 μg. Also Wadström and Möllby (1971b, 1972) reported lethality for mice, rabbits, guinea-pigs (LD_{50} 0.25–10 μg) although at relatively high doses. In retrospect, it is impossible to assess the absolute contribution that small amounts of contamination with α-toxin had on these early tests, but there is no doubt that it was significant.

3.5.2. *Role of Beta-Lysin in Staphylococcal Pathogenesis*

Finally, the role of staphylococcal β-lysin in the pathogenesis of staphylococcal disease is poorly understood. If it can be considered as a lethal toxin at all, then it is considerably less potent than the α-toxin. There is no convincing evidence that β-lysin alone plays an important role in staphylococcal pathogenicity (Adlam *et al.*, 1977; Ward *et al.*, 1979). However, it may play a significant part in the potentiation of the effects of other staphylococcal toxins produced concurrently.

4. STAPHYLOCOCCAL GAMMA-TOXIN (LYSIN)

4.1. Description

The existence of staphylococcal γ-lysin was first suggested as early as 1938 by Smith and Price, yet it remained virtually undefined until the studies of Plommet and colleagues gave details for its successful production and purification in workable yields from strain Smith 5R

(Plommet and Bouillanne, 1966; Guyonnet, *et al.*, 1968; Guyonnet and Plommet, 1970; Bezard and Plommet, 1973).

Serological evidence suggests that it is produced commonly *in vivo* in bone lesions caused by *S. aureus*. It is immunogenic, cytolytic and cytotoxic and can be resolved into two components, I and II, which act synergistically to give toxic and hemolytic activity. Molecular weights of 29,000 and 26,000 and pI values of 9.8 and 9.9 have been reported for components I and II, respectively. Its activity, which is normally assessed by hemolysis of rabbit erythrocytes, is inhibited by sulfonated polymers such as agar and dextran sulfate.

4.2. PRODUCTION OF STAPHYLOCOCCAL GAMMA-LYSIN

No systematic studies have been done to determine factors which control the production of γ-toxin by staphylococci. Recent studies have utilized strain Smith 5R for toxin production in yeast diffusate–casein hydrolysate (CCY) medium (Guyonnet and Plommet, 1970; Plommet and Bouillane, 1966; Möllby and Wadström, 1971; Taylor and Bernheimer, 1974), often with an atmosphere of 80% (v/v) oxygen, 20% CO_2 (v/v). Fackrell and Wiseman (1976a) preferred a cellophane overlay method first used by Jackson (1963) for growth and toxin production, again using strain Smith 5R grown in an atmosphere of 10% (v/v) CO_2 in air, which was optimal for toxin production. This technique obviates the necessity for forced aeration, found by Möllby and Wadström (1971), to lower the titers of toxin in liquid cultures. The pH optimum for toxin production lies between 6 and 8, and toxin is produced, like α-toxin, in late exponential phase of growth, with comparatively small amounts being cell-associated. The importance of selecting rough hemolytic colonies and passaging them on sheep-blood–agar prior to the preparation of the inoculum for batch liquid culture was emphasized by Bezard and Plommet (1973) as an essential prerequisite for good toxin yields.

Because of the inhibition of gamma hemolytic activity by agar, surveys of staphylococcal isolates do not usually include specific screening for γ-toxin production. Hence there is a dearth of information on how widespread is the ability to produce γ-lysin among clinical isolates. Serological tests suggest that γ-toxin may be quite commonly produced by *S. aureus* strains isolated from clinical infections involving bone disease (Taylor *et al.*, 1975).

4.3. PURIFICATION AND CHARACTERIZATION OF STAPHYLOCOCCAL GAMMA-LYSIN

Purification methods for γ-lysin were reviewed in detail by Wiseman (1975) and more recently by Rogolsky (1979). The binding properties of hydroxylapatite were utilized by Guyonnet and Plommet (1970) to remove acidic pigmented material from the yeast extract diffusate before its incorporation into liquid medium used for toxin production. Gamma-lysin will bind to hydroxylapatite under conditions of low ionic strength (Guyonnet and Plommet, 1970; Bezard and Plommet, 1973) and utilizing this phenomenon, Plommet's group absorbed the lysin from culture supernatant fluids and succeeded in purifying it using a combination of hydroxylapatite chromatography and membrane ultrafiltration. Two distinct toxin components were recovered (γ_1 and γ_2) by elution with increasing ionic strength from a hydroxylapatite column. Each component was nonhemolytic alone, but both acted synergistically to give hemolytically active toxin. Taylor and Bernheimer (1974) confirmed these findings and went on to characterize their products further. Component I (γ_1) had a pI value of 9.8 and a molecular weight of 29,000, whereas component II (γ_2) had a pI value of 9.9 and a molecular weight of 26,000.

Möllby and Wadström (1971), using strain Smith 5R, failed to separate the toxin into two components when using isoelectric focusing on a broad gradient (pH 3–10) as a purification method. This is not surprising when the similarity in pI values of the two components is considered. Their product had a pI value of 9.5, a figure reasonably close to those reported by previous workers. In contrast, Fackrell and Wiseman (1976b), again using strain Smith 5R, but under different cultural conditions to those described above, used ultrafiltration and gel filtration chromatography to purify their toxin. The product, a single component, had a pI value of 6.0 and a molecular weight of 45,000, thus differing considerably from the toxins of both Taylor and Bernheimer (1974) and Möllby and Wadström (1971). This material had a sedimentation value of 2.6S and amino acid analysis gave low levels of methionine and histidine, while cysteine was completely absent.

Also in common with the α-and δ-lysins, their γ-lysin had high levels of aspartic acid and lysine. All the methionine was thought to be present as N-terminal residues.

At present, there appears to be general agreement on the following properties of γ-lysin:

(a) It is inactivated by agar and other sulfonated polymers.
(b) Hemolytic activity is inhibited by cholesterol and cholesterol esters.
(c) It is inactivated by heating at 60°C for 10 min.
(d) Both components are required for toxic and hemolytic activity.
(e) It preferentially lyses rabbit erythrocytes.
(f) It is inhibited by a variety of phospholipids and free fatty acids.
(g) It is antigenic.

4.4. BIOLOGICAL ACTIVITIES OF STAPHYLOCOCCAL GAMMA-LYSIN

4.4.1. Suggested Enzyme Activity

On circumstantial evidence, Fackrell and Wiseman (1976b) suggested that γ-lysin may have phospholipase activity. They reported the linear release of acid-soluble phosphorus and nitrogen from human erythrocyte membranes exposed to γ-lysin, but curiously, at different rates. In addition, the hemolytic activity of the toxin was sensitive to inhibition by EDTA, yet this was not relieved by the addition of up to 0.1 M Mg^{2+} or Ca^{2+} after removal of EDTA by dialysis. A requirement for Na^+ or K^+ ions was also reported for hemolytic activity.

No degradation of isolated membrane phospholipids by γ-lysin could be demonstrated, confirming the earlier observation of Taylor and Bernheimer (1974), nor was there any evidence of proteolytic activity. Since the work of Fackrell and Wiseman (1976b), there have been no further reports of enzymic activity.

4.4.2. Cell Damaging Activity

Cell-damaging activity at relatively high doses (700 HU ml^{-1}) was demonstrated *in vitro* in a study of the lytic effects of γ-lysin on human leucocytes (Fackrell and Wiseman, 1976b). A dose-related killing of C_6 cell line (human lymphoblasts) by γ-lysin, as assessed by dye exclusion, was also demonstrated in the same study. That relatively high doses of lysin were needed for cytopathic effect (200 HU ml^{-1}) was confirmed by Szmigielski *et al.* (1975), who studied the release of intracellular enzyme markers from rabbit polymorphs.

Gamma-lysin induced a similar pattern of release of lysosomal hydrolases from rabbit peritoneal granulocytes as did the α-toxin. Large amounts of acid phosphatase and lysozyme were released by both toxins, although more γ-lysin than α-toxin was required to induce the same level of damage. The lytic effect appeared to be relatively specific for lysosomes, since no appreciable release of catalase or alkaline phosphatase occurred, indicating the peroxisomes and specific granules were more resistant to these toxins.

The similarity in the type of membrane lesions induced by α-toxin and γ-lysin suggested by the study of Szmigielski *et al.* (1975) was confirmed by Thelestam and Möllby (1979), who studied the release patterns of different sized cytoplasmic markers from diploid human embryonic lung fibroblasts. Both α-toxin and γ-lysin caused the selective release of the smallest marker (α-amino isobutyric acid, MW = 103), although the high sensitivity of this assay system allowed differentiation of the two toxins on the basis of release of RNA label at high toxin concentrations. It was concluded that γ-lysin caused only subtle changes in membrane permeability, as evidenced by AIB leakage, and α-toxin caused small functional holes (∼0.5 nm diameter) in the membrane.

4.5. *In vivo* EFFECTS OF STAPHYLOCOCCAL GAMMA-LYSIN

The γ-lysin of Fackrell and Wiseman (1976b) was lethal for guinea-pigs when 50 μg was administered by intracardial injection, but had no effect on rabbits or mice under similar conditions. Guinea-pigs on autopsy showed massive haemorrhage of the kidneys and serosal surfaces of the intestines, with frank lysis in the major blood vessels.

In an earlier publication Wiseman (1975) reported that 100 μg of γ-lysin injected subcutaneously into rabbits or guinea-pigs was without effect. The same dose administered intraperitoneally to mice also appeared innocuous. This contrasts with the earlier report of Guyonnet (1970), who demonstrated the toxicity of γ-lysin for mice, and that of Wadström and Möllby (1972) who showed lethality in mice and rabbits. Some reservation is advisable when interpreting toxicity tests, since Guyonnet (1970) reported a lack of parallelism between hemolytic activity and toxicity when the ratios of two components of the toxin were varied.

Gamma-lysin production *in vitro* is common in human coagulase-positive strains (Jackson, 1963) and recent reports (Taylor and Plommet, 1973; Taylor *et al.*, 1975) show that elevated titers of antibodies to γ-lysin are present in patients with staphylococcal bone disease. Increased titers of anti-γ-toxin antibodies correlate closely with the establishment of experimentally induced staphylococcal osteomyelitis in rabbits (Kurek *et al.*, 1977). Evidence favoring a role for γ-toxin in staphylococcal bone disease is at best circumstantial; it does seem beyond doubt that γ-lysin is produced *in vivo* in staphylococcal bone lesions. As might be expected, in experimental infections there was no apparent correlation between the severity of the lesion and the increase in the anti-γ-toxin titer (Kurek *et al.*, 1977).

Gamma-lysin is one of the most poorly defined of the staphylococcal toxins, and more data is needed before any attempt can be made to define its mode of action and its significance in staphylococcal pathogenicity.

5. STAPHYLOCOCCAL DELTA-LYSIN (TOXIN)

5.1. DESCRIPTION

Delta-lysin (toxin) is produced by most (97%) pathogenic strains of coagulase-positive staphylococci (Elek, 1959; Jeljaszewicz, 1972), and a high proportion (50–70%) of coagulase-negative isolates (Gemmell *et al.*, 1976). Present evidence suggests that the lysins from these two groups of strains are immunologically identical whether they are from human sheep or rabbit origin, but that they are only partially cross-reactive with strains of canine origin (Turner and Pickard, 1979).

Delta-lysin is an immunogenic exoprotein consisting of 26 amino acid residues and has a molecular weight of 2,977 (Fackrell and Wiseman, 1974). Both acidic (pI 5.5) and basic (pI 9.5) forms occur after isoelectric focusing. The lysin has a wide spectrum of activity, affecting most cell types that have been tested, and is thought to damage cell membranes or membrane-bounded organelles by virtue of its surface activity. It is inactivated by phospholipids and normal serum showing common features with staphylococcal α-, γ- and leucocidal toxins. Specific hemolytic activity is relatively low when compared with the other staphylococcal lysins, but the range of activity is very broad, as would be expected of a surfactant.

The toxin is reported to be lethal for laboratory animals, but only at relatively high doses (10–100 mg). It causes erythema after intradermal injection into the rabbit, and results in increased vascular permeability.

5.2. PRODUCTION OF STAPHYLOCOCCAL DELTA-LYSIN

In the main, two methods have been commonly employed as a basis for production of δ-lysin, either the cellophane overlay method or the liquid shake culture in modifications of casein hydrolysate–yeast extract diffusate medium (for review see Wiseman, 1975). No definitive data are available on cultural conditions controlling δ-lysin production and release, although oxygen tension appears to be an important factor (Turner, 1978a).

5.3. PURIFICATION OF STAPHYLOCOCCAL DELTA-LYSIN

Several new methods for the purification of δ-lysin were published in the early seventies, two depending on the pronounced adsorption of the lysin to the inorganic matrices of alumina (Kantor *et al.*, 1972) or hydroxylapatite (Kreger *et al.*, 1971), and one utilizing the unusual differential solubility of the lysin in organic solvents of differing polarity (Heatley, 1971). The introduction of these relatively simple procedures helped to resolve some of the earlier conflicting reports on the properties of the lysin (Wiseman, 1970), which no doubt partly reflected the levels of different biologically-active products copurifying with the lysin. Using the method of Kreger *et al.*, (1971), but with an additional final isoelectric focusing step, Chao and Birkbeck (1978) produced lysin with a high hemolytic specificity towards fish erythrocytes, an assay which clearly distinguishes the hemolytic activity due to α, β- and δ-lysins.

5.4. PHYSICOCHEMICAL PROPERTIES OF STAPHYLOCOCCAL DELTA-LYSIN

5.4.1. *Molecular Weight and Isoelectric Point*

Chao and Birkbeck (1978) found that all the lytic activity against fish erythrocytes focused as a single component with a pI value of 4.5, close to the value reported by Kantor *et al.* (1972) for their lysin which was focused in the presence of low concentrations of Tween 80. Without Tween 80, three hemolytic peaks with pI values of 4.65, 6.7 and 9.0 were obtained, each containing approximately equal amounts of hemolytic activity.

Both Kreger *et al.* (1971) and Turner (1978b) reported anionic and cationic forms of lysin in their purified preparations (pI values of 5.0 and 9.5; 4.5 and 9.5 respectively), and in both instances refocusing of the cationic form yielded cationic and anionic lysin; refocusing of the anionic forms however, did not result in the appearance of further cationic lysin.

Recently, Fitton *et al.* (1980) reported the amino acid sequence of δ-lysin prepared by the Heatley method (Heatley, 1971) and stated that a pI value of 5.5 would be compatible with the proposed structure of the lysin where the amino terminus is *N*-formulated. The significance of the reported basic forms of the lysin is unclear, but they may partly reflect the methods used for determination of pI (column electrofocusing), where lysin is exposed to extremes of pH. Whatever their significance, it seems likely that both basic and acidic forms of the lysin have similar properties.

The most reliable value for minimum molecular weight of δ-lysin is 2,977, calculated from the recently published sequence of this 26 amino acid residue peptide from strain 168X (Fitton *et al.*, 1980). Minor variations at positions 10, 11, 17 and 18 are apparent in the sequence from toxin isolated from canine strains.

The widely different published values for molecular weight (5,000 to 7.4×10^8) of δ-lysin by different groups (see Table 8) almost certainly reflects various degrees of aggregation of the toxin, perhaps promoted in some instances by low levels of impurities (for review see Wiseman, 1975).

5.4.2. *Amino Acid Composition and Tertiary Structure*

From amino acid analyses and the demonstrated surface activity of δ-lysin, Bernheimer (1974) speculated that if the relatively large number of hydrophobic residues were localized in one region of the molecule, then this would result in amphipathic properties, similar to those previously demonstrated for melittin, the major amphipathic peptide from bee venom (see Fig. 2), and would add substantial weight to the postulated detergent-like mode of cytolysis proposed for this lysin. From the published amino acid sequence of δ-lysin (Fitton *et al.*, 1980) there appears to be no such concentration of hydrophobic residues in one region of the molecule, unlike melittin which is linearly amphipathic with residues 1–20 largely hydrophobic and 21–26 polar in properties (Fig. 2). Nevertheless, Fitton *et al.* (1980) conclude that when the sequence of the two molecules are compared and the common properties are taken into account, a common structural basis for their membrane-damaging action is likely.

TABLE 8. *Some Characteristics of Purified Staphylococcal Delta-Lysin*

References	Strain organism	Molecular weight	Sedimentation coefficient ($S_{20,w}$)	Isoelectric point (pI)	Specific hemolytic activity (units mg^{-1} protein or N)
Jackson & Little (1958)	1363, 2426, 2428, 2429	—*			3200
Yoshida (1963)	Foggie	68–150,000	6.1	—	120–400
Kayser & Raynaud (1965)	—	12,000	1.4; 5.5	—	—
Hallander (1968)	—	200,000		—	—
Caird & Wiseman (1970)	E-delta	200,000	2.8; 9.8	—	12,000
Maheswaran & Lindorfer (1970)	—	—		(i) 3.32 (ii) 3.75 (iii) 8.45	—
Möllby & Wadström (1970)	—	—		9.6	250–300
Heatley (1971)	186x†	—	4.9	—	
Kapral & Miller (1971)	PG114	—		—	400‡; 200§
Kreger et al. (1971)	Wood 46M¶	—	4.9; 11.9	(i) 9.5 (ii) 5.0	400‡; 200§
Kantor et al. (1972)	Wood 46M¶	103,000	6.04	(i) 4.65 (ii) 6.7 (iii) 9.0	75
Turner (1978b)	CN 4108 (Newman D2)	82,000	—	4.5; 9.5	150–200
	CN 7450	10,000	—	7.8	200
Fitton et al. (1980)	168x	2,977	—	—	—

*Not reported.
†Derived from Newman by subculture.
‡Insoluble δ-lysin.
§Soluble δ-lysin.
¶Derived from Wood 46 using u.v. irradiation.

	1	5	10	15	20	25

δ-lysin: H₃N-Met-Ala-Gln-Asp-Ile-Ile-Ser-Thr-Ile-Gly-Asp-Leu-Val-Lys-Trp-Ile-Ile-Asp-Thr-Val-Asn-Lys-Phe-Thr-Lys-Lys-COO

     (+)   (−)   (−)   (+)   (−)   (+)   (−) (−)(−)

                  (+)   (+) (+) (+) (+)

Melittin: (+)H₃N-Gly-Ile-Gly-Ala-Val-Leu-Lys-Val-Leu-Thr-Thr-Gly-Leu-Pro-Ala-Leu-Ile-Ser-Trp-Ile-Lys-Arg-Lys-Arg-Gln-Gln-CONH₂

	1	5	10	15	20	25

Fig. 2. Primary structure of staphylococcal δ-lysin and comparison with bee venom melittin. Groups likely to be charged at **pH 6.8 are indicated.** From Fitton *et al.* (1980).

It seems improbably, however, that δ-lysin will share common features of secondary structure with melittin, which is thought to insert into the membrane by a wedge-like mechanism (Dawson *et al.*, 1978). The distribution of charged residues in the two molecules is considerably different, as well as δ-lysin lacking a central proline residue, essential for the hinge of the melittin wedge. From the frequency of distribution of charged residues in the δ-lysin sequence, it is tempting to speculate that the lysin may form an α-helical structure with the charged residues resulting in a distinctly polar side to an otherwise hydrophobic rod (Freer and Birkbeck, 1982). Similar regular distributions of polar and nonpolar residues are found in the α-helical region of Braun's murein lipoprotein (Inouye, 1974).

5.4.3. *Stability of Staphylococcal Delta-Lysin*

One of the unique features of the lysin is its heat stability (Marks and Vaughan, 1950), the lysin losing less than half of its hemolytic activity after exposure to 90°C for 10 min (Kantor *et al.*, 1972). Additional features which characterize the lysin are its high surface activity, its solubility in chloroform: methanol (2:1) and its amino acid composition with the absence of proline, cysteine, histidine, arginine and tyrosine (Freer and Arbuthnott, 1976).

In common with staphylococcal α- and β-lysins, δ-lysin is inactivated by exposure to phospholipids. This is also reflected in its inactivation by normal human serum, here interacting with the phospholipid components of the α- and β-lipoproteins (Whitelaw and Birkbeck, 1978).

5.5. BIOLOGICAL ACTIVITIES OF STAPHYLOCOCCAL DELTA-LYSIN

5.5.1. *Cytolytic Activity*

The biological and physicochemical properties of δ-lysin are consistent with it being a surface-active agent. Highly purified toxin is cytolytic to a wide variety of membrane systems including bacterial protoplasts and spheroplasts, erythrocytes, tissue cultured cells, lysosomes and liposomes (Kreger *et al.*, 1971). Moreover, its action is characterized by a rapid rate of lysis and the absence of a lag phase (Wadström and Möllby, 1972; Thelestam *et al.*, 1973). For instance, the toxin had an instantaneous effect on the cell-membrane of human embryonic diploid lung fibroblasts as shown by the release of radioactively labeled nucleotides (MW < 1000). Within 2 min of addition of 0.5–1.0 hemolytic units of toxin to cells at 37°C, 70–80% of maximum release of nucleotides had occurred. Thelestam and Möllby (1975a) then showed that δ-toxin resembled bee venom melittin in its action. Both these agents, on initial contact with the membranes, caused preferential release of low molecular weight markers (< 1000), higher molecular weight labeled RNA (> 200,000) being released only after prolonged incubation or by treatment with increased doses of toxin. This pattern of release contrasts with that of Triton-X100, which rapidly released both low and high molecular weight markers.

When considering functional lesions in toxin-treated cells, it is interesting to note the finding of Durkin and Shier, (1981) that polypeptide toxins can activate endogenous phospholipases A_2 in the membrane of 3T3-4a mouse fibroblasts, generating, in turn, lysophospholipids and free fatty acids, both of which can lead to cytolysis by detergent-like effects. Moreover, Durkin and Shier (1980) have shown that this susceptibility is modulated by the cell cycle, with increased resistance to the lysin in the mitotic phase. Interestingly, this cyclic variation in sensitivity is not evident when melittin is the lytic agent.

The surface activity of δ-lysin, was commented on by Heatley (1971), who noted changes in the contact angle of water drops on a hydrophobic substrate after the addition of δ-lysin. Later, it was the subject of a detailed study by Colacicco *et al.* (1977), who showed that at air/water interfaces, the toxin formed a lipid-like film when spread from chloroform: methanol. But when spread from water, it behaved like a protein in that surface pressure and surface potential decreased linearly as the pH value was increased between 2 and 12. The high surface potentials obtained could indicate that the toxin possessed a net positive charge on the water surface or that the toxin molecules pack densely in the manner of hydrophobic lipid-like structures, or indeed that both situations hold.

5.5.2. *In-vivo Effects*

Kapral and coworkers (Kapral *et al.*, 1976; O'Brien and Kapral, 1976) recently reported a series of studies showing that purified δ-lysin preparations inhibited water absorption in guinea-pig (and rabbit) small intestine, with an associated but delayed increase in the level of cyclic AMP (cAMP) demonstrated in the guinea-pig ileum tissue. This effect, sensitive to the presence of lecithin which is an inhibitor of δ-lysin, is reminiscent of the effects caused by cholera toxin, which elevates the level of cAMP by activation of adenyl cyclase in the intestinal epithelial cells. The increase in cAMP noted by Kapral was, however, considerably delayed, occurring about one hour after administration of the toxin, thus differing from the cholera toxin effects. That the mechanism of elevation of cAMP was different in the two instances was confirmed by a complete lack of any cAMP-mediated morphological changes in Y-1 adrenal cells (cell rounding effect) or in chinese hamster ovary cells (spindling) after treatment with δ-lysin (O'Brien and Kapral, 1977). Such alterations in cell morphology result if there is a stimulation of adenyl cyclase, as is the case with cholera toxin. O'Brien *et al.* (1978) later showed that the immediate effect of δ-lysin in the guinea-pig ileum was to cause a rapid increase in the ion flux across the mucosal membranes, thus differing fundamentally from the primary effect of cholera toxin. Increase in ion flux was thought to arise by a direct stimulatory effect of δ-lysin on membrane ion pumps.

Other reported biological activities of δ-lysin include its lethality for laboratory animals at high doses (10–100 mg) (Kreger *et al.*, 1971), a property which is by no means universally accepted by all groups of workers. Doubt stems from the fact that levels of contamination by α-toxin as low as 0.1 % could account for such lethal effects. Highly purified δ-lysin is also responsible for erythema when given intradermally in rabbits, but very high doses are required to cause dermal necrosis inside the erythematous zone (Kreger *et al.*, 1971; Turner, 1978b), increase in vascular permeability also results from intradermal injection of this toxin.

6. STAPHYLOCOCCAL LEUCOCIDIN

6.1. Description

Leucocidin (Panton–Valentine leucocidin), first described as an extracellular leucocyte toxin (Panton and Valentine, 1932) and produced by *S. aureus* consists of two components designated S and F which are both required and act synergistically to give leucotoxic activity. Molecular weights of 32,000 and 31,000 and pI values of 9.08 and 9.39 for crystalline F and S components respectively were recently reported by Noda *et al.* (1980a,b).

Work prior to 1970 on this toxin complex was pioneered by A. M. Woodin and colleagues and the most authoritative and complete reviews of its nature and activities are those of Woodin (1970, 1972). Leucocidin acts on a remarkably narrow range of cell types being restricted to polymorphonuclear leucocytes (Gladstone and van Heyningen, 1957), macrophages (Woodin, 1959) and mast cells (Kwarecki *et al.*, 1968) of both man and rabbit. Recently, it has been shown to be a potent dermonecrotizing agent in the rabbit (Ward and Turner, 1980).

6.2. Production of Staphylococcal Leucocidin

Woodin (1970) reported that good yields of toxin were obtained from strain V8 grown on a medium consisting of a mixture of amino acids, mineral salts, lactate, glycerophosphate and yeast extract diffusate. Using a modification of the medium described by Gladstone and van Heyningen (1957), Woodin (1970) reported yields of 50 mg l^{-1} of each of the S and F components, which together accounted for up to 20 % of the soluble protein in the culture fluid after 8–10 hr growth in an aerated fermentor. Strain V8, which produces relatively good yields of leucocidin, has been used in most studies on this toxin, usually grown in a medium based on the yeast diffusate recipe described above.

6.3. PURIFICATION OF STAPHYLOCOCCAL LEUCOCIDIN

S and F components can be recovered from the cell free culture fluid by 'salting out' with ammonium sulfate (Woodin, 1959; 1960) or with $ZnCl_2$ (Noda et al., 1980b). After dialysis, the crude toxin is purified further by a series of chromatography steps including separations on columns of calcium phosphate and two steps on carboxymethyl cellulose which result in separation of the S (slow eluting) and F (fast eluting) components. Each is then further purified on Dowex and Amberlite ion exchange resins before being crystallized, although the crystalline S component still carries some impurities (Woodin, 1959, 1960).

Noda et al. (1980b) used a different purification procedure after 'salting out' which included chromatography on carboxymethyl Sephadex, Sephadex G100 gel filtration and starch zone electrophoresis before final crystallization of S and F components by dialysis against ammonium sulfate.

6.4. PHYSICOCHEMICAL PROPERTIES OF STAPHYLOCOCCAL LEUCOCIDIN

6.4.1. Molecular Weight and Isoelectric Point

From sedimentation and diffusion constants determined at pH 5.0 by ultracentrifugation, the molecular weights of the F and S components were reported by Woodin (1960) as 32,000 and 38,000 daltons. Toxin prepared by Noda et al. (1980b) was analysed by sodium dodecyl sulfate polyacrylamide gel electrophoresis and molecular weights for F and S components of 32,000 and 31,000 respectively were reported. Both F and S components were polydispersed in sucrose gradient centrifugation and had mean S values of 3.0 in both cases (Woodin, 1960). The isoelectric point for a mixture of the F and S components, present as a single band of activity after electrophoretic separation of proteins in staphylococcal culture filtrates was reported as 9.0 by Wadström (cited as unpublished observation by Woodin, 1970). In a more recent study, Noda et al. (1980b) reported pI values of 9.08 and 9.39 for the crystalline F and S components respectively.

No information is published on the amino acid composition, secondary or tertiary structure of either of the components.

6.4.2. Stability

A fraction of both components undergoes reversible polymerization in low ionic strength media and Woodin believed that this reflected the existence of a mixture of different conformers in each component (Woodin and Wieneke, 1966). The leucocidin complex is relatively labile and almost all activity is lost rapidly ($\sim 10\,min$) at 60°C (Gladstone and van Heyningen, 1957) and less so at room temperature or at 4°C, with a half-life at this temperature (4°C) of approximately 3 days. However, it can be stored at -20°C or lyophilized without appreciable loss of activity (Jeljaszewicz, et al., 1976).

6.5. BIOLOGICAL ACTIVITY OF STAPHYLOCOCCAL LEUCOCIDIN

6.5.1. Interaction with Membranes Leading to Cytolysis

The biological activities and postulated mode of action of leucocidin have been the subject of recent reviews by Jeljaszewicz et al. (1978) and McCartney and Arbuthnott (1978) and a brief summary of the activities is presented here.

When susceptible rabbit leucocytes are exposed to leucocidin in vitro at sublytic concentrations, a progression of morphological changes occur rapidly and include loss of pseudopodia with immobilization, degranulation and rupture of the nucleus. Increasing the concentration of the toxin complex results in complete lysis of the cells.

The presence of calcium ions is essential for these changes and cells are protected from the action of the toxin when ethylenediamine tetraacetate is present (Woodin, 1972). The mode of action of the toxin proposed by Woodin (1970) involves the synergistic action of the F and S components on the leucocyte membrane to produce a channel permeable to cations. Trisphosphoinositide, a minor phospholipid component of the membrane, plays a key role in the process and may account in some way for the specificity of the toxin. Since this lipid also occurs in the membranes of nonsusceptible erythrocytes, the presence of triphosphoinositide *per se* is not sufficient to account for susceptibility but its accessibility at the cell surface may differ in different membranes. It was estimated that the outer leaflet of the leucocyte membrane contains approximately 1 % triphosphoinositide (Woodin, 1970).

According to Woodin, the following sequence of events may account for the synergism between the F and S component of leucocidin. Entry of part of the F component into a region of low dielectric constant in the membrane leads to a change in F to a more expanded conformation which interacts with esterified fatty acid chains in a membrane phospholipid. This complex then allows adsorption of the S component onto the altered surface of the F component, and results in S interacting with the exposed inositol triphosphate of triphosphoinositide which, in turn, leads to the formation of a channel permeable to electrolyte. The consequent loss of the region of low dielectric constant induces a reversal of the earlier conformational change and desorption of both inactivated F and S components from the membrane. Finally the conformation of triphosphoinositide is restored to its original state with the expenditure of ATP. The perturbation of the membrane by leucocidin results in stimulation of the K^+- sensitive acylphosphatase and adenylate cyclase which, in turn, leads to impairment of the sodium–potassium pump. A more detailed discussion of data relating to the biological activity of leucocidin appears in the excellent review by Rogolsky (1979).

In recent binding studies, Noda *et al.* (1980a) failed to confirm the earlier observations of Woodin and Wieneke (1966) and Woodin (1970) which lead to the above hypothesis. Noda *et al.* (1980a) found that pretreatment of rabbit leucocytes with the S component resulted in rapid lysis of the leucocytes after addition of F. They interpreted this as strong evidence that the S component binds to leucocytes before F is bound and also suggest that F may bind preferentially to the palmitoyl moiety of phosphatidyl choline. On testing inhibition of leucocyte activity by competitive binding studies between S and various glycosphingolipids and phospholipids, the most potent inhibitor of S binding was GM_1 ganglioside, the inhibition being eleviated by cholera toxin fragment B which shares this binding moiety.

The mode of action of leucocidin involves ᐧ complex sequence of interactions at the membrane surface, which are by no means clearly defined. Further work is necessary before we understand the molecular basis for the induced permeability changes and specificity of this toxin.

6.5.2. *Role in Pathogenicity*

Leucocidin is not regarded as a lethal toxin, but when injected into rabbits, significant changes in the kinetics and the functional state of granulocytes in the peripheral blood result. Its role in pathogenesis is far from clear, yet there is no doubt that it is produced *in vivo* during staphylococcal infection, since antibodies against it are frequently found in the sera of patients with chronic infections. However, in a recent study of experimental staphylococcal mastitis (a naturally occurring staphylococcal infection in farmed rabbits) in the rabbit, Adlam *et al.* (1980) found that no protection was afforded by prior immunization with leucocidin, in spite of high levels of circulating anti-PV leucocidin in the serum.

7. STAPHYLOCOCCAL EPIDERMOLYTIC TOXINS

7.1. Discovery of Epidermolytic Toxin

In 1970, Drs Marian Melish and Lowell Glasgow, then working in Rochester, New York, published their seminal paper on the pathogenesis of the disease syndrome that they termed the Staphylococcal Scalded Skin Syndrome (SSSS). This term was introduced to describe the spectrum of response to epidermolytic strains of *S. aureus* and includes Ritter's disease, staphylococcal TEN (Toxic Epidermal Necrolysis), bullous impetigo and the generalized erythematous rash without epidermolysis. Lyell (1981), however, takes the view that the term SSSS should be reserved for the extensive scalding manifestations.

In their study, Melish and Glasgow (1970) investigated 17 patients aged from 5 days to 5 years. Phage group II staphylococci isolated from all 17 cases, when injected subcutaneously or intraperitoneally into newborn mice at sublethal doses, uniformly produced reaction strikingly similar to SSSS in young children. By 12–16 hr after injection, the skin became loosened when gently stroked (a positive Nikolsky sign). Within a few hours bullae were evident and the skin began to peel, revealing a moist bright red glistening surface underneath. Fluid aspirated from the lesions was consistently sterile and on histopathological examination, and intraepidermal cleavage plane was seen at the level of the stratum granulosum.

Melish and Glasgow correctly recognized the significance of their observations in relation to the pathogenesis of SSSS and postulated '. . . a soluble product induces the dermatologic manifestations of this disease'. Confirmation of this hypothesis required the isolation of the putative toxin and this was soon reported by several authors (Melish *et al.*, 1970; Kapral and Miller, 1971; Arbuthnott *et al.*, 1971). The extracellular factor responsible for epidermal splitting is now known as epidermolytic toxin [exofiliative toxin (ET)]. The toxin causes extensive epidermal splitting (epidermolysis) in neonatal mice and the experimental disease resembles closely the disease in humans (Faden *et al.*, 1974). These early observations triggered an explosion of interest and within the next few years a large number of publications covering many aspects of ET appeared in the bacteriological, dermatological and pediatric literature, and it was some time before a coherent picture emerged. The situation was complicated further by the subsequent realization that two different serotypes of ET, having different physicochemical properties, exist (Kondo *et al.*, 1974). The literature has been reviewed comprehensively by Elias *et al.* (1977) and Rogolsky (1979).

7.2. Production and Assay

Factors affecting the production of ET in culture are still poorly understood. Melish *et al.* (1972) reported that several media failed to support toxin production *in vitro* and they resorted to culturing toxinogenic strains in dialysis sacs, containing tissue culture medium, implanted in the peritoneal cavities of rats. Their failure to achieve toxin production *in vitro* was probably due to the fact that they did not supplement the atmosphere with CO_2 during growth. Most other groups used *in vitro* methods, employing complex media in semi-solid agar or liquid shake cultures in the presence of CO_2 at a concentration of 10–20% (v/v) in the gaseous atmosphere. Arbuthnott *et al.* (1974) subsequently found that high yields of ET could be produced in the absence of added CO_2 using a yeast diffusate–casamino acids medium originally developed for α-toxin production by Bernheimer and Schwartz (1963).

The biological assay for ET involves the subcutaneous injection of up to 0.1 ml of test sample in groups of 2–4-day-old suckling mice. The unit of ET activity is defined as the lowest dose causing epidermal splitting within 3–6 hr after challenge. The presence in crude or partially purified toxin preparations of contaminating amounts of the lethal and necrotizing α-toxin, which is produced by over 90% of *S. aureus* strains, often complicates the bioassay; α-toxin causes a pronounced reddening of the skin, followed by death within a few hours. These effects can be avoided by neutralizing the α-toxin with an excess of α-antitoxin. As the minimum effective dose of ET is approximately 0.3–0.5 μg (Arbuthnott *et al.*, 1974; Wuepper *et al.*, 1976) and the maximum volume that can be injected is 0.1 ml, the mouse test will detect only concentrations of toxin exceeding 3–5 μg ml^{-1}. Radial immunodiffusion assays for ET have about the same sensitivity as the mouse assay (Wuepper *et al.*, 1976). However the sensitivity of radioimmunoassay is considerably higher; Wuepper *et al.* (1976) reported a sensitivity of 20 ng ml^{-1} and Melish *et al.* (1981), using a competitive binding assay, were able to detect amounts down to 100 pg ml^{-1}. Although sensitive immunological assays are extremely useful, it should be noted that toxic activity can be assayed only by skin tests in sensitive species or by the appearance of epidermal splitting in skin organ cultures (McCallum, 1972; Elias *et al.*, 1976).

7.3. PURIFICATION AND CHARACTERIZATION

Between 1972 and 1976, six groups published findings of purification studies (Melish *et al.*, 1972; Kondo *et al.*, 1973; Arbuthnott *et al.*, 1974; Johnson *et al.*, 1975; Dimond and Wuepper, 1976; Wiley *et al.*, 1976). Molecular weight estimates were in the range 24,000–32,000 and there were conflicting opinions about heat sensitivity, metal ion dependence and the existence of multiple forms detected by electrophoresis and isoelectric focusing. The results obtained in different laboratories have been reviewed in detail recently (Rogolsky, 1979). Some of these discrepanices were resolved when it was shown that at least two serotypes of ET exist that differ in heat stability (Kondo *et al.*, 1974) and that epidermolytic strains of *S. aureus* may produce either or both of these serotypes (Kondo *et al.*, 1975; Arbuthnott and Billcliffe, 1976). More recently these serotypes, which have been designated variously as ExA and ExB, TA and DI, and serotype i and ii toxins, have been analyzed in detail (Kondo *et al.*, 1976; Johnson *et al.*, 1979; Bailey *et al.*, 1980). Based on an assessment of the amino acid compositions obtained in different laboratories, Bailey *et al.* (1980) concluded that the TA- and DI-type toxins of Johnson *et al.* (1979) are very similar to the type i and type ii toxins of Bailey *et al.* (1980). TA-type toxin and type i toxin have the same N- and C-terminal amino acids (glutamic acid and lysine respectively) and they have very similar amino acid analyses (Table 9). Also the DI-type toxin and type ii toxin are obviously similar, each having lysine at the N- and C-termini. The main difference is in the tryptophan content of the DI and type ii toxins; Johnson *et al.* (1979) reported one mol tryptophan, whereas type ii toxin contained no tryptophan (Bailey *et al.* 1980). A possible explanation for this lies in the reported contamination of DI-toxin with small amounts of TA-toxin. These findings, taken together with the fact that the DI and type ii toxins are controlled by plasmid encoded genes and that TA and type i toxin appear to be encoded by chromosomal genes, argue strongly in favor of the probable identity of these toxin serotypes, respectively.

The amino acid compositions of Kondo's ExA and ExB forms of ET (Kondo *et al.*, 1976) apparently differ from the TA/type i and DI/type ii toxins. However, Bailey *et al.* (1980) argue that internal evidence based on a comparison of native toxins and nitrotoxoids (see Kondo *et al.*, 1976) suggests that this difference is due mainly to contamination of ExA and ExB with glycine. It seems likely, that each of the three research groups has isolated the same two serotypes of ET. Moreover, through an exchange of toxin preparations and antisera, it has been possible to show that TA, type i and ExA toxins cross-react immunologically as do DI,

TABLE 9. *Amino Acid Composition of Epidermolytic Toxins (Residues per Molecule ET)*

Amino acid	Type i toxin Bailey *et al.* (1980)	TA-toxin Johnson *et al.* (1979)	Type ii toxin Bailey *et al.* (1980)	DI toxin Johnson *et al.* (1979)
Tryptophan	1.19	1	0	1
Lysine	23.9	22	24.2	22
Histidine	7.26	7	7.26	5
Arginine	10.2	9	6.98	5
Aspartic acid	38.0	34	34.2	29
Threonine	13.7	12	14.1	12
Serine	18.3	17	19.3	17
Glutamic acid	28.1	27	28.1	26
Proline	11.8	10	13.8	12
Glycine	28.9	24	25.9	21
Alanine	10.7	8	17.9	13
Cystine	0 (<0.14)	0	0 (<0.02)	0
Valine	18.4	13	10.2	9
Methionine	1.23	1	1.07	1
Isoleucine	17.7	17	18.5	17
Leucine	19.1	15	19.6	16
Tyrosine	12.0	11	16.5	13
Phenylalanine	9.78	9	11.1	9

type ii and ExB toxins (Melish, personal communication). This of course in no way excludes the possibility that additional new serotypes will be found. Following the nomenclature used for the staphylococcal enterotoxins, it is to be hoped that serotypes will be designated in a common way using an alphabetical notation. Thus, the two serotypes described so far would be designated ETA and ETB; this is the notation that will be used throughout this section. The main properties of ETA and ETB are summarized in Table 10.

It is not yet possible to explain the discrepancies in values reported for the molecular weight of the toxin(s). Johnson *et al.* (1979) estimated a value of 26,500 for TA toxin (ETA) and 26,000 for DI-toxin (ETB) by SDS polyacrylamide gel electrophoresis, whereas Bailey *et al.* (1980) reported values of 30,000 and 29,500 for ETA and ETB respectively. The latter found that cyanogenbromide digestion of each toxin yielded two peptide fragments. The larger of these fragments in each case had a molecular weight of 22,000, while the smaller fragment from ETB is slightly larger (8,400) than that from ETA (7,800).

Tryptic peptide maps for ETA and ETB revealed only four out of thirty spots to be identical (Bailey *et al.*, 1980). This suggests that at most there is limited similarity at the level of amino acid sequence. The amino acid sequence of the first 26 and 23 residues of ETA and ETB respectively were determined by Johnson *et al.* (1979) and are shown in Table 11. A direct comparison of these sequences showed little obvious homology. However, a one residue shift of ETA creates greater homology with eight residues of ETA now being common to ETB. Johnson *et al.* (1979) also point out that the shift results in eight other positions having amino acids whose codons differ by only a single nucleotide change. The question of the degree of relatedness between ETA and ETB awaits further information on the amino acid sequence and the genetic control of production of the toxins.

It has been shown that approximately 50 % of phage group II staphylococci produce ET (Kapral, 1974; Galinski, 1976). Some nonphage group II strains isolated from superficial skin lesions also produce ET, and it was reported by Kondo *et al.* (1975) for Japanese isolates that most nongroup II strains produce only ETB, whereas group II strains produce either ETA alone or a mixture of ETA and ETB. However, in a survey of 116 strains isolated in Britain and Ireland, de Azavedo and Arbuthnott (1981) found that the ability to produce ETA and ETB was not confined to particular phage groups.

7.4. Genetic Control of Production of Epidermolytic Toxin

Rogolsky and his coworkers, in a series of studies, have attempted to resolve the genetic basis for ET production in *S. aureus* (Rogolsky *et al.*, 1974, 1976; Warren *et al.*, 1974, 1975; Wiley and Rogolsky, 1977), and this aspect has been comprehensively reviewed recently (Rogolsky, 1979). They set out to investigate the suggestion by Melish *et al.* (1972) that ET formation may be under the control of a bacteriophage. Such a relationship was excluded on several grounds and in the course of phage curing experiments, it was noted that ethidium bromide 'cured' cells of one strain, from which temperate phage was not eliminated, had lost the ability to produce ET. Furthermore, the capacity to produce ET was either completely or

TABLE 10. *The Properties of Staphylococcal Epidermolytic Toxins*

Property	ETA	ETB
Molecular weight	30,000*	29,500*
	26,500†	26,000†
Isoelectric point	7.0*	6.95*
Heat sensitivity	Heat stable‡	Heat labile‡
N-terminal amino acid	Glutamic*,†	Lysine*,†
C-terminal amino acid	Lysine*,†	Lysine*,†
No. of tryptic peptides	33*	27*
Genetic control	Chromosomal§,¶	Plasmid§,¶

*Bailey *et al.* (1980).
†Johnson *et al.* (1979).
‡Kondo *et al.* (1974).
§Rogolsky *et al.* (1976).
¶O'Reilly *et al.* (1981).

TABLE 11. *Comparisons of the Amino Terminal Sequences of Toxins TA and DI**

Strain							Residue No							
	1	2	3	4	5	6	7	8	9	10	11	12	13	14
DI	Lys	Glu	Tyr	**Ala**	Ala	Glu	Glu	Ile	**Arg**	Lys	**Leu**	**Lys**	Glu	Lys
TA		Glu	Val	**Thr**	Ala	Glu	Glu	Ile	**Lys**	Lys	**His**	**Glu**	Glu	Lys
Strain	15	16	17	18	19	20	21	22	23	24	25	26		
DI	Phe	**Glu**	Val	Pro	Pro	Thr	**Asp**	Lys	**Glu**	**Leu**	Tyr	Tyr		
TA	Trp	**Asp**	Lys	Tyr	Tyr	Gly	**Val**	X	Asx	**Phe**	Tyr			

*A single unit shift produces the indicated homology. Identical residues are boxed and residues whose codons differ by one nucleotide are in boldface.
From Johnson *et al.* (1979).

partly lost by some strains when they were grown at high temperatures or in the presence of ethidium bromide or SDS, which suggested that a plasmid might be implicated in the expression of the toxin (Rogolsky et al., 1974). Many toxin producing strains also produced a bacteriocin and in some cases, the elimination of bacteriocin correlated with loss of ET production suggesting that both determinants might be linked on the same plasmid (Warren et al., 1974). Later experiments showed that purified ET had no bacteriocin activity and that bacteriocin had no ET activity (Rogolsky and Wiley, 1977); these products were thus distinct entities. Further evidence in support of the extrachromosomal nature of the ET gene was obtained by dye-buoyant density centrifugation of cell lysates. This led to the identification of a plasmid of '56S' in a covalently closed circular form in two strains that correlated with the ET and bacteriocin markers (Warren et al., 1975).

However, the majority of the strains examined by Rogolsky and his coworkers were only partially cured of ET production by the elimination of the '56S' plasmid (Rogolsky et al., 1974, 1976). This suggested that in some strains both plasmid and chromosomal determinants might be involved in ET synthesis. Kayhani et al. (1975) and Rosenblum and Tyrone (1976) then reported that strains exist that possess only chromosomal determinants for toxin production. The results of DNA–DNA hybridization experiments with purified ET plasmid DNA and chromosomal DNA from a strain in which the ET genes were chromosomally located, suggested that the plasmid and chromosomal determinants were not homologous (Rogolsky, 1979).

Purified ET preparations from strains or cured derivatives that produced plasmid encoded toxin, or chromosomally encoded toxin, when examined by thin-layer gel isoelectric focusing, each showed single protein bands that differed slightly in pI. ET preparations from strains that produced both plasmid- and chromosomally-encoded toxins contained both protein bands (Wiley and Rogolsky, 1977). In the same study it was also found that the plasmid- and chromosomally-determined ET were immunologically distinct. So far it has not been possible to map the loci for the chromosomally-determined toxin.

Recently, Warren (1980) has reported an analysis of the molecular relationships between the plasmids isolated from seven strains that produce ETB. Six of the strains contained a large plasmid (40.5 kilobases) that carries the genes for ETB and bacteriocin production. Restriction enzyme analysis of plasmids from these strains showed a similar pattern of restriction fragments indicating that they were closely related. The findings of Wiley and Rogolsky (1977) and of Warren (1980) have been confirmed and extended by O'Reilly et al. (1981) who studied the plasmids of epidermolytic strains of S. aureus. The plasmid content of 34 strains, representing different phage groups and isolated from different hospitals in Britain, Ireland and the United States, was determined using the gel electrophoresis technique for plasmid DNA. The results strongly suggest that ETA and ETB are specified by genetic determinants on different replicons. Strains that formed ETA when cured of all detectable plasmids or which were naturally devoid of extrachromosomal DNA, retained the ETA phenotype. By contrast, ETB was invariably plasmid-controlled being eliminated from all the strains tested when they were grown under conditions which promoted loss of plasmids. ETB production was correlated with the presence of a 42 kilobase plasmid.

O'Reilly et al. (1981) also reported that most epidermolytic strains also formed a bacteriocin (Bac$^+$) and that in strains that produced ETB, the ETB determinant and Bac$^+$ were associated with the same 42 kilobase plasmid. However some strains that produced only ETA were also Bac$^+$ and again a 42 kilobase plasmid was associated with the Bac$^+$ phenotype. Restriction enzyme analysis of preparations of 42 kilobase plasmid DNA from strains of differing phenotype and from different parts of the world revealed that the plasmids are very closely related. Each plasmid shared 19 of 22 fragments generated by cleavage with the restriction endonuclease HindIII. More recently Warren (1980) has presented a restriction map of the phage group II S. aureus ET plasmid pRN001 and the way is now open to further characterize the genetic control of ETB by cloning techniques.

7.5. Mode of Action of Epidermolytic Toxin

The molecular basis of the action of ET remains unknown at present and, in characterization of the toxin, this remains the most challenging problem. Both ETA and ETB cause the same histological changes in sensitive skin, namely, separation of cells in the stratum granulosum with the resulting formation of an intraepidermal cleft. Like many other bacterial toxins, ET exhibits species specificity and of the animal species tested only humans, mice, monkeys and golden hamsters are sensitive to toxin action (Elias *et al.*, 1976; Fritsch *et al.*, 1979). Most experimental work has been done using the mouse. Initially it was thought that only newborn mice less than six days old were susceptible to ET. However, epidermal splitting can be demonstrated in the skin of adult mice. Though this is difficult to demonstrate in haired areas of adult mouse skin, there is no doubt that the glabrous (nonhaired) surfaces of adult mice are sensitive (Elias *et al.*, 1974) as is the skin of adult hairless mice (Kapral and Miller, 1972; Arbuthnott *et al.*, 1973).

The ultrastructural changes in the epidermis that follow administration of ET have been well documented and have been reviewed by Rogolsky (1979). The time required for the development of epidermal splitting is dose dependent and it is interesting to note that Dimond and Wuepper (1976) observed that large doses of toxin caused a positive Nikolsky sign in one day old mice within 10 min. The first ultrastructural change involves the formation of fluid filled gaps between cells in the stratum granulosum along a horizontal cleavage plane with the accompanying disappearance of the small vesicles normally present in the intercellular space (Lillibridge *et al.*, 1972; Elias *et al.*, 1975; McLay *et al.*, 1975).

Thus far, the primary cause of these structural changes has not been determined. Cells in the region of the epidermal split did not show cytolysis nor was there removal of the mucopolysaccharide of the glycocalyx on the surface of the cells (Elias *et al.*, 1975). Wuepper *et al.* (1975) excluded the possibility that a complement-mediated cytotoxic effect was involved, as C3 and C5 deficient mice were as sensitive to ET as control animals. This group also showed that hairless, athymic, adult mice were susceptible to ET, indicating that immunocompetent thymocytes are not required for the action of the toxin.

Elias *et al.* (1976) conducted an interesting study of the action of ET on *in vitro* organ cultures of skin from sensitive and resistant species. When pieces of full-thickness mouse skin (sensitive) and rat skin (resistant) were coincubated in organ cultures containing ET, only the mouse skin showed epidermal splitting, suggesting that rat skin does release an inhibitor of ET. Also, rat plasma did not inhibit the splitting of mouse skin by ET. In experiments in which sheets of rat dermis were overlayed with sheets of mouse epidermis, the mouse epidermis remained sensitive to ET; also rat epidermis overlayed on mouse dermis remained resistant to the action of the toxin. These results indicate that the dermis is not responsible for resistance of rat skin *in vitro* and that activation of ET by the dermis is not a prerequisite for its action on mouse skin.

Several groups (Wuepper *et al.*, 1975; McLay *et al.*, 1975; Elias *et al.*, 1977) followed up an early suggestion by Lillibridge *et al.* (1972) that the disappearance of intercellular vesicles which accompanies epidermal splitting might result in the release of a proteolytic enzyme that could be involved in cell separation but they failed to detect inhibition of epidermal splitting by protease inhibitors. Also, there is as yet no convincing evidence for the existence of a specific receptor for the toxin in mouse skin (Baker *et al.*, 1978), although Kondo and Sakurai (1981) have recently described the partial characterization of an inhibitor of ET isolated by extraction of mouse skin with SDS.

At present any proposed mechanism for the action of ET must remain speculative. There are several possibilities and these must be the subject of further research in this area. Three such possible mechanisms are as follows:

1. ET may associate weakly and perhaps reversibly with a component on the surface of suceptible cells and this interaction could trigger the secretion of fluid into the intercellular space. Such a weak association might be difficult to demonstrate in binding studies.
2. ET may have an as yet unidentified enzymic action on key components involved in the adherence of adjacent cells.
3. Disruption of the vesicles in the intercellular space could lead to alteration of the cohesive forces that bind cells together perhaps as a result of indirect changes in surface components involved in adherence.

8. THE STAPHYLOCOCCAL ENTEROTOXINS

8.1. DESCRIPTION

The enterotoxins of *S. aureus* form a group of six serologically distinct extracellular proteins, designated A, B, C_1, C_2, D and E that are recognized as the causative agents of staphylococcal food poisoning. Very recently, a seventh enterotoxin (F), which may be of importance in the pathogenesis of the staphylococcal toxic shock syndrome, has been described (Bergdoll *et al.*, 1981).

Ingestion of preformed enterotoxin in contaminated food leads to the rapid development (within 2–6 hr) of the symptoms of vomiting and diarrhoea that are characteristic of staphylococcal food poisoning. The illness is usually mild, lasting only for up to 24 hr. The incidence of the disease is difficult to determine because it is not notifiable and many cases probably go unrecognized. However, from an analysis of recorded food-borne outbreaks (Turnbull, 1979) it appears that the incidence of staphylococcal food poisoning varies widely in different countries (Table 12). In some areas it accounted for more than 50 per cent of total outbreaks of food poisoning. Strains of *S. aureus* that produce enterotoxin A, or a mixture of enterotoxins A and D have been found in 69 per cent of reported outbreaks in the USA and UK; strains producing enterotoxin D alone or together with enterotoxin C account for 10 per cent of outbreaks; those that produce only enterotoxin B are found rarely (Casman *et al.*, 1967; Gilbert and Wieneke, 1973).

There is a very extensive literature on the topic of staphylococcal enterotoxins and it is not possible to include a comprehensive review in this section. Rather it is intended to summarize the main developments that have occurred in the last two decades in the knowledge of detection, production, chemical characterization and biological properties of this group of toxins. More detailed information can be obtained from the comprehensive reviews of Bergdoll (1970, 1972, 1983) who with his colleagues at the Food Research Institute (F.R.I.) Wisconsin, has played a major role in pioneering this field.

8.2. DETECTION OF ENTEROTOXINS

Until recently the lack of sensitive methods for detecting staphylococcal enterotoxins has proved a limiting factor in research in this area. This has affected the ability to detect enterotoxin in food, the assessment of the incidence of toxin producing strains of *S. aureus* and studies of the mode of action of enterotoxin. Biological assays have proved to be a particular problem. Although a variety of animals react to enterotoxin, most species, such as pigs, dogs, cats and kittens are relatively insensitive. Also rodents, which lack a vomiting reaction, are of little value. The most reliable test is the feeding of enterotoxin to young rhesus monkeys (Bergdoll, 1972). In this test, in which up to 50 ml of toxin solution can be administered by catheter, the ED_{50} is about 5 μg enterotoxin per dose. However, to provide

TABLE 12. *Incidence of Staphylococcal Food Poisoning in Different Countries**

Reporting centre	Staphylococcal food poisoning as per cent of total food poisoning outbreaks
England and Wales (1969–1976)	2.6
Scotland (1973–1977)	4.2
USA (1972–1976)	32.6
Canada (1973–1975)	44.7
Australia (1967–1971)	27.3
Japan (1969–1975)	28.4
Hungary (1960–1968)	56.1
Finland (1965–1974)	50.6

*From Turnbull (1979).

reliable results, six animals are required to test a given sample and the expense involved, together with the difficulty in obtaining monkeys, greatly limits the use of this bioassay.

Not surprisingly, there has been great reliance on serological tests, employing specific antisera raised against purified enterotoxins. Until the recent introduction of highly sensitive radioimmunoassay (RIA) and enzyme linked immunosorbent assay (ELISA), most workers have made use of precipitin tests or hemagglutination tests. The single gel diffusion test has a sensitivity of $1-2 \mu g \, ml^{-1}$ and the microslide double gel diffusion test has a sensitivity of $0.1 \mu g \, ml^{-1}$ (Casman and Bennet, 1963; Hall *et al.*, 1965). In both cases several days of incubation may be necessary to detect low concentrations. Serological tests based on hemagglutination or hemmagglutination inhibition were introduced for enterotoxin B (Morse and Mah, 1967; Johnson *et al.*, 1967) and a reverse passive hemagglutination assay gave a sensitivity of $0.0015 \mu g \, ml^{-1}$ (Silverman *et al.*, 1968). RIA (Miller *et al.*, 1978) and ELISA (Stiffler–Rosenberg and Fru, 1978) techniques have increased the sensitivity of detection so that a 1.0 ng sample or less can be detected.

8.3. PRODUCTION OF ENTEROTOXINS

Early work on factors influencing production of enterotoxins is difficult to assess due to the lack of adequate methods of detection and because the existence of several different enterotoxins was not recognized until the work of Bergdoll *et al.* (1959). Also, most work has been done with enterotoxin B because relatively large amounts of toxin are released by producing strains. To some extent the choice of medium is dictated by the purpose of the study; for instance, a medium suitable for screening strains may not be the best medium for purification work.

Brain Heart Infusion (BHI) broth (Casman and Bennet, 1963) has been widely used, though some workers reported variable yields with this medium. For instance, Reiser and Weiss (1969) pointed out that the yield was influenced by the brand and possibly the lot of BHI used. Of various media based on protein digests, Bergdoll and his coworkers at F.R.I. selected Protein Hydrolysate Powder (PHP) (Mead Johnson International, Evansville, Indiana) supplemented with niacin and thiamin which gave consistent yields of all the enterotoxins (Bergdoll, 1972). A cheaper medium comprising a mixture of 3 % PHP and 3 % N–Z Amine (NAK) (Humko Sheffield Chemical, Norwich, NY) gave comparable results (Bergdoll, 1972). The importance of strain variation was emphasized by Jarvis *et al.* (1973) who studied the production of enterotoxins A, B and C under conditions of controlled pH and aeration. This group also obtained better toxin production in a defined amino acid medium than in casein hydrolysate and found that, in fermenter cultures, a pH of 6.5 favored toxin production.

The effect of glucose on enterotoxin B production has been studied in some detail. Morse *et al.* (1969) reported that, in the presence of glucose, enterotoxin B was produced only when glucose was depleted and concluded that toxin synthesis is regulated by catabolite repression. Later studies (Morse and Baldwin, 1973) suggested that a functional electron transport system was involved in regulating the degree of glucose and pyruvate repression. While accepting that glucose exerts a repressive effect on the synthesis of enterotoxin B, Iandolo and Shafer (1977) concluded that the mode of regulation by glucose was not consistent with catabolite repression.

In a general assessment of enterotoxin synthesis, Bergdoll *et al.* (1974a) pointed out that the mechanism of synthesis of enterotoxin A may differ from that of enterotoxins B and C. Enterotoxin A-producing colonies typically gave uniform small haloes of immunoprecipitate on antiserum-containing agar, but strains producing enterotoxins B and C gave colonies that differed widely in the diameter of the ring of precipitate produced. Also enterotoxin A production tended to be stable and at a low level, whereas colonies producing high levels of enterotoxins B and C could be selected but were unstable on subculture. Moreover Czop and Bergdoll (1970), in a study of L forms of enterotoxin A, B and C producing strains, observed that enterotoxin production was sustained only by L forms of enterotoxin A producing strains. This finding taken together with the results of Friedman (1968), who reported that detergents and agents that specifically block cell wall synthesis also inhibit enterotoxin B formation, suggested that enterotoxin B and C production may be associated in some way with the cell surface. In this regard it is interesting to note that up to 67 per cent of cell associated enterotoxin B was surface-bound, being located external to the cytoplasmic membrane (Miller and Fung, 1976).

There have been some studies of enterotoxin production in synthetic media (Wu and Bergdoll, 1971). A minimal medium that supported growth and enterotoxin B production consisted of three amino acids (arginine, cystine and phenylalanine), six inorganic salts and four vitamins with glutamate as the energy source (Mah et al., 1967); there was an additional requirement for proline and valine when glucose was used as the energy source. Bergdoll et al. (1974a) in reconsidering the early work of Surgalla (1947), which was done with strains later shown to be enterotoxin A producers, concluded that the minimal requirements for enterotoxin A production were three amino acids (cystine, arginine and proline), ammonium sulfate and three vitamins. However, when different permutations of mixtures containing 18 amino acids were used to study enterotoxin production, the interactions between different amino acids proved to be extremely complex (Bergdoll et al., 1974a).

8.3.1. Genetic Control of Enterotoxin Production

The genetic control of enterotoxin B production has been examined by several workers in some detail. This aspect first attracted attention because of the apparent association between enterotoxin B production and methicillin resistance in hospital isolates. The initial findings of Dornbusch et al. (1969) and Dornbusch and Hallander (1973) pointed to a plasmid location for the enterotoxin B gene in the methicillin resistant strain DU-4196. Also Shalita et al. (1977) strongly implicated the involvement of a small plasmid (pSN2) in enterotoxin B production. However, in food poisoning strains, the genetic control of enterotoxin B appeared to be chromosomal (Shafer and Iandolo, 1978). The same authors (Shafer and Iandolo, 1979) working with methicillin resistant (MecR) strains observed that the entB gene occupied either a plasmid or chromosomal locus but was not physically linked to the mec gene. These various observations have been reconciled by Dyer and Iandolo (1981). The small plasmid pSN2 does not contain the structural gene for enterotoxin B but it encodes for a regulatory function which can control the synthesis of enterotoxin B in both plasmid-bearing and chromosomal producers. In the latter strains, it is proposed that pSN2 becomes integrated into the chromosome.

8.4. Characterization of Enterotoxins

With the exception of enterotoxin B which is produced in large amounts (up to $500 \mu g \, ml^{-1}$) enterotoxin yields tend to be low (around $5 \mu g \, ml^{-1}$) and large volumes of culture are required for purification. After an initial concentration step using carbowax 20 M, ion exchange chromatography gel filtration was used successfully for purification. Each of the known serotypes of enterotoxin have been obtained in highly purified form and they have been well characterized (Table 13). The chemical properties of the enterotoxins have been reviewed in some detail by Bergdoll et al. (1974b).

The proteins are of similar molecular weight and are easily soluble in water and salt solutions. They are relatively resistant to proteolytic enzymes and to heat. For example heating at 100°C for 130 min is required to give 95 per cent inactivation of a $20 \mu g \, ml^{-1}$ solution of enterotoxin A.

The amino acid compositions of enterotoxins A, B, C_1, C_2 and E are shown in Table 14. The most striking features are: (i) the high content of lysine, aspartic acid and tyrosine present in all of them, and (ii) enterotoxins A and E are similar in methionine, leucine and arginine content and differ in this regard from enterotoxins B, C_1 and C_2.

The amino acid sequence of enterotoxin B was found to consist of 239 amino acids (Huang and Bergdoll, 1970). Half-cystine residues found at positions 92 and 112 form a disulfide bridge, and Bergdoll et al. (1974b) have suggested that the primary structure in this region

TABLE 13. *Physicochemical Properties of Staphylococcal Enterotoxins*[*]

Property	Enterotoxin					
	A[a]	B[b]	C[c]$_1$	C[d]$_2$	D[e]	E[f]
Emetic dose for monkey (μg)	5	5	5	5–10	—	—
Sedimentation coefficient ($S_{20,w}$)	3.03	2.89	3.0	2.9	—	2.6
Molecular weight	27,800	28,366[g]	26,000	34,100	27,300	29,600
Isoelectric point	7.26	8.6	8.6	7.0	7.4	7.0
C-terminal residue	Serine	Lysine	Glycine	Glycine	Lysine	Threonine
N-terminal residue	Alanine	Glutamic acid	Glutamic acid	Glutamic acid	Serine	—

[a]Schantz *et al* (1972); [b]Schantz *et al.* (1965); [c]Borja and Bergdoll (1967); [d]Avena and Bergdoll (1967); [e]Chang and Bergdoll (1979); [f]Borja *et al.* (1972); [g]Dayhoff (1972) (determined from the amino acid sequence of Huang and Bergdoll, 1970).
[*]Modified from Bergdoll *et al.* (**1974b**).

TABLE 14. *Amino Acid Composition of the Enterotoxins* (g/100 g protein)[¶]

Amino acid	Enterotoxin				
	A[*]	B[†]	C$_1$[‡]	C$_2$[‡]	E[§]
Lysine	11.26	14.85	14.43	13.99	10.83
Histidine	3.16	2.34	2.91	2.87	3.04
Arginine	4.02	2.69	1.71	1.75	4.50
Aspartic acid	15.53	18.13	17.85	18.38	15.10
Threonine	5.96	4.50	5.31	5.80	6.36
Serine	2.99	4.05	4.58	4.81	4.72
Glutamic acid	12.36	9.45	8.95	8.93	12.15
Proline	1.35	2.11	2.16	2.23	1.93
Glycine	2.96	1.78	2.99	2.90	4.10
Alanine	1.94	1.32	1.85	1.61	2.38
Half-cystine	0.66	0.68	0.79	0.74	0.81
Valine	4.93	5.66	6.50	5.87	4.36
Methionine	0.96	3.52	3.20	3.60	0.45
Isoleucine	4.11	3.53	4.09	4.02	4.30
Leucine	9.78	6.86	6.54	6.13	10.08
Tyrosine	10.63	11.50	9.80	10.27	9.79
Phenylalanine	4.31	6.23	5.35	5.25	4.47
Tryptophan	1.46	0.95	0.99	0.84	1.51
Amide NH$_3$	1.80	1.66	1.71	1.62	1.66
TOTAL	98.37	100.15	100.00	99.99	100.88

[*]Schantz *et al.*, 1972.
[†]Bergdoll *et al.*, 1965.
[‡]Huang *et al.*, 1967.
[§]Borja *et al.*, 1972.
[¶]From Bergdoll *et al.* (1974b).

may be common to all of the enterotoxins. Reduction of the disulfide bridge and subsequent alkylation of the –SH groups did not affect the physical or emetic properties of the toxin. Acetylation of enterotoxins B and C with acetylimidazole and nitration with tetranitromethane indicated that there were 5–6 'free' tyrosyl residues (Borja, 1969; Borja and Bergdoll, 1969; Chu, 1968). Modification of these residues had no effect on the toxic or immunological properties of toxin. However, in the unfolded state in the presence of 5 M guanidine hydrochloride, all the tyrosyl residues were accessible to acetylation and this resulted in complete loss of activity. Also, modification of the methionine residues in enterotoxin B (Chu and Bergdoll, 1969) showed that emetic activity was lost when six of the eight residues reacted. Similarly it required modification of 31–32 of the 33 carboxyl groups in the enterotoxin B molecule to inactivate toxin (Chu and Crany, 1969). The free amino groups could be guanidinated with little change in conformational or biological properties (Spero *et al.*, 1971). However, removal of the ε-amino groups or neutralization of the positive charge on the molecule resulted in inactivation.

Multiple forms of the enterotoxins have been reported in several isoelectric focusing studies (Chang and Dickie, 1971a,b; Chang *et al.*, 1971; Dickie *et al.*, 1972; Schantz *et al.*, 1972; Yotis *et al.*, 1974). The evidence available indicates that this heterogeneity is due to deamidation of the protein that occurs during culture or in the procedures used in purification. In a study of the secondary structure of enterotoxins A, B and C, Middlebrook *et al.* (1980) showed that the circular dichroisms of enterotoxins B and C were similar and that both differed from enterotoxin A. The analysis suggested that the enterotoxin molecules contained little α-helix. For example, it was computed that for enterotoxin B, 29 amino acid residues were in α-helices, 71 in β-pleated sheets, 88 in β-turns and 55 in aperiodic conformation.

8.4.1. *Immunological Cross-reaction Between Enterotoxins*

The existence of different serotypes of staphylococcal enterotoxins was established when Bergdoll *et al.* (1959) showed that antiserum to highly purified enterotoxin B did not neutralize the enterotoxins produced by a number of strains of *S. aureus*. Specific antibodies are now available for enterotoxins A–E. However there is a considerable amount of evidence that indicates varying degrees of immunological relatedness between certain enterotoxins. Initially enterotoxins C_1 and C_2 were thought to differ only in their isoelectric points. However, Bergdoll *et al.* (1974b) concluded from double diffusion tests that, although the major antigenic sites of these toxins are identical, each toxin possesses a minor specific antigenic site. Also, it was noted that enterotoxin E was neutralized by anti A antiserum but not by antiserum to B or C.

Recently it was reported (Lee *et al.*, 1980) that enterotoxin C_1 and C_2 elicit both specific and cross-reacting antibodies. Similarly, enterotoxin B elicited specific antibodies but in some rabbits it induced the formation of antibodies that react with enterotoxins B, C_1 and C_2. Specific and common antibodies for enterotoxins A and E were isolated by affinity chromatography (Lee *et al.*, 1978); the specific antibodies reacted only with homologous enterotoxin preparations whereas the common antibodies reacted with both enterotoxins A and E in immunodiffusion tests.

A different approach to the analysis of similarities and differences between enterotoxins was adopted by Spero and coworkers (see, for example, Spero and Morlock, 1978, 1979). They found that enterotoxins B and C_1 could be cleaved by trypsin to yield large well defined polypeptide fragments. In the case of enterotoxin C_1 there was two trypsin cleavage sites, one internal to and the other external to the disulfide loop. Analysis of the three peptide fragments produced (MW = 6,500, 4,000 and 19,000, respectively) suggested that two major antigenic determinants were located on the 19,000 dalton component and one antigenic site on the 6,500 dalton component. The 19,000 dalton fragment also contained the site of emetic activity while mitogenic activity was restricted to the 6,500 dalton fragment. A similar analysis of enterotoxin B revealed a single trypsin cleavage site. In this case both fragments (MW = 11,500 and 17,000 respectively) contained antigenic sites. It was proposed that sites on the N-terminal polypeptide fragments of enterotoxins B and C_1 were responsible for the cross-reactions between these enterotoxins.

8.5. Mode of Action of Staphylococcal Enterotoxins

The symptoms of staphylococcal food poisoning are well defined (Bergdoll, 1972). The main symptoms are vomiting and diarrhoea which develop between 1–6 hr after ingestion of contaminated food. Accompanying symptoms include salivation, nausea, retching and abdominal cramps. In severe cases there may be marked prostration, a drop in blood pressure and there may be either fever or sub-normal temperature; blood and mucus may appear in the stools and vomitus.

The explanation of this symptomatology in cellular and molecular terms remains vague. At least part of the reason for this situation is the difficulty of devising appropriate animal models. Some species, such as the cat and the dog, are relatively insensitive to intragastric administration of enterotoxin and, as pointed out earlier, rodents lack a vomiting mechanism. Accordingly, much work has had to be carried out using rhesus monkeys.

Unlike the enterotoxins produced by other enteric pathogens, the action of staphylococcal enterotoxins is not restricted to the gastrointestinal tract. Enterotoxin administered intravenously induces vomiting and diarrhoea. Indeed lower doses are required by the intravenous route than by the intragastric route.

A study of emesis in monkeys (Sugiyama and Hayama, 1965) suggested that the site of emetic action was in the abdominal viscera and that the sensory stimulus for this action reached the vomiting centre of the CNS via the vagus nerves. However, a specific organ was not identified as the locus of emetic action.

Following these observations, there has been a tendency to regard staphylococcal enterotoxins as neurotoxins. This is misleading as there is evidence that the enterotoxins have a spectrum of biological effects. For instance, in experiments designed to study diarrhoea in dogs receiving large doses of enterotoxin, Shemano *et al.* (1967) suggested that diarrhoea could be attributed, at least in part, to inhibition of water absorption from the intestinal lumen, or to increased transmucosal fluid flux or to both these effects. Also, Kent (1966) studied acute gastroenteritis produced in the monkey by administration of a large dose (150 μg) of enterotoxin B; at 4–8 hr the jejunal mucosal surface showed development of long crypts and short villi. Using similar large doses, Merril and Sprintz (1968) reported that the most pronounced toxin-induced changes were at the villus crest. Electronmicroscopic studies indicated that mitochondria of villus and crypt epithelial cells underwent degeneration.

The action of staphylococcal enterotoxin on the intestine, in species other than the monkey, has been investigated by a few workers. Sullivan and Asano (1971) reported a brief and transient inhibition of intestinal water absorption by enterotoxin B in the rat, and altered ion transport and electrical properties in the flounder intestine treated with enterotoxins A, B and C was reported by Huang *et al.* (1974). However, in the course of studying the effect of δ-toxin on water absorption, Kapral *et al.* (1976) noted that enterotoxin B at a dose of 5 μg ml^{-1} had no effect on guinea-pig ileum. This confirmed the work of Koupal and Deibel (1977) that purified preparations of staphylococcal enterotoxins failed to elicit a positive ileal loop test in the rabbit. Interestingly, however, these workers described an exoprotein produced by strain 100 that was active in this system. Moreover, the enterotoxinogenic effect of this factor was neutralized by antiserum to enterotoxin A and the suggestion that the factor could be an altered form of enterotoxin A remains to be investigated.

A variety of other biological effects have been described, including leucocytosis following administration of enterotoxin at a dose of 5–10 μg *per os* to monkeys (Sugiyama and McKissic, 1966) and death after introduction of very large doses (1 mg kg^{-1}) of enterotoxin B intravenously in monkeys. In a further study of the lethal effect, Liu *et al.* (1978) attributed death to pulmonary dysfunction and terminal pulmonary edema.

There is little evidence that the enterotoxins exhibit general cytotoxic effects in tissue culture, though Schaeffer (1970) reported a cell damaging effect at high concentrations (100 μg ml^{-1}). A number of cell types were affected after 8 hr contact with enterotoxin B in medium containing human serum but *not* in the presence of calf serum. More importantly there have been several reports of the mitogenic action of enterotoxins on lymphocytes (Peavy *et al.*, 1970; Kaplan, 1972; Smith and Johnson, 1975; Warren, J. R. *et al.*, 1975; Warren, J. R. 1977). Recently Langford *et al.* (1978b) found that enterotoxin A stimulated maximum DNA and immune interferon synthesis in human peripheral lymphocytes at concentrations of 3.5×10^{-13} to 3.5×10^{-10} M, placing this toxin in a potency range equivalent to that of the hormones.

As enterotoxigenic strains are commonly isolated from purulent staphylococcal lesions, it is possible that the enterotoxins play an important role in modulating the immune response at the site of infection. This aspect as well as studies of emetic and diarrhoeagenic properties of staphylococcal enterotoxins merits further study.

9. STAPHYLOCOCCAL TOXINS AND THE TOXIC SHOCK SYNDROME

In 1978, Todd *et al.* described a severe acute disease in seven children (aged 8–17 years) associated with phage group I staphylococci. The main features of the disease which they termed Toxic Shock Syndrome (TSS) were: high fever, low blood pressure, a scarlatiniform rash, edema of the extremities and shock. One patient died, and all survivors developed desquamation of affected skin and peeling of palms and soles during convalescence. By September 1980, 229 cases of TSS had been reported to the Centres of Disease Control (CDC) in the United States; 95 per cent of these were in women with a mortality of 8 per cent. The clinical criteria for diagnosis of the disease (Davis *et al.*, 1980), all of which must be present, are as follows: fever above 38.9°C, documented hypotension or orthostatic dizziness, diffuse or palmar erythroderma followed by desquamation of the skin of the hands and feet, hyperemia of the conjuctiva or the mucous membranes of the oropharynx or vagina; and multisystem dysfunction which must include four of the following: vomiting or diarrhoea, alterations in consciousness, impaired renal function, impaired hepatic function, thrombocytopenia, elevated muscle creatine phosphokinase, cardiopulmonary dysfunction and decreased serum calcium and phosphate.

The overwhelming number of cases occurred in women during menstruation. A nationwide investigation initiated by CDC, Atlanta, revealed a strong association with vaginal tampons and confirmed the association with the presence of *S. aureus* in cervical and vaginal swabs. Although the association with tampons is striking, it should be noted that TSS has occasionally been associated with *S. aureus* infection in extragenital sites (Todd *et al.*, 1978; Davis *et al.*, 1980). More recent data shows that an increasing proportion (13.2 per cent) of reported cases of TSS are not associated with menstruation (Reingold *et al.*, 1982). The role of tampons and the factors that precipitate the occurrence of TSS in certain individuals is not yet fully understood.

The absence of septicemia in TSS, taken together with the symptomatology of the disease, suggests the involvement of a staphylococcal toxin(s) in its pathogenesis. Again, because of the clinical symptoms, attention has focussed on staphylococcal products that have pyrogenic and/or enterotoxigenic properties.

In 1978, Dr. Patrick Schlievert and his coworkers, a team with considerable experience in the field of streptococcal pyrogenic exotoxins, began to investigate the production of pyrogenic exotoxin by a strain of *S. aureus* isolated from a patient with Kawasaki's disease. Their publication (Schlievert *et al.*, 1979b) described a factor, Pyrogenic exotoxin A (PEA), that caused fever in rabbits and mice and enhanced the susceptibility of these animals to endotoxin; PEA was also mitogenic. It had a molecular weight of 12,000 and an isoelectric point of 5.3. This study was followed up by the description of two additional serologically distinct staphylococcal pyrogenic exotoxins (PEB and PEC) (Schlievert, 1980; Schlievert *et al.*, 1981).

The association of pyrogenic exotoxins with TSS was studied (Schlievert, *et al.*, 1981). No association was found for PEA and PEB but a positive association was observed for PEC; all of 28 isolates from patients with TSS but only 5 of 16 control isolates produced PEC, which was detected by its characteristic pI of 7.2 in thin layer isoelectric focusing gels. The molecular weight was estimated to be 22,000 and purified PEC was pyrogenic in rabbits; it also potentiated the lethal effect of endotoxin and was mitogenic. Because of strong association with TSS, Schlievert *et al.* (1981) considered PEC to be a useful marker for identifying strains of *S. aureus* capable of causing TSS. However, the purified toxin did not reproduce the full spectrum of symptoms of TSS in experimental animals. Recently Schlievert (1983) has shown that injection of sublethal amounts of PEC together with endotoxin in rabbits suppresses the complement fixing antibody response to sheep erythrocytes and also suppresses clearance of colloidal carbon by the reticuloendothelial system. On the basis of this, he has postulated that in TSS, PEC is involved in suppression of the immune response to gram-negative bacteria and furthermore in failure to clear endotoxin thus allowing host susceptibility to endotoxic shock. In a comparison of 15 isolates from TSS and 18 vaginal isolates from women without TSS, Barbour (1981) observed that all the TSS isolates and 50 per cent of non-TSS isolates produced a protein with a pI of 7.0 and a molecular weight of 22,000 which could be identical with PEC.

Some of the symptoms of TSS also resemble the effects of staphylococcal enterotoxins (see Section 8). This prompted Bergdoll and his coworkers (Bergdoll *et al.*, 1981) to assess the production of enterotoxins by strains from TSS patients. It was found that 93.8 per cent of 65 such isolates produced an enterotoxin-like protein which was serologically distinct from the known enterotoxins and this factor has been designated enterotoxin F; only 4.6 per cent of 87 *S. aureus* strains from other sources were found to produce this toxin.

Enterotoxin F was purified by a combination of ion exchange chromatography and gel filtration and the degree of purity, as determined by polyacrylamide gel electrophoresis, was estimated to be greater than 95 per cent. The molecular weight was reported as 20,000 and the isoelectric point was 6.8. Studies of the biological properties of enterotoxin F are as yet incomplete, but Bergdoll *et al.* (1981) found that it caused emesis in monkeys when administered intragastrically.

In our laboratory, 17 isolates from TSS patients in Britain were examined. They belonged to phage group I, a characteristic of TSS strains, and were resistant to penicillin, cadmium and arsenate (de Saxe *et al.*, 1982a). It was found that 15 isolates (88 per cent) produced a protein with a pI of 7.3 which we designated Toxic Factor (TF). A relatively large proportion (33 per cent) of our 49 control strains also produced TF and we noted that control strains which had been matched to TSS strains on the basis of phage type and antibiotic/heavy metal ion resistance showed a higher frequency of TF production (de Saxe *et al.*, 1982b). Kreisworth *et al.* (1982) however, have shown that the toxin gene is not linked to any of these three resistance traits. We also found that TSS strains were generally less haemolytic than control strains and this finding has been confirmed by other workers (Barbour, 1981; Chow *et al.*, 1983).

TF was purified by preparative isoelectric focusing and the degree of purity, as estimated by polyacrylamide gel electrophoresis, was estimated to be greater than 98 per cent. The molecular weight was estimated at 23,000 and the protein was resistant to heating; the amino acid composition differed from other known staphylococcal toxins. TF induced a shock-like syndrome in rabbits when injected intravenously, intradermally or *in utero* and single doses of greater than 20 μg were lethal in rabbits; mice, rats, hamsters, guinea-pigs and cats were resistant to 100 μg TF. Purified TF also caused enhanced capillary permeability and in common with PEC, was mitogenic, weakly pyrogenic and acted synergistically with endotoxin to enhance lethality in rabbits (de Azavedo *et al.*, 1984). TF and enterotoxin F show immunological identity and Notermans (1983) has also shown that partially purified enterotoxin F is lethal in rabbits. These findings indicate that PEC, enterotoxin F and TF are in fact the same protein. The role of such factors in TSS as well as the cell-associated protein antigens described by Cohen and Falkow (1981) remain to be determined. Indeed the complex interactions of host, tampon, colonizing *S. aureus* and toxic products presents a challenging and important medical problem.

10. CONCLUDING REMARKS

In assessing the past 25 years of research on staphylococcal toxins, undoubtedly the greatest success has been achieved in the area of physicochemical characterization. The application of increasingly powerful techniques of protein purification has enabled almost all of the toxins covered in this review to be isolated in highly purified form. Detailed analysis of the molecular structure is now at a fairly advanced stage for several toxins (α-toxin, δ-toxin, epidermolytic toxin and the enterotoxins).

Though our knowledge of the range of biological effects of staphylococcal toxins has advanced considerably, the molecular basis of action continues to present a challenge. The enzymic mode of action of β-toxin has been unequivocally established and there is general agreement about the detergent-like properties of δ-toxin. We are tantalizingly close to an answer to the mode of action of α-toxin and this problem should be solved soon. However, in the case of γ-toxin, leucocidin, epidermolytic toxin and the enterotoxins, the molecular basis of action continues to pose fascinating problems.

Analysis of the genetic regulation of exotoxin production in *S. aureus* is also a challenging area of future research. There has been some progress in determining the genetic location of certain toxin genes (e.g. epidermolytic toxin, enterotoxin B and α-toxin), but our knowledge is in its infancy. Progress will depend on how easily recombinant DNA techniques can be applied to *S. aureus*. So far this has proved technically much more difficult than in Gram-negative organisms.

Steady progress is being made on our understanding of the role of staphylococcal toxins in pathogenesis. The enterotoxins are clearly responsible for the symptoms of food poisoning and epidermolytic toxin for the epidermal splitting that is characteristic of blistering diseases of the skin. Work with experimental infections has also established the role of α-toxin in causing local necrosis. Similar studies suggest that, if β-toxin, δ-toxin and leucocidin have a role, it is likely to be subtle and part of a multifactorial interaction between the host and the staphylococcus.

The clinical features of the recently described Toxic Shock Syndrome suggest the involvement of a potent toxin, or combination of toxic factors. That enterotoxin F or pyrogenic exotoxin C may be implicated in TSS is certainly suggested by recent work. Indeed, this work may point to a wider role for the enterotoxins. The fact that enterotoxins are potent mitogens and are also pyrogenic suggests that they may be involved in diseases other than food poisoning.

ACKNOWLEDGEMENT

We are grateful to Gillian Johnston for typing the manuscript.

REFERENCES

ABBAS-ALI, B. and COLEMAN, G. (1977a) Nutritional shifts and their effect on the secretion of extracellular proteins by *Staphylococcus aureus* (Wood 46). *Biochem. Soc. Trans.* **5**: 420–422.

ABBAS-ALI, B. and COLEMAN, G. (1977b) The characteristics of extracellular protein secretions by *Staphylococcus aureus* (Wood 46) and their relationship to the regulation of α-toxin formation. *J. Gen. Microbiol.* **99**: 277–282.

ADLAM, C., WARD, P. D., MCCARTNEY, A. C., ARBUTHNOTT, J. P. and THORLEY, C. M. (1977) Effect of immunization with highly purified alpha- and beta-toxins on staphylococcal mastitis in rabbits. *Infect. Immun.* **17**: 250–256.

ADLAM, C., WARD, P. D. and TURNER, W. H. (1980) Effect of immunization with highly purified Panton–Valentine leucocidin and delta-toxin on staphylococcal mastitis in rabbits. *J. Comp. Path.* **90**: 265–274.

ARBUTHNOTT, J. P. (1970) Staphylococcal α-toxin. In: *Microbial Toxins*, Vol. III, *Bacterial Protein Toxins*, pp. 189–232, MONTIE, T. C., KADIS, S. and AJL, S. J. (Eds). Academic Press, New York.

ARBUTHNOTT, J. P. and BILLCLIFFE, B. (1976) Qualitative and quantitative methods for detecting staphylococcal epidermolytic toxin. *J. Med. Microbiol.* **9**: 191–201.

ARBUTHNOTT, J. P., FREER, J. H. and BERNHEIMER, A. W. (1967) Physical states of staphylococcal α-toxin. *J. Bact.* **94**: 1170–1177.

ARBUTHNOTT, J. P., KENT, J., LYELL, A. and GEMMELL, C. G. (1971) Toxic epidermal necrolysis produced by an extracellular product of *S. aureus. Br. J. Derm.* **85**: 145–149.

ARBUTHNOTT, J. P., KENT, J. and NOBLE, W. C. (1973) The response of hairless mice to staphylococcal epidermolytic toxin. *Br. J. Derm.* **88**: 481–485.

ARBUTHNOTT, J. P., BILLCLIFFE, B. and THOMPSON, W. D. (1974) Isoelectric focusing studies of staphylococcal epidermolytic toxin. *FEBS Letts* **46**: 92–95.

AVENA, R. M. and BERGDOLL, M. S. (1967) Purification and some physicochemical properties of enterotoxin C. *Staphylococcus aureus* strain 361. *Biochemistry* **6**: 1474–1480.

AVIGAD, L. S. and BERNHEIMER, A. W. (1978) Inhibition of haemolysins by zinc and its reversal by histidine. *Infect. Immun.* **19**: 1101–1103.

DE AZAVEDO, J. and ARBUTHNOTT, J. P. (1981) Prevalence of epidermolytic toxin in clinical isolates of *Staphylococcus aureus. J. Med. Microbiol.* **14**: 341–344.

DE AZAVEDO, J. C., HARTIGAN, P. J. and ARBUTHNOTT, J. P. (1984) Toxins in relation to Staphylococcal toxic shock syndrome. pp 331–338 in *Bacterial Protein Toxins.* ed. J. ALOUF, F. FEHRENBACH, J. H. FREER and J. JELJASZEWICZ. Academic Press. London.

BAILEY, C. J., DE AZAVEDO, J. and ARBUTHNOTT, J. P. (1980) A comparative study of two serotypes of epidermolytic toxin from *Staphylococcus aureus. Biochim. biophys. Acta* **624**: 111–120.

BAKER, D. H., DIMOND, R. L. and WUEPPER, K. D. (1978) The epidermolytic toxin of *S. aureus*. Its failure to bind to cells and its detection in blister fluids of patients with bullous impetigo. *J. Invest. Derm.* **71**: 274–275.

BARBOUR, A. G. (1981) Vaginal isolates of *Staphylococcus aureus* associated with toxic shock syndrome. *Infect. Immun.* **33**: 442–449.

BAREI, G. M. and FACKRELL, H. B. (1979) The binding of fluorescein-labelled staphylococcal alpha toxoid to erythrocytes. *Can. J. Microbiol.* **25:** 1219–1226.

BERGDOLL, M. S. (1970) Enterotoxins In: *Microbial Toxins* Vol. **III.** *Bacterial Toxins*, pp. 265–326, MONTIE, T. C., KADIS, S. and AJL, S. J. (Eds). Academic Press. New York.

BERGDOLL, M. S. (1972) The enterotoxins. In: *The Staphylococci*, pp. 301–331, COHEN, J. O. (Ed). John Wiley, New York.

BERGDOLL, M. (1983) Enterotoxins. In: *Staphylococci and Staphylococcal Infections*, Vol. **II,** EASMON, C. and ADLAM, C. (Eds). Academic Press. New York.

BERGDOLL, M. S., SURGALLA, M. J. and DACK, G. M. (1959) Staphylococcal enterotoxin. Identification of a specific precipitating antibody with enterotoxin-neutralizing property. *J. Immun.* **83:** 334–338.

BERGDOLL, M. S., CHU, F. S., HUANG, I.-Y., ROWE, C., and SHIH, T. (1965) Staphylococcal enterotoxin B—III. The physicochemical properties and the N- and C-terminal amino acid sequences. *Archs Biochem. Biophys.* **112:** 104–110.

BERGDOLL, M. S., CZOP, J. K. and GOULD, S. S. (1974a) Enterotoxin synthesis by the staphylococci. In: *Recent Advances in Staphylococcal Research*, pp. 307–316, YOTIS, W. W. (Ed.). *Ann. N.Y. Acad. Sci.*, Vol. **236.**

BERGDOLL, M. S., HUANG, I. Y. and SCHANTZ, E. J. (1974b) Chemistry of the staphylococcal enterotoxins. *J. Agric. Food Chem.* **22:** 9–13.

BERGDOLL, M. S., CROSS, B. A., REISSER, R. F., ROBBINS, R. N. and DAVIS, J. P. (1981) A new staphylococcal enterotoxin, enterotoxin F, associated with toxic-shock-syndrome *Staphylococcus aureus* isolates. *Lancet* **ii:** 1017–1021.

BERNHEIMER, A. W. (1974) Interactions between membranes and cytolytic bacterial toxins. *Biochim. biophys. Acta* **344:** 27–50.

BERNHEIMER, A. W. and AVIGAD, L. S. (1980) Inhibition of bacterial and other cytolysins by glycophorin. *FEMS Letts* **9:** 15–17.

BERNHEIMER, A. W. and SCHWARTZ, L. L. (1963) Isolation and composition of staphylococcal alpha toxin. *J. Gen. Microbiol.* **30:** 455–468.

BERNHEIMER, A. W., AVIGAD, L. S. and KIM, K. S. (1974) Staphylococcal sphingomyelinase (beta haemolysin) *Ann. N.Y. Acad. Sci.* **236:** 292–306.

BEZARD, G. and PLOMMET, M. (1973) Production de la toxine staphylococcique Gamma brute. *Ann. Rech. Veter.* **4:** 355–358.

BHAKDI, S., FÜSSLE, R. and TRANUM–JENSEN, J. (1981) Staphylococcal α-toxin: Oligomerization of hydrophilic monomers to form amphiphilic hexamers induced through contact with deoxycholate detergent micelles. *Proc. Natl. Acad. Sci. U.S.A.* **78:** 5475–5479.

BIGGER, J. W., BOLAND, C. R. and O'MEARA, R. A. Q. (1927) A new method of preparing staphylococcal haemolysin. *J. Path. Bact.* **30:** 271–277.

BJORKLIND, A. and ARVIDSON, S. (1980) Mutants of *Staphylococcus aureus* affected in the regulation of exoprotein synthesis. *FEMS Letts* **7:** 203–206.

BLAIR, J. E. and CARR, M. (1961) Lysogeny in staphylococci. *J. Bact.* **82:** 987–993.

BORJA, C. R. (1969) Staphylococcal enterotoxin C—I. Phenolic hydroxyl ionization. *Biochemistry* **8:** 71–75.

BORJA, C. R. and BERGDOLL, M. S. (1967) Purification and partial characterization of enterotoxin C produced by *Staphylococcus aureus* strain 137. *Biochemistry* **6:** 1467–1473.

BORJA, C. R. and BERGDOLL, M. S. (1969) Staphylococcal enterotoxin C—II. Some physical, immunological and toxic properties. *Biochemistry* **8:** 75–79.

BORJA, C. R., FANNING, E., HUANG, I.-Y. and BERGDOLL, M. S. (1972) Purification and some physicochemical properties of staphylococcal enterotoxin E. *J. Biol. Chem.* **247:** 2456–2463.

BRETSCHER, M. S. (1972) Asymmetrical lipid bilayer structure for biological membrane. *Nature, New Biol.* **236:** 11–12.

BROWN, D. R. and PATEE, P. A. (1980) Identification of a chromosomal determinant of alpha-toxin production in *Staphylococcus aureus. Infect. Immun.* **30:** 36–42.

BRYCE, L. M. and ROUNTREE, P. M. (1936) The production of β-toxin by staphylococci. *J. Path. Bact.* **86:** 702–707.

BUCKELEW, A. R. and COLACICCO, G. (1971) Lipid monolayers: interactions with staphylococcal α-toxin. *Biochim. biophys. Acta* **233:** 7–16.

CAIRD, J. D. and WISEMAN, G. (1970) Purification of the delta-toxin of *Staphylococcus aureus. Can. J. Microbiol.* **16:** 703–708.

CASMAN, E. P. and BENNET, R. W. (1963) Culture medium for the production of staphylococcal enterotoxin A. *J. Bact.* **86:** 18–23.

CASMAN, E. P., BENNET, R. W., DORSEY, A. E. and ISSA, J. A. (1967) Identification of a fourth staphylococcal enterotoxin, enterotoxin D. *J. Bact.* **94:** 1875–1882.

CASSIDY, P. and HARSHMAN, S. (1976a) Purification of Staphylococcal alpha toxin by adsorption chromatography on glass. *Infect. Immun.* **13:** 982–986.

CASSIDY, P. and HARSHMAN, S. (1976b) Iodination of a tyrosyl residue in staphylococcal α-toxin. *Biochemistry* **15:** 2342–2348.

CASSIDY, P. and HARSHMAN, S. (1976c) Studies on the binding of staphylococcal ^{125}I-labeled α-toxin to rabbit erythrocytes. *Biochemistry* **15:** 2348–2355.

CASSIDY, P. and HARSHMAN, S. (1979) Characterisation of detergent-solubilized iodine ^{125}I-labeled α-toxin bound to rabbit erythrocytes and mouse diaphragm muscle. *Biochemistry* **18:** 232–236.

CASSIDY, P., HOAR, P. E. and KERRICK, W. G. I. (1978) Tension development in rabbit ileum smooth muscle skinned by staphylococcal α-toxin: activation by Ca^{2+} and Sr^{2+}, irreversible activation in presence of ATP *Biophys. J.* **21:** 11a.

CASU, A., NANNI, G., MARINARI, N. M., PALA, V. and MONACELLI, R. (1969) Structure of membranes—Note V: Sphingomyelin detection by immune reaction on the surface of sheep erythrocytes. *Ital. J. Biochem.* **18:** 154–165.

CHANG, P.-C. and BERGDOLL, M. S. (1979) Purification and some properties of staphylococcal enterotoxin D. *Biochemistry* **18:** 1937–1942.

Chang, P.-C. and Dickie, N. (1971a) Fractionation of staphylococcal enterotoxin B by isoelectric focusing. *Biochim. biophys. Acta* **236**: 367–375.

Chang, P.-C. and Dickie, N. (1971b) Heterogeneity of staphylococcal enterotoxin B. *Can. J. Microbiol.* **17**: 1479–1481.

Chang, P.-C., Dickie, N. and Thatcher, F. S. (1971) Hydroxyapatite column chromatography of enterotoxin B. *Can. J. Microbiol.* **17**: 296–297.

Chao, L. P. and Birkbeck, T. H. (1978) Assay of staphylococcal δ-haemolysin with fish erythrocytes. *J. Med. Microbiol.* **11**: 303–313.

Chesbro, W. R. and Kucic, V. (1971) Beta haemolysin: a persistent impurity in preparation of staphylococcal nuclease and enterotoxin. *Appl. Microbiol.* **22**: 233–241.

Chesbro, W. R., Heydrick, F. P., Martineau, R. and Perkins, G. N. (1965) Purification of staphylococcal beta haemolysin and its action on staphylococcal and streptococcal cell walls. *J. Bact.* **89**: 378–389.

Chow, A. W., Gribble, M. J. and Bartlett, K. H. (1983) Characterization of the haemolytic activity of *Staphylococcus aureus* strains associated with Toxic Shock Syndrome. *J. Clin. Microbiol.* **17**: 524–528.

Chu, F. S. (1968) Hydrogen ion equilibria of staphylococcal enterotoxin B. *J. Biol. Chem.* **243**: 4342–4349.

Chu, F. S. and Bergdoll, M. S. (1969) Studies on the chemical modification of staphylococcal enterotoxin B—I. Alkylation and oxidation of methionine residues. *Biochim. biophys. Acta* **194**: 279–286.

Chu, F. S. and Crany, E. (1969) Studies on the chemical modification of staphylococcal enterotoxin B—II. Carboxyl residues. *Biochim. biophys. Acta.* **194**: 287–292.

Cohen, M. L. and Falkow, S. (1981) Protein antigens from *Staphylococcus aureus* strains associated with toxic shock syndrome. *Science* **211**: 842–844.

Colacicco, G. and Buckelew, A. R. (1971) Lipid monolayers: Influence of lipid film and urea on the surface activity of staphylococcal α-toxin. *Lipids* **6**: 546–553.

Colacicco, G., Basu, M. K., Buckelew, A. R. and Bernheimer, A. W. (1977) Surface properties of membrane systems. Transport of staphylococcal δ-toxin from aqueous to membrane phase. *Biochim. biophys. Acta* **465**: 378–390.

Coleman, G. (1981) Pleiotropic compensation in the regulation of extracellular protein formation by a low α-toxin producing variant of *Staphylococcus aureus* (Wood 46). *J. Gen. Microbiol.* **122**: 11–15.

Coleman, G. and Abbas-Ali, B. (1979) Comparison of the patterns of increase in α-toxin and total extracellular protein by *Staphylococcus aureus* (Wood 46) grown in media supporting widely differing growth characteristics. *Infect. Immun.* **17**: 278–281.

Coleman, G., Brown, S. and Stormonth, D. A. (1975) A model for the regulation of bacterial extracellular enzyme and toxin biosynthesis. *J. Theor. Biol.* **52**: 143–148.

Colley, C. M., Zwaal, R. F. A., Roelofsen, B. and van Deenen, L. L. M. (1973) Lytic and nonlytic degradation of phospholipids in mammalian erythrocytes by pure phospholipases. *Biochim. biophys. Acta* **307**: 74–82.

Cooper, L. Z., Madoff, M. A. and Weinstein, L. (1966) Heat stability and species range of purified staphylococcal alpha toxin. *J. Bact.* **91**: 1686–1692.

Coulter, J. R. (1966) Production, purification and composition of staphylococcal α-toxin. *J. Bacteriol.* **92**: 1655–1662.

Czop, J. K. and Bergdoll, M. S. (1970) Synthesis of enterotoxin by L-forms of *Staphylococcus aureus*. *Infect. Immun.* **1**: 166–168.

Dalen, A. B. (1975) Multiple forms of staphylococcal α-toxin. *Acta Path. Microbiol. Scand., Sect. B.* **83**: 561–568.

Dalen, A. B. (1976a) Proteolytic degradation of staphylococcal α-toxin. *Acta Path. Microbiol. Scand. Sect. B.* **84**: 309–314.

Dalen, A. B. (1976b) A simple procedure for the purification of staphylococcal α-toxin. *Acta Path. Microbiol. Scand., Sect B.* **84**: 326–332.

Dalen, A. B. (1976c) Spontaneous α-toxin mutants of *Staphylococcus aureus*. *Acta Path. Microbiol. Scand., Sect. B.* **84**: 333–338.

Davis, B. D. and Tai, P.-C. (1980) The mechanism of protein secretion across membranes. *Nature,* **283**: 433–438.

Davis, J. P., Chesney, P. J., Wand, P. J. and La Venture, M. and the Investigation and Laboratory Team (1980) Toxic shock syndrome: epidemiologic features, recurrence, risk factors and prevention. *New Eng. J. Med.* **303**: 1429–1435.

Dawson, C. R., Drake, A. F., Helliwell, J. and Hider, R. C. (1978) The interaction of bee melittin with lipid bilayer membranes. *Biochim. biophys. Acta.* **510**: 75–86.

Day, S. E. J. (1983) *In* A System for the study *in vivo* of staphylococcal populations and the ensuing host response. Ph.D. thesis. Trinity College Dublin.

Day, S. E. J., Vasli, K. K., Russell, R. J. and Arbuthnott, J. P. (1980) A simple method for the study *in vivo* of bacterial growth and accompanying host response. *J. Infect.* **2**: 39–51.

Dayhoff, M. ed. (1972) Data section. In: *Atlas protein Sequence Structure*, **5**: D227. National Biomedical Research Foundation, Washington, D.C.

Demel, R. A., Guerts van Kessel, W. S. M., Zwaal, R. F. A., Roelofsen, B. and van Deenen, L. L. M. (1975) Relation between various phospholipase actions on human red cell membranes and the interfacial phospholipid pressure in monolayers. *Biochim. biophys. Acta* **406**: 97–107.

Dickie, N., Yano, Y., Robern, H. and Stavric, S. (1972) On the heterogeneity of staphylococcal enterotoxin C_2. *Can. J. Microbiol.* **18**: 801–804.

Dimond, R. L. and Wuepper, K. D. (1976) Purification and characterization of a staphylococcal epidermolytic toxin. *Infect. Immun.* **13**: 627–633.

Doery, H. M., Magnuson, B. J., Cheyne, I. M. and Galasekharam, J. (1963) A phospholipase in staphylococcal toxin which hydrolyses sphingomyelin. *Nature (Lond.)* **198**: 1091–1092.

Doery, H. M., Magnusson, B. J., Galasekharam, J. and Pearson, J. E. (1965) The properties of phospholipase enzymes in staphylococcal toxins. *J. Gen. Microbiol.* **40**: 283–296.

Dornbusch, K. and Hallander, H. O. (1973) Transduction of penicillinase production and methicillin resistance-enterotoxin B production in strains of *Staphylococcus aureus*. *J. Gen. Microbiol.* **76**: 1–11.

Dornbusch, K., Hallander, H. O. and Lofquist, F. (1969) Extrachromosomal control of methicillin resistance and toxin production in *Staphylococcus aureus*. *J. Bacteriol.* **98**: 351–358.

DUNCAN, J. L. and CHO, G. J. (1971) Production of staphylococcal alpha toxin—I. Relationship between cell growth and toxin formation. *Infect. Immun.* **4:** 456–461.

DURKIN, J. P. and SHIER, W. T. (1980) Cell-cycle resistance to staphylococcal delta toxin-induced lysis of cultured cells. *Biochim. biophys. Res. Commun.* **94:** 980–987.

DURKIN, J. P. and SHIER, W. T. (1981) Staphylococcal delta toxin stimulates endogenous phospholipase A_2 activity and prostaglandin synthesis in fibroblasts. *Biochim. biophys. Acta* **663:** 467–479.

DYER, D. W. and IANDOLO, J. J. (1981) Plasmid-chromosomal transition of genes important in staphylococcal enterotoxin B expression. *Infect. Immun.* **33:** 450–458.

ELEK, S. D. (1959) *Staphylococcus pyogenes* and its Relation to Disease, p. 239, Livingstone, London.

ELEK, S. D. and LEVY, E. (1950) Distribution of haemolysins in pathogenic and non-pathogenic staphylococci. *J. Path. Bact.* **62:** 541–554.

ELIAS, P. M., MITTERMAYER, H., TAPPEINER, G., FRITSCH, P. and WOLFF, K. (1974) Staphylococcal toxic epidermal necrolysis (TEN): The expanded mouse model. *J. Invest. Dermatol.* **63:** 467–475.

ELIAS, P. M., FRITSCH, P., DAHL, M. V. and WOLFF, K. (1975) Staphylococcal exfoliative toxin: pathogenesis and subcellular site of action. *J. Invest. Derm.* **65:** 501–512.

ELIAS, P. M., FRITSCH, P. and MITTERMAYER, G. (1976) Staphylococcal toxic epidermal necrolysis: species and tissue susceptibility and resistance. *J. Invest. Derm.* **66:** 80–89.

ELIAS, P. M., FRITSCH, P. and EPSTEIN, E. H. (1977) Staphylococcal scalded skin syndrome. Clinical features, pathogenesis and recent microbiological and biochemical developments. *Archs. Derm.* **113:** 207–219.

FACKRELL, H. B. (1973) Studies with gamma haemolysin of *Staphylococcus aureus*. Ph.D. thesis, University of Mannitoba, Winnipeg, Canada.

FACKRELL, H. B. and WISEMAN, G. M. (1974) Immunogenicity of the delta haemolysin of *Staphylococcus aureus*. *J. Med. Microbiol.* **7:** 411–414.

FACKRELL, H. B. and WISEMAN, G. M. (1976a) Production and purification of the gamma haemolysin of *Staphylococcus aureus* 'Smith 5R'. *J. Gen. Microbiol.* **92:** 1–10.

FACKRELL, H. B. and WISEMAN, G. M. (1976b) Properties of the gamma haemolysin of *Staphylococcus aureus* 'Smith 5R'. *J. Gen. Microbiol.* **92:** 11–24.

FADEN, H., BURKE, J., EVERETT, J. and GLASGOW, L. A. (1974) Nursery outbreak of staphylococcal scalded skin syndrome due to group 1 *S. aureus*. *Pediat. Res.* **8:** 424.

FITTON, J. E., DELL, A. and SHAW, W. V. (1980) The amino acid sequence of the delta haemolysin of *Staphylococcus aureus*. *FEBS Letts* **115:** 209–212.

FORLANI, L. A., BERNHEIMER, A. W. and CHIANCONE, E. (1971) Ultracentrifugal analysis of staphylococcal alpha toxin. *J. Bact.* **106:** 138–142.

FREER, J. H. and ARBUTHNOTT, J. P. (1976) Biochemical and morphologic alterations of membranes by bacterial toxins. In: *Mechanisms in Bacterial Toxinology*, pp. 169–193, BERNHEIMER, A. W. (Ed.). Wiley, New York.

FREER, J. H. and BIRKBECK, T. H. (1982) Possible conformation of delta-lysin, a membrane-active peptide of *Staphylococcus aureus*. *J. Theor. Biol.* **94:** 535–540.

FREER, J. H., ARBUTHNOTT, J. P. and BERNHEIMER, A. W. (1968) Interaction of staphylococcal α-toxin with artificial and natural membranes. *J. Bact.* **95:** 1153–1168.

FREER, J. H., ARBUTHNOTT, J. P. and BILLCLIFFE, B. (1973) Effects of staphylococcal α-toxin on the structure of erythrocyte membranes: a biochemical and freeze-etching study. *J. Gen. Microbiol.* **75:** 321–332.

FRIEDMAN, M. E. (1968) Inhibition of Staphylococcal enterotoxin B formation by cell wall blocking agents and other compounds. *J. Bact.* **95:** 1051–1055.

FRITSCH, P. O., KAASERER, G. and ELIAS, P. M. (1979) Action of staphylococcal epidermolysin: further observations on its species specificity. *Archs Dermatol. Res.* **264:** 287–291.

FRITSCHE, D. and ZITZ, M. (1973) The effect of uptake of free fatty acids on the growth and the β-haemolysin production of *Staphylococcus aureus*. *Med. Microbiol. Immun.* **158:** 185–191.

FÜSSLE, R., BHAKDI, S., SZIEGOLEIT, A., TRANUM–JENSEN, J., KRANZ, T. and WELLENSIEK, H.-J. (1981) On the mechanism of membrane damage by Staphylococcus aureus α-toxin. *J. Cell. Biol.* **91,** 83–94.

GALINSKI, J. (1976) Exfoliatin production by *Staphylococcus aureus* of phage group II. In: *Staphylococci and Staphylococcal Diseases*, pp. 517–521, JELJASZEWICZ, J. (Ed.). *Zbl. Bakt., Suppl. 5*. Gustav Fischer Verlag, Stuttgart.

GEMMELL, C. G., THELESTAM, M. and WADSTRÖM, T. (1976) Toxigenicity of coagulase-negative staphylococci. In: *Staphylococci and staphylococcal diseases*, pp. 133–136, JELJASZEWICZ, J. (Ed.). *Zbl. Bakt., Suppl. 5*. Gustav Fischer Verlag, Stuttgart.

GILBERT, R. J. and WIENEKE, A. A. (1973) Staphylococcal food poisoning with special reference to the detection of enterotoxin in food. In: *The Microbiological Safety of Food*, p. 273. HOBBS, B. C. and CHRISTIAN, J. H. B. (eds). Academic Press, London and New York.

GLADSTONE, G. P. (1938) The production of staphylococcal α-haemolysin in a chemically defined medium. *Br. J. Exp. Path.* **19:** 208–226.

GLADSTONE, G. P. and VAN HEYNINGEN, W. E. (1957) Staphylococcal leucocidins. *Br. J. Exp. Path.* **38:** 123–127.

GLENNY, A. T. and STEVENS, N. F. (1935) Staphylococcus toxins and antitoxins. *J. Path. Bact.* **40:** 201–210.

GOODE, R. L. and BALDWIN, J. N. (1973) Purification of staphylococcal α-toxin by electrofocusing. *Preparative Biochem.* **3:** 349–361.

GOODE, R. L. and BALDWIN, J. N. (1974) Comparison of purified alpha toxins from various strains of *Staphylococcus aureus*. *Appl. Envir. Microbiol.* **28:** 86–90.

GOSHI, K., CLUFF, L. E. and NORMAN, P. S. (1963) Studies on pathogenesis of staphylococcal infection—V. Purification and characterisation of staphylococcal alpha haemolysin. *Bull. Johns Hopkins Hosp.* **112:** 15–30.

GOW, J. A. and ROBINSON, J. (1969) Properties of purified beta haemolysin. *J. Bact.* **97:** 1026–1032.

GUYONNET, F. (1970) Toxicite de la toxine gamma de *Staphylococcus aureus* pour la souris. *Ann. Rech. Veter.* **1:** 155–160.

GUYONNET, F. and PLOMMET, M. (1970) Hemolysine gamma de *Staphylococcus aureus*: purification et propriétés. *Ann. Inst. Pasteur* **118:** 19–33.

GUYONNET, F., PLOMMET, M. and BOUILLANNE, C. (1968) Purification de l'hemolysine gamma de *Staphylococcus aureus*. *C.R. Acad. Sci.* **267:** 1180–1182.

Hall, H. E., Angelotti, R. and Lewis, K. H. (1965) Detection of staphylococcal enterotoxins in food. *Hlth Lab. Sci.* **2:** 179–191.

Hallander, H. O. (1968) Characterisation and partial purification of staphylococcal delta lysin. *Acta Path. Microbiol. Scand.* **72:** 586–600.

Haque, R. U. and Baldwin, J. N. (1969) Purification and properties of staphylococcal beta-haemolysin—II. Purification of beta haemolysin. *J. Bact.* **88:** 1304–1309.

Harshman, S., (1979) Action of staphylococcal α-toxin on membranes: Some recent advances. *Molec. Cell. Biochem.* **23:** 143–152.

Heatley, N. G. (1971) A new method for the preparation and some properties of staphylococcal delta-haemolysin. *J. Gen. Microbiol.* **69:** 269–278.

Hendricks, C. W. and Altenbern, R. A. (1968) Studies on the synthesis of staphylococcal alpha toxin. *Can. J. Microbiol.* **4:** 1277–1281.

Heydrick, F. P. and Chesbro, W. R. (1962) Purification and properties of staphylococcal beta toxin. *Bact. Proc.* p. 63.

Huang, I.-Y. and Bergdoll, M. S. (1970) The primary structure of staphylococcal enterotoxin B—I. Isolation, composition, and sequence of tryptic peptides from oxidised enterotoxin B. *J. Biol. Chem.* **245:** 3493–3510.

Huang, I.-Y., Shih, T., Borja, C. R., Avena, R. M. and Bergdoll, M. S. (1967) Amino acid composition and terminal amino acids of staphylococcal enterotoxin C. *Biochemistry* **6:** 1480–1484.

Huang, K.-C., Chen, R. S. T. and Rent, W. R. (1974) Effect of staphylococcal enterotoxins A, B and C on ion transport and permeability across the flounder intestine. *Proc. Soc. Exp. Biol.* **147:** 250–254.

Iandolo, J. J. and Shafer, W. M. (1977) Regulation of staphylococcal enterotoxin B. *Infect. Immun.* **16:** 610–616.

Inouye, M. (1974) A Three-dimensional assembly model of a lipoprotein from the *Escherichia coli* outer membrane. *Proc. Natn. Acad. Sci. U.S.A.* **71:** 2396–2400.

Jackson, A. W. (1963) Staphylococcal gamma lysin and its differentiation from delta-lysin. In: *Recent progress in Microbiology*: Symposia. Gibbons, N. E. (ed.). University of Toronto Press, Toronto. (Cited by Wiseman, G., 1975).

Jackson, A. W. and Little, R. M. (1958) Staphylococcal toxins—III. Partial purification and some properties of delta-lysin. *Can. J. Microbiol.* **4:** 453–461.

Jackson, A. W. and Mayman, D. (1958) Staphylococcal toxins—IV. Factors affecting haemolysis by β-lysin. *Can. J. Microbiol.* **4:** 477–486.

Jarvis, A. W., Laurence, R. C. and Pritchard, G. G. (1973) Production of staphylococcal enterotoxins A, B and C under conditions of controlled pH and aeration. *Infect. Immun.* **7:** 847–854.

Jeljaszewicz, J. (1972) Toxins (Haemolysins). In: *The Staphylococci*, p. 250, Cohen, J. O. (ed.). Wiley, New York.

Jeljaszewicz, J., Szmigielski, S. and Grojec, P. (1976) Staphylococcal leucocodin: stimulatory effect on granulopoiesis disturbed by cytostatic agents and review of the literature. In: *Staphylococci and Staphylococcal Disease*, pp. 639–657, Jeljaszewicz, J. (ed.). Gustav Fischer Verlag, Stuttgart.

Jeljaszewicz, J., Szmigielski, S. and Hryniewicz, W. (1978) Biological effects of staphylococcal and streptococcal toxins. In: *Bacterial Toxins and Cell Membranes*, pp. 185–227, Jeljaszewicz, J. and Wadström, T. (eds). Academic Press, London.

Johnson, A. D., Metzger, J. F. and Spero, L. (1975) Production, purification and chemical characterisation of *S. aureus* exfoliative toxin. *Infect. Immun.* **12:** 1206–1210.

Johnson, A. D., Spero, L., Cades, J. S. and De Cicco, B. T. (1979) Purification and characterisation of different types of exfoliative toxin from *S. aureus. Infect. Immun.* **24:** 679–684.

Johnson, H. M., Hall, H. E. and Simon, M. (1967) Enterotoxin B: serological assay in cultures by passive haemagglutination. *Appl. Microbiol.* **15:** 815–818.

Kantor, H. S., Temples, B. and Shaw, W. V. (1972) Staphylococcal Delta haemolysin: purification and characterization. *Archs Biochem. Biophys.* **151:** 142–156.

Kaplan, J. (1972) Staphylococcal enterotoxin B induced release of macrophage inhibition factor from normal lymphocytes. *Cell Immun.* **3:** 245–252.

Kapral, F. A. (1974) *Staphylococcus aureus*: some host–parasite interactions. *Ann. N.Y. Acad. Sci.* **236:** 267–276.

Kapral, F. A. and Miller, M. M. (1971) Product of *S. aureus* responsible for the scalded skin syndrome. *Infect. Immun.* **4:** 541–545.

Kapral, F. A. and Miller, M. M. (1972) Skin lesions produced by *S. aureus* exfoliatin in hairless mice. *Infect. Immun.* **6:** 877–879.

Kapral, F. A., O'Brien, A. D., Ruff, P. D. and Drugan, W. J. (1976) Inhibition of water absorption in the intestine by *S. aureus* δ-toxin. *Infect. Immun.* **13:** 140–145.

Kates, M. and James, A. T. (1961) Phosphatide components of fowl blood cells. *Biochim. biophys. Acta* **50:** 478–485.

Kato, I. (1979) Inhibitory effect of a lethal toxic fragment of staphylococcal α-toxin of cyclic AMP-dependent protein kinase activity. *Biochim. biophys. Acta* **570:** 388–396.

Kato, I. and Naiki, M. (1976) Ganglioside and rabbit erythrocyte membrane receptor of staphylococcal alpha toxin. *Infect. Immun.* **13:** 289–291.

Kato, I. and Watanabe, M. (1980) Chemical studies on staphylococcal alpha toxin and its fragments. *Toxicon* **18:** 361–365.

Kato, I., Sakoda, K., Saito, M., Suzuki, U. and Watanabe, H. (1975a) Studies on the haemolytic action of staphylococcal alpha toxin. *Jap. J. med. Sci. Biol.* **28:** 332–334.

Kato, I., Sakoda, K., Saito, M., Suzuki, U. and Watanabe, H. (1975b) Inhibitory effect of flavin mononucleotide on the haemolysis of rabbit erythrocytes by staphylococcus alpha-toxin. *Infect. Immun.* **12:** 696–697.

Kato, I., Sakoda, K., Saito, M. and Suzuki, Y. (1977) Effects of lectins on the hemolysis of rabbit erythrocytes by staphylococcal alpha toxin. *Microbiol. Immunol.* **21:** 517–524.

Kato, I., Watanabe, H. and Kumazawa, N. H. (1979) Inhibition of adenosine-3′,5′-monophosphate-dependent protein kinase by staphylococcal alpha-toxin. *Infect. Immun.* **24:** 286–288.

Kayser, A. and Raynaud, M. (1965) Etude d'une deuxieme hemolysine (distincte de l'hemolysine Alpha) présents dans les filtrats de culture de la souche Wood 46 de *Staphylococcus aureus* (Hemolysine G ou Delta). *Anns Inst. Pasteur, Paris* **108:** 215–233.

KAYHANI, M. M., ROGOLSKY, M., WILEY, B. B. and GLASGOW, L. A. (1975) Chromosomal synthesis of staphylococcal exfoliative toxin. *Infect. Immun.* **12**: 289–291.

KEHOE, M., DOUGAN, G., FOSTER, T. J., KENNEDY, S., DUNCAN, J., TIMMIS, K., GREY, G. and FAIRWEATHER, N. (1984) Genetic analysis of toxins from Gram positive cocci. pp 47–54, in *Bacterial Protein Toxins*. J. E. ALOUF, F. J. FEHRENBACH, J. H. FREER and J. JELJASZEWICZ. Ed. Academic Press. London.

KENT, T. H. (1966) Staphylococcal enterotoxin gastroenteritis in rhesus monkeys. *Ann. J. Path.* **48**: 387–399.

KINSMAN, O. and ARBUTHNOTT, J. P. (1980) Experimental staphylococcal infections in newborn mice: inhibition of weight gain as an index of virulence. *J. Med. Microbiol.* **13**: 281–290.

KINSMAN, O., JONSSON, P., HARALDSON, I., LINDBERG, M., ARBUTHNOTT, J. P. and WADSTROM, T. (1980) Decreased virulence of alpha-haemolysin negative and coagulase negative mutants of *S. aureus* in experimental infections in mice. *In* Proceedings of IVth International Symposium on Staphylococci and Staphylococcal Infections. Gustav Fischer Verlag, Stuttgart. pp. 651–659.

KLEINIG, H., ZENTGRAF, H., COMES, P. and STADLER, J. (1971) Nuclear membranes and plasma membranes from hen erythrocytes—III. Lipid composition. *J. Biol. Chem.* **246**: 2996–3000.

KONDO, I. and SAKURAI, S. (1981) Research on the receptor for staphylococcal exfoliatin. In: *Staphylococci and Staphylococcal Infection*, pp. 311–317, JELJASZEWICZ, J. (Ed.). *Zbl. Bakt., Suppl. 10*, Gustav Fischer Verlag, Stuttgart.

KONDO, I., SAKURAI, S. and SARAI, Y. (1973) Purification of exfoliatin produced by *S. aureus* of bacteriophage group II and its physicochemical properties. *Infect. Immun.* **8**: 156–164.

KONDO, I., SAKURAI, S. and SARAI, Y. (1974) New type of exfoliatin obtained from staphylococcal strains belonging to phage groups other than group II isolated from patients with impetigo and Ritters disease. *Infect. Immun.* **10**: 851–861.

KONDO, I., SAKURAI, S., SARAI, Y. and FUTAKI, S. (1975) Two serotypes of exfoliatin and their distribution in staphylococcal strains isolated from patients with staphylococcal scalded skin syndrome. *J. Clin. Microbiol.* **1**: 397–400.

KONDO, I., SAKURAI, S. and SARAI, Y. (1976) Staphylococcal exfoliatin A and B. In: *Staphylococci and Staphylococcal Diseases*, pp. 489–498, JELJASZEWICZ, J. (Ed.). *Zbl. Bakt. Suppl. 5*, Gustav Fischer Verlag, Stuttgart.

KOUPAL, A. and DEIBEL, R. H. (1977) Rabbit intestinal fluid accumulation by an enterotoxigenic factor of *Staphylococcus aureus*. *Infect. Immun.* **18**: 298–303.

KREGER, A. S., KIM, K. S., ZABORETZKY, F. and BERNHEIMER, A. W. (1971) Purification and properties of staphylococcal delta hemolysin. *Infect. Immun.* **3**: 449–465.

KREISWORTH, B. N., NOVICK, R. P., SCHLIEVERT, P. M. and BERGDOLL, M. (1982) Genetic studies on staphylococcal strains from patients with toxic shock syndrome. *Ann. Int. Med.* **96**: 974–977.

KUMAR, S., LOCKEN, K., KENYON, A. and LINDORFER, R. K. (1962) The characterisation of staphylococcal toxins—II. The isolation and characterisation of a homogeneous staphylococcal protein possessing alpha haemolytic, dermonecrotic, lethal and leucocidal activities. *J. Exp. Med.* **115**: 1107–1115.

KUREK, M., PRYJMA, K., BARTKOWSKI, S. and HECZKO, P. B. (1977) Anti-staphylococcal gamma haemolysin antibodies in rabbits with staphylococcal osteomylitis. *Med. Microbiol. Immun.* **163**: 61–65.

KWARECKI, K., SZMIGIELSKI, S., JELJASZEWICZ, J. and ZAK, C. (1968) Injury of rat peritoneal mast cells *in vivo* by staphylococcal alpha haemolysin and leukocidin. *J. Infect. Dis.* **118**: 361–364.

LANGFORD, M. P., STANTON, G. T. and JOHNSON, H. M. (1978a) Biological effects of staphylococcal enterotoxin A on human peripheral lymphocytes by products of staphylococci. *Br. J. Haemat.* **11**: 421–431.

LANGFORD, M. P., STANTON, G. J. and JOHNSON, H. M. (1978b) Biological effects of staphylococcal enterotoxin A on human lymphocytes. *Infect. Immun.* **22**: 62–68.

LEE, A. C.-M., ROBBINS, R. N. and BERGDOLL, M. S. (1978) Isolation of specific and common antibodies to staphylococcal enterotoxins A and E by affinity chromatography. *Infect. Immun.* **21**: 387–391.

LEE, A. C.-M., ROBBINS, R. N., REISSER, R. F. and BERGDOLL, M. S. (1980) Isolation of specific and common antibodies to staphylococcal enterotoxins B, C_1 and C_2. *Infect. Immun.* **27**: 431–434.

LILLIBRIDGE, C. B., MELISH, M. E. and GLASGOW, L. A. (1972) Site of action of exfoliative toxin in the staphylococcal scalded skin syndrome. *Pediatrics* **50**: 728–738.

LIU, C. T., DE LAUTER, R. D., GRIFFIN, M. J. and HADICK, C. L. (1978) Effects of staphylococcal enterotoxin B on the functional and biochemical changes of the lung in rhesus monkeys. *Toxicon* **16**: 543–550.

LO, C. Y. and FACKRELL, H. B. (1979) Immunological evidence that staphylococcal alpha toxin is orientated on membranes. *Can. J. Microbiol.* **25**: 686–692.

LOMINSKI, I., ARBUTHNOTT, J. P. and SPENCE, J. B. (1963) Purification of staphylococcal alpha toxin. *J. Path. Bact.* **86**: 258–262.

LOW, D. K. R. and FREER, J. H. (1977a) The purification of β-lysin (sphingomyelinase C) from *Staphylococcus aureus*. *FEMS Letts* **2**: 139–143.

LOW, D. K. R. and FREER, J. H. (1977b) Biological effects of highly purified β-lysin (sphingomyelinase C) from *Staphylococcus aureus*. *FEMS Letts* **2**: 133–138.

LOW, D. K. R., FREER, J. H., ARBUTHNOTT, J. P., MÖLLBY, R. and WADSTRÖM, T. (1974) Consequences of sphingomyelin degradation in erythrocyte ghost membranes by staphylococcal beta-toxin (sphingomyelinase C). *Toxicon* **12**: 279–285.

LYELL, A. (1981) Clinical aspects of epidermolytic toxins of *Staphylococcus aureus*. In: *The Staphylococci, Proceedings of The Alexander Ogston Centenary Conference*, pp. 119–124, MACDONALD, A. and SMITH, G. (Eds). Aberdeen University Press.

McCALLUM, H. M. (1972) Action of staphylococcal epidermolytic toxin on mouse skin in organ culture. *Br. J. Derm.* **86**: Suppl. 8: 40–41.

McCARTNEY, A. C. and ARBUTHNOTT, J. P. (1978) Mode of action of membrane-damaging toxins produced by staphylococci. In: *Bacterial Toxins and Cell Membranes*, pp. 89–127, JELJASZEWICZ, J. and WADSTRÖM, T. (Eds). Academic Press, London.

McCLATCHY, J. K. and ROSENBLUM, E. D. (1966) Genetic recombination between alpha-toxin mutants of *Staphylococcus aureus*. *J. Bact.* **92**: 580–583.

McLAY, A. L. C., ARBUTHNOTT, J. P. and LYELL, A. (1975) Action of staphylococcal epidermolytic toxin on mouse skin: an electron microscopic study. *J. Invest. Derm.* **65**: 423–428.

McNIVEN, A. C. and ARBUTHNOTT, J. P. (1972) Cell associated alpha-toxin from *Staphylococcus aureus*. *J. Med. Microbiol.* **5**: 123–127.

MADOFF, M. A. and WEINSTEIN, L. (1962) Purification of staphylococcal alpha haemolysin. *J. Bact.* **83**: 914–918.

MAH, R. A., FUNG, D. Y. C. and MORSE, S. A. (1967) Nutritional requirements of *Staphylococcus aureus* S-6. *Appl. Microbiol.* **15**: 866–870.

MAHARAJ, I. and FACKRELL, H. B. (1980) Rabbit erythrocyte band 3: a receptor for staphylococcal alpha toxin. *Can. J. Microbiol.* **26**: 524–531.

MAHESWARAN, S. K. and LINDORFER, R. K. (1970) Purification and partial characterisation of staphylococcal delta haemolysin. *Bact. Proc.* p. 78.

MAHESWARAN, S. K., SMITH, K. L. and LINDORFER, R. K. (1967) Staphylococcal beta haemolysin—I. Purification of beta haemolysin. *J. Bact.* **94**: 300–305.

MARKS, J. and VAUGHAN, A. C. T. (1950) Staphylococcal δ-haemolysin. *J. Path. Bact.* **62**: 597–615.

MELISH, M. E. and GLASGOW, L. A. (1970) The staphylococcal scalded skin syndrome: development of an experimental model. *New Eng. J. Med.* **282**: 1114–1119.

MELISH, M. E., GLASGOW, L. A. and TURNER, M. D. (1970) Staphylococcal scalded skin syndrome: experimental model and isolation of a new exfoliative toxin. *Pediat. Res.* **4**: 378.

MELISH, M. E., GLASGOW, L. A. and TURNER, M. D. (1972) The staphylococcal scalded skin syndrome: isolation and partial characterisation of the exfoliative toxin. *J. Infect. Dis.* **125**: 129–140.

MELISH, M. E., CHEN, F. S., SPROUSE, S., STUKEY, M. and MURATA, M. S. (1981) Epidermolytic toxin in staphylococcal infection: Toxin levels and host response. In: *Staphylococci and Staphylococcal Infections*, pp. 287–299, JELJASZEWICZ, J. (Ed.). *Zbl. Bakt.*, *Suppl. 10*, Gustav Fischer Verlag, Stuttgart.

MIDDLEBROOK, J. L., SPERO, L. and ARGOS, P. (1980) The secondary structure of staphylococcal enterotoxins A, B and C. *Biochim. biophys. Acta* **621**: 233–240.

MERRIL, T. G. and SPRINTZ, H. (1968) The effect of staphylococcal enterotoxin on the fine structure of the monkey jejunum. *Lab. Invest.* **18**: 114–123.

MILLER, R. D. and FUNG, D. Y. C. (1976) The occurrence of cell-associated enterotoxin B in *Staphylococcus aureus*. *Can. J. Microbiol.* **22**: 1215–1221.

MILLER, B. A., REISER, R. F. and BERGDOLL, M. S. (1978) Detection of staphylococcal enterotoxins A, B, C, D and E in foods by radioimmunoassay, using staphylococcal cells containing protein A as immunoadsorbent. *Appl. Envir. Microbiol.* **36**: 421–426.

MÖLLBY, R. and WADSTRÖM, T. (1970) Studies on haemolysins from *Staphylococcus aureus* by the method of isoelectric focusing. In: *Protides of the Biological Fluids* **17**, pp. 465–469. PEETERS, H. (Ed.). Pergamon Press, Oxford.

MÖLLBY, R. and WADSTRÖM, T. (1971) Separation of gamma haemolysin from *Staphylococcus aureus* Smith 5-R. *Infect. Immun.* **3**: 633–635.

MORSE, S. A. and BALDWIN, J. N. (1973) Factors affecting the regulation of staphylococcal enterotoxin B. *Infect. Immun.* **7**: 839–846.

MORSE, S. A. and MAH, R. A. (1967) Microtiter haemagglutination-inhibition assay for staphylococcal enterotoxin B. *Appl. Microbiol.* **15**: 58–61.

MORSE, S. A., MAH, R. A. and DOBROGOSZ, W. J. (1969) Regulation of staphylococcal enterotoxin B. *J. Bact.* **98**: 4–9.

NODA, M., KATO, I., HIRAYAMA, T. and MATSUDA, F. (1980a) Fixation and inactivation of staphylococcal leukocidin by phosphatidylcholine and ganglioside GM_1, in rabbit polymorphonuclear leukocytes. *Infect. Immun.* **29**: 678–684.

NODA, M., HIRAYAMA, T., KATO, I. and MATSUDA, F. (1980b) Crystallization and properties of staphylococcal leukocidin. *Jap. J. Bact.* **35**: 137–144.

NOTERMANS, S., VAN LEEUWN, W. J., DUFRENNE, J. and TIPS, P. D. (1983) Serum antibody to enterotoxin produced by *Staphylococcus aureus* with special reference to enterotoxin F and toxic shock syndrome. *J. Clin. Microbiol.* **18**: 1055–1060.

O'BRIEN, A. D. and KAPRAL, F. A. (1976) Increased cyclic adenosine-3′,5′-monophosphate content in guinea-pig ileum after exposure to *Staphylococcus aureus* delta toxin. *Infect. Immun.* **13**: 152–162.

O'BRIEN, A. D. and KAPRAL, F. A. (1977) Effect of *Staphylococcus aureus* delta-toxin on chinese hamster ovary cell morphology and Y-1 adrenal cell morphology and steroidogenesis. *Infect. Immun.* **16**: 812–816.

O'BRIEN, A. D., McCLUNG, W. J. and KAPRAL, F. A. (1978) Increased tissue conductance and ion transport in guinea-pig ileum after exposure to *Staphylococcus aureus* delta-toxin *in vitro*. *Infect. Immun.* **21**: 102–113.

OMURA, S. (1976) The antibiotic cerulenin, a novel tool of biochemistry as an inhibitor of fatty acid synthesis. *Bact. Rev.* **40**: 681–697.

O'REILLY, M., DOUGAN, G., FOSTER, T. J. and ARBUTHNOTT, J. P. (1981) Plasmids in Epidermolytic strains of *Staphylococcus aureus*. *J. Gen. Microbiol.* **124**: 99–107.

PANTON, P. M. and VALENTINE, F. C. O. (1932) Staphylococcal toxin. *Lancet* **ii**: 506–508.

PEAVY, D. L., ALDER, W. H. and SMITH, R. T. (1970) The mitogenic effects of endotoxin and staphylococcal enterotoxin B on mouse spleen cells and human peripheral lymphocytes. *J. Immunol.* **105**: 1453–1458.

PETRINI, B. and MÖLLBY, R. (1981) Activation of human lymphocytes *in vitro* by membrane-damaging toxins from *Staphylococcus aureus*. *Infect. Immun.* **31**: 952–956.

PHIMISTER, G. M. and FREER, J. H. (1984) Binding of ^{125}I-Alpha toxin of *Staphylococcus aureus* to erythrocytes. *J. Med. Microbiol.* **18**: 197–204.

PLOMMET, M. and BOUILLANNE, C. (1966) Production des hemolysines staphylococciques delta et gamma. *Anns Biol. Anim. Biochim. Biophys.* **6**: 529–532. (Cited by BEZARD and PLOMMET, 1973).

PORCELLI, L. J., SMALL, E. D. and BREWER, J. M. (1978) Origin of multiple species of yeast enolase A on isoelectric focussing. *Biochem. Biophys. Res. Commun.* **82**: 316–321.

RASMUSSEN, E. (1975) Toxic epidermal necrolysis. *Archs. Dermatol.* **111**: 1135–1139.

REINGOLD, A. L., SHANDS, K. N., DAN, B. B. and BROOME, C. V. (1982) Toxic Shock Syndrome not associated with menstruation. *Lancet* i: 1–4.

REISER, R. F. and WEISS, K. F. (1969) Production of staphylococcal enterotoxins A, B and C in various media. *Appl. Microbiol.* 18: 1041–1043.

ROBINSON, J. and THATCHER, F. S. (1963) Studies with staphylococcal toxins—VII. Separation of a proteolytic enzyme from alpha haemolysin. *Can. J. Microbiol.* 9: 697–702.

ROBINSON, J., THATCHER, F. S. and GAGNON, J. (1958) Studies with staphylococcal toxins—IV. The purification and metallic requirements of specific haemolysins. *Can. J. Microbiol.* 4: 345–361.

ROGOLSKY, M. (1979) Nonenteric toxins of *Staphylococcus aureus*. *Microbiol. Rev.* 43: 320–360.

ROGOLSKY, M. and WILEY, B. B. (1977) Production and properties of a staphylococcin genetically controlled by the staphylococcal plasmid for exfoliative toxin synthesis. *Infect. Immun.* 15: 726–732.

ROGOLSKY, M., WARREN, R., WILEY, B. B., NAKAMURA, H. T. and GLASGOW, L. A. (1974) Nature of the genetic determinant controlling exfoliative toxin production in *Staphylococcus aureus*. *J. Bact.* 117: 157–165.

ROGOLSKY, M., WILEY, B. B. and GLASGOW, L. A. (1976) Phage group 2 staphylococcal strains with chromosomal and extrachromosomal genes for exfoliative toxin production. *Infect. Immun.* 13: 44–52.

ROSENBLUM, E. D. and TYRONE, S. (1976) Chromosomal determinants for exfoliative toxin production in two strains of staphylococci. *Infect. Immun.* 14: 1259–1260.

ROUSER, G., NELSON, G. J., FLEISCHER, S. and SIMON, G. (1968) Lipid composition of animal cell membranes, organelles and organs. In: *Biological Membranes—Physical Fact and Function*, pp. 5–69, CHAPMAN, D. (Ed.). Academic Press, New York.

SALEH, F. A. K. and FREER, J. H. (1984) Inhibition of secretion of Staphylococcal alpha toxin by cerulenin. *J. Med. Microbiol.* 18: 205–216.

DE SAXE, M. J., WIENEKE, A., DE AZAVEDO, J. and ARBUTHNOTT, J. P. (1982a) Toxic Shock Syndrome in Britain. *Brit. Med. J.* 284: 1641–1642.

DE SAXE, M. J., WIENEKE, A., DE AZAVEDO, J. C. and ARBUTHNOTT, J. P. (1982b) Staphylococci associated with toxic shock syndrome in the United Kingdom. *Ann. Intern. Med.* 96: 991–996.

SCHAEFFER, W. L. (1970) Interaction of staphylococcal enterotoxin B with cell cultures—I. Effect of serum and testing procedures. *Infect. Immun.* 1: 455–458.

SCHANTZ, E. J., ROESSLER, W. G., WAGMAN, J., SPERO, L., DUNNERY, D. A. and BERGDOLL, M. S. (1965) Purification of staphylococcal enterotoxin B. *Biochemistry* 4: 1011–1016.

SCHANTZ, E. J., ROESSLER, W. G., WOODBURN, M. J., LYNCH, J. M., JACOBY, H. M., SILVERMAN, S. J., GORMAN, J. C. and SPERO, L. (1972) Purification and some chemical properties of staphylococcal enterotoxin A. *Biochemistry* 11: 360–366.

SCHLIEVERT, P. M. (1980) Purification and characterization of staphylococcal pyrogenic exotoxin type B. *Biochemistry* 19: 6204–6208.

SCHLIEVERT, P. M. (1983) Alteration of immune function by staphylococcal pyrogenic exotoxin type C: Possible role in toxic shock syndrome. *J. Infect. Dis.* 147: 391–398.

SCHLIEVERT, P. M., SCHOETTLE, D. J. and WATSON, D. W. (1979a) Non-specific T-lymphocyte mitogenesis by pyrogenic exotoxins from group A streptococci and *Staphylococcus aureus*. *Infect. Immun.* 25: 1075–1077.

SCHLIEVERT, P. M., SCHOETTLE, D. J. and WATSON, D. W. (1979b) Purification and physicochemical and biological characterization of a staphylococcal pyrogenic exotoxin. *Infect. Immun.* 23: 609–617.

SCHLIEVERT, P. M., SHANDS, K. N., DAN, B. D., SCHMID, G. P. and NISHIMURA, R. D. (1981) Identification and characterization of an exotoxin from *Staphylococcus aureus* associated with toxic shock syndrome. *J. Infect. Dis.* 143: 509–516.

SHAFER, W. M. and IANDOLO, J. J. (1978) Chromosomal locus for staphylococcus enterotoxin B. *Infect. Immun.* 20: 273–278.

SHAFER, W. M. and IANDOLO, J. J. (1979) Genetics of staphylococcal enterotoxin B in methicillin-resistant isolates of *Staphylococcus aureus*. *Infect. Immun.* 25: 922–911.

SHALITA, Z., HERTMAN, I. and SARID, S. (1977) Isolation and characterisation of a plasmid involved with enterotoxin B production in *S. aureus*. *J. Bacteriol.* 129: 317–325.

SHEMANO, I., HITCHENS, J. T. and BEILER, J. M. (1967) Paradoxical intestinal inhibitory effects of staphylococcal enterotoxin. *Gastroenterology* 53: 71–77.

SILVERMAN, S. J., KNOTT, A. R. and HOWARD, M. (1968) Rapid sensitive assay for staphylococcal enterotoxin and a comparison of serological methods. *Appl. Microbiol.* 16: 1019–1023.

SIX, H. and HARSHMAN S. (1973a) Purification and properties of two forms of staphylococcal α-toxin. *Biochemistry* 12: 2672–2677.

SIX, H. and HARSHMAN, S. (1973b) Physical and chemical studies on staphylococcal α-toxins A and B. *Biochemistry* 12: 2677–2683.

SLANETZ, L. W. and BARTLEY, C. H. (1953) The diagnosis of staphylococcal mastitis with special reference to the characteristics of mastitis staphylococci. *J. Infect. Dis.* 92: 135–151.

SMITH, B. G. and JOHNSON, H. M. (1975) The effect of staphylococcal enterotoxins on the primary *in vitro* immune response. *J. Immunol.* 115: 575–578.

SMITH, D. D. (1962) Experimental infection in mice. *J. Path. Bact.* 84: 359–365.

SMITH, L. M. and PRICE, S. A. (1938) Staphylococcus γ-haemolysin. *J. Path. Bact.* 47: 379–393.

SMYTH, C. J., MÖLLBY, R. and WADSTRÖM, T. (1975) Phenomenon of Hot–Cold haemolysis: Chelator-induced lysis of sphingomyelinase-treated erythrocytes. *Infect. Immun.* 12: 1104–1111.

SPERO, L. and MORLOCK, B. A. (1978) Biological activities of the peptides of staphylococcal enterotoxin C formed by limited tryptic hydrolysis. *J. Biol. Chem.* 253: 8787–8791.

SPERO, L. and MORLOCK, B. A. (1979) Cross-reactions between tryptic peptides of staphylococcal enterotoxins B and C_1. *J. Immunol.* 122: 1285–1289.

SPERO, L., JACOBY, H. M., DALIDOWICZ, J. E. and SILVERMAN, S. J. (1971) Guanidination and nitroguanidination of staphylococcal enterotoxin B. *Biochim. biophys. Acta* 251: 345–354.

SPETH, V., WALLACH, D. F. H., WEIDEKAMM, E. and KNUFFERMANN, H. (1972) Micromorphologic consequences following perturbation of erythrocyte membranes by trypsin, phospholipase A, lysolecithin, sodium dodecyl sulphate and saponin. A correlated freeze-etching and biochemical study. *Biochim. biophys. Acta* **255:** 386–394.

Stiffler–Rosenberg, G. and Fey, H. (1978) Simple assay for staphylococcal enterotoxin A, B and C: modification of enzyme linked immunosorbent assay. *J. Clin. Microbiol.* **8:** 473–479.

Sugiyama, H. and Hayama, T. (1965) Abdominal viscera as site of emetic action for staphylococcal enterotoxin in the monkey. *J. Infect. Dis.* **115:** 330–336.

Sugiyama, H. and McKissic, E. M. (1966) Leucocytic response in monkeys challenged with staphylococcal enterotoxin. *J. Bact.* **92:** 349–352.

Sullivan, R. and Asano, T. (1971) Effects of staphylococcal enterotoxin B on intestinal transport in the rat. *Ann. J. Physiol.* **220:** 1793–1797.

Surgalla, M. J. (1947) A study of the production of staphylococcal enterotoxin in defined media. *J. Infect. Dis.* **81:** 97–111.

Szmigielski, S. and Harshman, S. (1978) Enhancement of haemolytic and cytotoxic activity of staphylococcal α-toxin *in vitro* by incubation with cultured fibroblasts. *Zbl. Bakt. Hyg., 1 Abt. Orig. A.* **240:** 297–301.

Szmigielski, S., Kwarecki, K., Jeljaszewicz, J., Möllby, R. and Wadström, T. (1973) Alpha toxin and leukocidin effects on granulopoiesis. In: *Staphylococci and Staphylococcal Infections*, pp. 202–208, Jeljaszewicz, J. (Ed.). Polish Medical Publishers.

Szmigielski, S., Jeljaszewicz, J., Kobus, M., Luczak, M., Ludwicka, A., Möllby, R. and Wadström, T. (1975) Cytotoxic effects of staphylococcal alpha-, beta- and gamma-hemolysin. In: *Staphylococci and Staphylococcal Infections*, pp. 691–705, Jeljaszewicz, J. (Ed.). *Zbt. Bakt., Suppl. 5.* Gustav Fischer Verlag, Stuttgart.

Szmigielski, S., Blankenship, M., Robinson, J. P. and Harshman, S. (1979) Injury of myelin sheaths in isolated rabbit vagus nerves by α-toxin of *Staphylococcus aureus. Toxicon* **17:** 363–371.

Taylor, A. G. and Bernheimer, A. W. (1974) Further characteristics of staphylococcal gamma-haemolysin. *Infect. Immun.* **10:** 54–59.

Taylor, A. G. and Plommet, M. (1973) Anti gamma-haemolysin as a diagnostic test in staphylococcal osteomyelitis. *J. Clin. Path.* **26:** 409–412.

Taylor, A. G., Cook, J., Fincham, W. J. and Millard, F. J. C. (1975) Serological tests in the differentiation of staphylococcal and tuberculous bone disease. *J. Clin. Path.* **28:** 284–288.

Thelestam, M. and Möllby, R. (1975a) Determination of toxin induced leakage of different size nucleotides through the plasma membrane of human diploid fibroblasts. *Infect. Immun.* **11:** 640–648.

Thelestam, M. and Möllby, R. (1975b) A sensitive assay for detection of toxin induced damage to the cytoplasmic membrane. *Infect. Immun.* **12:** 225–232.

Thelestam, M. and Möllby, R. (1979) Classification of Microbial, plant and animal cytolysins based on their membrane-damaging effects on human fibroblasts. *Biochim. biophys. Acta* **557:** 156–169.

Thelestam, M., Möllby, R. and Wadström, T. (1973) Effects of staphylococcal alpha-, beta-, delta- and gamma-hemolysins on human diploid fibroblasts and HeLa cells: Evaluation of a new quantitative assay for measuring cell damage. *Infect. Immun.* **8:** 938–946.

Todd, J., Fishaut, M., Kapral, F. and Welch, T. (1978) Toxic-shock syndrome associated with phage-group I staphylococci. *Lancet* **ii:** 1116–1118.

Turnbull, P. C. B. (1979) Food poisoning with special reference to salmonella—its epidemiology, pathogenesis and control. *Clin Gastroenterol.* **8:** 663–714.

Turner, W. H. (1978a) The effect of medium volume and yeast extract diffusate on δ-hemolysin production by five strains of *Staphylococcus aureus. J. Appl. Bact.* **45:** 291–296.

Turner, W. H. (1978b) Purification and characterisation of an immunologically distinct delta-hemolysin from a canine strain of *Staphylococcus aureus. Infect. Immun.* **20:** 485–494.

Turner, W. H. and Pickard, D. J. (1979) Immunological relationship between delta-hemolysins of *Staphylococcus aureus* and coagulase-negative strains of staphylococci. *Infect. Immun.* **23:** 910–911.

Voureka, A. (1952) Induced variations in a penicillin-resistant staphylococcus. *J. Gen. Microbiol.* **6:** 352–360.

Wadström, T. (1968) Studies on extracellular proteins from *Staphylococcus aureus*—IV. Separation of alpha toxin by isoelectric focusing. *Biochim. biophys. Acta* **168:** 228–242.

Wadström, T. and Möllby, R. (1971a) Studies on extracellular proteins from *Staphylococcus aureus*—IV. Production and purification of beta lysin in large scale. *Biochim. biophys. Acta* **242:** 288–307.

Wadström, T. and Möllby, R. (1971b) Studies on extracellular proteins from *Staphylococcus aureus*—VII. Studies on β-haemolysin. *Biochim. biophys. Acta* **242:** 308–320.

Wadström, T. and Möllby, R. (1972) Some biological properties of purified staphylococcal haemolysins. *Toxicon* **10:** 511–519.

Walbum, L. E. (1921) Action de la staphylolysine sur les globules de chèvre. *C.R. Seanc. Soc. Biol.* **85:** 1205–1206.

Ward, P. D. and Turner, W. H. (1980) Identification of staphylococcal panton–valentine leukocidin as a potent dermonecrotic toxin. *Infect. Immun.* **28:** 393–397.

Ward, P. D., Adlam, C., McCartney, A. C., Arbuthnott, J. P. and Thorley, C. M. (1979) A histopathological study of the effects of highly purified staphylococcal alpha- and beta-toxins on the lactating mammary glands and skin of the rabbit. *J. Comp. Path.* **89:** 169–177.

Warren, J. R. (1977) Mitogenic stimulation of murine spleen cells by brief exposure to *Staphylococcus aureus* enterotoxin B. *Infect. Immun.* **18:** 99–101.

Warren, J. R., Leatherman, D. L. and Metzger, J. F. (1975) Evidence for cell receptor activity in lymphocyte stimulation by staphylococcal enterotoxin. *J. Immunol.* **115:** 49–53.

Warren, R. L. (1980) Exfoliative toxin plasmids of bacteriophage group 2 *Staphylococcus aureus*: sequence homology. *Infect. Immun.* **30:** 601–606.

Warren, R., Rogolsky, M., Wiley, B. B. and Glasgow, L. A. (1974) Effect of ethidium bromide on elimination of exfoliative toxin and bacteriocin production in *S. aureus. J. Bact.* **118:** 980–985.

Warren, R., Rogolsky, M., Wiley, B. B. and Glasgow, L. A. (1975) Isolation of extrachromosomal DNA for exfoliative toxin production from phage group II. *S. aureus. J. Bact.* **122:** 99–105.

WATANABE, M. (1976) Studies on the staphylococcal toxins: crystallization and some characteristics of staphylococcal α-toxin. *Bull. Azabu. Ret. Coll.* **1**: 151–162.

WATANABE, M. and KATO, I. (1974) Purification and some properties of staphylococcal α-toxin. *J. Exp. Med.* **44**: 165–178.

WATANABE, M. and KATO, I. (1978) Purification and some properties of a lethal toxic fragment of staphylococcal α-toxin by tryptic digestion. *Biochim. biophys. Acta* **535**: 388–400.

WEISSMANN, G., SESSA, G. and BERNHEIMER, A. W. (1966) Staphylococcal α-toxin: effects on artificial lipid spherules. *Science* **154**: 772–774.

WHELLER, D. (1975) Pleiotropic mutation of several pathogenicity factors in *Staphylococcus aureus*. *Proc. Soc. Gen. Microbiol.* **2**: 42–43.

WHITELAW, D. D. and BIRKBECK, T. H. (1978) Inhibition of staphylococcal delta-haemolysin by serum lipoproteins. *FEMS Letts* **3**: 335–338.

WILEY, B. B. and ROGOLSKY, M. (1977) Molecular and serological differentiation of staphylococcal exfoliative toxin synthesised under chromosomal and plasmid control. *Infect. Immun.* **18**: 487–494.

WILEY, B. B., GLASGOW, L. A. and ROGOLSKY, M. (1976) Staphylococcal scalded skin syndrome: development of a primary binding assay for human antibody to the exfoliative toxin. *Infect. Immun.* **13**: 513–520.

WISEMAN, G. M. (1965) Some characteristics of the beta-hemolysin of *Staphylococcus aureus*. *J. Path. Bact.* **89**: 187–207.

WISEMAN, G. M. (1970) The beta- and delta-toxins of *Staphylococcus aureus* In: *Microbial Toxins III Bacterial Protein Toxins*, pp. 253–262. MONTIE, T. C., KADIS, S. and AJL, S. J. (Eds). Academic Press, New York.

WISEMAN, G. M. (1975) The haemolysins of *Staphylococcus aureus*. *Bact. Rev.* **39**: 317–344.

WISEMAN, G. and CAIRD, J. D. (1967) The nature of staphylococcal beta haemolysin—I. Mode of action. *Can. J. Microbiol.* **13**: 369–376.

WISEMAN, G. M. and CAIRD, J. M. (1970) Mode of action of the alpha toxin of *Staphylococcus aureus*. *Can. J. Microbiol.* **16**: 47–50.

WISEMAN, G. M. and CAIRD, J. D. (1972) Further observations on the mode of action of the alpha toxin of *Staphylococcus aureus* "Wood 46". *Can. J. Microbiol.* **18**: 987–992.

WISEMAN, G. M., CAIRD, J. D. and FACKRELL, H. B. (1975) Trypsin-mediated activation of the α-haemolysin of *Staphylococcus aureus*. *J. Med. Microbiol.* **8**: 29–38.

WITTE, W. (1976) Control of α-haemolysin formation by plasmids in distinct strains of *Staphylococcus aureus*: influence of erythromycin, rifampicin and streptomycin. In: *Staphylococci and Staphylococcal Disease*, pp. 297–305, JELJASZEWICZ, J. (Ed.). Gustav Fischer Verlag, Stuttgart.

WOODIN, A. M. (1959) Fractionation of the two components of leukocidin from *Staphylococcus aureus*. *Biochem. J.* **73**: 225–237.

WOODIN, A. M. (1960) Purification of the two components of leucocidin from *Staphylococcus aureus*. *Biochem. J.* **75**: 158–165.

WOODIN, A. M. (1970) Staphylococcus leukocidin. In: *Microbial Toxins*. Vol III, pp. 327–356, MONTIE, T. C., KADIS, S. and AJL, S. J. (Eds). Academic Press, London.

WOODIN, A. M. (1972) Staphylococcal Leucocidin In: *The Staphylococci*, pp. 281–299, COHEN, J. O. (Ed.). Wiley Interscience, New York.

WOODIN, A. M. and WIENEKE, A. A. (1966) The interaction of leucocidin with the cell membrane of the polymorphonuclear leucocyte. *Biochem. J.* **99**: 479–492.

WU, C. H. and BERGDOLL, M. S. (1971) Stimulation of enterotoxin B production—II. Synthetic medium for staphylococcal growth and enterotoxin B production. *Infect. Immun.* **3**: 784–792.

WUEPPER, K. D., BAKER, D. H. and DIMOND, R. L. (1976) Measurement of *S. aureus* epidermolytic toxin: a comparison of bioassay, radial immunodiffusion and radioimmunoassay. *J. Invest. Derm.* **67**: 526–531.

WUEPPER, K. D., DIMOND, R. L. and KNUTSON, D. D. (1975) Studies of the mechanism of epidermal injury by a staphylococcal epidermolytic toxin. *J. Invest. Derm.* **65**: 191–200.

YOSHIDA, A. (1963) Staphylococcal delta-haemolysin—I. Purification and chemical properties. *Biochim. biophys. Acta* **71**: 544–553.

YOSHIKAWA, M., MATSUDA, F., NAKA, M., MUROFUSHI, E. and TSUNEMATSU, Y. (1974) Pleiotropic alteration of activities of several toxins and enzymes in mutants of *Staphylococcus aureus*. *J. Bacteriol.* **119**: 117–122.

YOTIS, W. M., CATSIMPOOLAS, N., BERGDOLL, M. S. and SCHANTZ, E. J. (1974) Scanning density gradient isoelectric focusing of *Staphylococcus aureus* enterotoxins B and C₁. *Infect. Immun.* **9**: 974–976.

ZWAAL, R. F. A., ROELOFSEN, B. and COLLEY, C. M. (1973) Localization of red cell membrane constituents. *Biochim. biophys. Acta* **300**: 159–182.

ZWAAL, R. F. A., ROELOFSEN, B., COMFURIUS, P. and VAN DEENEN, L. L. M. (1975) Organisation of phospholipids in human red cell membranes as detected by the action of various purified phospholipases. *Biochim. biophys. Acta* **406**: 83–96.

CHAPTER 27

STREPTOCOCCAL TOXINS
(STREPTOLYSIN O, STREPTOLYSIN S, ERYTHROGENIC TOXIN)

JOSEPH E. ALOUF

Institut Pasteur Paris, France

1. INTRODUCTION

More than twenty extracellular proteins or peptides are produced by the micro-organism *Streptococcus pyogenes* group A into their environment whether culture medium or host (essentially man) tissues. This impressive multiplicity of macromolecular substances released upon bacterial growth is detected by submitting concentrate culture supernatant fluid to polyacrylamide gel electrophoresis (Alouf and Raynaud, 1973; Linder, 1979), isoelectric focusing in a pH gradient (Smyth and Fehrenbach, 1974) and immunodiffusion or immunoelectrophoresis in gel media against human sera or gamma-globulins (Fig. 1) (Harris *et al.*, 1955; Halbert 1958, 1963; Hanson and Holm, 1961; Holm and Möller, 1971; Alouf and Raynaud, 1973; Alouf *et al.*, 1978), and immune sera raised in animals (Hanson, 1959; Alouf *et al.*, 1965). Some of these extracellular products are identifiable as toxins, mitogens or enzymes (Fig. 2) while others are still without known biological activity.

The streptococcal toxins which are the subject of the chapter are streptolysin O (SLO), streptolysin S (SLS) and erythrogenic toxin (ET). SLO is an immunogenic, 65,000-dalton protein and SLS a non-immunogenic peptide associated to an inducer (RNA, serum components, detergents). Both toxins are very potent cytolytic agents especially on erythrocytes (hemolysis). ET which is also known as scarlatinal toxin or streptococcal pyrogenic exotoxin (Kim and Watson, 1972) is a protein which exhibits a great diversity of interesting biological effects *in vivo*. Its lethal potency on animals is low. Three antigenically distinct forms (A, B, C) are known. Several excellent reviews have been published in the past few years on one or several aspects of SLO (Halbert, 1970; Bernheimer, 1972, 1974, 1976; Duncan, 1975; Alouf, 1977; Smyth and Duncan, 1978; Jeljaszewicz *et al.*, 1978), SLS (Ginsburg, 1970; Okamoto, 1976; Okamoto *et al.*, 1978; Jeljaszewicz *et al.*,

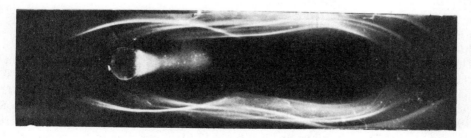

FIG. 1. Immunoelectrophoretic analysis of concentrate culture fluid of a group A streptococcal strain. The central well contains the concentrated streptococcal material. The trough contains human γ-globulins (see Alouf *et al.*, 1978).

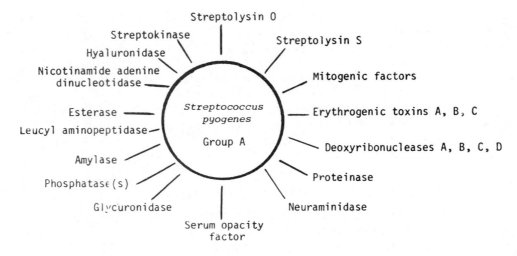

FIG. 2. Extracellular macromolecular substances identified in culture fluids of group A
streptococci.

1978) and ET (Watson and Kim, 1970; Kim and Watson, 1972). This review will therefore summarize the current status of information on the chemistry, physicochemical properties, biological effects and mode of action of these toxins and will concentrate on more recent studies with particular emphasis on the pharmacological properties on intact animal and isolated organs or tissues. I will try to state where evidence is still incomplete or lacking and discuss the clinical significance of these toxins which is still a vexed question. Several statements have been proposed suggesting a role for SLO, SLS and ET in the non suppurative sequelae of streptococcal infections such as: rheumatic fever, glomerulonephritis, chorea and scarlet fever. In order to clarify further the possible involvement of these toxins in these diseases, such a review may prove useful in promoting future investigations.

2. STREPTOLYSIN O

2.1. DEFINITION

Streptolysin O may be defined as a toxic immunogenic protein released in the extracellular medium by most strains of group A and many strains of groups C and G streptococci particularly those causing human infections. The toxin is cytolytic or cytotoxic on eukaryotic cells including erythrocytes from mammals and other species (hemolysis) whereas prokaryotic cells (bacterial protoplasts or spheroplasts) are unsensitive. This cytolysin is lethal to laboratory animals and has very potent cardiotoxic properties: the biological activity of SLO is lost by oxidation and restored upon reduction by reducing agents such as thiols or hydrosulfite.

2.2. HISTORICAL BACKGROUND

The hemolytic activity toward red blood cells discovered by Marmorek (1895) in the filtrates of certain streptococcal cultures was shown by Todd (1932, 1938a) and Weld (1935) to be due to two distinct hemolysins named oxygen-labile streptolysin O to indicate the sensitivity of one of them to oxidation and oxygen-stable streptolysin S to indicate the stability to oxidation of the other hemolysin and its production in serum-containing media. The reversible inactivation of SLO on standing in the presence of air or oxygen which was first recognized by Neill and Mallory (1926) is an essential characteristic of this toxin. The zone of β-hemolysis surrounding colonies of *Streptococcus pyogenes* on blood agar plates is primarily due to the mediation of SLS since SLO becomes oxidized. However deep colonies are hemolytically active through both toxins (Halbert, 1970). A second essential feature of SLO is the inhibition of its hemolytic effect by minute amounts of cholesterol (Hewitt and Todd, 1939) and other sterols having a 3β-hydroxy group on carbon 3 of the A ring of the cyclopentanoperhydrophenanthrene nucleus and a lateral hydrophobic side chain at carbon 17 as first shown by Howard *et al.* (1953). The other toxic effects (lethality, cardiotoxicity and cytolysis on other eukaryotic cells) are also suppressed by cholesterol and related sterols (see Bernheimer, 1976). Toxin interaction with sterols and its relevance to the mode of action of SLO at the cellular level are discussed in detail in another section of this review.

2.3. RELATEDNESS OF STREPTOLYSIN O TO OTHER CYTOLYTIC TOXINS

SLO is the prototype of a group of fifteen bacterial cytolytic protein toxins (Table 1) elaborated by gram-positive bacteria of the species *Streptococcus, Clostridium, Bacillus* and *Listeria* (Bernheimer, 1976; Alouf, 1977; Smyth and Duncan, 1978). These toxins share a number of common properties: they are antigenically related as shown by cross-neutralization and immunoprecipitation (Fig. 3, Bernheimer, 1976; Cowell and Bernheimer, 1977; Alouf *et al.*, 1977); their cytolytic and other biological effects are lost by oxidation and restored by SH-compounds and other reducing agents; these toxins are inactivated by cholesterol and certain related sterols. This group of oxygen-labile cytolytic toxins has been named sulfhydryl-activated toxins (Bernheimer, 1976) or thiol-activated cytolysins (Smyth and Duncan, 1978). The mechanism of action of these toxins is very likely identical or at least closely similar.

2.4. PRODUCTION OF STREPTOLYSIN O

Culture supernatant fluids are the starting material for toxin production as SLO is an extracellular toxin (Raynaud and Alouf, 1970) released during the exponential and stationary phases of bacterial growth. Cellular location of SLO before release appears essentially periplasmic (Calandra and Theodore, 1975). SLO is synthetized in chemically defined media (see Bernheimer, 1954; Alouf and Dassy, unpublished results). However much better yields are obtained in media prepared by dialysis of peptones casein hydrolysate (Trypticase) supplemented with yeast extract. Complete media such as Todd-Hewitt broth should not be used for purification purposes because of the presence of large molecular weight peptides. Glucose is necessary (0.5–1%) for optimal production.

TABLE 1. *Gram-Positive, Bacterial Species Producing the Immunologically and Chemically Related Sulfhydryl Dependent ('Oxygen-Labile') Cytolytic Toxins*

Family	Genus	Species	Toxin
Streptococcaceae	Streptococcus	*S. pyogenes*	Streptolysin O
		S. pneumoniae	Pneumolysin
Bacillaceae	Bacillus	*B. cereus*	Cereolysin
		B. thuringiensis	Thuringiolysin O
		B. alvei	Alveolysin
		B. laterosporus	Laterosporolysin
	Clostridium	*C. bifermantans (sordellii)*	Bifermentolysin
		C. botulinum	Botulinolysin
		C. histolyticum	ϵ-Toxin (Histolyticolysin)
		C. novyi type A (*oedematiens*)	γ-Toxin (Oedematolysin O)
		C. perfringens	θ-Toxin (Perfringolysin O)
		C. septicum	Septicolysin O
		C. tetani	Tetanolysin
		C. chauvoei	Chauveolysin
Lactobacillaceae	Listeria	*L. monocytogenes*	Listeriolysin

Bernheimer (1976), Alouf (1977).

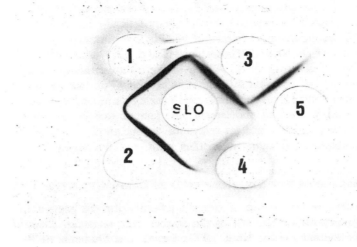

FIG. 3. Cross-reactivity between streptolysin O and the SH-activated toxin, alveolysin from *Bacillus alvei* (see Alouf *et al.*, 1977). Central well: SLO; Wells 1 and 2: human γ-globulins; Wells 3 and 4: hyperimmune anti SLO sera; Well 5: alveolysin.

However as lactic acid is produced during growth, the pH should be always maintained between 6.8 and 7.4 to avoid toxin destruction by acidity and (or) by proteolysis by the streptococcal proteinase which is released into the medium when pH drops below 6.7 (Cohen, 1969). Most work on toxin production and purification has been carried out by batchwise cultures. The peak of SLO occurs between 6–12 hr (Alouf and Raynaud, 1965, 1973; Halbert, 1970). All types A, C and G strains appear to produce a toxin which is identical biologically and immunochemically (Halbert, 1970). Individual strains vary considerably in their quantitative ability to produce SLO in suitable media.

The best yields (500–1000 hemolytic units/ml) in optimal culture conditions have been obtained with the following strains: C 203 S type 3 (Bernheimer *et al.*, 1942; Halbert, 1958; Smyth and Fehrenbach, 1974) Richards type 3 (Duncan and Schlegel, 1975), Kalback's S 84 type 3 (Alouf and Raynaud, 1965, 1973; Holm and Möller, 1971), strain 814, type 4 (Alouf *et al.*, 1978).

The production of SLS by these strains may be avoided if culture media are free from SLS-inducers (serum components, yeast RNA active fraction, detergents). This is the case for the dialyzed medium described elsewhere (Alouf and Raynaud, 1973). The SLS⁻ mutant C 203 U derived from C 203 S strain (Bernheimer, 1954) has also been successfully employed for SLO production and purification by Shany *et al.* (1973) and Linder (1979).

SLO may be produced by bacterial cultivation in fermentors under pH control (see Halbert, 1970; Shany *et al.*, 1973). This technique has also been employed in our laboratory in 15-liter effective growth volume with good yields (Alouf and Dassy, unpublished data) provided the culture is not aerated and the pH automatically maintained at 7.0–7.2 by addition of 0.5 N, NaOH.

The physiological and genetic regulation of SLO biosynthesis and excretion as well as its possible biological function in the metabolism of the bacterial cell remains unknown. A comparative study of C 203 U strain which produces 500 HU/ml and a spontaneous non toxinogenic mutant isolated in our laboratory (C 203 U/IP) which does not excrete detectable SLO did not show any significant differences as regards growth kinetics, the pattern of extracellular products tested by immunochemical analysis as described in Fig. 1 and the production of nicotinamide adenine dinucleotide glycohydroxylase which is known to be released closely associated to SLO (Smyth and Fehrenbach, 1974; Shany *et al.*, 1973). However the mutant did not release the SH-dependent streptococcal proteinase. Whether SLO synthesis could be coded by plasmid genes as it is the case for some

TABLE 2. *Inhibitory Effects of some Antibiotics on the Production of Streptolysin O and other Extracellular Proteins by S. pyogenes*

Toxins or Enzymes	no antibiotic	Yield* in presence of			
		lincomycin	clindamycin	erythromycin	chloramphenicol
Streptolysin O	128	< 4	< 4	128	128
Streptolysin S	512	< 4	< 4	512	512
DNase	1024	< 2	< 2	128	128
NADase	512	< 2	< 2	256	256
Serum-opacity factor	32	< 2	< 2	16	16

*Highest dilution just showing activity.
From Gemmel and Abdul Amir (1979)

bacterial toxins such as *Streptococcus faecalis* hemolysin (Frazier and Zimmerman, 1977). *E. coli* hemolysin and enterotoxins (Gyles *et al.*, 1974) and staphylococcal dermoexfoliative toxin (Wiley and Rogolsky, 1977) is also unknown. Experiments in our laboratory (Alouf, and Geoffroy, unpublished data) of strain cultivation under conditions described for curing bacteria from plasmids (ethidium bromide, temperature at 41°C) did not appear to affect toxin production.

The intracellular events involved in SLO biosynthesis and excretion remain to be established. Interesting experiments were reported by Fox (1961) who observed *de novo* synthesis of SLO and proteinase by non-proliferating streptococci provided the reaction mixture in which the cells were suspended contained peptides, free amino acids and glucose. The peptides stimulated the incorporation of counts from radioactive amino acids into SLO. This process was inhibited by chloramphenicol.

The effects of sub-inhibitory concentration of some antibiotics on the formation of SLO and other streptococcal extracellular products (SLS, DNase, NADase, serum-opacity factor) or cellular antigens (M and T proteins and carbohydrate C) have recently been investigated by Gemmell and Abdul-Amir (1979).

As shown in Table 2, none of the major extracellular toxins or enzymes was expressed in the presence of lincosamine antibiotics (lincomycin and clindamycin). In the presence of chloramphenicol and erythromycin, however SLO and SLS production was not affected whereas that of DNase, NADase and the serum-opacity factor were partially inhibited. Expression of cellular M and C antigens was also inhibited by the lincosamines.

New experiments in this field, in the light of the recent development of the studies in the secretion of extracellular products and the existence of internal hydrophobic signal sequence (see Newark, 1979) will likely be rewarding.

2.5. ASSAY OF STREPTOLYSIN O

The quantitative determination of SLO in crude or purified material is usually based on the estimation of the hemolytic activity of the toxin expressed as hemolytic units (HU) per ml of toxin solution (Herbert, 1941). The HU is arbitrarily defined as that smallest amount (highest dilution) of toxin previously activated (see Bernheimer and Avigad, 1970) that will liberate half the hemoglobin (50% lysis) from a suspension of washed erythrocytes (usually sheep or rabbit) under fixed conditions of time, temperature, ionic environment and red blood cell concentration. As shown in Table 3, the HU employed is unfortunately not identical in all instances, the parameters of the assay system being different depending on laboratories. An agreement for a unified titration system by all investigators studying SLO and related toxins is highly desirable in order to facilitate the comparison of experimental data. However in spite of this situation the figures found in the literature are at least roughly comparable (Bernheimer, 1972).

A detailed description of our assay system of SLO on rabbit erythrocytes as well as the rationale, limitations and requirements for accurate determination of the hemolytic activity have been reported elsewhere (Alouf *et al.*, 1965; Alouf and Raynaud, 1968c). For

TABLE 3. *Some Parameters of Assay System at 37° of Streptolysin O from Various Laboratories*

Reaction mixture Volume (ml)	Erythrocyte suspension (vol. and %)		Buffer	Incubation time (min)	References
2	1 ml 2.25%	RRBC	PBS pH 6.5	30	Herbert (1941)
1.6	0.4 ml 4%	RRBC	PBS + BSA pH 6.7	60	Halbert et al. (1955)
1.5	0.5 ml 2.25%	RRBC	PBS + BSA pH 6.5	45	Alouf et al. (1965)
1.5	0.5 ml 5%	SRBC	PBS + BSA pH 6.5	45	Alouf et al. (1977)
2	1 ml 2%	RRBC	PBS + BSA pH 6.4	45	Kanbayashi et al. (1972)
4	2 ml 0.7%	RRBC	PBS pH 6.5	30	Duncan (1974)
2	1 ml 0.7%	RRBC	PBS + BSA pH 7	30	Grushoff et al. (1975)
2	1 ml 1%	SRBC	PBS pH 6.8	30	Smyth & Fehrenbach (1974)
5.5	0.5 ml 3%	SRBC	PBS pH 6.5	75	Calandra & Theodore (1975)
2	2 ml 2%	RRBC	Saline pH ?	45	Ricci et al. (1978)

Abbreviations: RRBC, rabit red blood cells; SRBC, sheep red blood cells; PBS, phosphate buffered saline; BSA, bovine serum albumin.

practical reasons we use at present 5% sheep erythrocytes standardized suspensions (6×10^8 cells/ml) instead of 2.25% rabbit erythrocyte suspension (Alouf et al., 1977). However, either sheep or rabbit cells suspensions are always standardized so that 0.5 ml lysed by adding 14.5 ml of 0.1% sodium carbonate solution gives an optical absorbance of 0.200 at 541 nm in a Beckman spectrophotometer in a 10-mm light path cuvette. Under these conditions one HU of SLO in the sheep assay system is equivalent to 2 HU in the rabbit system.

SLO may also be determined through the measurement of its combining titer with corresponding antibodies as described elsewhere (Alouf et al., 1965). The combining unit of toxin (Lh T) is defined as that amount of SLO which in the presence of 1 international unit of anti-SLO lyses under the experimental conditions described 50% of the standard cell suspension. 1 Lh T unit of SLO is equivalent on average to 50 HU in the rabbit cells assay system or 25 HU in the sheep cells assay system. This technique is particularly suitable for the determination by a classical blind-test procedure of partially active or completely inactive SLO toxoids (or cross-reacting material) devoid of hemolytic activity (Alouf et al., 1965).

Finally, the determination of antistreptolysin O activity of immune sera or isolated immunoglobins are determined by the well-known techniques used in clinical immunology (see Alouf et al., 1965, 1978; Klein, 1976). The titers of test sera are determined with SLO preparation of known combining titer evaluated by reference to a standard antiserum.

2.6. Purification of Streptolysin O

The isolation of SLO from the culture fluid to an apparent pure state assessed by physical (SDS-polyacrylamide gel electrophoresis) and immunochemical criteria for protein homogeneity is a difficult task owing to the multiplicity of extracellular components, in the crude material, the low amount of SLO released (2 to 5% of total exoproteins) and its tendency to undergo irreversible denaturation even when manipulations are carefully conducted in the cold. These difficulties explain the failure of the first investigators (Smythe and Harris, 1940; Herbert and Todd, 1941) to obtain reasonably purified preparations. Appreciable progress was made in the sixties by the groups of Halbert and Alouf and Raynaud when chromatographic and continuous flow electrophoresis techniques became employed. Highly purified preparations with specific activities of about 250,000 HU per mg protein were obtained (see Halbert, 1970). However they remained contaminated with low amounts of one to three additional streptococcal proteins one of them being nicotinamide adenine dinucleotide glycohydrolase (NADase–EC. 3.2.2.5). In most, if not all conventional purification procedures described, this enzyme exhibits a tendency to co-purify with SLO as observed by many investigators (Alouf and Raynaud, 1973; Shany et al., 1973; Smyth and Fehrenbach, 1974; Grushoff et al., 1975). However physical separation of SLO and NADase has been achieved by these authors using isoelectric focusing (see Fig. 4) or chromatography on carboxymethyl-Sephadex.

Despite the difficulties mentioned above, SLO has been successfully purified to apparent homogeneity in several laboratories by combination of a multiplicity of conventional procedures including salting-out, ion-exchange chromatography, gel filtration and isoelectric focusing or preparative acrylamide gel electrophoresis (Van Epps and Andersen, 1973; Alouf and Raynaud, 1973; Duncan and Schlegel, 1975). The toxin isolated by Duncan and Schlegel had a specific activity of approximately 200,000 HU per mg protein and gave a single band on disc gel electrophoresis. A single band was also detected by this technique and by immunodiffusion for the preparation purified by Van Epps and Andersen. However the specific activity of the toxin was not reported. Toxin purification to apparent homogeneity in our laboratory has been described (Alouf and Raynaud 1973) and was later slightly improved by Alouf, Geoffroy and Prigent* as summarized in

*(1977, unpublished)

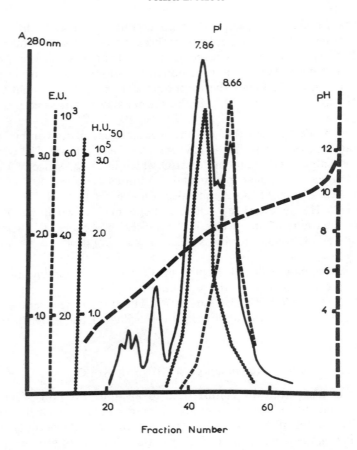

Fig. 4. Isoelectric focusing of a mixture of streptolysin O and NADase; pI, SLO: 7.86; pI,
NADase 8.66. (Alouf, Geoffroy and Prigent, 1977, unpublished.)

Table 4 to allow simultaneous isolation of purified NADase. The best specific activity
found for SLO was around 4×10^5 HU (rabbit)/per mg protein. Nevertheless if one
takes into consideration the partial denaturation of the toxin undergone during the
purification process, we may assume that the actual specific activity of SLO should be
about 10^6 HU per mg protein (rabbit assay system).

However in all instances toxin-purification by the conventional procedures is tedious
and the yields are poor ($\simeq 5\%$). This situation has recently led to devise specific methods
of toxin purification in two laboratories. The procedure reported by Linder (1979) is a
rapid 5-step method based on immunoaffinity chromatography of SLO by using antiteta-
nolysin as immunoadsorbent for SLO which is antigenically related to tetanolysin an
SH-activated cytolysin released by *Clostridium tetani*. The SLO preparation obtained was
80% pure (specific activity 108711 HU per mg protein) and contained two minor components of lower molecular weight as evidenced by polyacrylamide gel electrophoresis.

Another approach has been devised in our laboratory for SLO (Prigent *et al.*, 1978)
and extended later (Alouf and Geoffroy, in preparation) to other SH-activated toxins
as alveolysin and perfringolysin. The procedure is based on the selective isolation of
SH-proteins as reported for a variety of SH-enzymes (Brocklehurst *et al.*, 1974) by
covalent chromatography on sulfhydryl-agarose gels involving a thiol-disulfide reaction
according to the scheme described in Fig. 5.

The crude material to be fractionated is first reduced after suitable concentration and
those proteins containing a thiol group are retained in the SH-agarose column. A covalent bond is formed between the SH-proteins and the solid support which is then split

TABLE 4. *Schematic Diagram For The Isolation of Streptolysin O and NADase**

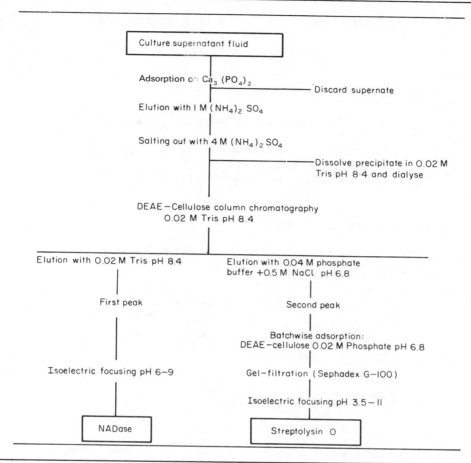

*Procedure devised by Alouf, Geoffroy and Prigent (1977, unpublished) modifying that reported by Alouf and Raynaud (1973).

with excess of dithiothreitol after the unretained material has been washed out. The gels used were agarose-glutathione-2-pyridyl disulfide (activated Thiol-Sepharose 4B) or Thiopropyl-6B Sepharose in PBS buffer pH 6.0. The former proved more suitable for SLO purification and the latter for alveolysin and perfringolysin.

The whole procedure for SLO involved five steps with a final yield of 20%. The toxin obtained was homogeneous.

2.7. PHYSICAL CHARACTERISTICS OF STREPTOLYSIN O

The data concerning the molecular weight and isoelectric points (pI values) of SLO have been reviewed by Bernheimer (1974, 1976) and Smyth and Duncan (1978). The values determined in the past decade on toxin preparations purified to a high extent and carefully studied as regards the molecular weights and pI show discrepancies which however on careful analysis lead to a reasonable evaluation of the actual values of these physical parameters.

A molecular weight of 60,500–61,000 was calculated from sedimentation velocity and gel filtration by Van Epps and Andersen (1969) who also found that both oxidized and reduced forms of SLO had the same sedimentation coefficient (3.7 S) indicating a little or no change in size or shape associated with toxin activation. Recent estimates of the

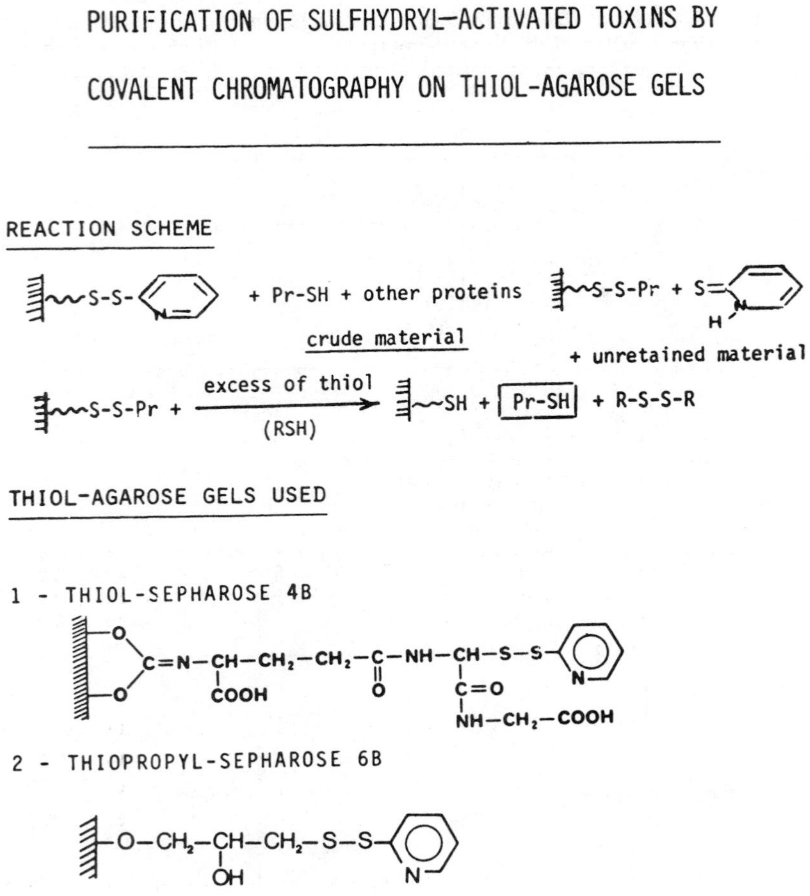
PURIFICATION OF SULFHYDRYL-ACTIVATED TOXINS BY
COVALENT CHROMATOGRAPHY ON THIOL-AGAROSE GELS
REACTION SCHEME
+ Pr-SH + other proteins
crude material
+ unretained material
excess of thiol
(RSH)
Pr-SH
+ R-S-S-R
THIOL-AGAROSE GELS USED
1 - THIOL-SEPHAROSE 4B
2 - THIOPROPYL-SEPHAROSE 6B

FIG. 5. Purification of SLO and related toxins by covalent chromatography.

molecular weight of various highly purified SLO preparations in our laboratory gave values of 55,000 by gel filtration and 70,000-75,000 by SDS-polyacrylamide gel electrophoresis. Molecular weights of 67,000–69,000 were reported by the latter procedure by Shany *et al.* (1973) whereas a value of 53,000 was found by the former technique by Calandra and Theodore (1975). We have now good evidence (Alouf and Geoffroy, to be published) that SLO has hydrophobic properties and is somewhat retained by dextran gels. This behavior may explain the lower values found by gel filtration techniques.

Linder (1979) has recently reported a value of 56,000 by polyacrylamide gel electrophoresis. In an earlier work we found a value of 55,000 by ultracentrifugation in guanidinium chloride-2-mercaptoethanol (Alouf and Raynaud, 1973). The 'heavy form' reported in the same work is very likely due to aggregation of SLO as also described by other investigators (Bernheimer, 1972; Calandra and Theodore, 1975). The same phenomenon has been shown to occur for the related toxins, cereolysin and perfringolysin (Smyth and Duncan, 1978). In short on the basis of the data hitherto obtained, we may assume that the molecular weight of SLO falls very likely within the value 67,000 $\pm$ 5000. It is to be noted that the discrepancies among the values reported may not only stem from the methods employed in the measurement of the molecular weight but could also be due to other factors. Possible nicking by the streptococcal proteinase which may cleave a peptide from the native toxin could explain the lower values reported. In contrast, the high values could be due to small peptides from the medium or from other streptococcal protein(s) which may co-purify with the toxin. This possibility is

TABLE 5. *Isoelectric Points of Streptolysin O and NADase Determined on Various Preparations by Density Gradient Isoelectric Focusing*

		pI values		
		SLO		NADase
1.	Crude preparation (concentrate culture fluid)			
	(a) in presence of 2-mercaptoethanol	6.0	<u>8.0</u>	8.4
	(b) in absence of 2-mercaptoethanol	<u>5.95</u>	7.5	n.d.
2.	Concentrate culture filtrate from dialysed proteose-peptone medium		<u>7.8</u>	8.5
3.	Partially purified (10%) preparation			
	(a) in presence of 2-mercaptoethanol	6.1	<u>7.6</u>	8.7
	(b) in absence of 2-mercaptoethanol	<u>6.0</u>		8.7
4.	Unreduced partially purified (50%) preparation from undialyzed proteose-peptone medium	<u>6.1</u>	8.2	8.6
5.	Previous pI 6.1 pool peak reduced with 2-mercaptoethanol		7.6	
6.	Highly purified reduced SLO preparation (last step of Table 4 process and Figure 5)		7.8	

pH determinations were carried out at + 4°C on effluents from 110-ml LKB column (Alouf, Geoffroy and Prigent, 1977, unpublished). The major hemolytic component underlined. Reduction was undertaken by adding 2-mercaptoethanol (0.02M final concentration).

substantiated by the finding of abnormal amounts of collagen amino-acids upon amino-acids analysis of some SLO samples purified from culture media containing meat peptones (Alouf, unpublished). As mentioned previously NADase (mol. wt. $\simeq$ 55,000) may also remain associated to SLO unless careful means of separation is being employed (see Fig. 4).

The pI values of SLO have been determined in several laboratories by gradient isoelectric focusing on preparations of various degrees of purity. A variety of different pI values were reported and in all cases marked charge heterogeneity was found. Smyth and Fehrenbach (1974) detected two SLO forms of pI 6.0/6.1 (major form) and 7.5/7.6 (minor form) respectively on concentrated culture supernatant fluids from streptococci of groups A, C and G. Similar pI values of 6.1 and 7.55 were reported by Shany et al. (1973) on a partially purified preparation. However, the relative distribution of the two components differed. These data are in good agreement with the pI of 7.5 reported by Halbert (1970) on a nonpurified preparation and the pI of 5.8 found by this author in the presence of 1 M glycine. Two forms of pI 7.2 (major) and 6.5 (minor) were found for the highly purified SLO obtained in our laboratory (Alouf and Raynaud, 1973). We have also shown that the pIs of lower values (5.5–5.9) irregularly found corresponded to toxoided forms of SLO.

The occurrence of multiple forms has been reported for many toxins and enzymes and their significance discussed in detail by Wadström et al. (1974), Arbuthnott et al. (1975) and Smyth and Duncan (1978). Some of the possible causes of heterogeneity could be due to artefacts of chemical modifications or environmental effects. In the very case of SLO, we have previously suggested (Alouf and Raynaud, 1973) that differences in the degrees and methods of purification of the preparations used for isoelectric focusing could partly explain the heterogeneity observed and the discrepancies concerning the pI values reported by different laboratories. This contention is supported by recent experiments in our laboratory concerning pI determination on different SLO preparations. As summarized in table 5, the apparent pI and relative distribution of SLO was greatly affected by several factors such as: the state of purity of the preparation, the medium used for toxin production whether dialyzed or undialyzed and the oxidation-reduction state. The latter factor has also been shown to affect the pI value of cereolysin and perfringolysin (see Smyth and Duncan, 1978). The toxin of high specific activity separated at the last step of

Table 6. *Some Characteristics of Streptolysin O*

Molecular weight (SDS–Page)	67,000 ± 5,000
Isoelectric point	7.8
Hemolytic units (HU) per mg protein*	400,000
One HU is equal to 2.5 ng of protein or 1.5×10^{-2} pmole	
LD_{50} (i.v.) in μg of protein:	
20-g mouse	0.2 μg
250-g guinea-pig	6
2-kg rabbit	3
Minimum lethal dose for 9-day-old embryonated hen egg	2.10^{-2} μg

Amino acid composition (<u>Best</u> whole numbers of residues)**

Aspartic acid	76	Isoleucine	24
Threonine	33	Leucine	23
Serine	38	Tyrosine	15
Glutamic acid	48	Phenylalanine	16
Proline	19	Histidine	7
Glycine	27	Lysine	57
Alanine	42	Arginine	18
Valine	42	Half-cystine	n.d.
Methionine	n.d.	Tryptophane	n.d.

*Assay system on rabbit erythrocytes as described by Alouf et al. (1965).
This value is the <u>best</u> experimental one found at the end of the purification process. However, if one takes into consideration the partial denaturation of the toxin which occurs during purification, one may calculate that, the actual specific activity of SLO should be about 10^6 HU/mg protein.
**Alouf and Geoffroy (unpublished data, see text).

the purification process summarized in Table 4 shows only one hemolytic peak of pI 7.8 (Fig. 4) whereas accompanying NADase had a pI of 8.66. In conclusion, the various data reported by the different laboratories lead to infer that the actual pI of SLO is around 7.6–7.8. Whether the isoelectric point of the toxin could differ depending on the producing strain is unknown. Finally, it is to be noted that variation in pI may also originate from a possible nicking or partial proteolysis by streptococcal proteinase.

2.8. Chemical Characteristics

2.8.1. *Amino Acid Composition*

No amino acid analysis of the SLO preparations purified by the authors mentioned above has been reported to our knowledge. A tentative partial analysis (Table 6) has been carried out recently in our laboratory on a toxin sample purified by the conventional procedure of Table 4. Other analyses are in progress on SLO samples purified by the thiol-agarose procedure.

Amino acid analyses of cereolysin, perfringolysin and listeriolysin have been reported (see Smyth and Duncan, 1978).

2.8.2. *Activation by Reducing Agents*

SLO and the related 'oxygen-labile' cytolysins can be reversibly oxidized and reduced as shown in early studies (Neill and Mallory, 1926; Smythe and Harris, 1940; Herbert and Todd, 1941) and confirmed later by many authors (see Halbert, 1970; Bernheimer, 1976; Alouf, 1977; Smyth and Duncan, 1978). The cytolytic and other biological activities of SLO are lost upon exposure to atmospheric O_2 or by treatment with mild oxidizing agents (H_2O_2, $K_3Fe(CN)_6$, iodine). These activities are rapidly restored by adding reducing agents such as hydrosulfite or thiols. These properties led to the assumption by Herbert and Todd (1941) that SLO is a protein containing at least one disulfide bond in the oxidized (biologically inactive) state which can be reduced into free -SH groups in the biologically active state. This situation can be summarized as follows (but does not correspond to the actual stoichiometry of the reaction as still no data are available about the number of cysteine residues in SLO):

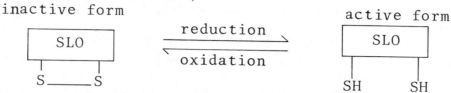

Cowell *et al.* (1976) detected two half-cystine residues per molecule of cereolysin thereby providing the first chemical evidence for substantiation of the sulfhydryl mechanisms of activation (Smyth and Duncan, 1978) of an SLO-like toxin. Recently Alouf and Geoffroy found four half-cystine residues per molecule of alveolysin (article in preparation).

The reduction of SLO by various agents has been studied in detail. Herbert and Todd (1941) reported for the partially purified SLO obtained at that time that SLO was activated to the same extent by inorganic (H_2S, $Na_2S_2O_4$, Na_2SO_3) as well as organic reducing agents (cysteine, 2-mercaptopropionic acid, thiolacetic acid, reduced gluta-thione). In contrast, important differences in the degree of activation of a crude commercial SLO preparation by six different straight-chain thiols were reported by Rahman *et al.* (1969) and Rahman-Gauthier *et al.* (1971). This finding was not confirmed by Bernheimer and Avigad (1970) who found the same maximal activation of a relatively crude SLO preparation by similar or identical straight-chain thiols. These discrepancies may be relevant to pH as suggested by these authors and/or to the crude state of the preparations used. Recent observations in our laboratory on the reducing effects of dithiothreitol (DTT) on highly purified SLO is in agreement with the possible role of pH. The activation was maximal at pH 7.6 and very poor at pH 6.0.

Rahman's group also reported that no reactivation was observed with four aromatic compounds carrying one or two thiol groups. These results are unlike our finding that aromatic thiols such as thio-2-naphtol and p-thiocresol dissolved in petroleum ether reactivate SLO (Prigent *et al.*, 1978).

Crude reduced or partially purified SLO material undergoes reversible oxidation upon storage or during the purification process. As noted by Halbert (1970) and verified in several instances over 95–98% of the molecules may become oxidized. In contrast, the oxidation of purified reduced SLO without irreversible loss of activity is difficult. It does not take place readily upon storage in air and even in under a current of pure oxygen (Alouf, unpublished data). In addition, denaturation is observed particularly for dilute toxins solutions (Van Epps and Andersen, 1971). Oxidants such as hydrogen peroxide are sometimes effective (Alouf and Raynaud, 1968a) but irreversible loss may also take place. Periodate oxidation causes complete and irreversible loss of activity (Van Epps and Andersen, 1971).

We have recently found in our laboratory that purified reduced SLO could be reversibly oxidized by treatment with either oxidized dithiothreitol (DTT$_{ox.}$) at pH 7.6 or 2,2'-dipyridyl disulfite at pH 6.0:

The reduced active form is readily restored by treatment with any suitable thiol.

Thiol-blocking agents inhibit the biological activity of SLO as shown by treatment of reduced toxin with phenylmercuric-chloride (Smythe and Harris, 1940), p-chloromercuribenzoate (Stock and Uriel, 1961; Alouf and Raynaud, 1968c) and some heavy metals ions (Van Epps and Andersen, 1971). Inhibition by mercuric components could be reversed by adding thiols. The activity is also lost by alkylation with iodoacetamide or monoiodoacetic acid (Smythe and Harris, 1940; Herbert and Todd, 1941; Van Epps and Andersen, 1971).

2.9. BIOLOGIC EFFECTS OF STREPTOLYSIN O

The effects of SLO have been studied during the past forty years at various levels: whole organism, isolated organs or tissues, cell systems and subcellular organelles. A great number of the investigations on the toxic, pharmacologic and cytolytic effects of SLO were unfortunately carried out (not only prior to 1960 but even more recently) with crude or partially purified preparations of unknown complexity. These preparations were contaminated by other streptococcal components endowed with a variety of biological effects (Fig. 2). However despite this situation, the results obtained with highly purified preparations on the one hand and indirect lines of evidence (inhibition by cholesterol or low activity of crude unreduced preparations) on the other hand permit to infer that the toxic or pharmacologic phenomena observed are due to SLO *per se* except as regards quantitative data (dose–response relationship).

2.9.1. *Toxic and Pharmacologic Effects on Whole Living Organisms*

2.9.1.1. *Lethality.* Mice, rats, guinea pigs, rabbits and cats were shown to be rapidly killed by intravenous injection of activated SLO (Todd, 1938b; Herbert and Todd, 1941; Howard and Wallace, 1953b; Bernheimer, 1954; Halbert *et al.*, 1961; Alouf and Raynaud, 1973). The values of the LD_{50} by the i.v. route has been determined in mouse (0.2 μg), guinea-pig (6 μg) and rabbit (2 μg) by Alouf and Raynaud (1973) with highly purified SLO (see Table 6). These authors also found that the minimal lethal dose for the 9-day-old embryonated hen egg was 20 ng of protein. The LD_{50} for the mouse with the most active preparation of Halbert was 1–2 μg (Halbert, 1970). It has been reported by Howard and Wallace (1953b) that on a weight basis the mouse was about 30 times as resistant as the other species, a difference that paralleled the resistance of mouse erythrocytes as compared to those of rabbits and guinea pigs (Howard and Wallace, 1953a). However crude SLO preparation was used by these authors and when the data obtained with highly purified SLO are compared, the difference between the LD_{50} per unit weight for the mouse and that for the other species tested was of a much lower order ($\simeq 2$ fold) (Table 6). Routes of administration other than intravenous have not been investigated in detail. However, they appear to be not nearly as lethal (Halbert, 1970). Oxidized SLO is much less toxic than the reduced activated form. Whether some further reductions occurs *in vivo* is likely.

The titration of lethal activity tends to show sharp endpoints. Death occurs in mice or rabbits within seconds or minutes depending on doses. With several multiples of a lethal dose, death is almost instantaneous. At dose levels which kill only a portion of the animals, death will generally occur within minutes or survival will be indefinite (Barnard and Todd, 1940; Halbert *et al.*, 1963b).

2.9.1.2. *Clinical symptoms.* A variety of physiopathological manifestations are observed upon i.v. or i.p. injection of lethal or sublethal doses of SLO in rabbits or mice (see review by Halbert, 1970; Ginsburg, 1972; Bernheimer, 1976). In both species, generalized tonic and clonic motor convulsion with the head in extreme extension followed toxin injection within as short a time as 10 seconds up to 10–15 min. The electroencephalogram in rabbits did not show patterns of convulsive discharges followed by E.E.G. silence between the attacks of clonic and tonic convulsions indicating that the central nervous system was not directly involved in seizures begun by the SLO injections (Halbert *et al.*, 1961). Blood pressure drop, cessation of respiration and micturation also rapidly occurred. Pulmonary oedema or haemorrhage as evidenced by nasal frothing as well as general venous congestion were observed (Barnard and Todd, 1940; Halpern and Rahman, 1968). Halpern *et al.* (1969) reported the same symptoms as well as modification of coagulation factors favoring massive intravascular thrombosis in the chambers of the heart in the great veins. With large doses of toxin the heart was found at systolic standstill. According to these authors in mice dying within 30 seconds, the earliest lesion was a general congestion of the small terminal vessels with marked edema of the interfascicular space. The fine structure of the cardiac cell was, however, preserved. In spite of the distention by edema of the intracellular space, no abnormality of the nucleus, mitochondria or myofibrils was observed. The fine structure of the capillaries seemed to be preserved. For those mice which survived for more than 2 min, lesions of the heart were clearly apparent and zones of necrosis were found. Much cells lost their usual affinity for dye and were invaded by granular leukocytes. In rabbits, the toxin caused a general depression, frequent and deep respiration, diarrhoea and pronounced pyrexia. A temperature drop below 36°C, diarrhoea and abrupt fall of blood pressure were the signs of imminent death (Rašková and Vaněček, 1964).

2.9.1.3. *Cardiotoxic effects.* The almost instantaneous lethal effects of SLO on laboratory animals is to be largely attributed to the direct cardiotoxicity of the toxin as shown *in vivo* and also *in vitro* (see section 2.9.2.) on isolated heart and deriving tissues. Electrocardiogram tracings in rabbits and mice given lethal doses of SLO revealed profound disorganization of heart function characterized by conduction defects and ventricular automatism (Halbert et al., 1961, 1963a,b; Halpern and Rahman, 1968; Halpern et al., 1969). The injection of $3-6\,LD_{50}$ in rabbit induced extremely rapid transition from a normal sinus rhythm to ventricular arrhythmia ending by ventricular fibrillation and standstill. These events occurred within 2–4 seconds following the injection. This period is that required for the dose to reach the heart from the peripheral vein (Halbert et al., 1961). For smaller but still lethal doses the changes were not always the same. Common alteration were AV nodal rhythm, depression of the ST segment and T wave elevation or depression, PQ and QRS prolongation and decrease in the amplitude of the P waves and QRS complex. These changes were followed by ventricular extrasystoles, ventricular tachycardia and flutter, fibrillation and standstill. Similar electrocardiographic patterns were observed in mice (Halbert et al., 1963a; Halpern and Rahman, 1968; Halpern et al., 1969) and more recently in rats (Gupta and Gupta, 1979). Halpern and Rahman (1968) found that mice given large lethal doses of SLO exhibited immediate and intense brachycardia followed in some cases by temporary arrest. Progressive arterioventricular dissociation implicated the conductile tissue.

The possible mechanism(s) of the cardiotoxicity of SLO are still not entirely clear and will be discussed in Section 2.9.2.1. However, on the basis of the *in vivo* observations on heart functions (see Halbert, 1970) it has been suggested that the extremely rapid cardiac alterations elicited by SLO might result from the release of vasoactive substances rather than from the direct action of the protein itself. This assumption appeared substantiated by the observation that smaller lethal or sublethal doses immediately produced a pronounced but transient sinus bradycardia followed by temporary or permanent recovery (Halbert et al., 1961). To explore the possibility of the release of small molecular weight pharmacologically active effectors, Halbert et al. (1963a) studied the effectiveness of various pharmacological blocking agents in protecting against the putative effectors responsible for the i.v. effects of SLO. These authors found that several antiserotonin drugs of different chemical families (lysergic acid derivatives, thioridazine) afforded protection against the acute lethal toxicity of SLO. However other serotonin agents, and other drugs, did not show protective effects. It was concluded that there was little correlation between protection and antiserotonin activity. In addition, serotonin was not very toxic to rabbits and mice, so it appeared unlikely that the acute toxicity of SLO could be accounted for entirely by the release of this amine.

Besluau et al. (1979) reported recently that prometazine and chlorpromazine protected mice against the lethal effects of $3\,LD_{50}$ of toxin. These prevented cardiotoxic effects and damage of vascular and pulmonary endothelium, probably by their stabilizing effect on cell membranes. The possible role of intravascular hemolysis and plasma K^+ ions in the cardiotoxic effects of SLO has been investigated (Halbert et al., 1963a). However as noted by Bernheimer (1954), Rašková and Vaněček (1964) and Halbert (1970) the degree of intravascular hemolysis although sometimes considerable and rapid with the high plasma K^+ levels is insufficient to account for death. Furthermore a number of discrepancies were found between the plasma K^+ levels and the electrocardiographic findings during the *in vivo* studies (Halbert, 1970). It is also to be noted that the protective antiserotonin drugs against SLO toxicity did not appear to be associated with a significant interference with intravascular hemolysis. In addition, these drugs did not show protection against experimental KCl toxicity in mice.

2.9.1.4. *Effects on the central nervous systems (CNS).* Electroencephalographic (E.E.G.) tracings taken in parallel with the electrocardiograms revealed that alterations of the CNS patterns only occurred long after the heart had stopped functioning adequately and well after the blood pressure had fallen to almost zero (Halbert et al., 1961).

Rašková and Vaněček (1964) reported the effects of crude SLO concentrate on the CNS of unanesthetized cat by intracerebroventricular injection. Numerous behavioral changes somewhat like those Nydenham's chorea were observed, particularly changes in motility. Dogs and rabbits were similarly challenged recently with partially purified SLO (Gupta, 1979; Gupta and Srimal, 1979). Neuroexcitatory effects were observed. The rabbits exhibited at low doses tachypnea and mydriasis, spasticity of forelimbs and contralateral bending of neck followed by contralateral stereotyped circular movements. The same behavioral effects were found in dogs with excessive salivation, facial clonus and tremors of the limbs. For higher doses the animals developed generalized convulsions, spastic quadriparesis with rigidity of neck and back (opisthothonos) leading to respiratory arrest and death within 3–5 hr after the injection.

Intraventricular administration of SLO in doses of 0.05 and 0.1 per kg did not produce any electroencephalographic changes. However, at a dose of 0.2 HU per kg, an immediate stimulation of the E.E.G. pattern was obtained. The electrical discharges comprised high frequency and low voltage waves which persisted for about 20 min followed by return of the E.E.G. to normal awake pattern (30–45 min); thereafter the E.E.G. showed a sleep pattern (60 min). Pretreatment of animals with varying doses of dexamethasone or antistreptolysin O provided protection against the neuroexcitatory effects of challenging SLO. Pentobarbitone sodium rapidly antagonised the excitatory effects of the toxin. In contrast, 6-hydroxydopamine did not abolish the effects of SLO on the central nervous system. This suggests that this effect is not mediated via the release of catecholamines in the brain. Rapid onset of neurostimulation evoked by SLO leads to suggest that it may be acting directly on neurones. The failure of SLO to induce any neurostimulation in rabbits pretreated with dexametasone, a substance known to stabilize the cell membrane and lysosomal membrane is consistent with this contention.

Since a causal relationship between Sydenham's chorea and streptococcal infections has been proposed (Taranta, 1959), it is tempting to suggest on the basis of the neurostimulatory effects of SLO that this toxin may be involved in the causation of chorea during acute rheumatic fever in man. However, detailed neuropharmacological studies are required to prove this contention (Gupta and Srimal, 1979).

2.9.1.5. *Induction by SLO of non specific inhibitory plasma components.* Mice injected intravenously with small non toxic doses of SLO become refractory for about 2 days to a subsequent lethal dose. This unsensitivity is not due to antibodies but to the development of a new or altered lipoprotein in the serum (Rowen and Bernheimer, 1956). This component has been purified over 300-fold (Rowen, 1963). A new acute phase protein (α_2-globulin) distinct from C-reactive protein and lipoprotein have also been detected in the sera of mice receiving sublethal doses of SLO and other toxic or infectious agents (Rowen and Wiest, 1965). This phenomenon may be a manifestation of a physiologic response of the host to deleterious agents.

2.9.2. *Effects* In Vitro *on Tissue Targets*

SLO being *a pantropic* toxin, virtually every organ, tissue or cell from eukaryotic organisms may be affected by the toxin. However, the cytopathogenic effects will be different depending on whether the doses of toxin which come into contact with the cells are lytic or sublytic.

2.9.2.1. *Interaction with isolated organs.*

i. *Effects on heart.* The cardiotoxicity of SLO is one of the prominent features of this toxin. This property is shared by relatively few bacterial toxins. This is the case of the other members of the group of SH-activated toxins insofar as other members have been tested (listeriolysin, pneumolysin, tetanolysin; see review in Bernheimer, 1976) and *Vibrio parahaemolyticus* thermostable hemolysin (Honda *et al.*, 1976).

Cardiotoxicity of SLO *in vitro* was first demonstrated on the isolated frog heart (Bernheimer and Cantoni, 1945, 1947; Cantoni and Bernheimer, 1945, 1947). The toxins induced systolic contracture in an unusual way. Perfusion of a first dose of SLO through the heart had no evident effect but after a brief washing, a second small dose produced the contracture.

The direct toxicity of small amounts of toxin was subsequently shown *in vitro* with relatively crude preparations on isolated perfused mammalian hearts of guinea pig, rabbit and rat by Vaněček (see Rašková and Vaněček, 1964; Kellner *et al.*, 1956). More purified preparations were used later by Coraboeuf and Goullet (1963), and Halpern and Rahman (1968) on perfused rat heart. In all instances the observations were similar. Permanent and irreversible standstill accompanied by a profound but transitory reduction in coronary flow resulted from exposure to small amounts of the toxin (Kellner *et al.*, 1956). As noted by Halbert (1970) unlike the amphibian hearts, the first exposure of mammalian beating hearts to SLO produced cardiac standstill within 2–3 min with as low as 5–50 ng of toxin indicating that SLO is an extremely potent cardiotoxic agent. Halpern and Rahman (1968) also found rapid arrest of beating isolated rat heart perfused with as low as 50 HU ($\simeq$ 100 ng) of toxin. Electrocardiographic changes such as QRS inhibition, extrasystoles and fibrillation were similar to those seen *in vivo* after injection of SLO. In all cases the ventricles stopped beating before the auricles.

Toxin effects were also studied by these authors on isolated right rabbit auricle, biauricular preparations of the rat heart and strips of human auricular myocardium. The decrease and arrest of the contractile force was observed in all instances with generally little effect on the rhythm. Coraboeuf and Goullet (1963) reported initial positive inotropic (cardiotonic) effect on rat heart perfused with SLO through the coronary route before observing the subsequent disruption of heart function. The same early cardiotonic effect was elicited by the toxin on myocardiac ventricular strips bathing in a physiological fluid.

In short, these *in vitro* results clearly indicate a direct toxic effect on myocardial and (or) nervous intracardial tissue as well as toxin penetration into structures through a mechanism which could not be simple diffusion.

The site of SLO toxicity for the perfused hearts from mammalian species was appreciably clarified by Reitz *et al.* (1968) and Thompson *et al.* (1970). The former workers reported an analysis of the toxic action of purified SLO on the isolated heart and separate cardiac tissue of the guinea pig. They showed that the toxic response consisted of two separate and distinct phases. There is initially a rapid but transient decrease in the rate and amplitude of concentration associated with the release of acetylcholine from the atria. These events are superimposed on the second phase, a gradual, irreversible decline in ventricle contractility.

Tests on spontaneously beating isolated atrial pairs show that the toxin induces a dose-dependent, reversible, decline in rate and amplitude which is accompanied by a marked, but transient, increase in the velocity of repolarization of the intracellular potential. The atrial reactions (tachyphylaxis) were completely blocked by atropine and potentiated by eserine (physostigmine). Acetylcholine was detected in the perfusates obtained by incubating a large pool of atrial tissue with active toxin, supporting the inference that the transient mechanical and electro-physiological reactions to toxin might be consequences of the release of acetylcholine from these tissues by the active toxin.

At ventricular standstill, the atria continue to beat spontaneously in a normal way. Isolated ventricule strips prepared from such preparations can be driven electrically, and their behavior is functionally indistinguishable from that of similar preparations made from normal hearts.

Since the driven ventricle strip was mechanically and electrophysiologically insensitive to SLO, the irreversible changes in the whole heart must have occurred because of a defect in the atrioventricular conduction system. Such a conclusion was also independently inferred by Halpern and Rahman (1968) who reported damage of conduction systems by SLO in perfused rat heart. It was also shown by Goullet et al. (1963) that contractions of electrically stimulated isolated rat ventricle strips were not inhibited by SLO.

In conclusion, it appears clearly established that the irreversible damage of the heart is due to the disturbance of atrioventricular conduction system while atria are reversibly depressed via the release of acetylcholine. However, the exact nature of the former irreversible damage is still not clarified.

It is to be noted that Goullet et al. (1968) reported contracture and cardiac arrest of 3-day-old chicken embryo heart as well as the decrease and arrest of the beating of atrial and ventricular fragments of this heart. Since at this stage of development, cardiac innervation and vascularization are still not established, one may conclude that SLO acts directly on myocardial tissue.

In addition to the direct in vivo or in vitro toxicity of SLO analyzed above, a distinct harmful effect of SLO on the heart may potentiate and aggravate toxin action. It has been demonstrated (Prager and Feigen, 1970; Feigen et al., 1974; Hadji, 1979) that in guinea pigs previously sensitized by an active immunization or perfusion of isolated auricles, the introduction of SLO produces a typical anaphylactic response with increased rate and amplitude of atrial contraction resulting from the liberation of large quantities of histamine. This immunological mechanism was shown to be mediated by both homocytotropic and heterocytotropic antibodies to SLO.

The toxicity of SLO for beating mammalian heart cells in tissue culture was studied by light and electron microscopic techniques by Thompson et al. (1970) in the hopes of shedding light on the cardiotoxicity at the cellular level. Pulsating mammalian myocardial cells were found to be highly susceptible to rapid destruction by SLO. Cessation of beating occurred almost immediately followed within minutes by multiple cell membrane bleb formation observed under phase contrast microscopy. Parallel with these changes the cytoplasm became intensely granular and the nuclear membrane appeared thickened. The endoplasmic reticulum was quite swollen and its contents were considerably condensed.

The blebs observed under phase contrast could be resolved by electron microscopy as protrusions of the plasmalemma into which there was comparatively sparse leakage of organelles from the cytoplasm. No evidence of cell membrane rupture was seen. However, the most dramatic and unusual early alteration of cardiac cells was strikingly manifested in the endoplasmic reticulum. The cisternae were considerably swollen and the contents became condensed. There was widespread vacuolation of the cytoplasm accompanied by similar changes in the mitochondria with some swelling of the cristae. Golgi complex was also vacuolated. The nuclear envelope remained intact and its apparent thickening observed by phase-contrast microscopy was seen to be due to the piling up of dense material (presumably chromatin) against the inner side of the nuclear envelope. Similar lesions were reported by Halpern et al. (1969). The study of the effects of the toxin on kidney or endothelial cells has shown similar blebs but their number was much less than those observed on myocardial cells (Thompson et al., 1970). It is conceivable that this is a reflection of the number of 'attack' sites on the cell membrane.

The cytological changes observed are similar to those elicited by SLO on other cells as described in another section.

ii. *Effects on other organs or tissues.* A variety of tissues has been challenged with crude or partially purified SLO preparations (see reviews by Rašková, 1964; Rašková and Vaněček, 1964; Halbert, 1970; Ginsburg, 1972). The effects reported include dermal necrosis, blood vessel contraction, increased capillary permeability in rabbit, disturbances in nerve conduction and bile secretion. Crude SLO preparations added to the bath fluid was shown to produce a slow contraction of isolated rat uterus. The effect was not antagonized by atropine or antihistaminics and only partly by 5-hydroxy-tryptamine antagonists. However, the chemical complexity of most of the preparations suggests that factors other than SLO were also active in some of the processes described.

2.9.3. *Action on Isolated Eukaryotic Cell Suspensions or Tissue Cultures*

Mammalian and other eukaryotic cells tested so far have been shown to be killed by SLO. In most cases, cell death is accompanied by cell lysis indicating dramatic damage of the cytoplasmic membrane of target cells. As shown in a next section, membrane cholesterol is the binding site and the target of the toxin.

This property explains the insensitivity to SLO of prokaryotic cells (bacterial protoplasts and spheroplasts and saprophytic mycoplasma) which unlike eukaryotic cells lack cholesterol in their cell membranes (see Bernheimer, 1974). In contrast, parasitic species of mycoplasma known to have sterol-containing membranes are lysed by SLO. Primitive cells such as free-living protozoa and *Arbaccia* eggs were unaffected by this toxin (Bernheimer, 1954).

2.9.3.1. *Effects on erythrocytes* ('*hemolysis*').
The cytolytic effects and mode of action of SLO have been studied primarily on mammalian erythrocytes inasmuch as this toxin was first discovered as a result of its hemolytic activity (Marmorek, 1895). This activity is the most characteristic biological property of SLO and related SH-activated cytolysins which rate among the most potent bacterial cytolytic toxins along with staphylococcal β-toxin and SLS (see Alouf, 1977; McCartney and Arbuthnott, 1978; Smyth and Duncan, 1978). One HU of SLO (equivalent to about 1 ng of native protein) lyses by definition 7.5×10^7 rabbit erythrocytes at 37°C (Alouf *et al.*, 1965). Assuming a molecular weight of 70,000 daltons for SLO (1 ng = 1.42×10^{-5} nmole) one may calculate that about 100 molecules suffice to lyse one erythrocyte. Comparatively as high as 10^8 molecules of sodium dodecyl sulfate, lysolecithin or polyene antibiotics which have some common biological properties with the SH-activated toxins are required for lysis of one red blood cell (Alouf and Raynaud, 1968a).

The comparative susceptibility of erythrocytes from various poikilothermic or homeothermic animal species has been studied in several laboratories (Howard and Wallace, 1953a; Schwab, 1956; Alouf, 1967, 1977; Klein *et al.*, 1968). As shown in Table 7 the cells of all mammalian, amphibian and avian species examined were lysed by SLO. In contrast to staphylococcal and other cytolysins (Alouf, 1977; McCartney and Arbuthnott, 1978) the relative susceptibility of erythrocytes to lysis by SLO was roughly of the same order (two to four-fold differences are considered not really significant because of variation in the parameters of each hemolytic system) except for murine erythrocytes which were 25 to 35-fold more resistant. This resistance was also observed towards the SLO-like toxins perfringolysin and tetanolysin (see Smyth and Duncan, 1978) although to a less pronounced degree. The possible reasons of mouse cells resistance are discussed in another section. However it is difficult to find any correlation between resistance and either erythrocyte diameter or total cholesterol content of erythrocyte membrane (Smyth and Duncan, 1978). Finally it is to be noted that according to Howard and Wallace (1953a), 50% lysis of rabbit RBC required 1 HU, whereas sheep and human RBC required 0.75 and 0.25 HU respectively. These results do not agree with those found in our laboratory (Alouf, 1967, 1977) and the data of Klein *et al.* (1968) who reported that

TABLE 7. *Comparative Susceptibility of Erythrocytes of Various Animal Species to Hemolysis by Streptolysin O*

Animal species	Number of HU for 50% lysis		
	(a)	(b)	(c)
Mammalian species			
Rabbit	1	1	1
Guinea pig	1	1	0.8
Hamster	1.5	—	—
Mouse	> 32	> 50	> 5
Rat	2	—	—
Ferret	—	1.2	—
Sheep	0.75	1.2	1
Ox	0.75	1.1	—
Goat	1.5	—	—
Horse	0.75	1.1	0.9
Dog	0.75	1.2	1
Pig	0.75	—	—
Cat	1	—	—
Monkey	—	1.5	
Human	0.25	1	1.1
Other species			
Pigeon	1.5	—	—
Duck	1	—	—
Chicken	5	0.9	> 10
Frog	2	—	—

(a) Howard and Wallace (1953a), (b) Alouf (1967, 1977), (c) Schwab (1956)

sheep RBC are the most resistant and rabbit RBC the less resistant to lysis as compared to human cells.

2.9.3.2 *Cytolytic effects on other eukaryotic cells.* A wide variety of cells as well as membrane-bound cytoplasmic organelles have been shown to be damaged *in vitro* by SLO similarly to erythrocytes. Striking cytopathogenic effects culminating in cell death and lysis were observed on rabbit leukocytes and alveolar macrophages (Todd, 1942; Bernheimer and Schwartz, 1960; Hirsch *et al.*, 1963; Zucker-Franklin, 1965), mouse peritoneal macrophages (Fauve *et al.*, 1966), chicken fibroblasts, human amnion cells and Ehrlich ascites tumor cells (Ginsburg and Grossowicz, 1960) human spermatozoa (Ginsburg, 1972) and platelets from various species (Merucci *et al.*, 1964; Bernheimer and Schwartz, 1965; Launay and Alouf, 1979). SLO was also found cytotoxic on a variety of tissue cultures *in vitro* such as rabbit kidney cells, HeLa and KB cells (Alouf, 1967; Mastroeni *et al.*, 1969; Duncan and Buckingham, 1977), L-cell fibroblasts (Duncan and Buckingham, 1978) and human diploid fibroblasts (Thelestam and Möllby, 1979).

Optical and electron microscopy of target cells submitted to lethal doses of SLO showed striking cell damage as evidenced by the almost instantaneous swelling of the cell, with numerous spherical cytoplasmic blebs vacuolization, leakage of intracellular substances, disruption of cytoplasmic organelles (mitochondria, lysosomes, other bodies). These changes supported other experimental indications that SLO acts primarily through physical disruption of cytoplasmic membrane and that similar surrounding intracellular organelles.

Interesting findings were reported in a cinemicro-photographic study of the toxic action of SLO rabbit polymorphonuclear leucocytes and alveolar macrophages (Hirsch *et al.*, 1963). The effects on leucocytes resulted in rapid and extensive lysis of cytoplasmic granules into the cell sap. Within a few minutes following degranulation, the leucocytes rounded up, filamentous processes appeared on the cell membrane the cytoplasm liquefied and the nuclear lobes swelled and fused. Exposure of rabbit macrophages to SLO also resulted in lysis of granules soon followed by alteration in the cytoplasm and membranes. Similar findings were reported for mouse macrophages (Fauve et al., 1966). Characteristic for SLO action on white blood cells is an apparent 'all or none' effect: some cells in suspension are completely disrupted by the toxin whereas others in their immediate vicinity are not affected at all.

Electron microscopic study of the degranulation of leucocytes treated with SLO revealed marked changes in subcellular architecture preceding visible damage or rupture of cellular membranes; especially characteristic was clumping of intracytoplasmic organelles and their intracellular translocation (Zucker-Franklin, 1965).

SLO was shown to release lysosomal and mitochondrial enzymes into the supernatants of granular fractions from rabbit liver, heart, spleen and lymph nodes (Weissman et al., 1963; Keiser et al., 1964). Mitochondrial swelling was shown to occur prior to lysis. The isolated leucocyte granules suspended in sucrose were also disrupted by SLO with release of their intragranular content (Weissman et al., 1964).

The lysosomal enzymes released by SLO may be responsible for the subsequent damage seen in various other cell structures.

Partially purified SLO was shown to be lytic on human and rabbit platelets (Merucci et al., 1964; Bernheimer and Schwartz, 1965). Recently a detailed biochemical and ultrastructural study of the disruption of human rabbit and guinea-pig platelets by highly purified SLO was reported (Launay and Alouf, 1979). The platelets appeared very sensitive to SLO. About 15 molecules of toxin were sufficient to lyse one cell. The cytoplasmic membrane was disrupted at several discrete loci as shown by electron microscopy with almost complete leakage of cytoplasmic material. Intracellular organelles were also disrupted or damaged. Cell damage was also reflected by the clearing of cell suspensions and the release of cytosol material such as lactate dehydrogenase. Evidence for organelle lysis was given by the liberation of serotonin, monoamine oxidase and glutathione peroxidase which are respective markers of dense bodies, mitochondrial external membrane and dense tubular system. No platelet aggregation or shape change was elicited by SLO. The ghosts resulting from platelet lysis retained properties of the native membrane such as aggregability and serotonin uptake. Dense bodies were easily separated after gentle disruption of the plasmic membrane by small amounts of toxin. Platelet lysis by SLO proved a useful procedure for the determination of protein content, enzyme activities and serotonin assay on the same lysate in contrast to usual methods.

2.9.3.3. *Subtle cytological alterations by SLO at sublytic levels.* Several investigations have examined the cellular effects produced by sublytic concentrations of toxin on various mammalian cells. Van Epps and Andersen (1974) observed inhibition by low amounts of SLO of the chemotaxis and mobility of neutrophilic leucocytes of man, baboon and sheep but not of rabbits. The possible involvement of immune mediators was excluded.

A similar inhibition of leucocyte locomotion and chemotaxis was also reported for the SLO-like toxin perfringolysin (Wilkinson, 1975). The effects of low concentrations of toxin was studied on human lymphocytes (Andersen and Cone, 1974; Andersen and Amirault, 1976). The toxin was a very effective inhibitor of phytohemagglutinin-induced lymphocyte transformation when the cells were first treated by SLO. It was suggested that SLO may interfere with the lectin receptor sites on the lymphocyte membrane. Specific stimulation of lymphoid cells by purified protein derivative was also suppressed by the toxin indicating that T-lymphocytes were affected. It was also shown that sheep erythrocyte-lymphocyte rosette (E-rosette) formation was inhibited by incubating lymphocytes with sublytic concentrations of SLO. This finding suggests alteration of erythrocyte receptor site on the surface of T-lymphocytes. A reduction in phagocytosis by mouse macrophages treated with SLO or SLS under similar conditions was reported (Ofek et al., 1972). All of the effects produced reflected subtle membrane damage of target cells. Such membrane changes were also illustrated by the impairment of the transport of amino-acids, nucleosides and glucose analogs in HeLa cells treated with sublethal concentrations of SLO. After treatment in such conditions the cells recovered their ability to transport α-aminoisobutyric acid in about 4 hr (Duncan and Buckingham, 1977; Smyth and Duncan, 1978). Subtle membrane damage produced by SLO and a variety of cytolytic and other membrane damaging agents has been studied on human diploid fibroblasts by measuring the leakage of various radioactive markers of different sizes from the cells (see Thelestam and Möllby, 1979). The differential release of these markers presumably reflected the size of the membrane lesions ('functional holes') produced by the cytolysin.

A detailed discussion of this methodology as regards SH-activated toxins was reported by Smyth and Duncan (1978).

2.10. Interaction of Streptolysin O with Cholesterol and Related Sterols

2.10.1. *Inhibition of Hemolytic and Other Biological Properties*

Hewitt and Todd (1939) first showed that very low amounts of cholesterol inhibit the hemolytic effects of SLO and this has been confirmed a great many times. This property is shared by all SH-activated cytolysins (Bernheimer, 1974, 1976; Alouf, 1977; Smyth and Duncan, 1978). Aqueous dispersions of cholesterol not only inhibit hemolysis but prevent other biologic effects of the toxin such as lethality, cardiotoxicity, lysis of lysosomes (see Bernheimer, 1966) and inhibition of chemotaxis and motility of leucocytes (Van Epps and Andersen, 1974).

2.10.2. *Strereospecificity of Sterol Effect*

Howard *et al.* (1953) investigated the effects of various sterols related to cholesterol and established that inhibition was effective only for those molecules having a β-hydroxyl group on carbon 3 of the steroid nucleus and a hydrophobic group at position 18. Similar findings were reported by Badin and Barillec (1968).

Detailed studies on the structural requirements and the stereochemical criteria necessary for sterol inhibition of SLO activity were undertaken with a wide range of compounds by Watson and Kerr (1974) Prigent and Alouf (1976) and Alouf and Geoffroy (1979). As one may infer from Table 8 and Fig. 6 the structural requirements are the following.

2.10.3. *Presence of a 3β-(Equatorial)Hydroxy Group on Ring A of the Cyclopentanoperhydrophenanthrene Nucleus*

This strict stereochemical and chemical requirement is illustrated by the ineffectiveness of any steroid having a modified 3β–OH group either by suppression (cholestane), oxidation (cholestanone), esterification (cholesterol acetate, 3-chlorocholestene) or epimerization into α position (epicholesterol with 3α-axial OH group).

Alouf and Geoffroy (1979) reported that in contrast to cholesterol the thiol analog of this sterol (thiocholesterol) (Fig. 7) did not interact with SLO, indicating a strict specificity of the oxygen atom of the 3β–OH group for toxin interaction. Although the –SH group possesses steric and chemical properties similar to the –OH group it differs in some physical and chemical properties. The lack of reactivity of thiocholesterol can be ascribed to the change in the geometry of the active 3β grouping i.e. the increase in radius of 0.4 Å and the change in the bond angle due to the sulfur atom. One consequence is that the dissociation energy of the –SH bond is less and the bond length longer than that of the –OH bond. In addition thiols differ from their oxygen counterparts in that they do not form notable hydrogen bonds. Whether such bonds are involved in cholesterol-toxin interaction is still unknown. It is interesting to note that most 3β-hydrosteroids and steroids are precipitated by digitonin whilst most 3α-hydrosteroids lacking a hydroxyl group at C-3 are not precipitated. Thiocholesterol was also found to be unable to fulfill the function of the –OH group to precipitate digitonin (see Alouf and Geoffroy, 1979).

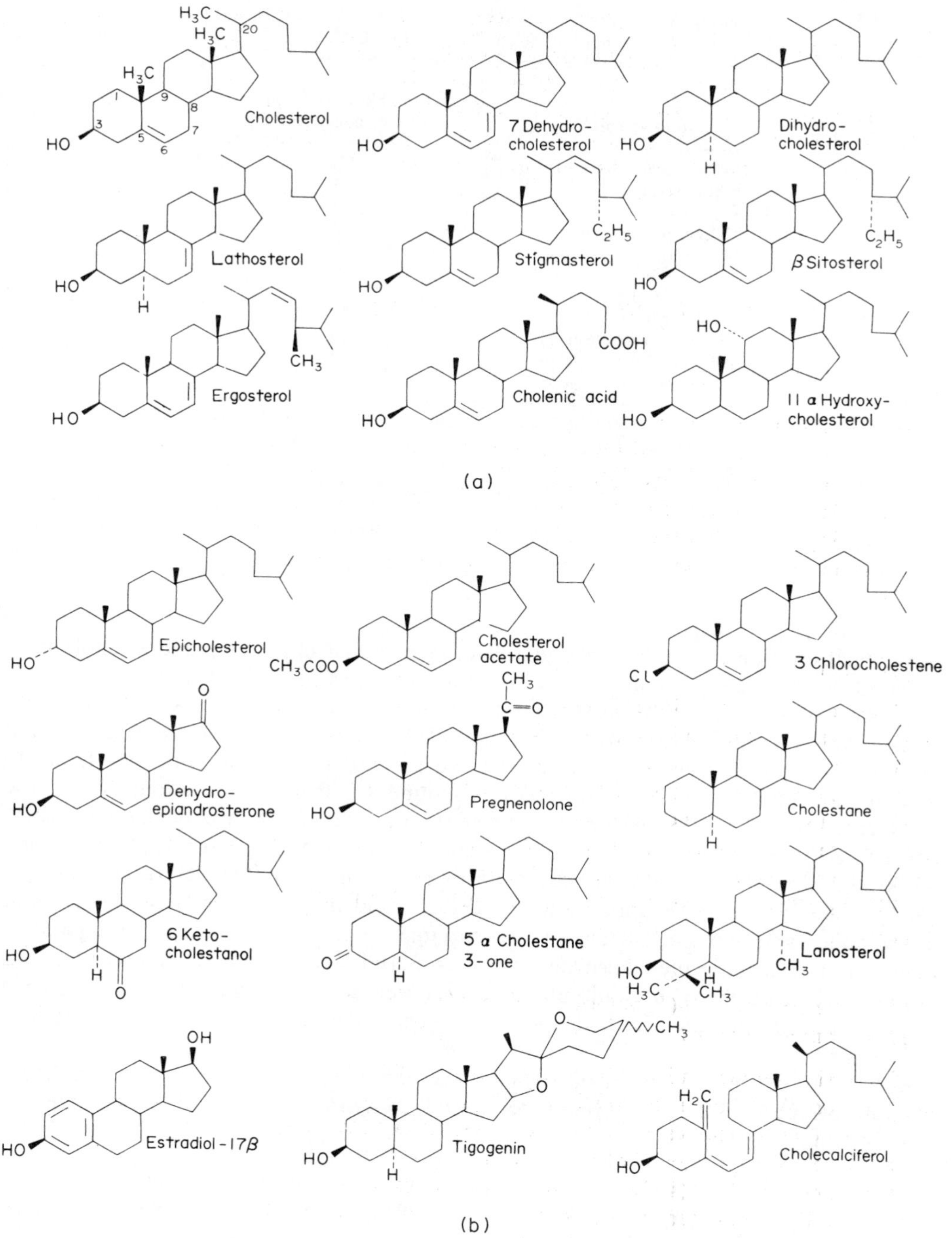

(a)

(b)

FIG. 6. Some steroids tested for inhibitory effects on streptolysin O activity. (a) Inhibitory steroids; (b) non inhibitory steroids.

2.10.4. *Presence of a Lateral Aliphatic Side Chain of Suitable Size at Carbon 17*

Suppression, shortening or lengthening of the hydrophobic isooctyl side chain of cholesterol or the introduction of functional groups on it greatly affect or suppress the inhibitory effect as in the case of dehydroepiandrosterone which lacks side chain and tigonenin which has a complex cyclic structure instead of an aliphatic side chain. Modification of the eight-carbon chain by introduction of an ethyl group at C–24 (β-sitosterol) is

TABLE 8. 50% *Inhibitory Dose of Various Sterols upon the Hemolytic Activity of Streptolysin O* (PRIGENT et al., 1976).

Inhibitory sterols	Inhibitory dose 50 ng sterol/hemolytic unit
7-Dehydrocholesterol	3
Cholesterol	5
Coprostanol	7
Dihydrocholesterol	10
Sitosterol	10
Lathosterol	10
Stigmasterol	15
Cholenic acid	20
11α-hydroxycholesterol	20
20α-hydroxycholesterol	50
Ergosterol	50

Steroids were dispersed in phosphate buffered saline pH 6.8. The values of ID$_{50}$ of the sterols employed have been determined by plotting residual activity of streptolysin O versus sterol concentration. Any steroid, the inhibitory effect of which was 50-fold less than that of cholesterol (250 ng per HU) was considered as non inhibitory. Non inhibitory sterols are shown in Fig. 6.

not critical since only a 2-fold decrease of the inhibitory effect as compared to cholesterol is found. When the side chain has an extra double bond at C22–23 and either $-C_2H_5$ (stigmasterol) or $-CH_3$ (ergosterol) group the inhibitory effect becomes 3-fold and 10-fold weaker. Watson and Kerr (1974) reported that desmosterol (double bond at C 24–25) and fucosterol (=CH–CH$_3$ group) were as effective as cholesterol. However they failed to demonstrate inhibition with stigmasterol as found by Prigent and Alouf (1976) and Howard *et al.* (1953). The discrepancy remains unexplained. With cholenic acid which has a 5-carbon chain ending by a carboxyl group at C–25, Watson and Kerr observed a weak inhibitory effect (which was also confirmed by Prigent and Alouf). In contrast, the methyl ester was inactive. Inhibition by cholenic acid indicates that a non polar side chain appears to be not absolutely critical for chain attachment to corresponding region(s) of SLO molecules. According to Watson and Kerr (1974) attachment may take place in this case through Coulomb forces between the C–17 side chain and ionized groups on SLO molecule. For hydrophobic side chain the interaction is probably by Van der Waals forces.

Clearly spatial orientation is important since compounds structurally very similar to cholesterol such as 25-hydroxycholesterol and 26-hydroxycholesterol were ineffective

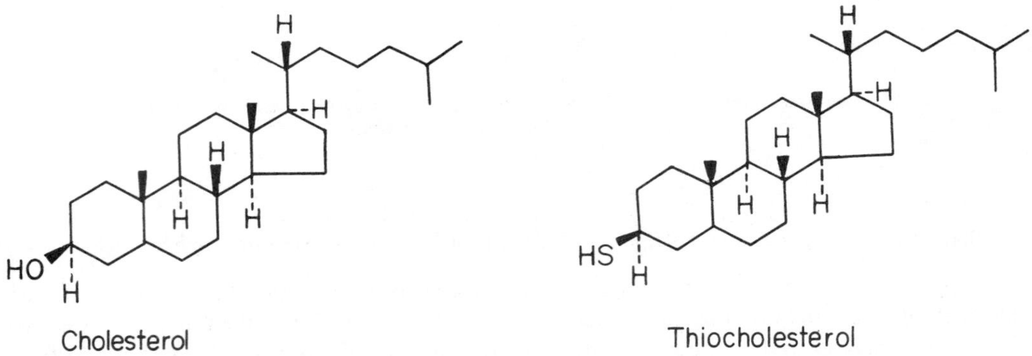

FIG. 7. Formulas of cholesterol and thiocholesterol.

(Watson and Kerr). Prigent and Alouf observed very poor inhibition with 20-α-hydroxy-cholesterol which differs from cholesterol by a hydroxyl group instead of a methyl group at C–20. Effective inhibition requires therefore the presence of this apolar group on the side chain.

2.10.5. *Intact B Ring*

This requirement is illustrated by the failure of cholecalciferol to inhibit toxin activity. This secosteroid which has both hydroxyl group and isooctyl side chain has no longer the conformation of a steroid nucleus due to the rupture of B ring.

In contrast the saturated or unsaturated state of intact B ring and the positions of double bonds are not critical for inhibition. Dihydrocholesterol (saturated ring) and lathocholesterol (C–7, 8 double bond) are a little weaker than cholesterol, whereas 7-dehydrocholesterol (C–5, 6; 7, 8 double bond) was more inhibitory. On the other hand, the stereochemical relationships of rings A and B to each other are also not critical. The 5β *cis* and the 5α *trans* (planar) steroids such as coprostranol and dihydrocholesterol respectively, originating from the presence of a chiral center at carbon 5 are both inhibitory. In contrast, only planar steroids inhibit polyene antibiotics.

The three above-mentioned criteria are minimal ones and have to be fulfilled simultaneously. In general, any additional group either polar or apolar at various positions decreases or suppresses the inhibitory potency. Moreover, in a steroid molecule differing in several respects from cholesterol, no mutual compensations occurs between the different additional groups to create or enhance inhibitory effect. This seems the case for inhibitory steroids such as 6 ketocholestanol and lanosterol. The latter has two methyl groups at C–4 contiguous to the 3β–OH group.

The structural requirements appear of great biological significance. It is well known that polyene antibiotics which also change the membrane permeability of eucaryotic cells and lead to cell lysis are inhibited by sterols meeting the same structural requirements found for SLO and the SH-activated toxins (see Norman *et al.*, 1976). Sterol-polyene interaction results in the formation of hydrophobic complexes in strict stoichiometric ratios. It has also been shown that many Mycoplasma strains require an external source of sterol for growth. Effective sterols are those containing the cholestane ring system (A/B *trans*), an unsubstituted 3β–OH group and branched aliphatic side chain eight or more carbon atoms in length (Odriozola *et al.*, 1978). Similar structural features appear to be necessary for regulatory functions (e.g. solute permeability, stability and viscosity) of sterols in biological or artificial membranes (Demel and deKruyff 1976, Lee 1977).

2.10.6. *Characteristics of Sterol-Streptolysin O Interaction*

Evidence supporting the idea of complex formation between SLO and cholesterol (or other inhibitory sterols) has been obtained through different approaches.

2.10.6.1. *Interaction in agar gels.* Insoluble sterol-toxin complexes were shown (Fig. 8) to occur by diffusion of SLO into cholesterol and other inhibitory sterols incorporated in an agar gel (Prigent and Alouf, 1976; Alouf and Geoffroy, 1979). A similar precipitation pattern was found under the same conditions with digitonin (Alouf, 1977).

Complex formation appears to be a specific phenomenon as non-inhibitory sterols (except lanosterol) did not give insolubilization under the same conditions.

2.10.6.2. *Electron microscope studies.* The formation of SLO-cholesterol complex is also supported by the electron microscope study by Duncan and Schlegel (1976) of the effect of the toxin on rabbit erythrocyte membrane, cholesterol-containing liposomes and cholesterol-lipid dispersion. When erythrocytes were treated with SLO and examined by electron microscopy, rings and 'C'-shaped structures were observed in the cell membrane. The rings had an electron-dense center, 24 nm in diameter, and the overall diameter of

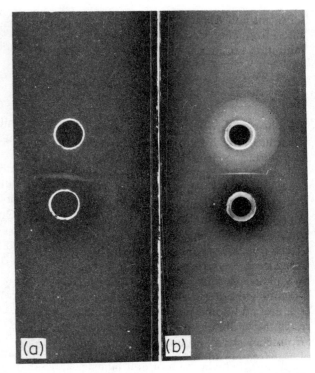

Fig. 8. Immunodiffusion of streptolysin O in sterol-containing agar gels. Left (a): thiocholesterol gel (100 μg/ml); Right (b): cholesterol gel (100 μg/ml). Upper well: 10 μl of streptolysin O (15,000 HU/ml) in PBS pH 6.8; bottom well: 10 μl of antistreptococcal γ-globulins (600 combining units/ml). A toxin-antitoxin precipitation zone similar to plate b was found in sterol-free gel. No toxin-antitoxin precipitation zone forms when cholesterol concentration exceeds 300 μg/ml of gel. See Alouf and Geoffroy (1979).

the structure was 38 nm. The ring structures were also observed on lecithin-cholesterol-dicetylphosphate liposomes. The crucial role of cholesterol in the formation of rings and C's was demonstrated by the fact that these structures were present in the toxin-treated cholesterol dispersions, but not in lecithin-dicetylphosphate dispersions nor in the SLO preparations alone. The importance of cholesterol was also shown by the finding that no rings were present in membranes or cholesterol dispersions which had been treated with digitonin before SLO was added.

Based upon their uniformity, the identity in lengths of the C-shaped structures and the circumferences of rings, and the calculated length of unfolded α-helix SLO, Duncan and Schlegel propose that interaction with and adsorption of cholesterol by SLO results in an unfolding of the toxin molecule and stabilization of the α-helix: 'sticky' ends of the C-shaped structures close to produce rings; dimers produce S-shaped forms as well. The resultant high concentrations of cholesterol at these loci on a membrane surface, therefore, may weaken the site sufficiently to produce membrane disorganization. Although the rings do not appear to be 'holes' in the membrane, a model was proposed which suggests that cholesterol molecules are sequestered during ring and C-structure formation, and that this process plays a role in SLO-induced hemolysis. Very similar ring- and arc-shaped structures in erythrocyte membrane, liposomes, lipid dispersions containing cholesterol and cholesterol dispersions have been found with other bacterial SH-activated toxins such as perfringolysin (Smyth et al., 1975; Mitsui et al., 1979a,b) and cereolysin (Cowell et al., 1978) as well as with the SH-activated toxin (metridiolysin) from the sea anemone *Metridium senile* (Bernheimer et al., 1979). In all cases rings and arcs are interpreted as toxin-cholesterol complexes.

However such structures have also been reported in cereolysin or perfringolysin preparations (but not SLO) at high protein concentration in the absence of added cholesterol.

The possible explanations proposed are trace contamination with cholesterol from initial culture medium or glassware during purification and (or) aggregation (Smyth *et al.*, 1975; Alouf, 1977; Cowell *et al.*, 1978). According to Mitsui *et al.* (1979b), some kinds of rings in the case of prefringolysin may be due to the toxin-phosphotungstic acid complexes produced during specimen preparation on a grid in vacuo.

2.10.6.3. *Dispersing effects of streptolysin O on cholesterol suspensions.* We recently observed in this laboratory that the granular heterogeneous aspect of cholesterol suspensions (1 mg/ml) in isotonic phosphate buffer pH 6.8 was strikingly changed into an apparently homogeneous dispersed phase upon mixing with 30 μg of SLO or alveolysin. Heat-denatured toxin preparation did not exhibit the dispersing effect (Fig. 9).

2.10.6.4. *Evidence for toxin binding by cholesterol.* Smyth and Duncan (1978) referred to unpublished data on ^{14}C-cholesterol binding to SLO and cereolysin. Recently direct evidence of the binding of the SH-activated toxins, SLO, alveolysin and pneumolysin by cholesterol was reported for the first time by Johnson *et al.* (1980).

Studies of cholesterol binding are hampered by the limited solubility of this compound, its tendency to form micelles and to stick to the walls of glassware and other materials. Johnson and co-workers have taken advantage of the fact that when solutions of cholesterol in phosphate buffer are added to Sephadex or Sephacryl columns, the free cholesterol sticks to the gel and only cytolysin-bound cholesterol is eluted with buffer (Fig. 10). The existence of a cytolysin-cholesterol complex was evidenced by the fact that after combination of cytolysin and cholesterol the properties of cholesterol were changed in that it was readily eluted from the Sephadex, and the properties of the cytolysin

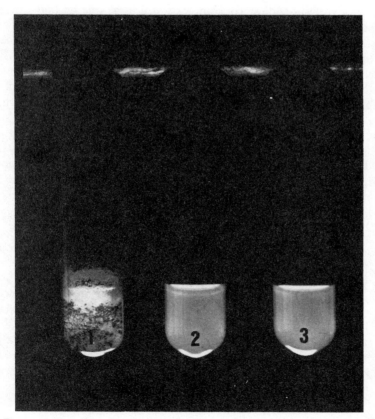

FIG. 9. Detergent like effect of SH-activated toxins on cholesterol dispersions. (1) Cholesterol dispersion (1 mg/ml) in PBS pH 6.8; (2), (3) The same dispersion after adding streptolysin O or alveolysin (10^3 hemolytic units).

GEL-FILTRATION OF CYTOLYSIN-CHOLESTEROL MIXTURE

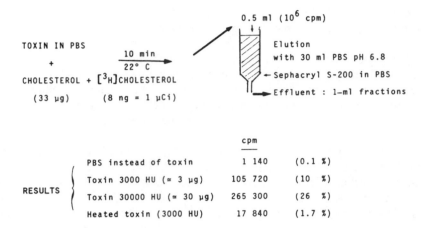

TOXIN IN PBS

+ $\xrightarrow[\text{22° C}]{\text{10 min}}$

CHOLESTEROL + [^{3}H]CHOLESTEROL

(33 μg)   (8 ng = 1 μCi)

0.5 ml (10^6 cpm)

Elution
with 30 ml PBS pH 6.8

← Sephacryl S-200 in PBS

→ Effluent : 1-ml fractions

		cpm	
	PBS instead of toxin	1 140	(0.1 %)
	Toxin 3000 HU (≈ 3 μg)	105 720	(10 %)
RESULTS	Toxin 30000 HU (≈ 30 μg)	265 300	(26 %)
	Heated toxin (3000 HU)	17 840	(1.7 %)

Non-eluted radioactivity : quantitatively recovered by washing
with Triton X-100

FIG. 10. Behavior of streptolysin O-cholesterol mixtures on Sephacryl gels.

changed in that it was no longer hemolytic. The results obtained with Sephacryl 200 indicated that the cytolysin-cholesterol complex was a large one (in that it was excluded) and must consist of more than one molecule of lysin and one molecule of cholesterol. Because the solutions of cholesterol used in these experiments contained micelles, it was not possible to establish a molar ratio for cytolysin-cholesterol interaction. Binding also occurred at sub-micellar concentrations but the difficulties of working at this level were considerable. It was impossible under these conditions to examine the binding reaction over a range of concentrations of toxin and cholesterol sufficient to establish molar ratios or affinities.

In addition, the specificity of the system toward other steroids—this is, epi-cholesterol non-competing and 7-dehydrocholesterol strongly competing reflected exactly the pattern described by Prigent and Alouf (1976) with respect to their effects on hemolytic activity of SLO. It therefore appears that SLO and related SH-activated toxins are

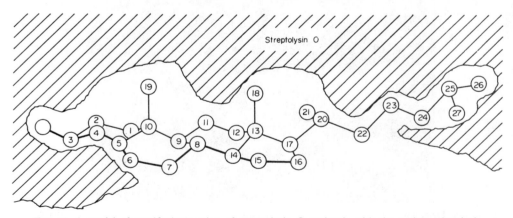

FIG. 11. A model of specific interaction of streptolysin O molecule with the various chemical groups of cholesterol molecule.

steroid-binding prokaryotic proteins. The stereochemical and structural requirements for sterol interaction with these proteins lead us to propose a model (Fig. 11) for toxin binding. The topology of protein-sterol contact takes into consideration the various chemical groups or atoms instrumental for toxin interaction with the steroid molecule as inferred from inhibition studies.

2.10.7. *Interaction of Streptolysin O With Cholesterol-Containing Liposomes or Lipid Dispersions*

Besides the electron microscope studies of this interaction mentioned above a number of studies of toxin interaction with liposomes or lipid dispersions containing varying amounts of cholesterol have been reported. Liposomes prepared from total lipid extract of sheep erythrocytes which contain cholesterol have been shown to fix SLO (Fehrenbach, 1977). Competition for toxin fixation between liposomes and sheep erythrocytes was also observed. It is to be noted that Shany et al. (1974) observed similar results with cereolysin one of the SLO-like SH-activated toxins. Liposomes composed of both lecithin and cholesterol inhibited the hemolytic activity of cereolysin and saponin whereas liposomes containing lecithin only did not. Incubation of cereolysin or SLO with untreated erythrocyte membrane caused complete inhibition of hemolytic activity whereas incubation with erythrocyte membranes pretreated with cereolysin, SLO, filipin or alfalfa saponin did not. Incubation of cereolysin or streptolysin O with erythrocyte membranes pretreated with soybean saponin resulted in complete inhibition of hemolysis. The results provide strong support for the idea that alfalfa saponin, filipin and SLO share a common membrane binding site and the binding site is cholesterol.

The inhibition of SLO activity by cholesterol-lecithin dispersion was studied by Delattre et al. (1973) as a function of the lecithin-sterol ratio (R). Inhibition increased for $R = 0.1$ up to 0.5 and decreased beyond this ratio until 1.2 since inhibition was no longer observed. This finding is consistent with cholesterol masking by phospholipids for high content of the latter whereas at low ratios inhibition was optimal as compared to cholesterol alone owing likely to a better dispersion and therefore availability of cholesterol to toxin molecules.

SLO binding by erythrocyte ghosts and lipoproteins was also shown to be dependent on cholesterol content (Badin and Denne, 1978). Recently, Delattre et al. (1979) reported a detailed study of the inhibition of SLO by phospholipid-cholesterol liposomes of different chemical nature and molar ratios. Toxin binding (equated with inhibition) was shown to vary between 0–100% depending on the nature of the phospholipid and the phospholipid/sterol molar ratio. In phosphatidylcholine (P-choline) and sphingomyelin liposomes, no sterol was found to be available for SLO binding at ratios equal or above 1.5, whereas, sterol was almost totally available when the ratio was below 1.

In P-serine liposomes, cholesterol remained largely but not completely available for SLO binding at any ratio up to 3. In phosphatidic acid and P-ethanolamine liposomes, cholesterol was largely, if not totally, available for binding at all the ratios studied.

Incorporation of phosphatidic acid into inactive P-choline liposomes with a phospholipid/sterol ratio at 2 restored some cholesterol availability for SLO binding, whereas, P-ethanolamine had no effect. Several hours incubation of inactive P-choline liposome ($r = 2$) with phospholipase D at pH 5.6 in presence of trace of ethanol also restored some SLO binding activity to the liposomes. It was therefore suggested that the choline group plays a major role in masking the reactivity of liposome cholesterol. Electron microscopy studies of P-choline-sterol liposomes showed that the suspension structure considerably depended on the molar ratio of the components. Liposomes were vesicular at ratio > 1 and mainly tubular at ratios below 1. SLO did not alter the structure of liposomes with $r = 2$ evidently because of the lack of toxin binding to cholesterol, whereas, it rapidly destroyed the structure of P-choline/sterol liposomes with $r = 1$ or lower than 1. During this process, SLO-sterol complexes appeared on the grid, often with the characteristic aspect of networks of juxtaposed hexagones disseminated among the liposome fragments.

It is to be noted that no disruption of liposomes by SLO as evidenced by the release of internal markers was observed by Duncan and Schlegel (1975). According to Smyth and Duncan (1978) the compositional or configurational requirements for SLO activity were not met in these preparations. In contrast, Prigent and Alouf (1978) observed that liposomes made up of phosphatidylcholine-cholesterol-phosphatidic acid (1.2:1:0.1) including ^{14}C-arginine as a tracer were disrupted as evidenced by the release of ^{14}C-arginine. This lytic action depends on the dose of toxin and on temperature. The presence of cholesterol was required.

Those liposomes which do not include this sterol do not react with the toxin. The same holds true if other sterols (ergosterol, stigmasterol, lanosterol) were substituted for cholesterol.

No binding of ^{125}I-SLO on cholesterol-free liposomes was observed. Toxin-fixation was shown to be strictly dependent on sterol content in the liposomes.

2.10.8. *Effect of Cholesterol on the Immunogenicity of Streptolysin O*

Early brief work by Turner and Pentz (1950) indicated that the cholesterol-neutralized SLO was as immunogenic in rabbits as free SLO. This view has been recently challenged by Kaplan and Wannamaker (1976) in a detailed study. It was shown that lipids extracted from rabbit skin block the hemolytic capacity of SLO and also suppress the neutralizing antibody response to this streptococcal extracellular antigen in rabbits immunized intravenously. The modification in antibody response was specific for SLO; the antibody responses to streptococcal DNase B and to streptococcal NADase were not affected. Cholesterol, a lipid present in abundance in skin, had a similar specific effect on the antigenicity of SLO and may be the component responsible for the demonstrated effects of these lipid extracts of skin. *In vitro* experiments indicate that lipid extracts of rabbit skin have a greater capacity to block the hemolytic capacity of SLO than do lipid extracts of rabbit heart, kidney, lung, liver, or spleen. These data support the view that the feeble anti-SLO response observed in patients with streptococcal pyoderma is a result of the abundance of a local lipid inhibitor, such as cholesterol, in the skin. They may also bear on the pathogenesis of rheumatic fever, a complication which apparently does not occur following group A streptococcal pyoderma but could be initiated by SLO (see Wannamaker, 1973).

2.11. MECHANISM OF ACTION OF THE MEMBRANE-DAMAGING ACTION OF STREPTOLYSIN O

As may be inferred from the preceding sections a great progress was accomplished in the past decade toward the understanding of the mechanism of action of SLO and more generally SH-activated toxins at the molecular level. Several approaches were particularly useful for this progress. Recent reviews reported the achievements in this respect (Bernheimer, 1974, 1976; Duncan, 1975; Alouf, 1977; Smyth and Duncan, 1978). We shall summarize here the main conclusions of our present knowledge on the mechanism of the lytic process. This mechanism was essentially studied on erythrocytes which have been taken as a very convenient model for the study of toxin action at membrane level.

2.11.1. *Characteristics of the Hemolytic Process*

The kinetics of SLO-induced hemolysis has been examined in detail by Alouf and Raynaud (1968a,b,c) and Kanbayashi *et al.* (1972). Studies of the time course of hemolysis as a function of toxin concentration generated a family of sigmoid-shaped curves. A pre-lytic lag period was followed by a non linear release of hemoglobin. A mathematical study of the rates of this release as well as that of various parameters of the lytic curve as a function of toxin concentration, temperature and erythrocyte concentration was described (Alouf and Raynaud, 1968b). The results obtained were consistent with a multi-hit process which was also suggested by the studies of Kanbayashi *et al.* (1972) and Duncan *et al.* (1976) and the mathematical analysis of lysis data by Inoue *et al.* (1976). In a study by Duncan (1974) the kinetics of hemoglobin and $^{86}Rb^+$ release under the action of SLO was investigated. Both components were lost at the same rate from the treated cells, and the addition of large molecules (albumin) to the suspending medium did not retard the escape of these substances. The results indicated that a colloid-osmotic process is not involved in SLO hemolysis. This finding suggests that the functional membrane lesion produced by the toxin are sufficiently large to allow simultaneous escape of Rb^+ and hemoglobin (effective radius greater than 3.5 nm).

The interaction of unlabeled and ^{125}I-labeled SLO and its formaldehyde toxoid with rabbit erythrocytes was studied in detail in the cold and at 37°C under several conditions by Alouf and Raynaud (1968a,c) and Prigent *et al.* (1974). It was clearly established that the lytic process involves two sequential steps. The first step consists of toxin fixation on its binding site at the surface of the cytoplasmic membrane. Toxin binding was found temperature-independent since fixation was almost instantaneous and irreversible at 0°C. The second step involves membrane damage as evidenced by the release of hemoglobin. It is relatively slow and is temperature-dependent; it does not take place at 0°C (for moderate concentrations of SLO). This property permits the dissociation of the two steps and allows their study separately.

Only reduced SLO or toxoid could specifically bind onto its membrane receptor. Oxidized SLO molecules do not bind. This explains their inactivity. Once binding of the toxin had occurred further lysis was not prevented by adding cholesterol or SH-compounds blocking agents as it is the case when these reagents added to the toxin prior to interaction with target cells. In contrast, Alouf and Raynaud (1968b,c) and Prigent *et al.* (1974) found that some kinds of neutralizing anti-SLO antibodies from horse sera or human myeloma prevented subsequent hemolysis after reduced SLO has become fixed to them at 0°C. However other neutralizing antibodies from horse or human sera were found to be active on the first stage of the lytic process by preventing toxin fixation on cell surface but did not prevent cell lysis after toxin binding. These two types of 'anti-lytic' and 'anti-fixation' antibodies are likely directed toward two regions of SLO molecule involved in the lytic process as detailed below (see Fig. 12).

Of interest was the observation that different sera varied considerably in their potency for neutralizing such erythrocyte-fixed SLO indicating that hyperimmune sera contained various proportions of the two types of anti-SLO antibodies.

From Arrhenius plot the activation energy from hemolysis was rather high (33700 cal/mol) as determined by Alouf and Raynaud (1968b). A value of 40,000 cal/mol was found by Bernheimer (see Smyth and Duncan, 1978) between 0 and 15°C. This may reflect a phase transition of the membrane lipids from a more fluid to a highly ordered state in the region of the site of toxin action.

Many other characteristics of SLO-induced hemolysis have been summarized by Smyth and Duncan (1978). Whereas intact-SH groups on the toxin molecule are necessary for binding, the same is not true for the target cell. Erythrocytes on which sulfhydryl groups had been alkylated with iodoacetamide (Van Epps and Andersen, 1971) or blocked with N-ethyl-maleimide (Oberley and Duncan, 1971) remained completely susceptible to SLO action, suggesting that S-S bond formation between toxin and membrane peptides is not important in binding. Similarly, erythrocytes which had been treated with proteolytic enzymes to remove the external proteins exposed on the surface of the cell membrane remained completely susceptible to SLO (Oberley and Duncan, 1971). The binding of SLO at 0°C was shown to be independent of pH and ionic strength (Oberley and Duncan, 1971). One interpretation of these findings is that interactions other than electrostatic forces between the toxin molecule and the cell membrane may be important in the initial binding step. Repeated washing of sensitized erythrocytes (erythrocytes with bound toxin at 0°C) did not remove SLO (Alouf and Raynaud, 1968c), but Kanbayashi *et al.* (1972) found that SLO could be transferred from one cell to another. Sensitized erythrocytes were washed at 4°C, and incubated with varying amounts of fresh

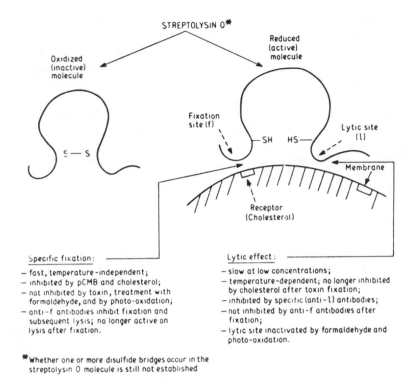

STREPTOLYSIN O*

Oxidized
(inactive)
molecule

Reduced
(active)
molecule

Fixation
site (f)

Lytic site
(l)

S — S

—SH   HS—

Membrane

Receptor
(Cholesterol)

Specific fixation:
- fast, temperature-independent;
- inhibited by pCMB and cholesterol;
- not inhibited by toxin, treatment with formaldehyde, and by photo-oxidation;
- anti-f antibodies inhibit fixation and subsequent lysis; no longer active on lysis after fixation.

Lytic effect:
- slow at low concentrations;
- temperature-dependent; no longer inhibited by cholesterol after toxin fixation;
- inhibited by specific (anti-l) antibodies;
- not inhibited by anti-f antibodies after fixation;
- lytic site inactivated by formaldehyde and photo-oxidation.

*Whether one or more disulfide bridges occur in the streptolysin O molecule is still not established

FIG. 12. Speculative model of streptolysin O molecule interaction with erythrocyte membrane
(Alouf, 1977).

red cells at 37°C. The addition of increasing amounts of fresh red cells resulted in the release of more hemoglobin than could be accounted for by the lysis of the sensitized cells, suggesting that some toxin molecules had been transferred from the sensitized cells to the fresh cells, and demonstrating that more toxin bound to the membrane than necessary to lyse the cell. Oberley and Duncan (1971) demonstrated that the hemolytic process (following SLO binding) was inhibited by low pH and high ionic strength. In addition, haemolysis by SLO have been shown to be inhibited by low concentrations of divalent cations (Van Epps and Andersen, 1971). Oberley and Duncan (1971) demonstrated that cells protected against hemolysis by low concentrations of divalent cations, lysed when they were resuspended in isotonic saline. No lysis occurred, however when the protected cells were resuspended in saline containing anti-streptolysin O antibody. These experiments demonstrated that divalent cations did not prevent or reverse the binding of SLO to the erythrocytes, nor did the cations inactivate the toxin. The ability of antitoxin to prevent cell lysis after removal of the divalent cations indicated that the cell membrane was not irreversibly damaged by the toxin during the incubation. Thus, it seems that divalent cations inhibit a stage in the hemolytic process but prior to the action of the toxin which results in irreversible damage to the cell membrane.

2.11.2. Nature of Toxin Binding Site

From the various biological and biochemical results concerning the relationship of cholesterol to the biological activity of SLO and the other SH-activated toxins reported in the preceding paragraphs, it appears beyond any doubt that membrane cholesterol is the binding site and (or) target of toxin action at the surface of the cytoplasmic membrane of eukaryotic cells (Bernheimer, 1974, 1976; Alouf, 1977; Smyth and Duncan, 1978; Cowell and Bernheimer, 1978). It is well established now that this sterol is present in all eukaryotic cells as a fundamental constituent of their membrane playing a critical role as a condensing agent in the bilayer structure and then instrumental for ensuring membrane stability.

New support to this concept was recently afforded by Duncan and Buckingham (1978) by treatment of L cell fibroblasts which certain oxygenated derivatives of cholesterol which are known to inhibit cholesterol biosynthesis in mammalian cells. After incubation in the presence of 20-α-hydroxycholesterol or 25-α-hydroxycholesterol for 18 hr the cells became increasingly resistant to SLO. Maximum resistance to toxin was obtained by incubating for 48 hr in 0.25 μg/ml 25-hydroxycholesterol; under these conditions, the cells were 10–50 times more resistant than were untreated controls. In contrast to control cultures, most of the toxin activity remained in the medium after being incubated with hydroxycholesterol-treated cultures. The results indicated that less toxin binds to the resistant cells, and suggest that a reduction in membrane cholesterol content may account for resistance to streptolysin O.

Similar results were reported by Cowell and Bernheimer (1978) for the SH-activated toxin cereolysin. Treatment of erythrocyte membranes and *Acholeplasma laidlawii* cells containing cholesterol with cholesterol oxidase which converts cholesterol to Δ4-choles-tone abolished the ability of these membranes to bind the toxin and inhibited its hemolytic activity.

The relative resistance of mouse erythrocytes to SLO was also recently investigated by Fehrenbach and Templefeld (1979) in the light of membrane cholesterol content.

The ratio of cholesterol/phospholipid in total lipid extracts of human (HRBC), sheep (SRBC), rabbit (RRBC) and mouse erythrocytes (MRBC) was determined. The cholesterol/phospholipid quotient of MRBC) was determined. The cholesterol/phospholipid quotient of MRBC with Q = 1, was higher if compared with those of HRBC, SRBC and RRBC which amounted to 0.6, 0.5 and 0.7 respectively.

Binding studies with ^{125}I-streptolysin revealed that the amount of toxin fixed to MRBC and liposomes, prepared from cell total lipid extracts, was less than 25% of the values found for HRBC, SRBC and RRBC. Calculated from double labelling experiments the molecular binding ratio was 15, 15 and 12 ^{125}I-toxin molecules/liposome for HRBC-, SRBC- and RRBC-extracts whereas for MRBC-extracts the value was 3 molecules/liposome. The relative resistance of mouse erythrocyte was then due to the low binding capacity of MRBC membranes for SLO though their relative cholesterol content is higher than that of other mammalian erythrocytes. It appeared plausible that the mobility, accessibility and distribution of cholesterol in natural and artificial membrane is strongly influenced through the presence and composition of individual lipid constituents of the membrane. Therefore, the binding of SLO to membranes is dependent on the molecular interaction of cholesterol with individual lipid constituents.

2.11.3. *Mechanism of Membrane Disruption by Streptolysin O*

Although the membrane-binding site of the toxin is well characterized, it is still not known how SLO and related toxins produce membrane changes which result in lysis or death of sensitive cells. In an electron-microscope study Dourmashkin and Rosse (1966) reported that SLO produced what were described as 50-nm 'holes' in the erythrocyte membrane.

In 1974 Bernheimer proposed that lysis of cells by SLO may be due to the escape of molecules through these holes which could be lined by cholesterol-SLO complexes. Besides SLO, ring structures have been seen in membranes treated with perfringolysin and cereolysin as mentioned in a previous section. SLO and perfringolysin have been shown to form ring structures, along with arc-shaped structures, after interaction with cholesterol. Despite these findings there was no evidence to show that these structures actually produced functional pores in membranes, and it is not clear what role the ring and arcs have in the lytic mechanism of thiol-activated toxins. Using freeze fracture electron microscopy, Cowell *et al.* (1978) indicated that the structures observed for cereolysin are not transverse holes in the membrane.

The structural alterations produced were seen only in the outer half of the hydrophobic layer of the membrane and no changes were observed in the inner half of bilayer. A similar conclusion concerns very likely SLO and the other SH-activated toxins. The structures observed are rather considered as polymerized forms of the toxin. It was suggested (Bernheimer, 1974; Prigent and Alouf, 1976; Alouf, 1977; Cowell et al., 1978) that the toxin binds to cholesterol in the membrane, the toxin cholesterol complexes aggregate in the plane of the membrane and cause lysis because of increased membrane disorganization due to the removal of cholesterol from its normal interaction with phospholipids. The formation by cereolysin of apparent aggregated areas in the hydrophobic core of the membrane is consistent with this theory. If the rings and arcs formed by interaction of thiol-activated toxins with cholesterol are eventually found to be composed of cholesterol and toxin molecules, this would obviously add support to the above theory. These structures have never been isolated or chemically defined with any of the lytic agents known to form them.

According to Smyth and Duncan (1978) the following course of events may be envisaged for hemolysis (cytolysis) by the SH-activated cytolysins. The toxin molecules interact with cholesterol at the surface (or accessible at the surface) of a membrane. This interaction may be hydrophobic in nature although hydrogen bonding between amino acids of the cytolysin and the 3β-OH groups of the cholesterol molecules may also contribute. At $0°C$ (or below the phase transition temperature of phospholipids from natural membranes) primary toxin-cholesterol complexes of unknown stoichiometry form. The formation of such complexes produces no visible structural alterations in the membrane, nor does the "sensitized" membrane appear to be weakened or damaged as shown by osmotic fragility determinations (Duncan, unpublished data). The toxin molecule in the primary complex remains susceptible to antitoxin neutralization, but it can no longer be inactivated by the addition of exogenous cholesterol.

After binding (primary complex formation), warming of 'sensitized' cells to $37°C$ may lead to an aggregation of the primary toxin-cholesterol complexes which are dispersed over the membrane at $0°C$. Alternatively, the temperature-dependent step may result in the sequestration of cholesterol around extended (or circularized) toxin molecules (Duncan and Schlegel, 1975). According to either interpretation, the rings and arc-shaped structures represent aggregates of one or more toxin molecules with membrane cholesterol. This proposal suggests, therefore, that the SH-activated cytolysins sequester or 'extract' cholesterol from certain regions of the membrane, thereby permitting a lipid phase-transition to occur in those areas. Based on studies of the effects of cholesterol on phospholipid phase transitions in natural and artificial membranes the withdrawal of cholesterol from its interaction with phospholipids would be expected to result in increased disorder and mobility of the hydrocarbon chains of the phospholipids above their phase-temperature. The phospholipid molecules, occupying an increased molecular area, would be less condensed and as a result, the membrane in these regions would be in a more fluid state (see Demel and de Kruyff, 1976; Lee, 1977; Huang, 1977; Martin and Yeagle, 1978).

Other biological agents known to complex or interact with cholesterol produce lysis e.g. saponin, digitonin, filipin and other polyene antibiotics, and some of these compounds have been shown to reverse the effects which cholesterol is known to have on phase transition and membrane permeability (Demel and de Kruyff, 1976; Norman et al., 1976).

As stated by Smyth and Duncan (1978) the model proposed by us (Alouf, 1977; (Fig. 12) does not conflict with the events envisaged above. On the basis of experimental data (Alouf, 1968a,b,c; Prigent et al., 1974), one may consider the occurrence of two topologically distinct sites on SLO molecule relatively distant one from another i.e. a fixation site termed f which recognizes and binds to the membrane target or receptor, namely cholesterol, and a lytic site termed l which is involved in triggering cell damage. The idea of different topological sites is supported by the demonstration of specific anti-f and anti-l antibodies (Prigent et al., 1974). Binding of anti-l antibodies to membrane-bound SLO may prevent secondary aggregation of toxin-cholesterol complexes above the phase-transition temperature by steric hindrance. Alternatively if the *l* site is actively involved in promoting or directing sequestration of cholesterol, its neutralization would inhibit this secondary reaction. It could be possible that after toxin fixation on cholesterol some penetration of a hydrophobic region of SLO molecule comprising the '*l*' site into the bilayer takes place. This event will be rather slow and temperature-dependent and will correspond to the lytic phase of the process. Anti-*l* antibodies will prevent such a penetration. This view is consistent with the finding that anti-*l* antibodies no longer block the lytic phase if added too late (1 hr) after toxin binding in the cold on target cells.

2.11.4. *Possible Role of Streptolysin O in Human Disease*

The rapid proliferation of streptococci at the portal of entry in the host (the throat in major cases) can be expected to lead to the production of relatively high amounts of SLO (and other toxins such SLS and ET as well as hydrolytic enzymes). It is still not clear what could be the possible pathological consequences of the release of SLO in surrounding tissues and its eventual spread through the blood stream and lymphatics. In this case, it may cause cellular damage at tissue sites remote from the portal of entry of the microorganism (Ginsburg, 1972). Patients infected with group A streptococci develop antistreptolysin O antibodies which reflect the production of this toxin in the patient. Anti-SLO titer increases during acute rheumatic fever and post-streptococcal glomerulonephritis.

The various clinical aspects of these phenomena have been reviewed by Halbert (1970) and Wannamaker (1973). Both investigators do not rule out the possibility that SLO is necessary to initiate the rheumatic process. According to Halbert, during the streptococcal infection an abundance of SLO (and other extracellular products) are released into the tissues and the circulation. The secreted SLO combines with antibody immediately and circulates as an antigen-antibody complex. An equilibrium becomes established between continued secretion of streptolysin and further development of antistreptolysin during the period of invasion by streptococci. Because of the well established, small, but definite *in vivo* dissociation of antigen-antibody complexes, the SLO-anti-SLO complex could act as the source for the slow release of active SLO. This latter, having a higher degree of predilection for certain tissues (e.g. heart, etc...) accumulates on or in the susceptible tissue cells until a toxic level is reached. At this point in time, the overt symptoms of rheumatic fever would begin. Symptoms and damage would continue as long as significant amounts of streptolysin-antistreptolysin complexes were present to supply a source of streptolysin.

It has also been suggested by Van Epps and Andersen (1974) that the chemotactic suppression of white blood cells by low doses of SLO may be a factor in the increasing pathogenicity of group A streptococci in humans.

3. STREPTOLYSIN S

Comprehensive reviews on streptolysin S (SLS) have been published in the past years (Ginsburg, 1970, 1972; Bernheimer, 1972; Okamoto, 1976; Okamoto *et al.*, 1978; Jeljaszewicz *et al.*, 1978) therefore we shall only briefly summarize here the main properties of this highly potent cytolytic toxin and deal with new recent findings concerning its chemical and biological properties.

3.1. DEFINITION

Streptolysin S is the non-immunogenic oxygen-stable cytolysin produced by streptococci which is responsible for zones of beta-hemolysis surrounding colonies on bloodagar media. This toxin is composed of a polypeptide moiety associated to a carrier. It is only active in the carrier-bound state. It appears that a variety of unrelated carrier substances can induce the release of active cytolysin by streptococci. These carriers are serum albumin, α-lipoprotein, RNA, ribonuclease-resistant core RNA, Trypan blue and some non-ionic detergents such as Tween 40, 60 and 80 and Triton X-205. SLS is a very potent cytolytic agent active on eucaryotic as well as procaryotic cells (bacterial protoplasts and spheroplasts). SLS appears to be endowed with antitumor activity.

3.2. Discovery and Historical Background

It was demonstrated originally by Weld (1934, 1935) that streptococci produce appreciable amounts of hemolytic and lethal toxin upon shaking the cells derived from young cultures in the presence of heat-inactivated horse serum. The hemolytic toxin so obtained was designated streptolysin S by Todd (1938a), in order to differentiate it from the oxygen-labile hemolytic toxin, streptolysin O (SLO) which is produced independently of the presence of serum. SLS also known as oxygen-stable hemolysin was thereafter characterized more completely by Herbert and Todd (1944). In 1940 Okamoto (see Okamoto, 1976) discovered that yeast nucleic acid caused a thousandfold increase in the production of SLS in broth culture fluid of streptococci. Subsequently, Bernheimer and Rodbart (1948) studied the factors affecting the formation of SLS in cultures containing RNA. They found that it was possible to form SLS through the interaction of RNA and resting streptococci, that is, by employing the system used by Weld but substituting RNA for serum. It was also established that sodium nucleate digested by ribonuclease was more effective than the native nucleate employed by Okamoto and that, in the presence of this factor maltose promoted the production of SLS. The addition of these two factors to the synthetic medium previously described by Bernheimer et al. (1942) resulted in the production of highly potent filtrates of SLS.

A great contribution to our understanding of SLS was made by Ginsburg and coworkers (see Ginsburg, 1970) who found that besides serum and RNA, other substances such as Tweens, Triton X-205 or trypan blue can also induce SLS formation. They characterized the active fractions from sera responsible of SLS induction. They also established that the lytic moiety of RNA-streptolysin or that of albumin-streptolysin could be transferred to Tween or Triton. They further showed that the hemolytic activity of albumin-streptolysin was transferable to RNA and vice versa. Their findings led to the simplifying concept that RNA, Tween, albumin, etc. . . function as carriers for a hemolytic moiety which, under appropriate conditions, can be transferred from one carrier to another. As noted by Bernheimer (1972) no one has ever succeeded in isolating in active form the hemolytic moiety by itself, that is, free of a carrier. It may indeed prove impossible to do so because the experience of several investigators suggests the active moiety undergoes rapid decay when the complex is treated in ways designed to remove or destroy only the carrier.

Non extracellular forms of SLS-like material were also demonstrated. An intracellular form was described by Schwab (1956) which was released by prolonged sonication of the cocci. The hemolysin was found to be similar to RNA-core SLS in stability, kinetics of hemolysis and sensitivity to inhibitors but different in monovalent ions effects and susceptibility of erythrocytes of different species. The intracellular toxin was also studied by Taketo and Taketo (1964) who extracted it by sonicating or grinding of streptococcal cells (see Calandra and Oginsky, 1975).

On the other hand a cell-bound hemolysin demonstrated only with intact streptococci was shown by Ginsburg and coworkers to be present in strains capable of producing extracellular SLS (see Ginsburg, 1970). The cell bound-toxin was shown to be released from the streptococcal cells by certain detergents and by α-lipoproteins. It was likely that this hemolysin represents SLS attached to the bacterial cell surface.

A detailed study of the cellular forms of SLS has been undertaken by Calandra and Oginsky (1975) and Calandra et al. (1976). These investigations, as summarized by Jeljaszewicz et al. (1978), revealed the existence of intracellular hemolysins, of which two seem to function as SLS precursors. One of them, named 'labile active cellular hemolysin', is released from cells by phage associated lysin (muralysin) and is stabilized by the RNA-core, whereas the second, termed 'latent hemolysin', is activated by sonic treatment in the presence of RNA-core. The application of sonication or a grinding technique releases one of these hemolysins. Latent hemolysin is a large molecular weight substance, and during its activation disaggregation or fragmentation takes place. Activated intracellular hemolysin exhibits properties of RNA-core hemolysin, and both can be inhibited by early addition of glucose to the culture. The inhibitory effect of glucose was earlier described by Bernheimer (1948) and Taketo and Taketo (1964). The introduction of glucose after initiation of production of both hemolysins results only in inhibition of intracellular hemolysin (Calandra and Oginsky, 1975). In a subsequent study (Calandra et al., 1976) it has been demonstrated that latent hemolysin is produced by all group A strains excreting streptolysin S. Strains which are streptolysin S-negative do not elaborate hemolysin. Liberation of free streptolysin S into basal Bernheimer's medium without RNA leads to the disappearance of the cellular precursor. Incubation of group A streptococci under the same conditions leads to a decrease, although to a lesser degree, of latent hemolysin production. Addition at that stage of RNA results in the appearance of small amounts of streptolysin S. Based on these findings, the authors conclude that latent hemolysin is a precursor of extracellular streptolysin S (Calandra et al., 1976).

3.3. PRODUCTION OF STREPTOLYSIN S

Most work on SLS has been done using streptococci belonging to Lancefield group A. As reported by Ginsburg (1970) over 95% of group A, C and G tested produced serum or RNA-toxin. Production of the hemolysin by certain strains from groups belonging to groups E, H and L was also reported. In contrast, SLS does not appear to be produced by groups B and D (enterococci). It is still not demonstrated whether SLS is produced *in vivo* during streptococcal infections (Ginsburg, 1970; Jeljaszewicz et al., 1978).

3.3.1. *Obtention of Extracellular SLS*

Most commonly extracellular SLS is obtained as 'RNA-core SLS' produced on incubation of resting cells of group A streptococci in pH 7.0 phosphate buffer containing Mg_2^+, maltose, RNA-core and cysteine or thioglycolate (see references in Calandra and Oginsky, 1975).

The production of SLS induced by other chemical substances is described by Ginsburg et al. (1963).

3.3.2. *Obtention of Cellular SLS*

Several procedures have been described for the obtention of cellular hemolysins such as sonication or grinding of streptococcal cells or treatment with phage-derived muralysin (see Calandra and Oginsky, 1975; and Calandra et al., 1976).

3.3.3. *Synthesis of SLS by Streptococci*

Several studies have been undertaken on *in vitro* formation of SLS by growing cells, resting cells protoplasts, protoplast membranes and cell-free systems. These studies have been reviewed by Ginsburg (1970).

3.4. PURIFICATION OF STREPTOLYSIN S

Early attempts at purifying SLS were reported by a number of authors (see reviews by Bernheimer, 1954, 1972; Ginsburg, 1970). Great difficulties were however encountered and the preparations obtained were of low purity. A great step was made by Koyama

(1963) and Koyama and Egami (1963) who obtained a purified SLS to a point at which the result of chemical analyses were likely to be meaningful. These investigators used extensively purified oligoribonucleotide to induce SLS and purified the hemolysin through two-zone electrophoresis in starch blocks followed by DEAE-cellulose chromatography. The overall yield was reported as 15% and the specific activity of the preparation was 2×10^6 HU per mg protein. The purified material was composed on an oligonucleotide and a polypeptide in a molar ratio of 3.1 : 1.

Bernheimer (1967) estimated the sedimentation coefficient of RNA-core hemolysin as determined by sucrose-gradient centrifugation to be about 2.4; the molecular weight determined by gel filtration was 12,000 daltons.

Calandra and Oginsky (1975) submitted various SLS preparations to Sephadex G-100 chromatography and estimated the molecular weight of RNA-core SLS as 18,500. In contrast they found that SLS hemolysins from sonication supernatant and 'cellular potential hemolysin' eluted in the void volume indicating molecular weights greater than 200,000.

A purification of RNA-core SLS was reported by Hryniewicz et al. (1977) with a specific activity of about 0.07 μg protein per hemolytic unit (HU). This preparation was shown to have an apparent weight of 20,000 daltons in the presence of 6 M urea and 40,000 in the absence of this agent indicating aggregation of the toxin molecule.

It appears that the major problems encountered by the above-mentioned investigators is the instability of the toxin through the prolonged manipulation steps. These difficulties were recently overcome by Lai et al. (1978) who reported improved purification and characterization of RNA-core SLS with a specific activity (1.2×10^7/HU mg protein) at least 6 times greater than that reported before (Koyama and Egami, 1963; Bernheimer, 1972). The purification process was rapid and involved four steps consisting of gel-filtration on Sephadex G-75, DEAE-cellulose, chromatography and two gel-filtrations on Sephadex G-75 in the presence of 6M guanidine hydrochloride. The use of ammonium acetate in potassium buffer throughout purification procedure proved instrumental for toxin stability.

3.5. Molecular Properties of Streptolysin S

The SLS preparation obtained by Lai et al. (1978) confirmed previous findings that the active hemolysin in a complex consisting of a polypeptide moiety associated to an oligonucleotide. Both moieties were found in a dimeric form in the toxin. The apparent molecular weight of SLS and carrier oligonucleotide were estimated at 15,000 and 7,100 respectively. The oligonucleotide is a 10-nucleotide moiety (m.w. about 3500) having the composition A:U:G:C = 10:13.2:35:5.6. In agreement with the finding of Koyama and Egami (1963) the guanosine content is unusually high.

The peptide which constitutes the specific active principle of SLS was shown to contain 32 amino acids in agreement with the size (28 residues) proposed by Bernheimer (1972) based on Koyama's data and molecular weight determination. Its amino-acid composition was peculiar as compared to usual proteins including many bacterial protein cytolysins since six amino acids were lacking: histidine, arginine, cysteine, valine, methionine and isoleucine.

As noted by Bernheimer and Avigad (1979) the amino acid composition of SLS is somewhat similar to mellitin, the cytolytic polypeptide of bee venom which lacks six of the usual amino acids (Yunes et al., 1977), to staphylococcal delta toxin which lacks five (Kantor et al., 1972) and to pleurotolysine, a cytolytic protein from the edible mushroom Pleurotus ostreatus which lacks seven (Bernheimer and Avigad, 1979). The latter cytolysin has a molecular weight of 12,050 and apparently gives rise to dimers as found for SLS. The polypeptide moiety of SLS exhibited a high content of glycine and proline (Lai et al., 1978) suggestive of a collagen-type structure. The peptide nature of the active principle of SLS was confirmed by studies of the effects of various hydrolytic enzymes on the toxin. Only endoproteinases (pronase, chymotrypsin and subtilisin) were found to inactivate the hemolysin. The exoproteinases were inactive. These results indicated that neither the NH_2- nor the COOH- terminal residue in the active moiety was accessible to these proteinases.

Koyama (1963) and Hryniewicz (see Jeljaszewicz et al., 1978) demonstrated resistance of SLS to numerous ribonucleases as also shown by Lai et al. (1978). These results may be explained by possible masking of the carrier molecule when attached to the active polypeptide thus making SLS unsensitive to these enzymes. Finally a remarkable property of the toxin is its stability in 6M-guanidinine hydrochloride for several hours in the cold.

3.6. BIOLOGICAL PROPERTIES OF STREPTOLYSIN S

SLS appears as a very potent membrane-damaging agent. It lyses a wide variety of living cells. Its lytic spectrum is somewhat broader than SLO, it is lytic or cytotoxic not only for eukaryotic cells but also for wall-less forms of some bacteria notably protoplasts and L-forms from various species (see Bernheimer, 1972). All eukaryotic cells tested were found damaged: erythrocytes, lymphocytes, polymorphonuclear leucocytes, platelets, various tissue culture cells and tumor cells. Intracellular organelles such as mitochondria and lysosomes are also disrupted by SLS (see for references: Ginsburg 1970, 1972; Bernheimer, 1972; Freer and Arbuthnott, 1976; Okamoto, 1976; Okamoto et al., 1978; Jeljaszewicz et al., 1978).

3.6.1. Hemolytic Effects of Streptolysin S

The highest specific activities reported for SLS are 2×10^6 HU/mg (Koyama and Egami, 1963) and 1.2×10^7 HU/mg (Lai et al., 1978). Thus by weight SLS is one of the most potent bacterial hemolysins.

The kinetics of SLS-induced hemolysis has been studied by several investigators (Bernheimer, 1948; Cinader and Pillemer, 1950; Koyama, 1965; Duncan and Mason, 1976; Hryniewicz et al., 1977). Early work investigated several features of the kinetic process: prolonged lag period, heat of activation of about 17,900 cal/mole, sigmoidal time dilution curves, hemolysin rate as a function of toxin and erythrocyte concentration, etc.

Elias et al. (1966) and Bernheimer (1972) demonstrated that the hemolytic activity of SLS was inhibited by relatively low concentrations of several phospholipids including phosphatidyl choline, phosphatidyl ethanolamine and phosphatidic acid. The latter was the most potent inhibitor. It was also found by Elias et al. that SLS became irreversibly bound to erythrocytes and to red cell ghosts, and that pretreatment of the latter with phospholipase C reduced the amount of streptolysin S that became bound. On the basis of these results it seems likely that the phospholipids of cell membranes are the constituents specifically involved in the biological action of streptolysin S.

This conclusion is also suggested by the finding that liposomes composed of phosphatidylcholine, together with small amounts of cholesterol and dicetyl phosphate were disrupted by SLS (Bangham et al., 1965). Similar liposomes lacking cholesterol were also destroyed. It is to be noted that SLS has no known enzymatic activity including phospholipase activity.

Aniline dyes are strongly inhibitory. Trypan blue in a concentration of 13 µg/ml abolished the action of SLS (Ginsburg, 1970). The mechanism of this phenomenon is not known.

Several lines of evidence suggest that SLS produces more subtle changes than SLO at the membrane surface of target erythrocytes. Electron-microscope studies unlike SLO do not show structure changes on red blood cells (Dourmashkin and Rosse, 1966). Studies of marker release from human diploid fibroblasts (see Thelestam and Möllby, 1979) challenged with SLS caused the egress of α-isoaminobutyric acid which is a low molecular weight molecule whereas nucleotides were not liberated. This may indicate that SLS creates small functional 'holes' in contrast to SLO and other cytolytic agents. According to Bernheimer (1972) SLS probably brings about a relatively subtle alteration in the organization of the lipid and/or protein molecules comprising the membrane, an alteration which abolishes selective permeability, thereby permitting free passage of ions. The retained hemoglobin exerts osmotic pressure which draws water into the cell causing increased cell volume and rupture of the membrane. Thus lysis by SLS involves an osmotic mechanism and is similar in this respect to several other hemolytic systems as those involving staphylococcal α-toxin or *Clostridium septicum* hemolysin. That SLS-induced lysis is a colloid-osmotic process is well documented by the recent studies of Duncan and Mason (1976) on rabbit erythrocytes and Hryniewicz et al. (1977) on human erythrocytes as shown by the release of ^{86}Rb prior to the escape of hemoglobin from the cells.

As noted by Bernheimer SLS possesses certain features common to two other lysins of bacterial origin: surfactin which is responsible for the zone of hemolysis around colonies of *Bacillus subtilis*, and staphylococcal δ-toxin. Surfactin is a heptapeptide linked to a derivative of tetradecanoic acid while staphylococcal δ-toxin is either a polypeptide or a small protein, or an aggregate of small proteins (Kantor et al., 1972). Surfactin and probably also δ-toxin, tends to undergo self-aggregation and there are suggestions that the latter may bind to carrier proteins. The active moiety of all three agents is or contains an oligopeptide or polypeptide. None of them gives rise to neutralizing antibody; in fact, they appear not to be immunogenic at all. All three, in contrast to certain other hemolysins, will lyse several kinds of bacterial protoplasts. The hemolytic action of each is inhibited by phosphatides. In terms of specific lytic activity, however, SLS is very powerful while surfactin and δ-toxin are comparatively feeble and it may be that the mechanisms of lysis are quite different.

3.6.2. *Effects on Cells Involved in the Immune Response*

Recent studies by Hryniewicz and Pryjma (1977, 1978) have shown that lymphoid cells concerned in immune reactions were susceptible to various degrees to SLS. Lymphocytes appeared to be the most sensitive to the cytotoxic action of SLS as measured by ^{51}Cr release assay and Trypan blue exclusion test. Of particular interest was the finding that T lymphocytes (human, mice) were much more affected than B lymphocytes.

Mouse bone marrow cells were much more resistant than cells obtained from the thymus. The number of human lymphocytes forming nonimmune rosettes with sheep red blood cells (SRBC) was substantially reduced after treatment of lymphocytes with SLS, and a lower concentration was required than that needed to obtain comparable loss of viability.

The preferential killing of human T lymphocytes was shown by comparing the viability after treatment with SLS of cells fractionated into populations possessing or not possessing C3 receptors (which are characteristic for most B cells but only very occasionally for T cells). The susceptibility of T cells to the cytotoxic action of SLS does not appear to be a result of greater binding of this toxin to the surface of T cells since the preincubation of mouse bone marrow cells or thymocytes with SLS resulted in a greater loss of hemolytic activity in the case of bone marrow cells. Hirsch et al. (1963) suggested that the cytotoxic effect of SLS towards leukocytes may be due to autolysis after labilization of lysosomal membranes. A possibility also exists that the observed differences are related to the surface composition of both lymphocyte populations or to reported differences in enzymatic activity. It was also shown by Hryniewicz and Pryjma (1978) that human T-lymphocyte reactivity *in vitro* measured by thymidine incorporation and migration-inhibition factor production on stimulation with phytohemagglutinin were effectively blocked by pre-treatment with SLS as well as ability to form non-immune rosettes with sheep red blood cells (SRBC). The T cell-dependent and T cell-independent antibody response and the contact-sensitivity reaction were chosen for testing the action of SLS on T and B lymphocytes *in vivo*. *In vivo* treatment with SLS suppressed the T-dependent but not the T-independent response, suggesting that the function of B cells is not altered by SLS. The helper T-cells concerned in cooperation with B lymphocytes seem to be most likely target for SLS action *in vivo*, since the function of the memory T-cells and the T cells concerned in contact sensitivity were not affected. The secondary response of animals treated with SLS at the time of priming was not suppressed. However, when SLS was administered at the time of boost the secondary IgG response was diminished. The induction of contact sensitivity to oxazolone was not changed by SLS treatment. The possible impairment of macrophage function by SLS in T-cell dependent antibody response was also investigated. Thioglycollate-induced mouse-peritoneal-exudate cells were incubated with ^{51}Cr-labelled SRBC and subsequently incubated for 0.5 hr with SLS (final concentration of toxin 500 HU/ml). This was followed by transfer into syngeneic recipients. The plaque-forming cell response measured 4 days after transfer was not changed by pre-treatment with SLS, which strongly suggests that impairment of macrophage function is not responsible for decreased anti-SRBC response in SLS-treated animals. The data suggest that SLS can selectively suppress the function of the T cells concerned in cooperation with B cells, namely the helper T-cells.

3.6.3. Effects on Polymorphonuclear Leucocytes

The studies reported on SLS effects on leucocytes have been reviewed by Jeljaszewicz *et al.* (1978) Bernheimer and Schwartz (1960) and Hirsch *et al.* (1963) showed that SLS was cytotoxic and caused degranulation of intracellular organelles and changes in the cytoplasm. Ofek *et al.* (1972) reported that cell-bound hemolysin killed mouse peritoneal macrophages within 30 min whereas RNA-SLS or serum-SLS required 60–180 min for complete killing. Addition of 10% mouse or rabbit serum to RNA-SLS or cell-bound hemolysin delayed its cytotoxic action. This result illustrates the important role played by the carrier molecule. It has been shown (see Ginsburg, 1972) that the hemolytic moiety can be transferred from one carrier molecule into another depending on affinity of this moiety to the carrier and its concentration. Lower concentrations of SLS which killed only 5% of the macrophages produced a 50% inhibition of phagocytosis.

3.6.4. Effects on Other Cells

In addition to red and white blood cells, many other cells were shown to undergo lysis after exposure to SLS. This is the case for platelets (Bernheimer and Schwartz, 1965), Ehrlich ascites tumor cells (Ginsburg and Grossowicz, 1960), heart cells of the rabbit and rat, renal cells, McCoy, HeLa and KB cells (see Ginsburg, 1972).

3.6.5. Effects on Subcellular Organelles

SLS disrupts membrane-bound organelles such as lysosomes, nuclei and mitochondria (Weissmann *et al.*, 1963, 1964; Keiser *et al.*, 1964). This damage to membrane probably initiates secondary metabolic changes in cells which in turn result in cell death. An interesting study of RNA-SLS was reported on mouse liver mitochondria (Symington and Arbuthnott, 1972). Toxin preparation impaired the succinic- and cytochrome-oxidase activity of these organelles. The presence of cytochrome C prevented impairment and reversed the observable effects of the toxin on them. That SLS causes dislocation of the electron-transport between cytochrome C and oxygen may be of importance in the mechanism of pathogenicity of group A streptococci.

3.6.6. Antitumor Activity of Streptolysin S-Forming Streptococci

Living SLS-forming streptococci have been shown to have antitumor activity which has been reviewed by Okamoto (1976), and Okamoto *et al.* (1978). This activity was observed on a variety of animal tumors including carcinoma, sarcoma, hepatoma, fibrosarcoma and lymphatic leukemia. The antitumor properties appear to be due to two different effects, namely a direct cytotoxic effect on tumor cells and a host-mediated antitumor effect with probable involvement of immune response and reticuloendothelial system stimulating factor.

3.6.7. *Possible Pathogenic Effects of Streptolysin S*

According to Ginsburg (1972) the significance of SLS production by groups A, C and G streptococci in the pathogenesis of streptococcal disease and its sequelae is still not understood. Several experimental tissue lesions in animals have been shown to be elicited by various SLS preparations. In fact, it is still not known whether SLS is produced *in vivo*. As this toxin is not immunogenic the answer to this question remains difficult. As suggested by Jeljaszewicz *et al.* (1978), SLS may exert its cytolytic and lysosome-damaging activity especially at the site of a localized streptococcal lesion. Lack of antigenicity may enable its free circulation and thus disturbance of cells even in remote organs, especially since this toxin can occur in so many forms, such as cell-bound and intracellular precursor hemolysins, and also because of the ease with which the non specific carrier molecule can change.

4. ERYTHROGENIC TOXIN

4.1. DEFINITION

Erythrogenic toxin (ET) is a toxic, immunogenic, low-molecular weight single-chain protein released in the extracellular medium by group A streptococci. Three serologically distinct toxin types A, B, C have been identified and characterized biochemically and biologically. These toxins exhibit a multiplicity of biological properties and are pyrogenic in rabbits.

The terms 'streptococcal pyrogenic exotoxin' (SPE) has been proposed by Kim and Watson (1970) as more significant than erythrogenic toxin. According to these authors the skin rash appears to be the result of a secondary toxicity and probably is the least significant property of the toxins. Other synonyms in the literature are Dick toxin, scarlet fever toxin and streptococcal exotoxin. The terms ET or SPE will be used here depending on the works quoted.

4.2. HISTORICAL BACKGROUND

In 1924 G. F. and G. H. Dick reported that exotoxin called erythrogenic toxin responsible for the symptoms of scarlet fever in man was elaborated in broth cultures by hemolytic streptococci of scarlatinal origin. However it was established further that most Lancefield group A streptococci produce the toxin and not only the so-called scarlet fever strains.

Ten years later, Hooker and Follensby (1934) presented good evidence that more than one immunologically distinct toxin existed and described two types A and B. These investigators believed that a single toxinogenic strain could produce A or B or both and possibly a third type. This prediction was confirmed by Watson (1960) who reported the characterization of three types A, B and C. These types have been isolated and purified to homogeneity as discussed in another section. Comprehensive reviews and papers on erythrogenic toxins (SPE) have been published in the few past years (Watson and Kim, 1970; Kim and Watson, 1972; Jeljaszewicz *et al.*, 1978). Therefore this presentation will rather summarize the main properties of ET and will deal with the findings recently published.

4.2.1. *The Dick Reaction*

The detection of ET by the Dicks was based on the intradermal injection of culture filtrates (0.1 ml of a 1/1000 dilution) into certain healthy persons. Erythematous and edmatous skin reactions developed in the susceptible persons by 24 hr after injection and it was concluded that the resulting reactions was a local 'model' for the skin rash of scarlet fever. This so called positive Dick reaction has been widely held to be the manifestation of the primary toxicity of the erythrogenic toxin. The injection of larger doses induced a generalized reaction with fever, nausea, vomiting and a transient scarlatiniform rash (so-called miniature scarlet fever). Antitoxin neutralized the skin reactions. Persons with sufficient circulating antitoxin did not develop positive skin response (negative Dick reaction) and they were therefore not considered susceptible to scarlet fever. Antitoxin injected into the rash may neutralize the toxin within the skin and cause a local blanching of the rash (Schultz-Charlton test). An analogy was drawn with the Schick test for susceptibility to diphtheria toxin and the steady rise in the percentage of negatives during childhood was taken as evidence of the acquisition of active antitoxic immunity either by passing through an attack of scarlet fever or by having an inapparent infection.

A positive Dick reaction occurs most often in children and considerably less often in infants; it becomes progressively less common during adolescence and early adult life. Skin reactivity in laboratory animals is variable; young rabbits and guinea-pigs are usually insusceptible but become reactive after the injection of a small dose of toxin (see Boroff, 1951; Watson and Kim, 1970; Schlievert et al., 1979a).

As early as 1927 the view that the erythematous rash resulted from a direct (primary) toxic effect was challenged by Cook and Dochez and Stevens and by many workers later (see Schlievert et al., 1979a for references). These investigators emphasized the importance of delayed hypersensitivity (second toxicity) in the skin lesions. As stated by Schlievert et al. (1979a) the importance of age in developing scarlet fever is consistent with the delayed-hypersensitivity concept. Scarlet fever is not observed in infants and becomes more prevalent only after repeated streptococcal infections. Rantz et al. (1946) after testing a large number of men of military age, determined that positive Dick tests were infrequent in men from geographical areas with low incidences of streptococcal infections. These investigators concluded that the Dick reaction probably resulted from previous exposure, and therefore was the result of acquired hypersensitivity.

The work of Boroff (1951) and Kim and Watson (1970, 1972) also implicated delayed hypersensitivity in development of skin reactivity.

On the other hand, it was shown by Schwab et al. (1955) that group A streptococci grown in the skin of rabbits produce extracellular toxic products which were not highly lethal but could modify the host so that the tissues including the heart became vulnerable to damage by endotoxin and SLO. As described by Watson and Kim (1970) further investigation revealed that the toxic products were found associated to ETs, they were pyrogenic and exhibited three distinct immunologic types. These toxins were called pyrogenic exotoxins and their relationship to the erythrogenic toxins established.

In the light of all these findings a reinterpretation of the Dick test was recently published by Schlievert et al. (1979a). These investigators emphasized the fact that the primary toxicity alone as proposed by the Dicks is not responsible for rash development. SPEs failed to produce skin test reactions upon primary injection into non sensitized rabbits. As many investigators have equated SPEs with ETs the relationship of those two entities were reevaluated. According to Schlievert et al. ET may be defined more clearly as SPE enhancement of acquired hypersensitivity reactions to streptococcal products and the Dick test is a measure of SPE-enhanced hypersensitivity to streptococcal products. Since the enhancement of skin reactivity by SPE depends upon acquired hypersensitivity developed by the host to a streptococcal product, erythrogenic toxin should not be equated with SPE. Furthermore, erythrogenic toxin cannot be clearly defined unless the product to which the host was presensitized is known. In light of this, the use of SPE as a single toxic entity is preferred.

The biological effects of ET (or SPE) toxins on the host have been studied in detail during the past twenty years. These effects are numerous including pyrogenicity, enhancement of susceptibility to endotoxin shock, alteration of reticuloendothelial function and the blood – brain barrier, mitogenicity, immunosuppression and immunoenhancement.

4.3. PHAGE-DIRECTED SYNTHESIS OF ERYTHROGENIC TOXIN

It has been shown by Frobisher and Brown in 1927 and by Bingel in 1949 (cited by Zabriskie, 1964) that culture filtrates of scarlatinal strains of hemolytic streptococci could induce the formation of ET by non toxinogenic strains. In 1964, Zabriskie reported the conversion of a group A non-lysogenic, non toxinogenic strain (T25$_3$) to a toxin producer by infecting it with a phage (ϕ T 12) derived from a toxinogenic strain. A second serologically related phage was noted to convert strain T25$_3$ also. A virulent serologically unrelated phage had no effect on amounts of toxin produced by any of the strains studied. It was not known whether cured non lysogenic revertants of the converted strains became non toxinogenic.

The findings reported by Zabriskie were considered as evidence of true lysogenic conversion. In retrospect to Frobisher and Brown results were characteristic of a pseudo-lysogenic state as discussed by Barksdale and Arden (1974). The following comment was made by these investigators concerning 'lysogenic conversion for ET toxin': The simplest way to examine or screen for the expression of a particular phage gene is not by going through the elaborate routine of producing a lysogenic strain. What one wants to know is whether or not ϕ T12 carries information required for the synthesis of erythrogenic toxin. It should be a simple matter to obtain a virulent mutant of ϕ T12 (supposedly carrying the gene for the synthesis of erythrogenic toxin) and to examine the synthesis of erythrogenic toxin in one cycle of virus growth in the non scarlatinal strain of streptococcus T25$_3$. The results of such an experiment should lead to an unambiguous answer as to the role of ϕ T12 in the synthesis of erythrogenic toxin.

New investigations on phage-related toxinogenesis were reported recently by Nida et al. (1978) and Nida (personal communication). These authors devised an enzyme-linked immunosorbent assay as a method of detecting the toxin that is sensitive, specific and easily performed for the study of the genetic control of toxin synthesis and release. It is to be noted that Zabriskie used the rabbit skin test to demonstrate the presence or absence of ET. The results found by Nida and co-workers were as follows: Toxin production characteristics were determined for nine standard laboratory of S. pyogenes and 22 strains isolated from unrelated cases of scarlet fever. All 31 strains were found to be lysogenic, each phage lysate having a unique host-range. Twenty-four new lysogens were constructed and monitored for stability. They were stable for three months but by the end of the fourth month 75% of the clones had lost their phages. Eighteen of these cultures were tested and shown to have undergone toxinogenic conversion. Loss of the phage was accompanied by loss of toxin production. The phages were extremely delicate. Several phages were studied by electron microscopy and classified in the B1 morphological classification. Rabbit anti-ϕ T12 antiserum was produced which proved to be non-reactive with any of the other nine converting phages identified. DNA was isolated from four of the phages. The streptococcophage DNA and the lambda phage DNA standard migrated identically in agarose vertical slab gel electrophoresis. Restriction enzymes were not active in this system and absolute proof of the identity of the DNA samples was not accomplished. Analysis of the toxin production profiles revealed that the toxin types produced by the constructed lysogens were determined by the phage introduced. One of the conversion-pairs was shown to be a pseudolysogen. Evidence for the carrier state included non-inducibility and cratered and 'nibbled' colonies.

Toxigenic conversion of S. pyogenes by phages isolated from toxin-producing strains was shown to be a general case, accomplished by ten phages in five host recipients. The phages are related morphologically and are probably related by similar genome-size. They are all similarly delicate. Lack of identical host-range indicates each is unique. Lack of serological cross reaction of the other nine phages with anti-ϕT12-specific antibody indicates dissimilar coat-proteins. Toxin types produced by converted cultures are determined by the phage introduced. The question of disagreement between early publications

TABLE 9. *Production of Erythrogenic Toxins by Various* S. pyogenes *Group A Strains*

Antigen from strain number	Serotype of strain	Toxin detected*			Toxins reported in the literature
		A	B	C	
NY5 Dochez (ATCC 12351)	M12,T10	+	−	−	A,B,C
594	Not typable	+	−	−	A
T19 (089704; FU-7)	M19	−	+	−	B
T18 (T18P)	M18	−	−	+	C
C203U	M3,T1	+	+	+	C,D
64 × 402 (NCTC8301)	M23	−	+	−	...
402/C2034†	M23	−	+	+	...

Colon-Whitt *et al.* (1978)

*Double-diffusion test in agar: antigen = ammonium-sulphate precipitate of culture supernate; antiserum monospecific for toxin A, B or C; + = antigen detected, − = not detected.

†Strain 64 × 402 lysogenised by phage from strain C203U.

and the Zabriskie report was resolved. Conversion demonstrated by L. McKane* using his ϕT12^{vir} mutant and conversions characterized in the present research demonstrated that toxinogenic conversions of *S. pyogenes* follows the models of β phage and *C. diphtheriae* and of P22 and *S. typhimurium*; the converting gene is expressed by the prophage, the vegetative phage, and the virulent mutant phage. The location of the structural gene(s) for streptococcal exotoxins cannot be determined yet.

Recently, Colon-Whitt *et al.* (1978) reported that erythrogenic toxin B produced by strain 64 × 402 was not dependent on lysogeny but that toxin C in strain C 203 U may well be so dependent.

4.4. TOXIN PRODUCTION AND PURIFICATION

As shown in Table 9, toxins A, B and C may be produced simultaneously or separately depending on strains and very likely culture conditions as this could be for the NY-5 strain which has been the most widely used for toxin production and studies.

Attempts between 1930 and 1960 at purification of ET have been summarized by Watson and Kim (1970) and Kim and Watson (1972). Hartley, Pulvertaft and Veldee were able to precipitate and concentrate toxin by alcohol or tannic acid. The greatest progress during the fifties was made by Stock and co-workers who obtained a preparation containing 1.5×10^8 skin test doses (STD) per milligram. The molecular weight was 27,000. Hottle and Pappenheimer also isolated a purified protein toxin. Their preparations gave strong tests for protein. Like others, they found the preparations to be resistant to the proteolytic enzymes, pepsin, trypsin and papain. The floculation reaction as measured quantitatively was found to be specific for scarlet fever toxin and antitoxin. This material contained 1.3×10^8 skin test doses per milligram of nitrogen.

Stock and Lynn prepared concentrated type B toxin and found it to be protein in nature, precipitable by trichloroacetic acid. In contrast to toxin A, it was inactivated by trypsin confirming the observations of Hooker and Follensby (1934). A and B toxins were immunologically distinct as determined by floculation reactions with anti-A antitoxin and in agar gel diffusion methods. Mitrica *et al.* (1965) described a method for the crystallization of the toxin. Toxin recrystallized four times was electrophoretically homogeneous and contained 15.6% nitrogen. The activity was 1.04×10^9 STD/mg N as tested in New Zealand and chinchilla rabbits.

Type A toxin was purified to apparent homogeneity by Nauciel *et al.* (1968, 1969) from strain 594 by gel filtration and ion-exchange chromatography. The toxin had a molecular

*(according to a personal communication from K. Nida)

TABLE 10. *Physicochemical Characteristics of Streptococcal Erythrogenic (Pyrogenic) Exotoxins A, B, C*

	Toxin		
	A	B	C
Molecular weight	8000	17500	13200
Isoelectric point (s)	5.0	8.0	6.7
		8.4	
		9.0	

References: Schlievert *et al.* (1977), Barsumian *et al.* (1978a)

weight of 30,500 and amino acid composition was given. Two molecular forms were found attributed to binding of small molecules of different charges through a -SH group. Exposure to reducing agents induced conversion to a single form. Kim and Watson (1970) isolated type A toxin from the NY-5 strain by a series of ethanol precipitations. The material obtained had a molecular weight of about 29,000. It contained 80% protein and 20% hyaluronic acid. This material was however heterogeneous and consisted of different proteins as reported later by Cunningham *et al.* (1976). These investigators described the isolation of homogeneous type A toxin from the above-mentioned material by ion-exchange chromatography. More recently, type B toxin was isolated by Barsumian *et al.* (1978a) and type C by Schlievert *et al.* (1977) (Table 10). Type A toxin consisted of protein and 4 to 8% of hyaluronic acid. The molecular weight was 8,000 with a pI of 5.0. A microheterogeneity was found. It was later reported (Schlievert *et al.*, 1977; Barsumian *et al.*, 1978a) the obtention by isoelectric focusing of highly active homogeneous preparations free of hyaluronic acid. There was no evidence that hyaluronic acid contributed to the toxic activity, but toxins were more stable in the presence of it.

The discrepancy between the low molecular weight of toxin A found by these investigators and the higher values ($\simeq$ 30,000) reported previously (Kim and Watson, 1970; Nauciel *et al.*, 1968) remains unexplained. It is likely that the high molecular weight toxins are due to aggregation or association to other protein or non protein (hyaluronic acid) moieties.

Toxin B was found to be heterogeneous in charge. Three preparations, serologically identical as determined by immunodiffusion, had pIs of 8.0, 8.4 and 9.0. The molecular weight of each was 17,000. Only pI 8.4 toxin B was pyrogenic and unlike the others, enhanced the susceptibility of rabbits to lethal endotoxin shock. The inactive B fractions may be natural toxoids of the active pI 8.4 toxin. Amino-acid compositions of the three B toxins are similar. Like A and C toxin, they have no cysteine and only traces of methionine. All toxins are high in dicarboxylic acids and low in the aromatic amino-acids tyrosine and tryptophan.

Purified C toxin was homogeneous in immunodiffusion analysis and migrated as a single protein band (pI 6.7) in isoelectric focusing polyacrylamide gels and in sodium dodecylsulfate-polyacrylamide gels (molecular weight 13,000). C toxin was antigenically distinct from A and B toxins. Its amino-acid composition, like that of A and B toxins, was high in dicarboxylic acids, but it contained no lysine, arginine, histidine, tyrosine, tryptophan, cysteine, or methionine. N-terminal amino-acid analysis showed serine to be the terminal residue.

It was recently shown that type C toxin is a naturally phosphorylated protein (Schlievert *et al.* 1979b); It was established that adenosine monophosphate may function as a cofactor of type C toxin and contribute to the phosphate group required for biological activity. The toxin altered the permeability of the blood-brain barrier to endotoxin, several bacteria, as well as to itself. It did not alter the *in vivo* differential and total counts of peripheral blood leukocytes and did not elicit endogenous pyrogen release from leukocytes *in vitro*. *In vivo* peripheral blood platelet counts remained unchanged after toxin treatment. Cycloheximide pretreatment of rabbits did not inhibit fever production by type C toxin. In contrast to the hypothermia observed in mice treated with endotoxin intravenously, toxin C given intravenously to mice produced dose-dependent fever and enhanced susceptibility to lethal endotoxin shock. The abilities of the toxin to produce fever and enhance lethal shock were shown to be separate functions of the molecule; fever results from stimulation of the hypothalamus and enhancement appears not to involve the central nervous system.

Schlievert and Watson (1979) have shown that toxin-induced fever depended upon norepinephrine and stimulation of α-adrenergic receptors. Intracisternal injection of norepinephrine into rabbits already showing fevers due to the toxin resulted in further heightened fevers. Pretreatment of animals with either α-methyl tyrosine to deplete norepinephrine stores or phenoxybenzamine to block α-receptors depressed toxin-induced pyrogenicity. Pretreatment of animals with p-chlorophenylalanine to deplete serotonin stores accentuated fevers due to toxin and giving serotonin intracisternally to rabbits with fevers resulted in a significant drop in body temperature. This indicated serotonin exerted a negative effect on pyrogenicity. Isoproterenol and propranolol did not affect toxin C fever production.

4.5. Biological Properties of Erythrogenic (Streptococcal Pyrogenic) Exotoxins

A multiplicity of remarkable biological properties are associated to erythrogenic toxins (Table 11). Earlier work on these properties has been reviewed by Kim and Watson (1972) and Ginsburg (1972). New results have been reported during the past eight years and will be summarized here.

4.5.1. Pyrogenic Effects

Induction of fever in rabbits is a prominent and constant property of ET. The minimal pyrogenic dose at 3 hr of the purified preparation of Watson and Kim (1970) was 0.07 μg/kg by the i.v. route. Recent studies on toxin pyrogenicity was reported by Brunson and Watson (1974) and Schlievert and Watson (1978). The pyrogenic effect was neutralized by antitoxin when incubated with toxin *in vitro* before injection. Specificity of acquired pyrogenic immunity to each of toxins A, B or C was demonstrated by pyrogenic immunity cross-tests. The three types of ET were shown to induce Limulus amebocyte lysate gelation. This effect is much less pronounced when compared with the endotoxins of gram-negative bacteria, since as much as 100 μg of erythrogenic toxin is needed for a positive reaction (Brunson and Watson, 1974).

Schlievert and Watson (1978) reported that type C toxin produce fever by crossing the blood-brain barrier. The toxin directly stimulated the hypothalamic fever response con-

TABLE 11. *Biological Properties of Streptococcal Erythrogenic*
(Pyrogenic) exotoxins A, B, C

1.	Pyrogenicity.
2.	Skin reactivity (erythrogenic effect): erythema in humans and sensitized animals.
3.	Lethality (rabbit).
4.	Cytotoxicity and tissue (cardiac) damage.
5.	Enhanced susceptibility to endotoxin shock.
6.	Depression of reticuloendothelial functions
7.	Alterations of host antibody response to immunogens in rabbits and mice.
8.	Mitogenic activity on human and rabbit lymphocytes.

Watson and Kim (1970); Kim and Watson (1972); Cunningham and Watson (1978 a, b); Schlievert and Watson (1978); Barsumian *et al.* (1978, a, b); Schlievert *et al.* (1979, a, b, c); Cavaillon *et al.* (1979); Gray (1979).

trol center, thus bypassing a requirement for endogenous pyrogen release. It was detected in the cerebrospinal fluids of toxin-treated rabbits by drugs prevented the capacity of the toxin to enhance lethal endotoxin shock. However, phenoxybenzamine in combination with fluid replacement increased the survival rate of rabbits. It is proposed that toxin C may alter the endotoxin detoxification system, thus allowing endotoxin to persist in the circulation producing shock.

Hřibalová *et al.* (1979) investigated the role played by lymphocytes in the pyrogenic response to ET. Antilymphocyte serum inhibited the response to a subsequent i.v. injection of ET in rabbits. In contrast, the course of endotoxin fever remained uninfluenced by antilymphocyte serum. Pretreatment with this serum also inhibited the skin reaction after i.d. injection of ET. These findings are consistent with a mediating role of lymphocytes in the biological effects of ET. It is suggested by these investigators that ET elicits the release of endogenous pyrogen in contrast to the results reported by Schlievert and Watson (1978).

4.5.2. Enhancement of Lethal Endotoxin Shock

ET dramatically enhances the susceptibility of rabbits and other animals to endotoxin shock (see Watson and Kim, 1970). Application of this toxin to rabbits, mice and cynomolgus monkeys three hours before introduction of *Salmonella typhi* endotoxin largely increased susceptibility of these animals to endotoxin shock. For instance, monkeys not suceptible to doses of 2000 μg of ET and 8000 μg of endotoxin introduced separately, were killed by a dose of 500 μg of ET, followed by application of 2000 μg of endotoxin.

The most striking effects were observed in rabbits (Kim and Watson, 1972). Four different levels of the exotoxins (0.1, 1, 5 and 10 μg/ml) were injected intravenously, and 3 hr later, the rabbits were tested with endotoxins at four levels (0.1, 1, 5, and 10 μg/ml) given intravenously. Deaths were recorded over a 48 hour period. By graphic determination it was possible to estimate that the enhancement effect for endotoxin and exotoxin are greater than 100,000 and 1,000,000-fold respectively.

In a recent study of this effect, Schlievert and Watson (1978) suggest that the ability to enhance shock may result from alteration of a cell type in the liver because reticuloendothelial function is altered after treatment with ET.

4.5.3. Depression of Reticuloendothelial System (RES)

This effect of ET was reported by Hanna and Watson in 1965 who observed a depressed rate blood clearance of colloidal carbon in rabbits for 24 hr following treatment with ET type C. Recently, Cunningham and Watson (1978a) demonstrated the alteration of RES function elicited by type A as shown by studying the clearance of the particulate antigen, sheep red blood cells (SRBC) in syngeneic mice. The vascular clearance of ^{51}Cr-labeled SRBC was decreased and observed for doses ranging from 1 to 10 μg of toxin over a period of 3–24 hr. The depression was not due to a direct effect on macrophages.

Hribalova (1979) observed that i.v. injection of ET (30,000 STD per kg of rabbit or 20-g mouse) elicited biphasic change in carbon clearance rate—early depression followed by a stimulating phase—as has been described for Gram-negative endotoxins. Prolonged depression without a subsequent stimulation phase was obtained in mice by raising the ET dose. Pyrogenic tolerance to ET is not accompanied by accelerated carbon clearance and is not impaired by RES blockade. The possible mechanisms of this effect and tolerance to ET were discussed.

4.5.4. Immunosuppressive Effect on Antibody Response

A number of studies were conducted in the past fifteen years by Hanna and Watson on ET effects upon the antibody response (see ref. in Cunningham and Watson, 1978b). It was found that the toxin causes an early suppression (day 4–5) and late enhancement (day 10–15) of the antibody response to SRBC in rabbits, mice or cultures of mouse spleen cells. It was suggested that this two-phase effect may be associated with inhibition of phagocytosis. In such conditions, processing of antigen by macrophages may be slowed down or the phenomenon may be caused by differential susceptibility and rate of recovery of antibody producing B cells and T suppressor cells. The problem was further investigated by Hanna and Hale (1975) who speculated that erythrogenic toxin would either preferentially inactivate or inhibit the suppressor T cells allowing for unregulated expression of B cells.

Recently, Cunningham and Watson (1978b) reported the effect of the three types of ET on the antibody response to sheep erythrocytes in cultures of mouse spleen cells. Purified toxins types A, B and C shared the ability to suppress the day 4 direct plaque-forming cell response when added to cultures. Toxins A and C were most suppressive at concentrations of 0.1 to 1 ng per culture, while toxin B was active at 1 μg per culture. Pretreatment of mice with toxin A, 3 hr before removal of their spleens culture, also produced suppression. Cell populations were separated from spleens of normal and toxin-treated mice and recombined in culture to test the cellular site of action of toxin-mediated immunosuppression. When nonadherent cells (lymphocytes) and adherent cells (macrophages) from control and toxin-treated mice were separated and recombined, the plaque-forming cell response depended on the source of lymphocytes. Macrophages from toxin treated-mice functioned normally in the presence of control lymphocytes. In further experiments, toxin pretreatment failed to suppress the plaque-forming cell response of spleen cells that were T-cell depleted and reconstituted with control thymocytes. When the T-lymphocytes were removed from toxin-treated spleen cell suspensions, the remaining cells were able to respond normally to antigen if normal helper T-cells were provided. The results suggest that the suppressive activity of ET on antibody production is mediated by altered activity of T lymphocytes.

4.5.5. Mitogenic Properties

Supernatant fluids derived from the culture of a great number of growing group A *Streptococcus pyogenes* strains have been shown to induce non specific blast transformation *in vitro* of peripheral blood lymphocytes of man and rabbit. A similar mitogenic effect has also been reported for crude or partially purified extracellular materials such as streptolysin O (SLO), Varidase, a product containing streptokinase and deoxyribonuclease and streptolysin S (SLS) preparations constituted by a hemolysin-rich material released by resting streptococci. The SLS mitogen is distinct from the hemolysin (see Cavaillon *et al.* (1979) and Gray (1979) for references).

On the other hand, purified preparations of ET toxin were found to be strong nonspecific lymphocyte transforming substances (Kim and Watson, 1972; Nauciel, 1973; Hříbalová and Pospíšil, 1973) as measured by ^{3}H-thymidine incorporation. Kim and Watson (1972) reported that 50% transformation of human peripheral blood lymphocytes required only 0.00005 μg/ml of culture. Cavaillon *et al.* (1979) isolated two distinct, non specific, extracellular mitogenic proteins from culture fluid of a *Streptococcus pyogenes* group A strain by salting out with $(NH_4)_2SO_4$ and purified to apparent homogeneity by isoelectric focusing or CM-cellulose chromatography. The mitogen with pI 4.8 showed complete immunological cross-reaction with erythrogenic toxin. The other of pI 8.5 was immunologically different. Both were highly potent on human and rabbit peripheral blood lymphocytes as well as on rabbit thymocytes and splenocytes. These properties suggest that they are most likely T-cell mitogens. Their high potencies may be particularly useful in studying the functions of human and rabbit lymphocytes. These two mitogens were found to be much less active when tested on mouse splenocytes and thymocytes. The participation of adherent cells did not appear to be required for their action on lymphocyte transformation.

The relationship with ET of the potent mitogenic material on rabbit lymphocytes studied by Abe (1971a,b) is not known. However the strains used by this investigator releases ET. Two different stimulants were reported in this case. In contrast, the 17,500-dalton blastogen A isolated by Gray (1979) from the C 203 S strain was shown to be different from the three streptococcal erythrogenic (pyrogenic) toxins on the basis of electrophoretic and immunologic criteria.

Several investigators reported recent work on the mitogenicity of these toxins. Petermann et al. (1978) and Knöll et al. (1978) gave interesting data on the production of these toxins by various strains and groups and found that lymphocytes in the case of one donor could be stimulated by as less as 10^{-9} µg of toxin. Trebichavský et al. (1978) reported that rabbit peripheral blood, spleen and thymus lymphocytes were stimulated in vitro with ET. The ultrastructure of stimulated blast cells was described; the morphological features of these cells are similar to those of T-lymphoblasts. ^{3}H-thymidine incorporation into lymphocytes stimulated with ET or PHA was studied in correlation with blast formation.

Barsumian et al. (1978b) and Schlievert et al. (1979c) found similarly to Cavaillon et al. (1979) that toxins A, B and C as well as staphylococcal pyrogenic exotoxin were potent non specific T-lymphocyte mitogens. Macrophage (adherent cells) did not significantly affect the mitogenicity of these toxins. In some cases or for same animal species, mitogenicity appeared to be both non specific and specific (sensitized animals). It appeared also from the studies of Barsumain and co-workers that the mitogenic effects of the toxins may be independent of the immunosuppressive and immunoenhancing effects on antibody synthesis.

Streptococcal mitogens may prove interesting probes for the study of lymphocyte functions. They may also provide a new insight in the investigations concerning the mechanisms of streptococcal diseases and their sequelae.

4.5.6. Skin Reactions

Earlier work on skin reactivity induced by ET has been summarized by Watson and Kim (1970) and Kim and Watson (1972). A reaction was shown to be elicited by as low as 1 pg of toxin in man ($\simeq 10^9$ skin test doses/mg toxin). In rabbit and guinea pig one S.T.D. was equivalent to about 1 and 0.1 µg of toxin, respectively. However, the sensitivity is not only dependent upon the activity of toxin, but is also based on the immunological state of the host tested. Therefore the determination of S.T.D. is not the best method for quantitation of the primary activity of the toxin. A reinterpretation of the Dick Test was recently stated by Schlievert et al. (1979a) who demonstrated that in addition to the toxic reaction previously described ET enhances Arthus and delayed-hypersensitivity skin reactions.

REFERENCES

Abe, Y. (1971a) Lymphocyte stimulation with streptolysin O preparations. I. Purification of streptolysin O and the existence of two stimulants for rabbit lymphocytes cultured in vitro. Jap. J. Exp. Med. 41: 431–442.

Abe, Y. (1971b) Lymphocyte stimulation with streptolysin O preparations. II. Relationship between lymphocyte stimulating and hemolytic activities of purified streptolysin O. Jap. J. Exp. Med. 42: 131–137.

Alouf, J. E. (1967) Purification, physiochemical and biological properties of streptolysin O (in French). Doctoral dissertation, Paris University, No. A.O 1356 C.N.R.S. Library, Paris.

Alouf, J. E. (1977) Cell membranes and cytolytic bacterial toxins. In: Specificity and Action of Animal, Bacterial and Plant Toxins, pp. 221–270, Cuatrecasas, P. (Ed.), Chapman and Hall, London.

Alouf, J. E. and Raynaud, M. (1965) Un milieu simple pour la production de la streptolysine O de titre très élevé. Croissance et toxinogénèse sur ce milieu. Ann. Inst. Pasteur 108: 759–767.

Alouf, J. E. and Raynaud, M. (1968a) Action de la streptolysine O sur les membranes cellulaires. I. Fixation sur la membrane érythrocytaire. Ann. Inst. Pasteur 114: 812–827.

Alouf, J. E. and Raynaud, M. (1968b) Action de la streptolysine O sur les membranes cellulaires. II. Cinétique de la lyse érythrocytaire. Ann. Inst. Pasteur 115: 97–121.

Alouf, J. E. and Raynaud, M. (1968c) Some aspects of the mechanisms of lysis of rabbit erythrocytes by streptolysin O. In Current research on group A Streptococcus pp. 192–206, Caravano R. (Ed.) Excerpta Medica Foundation, Amsterdam.

ALOUF, J. E. and RAYNAUD, M. (1973) Purification and some properties of streptolysin O. *Biochimie* **55**: 1187–1193.

ALOUF, J. E. and GEOFFROY, C. (1979) Comparative effects of cholesterol and thiocholesterol on streptolysin O. *F.E.M.S. Microbiology Letters* **6**: 413–416.

ALOUF, J. E., VIETTE, M., CORVAZIER, R. and RAYNAUD, M. (1965) Préparation et propriétés de sérums de chevaux antistreptolysine O. *Ann. Inst. Pasteur* **108**: 476–500.

ALOUF, J. E., KIREDJIAN, M. and GEOFFROY C. (1977) Purification de l'hémolysine thiol-dépendante extracellulaire de *Bacillus alvei. Biochimie* **59**: 329–336.

ALOUF, J. E., DE ST-MARTIN, J. EYQUEM, A., GEOFFROY, C., JACQUEMOT, C. and DUPHOT, M. (1978) Titrage des anticorps sériques humains anti-exoprotéines du streptocoque du groupe A par microhémagglutination en plaque: corrélation avec les taux de l'antistreptolysine O et de divers antienzymes. *Ann. Microbiol. (Inst. Pasteur)* **129A**: 447–472.

ANDERSEN, B. R. and CONE, R. (1974) Inhibition of human lymphocyte blast transformation by streptolysin O. *J. Lab. Clin. Med.* **84**, 241–248.

ANDERSEN, B. R. and AMIRAULT, J. J. (1976) Decreased E-rosette formation following streptolysin O treatment. *Proc. Soc. Exp. Biol. Med.* **153**: 405–407.

ARBUTHNOTT, J. P., McNIVEN, A. C. and SMYTH, C. J. (1975) Multiple forms of bacterial toxins in preparative isoelectric focusing. In *Isoelectric focusing* pp. 212–239, ARBUTHNOTT, J. P. and BEELEY, J. A. (Eds), Butterworths, London.

BADIN, J. and BARILLEC, A. (1968) Effet des lipides de la β-lipoprotéine humaine normale sur le pouvoir hémolytique de la streptolysine O et de la digitonine. *Ann. Biol. Clin.* **26**: 213–229.

BADIN, J. and DENNE, M. A. (1978) A cholesterol fraction for streptolysin O binding on cell membrane and lipoproteins. I. Optimal conditions for the determination. *Cell Molec. Biol.* **22**: 133–143.

BANGHAM, A. D., STANDISH, M. M. and WEISSMANN G. (1965) The action of steroids and streptolysin S on permeability of phospholipids to cations. *J. Mol. Biol.* **13**: 253–259.

BARKSDALE, L. and ARDEN, S. B. (1974) Persisting bacteriophage infections, lysogeny and phage conversions. *Ann. Rev. Microbiol.* **28**: 265–299.

BARNARD, W. C. and TODD, E. W. (1940) Lesions in the mouse produced by streptolysins O and S. *J. Pathol. Bact.* **51**: 43–47.

BARSUMIAN, E. L., CUNNINGHAM, C. M., SCHLIEVERT, P. M. and WATSON, D. W. (1978a) Heterogeneity of group A streptococcal pyrogenic exotoxin type B. *Infect. Immun.* **20**: 512–518.

BARSUMIAN, E. L., SCHLIEVERT, P. M. and WATSON, D. W. (1978b) Non-specific and specific immunological mitogenicity by group A streptococcal pyrogenic exotoxins. *Infect. Immun.* **22**: 681–688.

BERNHEIMER, A. W. (1948) Properties of certain rapidly acting bacterial toxins as illustrated by streptolysin O and S. *Bacteriol. Rev.* **12**: 195–202.

BERNHEIMER, A. W. (1954) Streptolysins and their inhibitors. In *Streptococcal Infections* pp. 19–38, McCARTY, M. (Ed.) Columbia University Press, New York.

BERNHEIMER, A. W. (1966) Disruption of wall-less bacteria by streptococcal and staphylococcal toxins. *J. Bacteriol.* **91**: 1677–1680.

BERNHEIMER, A. W. (1967) Physical behavior of streptolysin S. *J. Bacteriol.* **93**: 2024–2025.

BERNHEIMER, A. W. (1972) Hemolysins of streptococci: characterization and effects on biological membranes. In *Streptococci and Streptococcal Diseases* pp. 19–31, WANNAMAKER, L. W. and MATSEN, J. M. (Eds), Academic Press, New York.

BERNHEIMER, A. W. (1974) Interactions between membranes and cytolytic bacterial toxins. *Biochim. Biophys. Acta* **344**: 27–50.

BERNHEIMER, A. W. (1976) Sulfhydryl-activated toxins, In *Mechanisms in Bacterial Toxinology.* pp. 85–97, BERNHEIMER A. W. (Ed) John Wiley and Sons, New York.

BERNHEIMER, A. W. and CANTONI, G. L. (1945) The cardiac action of preparations containing the oxygen labile hemolysin of *Streptococcus pyogenes.* I. Increased sensitivity of the isolated frog's heart to repeated application of the toxins. *J. Exptl Med.* **81**: 295–306.

BERNHEIMER, A. W. and CANTONI, G. L. (1947) The cardiac action of preparations containing the oxygen-labile hemolysin of *Streptococcus pyogenes.* III. Induction in mice of temporary resistance to the lethal effect of the toxin. *J. Exptl Med.* **86**: 193–202.

BERNHEIMER, A. W. and RODBART, M. (1948) The effect of nucleic acids and of carbohydrates on the formation of streptolysin S. *J. Exptl. Med.* **88**: 149–168.

BERNHEIMER, A. W. and SCHWARTZ, L. L. (1960) Leucocidal agents of hemolytic streptococci. *J. Path. Bact.* **79**: 37–46.

BERNHEIMER, A. W. and SCHWARTZ, L. L. (1965) Effects of staphylococcal and other bacterial toxins on platelets *in vitro. J. Path. Bact.* **89**: 209–223.

BERNHEIMER, A. W. and AVIGAD, L. S. (1970) Streptolysin O: activation by thiols. *Infect. Immun.* **1**: 509–510.

BERNHEIMER, A. W. and AVIGAD, L. S. (1979) A cytolytic protein from the edible mushroom *Pleurotus ostreatus. Biochim. Biophys. Acta* **585**: 451–461.

BERNHEIMER, A. W., AVIGAD, L. S. and KIM, K. S. (1979) Comparison of metridiolysins from the sea anemone with thiol-activated cytolysins from bacteria. *Toxicon* **17**: 69–75.

BERNHEIMER, A. W., GILLMAN, W., HOTTLE, G. A. and PAPPENHEIMER, A. M. JR (1942) An improved medium for the cultivation of hemolytic *Streptococcus. J. Bacteriol.* **43**: 495–498.

BESLUAU, D., GAUTHIER-RAHMAN, S. and HALPERN, B. (1979). The protective effect of some phenothiazine derivatives against streptolysin O. *Br. J. Pharmacol.* **67**: 173–177.

BOROFF, D. A. (1951) Allergenic property of scarlatinal toxin. *J. Bacteriol.* **62**: 627–631.

BROCKLEHURST, K., CARLSSON, J. KIERSTAN, M. P. J. and CROOK, E. M. (1974) Covalent chromatography by thiol-disulfide interchange. In *Methods in Enzymology* Vol. 22 pp. 531–534, JAKOBY, W. (Ed.), Academic Press, New York.

BRUNSON, K. W. and WATSON, D. W. (1974) Pyrogenic specificity of streptococcal exotoxins, staphylococcal exotoxins and gram-negative endotoxin. *Infect. Immun.* **10**: 347–351.

CALANDRA, G. B. and OGINSKY, E. L. (1975) Cellular streptolysin S-related hemolysins of group A *Streptococcus* C 203 S. *Infect. Immun.* **12**: 13–28.

CALANDRA, G. B. and THEODORE, T. S. (1975) Cellular location of streptolysin O. *Infect. Immun.* **12**: 750–753.

CALANDRA, G. B., WHITE, R. S. and COLE, R. M. (1976) Relationship of cellular potential hemolysis in group A streptococci to extracellular streptolysins. *Infect. Immun.* **13**: 813–817.

CANTONI, G. L. and BERNHEIMER, A. W. (1945) The cardiac action of preparations containing the oxygen-labile hemolysin of *Streptococcus pyogenes*. II. Inhibition of cardiotoxic effect by a substance released from the frog's heart. *J. Exptl Med.* **81**: 307–313.

CANTONI, G. L. and BERNHEIMER, A. W. (1947) The toxic action of preparations containing the oxygen-labile hemolysin of *Streptococcus pyogenes*. IV. Comparison of cardiotoxic action with that of saponin. *J. Pharmacol. Exptl Therap.* **91**: 31–38.

CAVAILLON, J. M., GEOFFROY, C. and ALOUF, J. E. (1979) Purification of two extracellular streptococcal mitogens and their effect on human, rabbit and mouse lymphocytes. *J. Clin. Lab. Immunol.* **2**: 155–163.

CINADER, B. and PILLEMER, L. (1950) The purification and properties of streptolysin S. *J. Exptl Med.* **92**: 219–237.

COHEN, J. O. (1969) Effect of medium composition and pH on the production of M protein and proteinase by group A streptococci. *J. Bacteriol.* **99**: 737–744.

COLON-WHITT, A., WHITT, R. S. and COLE, R. M. (1978) Production of an erythrogenic toxin (streptococcal pyrogenic exotoxin) by a non-lysogenised group A streptococcus. In *Pathogenic Streptococci* pp. 64–65, PARKER, M. T. (Ed.) Reedbooks Ltd, Chertsey, Surrey, United Kingdom.

CORABOEUF, E. and GOULLET, P. (1963) Quelques aspects de l'action de la streptolysine O sur le coeur isolé du rat. *J. Physiol.* (Paris) **55**: 232–233.

COWELL, J. L. and BERNHEIMER, A. W. (1977) Antigenic relationships among thiol-activated cytolysins. *Infect. Immun.* **16**: 397–399.

COWELL, J. L. and BERNHEIMER, A. W. (1978) Role of cholesterol in the action of cereolysin on membranes. *Arch. Biochem. Biophys.* **190**: 603–610.

COWELL, J. L., GRUSHOFF-KOSYK, P. S. and BERNHEIMER, A. W. (1976) Purification of cereolysin and the electrophoretic separation of the active (reduced) and inactive (oxidized) forms of the purified toxin. *Infect. Immun.* **14**: 144–154.

COWELL, J. L., KIM, K. S. and BERNHEIMER, A. W. (1978) Alteration by cereolysin of the structure of cholesterol-containing membranes. *Biochim. Biophys. Acta* **507**: 230–241.

CUNNINGHAM, C. M., BARSUMIAN, E. L. and WATSON, D. W. (1976) Further purification of group A streptococcal pyrogenic exotoxin and characterization of the purified toxin. *Infect. Immun.* **14**: 767–775.

CUNNINGHAM, C. M. and WATSON, D. W. (1978a) Alteration of clearance function by group A streptococcal pyrogenic exotoxin and its relation to suppression of the antibody response. *Infect. Immun.* **19**: 51–57.

CUNNINGHAM, C. M. and WATSON, D. W. (1978b) Suppression of antibody response by group A streptococcal pyrogenic exotoxin and characterization of the cells involved. *Infect. Immun.* **19**: 470–476.

DELATTRE, J., BADIN, J., CANAL, J. and GIRARD, M. L. (1973) Influence des lécithines sur le pouvoir inhibiteur du cholestérol vis-à-vis de la streptolysine O. *C.R. Acad. Sci.* Paris **277**: series D, 441–443.

DELATTRE, J., LEBSIR, R., PANOUSE-PERRIN, J. and BADIN, J. (1979) A cholesterol fraction for streptolysin O binding in cell membranes and lipoproteins. II Interaction of streptolysin O with phospholipid-cholesterol liposomes of different nature and molecular ratios. *Cell. Molec. Biol.* **24**: 157–166.

DEMEL, R. A. and DE KRUYFF, B. (1976) The function of sterols in membranes. *Biochim. Biophys. Acta* **457**: 109–132.

DICK, G. F. and DICK, G. H. (1924) A skin test for susceptibility to scarlet fever. *J. Am. Med. Assoc.* **82**: 265–266.

DOURMASHKIN, R. R. and ROSSE, W. F. (1966) Morphologic changes in the membranes of red blood cells undergoing hemolysis. *Am. J. Med.* **41**: 699–710.

DUNCAN, J. L. (1974) Characteristics of streptolysin O hemolysis: kinetics of hemoglobin and [86]rubidium release. *Infect. Immun.* **9**: 1022–1027.

DUNCAN, J. L. (1975) Streptococcal toxins, in *Microbiol.* p. 257–262 Schlessinger, D. (ed.), American Society for Microbiology, Washington, D.C.

DUNCAN, J. L. and SCHLEGEL, R. (1975) Effect of streptolysin O on erythrocyte membranes, liposomes, and lipid dispersions. A protein-cholesterol interaction. *J. Cell. Biol.* **67**: 160–173.

DUNCAN, J. L. and MASON, L. (1976) Characteristics of streptolysin S hemolysis. *Infect. Immun.* **14**: 77–82.

DUNCAN, J. L. and BUCKINGHAM, L. (1977) Effects to streptolysin O on transport of amino acids, nucleosides and glucose analogs in mammalian cells. *Infect. Immun.* **18**: 688–693.

DUNCAN, J. L. and BUCKINGHAM (1978) Increased resistance to streptolysin O in mammalian cells treated with oxygenated derivatives of cholesterol. *Infect. Immun.* **22**: 94–100.

ELIAS, N., HELLER, M. and GINSBURG, I. (1966) Bindings of streptolysin S to red blood cell ghosts and ghost lipids. *Israel J. Med. Sci.* **2**: 302–309.

FAUVE, R. M., ALOUF, J. E., DELAUNAY, A. and RAYNAUD, A. (1966) Cytotoxic effects *in vitro* of highly purified streptolysin O on mouse macrophages cultured in a serum-free medium. *J. Bacteriol.* **92**: 1150–1153.

FEHRENBACH, F. J. (1977) Interaction of streptolysin O with natural and artificial membranes. *Z. Naturforsch.* **32c**: 101–109.

FEHRENBACH, F. J. and TEMPELFELD, W. (1979) Relative resistance of mouse red blood cells to streptolysin O. In *Pathogenic streptococci* pp. 58–59, PARKER, M. T. (Ed.) Reedbooks Ltd, Chertsey, Surrey, United Kingdom.

FEIGEN, G. A., CONRAD, M. J., GERBER, J. D., SINGH, B. N. and HADJI, L. (1974) Analysis of the biphasic response in cardiac anaphylaxis to an active streptococcal toxin. *Int. Arch. Allergy Appl. Immunol.* **46**: 128–149.

Fox E. N. (1961) Peptide requirements for the synthesis of streptococcal proteins. *J. Biol. Chem.* **236**: 166–171.

Frazier, M. L. and Zimmerman, L. N. (1977) Genetic loci of hemolysin production in *Streptococcus faecalis* subsp. *zymogenes*. *J. Bacteriol.* **130**: 1064–1071.

Freer, J. H. and Arbuthnott, J. P. (1976) Biochemical and morphological alterations of membranes by bacterial toxins, pp. 170–193. In *Mechanisms in Bacterial Toxinology*, Bernheimer, A. W. (Ed.) John Wiley and Sons, New York.

Gemmel, C. G. and Abdul-Amir, M. K. (1979) Effect of certain antibiotics on the formation of cellular antigens and extracellular products by group A streptococci. In *Pathogenic streptococci* pp. 67–68, Parker, M. T. (Ed.) Reedbooks Ltd, Chertsey, Surrey, United Kingdom.

Ginsburg, I. (1970) Streptolysin S. In *Microbial toxins* pp. 99–171, Montie, T. C., Kadis, S. and Ajl, S. J. (Eds) Academic Press, New York.

Ginsburg, I. (1972) Mechanisms of cell and tissue injury induced by group A streptococci: relation to post-streptococcal sequelae. *J. Infect. Dis.* **126**: 294–340.

Ginsburg, I. and Grossowicz, N. (1960) Effect of streptococcal haemolysins on Ehrlich ascites tumour cells. *J. Path. Bact.* **80**: 111–119.

Ginsburg, I., Harris, T. N. and Grossowicz, N. (1963) Oxygen-stable hemolysins of group A streptococci I. The role of various agents in the production of the hemolysins. *J. Exptl Med.* **118**: 905–917.

Goullet, P., Coraboeuf, E. and Breton, D. (1963). Action d'une préparation de streptolysine O purifiée sur le tissu myocardique ventriculaire. *C.R. Acad. Sci.* Paris, **257**: 1735–1738.

Goullet, P., Obrecht-Coutris, G., Le Douarin, G. and Coraboeuf, E. (1968) Action de la streptolysine O sur le myocarde embryonnaire. *J. Physiol.* (Paris) **60** (suppl. 2): 451–452.

Gray, E. D. (1979) Purification and properties of an extracellular blastogen produced by group A streptococci. *J. Exptl Med.* **149**: 1438–1449.

Grushoff, P. S., Shany, S. and Bernheimer, A. W. (1975) Purification and properties of streptococcal nicotinamide adenine dinucleotide glycohydrolase. *J. Bacteriol.* **122**: 599–605.

Gupta, R. K. (1979) Effect of intracerebroventricular administration of streptolysin O on the behaviour of unanaesthetized rabbits and dogs. *Toxicon* **17**: 167–169.

Gupta, S. and Gupta, R. K. (1979) Disruption of electrocardiographic activity by streptolysin O in rats. *Toxicon* **17**: 664–667.

Gupta, R. K. and Srimal, R. C. (1979) Effect of intraventricular administration of streptolysin O on the electroencephalogram of rabbits. *Toxicon* **17**: 321–325.

Gyles, C., So, M. and Falkow, S. (1974) The enterotoxin plasmids of *E. coli. J. Infect. Dis.* **130**: 40–49.

Hadji, L. (1979) Etude immunopharmacologique de la réaction anaphylactique cardiaque à la streptolysine O. Doctoral dissertation, Paris IX University.

Halbert, S. P. (1955) The use of precipitin analysis in agar for study of human streptococcal infection. I. Oudin technic. *J. Exptl Med.* **101**: 539–556.

Halbert, S. P. (1958) The use of precipitin analysis in agar for the study of human streptococcal infections. III. The purification of some antigens detected by these methods. *J. Exptl Med.* **108**: 385–410.

Halbert, S. P. (1963) Naturally occurring human antibodies to streptococcal enzymes. *Ann. N.Y. Acad. Sci.* **103**: 1027–1051.

Halbert, S. P. (1970) Streptolysin O. In *Microbial Toxins*, Vol III, pp. 69–98, Montie, T. C., Kadis, S. and Ajl S. J. (Eds) Academic Press, New York.

Halbert, S. P., Bircher, R. and Dahle, E. (1961) The analysis of streptococcal infections. V. Cardiotoxicity of streptolysin O for rabbits *in vivo. J. Exptl Med.* **113**: 759–784.

Halbert S. P., Bircher, R. and Dahle E. (1963a) Studies on the mechanism of the lethal toxic action of streptolysin O and the protection by certain serotonin drugs. *J. Lab. Clin. Med.* **61**: 437–452.

Halbert, S. P., Dahle, E., Keatinge, S. and Bircher R. (1963b) Studies on the role of potassium ions in the lethal toxicity of streptolysin O. In *Recent Adv. Pharmacology Toxins*, pp. 439–453, Rásková, H. (Ed.) Pergamon Press, Oxford.

Halpern, B. N. and Rahman, S. (1968) Studies on the cardiotoxicity of streptolysin O. *Br. J. Pharmacol.* **32**: 441–452.

Halpern, B. N., Hollman, K. H., Rahman, S., Verley, J. M. (1969) Submicroscopical myocardial lesions produced by streptolysin O *in vivo. Israel J. Med. Sci.* **5**: 1138–1148.

Hanna, E. E. and Hale, M. (1975) Deregulation of mouse antibody-forming cells *in vivo* and in cell culture by streptococcal pyrogenic exotoxin. *Infect. Immun.* **11**: 265–272.

Hanna, E. E. and Watson, D. W. (1965) Host-parasite relationships among group A streptococci: III. Depression of reticuloendothelial function by streptococcal pyrogenic exotoxins. *J. Bact.* **89**: 154–158.

Hanson, L. Å. (1959) Immunological analysis of streptococcal antigens in human sera by means of diffusion-in-gel methods. *Int. Arch. Allergy* **14**: 279–291.

Hanson, L. Å. and Holm, S. E. (1961) Studies on the antigenic factors in a group A streptococcal culture filtrate. *Acta Path. Microbiol. Scand.* **52**: 59–70.

Harris, T. N., Harris, S. and Ogburn, C. A. (1955) Gel-precipitation of streptococcal culture supernates with sera of patients with rheumatic fever and streptococcal infection. *Proceed. Soc. Exptl Biol. Med.* **90**: 39–45.

Herbert, D. (1941) A simple colorimetric method for the estimation of haemolysis and its application to the study of streptolysin. *Biochem. J.* **35**: 1116–1123.

Herbert, D. and Todd, E. W. (1941) Purification and properties of a haemolysin produced by group A hemolytic streptococci (streptolysin O). *Biochem. J.* **35**: 1124–1139.

Herbert, D. and Todd, E. W. (1944) The oxygen-stable hemolysin of group A streptococci (streptolysin S). *Brit. J. Exptl Pathol.* **25**: 242–254.

Hewitt, L. F. and Todd, E. W. (1939) The effect of cholesterol and of sera contaminated with bacteria on the haemolysins produced by haemolytic streptococci. *J. Path. Bacteriol.* **49**: 45–51.

Hirsch, J. G., Bernheimer, A. W. and Weissmann G. (1963) Motion picture study of the toxic action of streptolysins on leucocytes. *J. Exptl Med.* **118**: 223–228.

Holm S. E. and Möller, Å. (1971) An immunodiffusion micromethod for comparative analysis of the haemolytic activity and antigenicity of streptolysin O. *Acta Path. Microbiol. Scand. section B* **79**: 73–78.

Honda, T., Goshima, K., Takeda, Y., Sugino, Y. and Miwatani, T. (1976) Demonstration of the cardiotoxicity of the thermostable direct hemolysin (lethal toxin) produced by *Vibrio parahaemolyticus*. *Infect. Immun.* **13**: 163–171.

Hooker S. B. and Follensby, E. M. (1934) Studies of scarlet fever. II. Different toxins produced by hemolytic streptococci of scarlatinal origin. *J. Immunol.* **27**: 177–193.

Howard, J. G. and Wallace, K. R. (1953a) The comparative resistances of the red cells of various species to haemolysins by streptolysin O and by saponin. *Br. J. Exptl Pathol.* **34**: 181–184.

Howard, J. G. and Wallace, K. R. (1953b) The comparative resistances of rabbits, guinea-pigs and mice to the lethal actions of streptolysin O and saponin. *Br. J. Exptl Pathol.* **34**: 185–190.

Howard, J. G., Wallace, K. R. and Wright, G. P. (1953) The inhibitory effects of cholesterol and related sterols on haemolysis by streptolysin O. *Br. J. Exptl Path.* **34**: 174–180.

Hřibalová, V. (1979) Effect of scarlet fever toxin on the phagocytic activity of the reticuloendothelial system. *Folia Microbiol.* **24**: 415–427.

Hřibalová, V. and Pospíšil, M. (1973) Lymphocyte-stimulating activity of scarlet fever toxin. *Experientia* **29**: 704–705.

Hřibalová, V., Castrovan A. and Pekarek, J. (1979) Influence of antilymphocyte and antipolymorphonuclear sera on the pyrogenic effect of scarlet fever toxin. *Folia Microbiol.* **24**: 428–434.

Hryniewicz, W., Szmigielski, S. and Janiak, M. (1977) Hemolysis induced by streptolysin S: kinetics of hemoglobin and [86]rubidium release. *Zblt. Bakt. Hyg. I. Abt A* **238**: 201–207.

Hryniewicz, W. and Pryjma, J. (1977) Effect of streptolysin S on human and mouse T and B lymphocytes. *Infect. Immun.* **16**: 730–733.

Hryniewicz, W. and Pryjma, J. (1978) Action of streptolysin S on cells concerned in the immune reaction. In *Pathogenic Streptococci* pp. 59–60, Parker, M. T. (Ed.) Reedbooks Ltd, Chertsey, Surrey, United Kingdom.

Huang, C. H. (1977) A structural model for the cholesterol-phosphatidylcholine complexes in bilayer membranes. *Lipids* **12**: 348–356.

Inoue, K., Akiyama, Y., Kinoshita, T., Higashi, T., Higashi, Y. and Amano, T. (1976) Evidence for one-hit theory in the immune bactericidal reaction and demonstration of a multi-hit response for hemolysis by streptolysin O and *Clostridium perfringens* theta-toxin. *Infect. Immun.* **13**: 337–344.

Jeljaszewicz, J., Szmigielski, S. and Hryniewicz, W. (1978) Biological effects of staphylococcal and streptococcal toxins. In *Bacterial toxins and cell membranes* pp. 185–227, Jeljaszewicz and Wadström, T. (Eds) Academic Press, New York.

Johnson, M. K., Geoffroy, C. and Alouf, J. E. (1980) The binding of cholesterol by sulfhydryl-activated cytolysins. *Infect. Immun.* **27**: 97–101.

Kanbayashi, Y., Hotta, M. and Koyama, J. (1972) Kinetic study of streptolysin O. *J. Biochem.* (Japan) **71**: 227–237.

Kantor, H. S., Temples, B. and Shaw, M. W. (1972) Staphylococcal delta-hemolysin: purification and characterization. *Arch. Biochem. Biophys.* **151**: 142–156.

Kaplan, E. L. and Wannamaker, L. W. (1976) Suppression of the antistreptolysin O response by cholesterol and by lipid extracts of rabbit skin. *J. Exptl Med.* **144**: 754–767.

Keiser, H., Weissman, G. and Bernheimer, A. W. (1964) Studies on liposomes. IV. Solubilisation of enzymes during mitochondrial swelling and disruption of liposomes by streptolysin S and other hemolytic agents. *J. Cell Biol.* **22**: 101–113.

Kellner, A., Bernheimer, A. W., Carlson, A. S. and Freeman, E. B. (1956) Loss of myocardial contractibility induced in the isolated mammalian hearts by streptolysin O. *J. Exptl Med.* **104**: 361–373.

Kim, Y. B. and Watson, D. W. (1970) A purified group A streptococcal pyrogenic exotoxin. *J. Exptl Med.* **131**: 611–628.

Kim, Y. B. and Watson, D. W. (1972) Streptococcal exotoxins. Biological and pathological properties. In: *Streptococci and Streptococcal diseases* pp. 33–50, Wannamaker, L. W. and Matsen, J. M. (Eds) Academic Press, New York.

Klein, G. C., Addison, B. V., Boome, J. S., and Moody, M. D. (1968) Effect of type of red blood cells on antistreptolysin O titer. *Appl. Microbiol.* **16**: 1761–1763.

Klein, G. C. (1976) Immune response to streptococcal infection. In: *Manual of Clinical Immunology* pp. 264–273, Rose N. R. and Friedman H. (Eds) American Society for Microbiology, Washington D.C.

Knöll, H., Petermann, F. and Köhler, W. (1978) Untersuchungen zur Mitogenität erythrogener Toxine. II. Mitteilung: Nachweis erythrogener Toxine in Kulturfiltraten von *Streptococcus pyogenes*. *Zbl. Bakt. Hyg. I. Abt. Orig. A* **240**: 466–473.

Koyama, J. (1963) Biochemical studies on streptolysin S formed in the presence of yeast ribonucleic acid. I. Properties of a polypeptide component and its role in the toxin activity. *J. Biochem.* (Japan) **54**: 146–151.

Koyama, J. (1965) Kinetic study on streptolysin S. *J. Biochem.* (Japan) **57**: 103–108.

Koyama, J. and Egami, F. (1963) Biochemical studies on streptolysin S formed in the presence of yeast ribonucleic acid. I. The purification and some properties of the toxin. *J. Biochem.* (Japan) **53**: 147–154.

Lai, C. Y., Wang, M-T., de Faria, J. B. and Akao, T. (1978) Streptolysin S: improved purification and characterization. *Arch. Biochem. Biophys.* **191**: 804–812.

Launay, J. M. and Alouf J. E. (1979) Biochemical and electronmicroscopic study of the cytolytic effect of streptolysin O on human and guinea pig platelets and their organelles. *Biochim. Biophys. Acta* **556**: 278–291.

Lee A. G. (1977) Lipid phase transitions and phase diagrams. II. Mixtures involving lipids. *Biochim. Biophys. Acta* **472**: 285–344.

Linder, R. (1979) Heterologous immunoaffinity chromatography in the purification of streptolysin O. *FEMS Microbiology Letters* **5**: 339–342.

MARMOREK, A. (1895) Le streptocoque et le sérum antistreptococcique. *Ann. Inst. Pasteur* **9**: 593–620.

MCCARTNEY, C. and ARBUTHNOTT, J. P. Mode of action of membrane-damaging toxins produced by staphylococci. In *Bacterial Toxins and Cell Membranes*, pp. 89–127, JELJASZEWICZ, J. and WADSTRÖM, T. (Eds), Academic Press, New York.

MARTIN, R. B. and YEAGLE, P. L. (1978) Models for lipid organization in cholesterol-phospholipid bilayers including cholesterol dimer function. *Lipids* **13**: 594–597.

MASTROENI, P., MISEFARI, A. and NACCI, A. (1969) Interaction between red cell and stroma and streptolysin O. Inhibition of cytotoxic activity. *Appl. Microbiol.* **17**: 650–651.

MERUCCI, P., VELLA, L. and CACCIAPUOTTI, B. (1964) Study of the lytic action of streptolysin O on rabbit platelets *in vitro* and *in vivo*. *Progress Immunobiol. Standard.* **1**: 127–129.

MITRICA, N., PLECEAS, P. and MESROBEANU, L. (1965) Crystallization of the Dick toxin. *Z. Immunitäts. Allergieforsch.* **129**: 78–83.

MITSUI, K., SEKIYA, T., NOZAWA, Y. and HASE, J. (1979a) Alteration of human erythrocyte plasma membranes by perfringolysin O as revealed by freeze-fracture electron microscopy. Studies on *Clostridium perfringens* exotoxins V. *Biochim. Biophys. Acta* **554**: 68–75.

MITSUI, K., SEKIYA, T., OKAMURA, S., NOZAWA, Y. and HASE, J. (1979b) Ring formation of perfringolysin O as revealed by negative stain electron microscopy. *Biochim. Biophys. Acta* **558**: 307–313.

NAUCIEL, C. (1973) Mitogenic activity of purified streptococcal erythrogenic toxin on lymphocytes. *Ann. Immunol. (Inst. Pasteur)* **124C**: 383–390.

NAUCIEL, C., RAYNAUD, M. and BIZZINI, B. (1968) Purification et propriétés de la toxine érythrogène du streptocoque. *Ann. Inst. Pasteur* **114**: 796–811.

NAUCIEL, C., BLASS, J., MANGALO, R. and RAYNAUD, M. (1969) Evidence for two molecular forms of streptococcal erythrogenic toxin. *Eur. J. Biochem.* **11**: 160–164.

NEILL, J. M. and MALLORY, T. B. (1926) Studies on the oxidation and reduction of immunological substances. *J. Exptl Med.* **44**: 241–260.

NEWARK, P. (1979) Pathways to secretion. *Nature* **281**: 629–630.

NIDA, S. K., HOUSTON, C. W. and FERRETTI, J. J. (1978) Erythrogenic toxin production by group A streptococci. In: *Pathogenic Streptococci*, pp. 64–65, PARKER M. T. (Ed) Reedbooks Ltd, Chertsey, Surrey, United Kingdom.

NORMAN, A. W., SPIELVOGEL, A. M. and WONG, R. C. (1976) Polyene antibiotic-sterol interaction. *Adv. Lipid Res.* **14**: 127–170.

OBERLEY, T. D. and DUNCAN, J. L. (1971) Characteristics of streptolysin O action. *Infect. Immun.* **4**: 683–687.

ODRIOZOLA, J. M., WAITZKIN, E., SMITH, T. L. and BLOCH, K. (1978) Sterol requirement of *Mycoplasma capricolum*. *Proc. Natl Acad. Sci.* **75**: 4107–4109.

OFEK, I., BERGNER-RABINOWITZ, S. and GINSBURG, I. (1972) Oxygen-stable hemolysins of group A streptococci. VIII. Leukotoxic and antiphagocytic effects of streptolysins S and O. *Infect. Immun.* **6**: 459–464.

OKAMOTO, H. (1976) Antitumor activity of streptolysin S-forming streptococci. In: *Mechanisms in Bacterial Toxinology*, pp. 237–257, BERNHEIMER, A. W. (Ed.), John Wiley and Sons, New York.

OKAMOTO, H., SHOIN, S. and KOSHIMURA, S. (1978) Streptolysin S-forming and antitumour activities of group A streptococci. In: *Bacterial Toxins and Cell Membranes*, pp. 259–289, JELJASZEWICZ J. and WADSTRÖM, T. (Eds.), Academic Press, New York.

PETERMANN, F., KNÖLL, H. and KÖHLER, W. (1978) Untersuchungen zur Mitogenität erythrogener Toxine. I. Mitteilung: Typenspezifisches Hemmung der mitogenen Aktivität erythrogener Toxine durch antitoxische Seren von Kaninchen. *Zbl. Bakt. Hyg., I Abt Orig.* A **240**: 366–379.

PRAGER, D. J. and FEIGEN, G. A. (1970) Response of the sensitized heart to oxidized and reduced streptolysin O. *Int. Arch. Allergy Appl. Immunol.* **38**: 175–184.

PRIGENT, D. and ALOUF, J. E. (1976) Interaction of streptolysin O with sterols. *Biochim. Biophys. Acta* **443**: 288–300.

PRIGENT, D., ALOUF, J. E. and RAYNAUD, M. (1974) Etude de la fixation de la streptolysine O radio-iodée sur les érythrocytes. *C. R. Acad. Sci.* **278** series D: 651–653.

PRIGENT, D., GEOFFROY, C. and ALOUF, J. E. (1978) Purification de la streptolysine O par chromatographie covalente sur gel de thiol-agarose. *C. R. Acad. Sci.* **287**, series D: 951–954.

PRIGENT, D. and ALOUF, J. E. (1978) Interaction de la streptolysine O avec les liposomes. (Colloque 'Microcapsules et liposomes' Châtenay-Malabry, Mai 1978). *Labo-Pharma, Problèmes et Techniques* No. 281, 910–913.

RAHMAN, S., REBEYROTTE, P., HALPERN, B. and BESLUAU, D. (1969) Kinetics of streptolysin O reactivation by different thiols. *Biochim. Biophys. Acta* **177**: 658–660.

RAHMAN-GAUTHIER, S., REBEYROTTE, P. and BESLUAU D. (1971) La réactivation de la streptolysine O par différents thiols et son incidence sur le dosage des antistreptolysines. *Revue Immunol.* Paris, **35**: 243–258.

RANTZ, L. A., BOISVERT, P. L. and SPINK, W. W. (1946) The Dick test in military personnel with special reference to the pathogenesis of the skin reaction. *N. Engl. J. Med.* **235**: 39–43.

RĂSKOVÁ, H. (1964) Les toxines microbiennes comme domaine de recherches pharmacologiques. *Actualités Pharmacologiques* (Paris) **17**: 71–84.

RĂSKOVÁ, H. and VANĚČEK, J. (1964) Pharmacology of bacterial toxins. *Pharmacol. Rev.* **16**: 1–45.

RAYNAUD, M. and ALOUF, J. E. (1970) Intracellular versus extracellular toxins. In: *Microbial Toxins*, Vol. 1, pp. 67–117, AJL S. J., MONTIE, T. C. and KADIS, S. (Eds), Academic Press, New York.

REITZ, B. A., PRAGER, D. J. and FEIGEN, G. A. (1968) An analysis of the toxic actions of purified streptolysin O on the isolated heart and separate cardiac tissues in the guinea pig. *J. Exptl Med.* **128**: 1401–1424.

RICCI, A., BERTI, B., MOAURO, C., PORRO, M., NERI, P. and TARLI, P. (1978) New hemolytic method for determination of antistreptolysin O in whole blood. *J. Clin. Microbiol.* **8**: 263–267.

ROWEN, R. (1963) Purification and characterization of an induced plasma lipoprotein that inhibits streptolysin O. *Proc. Soc. Exp. Biol. Med.* **114**: 183–187.

ROWEN, P. and BERNHEIMER, A. W. (1956) The toxic action of preparations containing the oxygen-labile

690   JOSEPH E. ALOUF

hemolysin of *Streptococcus pyogenes*. V. Mechanism of refractoriness of the lethal effect of the toxin. *J. Immunol.* **77**: 72–79.

ROWEN, R. and WIEST, M. (1965) A new acute phase protein elicited in mice by streptolysin O and other toxic or infectious agents. *J. Exptl Med.* **122**: 547–564.

SCHLIEVERT, P. M. and WATSON, D. W. (1978) Group A streptococcal pyrogenic exotoxin: pyrogenicity, alteration of blood-brain barrier, and separation of sites for pyrogenicity and enhancement of lethal endotoxin shock. *Infect. Immun.* **21**: 753–763.

SCHLIEVERT, P. M. and WATSON, D. W. (1979) Biogenic amine involvement in pyrogenicity and enhancement of lethal endotoxin shock by group A streptococcal pyrogenic exotoxin. *Proc. Soc. Exptl Biol. Med.* **162**: 269–274.

SCHLIEVERT, P. M., BETTIN, K. M. and WATSON, D. W. (1977) Purification and characterization of group A streptococcal pyrogenic exotoxin type C. *Infect. Immun.* **16**: 673–679.

SCHLIEVERT, P. M., BETTIN, K. M. and WATSON, D. W. (1979a) Reinterpretation of the Dick test: role of group A streptococcal pyrogenic exotoxin. *Infect. Immun.* **26**: 467–472.

SCHLIEVERT, P., BETTIN, K. M. and WATSON, D. W. (1979b) Natural phosphorylation of group A streptococcal pyrogenic exotoxin C. *Infect. Immun.* **26**: 585–589.

SCHLIEVERT, P., SCHOETTLE, D. J. and WATSON, D. W. (1979c) Non-specific, T lymphocyte mitogenesis by pyrogenic exotoxins from group A streptococci and *Staphylococcus aureus. Inject. Immun.* **25**: 1075–1077.

SCHWAB, J. H., WATSON, D. W. and CROMARTIE, W. J. (1955) Further studies of group A streptococcal factors with lethal and cardiotoxic properties. *J. Infect. Dis.* **96**: 14–18.

SCHWAB, J. H. (1956) An intracellular hemolysin of group A streptococci. II. Comparative properties of intracellular hemolysin, streptolysin S and streptolysin O. *J. Bacteriol.* **71**: 100–107.

SHANY, S., GRUSHOFF, P. S. and BERNHEIMER, A. W. (1973) Physical separation of streptococcal nicotinamide adenine dinucleotide glycohydrolase from streptolysin O. *Infect. Immun.* **7**: 731–734.

SHANY, S., BERNHEIMER, A. W., GRUSHOFF, P. S. and KIM, K. S. (1974) Evidence for membrane cholesterol as the common binding site for cereolysin, streptolysin O and saponin. *Molec. Cell Biochem.* **3**: 179–186.

SMYTH, C. J. and FEHRENBACH, F. J. (1974) Isoelectric analysis of haemolysins and enzymes from streptococci of groups A, C and G. *Acta Pathol. Microbiol. Scand. Sect. B* **82**: 860–874.

SMYTH, C. J. and DUNCAN, J. L. (1978) Thiol-activated (oxygen-labile) cytolysins. In: *Bacterial Toxins and Cell Membranes* pp. 129–183, JELJASZEWICZ, J. and WADSTRÖM, T. (Eds), Academic Press, New York.

SMYTH, C. J., FREER, J. H. and ARBUTHNOTT, J. P. (1975) Interaction of *Clostridium perfringens* theta-haemolysin, a contaminant of commercial phospholipase C with erythrocyte ghost membranes and lipid dispersions. A morphological study. *Biochim. Biophys. Acta* **382**: 479–493.

SMYTHE, C. V. and HARRIS, T. N. (1940) Some properties of a hemolysin produced by group A β-hemolytic streptococci. *J. Immunol.* **38**: 283–300.

STOCK, A. H. and URIEL, J. (1961) Electrophoretic mobility and detection of hemolytic activity of streptolysin O and S in agar-gel. *Nature* **192**: 435–436.

SYMINGTON, D. A. and ARBUTHNOTT, J. P. (1972) The action of streptolysin S on mouse liver mitochondria. *J. Med. Microbiol.* **6**: 225–234.

TAKETO, A. and TAKETO, Y. (1964) Biochemical studies on streptolysin S formation. I. Streptolysin S formation in cell free system. *J. Biochem. (Tokyo).* **56**: 552–561.

TARANTA, A. (1959) Relation of isolated recurrences of Sydenham's chorea to preceding streptococcal infections. *New Engl. J. Med.* **260**: 1204–1210.

THELESTAM, M. and MÖLLBY, R. (1979) Classification of microbial, plant and animal cytolysins based on their membrane-damaging effects on human fibroblasts. *Biochim. Biophys. Acta* **557**: 156–169.

THOMPSON A., HALBERT, S. P. and SMITH, U. (1970) The toxicity of streptolysin O for beating mammalian heart cells in tissue culture. *J. Exptl Med.* **131**: 745–763.

TODD, E. W. (1932) Antigenic streptococcal hemolysin. *J. Exptl Med.* **55**: 267–280.

TODD, E. W. (1938a) The differentiation of two distinct serological varieties of streptolysin, streptolysin O and streptolysin S. *J. Path. Bact.* **47**: 423–445.

TODD, E. W. (1938b) Lethal toxins of hemolytic streptococci and their antibodies. *Br. J. Exptl Pathol.* **19**: 367–378.

TODD, E. W. (1942) The leucocidin of group A hemolytic streptococci. *Brit. J. Exptl Pathol.* **23**: 136–145.

TREBICHAVSKÝ, I., HŘÍBALOVÁ, V. and POSPÍŠIL, M. (1978) *In vitro* lymphocyte stimulation with scarlet fever toxin. *Folia Biolog.* **24**: 101–106.

TURNER, G. S. and PENTZ, E. I. (1950) Effect of cholesterol on antigenicity of streptolysin O. *Proc. Soc. Exptl Biol. Med.* **131**: 169–171.

VAN EPPS, D. and ANDERSEN, B. R. (1969) Streptolysin O: sedimentation coefficient and molecular weight determinations. *J. Bacteriol.* **100**: 526–527.

VAN EPPS, D. and ANDERSEN, B. R. (1971) Streptolysin O. II. Relationship of sulfhydryl groups to activity. *Infect. Immun.* **3**: 648–652.

VAN EPPS, D. and ANDERSEN, B. R. (1973) Isolation of streptolysin O by preparative polyacrylamide gel electrophoresis. *Infect. Immun.* **7**: 493–495.

VAN EPPS, D. and ANDERSEN, B. R. (1974) Streptolysin O inhibition of neutrophil chemotaxis and mobility: non immune phenomenon with species specificity. *Infect. Immun.* **9**: 27–33.

WADSTRÖM, T., THELESTAM, M. and MÖLLBY, R. (1974) Biological properties of extracellular proteins from staphylococcus. *Ann. New York Acad. Sci.* **236**: 343–361.

WANNAMAKER, L. W. (1973) The chain that links the heart to the throat. *Circulation* **48**: 9–18.

WATSON, D. W. and KIM, Y. B. (1970) Erythrogenic toxins. In: *Microbial Toxins* Vol III, pp. 173–187, MONTIE, T. C., KADIS, S. and AJL, S. J. (Eds), Academic Press, New York.

WATSON, K. C. and KERR, E. J. C. (1974) Sterol structural requirements for inhibition of streptolysin O activity. *Biochem. J.* **140**: 95–98.

WATSON, K. C. (1960) Host-parasite factors in group A streptococcal infections: pyrogenic and other effects of immunologic distinct exotoxins related to scarlet fever toxins. *J. Exptl Med.* **111**: 255–260.

WEISSMANN, G., KEISER, H. and BERNHEIMER, A. W. (1963) Studies on lysosomes. III. The effects of streptolysin O and S on the release of acid hydrolases from a granular fraction of rabbit liver. *J. Exptl Med.* **118**: 205–222.

WEISSMANN, G., BECHER, B. and THOMAS, W. (1964) Studies on liposomes V. The effects of streptolysins and other hemolytic agents on isolated leucocyte granules. *J. Cell Biol.* **22**: 115–126.

WELD, J. T. (1934) The toxic properties of serum extracts of hemolytic streptococci. *J. Exptl Med.* **59**: 83–95.

WELD, J. T. (1935) Further studies with toxic serum extracts of hemolytic streptococci. *J. Exptl. Med.* **61**: 473–477.

WILEY, B. B. and ROGOLSKY, M. (1977) Molecular and serological differentiation of staphylococcal exfoliative toxin synthetized under chromosomal and plasmid control. *Infect. Immun.* **18**: 487–494.

WILKINSON, P. C. (1975) Inhibition of leukocyte locomotion and chemotaxis by lipid-specific bacterial toxins. *Nature* **255**: 485–487.

YUNES, R., GOLDHAMMER, A. R., GARNER, W. K. and CORDES, E. H. (1977) Phospholipases: mellitin facilitation of bee venom phospholipase A2-catalyzed hydrolysis of unsonicated lecithin liposomes. *Arch. Biochem. Biophys.* **183**: 105–112.

ZABRISKIE, J. B. (1964) The role of temperate bacteriophage in the production of erythrogenic toxin by group A streptococci. *J. Exptl. Med.* **119**: 761–779.

ZUCKER-FRANKLIN, D. (1965) Electron microscope study of the degranulation of polymorphonuclear leukocytes following treatment with streptolysin. *Am. J. Pathol.* **47**: 419–425.

CHAPTER 28

DIPHTHERIA TOXIN

Tsuyoshi Uchida

Research Institute for Microbial Diseases, Osaka University, Yamada-kami, Suita,
Osaka, 565, Japan

1. INTRODUCTION

Recent studies on the relationship between the structure and activity of diphtheria toxin, other bacterial toxins and plant toxins have shown that there are many similarities between toxic proteins (Collier, 1975; Pappenheimer, 1977; Olsnes *et al.*, 1974). Although it is known that diphtheria toxin inhibits protein synthesis of susceptible cells (Strauss and Hendee, 1959) by catalyzing ADP-ribosylation of elongation factor 2 (EF2) (Honjo *et al.*, 1968; Gill *et al.*, 1969a), for some time this enzymic activity of the toxin was thought to be unique, but several years ago, *Pseudomonas aeruginosa* exotoxin was also found to catalyze ADP-ribosylation of EF2 as diphtheria toxin does (Iglewski and Kabat, 1975). Recently colera toxin and LT toxin of *Escherichia coli* were shown to have enzymic activity which catalyzes ADP-ribosylation of GTP binding proteins regulating adenylate cyclase activity (Cassei and Pfeuffer, 1978; Gill and Merren, 1978). Thus, the ADP-ribosylation activity of toxins is now recognized not to be a unique activity of diphtheria toxin but to be an activity of some bacterial toxins and to be of general interest in the field of cell biology and bacteriology.

The mode of action of diphtheria toxin in cell cytoplasm is now fairly well understood, and there are many reviews on the structure and activity of diphtheria toxin (Collier, 1975; Pappenheimer, 1977). Moreover, making use of the actions of diphtheria toxin and serologically related proteins, these compounds have been applied in research on cell biology. The article describes the structure and activity of diphtheria toxin and cytochemical studies using diphtheria toxin and its fragments.

2. TOXIN PRODUCTION

Diphtheria toxin is synthesized on membrane bound ribosomes (Uchida and Yoneda, 1967; Smith *et al.*, 1980) and released extracellularly by diphtheria cells as a single polypeptide chain with a molecular weight of about 62,000 (Collier and Kandel, 1971; Gill and Dinius, 1971) by nontoxinogenic strains of *Corynebacterium diphtheriae* such as C7(−), after lytic infection (Matsuda and Barksdale, 1967) or after lysogenization with *β* phages (Barksdale and Pappenheimer, 1954; Freeman, 1951; Groman, 1953). The toxin gene can be expressed when it is carried by either a prophage or a nonintegrated phage as nonreplicating (Gill *et al.*, 1972) or replicating phage DNA. The question of whether the phage genome codes for the toxin or merely depressed a bacterial gene which can then synthesize the toxin has now been answered. *β* Phages carrying a mutated toxin gene were isolated after treatment of the phage with the mutagen nitrosoguanidine (Uchida *et al.*, 1971 and 1973a). Lysogens with the phage can produce nontoxic proteins with greatly reduced toxicity that cross-react with diphtheria toxin (Table 1). The toxin is synthesized in a cell-free system from *E. coli* using DNA from *β* phage (Murphy *et al.*, 1974). The toxin of the *β* phage genome was shown to be the structural gene for diphtheria toxin. The *tox* gene has been mapped (Holmes and Barksdale, 1970; Matsuda *et al.*, 1971; Singer, 1973; Laird and Groman, 1976).

TABLE 1. *Some Properties of CRMs**

	MW	Toxicity	Enzymic Activity		Binding to Receptor	Sizes of Main Tryptic Products
			Intact	Nicked		
Toxin	62,000	100	0	100	100	22,000 + 40,000
Toxoid	62,000	0	0	0	0	
Fragment A	22,000	0	100		0	
CRM22	22,000	0	100		0	
CRM30	30,000	0	30	100	0	22,000 + <10,000
CRM45	45,000	0	30	100	0	22,000 + 20,000
CRM176	62,000	0.5–1	0	10	100	22,000 + 40,000
CRM197	62,000	0	0	0	100	22,000 + 40,000
CRM228	62,000	0	0	0	20	22,000 + 40,000
A45–B176**	62,000	100		100	100	
A45–B197	62,000	100		100	100	
A45–B228	62,000	20		100	20	

A45 was obtained from CRM45 and was identical to fragment A of toxin.
B176 was obtained from CRM176.
* Modified from T. Uchida *et al.* (1973a) and A. M. Pappenheimer Jr. (1977).
** Hybrid toxin was formed from A45 and B176.

The yield of toxin by the bacterium is markedly affected by inorganic iron in the medium. Bacterial mutants which produce toxin at the normal level in the presence of excess iron were isolated (Kanei *et al.*, 1977). When β phage from the parent C7(β) was used to convert a cured strain of the mutant lysogenization, the resulting lysogenes produced toxin in the presence of iron, whereas when β phage from the mutant was lysogenized in the C7($-$) strain, the lysogens could not produce toxin in the presence of iron. A host bacterial factor(s) is involved in inhibition of toxin production by iron (Kanei *et al.*, 1977).

3. DIPHTHERIA TOXIN INHIBITS PROTEIN SYNTHESIS OF SUSCEPTIBLE CELLS BY CATALYZING ADP-RIBOSYLATION OF ELONGATION FACTOR 2

It was found that diphtheria toxin has cytotoxic activity on cultured cells and inhibits the incorporation of amino acids into the cells (Strauss and Hendee, 1959). Inhibition of protein synthesis was the earliest and more striking effect of the toxin (Strauss and Hendee, 1959; Strauss, 1960). The cultured cells exhibited a level of sensitivity corresponding to that of the parent animals (Solotorovsky and Gabliks, 1965). Susceptible eukaryotic cells include those of humans, monkeys, guinea-pigs, hamsters, chickens and rabbits etc. Cells derived from these animals are sensitive to the toxin; for example, established cell lines, such as HeLa, KB, FL (human), Vero, CV1, LLCMK2 (monkey kidney), BHK and CHO (hamster) are sensitive to the toxin. Rats and mice are insensitive to the toxin and thus L cells, Ehrlich's ascites tumor cells (mouse) and normal rat kidney (NRK) cells are also insensitive to the toxin. Rat and mouse cells are more than 10,000 times more resistant to the toxin than susceptible cells (Table 2).

The inhibition of protein synthesis in susceptible cells by the toxin provides a good system for studying the mode of action of diphtheria toxin, and study on the mode of action of the toxin has been focused on the mechanism of its inhibition of protein synthesis in the cells. Cell-free protein synthesizing systems have been used to study the detailed mechanism of inhibition of protein synthesis by the toxin.

Collier and Pappenheimer (1964) found that inhibition of protein synthesis by the toxin in a cell free protein synthesizing system of reticulocyte extracts required the cofactor NAD^+ (nicotinamide adenine dinucleotide).

Subsequently Collier (1967) showed that the target of the action of the toxin is elongation factor 2 (EF2), polypeptidyl-tRNA translocase. EF2 (MW $\sim$100,000) is required for

Table 2. *Comparison of Mammalian Cell Line Sensitivities to* Pseudomonas aeruginosa *Exotoxin (PAT) and Diphtheria Toxin (DT)**

| Cell line | | TCLD$_{50}$, ng/ml** | |
Name	Species source	PAT	DT
Henle 407	Human	0.70	0.20
WI-38	Human	1.5	0.20
HeLa	Human	14	1.5
KB	Human	3.0	0.3
WISH	Human	9.0	0.7
HEp-2	Human	8.0	0.3
LLC-MK2	Monkey	3.0	0.02
Vero	Monkey	15	0.01
BS-C-1	Monkey	50	0.01
HaK	Hamster	10	0.08
BHK-21	Hamster	5.0	0.2
Chick fibroblast	Chicken	2.0	0.15
Y-1	Rat	5.0	1×10^3
Morris heptoma	Rat	70	1×10^3
Glioma	Rat	3.0	1×10^3
L-929	Mouse	0.21	1×10^3
3T3	Mouse	0.15	1×10^3
Neuroblastoma	Mouse	60	1×10^3
S-180	Mouse	2.0	1×10^3
RAG	Mouse	3×10^2	1×10^3

* Modified from Middlebrook J. L. and Dorland R. B. *Can. J. Microbiol.*

** Tissue culture median lethal dose (TCLD$_{50}$) for each cell line as that concentration of toxin which produced 50% of the total change in cell protein (control minus maximum response plateau).

the translocation step of protein synthesis in which the ribosome is moved to the next codon on the mRNA after the peptide bond has been formed with the most recent amino acid to the chain, and in which the GTP is hydrolyzed to GDP (guanosine-5′-diphosphate).

In an elegant series of experiments, trypsin activated toxin was found to be enzymatically active by Honjo *et al.* (1968) and Gill *et al.* (1969a). In the presence of toxin, the adenosine diphosphate ribose moiety of NAD$^+$ was transferred to EF2 and nicotinamide was released into solution according to the following equation:

$$\text{(I)} \quad \text{NAD}^+ + \text{EF2} \leftrightharpoons \text{ADPR-EF2} + \text{nicotinamide} + \text{H}^+$$

The time course of ADP-ribosylation of EF2 was found to be the reciprocal of EF2 inactivation. The addition of nicotinamide to cell-free protein-synthesizing systems not only inhibits the toxin-catalyzed inactivation of EF2 *in vitro* but, in the presence of added toxin, high concentrations will shift the equilibrium to the left and reactivate ADPR-EF2. Under physiological conditions the equilibrium of the reaction lies far to the right. *In vitro* the equilibrium constant (K) has been determined to be 6.3×10^{-4} M. The pH optimum for the ADP-ribosylation of EF2 is 8.5 and 5.2 for the reverse reaction.

It has been shown that at least 75% of the EF2 in rat liver is bound to ribosomes. EF2 bound to ribosomes is resistant to ADP-ribosylation. The rate-limiting step in the toxin-catalyzed reaction may be the rate of release of EF2 from the ribosome. It has been found by Montanaro *et al.* (1971) and Bermek (1972) that EF2 inactivated by ADP-ribosylation still binds to risosomes in the presence of GTP, even though it does not participate in protein synthesis.

The treatment of ADPR-EF2 with snake venom phosphodiesterase cleaves adenosine-5′-phosphate (AMP) from the complex, leaving ribosephosphate covalently bound to EF2. This suggests that ADP-ribose is bound to EF2 through the ribose moiety of nicotinamide mononucleotide (NMN). Tryptic digestion of ^{14}C-ADPR-EF2, followed by

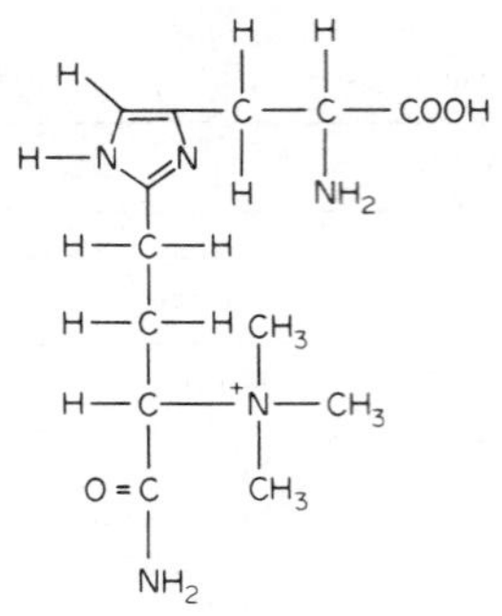

2−[3−(carboxyamido)−3−(trimethylammonio) propyl] histidine

FIG. 1. Structure of Diphthamide (Boldey *et al.*, 1979).

electrophoresis, has resolved one radioactive peptide of 13 amino acids with the following sequence: Phe-Asp-Val-His-Asp-Val-Thr-Leu-His-Ala-Ile-X-Arg.

ADP-ribose is bound to the unknown residue X. This residue is weakly basic and does not correspond to any amino acid commonly found in proteins. Recently Boldy *et al.* (1979) have elucidated the nature of the residue, for which the trivial name 'diphthamide' had been proposed (Structure depicted in Fig. 1).

It has been found recently that the ADP-ribosylation of EF2 by diphtheria toxin is not unique. Iglewski and Kabat (1975) have reported that *Pseudomonas aeruginosa* exotoxin catalyses an NAD-dependent inhibition of eukaryotic protein synthesis. The exotoxin has been shown to transfer the ADPR moiety of NAD and EF2; furthermore ADPR is covalently attached to the same tryptic peptide of EF2, as that in diphtheria toxin inactivated EF2.

A striking difference, however, has been observed in regards to the sensitivities of eukaryotic cells and animals to these toxins: rats and mice are sensitive to *P. aeruginosa* exotoxin whereas monkeys, guinea-pigs, hamsters and even humans are relatively resistant.

Resistant cells require 10,000–100,000 times more toxin than the sensitive cells to give equivalent levels of inhibition of protein synthesis; yet the rates of endocytosis in all these cell lines are almost identical (1–2% of cell-volume per hr at 30°C; Boquet and Pappenheimer, 1978). Toxin-resistant mutants of sensitive cell lines have been isolated in several laboratories (Moehring and Moehring, 1977; Moehring *et al.*, 1980; Gupta and Siminovitch, 1978; Draper *et al.*, 1979).

In mutants of one class, resistance has been shown to be at the membrane level. Draper *et al.* (1979) have described a mutant Chinese hamster V79 cell line in which resistance to diphtheria toxin results from a decrease in the cell surface receptor's affinity to diphtheria toxin, thus rendering it unable to facilitate the toxin's internalization.

In somatic cell mutations of one other class at least two types might effect the sensitivity of EF2 to ADP-ribosylation by diphtheria and also Pseudomonas toxins. One would be a mutation in the structural gene for EF2, and another would be a mutation altering a component of the post-translational modification system that directs the biosynthesis of X.

4. DIPHTHERIA TOXIN CONSISTS OF TWO FRAGMENTS A AND B

About 20 years ago diphtheria toxin was purified to crystalline form by starch block electrophoresis (Kato *et al.*, 1960) or DEAE column chromatography (Raynaud *et al.*, 1965). The toxin is produced by diphtheria bacilli in the form of a single polypeptide chain of 62,000 daltons with two disulfide bridges (Collier, 1975; Pappenheimer, 1977).

Such native form of toxin is named intact toxin. The intact toxin molecule is hydrolyzed easily by splitting the peptide bond in one of the disulfide bridges by mild treatment with trypsin or protease(s) in culture medium. This toxin form is named nicked toxin. Intact and nicked toxin have similar toxicities and show little or no enzymic activity. The nicked toxin is split by reduction of the disulfide bridges with a reducing agent into two peptides, which have been designated as fragment A (MW $\sim$22,000) and fragment B (MW $\sim$ 40,000). Fragment A is situated at the N-terminus (Michael et al., 1972) and has enzymic activity (Drazin et al., 1971; Gill and Pappenheimer, 1971) that catalyzes reaction I. Fragment A has also NAD^+-glycohydrolase activity (Kandel et al., 1974). The rate of hydrolysis of NAD^+ is several orders of magnitude slower than with EF2 as substrate. Intact toxin molecules are proenzymes and the molecules show enzymic activity only when treated with trypsin and then with a thiol reagent. On reduction of the disulfides with thiol the two fragments of nicked toxin remain attached by noncovalent bonds and can be separated from each other and purified only in the presence of thiol and under denaturing conditions. Fragment A has no effect when added to susceptible cells or animals because, although it is enzymically active, it cannot bind to the cell surface and thus cannot enter the cell cytoplasm. But when it is introduced artificially into viable cells, it kills the cells. The activity of fragment A is stable and shows little decrease on heating at 100°C at neutral pH or on exposure to pH 2–12 at room temperature. Fragment A is also fairly resistant to trypsin and chymotrypsin, especially in the presence of NAD (Kandel et al., 1974). The primary structure of fragment A has been determined, and from the data the molecular weight of fragment A was calculated as 21,150 (DeLange et al., 1976).

Fragment B has no ADP-ribosylating activity and it is not toxic, but it is needed for specific attachment of the toxin to receptors on sensitive cells (Uchida et al., 1972). Any possible role of fragment B in the process of entry of either intact toxin, nicked toxin, or fragment A into the cytosol remains to be determined. Fragment B is unstable, and becomes denatured and precipitated after dissociation of nicked toxin at neutral pH, but can be solubilized in borate buffer pH 8.0 (Zanen et al., 1976). Moreover it is rather sensitive to proteases.

Fragments A and B are immunologically distinct: on immunodiffusion against antitoxin, they do not cross-react (Fig. 2) (Pappenheimer et al., 1972). Antifragment A antibody inhibits the enzymic activity of isolated fragment A, but does not neutralize the action of the toxin in vivo (Pappenheimer et al., 1972; Yamaizumi et al., 1978a). Thus most of the antigenic determinants of fragment A seem to be masked in intact toxin; antifragment B antibody neutralizes the toxicity of the toxin in vivo by preventing its attachment to the surface of sensitive cells (Pappenheimer et al., 1972).

5. CROSS-REACTING MATERIALS (CRMs) OF TOXIN

Various proteins that cross-reacted immunologically with toxin but showed little or no toxicity were initially isolated by Uchida et al. (1971 and 1973a). Later some CRMs were also isolated by other laboratories (Laird and Groman, 1976; Holmes, 1976). These proteins were produced by diphtheria cells lysogenized with phages carrying mutation in the structural gene for the toxin, which were isolated as follows (Uchida et al., 1971 and 1973a): C7(β) cells were induced by irradiation with ultraviolet light. The cells were incubated for 15–20 min at 35°C, and then 30–60 μg/ml of nitrosoguanidine was added and incubation was continued for 150 min. The surviving phages were plated on C7($-$)$^{tox-}$, and resistant colonies were picked up from individual turbid plaques, then cultured and tested for toxicity. As expression of the toxin gene is not essential for phage multiplication, a relatively high proportion of phages with mutations of the toxin gene were obtained. When the modified toxin gene was expressed in a bacterial host, proteins with little or no toxicity that cross-reacted with diphtheria toxin were produced. These altered proteins (CRMs) have been particularly useful in studies on the interaction of

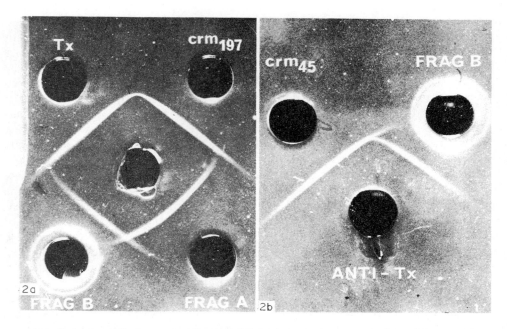

FIG. 2. Immunodiffusion against horse antidiptheria toxin in agar containing 0.5 M urea in buffered saline, from Pappenheimer *et al.* (1972).

diphtheria toxin with sensitive cells, on relationship between structure and activity of the toxin, and as tools in studies on cellular physiology.

As shown in Table 1, CRM22 (Uchida *et al.*, 1979), CRM30 and CRM45 are N-terminal fragments and are presumably products of a premature chain terminating mutation in the toxin gene. The molecular weights of these CRMs are less than that of the toxin (Uchida *et al.*, 1973a). CRM30 and CRM45 have full enzymic activity after activation with trypsin. The enzymic activity, molecular weight and isoelectric point of CRM22 is identical to those of fragment A. These CRMs have no toxicity because they lack all or part of the B fragment required for binding to the surface of sensitive cells.

CRM176, CRM197 and CRM228 have the same molecular weights as intact toxin and are immunologically identical to the toxin (Fig. 2). They are perhaps formed by missense mutations within the structural gene (Uchida *et al.*, 1973a). These CRMs, like intact toxin, are split into fragments A and B by treatment with trypsin and thiol. The A fragments of these CRMs are altered and thus have no enzymic activity (CRM197 and CRM228) or reduced enzymic activity (CRM176). CRM197 and CRM228 have no toxicity at all, while CRM176 shows about 0.5% of the toxicity of the intact toxin.

For examination of the function of the B fragment, toxic protein molecules were reconstituted from nontoxic mutant proteins with a defect in either the A or B region (Uchida *et al.*, 1972 and 1973c). CRM45, having a normal fragment A but lacking part of the B fragment, was mixed with CRM197. The mixture was treated with trypsin in the presence of a reducing agent, and then dialyzed to remove thiol and allow oxidation. In this way, fragment A from CRM45 and fragment B from CRM197 became linked covalently or noncovalently and the reconstituted molecules showed toxicity. The toxicity per microgram of CRM197 was proportional to the ratio of CRM45 to CRM197, indicating that the chance of B197 reassociating with A197 or A45 was random. Fully toxic molecules with the same toxicity as intact toxin were reconstituted at high ratios of A45 to B197 (24:1), thus B of CRM197 is functionally normal. The function of the B regions of CRM176 and CRM228 were determined in the same way. The function of B176 is normal but that of B228 is only about 15% of normal (Uchida *et al.*, 1973c).

CRM197 can compete with toxin for attachment to sensitive cells and thus block the inhibition by toxin of amino acid incorporation into cellular proteins (Fig. 3). The

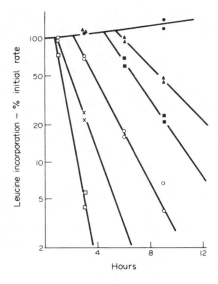

FIG. 3. Competition between toxin and cross-reacting material 197 for entry into HeLa cells. A HeLa cell suspension (2×10^5 cells per ml) in Eagle's medium containing 2% fetal calf serum was distributed among six spinner flasks. To all but the control flask, toxin + cross-reacting material 197 was added to a total concentration of 10^{-6} M. At intervals, 2-ml samples were withdrawn and pulse-labeled with [^{14}C]leucine for 1 hour in the usual manner. ●, control; □, toxin, 10^{-6} M; ×, toxin, 5×10^{-7} M + cross-reacting material 197, 5×10^{-7} M; ○, toxin, 1.7×10^{-7} M + cross-reacting material 197, 8.3×10^{-7} M; ■, toxin 7.1×10^{-8} M + cross-reacting material 197, 9.8×10^{-7} M; ▲, toxin, 3.5×10^{-8} M + cross-reacting material 197, 9.9×10^{-7} M. Uchida et al., (1973b).

blocking activity of CRM197 was compared with that of CRM228. The activity of CRM228 is about five times less than that of CRM197.

Studies on the mode of action of diphtheria toxin have been focused on the mechanism of inhibition of protein synthesis and have shown that the inhibition is due to NAD:EF2-ADP ribose transferase activity. Is this ribosylating activity essential for the lethal effect of toxin in animal? CRM197 has a fragment A without enzymic activity and a normal B fragment. This CRM has no lethal activity in sensitive animals. CRM176 has 8–10% of the enzymic activity of the A fragment and a normal B fragment; its lethal activity is about 0.5% of normal which is very low considering the enzymic activity of A176, because in preliminary experiments we found that A176 is much more easily degraded than fragment A of toxin in the cell cytoplasm. These properties of CRMs suggest that NAD:EF2-ADPR transferase activity is essential for the lethal activity of diphtheria toxin.

6. RECEPTORS AND BINDING OF TOXIN

Fragment A, CRM30 and CRM45 have enzymic activity but do not inhibit protein synthesis of sensitive cells. CRM197 can compete with toxin and block the action of toxin in cultured cells. Although EF2 in all eukaryotic cells is ADP-ribosylated (Pappenheimer and Gill, 1972) and thus protein synthesis can be inhibited by fragment A in the presence of NAD in extracts of these cells, only certain species of eukaryotic cells are sensitive to the toxin (Solotorovsky and Gabliks, 1965; Middlebrook and Dorland, 1977). These findings suggest that there are receptors for toxin on the surface of sensitive cells and that the toxin must be taken up by a specific active process.

When sensitive cells were treated with trypsin their sensitivity decreased to 10–30% of normal, but was restored to the normal level when the cells were incubated at 37°C for about 8 hr (Duncan and Groman, 1969; Moehring and Crispell, 1974; Mekada et al.,

1979). On the other hand, the sensitivity of cells was increased about three times by treatment with neuraminidase (Mekada *et al.*, 1979). Thus the receptors for the toxin may be glycoproteins. Recently it was found that a ^{125}I-labeled glycoprotein which reacts with the toxin has a molecular weight of 168,000 in sodium dodecylsulfate gel electrophoresis. This glycoprotein was found in sensitive lymph-node cells of guinea-pigs, but not in insensitive L cells (Proia *et al.*, 1979). It has not yet been determined whether the purified glycoprotein can bind to the toxin and block the action of the toxin in cultured cells.

Interspecies hybrid cells made by fusion of toxin-sensitive cells with toxin-resistant cells have been tested for sensitivity to toxin. Sensitivity to the toxin is dominant in heterokaryons. When heterokaryons were made by introducing chick embryo erythrocyte nuclei into toxin-resistant cells, these heterokaryons remain insensitive to the toxin until nucleoli appear in the erythrocyte nuclei, and then develop sensitivity to the toxin. Within three days after the appearance of nucleoli in the erythrocyte nuclei, all the heterokaryons become sensitive to the toxin (Dendy and Harris, 1973).

Hybrids between human cells and mouse cells usually eliminate human chromosomes preferentially and randomly. From studies on the chromosomes of the hybrid cells, the gene for sensitivity of human cells was located on human chromosome No. 5 (Creagan *et al.*, 1975).

Cell lines established from monkey kidney are much more sensitive to the toxin than HeLa cells. It was difficult to determine the specific binding of toxin to HeLa cells because of the high ratio of nonspecific association, but with highly sensitive Vero cells, specific binding of ^{125}I-toxin to the cells was clearly demonstrated (Middlebrook *et al.*, 1978). At 37°C, the amount of radioactive toxin associated with the cells increased for 1–2 hr, and then decreased to a steady state level. At 4°C, binding of toxin increased with time to a steady state and the maximum binding at this temperature was about twice that at 37°C. Unlabeled toxin or CRM197 can compete for the binding of radioactive toxin with cells (Fig. 4). A binding constant of $10^8 \, \text{M}^{-1}$ was calculated for the reversible reaction between CRM197 and receptors on sensitive cells (Ittelson and Gill, 1973). At 4°C, the association in Vero cells was $9 \times 10^8 \, \text{l mol}^{-1}$, and there were about $1–2 \times 10^5$ binding sites/cell. In HeLa cells, there were about 4×10^3 binding sites/cell (Boquet and Pappenheimer, 1978).

Adenine nucleotide blocks the action of diphtheria toxin (Middlebrook *et al.*, 1978). The nucleotides do not bind to receptors on the cell, but bind to the toxin. The binding

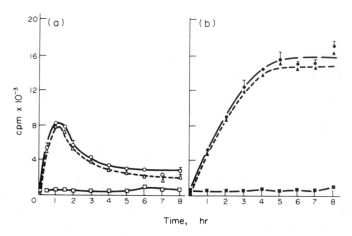

Fig. 4. Kinetics of ^{125}I-labeled diphtheria toxin-Vero cell association. ^{125}I-Toxin (0.6 μg/ml) or ^{125}I-toxin plus unlabeled toxin (6 μg/ml) was added to the cells. At the times indicated, triplicate samples were processed and counted. *Error bars* show standard errors of the mean, which if not shown, was smaller than the symbol. (a) 37°C: ^{125}I-toxin, ○; ^{125}I-toxin + unlabeled toxin, □; difference between ○ and □, △. (b) 4°C: ^{125}I-toxin, ●; ^{125}I-toxin + unlabeled toxin, ■; difference between ● and ■, ▲. Middlebrook *et al.* (1978).

entry of A176 into the cells is much faster than its rate of degradation. Thus it accumulates in the cells and the ratio of the amounts of the two proteins in the cytoplasm becomes the same in one week.

8. PASSAGE OF DIPHTHERIA TOXIN FRAGMENT A THROUGH THE CELL MEMBRANE

Diphtheria toxin binds to cell surface receptors of susceptible cells, then at least fragment A of the toxin reaches the cytoplasm to exert its lethal effect by inhibiting protein synthesis. It is uncertain whether the fragment A region penetrates the lipid bilayer of the cell membrane directly after binding of the toxin to the cell surface, or whether toxin molecules bound to the cell surface are internalized as endocytotic vesicles and fragment A then escapes degradation and is released into the cytoplasm. In either case, fragment A must penetrate the lipid bilayer to reach the cytoplasm. The hydrophobic region of the toxin and low pH conditions are probably essential in the initial stage of this penetration.

Methylamine and chloroquine prevent the action of diphtheria toxin in sensitive cultured cells, they do not affect the uptake of the toxin by the cells but block its degradation after its uptake (Leppla et al., 1980; Mekada et al., 1981). It is thought that the toxin enters sensitive cells by endocytosis and that this lysosomal processing is an essential step in penetration of fragment A into the cytoplasm. By adding methylamine, however, the cytotoxin action of ricin toxin was stimulated about 3–5 times. The actions of hybrid toxin ricin A-SS-*Wistaria floribunda* (WF) subunit and diphtheria A-SS-WF subunit were also both stimulated by methylamine (Mekada et al., 1981). The inhibition or stimulation by methylamine or chloroquine of the action of toxins depends upon the mode of initial binding of the toxins to the cell surface. At present it is difficult to be certain that lysosomal processing is actually an essential step in the mechanism by which fragment A of the toxin reaches the cytoplasm. Such lysosomal enzymes do not play an important role for penetration of the toxin, however acidic pH of lysosome vesicles is important for the penetration and both chloroquine and amines are known to increase the lysosomal pH. These agents inhibit infection of Semliki Forest virus to cells. If the pH is 6.0 or lower the virus infects the cell even in the presence of these agents, and fusion of the viral membrane and the lipid vesicle membranes occurs efficiently (Helenius et al., 1980). Diphtheria toxin acts on sensitive cells at low pH even in the presence of amines (Olsnes et al., 1974). Action of CRM45 on cells is blocked by amines, but this effect of amines is not observed in acidic condition. Although fragment A of hybrid toxins such as the A-SS-WF subunit, does not need acidic conditions for membrane penetration, fragment A of native toxin bound to sensitive cells must penetrate membranes by different ways because of a requirement for acidic conditions for membrane penetration to reach the cell cytoplasm (Uchida et al., 1978).

Two kinds of hybrid toxins, fragment A-SS-WF subunit and ricin A-SS-WF subunit, were formed using the intrinsic sulfhydrates of each protein. *Wistaria floribunda* lectin, which specifically binds to *N*-acetyl-D-galactosamine, consists of two identical subunits joined together covalently by a single disulfide bond (Kurokawa et al., 1976). The A chain of ricin toxin contains more hydrophobic amino acid residues than fragment A of diphtheria toxin (Funatsu et al., 1978; DeLange et al., 1976): hydrophobic residues are present in certain parts of the whole amino acid sequence of ricin A and especially in the C-terminus (Funatsu et al., 1978). The A chain of ricin has much higher affinity for lipids than the fragment A of diphtheria toxin or native toxin (Uchida et al., 1980). The toxicity of the hybrid ricin A-SS-WF, estimated by measuring inhibition of protein synthesis of cultured cells, was about 100–200 times that of the hybrid of diphtheria A-SS-WF (Uchida et al., 1980). Although fragment A of diphtheria toxin has no hydrophobic region, CRM45, which is a nontoxic form of the toxin (Uchida et al., 1971), has a hydrophobic region (Boquet et al., 1976) and lacks the C-terminal region of the toxin of molecular weight 17,000. The hydrophobic region of CRM45 is found in the B45-fragment. Though no hydrophobic region is exposed in the native form of diphtheria toxin, the toxin binds to receptors through its C-terminal part (MW $\sim 17,000$) and then undergoes a conformational change with exposure of its hydrophobic region. It is uncertain when the disulfide bridge linking fragment A and B is reduced. If the disulfide bridge is modified, but not cleaved by thiol, the protein has no toxicity (D. G. Gilliland and R. J. Collier, personal communication). As glycoproteins of the cell surface have some sulfhydryl groups, if reduction of the disulfide bridge occurs on the cell surface after binding of the toxin to receptors, the A and B fragments could remain to bind noncovalently with each other, and the hydrophobic region of the B fragment could still function in facilitating entry of the A fragment into the cytoplasm. It is not yet known how the hydrophylic fragment A passes though the lipid bilayer of the membrane to reach the cytoplasm. Intrinsic proteins may be involved in transport of such hydrophylic proteins in the membrane.

9. FRAGMENT A IN THE CYTOSOL

Although the mechanism of entry of diphtheria toxin into cells is not yet understood, it has been established that fragment A has potent enzymic activity and exerts its lethal effect by its enzymic activity in the cytoplasm. Fragment A has thus been used as a biological marker to establish methods for introducing macromolecules into the cytoplasm of living cells and to examine various aspects of cellular physiology.

Diphtheria toxin binds to and enters sensitive cells to kill them by inhibiting protein synthesis. Recently methods have been developed for introducing macromolecules into viable mammalian cells (Furusawa et al., 1976; Poste et al., 1976) and molecules can be introduced quantitatively by the erythrocyte ghost-fusion method using a fluorescence activated cell sorter (FACS) (Mekada et al., 1978). In this method human erythrocytes are suspended in phosphate buffered saline (PBS) containing a known number of molecules of fragment A with a constant amount of FITC-BSA (fluorescein isothiocyanate-bovine serum albumin) as a fluorescence marker. The erythrocytes are then first dialysed against a hypotonic solution and then against PBS. In this way fragment A and FITC-BSA are trapped within resealed erythrocyte ghosts. Since the concentration of fragment A enclosed in the ghost is the same as that in the mixture before dialysis, the number of molecules of fragment A trapped per ghost can be calculated from the initial concentration of fragment A. Using this method, fragment A and FITC-BSA were introduced into L cells by virus-mediated cell fusion of the cells with the ghosts, and the mononuclear recipients that had fused with only one erythrocyte ghost were separated in a FACS on the basis of their cell size and fluorescence intensity. After isolation of the cell population, the viability of cells containing known numbers of fragment A was examined by measuring colony-forming ability. The results showed that one molecule of fragment A was sufficient to kill a cell. When various numbers of fragment A176 molecules obtained from CRM176 were introduced into living cells in the same way, 100–200 molecules of fragment A176 were needed to kill the cell (Yamaizumi et al., 1978b).

When antifragment A antibody was introduced into toxin-sensitive cells by the same ghost-fusion method, the recipient cells were resistant to the action of the toxin (Yamaizumi et al., 1978a). Furthermore, using this system in which CRM176 acts on the sensitive cells containing antifragment A antibody, the efficiency of the antigen–antibody reaction within living cells and the functional stability of antibody was studied (Yamaizumi et al., 1979). When about 1,500 molecules of antifragment A antibody were introduced into toxin-sensitive Vero cells or FL cells, these cells became resistant to the toxin and formed normal colonies (Fig. 7). Transfer of about 300 molecules of A176 to cells containing antibody under these conditions resulted in quantitative precipitation in vitro in a molar ratio of antifragment A antibody to fragment A of eight to one. Thus, the antigen–antibody reaction took place in living cells as in a test tube. The functional stability of the antibody in cells was examined by exposing Vero cells containing subminimal amounts of anti-fragment A IgG to CRM176 at various times after introduction of

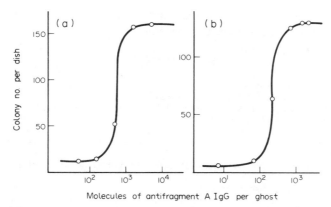

FIG. 7. Neutralization of Fragment A-176 with Anti-fragment A IgG inside cells. Plated FL cells (a) (600 cells per dish) and Vero cells (b) (800 cells per dish) were fused with red cell ghosts containing various numbers of molecules of antifragment A IgG. The cells were exposed to CRM 176 at 20 μg/ml for 11 hr (FL cells) or 400 μg/ml for 2 hr (Vero cells). After incubation in medium containing antitoxin for 1 day, they were cultured for a further 6 days in fresh medium. Colonies in duplicate dishes were counted after staining the cells with Giemsa. The number of molecules of antifragment A IgG trapped per ghost was estimated from the efficiency of incorporation of IgG by ghosts (Yamaizumi et al., 1978b), the proportion of specific antifragment A IgG in crude antifragment A IgG and the volume of ghosts (150 μm³). Yamaizumi et al (1979).

anti-fragment A IgG. More than 50% of the initial activity of the antibody to neutralize the action of CRM176 still remained after incubation for 20 hr (Yamaizumi et al., 1979).

Now that methods for introducing macromolecules into viable cells have been established, fragment A can be used as a biological marker for confirming that the molecules have reached the cell cytoplasm. A mixture of HVJ (Sendai virus) spike proteins, fragment A, lecithin and cholesterol was solubilized in a sucrose solution containing a nonionic neutral detergent, and liposomal vesicles containing fragment A were formed by removal of the detergent. The cytotoxicity to L cells of liposomes containing fragment A and associated with HVJ spikes was about 300 times that of similar liposomes without HVJ spikes, although the binding of liposomes without spikes to the cells was about 2–3 times greater than that of liposomes with spikes. These results suggest that the spike proteins associated with liposomes effectively transport fragment A trapped in the liposomes into the cell cytoplasm (Uchida et al., 1979). Reassembled HVJ envelopes containing CRM45 can be prepared, and are cytotoxic to mammalian cells (Uchida et al., 1977). But liposomes which contain surface-bound HVJ spikes are even more effective for introducing foreign proteins into cells than reassembled HVJ envelopes. This shows fragment A is a good marker protein to find the activity of fusion between liposomes and living cells by HVJ spikes.

10. CONCLUDING REMARKS

It is now thought that the NAD:EF2-ADP ribose transferase activity of fragment A is the lethal activity of the toxin for sensitive cultured cells and animals. Fragment A is easily obtainable from cultures of C7hm723(β22), which produce fragment A alone in the presence of excess iron. The properties of fragment A are now well known, fragment A is one of the best markers for confirming that foreign proteins have reached the cell cytoplasm after various treatments. Although much is known about the relation between the structure and activity of the toxin, information is still required on the structure–activity relation of fragment B of the toxin, especially in relation to the entry of the toxin into sensitive cells.

The mechanisms of uptake of toxin (fragment A) by sensitive cells have been studied, but little is yet known about them. Recently mutant cells that are resistant to the toxin have been isolated, and these should be useful in further studies on the uptake mechanisms and various aspects of cell physiology and molecular biology of mammalian cells. Thus studies on diphtheria toxin are now extending to new fields.

REFERENCES

Barksdale, W. L. and Pappenheimer, A. M. Jr. (1954) Phage–host relationships in nontoxinogenic and toxinogenic diphtheria bacilli. *J. Bacteriol.* **67**: 220–232.

Bermek, E. (1972) Formation of a complex involving ADP-ribosylated human translocation factor, guanosine nucleotide and ribosomes. *FEBS Lett.* **23**: 95–99.

Boldy, W., VanNess B. G. and Howard, J. B. (1979) The purification, properties and proposed structure of the novel amino acid in elongation factor 2 which is ADP-ribosylated by diphtheria toxin. Abstract of *Symposium on PolyADP ribose*.

Boquet, P. and Pappenheimer, A. M. Jr (1978) Interaction of diphtheria toxin with mammalian cell membranes. *J. biol. Chem.* **251**: 5770–5778.

Boquet, P., Silverman, M. S., Pappenheimer, A. M. Jr. and Vernon, W. (1976) Binding of Triton X-100 to diphtheria toxin cross-reacting material 45, and their fragments. *Proc. natn Acad. Sci. USA* **73**: 4449–4453.

Cassel, D. and Pfeuffer, T. (1978) Mechanism of cholera-toxin action: Covalent modification of the guanyl nucleotide-binding protein of adenylate cyclase system. *Proc. natn. Acad. Sci. USA* **75**: 2669–2673.

Collier, R. J. (1967) Effect of diphtheria toxin on protein synthesis: Inactivation of one of the transfer factors. *J. mol. Biol.* **25**: 83–98.

Collier, R. J. (1975) Diphtheria toxin: Mode of action and structure. *Bacteriol. Reviews* **39**: 54–85.

Collier, R. J. and Kandel, J. (1971) I. Thiol-dependent dissociation of a fraction of toxin into enzymically active and inactive fragments. *J. biol. Chem.* **246**: 1496–1503.

Collier, R. J. and Pappenheimer, A. M. Jr. (1964) Studies on the mode of action of diphtheria toxin. II. Effect of toxin on amino acid incorporation in cell free systems. *J. exp. Med.* **120**: 1019–1039.

Creagan, R. P., Chen, S. and Ruddle, F. H. (1975) Genetic analysis of the cell surface: Association of human chromosome 5 with sensitivity to diphtheria toxin in mouse–human somatic cell hybrids. *Proc. natn. Acad. Sci. USA* **72**: 2237–2241.

DeLange, R. J., Drazine, R. E. and Collier, R. J. (1976) Amino acid sequence of fragment A, an enzymically active fragment from diphtheria toxin. *Proc. natn. Acad. Sci. USA* **73**: 69–72.

Dendy, P. R. and Harris, H. (1973) Sensitivity to diphtheria toxin as a species-specific marker in hybrid cells. *J. Cell Sci.* **12**: 831–837.

Draper, R. K., Chin, D., Eurey-Owens, D., Scheffler, I. E. and Simon, M. I. (1979) Biochemical and genetic characterization of three hamster cell mutants resistant to diphtheria toxin. *J. Cell Biol.* **83**: 116–125.

Drazin, R. J., Kandel, J. and Collier, R. J. (1971) Structure and activity of diphtheria toxin. II. Attack by trypsin at a specific site within the intact molecule. *J. biol. Chem.* **246**: 1504–1510.

Duncan, J. L. and Groman, N. B. (1969) Activity of diphtheria toxin. II. Early events in the intoxication of HeLa cells. *J. Bacteriol.* **98**: 963–969.

Freeman, V. J. (1951) Studies on the virulence of bacteriophage-infected strains of *Corynebacterium diphtheriae*. *J. Bacteriol.* **61**: 675–688.

Funatsu, G., Yoshitake, S. and Funatsu, M. (1978) Primary structure of the A chain of ricin D. *Agric. Biol. Chem.* **42**: 501–503.

Furusawa, M., Yamaizumi, M., Nishimura, T., Uchida, T. and Okada, Y. (1976) Use of erythrocyte ghosts for injection of substances into animal cells by cell fusion. In: *Methods in Cell Biology*, XIV, pp. 73–80, Prescott, D. M. (ed).

Gill, D. M. and Dinius, L. L. (1971) Observations on the structure of diphtheria toxin. *J. biol. Chem.* **246**: 1485–1491.

Gill, D. M. and Merrin, R. (1978) ADP-ribosylation of membrane proteins catalyzed by cholera toxin: Basis of the activation of adenylate cyclase. *Proc. natn. Acad. Sci. USA* **75**: 3050–3054.

Gill, D. M. and Pappenheimer, A. M. Jr. (1971) Structure–activity relationships in diphtheria toxin. *J. biol. Chem.* **246**: 1492–1495.

Gill, D. M., Pappenheimer, A. M. Jr. and Baseman, J. B. (1969b) Studies on transferase II using diphtheria toxin. *Cold Spring Harbor Symp. Quant. Biol.* **34**: 595–602.

Gill, D. M., Pappenheimer, A. M. Jr., Brown, R. and Kurnick, J. J. (1969a) Studies on the mode of action of diphtheria toxin VII. Toxin-stimulated hydrolysis of nicotinamide adenine dinucleotide in mammalian cell extracts. *J. exp. Med.* **129**: 1–21.

Gill, D. M., Uchida T. and Singer, R. A. (1972) Expression of diphtheria toxin genes carried by integrated and nonintegrated phage beta. *Virology* **50**: 664–668.

Goor, R. S. and Maxwell, E. S. (1970) The diphtheria toxin-dependent adenosine diphosphate ribosylation of rat liver aminoacyl transferase II. *J. biol. Chem.* **245**: 616–623.

Groman, N. B. (1953) Evidence for the induced nature of the change from nontoxinogenicity to toxigenicity in *Corynebacterium diphtheriae* as a result of exposure to specific bacteriophage. *J. Bacteriol.* **66**: 184–191.

Gupta, R. S. and Siminovitch, L. (1978) Diphtheria-toxin-resistant mutants of CHO cells affected in protein synthesis: A novel phenotype. *Somatic Cell Genetics* **4**: 553–571.

Gupta, R. S. and Siminovitch, L. (1980) Diphtheria toxin resistance in chinese hamster cells: Genetic and biochemical characteristics of the mutants affected in protein synthesis. *Somatic Cell Genetics* **6**: 361–379.

Helenius, A., Karlenbeck, J., Simon, K. and Fries, E. (1980) On the entry of Semliki Forest virus into BHK-21 cells. *J. cell Biol.* **84**: 404–420.

Holmes, R. K. (1976) Characterization and genetic mapping of nontoxinogenic(*tox*) mutants of corynebacteriophage beta. *J. Virol.* **19**: 195–207.

Holmes, R. K. and Barksdale, L. W. (1970) Comparative studies with *tox*⁺ and *tox*⁻ corynebacteriophages. *J. Virol.* **5**: 783–794.

HONJO, T., NISHIZUKA, Y. and HAYAISHI, O. (1969) Adenosine diphosphoribosylation of aminoacyl transferase II by diphtheria toxin. *Cold Spring Harbor Symp. Quant. Biol.* **34**: 603–608.

HONJO, T., NISHIZUKA, Y., HAYAISHI O. and KATO, I. (1968) Diphtheria-toxin-dependent adenosine diphosphate ribosylation of aminoacyl transferase II and inhibition of protein synthesis. *J. biol. Chem.* **243**: 2553–3555.

IGLEWSKI, B. H. and KABAT, D. (1975) NAD-dependent inhibition of protein synthesis by *Pseudomonas aeruginosa* toxin. *Proc. natn. Acad. Sci. USA* **72**: 2284–2288.

ITTELSON, T. R. and GILL, D. M. (1973) Diphtheria toxin: Specific competition for cell receptors. *Nature, Lond.* **242**: 330–332.

IVINS, B., SAELINGER, C. B., BONVENTURE, P. F. and WOSCINSKI, C. (1975) Chemical modulation of diphtheria toxin action on cultured mammalian cells. *Infect. Immun.* **11**: 665–674.

KANDEL, J., COLLIER, R. J. and CHUNG, D. W. (1974) Interaction of fragment A from diphtheria toxin with nicotinamide adenine dinucleotide. *J. biol. Chem.* **249**: 2088–2097.

KANEI, C., UCHIDA, T. and YONEDA, M. (1977) Isolation of *Corynebacterium diphtheriae* C7(β) of bacterial mutants that produce toxin in medium with excess iron. *Infect. Immun.* **18**: 203–209.

KATO, I., NAKAMURA, H., UCHIDA, T., KOYAMA, J. and KATSURA, T. (1960) Purification of diphtheria toxin. II. The isolation of crystalline toxin–protein and some of its properties. *Jap. J. exp. Med.* **30**: 129–145.

KIM, K. and GROMAN, N. B. (1965a) Inhibition of diphtheria toxin action by ammonium salts and amines. *J. Bacteriol.* **90**: 1552–1556.

KIM, K. and GROMAN, N. B. (1965b) Mode of inhibition of diphtheria toxin by ammonium chloride. *J. Bacteriol.* **90**: 1557–1562.

KUROKAWA, T., TSUDA, M. and SUGINO, Y. (1976) Purification and characterization of a lectin from *Wistaria floribunda* seeds. *J. biol. Chem.* **251**: 5686–5693.

LAIRD, W. and GROMAN, N. B. (1976) Prophage map of converting corynebacteriophage beta. *J. Virol.* **19**: 208–219.

LEPPLA, S. H., DORLAND, R. B. and MIDDLEBROOK, J. L. (1980) Inhibition of diphtheria toxin degradation and cytotoxic action by chloroquine. *J. biol. Chem.* **255**: 2247–2250.

LORY, S. and COLLIER, R. J. (1980) Diphtheria toxin: Nucleotide binding and toxin heterogeneity. *Proc. natn. Acad. Sci. USA* **77**: 267–271.

MATSUDA, M. and BARKSDALE W. L. (1967) System for the investigation of the bacteriophage directed synthesis of diphtheria toxin. *J. Bacteriol.* **93**: 722–730.

MATSUDA, M., KANEI, C. and YONEDA, M. (1971) Temperature sensitive mutants of nonlysogenizing corynebacteriophage hv: Their isolation, characterization and relation to toxinogenesis. *Biken J.* **14**: 119–130.

MEKADA, E., UCHIDA, T. and OKADA, Y. (1979) Modification of the cell surface with neuraminidase increases the sensitivities of cells to diphtheria toxin and *Pseudomonas aeruginosa* exotoxin. *Exp. cell Res.* **123**: 137–146.

MEKADA, E., UCHIDA, T. and OKADA, Y. (1981) Methylamine stimulates the action of ricin toxin but inhibits that of diphtheria toxin. *J. biol. Chem.* in press.

MEKADA, E., YAMAIZUMI, M., UCHIDA, T. and OKADA, Y. (1978) Quantitative introduction of a given macromolecule into cells by fusion with erythrocyte ghosts using a fluorescence activated cell sorter. *J. histochem. Cytochem.* **26**: 1067–1073.

MICHAEL, A., ZANEN, J., MONIER, C., CRISPEELS, C. and DIRKX, J. (1972) Partial characterization of diphtheria toxin and its subunits. *Biochem. biophys. Acta* **257**: 249–256.

MIDDLEBROOK, J. L. and DORLAND, R. B. (1977) Response of cultured mammalian-cells to the exotoxins of *Pseudomonas aeruginosa* and *Corynebacterium diphtheriae*: Differential cytoxicity. *Can. J. Microbiol.* **23**: 183–189.

MIDDLEBROOK, J. L., DORLAND, R. B. and LEPPLA, S. H. (1978) Association of diphtheria toxin with Vero cells. *J. biol. Chem.* **253**: 7325–7330.

MOEHRING, T. J. and CRISPELL, J. P. (1974) Enzyme treatment of KB cells altered effect of diphtheria toxin. *Biochem. Biophys. Res. Comm.* **60**: 1446–1452.

MOEHRING, J. T. and MOEHRING, J. M. (1977) Selection and characterization of cells resistant to diphtheria toxin and Pseudomonas exotoxin A: Presumptive translational mutants. *Cell* **11**: 447–454.

MOEHRING, J. M., MOEHRING, T. J. and DANLEY, D. (1980) Posttranslational modification of elongation factor 2 in diphtheria toxin resistant mutants of CHO-K1 cells. *Proc. natn. Acad. Sci. USA* **77**: 1010–1014.

MONTANARO, L., SPERTI, S. and MATTIOLI, A. (1971) Interaction of ADP-ribosylated aminoacyl transferase II with GTP and with ribosomes. *Biochem. biophys. Acta* **238**: 493–497.

MURPHY, J. R., PAPPENHEIMER, A. M. JR. and deBORMS, S. T. (1974) Synthesis of diphtheria tox⁻ gene products in *Escherichia coli* extracts. *Proc. natn. Acad. Sci. USA* **71**: 11–15.

OLSNES, S., REFSNES, K. and PHIL, A. (1974) Mechanism of action of the toxic lectins abrin and ricin. *Nature (Lond.)* **249**: 627–631.

PAPPENHEIMER, A. M. JR. (1977) Diphtheria toxin. *Ann. Rev. Biochem.* **46**: 69–94.

PAPPENHEIMER, A. M. JR. and GILL, D. M. (1972) Inhibition of protein synthesis by activated diphtheria toxin. In: *Molecular mechanisms of antibiotic action on protein synthesis*, pp. 134–149, MUNOZ, E., GARCIA-FERRANDIZ, F. and VASQUEZ, D. (eds). Elsevier, Amsterdam.

PAPPENHEIMER, A. M., UCHIDA, T. and HARPER, A. A. (1972) An immunological study of the diphtheria toxin molecule. *Immunochemistry* **9**: 891–906.

POSTE, G., PAPAHADJOPOULOS, D. and VAIL, W. J. (1976) Lipid vesicles as carriers for introducing biologically active materials into cells, In: *Methods in Cell Biology*, **XIV**, pp. 34–72, PRESCOTT, D. M. (ed).

PROIA, R. L., HART, D. A., HOLMES, R. K., HOLMES, K. V. and EIDELS, L. (1979) Immunoprecipitation and partial characterization of diphtheria toxin-binding glycoproteins from surface of guinea pig cells. *Proc. natn. Acad. Sci. USA.* **76**: 685–689.

RAYNAUD, M., BIZZINI, B. and RELYVELD, E. H. (1965) Composition en amino-acides de la toxine diphtherique. *Bull. Soc. Chim. Biol.* **47**: 261–266.

SINGER, R. (1973) Temperature sensitive mutants of toxinogenic *corynebacteriophage beta*. I. Genetics. *Virology* **55**: 347–356.

SMITH, W. P., TAI, P. C., MURPHY, J. R. and DAVIS, B. D. (1980) A precursor in the cotranslational secretion of diphtheria toxin. *J. Bacteriol.* **141**: 184–189.

SOLOTOROVSKY, M. and GABLIKS, J. (1965) The biological action of diphtheria toxin in cell and tissue culture. In: *Cell culture in the study of bacterial disease*, pp. 5–15, SOLOTOROVSKY, M. (ed). Rutgers University Press, New Brunswick.

STRAUSS, N. and HENDEE, E. D. (1959) The effect of diphtheria toxin on the metabolism of HeLa cells. *J. exp. Med.* **109**: 144–163.

STRAUSS, N. (1960) The effect of diphtheria toxin on the metabolism of HeLa cells. II. Effect on nucleic acid metabolism. *J. exp. Med.* **112**: 351–359.

UCHIDA, T., GILL, D. M. and PAPPENHEIMER, A. M. JR. (1971) Mutation in the structural gene for diphtheria toxin carried by temperate phage beta. *Nature, New Biol.* **233**: 8–11.

UCHIDA, T., KIM, J., YAMAIZUMI, M., MIYAKE, Y. and OKADA, Y. (1979) Reconstitution of lipid vesicles associated with HVJ (Sendai virus) spikes. Purification and some properties of vesicles containing nontoxic fragment A of diphtheria toxin. *J. Cell Biol.* **80**: 10–20.

UCHIDA, T., MEKADA, E. and OKADA, Y. (1980) Hybrid toxin of the A chain of ricin toxin and s subunit of *Wistaria floribunda* lectin. Possible importance of hydrophobic region for entry of toxin into the cell. *J. biol. Chem.* **255**: 6687–6693.

UCHIDA, T., PAPPENHEIMER, A. M. JR. and GREANY, R. (1973a) Diphtheria toxin and elated proteins I. Isolation and some properties of mutant proteins serologically related to diphtheria toxin. *J. biol. Chem.* **248**: 3838–3844.

UCHIDA, T., PAPPENHEIMER, A. M. JR. and HARPER, A. A. (1972) Reconstitution of diphtheria toxin from two nontoxic cross-reacting mutant toxins. *Science* **175**: 901–903.

UCHIDA, T., PAPPENHEIMER, A. M. JR. and HARPER, A. A. (1973b) Diphtheria toxin and related proteins II. Kinetic studies on intoxication of HeLa cells by diphtheria toxin and related proteins. *J. biol. Chem.* **248**: 3845–3850.

UCHIDA, T., PAPPENHEIMER, A. M. JR. and HARPER, A. A. (1973c) Diphtheria toxin and related proteins. III. Reconstitution of hybrid diphtheria toxin from nontoxic mutant proteins. *J. biol. Chem.* **248**: 3851–3854.

UCHIDA, T., YAMAIZUMI, M., MEKADA, E., OKADA, Y., TSUDA, M., KUROKAWA, T. and SUGINO, Y. (1978) Reconstitution of hybrid toxin from fragment A of diphtheria toxin and a subunit of *Wistaria floribunda* lectin. *J. biol. Chem.* **253**: 6307–6310.

UCHIDA, T., YAMAIZUMI, M. and OKADA, Y. (1977) Reassembled HVJ (Sendai virus) envelopes containing nontoxic mutant proteins of diphtheria toxin. *Nature* **266**: 839–840.

UCHIDA, T. and YONEDA, M. (1967) Evidence for the association of membrane with the site of toxin synthesis in *Corynebacterium diphtheriae*. *Biochem. biophys. Acta* **145**: 210–213.

YAMAIZUMI, M., MAKEDA, E., UCHIDA, T. and OKADA, Y. (1978b) One molecule of diphtheria toxin fragment A introduced into a cell can kill the cell. *Cell* **15**: 245–250.

YAMAIZUMI, M., UCHIDA, T., MEKADA, E. and OKADA, Y. (1979) Antibodies introduced into living cells by red cell ghosts are functionally stable in the cytoplasm of the cells. *Cell* **18**: 1009–1014.

YAMAIZUMI, M., UCHIDA, T., OKADA, Y. and FURUSAWA, M. (1978a) Neutralization of diphtheria toxin in living cells by microinjection of antifragment A contained within resealed erythrocyte ghosts. *Cell* **13**: 227–232.

YAMAIZUMI, M., UCHIDA, T., TAKAMATSU, K., and OKADA, Y. in preparation.

ZANEN, J., MUYLDERMANS, G. and BEUGNIER, N. (1976) Competitive antagonists of the action of diphtheria toxin in HeLa cells *FEBS Lett.* **66**: 261–263.

CHAPTER 29

CONSTRUCTION AND PROPERTIES OF CHIMERIC TOXINS—
TARGET SPECIFIC CYTOTOXIC AGENTS *

SJUR OLSNES and ALEXANDER PIHL

Institute for Cancer Research at The Norwegian Radium Hospital, Montebello, Oslo, Norway

1. INTRODUCTION

The greatest problem in cancer chemotherapy is the lack of selectivity of the cytostatic drugs. In spite of tremendous efforts to develop agents suitable for chemical treatment of cancer, the success has so far been limited. None of the cytotoxic agents in current use act specifically on cancer cells.

A great deal of work has been aimed at increasing the specificity of the drugs. The high specificity of hormones and certain drugs involves their recognition and interaction with specific receptors on the cell surface or in the cytosol of the target cells. The interaction of a specific antibody with its antigen on the cell surface is also highly specific. For this reason many attempts have been made in recent years to utilize the selectivity of hormones and antibodies to direct various cytotoxic agents to defined groups of cells.

Much of previous work on antibody linked cytotoxic agents has involved the use of agents such as chlorambucil, methotrexate, daunomycin and adriamycin (see reviews by Gregoriadis, 1977, 1981 and by Ghose and Blair, 1978). A certain selective cytotoxic effect has indeed been obtained in these studies (Kulkarni *et al.*, 1981). However, the main short-coming of this approach is that the conventional cytotoxic agents act stoichiometrically rather than catalytically. Therefore a rather high number of such molecules is needed to achieve the desired cytotoxic effect. If the antibody used is directed against a cell surface antigen which occurs only in low number, it is difficult to deliver the required number of cytotoxic molecules to kill the cells. Clearly, a successful 'magic bullet' requires a very active 'warhead'.

A number of toxic proteins possess the required toxicity due to the fact that they have an enzymatically active A-chain which exerts the toxic effect. The presence in the cytosol of a single A-chain is sufficient to kill a cell. These toxins have one or more B chains which bind the toxins to cell surface receptors. Since receptors for the B-chain of these toxins are present on the surface of most cells of sensitive animals, the unmodified toxins show little selective toxicity.

Currently a number of laboratories are involved in constructing hybrid or chimeric toxins consisting of the enzymatically active moiety of such a protein toxin, linked to a binding moiety derived from a different source. As new binding moieties lectins, protein hormones or their subunits or antibodies or their fragments have been used. The availability of monoclonal antibodies has greatly increased the interest in this approach. Such chimeric toxins not only may have a high cell specificity, but they also have the added advantage that if the complexes are degraded and the enzymatically active A chains are released, they are virtually non toxic to cells. This is in contrast to conjugates involving conventional cytotoxic agents. If these are released from the complexes they will act non specifically. The present review will be restricted to chimeric toxins involving enzymatically active protein toxins.

*The manuscript was completed in February 1983.

2. STRUCTURE AND MECHANISM OF ACTION OF CYTOTOXINS INHIBITING PROTEIN SYNTHESIS

The successful construction of chimeric toxins requires an understanding of the structure and mechanism of action of the natural toxins from which the enzymatically active A-chains are derived. In particular, it is desirable to gain an understanding of the mechanism whereby the toxins are bound to the cell surface, and subsequently transferred to the cytosol. Unfortunately, the latter aspect is still inadequately understood.

Diphtheria toxin, *Pseudomonas aeruginosa* exotoxin A and the plant proteins, abrin, ricin, modeccin, and viscumin all have the general structure shown below

$$\left[\begin{array}{c}\text{enzymatically}\\ \text{active moiety}\end{array}\right]\!-\!S\!-\!S\!-\!\left[\begin{array}{c}\text{binding}\\ \text{moiety}\end{array}\right].$$

The two polypeptide chains which are joined by a disulfide bond have distinctly different functions. The binding moieties attach the toxins to cell surface receptors. The enzymatically active moieties inhibit protein synthesis.

Some of the important properties of these toxins are summarized in Table 1.

2.1. DIPTHERIA TOXIN AND *PSEUDOMONAS AERUGINOSA* EXOTOXIN A

These two toxins inhibit protein synthesis by the same mechanism. However, they differ in their specificity for cell surface receptors.

Diptheria toxin is synthesized as a single polypeptide chain (MW 62,000). It contains an arginine rich region which is easily cleaved by trypsin and several other proteolytic enzymes (Fig. 1). The two fragments are held together by a disulfide bond, but after reduction with 2-mercaptoethanol they can be separated (for review, see Collier, 1976; Pappenheimer, 1977). Also *Pseudomonas aeruginosa* exotoxin A (MW 72,000) is synthesized as a single chain (Iglewski and Sadoff, 1979).

Diphtheria toxin fragment A (MW 21,145) and exotoxin A from *Pseudomonas aeruginosa*, or a 45,000 daltons fragment of it, are enzymes catalyzing the reaction:

$$\text{NAD}^+ + \text{EF2} \rightleftharpoons \text{ADP-ribosyl-EF2} + \text{nicotinamide} + \text{H}^+.$$

The ADP-ribosylated elongation factor 2 retains its ability to bind to ribosomes in the presence of GTP, but it is unable to catalyze the translocation reaction of peptidyl-tRNA from the A site to the P site on the ribosomes and hence it stops the elongation cycle.

The equilibrium of the enzymatic reaction is strongly displaced to the right under the conditions prevailing in the cell. Under appropriate artificial conditions the reaction can, however, be driven in the reverse direction.

The covalent binding of ADP ribose to EF2 occurs at a unique site. EF2 contains here an unusual amino acid, diphthamide, not found in other proteins (Van Ness *et al.*, 1980). Diphthamide is synthesized by post-translational modifications of a histidine residue and several mutant cells lacking enzyme activities required for this modification have been isolated (Moehring *et al.*, 1980). Such mutants are resistant both to diphtheria toxin and to *Pseudomonas aeruginosa* exotoxin A. Mutant cells lacking the histidine residue to be modified have also been isolated (Moehring *et al.*, 1980).

Although highly active in cell free systems, the isolated A fragments are virtually non-toxic to cells and animals.

Diphtheria toxin B-fragment binds the toxin to specific receptors at the cell surface. Most cells of mammalian species are sensitive to diphtheria toxin, but cells from mice and rats are highly resistant. These cells are, however, sensitive to *Pseudomonas aeruginosa* exotoxin A. The nature of the receptors for the two toxins is not known.

The mechanism whereby the A chain of diphtheria toxin gains access to the cytosol, is still inadequately understood. It appears that the first step involves the binding of the toxin through its B chain to cell surface receptors, followed by receptor mediated endocytosis (Draper and Simon, 1980; Sandvig and Olsnes, 1980). The diphtheria toxin receptors play a

TABLE 1. *Some Properties of Enzymatically Active Toxins and their Constituent Peptide Chains*

| Toxin | Molecular weight | | | Binding parameters | | | ID_{50} after 20 hr M | Estimated number of toxin molecules bound at 50% inhibition of protein synthesis[a] |
	Whole	A	B	Cell	Number of binding sites/cell	Apparent K_a M^{-1}		
Diphtheria toxin	62,000	21,145	39,000	Vero	10^5	9×10^8	$\times 10^{-13}$	9
				HeLa	3×10^3	$\sim 10^8$	6×10^{-11}	19
Pseudomonas aeruginosa exotoxin A	72,000			CHO			10^{-12}	
Abrin	65,000	30,000	35,000	HeLa	3×10^7	1.5×10^7	10^{-11}	450^b
Ricin	62,057	30,625	31,422	HeLa	3×10^7	2×10^7	3×10^{-11}	1800^b
Modeccin	63,000	28,000	38,000	HeLa S$_3$	2×10^5	$\sim 10^8$	10^{-12}	20
Viscumin	60,000	29,000	34,000	Mouse 3T3			10^{-10}	
Shigella toxin	65,000	30,500	$5,000^c$	HeLa S$_3$	10^6	10^{10}	5×10^{-15}	27

[a] These values, calculated on the basis of measurements from different laboratories, should only be taken as rough approximations to indicate the relative efficiency of the toxins to internalize the enzymatically active part.

[b] Values corrected for the fact that about 90% of abrin and ricin added to cell cultures is bound to glycoproteins in the fetal calf serum in the medium.

[c] *Shigella* toxin contains 6–7 B-chains.

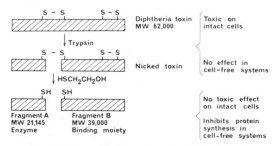

FIG. 1. Schematical structure of diphtheria toxin.

decisive role in the uptake mechanism. Thus, free diphtheria fragment A, which is internalized only by fluid phase pinocytosis, is almost non-toxic. It appears that the receptors for diphtheria toxin are far more efficient than the receptors for abrin and ricin in mediating toxin uptake. Thus, diphtheria toxin is as toxic to HeLa cells as abrin and ricin in spite of the fact that HeLa cells have only 3,000–4,000 receptors for diphtheria toxin and about 3×10^7 receptors for abrin and ricin (Table 1). It should be noted that the binding constants and the toxicity of the A chain in a cell free system are about the same for diphtheria toxin and abrin and ricin.

The B fragment of diphtheria toxin has a hydrophobic part which is believed to play a role in facilitating the entry of the A fragment or the whole toxin by interaction with the lipid membrane (Boquet et al., 1976, Lambotte et al., 1980).

Ammonium chloride, chloroquine and several amines inhibit the toxicity of diphtheria toxin. Recent work has shown that this effect can be abolished by exposing the cells to low pH for a short period of time (Draper and Simon, 1980; Sandvig and Olsnes, 1980). The results indicate that the uptake of diphtheria toxin requires low pH and probably occurs normally in the acidic intracellular vesicles. The protective effect of ammonium chloride is presumably due to its ability to raise the pH in lysosomes. Thus a variety of other compounds which increase the pH of intracellular vesicles also protect against diphtheria toxin (Sandvig et al. 1984). The lag time always seen between exposure of cells to diphtheria toxin and protein synthesis inhibition is also consistent with this.

When the cells are exposed to low pH, the uptake occurs very rapidly and apparently directly through the cell surface.

2.2. ABRIN, RICIN, MODECCIN, and VISCUMIN

The four plant toxins abrin, ricin, modeccin, and viscumin have similar structure and mechanism of action (see Olsnes and Pihl, 1976, 1982; Olsnes et al., 1982; Stirpe et al., 1982) (Fig. 2). The enzymatically active A-chains enter the cytoplasm and inactivate the 60S ribosomal subunit. The nature of the modification is not known. One A chain molecule of abrin and ricin is able to inactivate about 1,500 ribosomes per min in simple buffer solution. The toxin treated ribosomes have reduced ability to bind EF2, and it is likely that the modification involves the binding site for EF2 on the ribosome. In cell free systems a certain residual protein synthesizing activity remains, whereas in intact cells the protein synthesis comes to a complete halt.

The B chains of abrin, ricin, modeccin and viscumin are lectins with specificity for oligosaccharides with terminal galactose. Terminal sialic acid prevents binding of all four toxins to the penultimate galactose residue. Galactose and lactose are potent inhibitors of the binding of all four toxins to cells. Studies of resistant cell mutants indicate that abrin and ricin bind to the same receptors which are different from the receptors for modeccin. In all cases a multitude of cell surface glycoproteins and glycolipids may serve as binding sites.

Also in the case of abrin, ricin, modeccin and viscumin, binding to the cell surface receptors constitutes the first step in the uptake mechanism. The number of receptors for

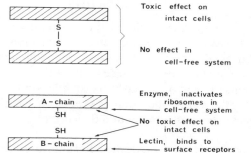

FIG. 2. Schematical structure of abrin, ricin and modeccin.

abrin and ricin is very high (about 3×10^7 per HeLa cell), whereas that for modeccin is about 2×10^5 per HeLa cell (Table 1). Since the association constants are about the same as for dipththeria toxin it is clear that at equal toxin concentrations a much larger concentration of toxin molecules occurs at the cell surface in the case of abrin and ricin than in the case of diphtheria toxin (Table 1). In spite of the fact that the A-chains are approximately equally efficient in inhibiting protein synthesis in a cell free system, the toxicity to HeLa cells is about the same for abrin, ricin and diphtheria toxin.

A temperature dependent lag time in the inhibition of protein synthesis is seen also for the plant toxins. This is consistent with the view that endocytosis is an obligatory process (Sandvig and Olsnes, 1979) although other mechanisms must also be involved. Thus, some resistant cell lines internalize toxins by adsorptive endocytosis at the same rate as the parent cells and the resistance seems to be due to a deficient transfer of receptor bound toxins through the lipid bilayer of the membrane (Sandvig *et al.*, 1978a).

Ammonium chloride and chloroquine protect cells against the toxic action of modeccin, but not against abrin and ricin (Sandvig *et al.*, 1979). The protective mechanism in the case of modeccin is clearly different from that operating in the case of diphtheria toxin. Thus, it could not be counteracted by exposure to low pH. Exposure to low pH did not decrease the lag time when cells were exposed to abrin, ricin or modeccin, in contrast to the situation with diphtheria toxin. Altogether these results indicate that abrin and ricin are taken up by a similar mechanism which differs from that operating in the case of modeccin and diphtheria toxin. There is, however, now convincing evidence that all toxins here discussed enter the cytosol from endocytotic vesicles (Sandvig and Olsnes, 1982). In some cases the entry may involve fusion of endocytotic vesicles with other vesicular compartments in the cell (Sandvig *et al.*, 1984).

2.3. SINGLE-CHAIN TOXIN-RELATED PROTEINS

In many plants, and particularly in their seeds, proteins are found which resemble the A chains of abrin, ricin and modeccin in properties and functions (Barbieri and Stirpe, 1982). In cell free systems they inhibit protein synthesis by the same mechanism and with the same activity as the A-chains of abrin and ricin. However, since they lack the binding moiety, they are non-toxic to intact cells. Such proteins have been isolated from poke weed (Obrig *et al.*, 1973), wheat germ (Roberts and Stewart, 1979), seeds of *Croton tiglium* (crotin), *Jatropha curcas* (curcin) (Stirpe *et al.*, 1976), *Momordica charantia* (Barbieri *et al.*, 1980), and other seeds (Gasperi Campani *et al.*, 1977). One such protein, gelonin, isolated from the seeds of *Gelonium multiflorum*, was shown to be toxic to cells when linked through a disulfide bond to concanavalin A (Stirpe *et al.*, 1980).

2.4. SHIGELLA TOXIN

Shigella toxin is a more complicated molecule than the toxins described above (Fig. 3). It has an enzymatically active A chain of molecular weight about 30,500 daltons which inactivates the 60S ribosomal subunit and inhibits the elongation of polypeptide chains (Olsnes *et al.*, 1981; Reisbig *et al.*, 1981). Interestingly, the A-chain can be proteolytically cleaved into two fragments, A_1 and A_2 joined by a disulfide bond. Only the free A_1 fragment formed after reduction of the disulfide bond possesses enzymatic activity. The binding moiety of the toxin appears to consist of about 6 B chains of molecular weight about 5,000 daltons.

Shigella toxin is highly selective in its mode of action and only a few primate epithelial cells have so far been found to be sensitive (Eiklid and Olsnes, 1980). The toxin is extremely potent to sensitive cells and 0.3 pg/ml culture medium kills 50 % of the HeLa S_3 cells overnight. The high toxicity is partly due to the high affinity of *Shigella* toxin to cell surface receptors ($K_a = 10^{10} M^{-1}$) and partly to efficient internalization of toxin molecules bound to the cell surface. *Shigella* toxin is extremely toxic to sensitive animals (Eiklid and Olsnes, 1983).

3. ALTERNATIVE LIGANDS

The choice of alternative ligand to replace the B-chain of the toxin will depend on the proposed use of the hybrid toxin.

3.1. LECTINS AND SPECIFIC SUGARS

By using lectins as binding moiety, information can be obtained on the role of different cell surface oligosaccharides in the uptake mechanism. Many lectins are available in high amounts and in pure state and a number of chimeric toxins using lectins as binding moieties have been prepared (see Table 2). The toxic effects can be prevented by adding competing sugars which prevent the binding of the lectin and hence of the chimeric toxin. Such chimeric toxins involving lectins may be useful tools in studying the factors influencing the penetration of the toxin moiety through the membrane. Also they may be used to select cell mutants lacking receptors for the respective lectin.

Fibroblasts carry a receptor for mannose 6-phosphate (for review, see Neufeld and Ashwell, 1980). This sugar is present on many lysosomal enzymes and fibroblasts are able to utilize this receptor to retrieve excreted enzymes from the culture medium. A toxin employing mannose 6-phosphate as binding moiety has been prepared (Youle *et al.*, 1979). Complexes binding to the receptor for desialylated glycoproteins present on hepatocytes have also been made (Cawley *et al.*, 1980a; Chang and Kullberg, 1982).

3.2. HORMONES

Protein hormones are bound to specific receptors on the surface of target cells. Such hormones are obvious candidates for construction of chimeric toxins. It is known that several of the hormones are internalized by adsorptive endocytosis and for several hormones

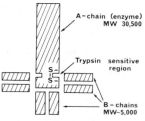

FIG. 3. Schematical structure of *Shigella* toxin.

intracellular hormone receptors have been detected. However, it is not yet clear whether these hormones actually reach the cytosol. The study of these questions is complicated by the lack of sensitive and convenient assays for the presence of the hormones in the cytoplasm. Chimeric toxins involving hormones a binding moieties may be useful as model systems as the presence of the toxic moiety in the cytosol can readily be measured by assaying the inhibition of protein synthesis.

Some hormones, like the glycoprotein hormones, have indeed a structure resembling that of the toxins discussed here, *viz.* a β-chain which binds to the cell surface and an α-chain which is required for the hormonal effect. Several protein hormones have already been used in the preparation of chimeric toxins (see Table 2).

3.3. ANTIBODIES

To achieve selective cell killing *in vivo*, the new ligand must bind exclusively or preferentially to the cell population in question. Probably the most versatile toxin-directing ligands are antibodies to cell surface antigens. Although antibodies bound to cell surface receptors may activate the complement system and thus kill the cell, it is well known that this does not always occur. Particularly antibodies to weak antigens not present in high density such as tumour associated antigens, often do not activate the complement system.

With the recent development of the 'hybridoma' technique a multitude of monoclonal antibodies to cell surface antigens have been made available in milligram quantities. Such antibodies may be highly concentrated in target organs (Scheinberg and Strand, 1983). Monoclonal antibodies specific for a variety of malignant cells have already been used to produce chimeric toxins (Gilliland *et al.*, 1980; Youle and Neville, 1980; Blythman *et al.*, 1981; Thorpe *et al.*, 1981; Raso *et al.*, 1982; Krolick *et al.*, 1981; Houston and Nowinski, 1981; Seto *et al.*, 1982; Bumol *et al.*, 1982). With this type of ligands selective killing of any cell carrying the specific surface antigen may be possible even in those cases where for some reason complement induced cell killing does not occur.

Experiments in cell culture have shown that a high binding constant of the ligand to the receptor and a high number of receptors on the surface of the target cells will increase the efficiency of the hybrid toxin. In cases where the appearance of resistant cell clones may be a problem, as in the treatment of malignant tumors, it may be advantageous to use two or more ligands which bind to the cells in question.

A special application of antibodies is to exploit the Fc-receptors present on a variety of cells including macrophages. Antibody-toxin complexes can be internalized by this route, as shown in this laboratory by Refsnes and Munthe–Kaas (1976).

Although it is questionable whether tumour specific antigens exist—they are usually embryonal antigens which are expressed during malignancy—tumor associated antigens may still represent targets for chimeric toxins. The possibility must, however, be borne in mind that the conjugate may also bind to and intoxicate other cells which express the antigen.

4. THE CONSTRUCTION OF CHIMERIC TOXINS

Many different approaches have been used in the construction of chimeric toxins. A brief discussion of the general strategies used and the coupling methods employed may be helpful.

4.1. COUPLING OF WHOLE TOXINS

The first chimeric toxins prepared involved the use of the whole toxins which were covalently linked to the new binding moieties.

Several authors have pointed out that the B-chains of the toxins may play a role in the entry mechanism beyond that of binding the toxin to surface receptors (Youle and Neville, 1979; Youle *et al.*, 1981). If this is the case, some advantage may be gained by retaining the

TABLE 2. *Properties of Toxic Chimeras*

Toxin moiety	Binding moiety	Test cells	Toxicity to cells with receptors for the new binding moiety		
			ID_{50} of toxin moiety alone (X) M	ID_{50} of conjugate (Y) M	Gain in activity (X/Y)
Abrin A	Ricin B	HeLa	$> 2 \times 10^{-7}$	2×10^{-11}	$> 10,000$
Ricin A	Abrin B	HeLa	$> 2 \times 10^{-7}$	2×10^{-11}	$> 10,000$
Ricin A	Diphtheria toxin B	Vero	$> 10^{-7}$	2×10^{-10}	> 500
Modeccin A	Ricin B	Vero	$> 10^{-7}$	2×10^{-11}	$> 5,000$
Ricin A	*Wistaria floribunda* subunit	FL-cells	$> 3 \times 10^{-7}$	8×10^{-10}	> 375
Diphtheria toxin A	*Wistaria floribunda* subunit	FL-cells	$> 3 \times 10^{-7}$	2×10^{-7}	> 1.5
Diphtheria toxin A	*Wistaria floribunda* subunit	L-cells	$\sim 5 \times 10^{-7}$	$\sim 3 \times 10^{-9}$	~ 150
Diphtheria toxin A	Concanavalin A	HeLa, SV3T3, CHO	10^{-6}	$2\text{–}6 \times 10^{-9}$	$100\text{–}1000$
Ricin A	Concanavalin A	BALB/3T3	$> 4 \times 10^{-9}$	8×10^{-10}	> 5
Gelonin	Concanavalin A	HeLa	$> 2 \times 10^{-7}$	8×10^{-9}	> 30
CRM 45	Ricinus agglutinin	L-cells	$\sim 10^{-9}$	$\sim 10^{-10}$	$8\text{–}10$
Ricin A	Asialofetuin	Hepatocytes	$\sim 10^{7}$	5×10^{-11}	1800
Ricin A	α_2-macroglobulin	Fibroblasts	1.3×10^{-6}	8.3×10^{-9}	> 165
Diphtheria toxin A	Asialoorosomucoid	Hepatocytes	$> 10^{-7}$	2×10^{-10}	> 500
Ricin	Monophosphopenta-mannose	Fibroblasts + lactose	$\sim 10^{-8}$	6×10^{-10}	~ 17
CRM 26	TRH	GH_3	$> 10^{-7}$	$> 10^{-7}$	—
CRM 45	TRH	GH_3	$> 6 \times 10^{-7}$	3×10^{-9}	> 200
Gelonin	Monophosphopenta-mannose	F-265		5×10^{-9}	
Ricin	Antiricin B	Macrophages		2×10^{-10}	
Diphtheria toxin A	Cholera toxin B	3T3	$> 10^{-6}$	3×10^{-10}	> 3000
Ricin A	EGF	Mouse 3T3	3.5×10^{-7}	4.5×10^{-11}	7800
Ricin A	EGF	Hepatocytes	3.5×10^{-7}	5×10^{-11}	7000
Diphtheria toxin A	EGF	Mouse 3T3	3.5×10^{-7}	$> 3 \times 10^{-8}$	—
Diphtheria toxin A	EGF	Hepatocytes	3.5×10^{-7}	5×10^{-11}	7000
Diphtheria toxin A	Insulin	Swiss 3T3	$> 6 \times 10^{-7}$	$\sim 10^{-7}$	> 6
Ricin A	hCG-β-chain	R_2C (Leydig)	$> 2 \times 10^{-6}$	$\sim 10^{-6}$	> 2

whole or part of the B-chain. However, this approach entails a number of difficulties as will be discussed below.

There is now convincing evidence that the enzymatic activity of the A-chain is only expressed when the A-chain is liberated. This constitutes no difficulty if a new binding moiety is conjugated to the B-chain of the toxin, as the A-chain can then be liberated by a reduction of the disulfide bond. However, in coupling experiments involving whole toxins it is usually not possible to avoid binding of the new moiety also to the A-chain. Moreover, cross linking between the A- and the B-chains of the toxins which would prevent the A-chain from being liberated is likely to occur unless special precautions are taken. Also, homopolymer formation is always a possibility in such experiments.

Another difficulty arising when whole toxins are coupled to new binding moieties is that the ability of the B-chain of the original toxin to bind to cell surface receptors is retained to a greater or lesser extent. This implies that even though the new carrier moiety may have a high binding specificity, the chimeric toxin will nevertheless tend to bind unspecifically by way of its B-chain. In principle it should be possible to reduce this non specific binding by modifying the B-chain prior to its coupling to the new binding moiety. Experiments in our laboratory (Sandvig *et al.*, 1978b) have shown that it is possible, by a number of chemical procedures, to inactivate preferentially the B-chains of abrin and ricin and reduce their binding to animal

Involving Lectins and Hormones

Toxicity of conjugate relative to native toxin %	Toxicity to cells lacking receptors for the new binding moiety			Reference
	Test cells	ID_{50} of conjugate (Z) M	Specificity factor (Z/Y)	
~ 100				Olsnes *et al.* (1974)
~ 100				Olsnes *et al.* (1974)
0.1				Sundan *et al.* (1982)
300–1,000				Sundan *et al.* (1983)
	FL-cells + GLcNAc	$> 2 \times 10^{-8}$	25	Uchida *et al.* (1980)
				Uchida *et al.* (1980)
	L-cells + GlcNAc	$\sim 10^{-7}$	~ 30	Uchida *et al.* (1978)
0.2–2				Gilliland *et al.* (1978)
50	BALB/3T3 + α-methylmannose		> 5	Yamaguchi *et al.* (1979)
0.1 (of ricin)	HeLa + α-methylmannose	$> 2 \times 10^{-7}$	> 30	Stirpe *et al.* (1980)
0.05 (of ricin)				Uchida *et al.* (1978)
	Rat heart cells	$> 10^{-8}$	200	Cawley *et al.* (1981b)
0.6				Martin and Houston (1983)
				Chang and Kullberg (1982)
50 (in absence) of lactose)	HeLa + lact.	10^{8}	~ 13	Youle *et al.* (1979)
				Bacha *et al.* (1983)
	Mouse 3T3	$> 10^{-7}$		Bacha *et al.* (1983)
	F-265 + Man 6P	$> 10^{6}$	200	Forbes *et al.* (1981)
0.01	HeLa cells	$> 2 \times 10^{-8}$	> 100	Refsnes and Munthe-Kaas (1976)
				Mannhalter *et al.* (1980)
53	3T3 + EGF	$> 2 \times 10^{-9}$		Cawley *et al.* (1980b)
				Cawley *et al.* (1981a)
				Cawley *et al.* (1980b)
				Simpson *et al.* (1982)
	IN-2	$> 10^{-7}$		Miskimins and Shimizu (1979)
< 0.1	L-cells	$> 2 \times 10^{-6}$	> 2	Oeltmann and Heath (1979)

cells without affecting appreciably the activity of the A-chains, as measured by the ability of the toxins to inhibit protein synthesis in a cell free system.

To avoid the formation of toxin polymers and cross linking between the A- and the B-chains of the toxins, Thorpe *et al.* (1978), Ross *et al.* (1980) and Thorpe and Ross (1982) used a mixed anhydride of chlorambucil to bind whole diphtheria toxin to anti (human lymphocyte) globulin or its F(ab')$_2$ fragment. The mixed anhydride of chlorambucil was first reacted with the antibody at 4°C. After removal of unreacted chlorambucil the modified protein was mixed with diphtheria toxin and the temperature was raised to 25–30°C to activate the mustard group of the chlorambucil which could then react with toxin to produce conjugates.

A coupling procedure which primarily involves the B-chain of abrin and ricin is the use of periodate oxidation. Abrin and ricin are glycoproteins. Most of the carbohydrates in ricin and all in abrin are present in the B-chain. Periodate oxidation of the terminal sugars of the oligosaccharide chains results in the formation of aldehyde groups which may be cross linked with free amino groups in the new binding protein. It was shown that careful oxidation with periodate did not strongly affect the enzymatic activity of the A-chain (Sandvig *et al.*, 1978b). Homopolymer formation could in this case be prevented by previous reductive methylation of the free amino groups in the toxin itself (Fig. 4). The methylation

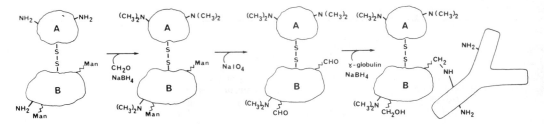

FIG. 4. Coupling of abrin to antibodies. Abrin was first treated with formaldehyde to methylate free amino groups and then treated with sodium periodate to oxidize the oligosaccharides linked to the B-chain to form free aldehyde groups (Sandvig *et al.*, 1978b). The toxin was then mixed with anti-TNP-immunoglobulin and stored at 4°C overnight to allow coupling to occur between the aldehyde groups on abrin B-chain and free amino groups on the immunoglobulin. The Schiff bases formed were reduced by sodium borohydride to stabilize the binding.

did not strongly reduce the toxic activity of abrin. This method was used to prepare complexes of abrin and anti-trinitrophenol antibodies (Olsnes, Sandvig, Refsnes and Pihl, unpublished results).

4.2. COUPLING OF TOXIN A-CHAINS

Since the use of whole toxins in the formation of chimeric toxins involves several drawbacks, most investigators have attempted to replace the B-chains of the toxins with a new binding moiety. It is then necessary to couple the A-chain to the new ligand through a disulfide bond to permit the liberation of the active free A-chain.

If the new binding moiety lacks free SH-groups which may be used for the formation of the disulfide bond, it is necessary to introduce artificially SH-groups into the proteins. Several procedures have been used for this purpose. Thus, SH-groups can be introduced by treatment with S-acetylmercaptosuccinic anhydride or by coupling to the binding moiety a disulfide which is subsequently reduced. For this purpose disulfides such as cystamine 3,3′ dimethyldithiobispropionate and N-succinimidyl-3-(2-pyridyldithiopropionate) (SPDP) have been used.

If both components to be linked together contain a free SH-group, disulfides may be obtained by oxidation of the SH-groups. In some cases this can be done simply by mixing the two proteins in equimolar amounts and dialyzing the mixture against buffer in the absence of reducing agents. Using this procedure, Olsnes *et al.* (1974) formed toxic hybrids of abrin A-chain and ricin B-chain, as well as of ricin A-chain and abrin B-chain. In both cases hybrid toxins were obtained in good yields. Later Funatsu *et al.* (1977) formed hybrids between the chains of ricin and ricinus agglutinin in a similar way. The reason for the good yield in these cases is probably that the new binding moiety is closely related to that being replaced, and that even before the disulfide bond is formed the new molecules form an unstable complex due to weak interactions between the protein chains.

The oxidation of thiols to disulfides is catalyzed by heavy metals and in particular by various heavy metal complexes. In cases where the proteins to be joined do not have a natural affinity for each other, disulfide formation can be induced by the presence of o-phenantroline and $CuSO_4$ (Freedman, 1979).

The yield of a chimeric toxin between diphtheria toxin fragment A and a subunit of *Wistaria floribunda* lectin was considerably increased by this procedure (Uchida *et al.*, 1978a).

A major problem in forming SS-bridges between proteins having low affinity for each other is that the yield of the desired heterodimer may be very low and that homodimer formation of the two proteins occurs to a much greater extent. To prevent such homodimer formation the disulfide bond is now frequently formed by an exchange reaction. In the synthesis of a conjugate of human placental lactogen and diphtheria toxin A fragment Chang and Neville (1977) utilized Swan's method for the synthesis of asymmetric disulfides:

$$RS^- + R'SSO_3^- \rightleftharpoons RSSR' + SO_3^{2-}$$

They developed a method to introduce an extrinsic S-sulfonate group into proteins according to the following reactions:

$$Protein-NH_2 + CH_3O-\overset{\overset{\displaystyle NH_2^+}{\|}}{C}(CH_2)_4-Br \longrightarrow Protein-NH-\overset{\overset{\displaystyle NH_2^+}{\|}}{C}(CH_2)_4-Br + CH_3OH$$

$$Protein-NH-\overset{\overset{\displaystyle NH_2^+}{\|}}{C}(CH_2)_4-Br + S_2O_3^{2-} \longrightarrow Protein-NH-\overset{\overset{\displaystyle NH_2^+}{\|}}{C}(CH_2)_4-SSO_3^- + Br^-$$

The hormone amino group was first amidinated by treatment with methyl-5-bromovalerimidate. The product was converted into S-sulfonated protein. Finally, diphtheria toxin fragment-A was added and the mixture was stored at 5°C in the absence of oxygen. This method prevented intramolecular cross linking as well as the formation of homopolymers and the yield of the desired conjugates was high. The procedure was later used by Oeltmann and Heath (1979a) to prepare toxic chimeras from ricin A-chain and the β-subunit of human chorionic gonadotropin. A similar exchange reaction was used by Masuho *et al.* (1979) to link diphtheria toxin A fragment to Fab′SH of IgG from antiserum against L 1210 cells. They first S-sulfonated the A-fragment and upon subsequent mixing with Fab′SH the desired hybrid was formed in good yield.

Raso and Griffin (1980) prepared chimeric toxins between ricin A-chain and the Fab′SH fragment of IgG against human immunoglobulin by a thiol disulfide exchange reaction. They first reacted the Fab′SH fragment with Ellman's reagent and then ricin A-chain was added. Complexes of Fab′ with ricin A chain were formed in good yield by the disulfide exchange:

A disulfide exchange reaction was also used by Gilliland *et al.* (1978) who coupled diphtheria toxin A-fragment to concanavalin A. The lectin was first coupled with cystamine using a carbodiimide (EDAC) as condensing agent. The protein disulfide was then mixed with diphtheria toxin A-fragment under conditions promoting disulfide exchange. Also in this case homopolymers were not formed and the yield of chimeric toxin was high (almost 50%). This method has later been used in the preparation of several other chimeric toxins in the same and other laboratories (Gilliland *et al.*, 1980; Miskimins and Shimizu, 1979; Shimizu *et al.*, 1980).

$$\text{Concanavalin A}-\overset{\overset{\text{O}}{\|}}{\text{C}}-\text{OH} \quad + \quad \begin{array}{l} {}^{+}\text{H}_3\text{NCH}_2\text{CH}_2\text{S} \\ \quad\quad\quad\quad | \\ {}^{+}\text{H}_3\text{NCH}_2\text{CH}_2\text{S} \end{array}$$

$$\Big\downarrow \text{EDAC}$$

$$\text{Concanavalin A}-\overset{\overset{\text{O}}{\|}}{\text{C}}-\text{NHCH}_2\text{CH}_2\text{S}-\text{SCH}_2\text{CH}_2\text{NH}_3^{+}$$

$$\Big\downarrow \quad + \quad \text{HS}-\boxed{\text{Fragment A}}$$

$$\text{Concanavalin A}-\overset{\overset{\text{O}}{\|}}{\text{C}}-\text{NHCH}_2\text{CH}_2\text{S}-\text{S}-\boxed{\text{Fragment A}}$$
$$+$$
$$\text{HSCH}_2\text{CH}_2\text{NH}_3^{+}$$

A slightly different procedure was used by Yamaguchi *et al.* (1979) who coupled ricin A-chain to concanavalin A. The lectin was coupled with 3,3′-dimethyldithiobis-propioimidate which was subsequently reduced. The SH-group was then blocked by reaction with Ellman's reagent. The disulfide bridge thus formed reacts easily with free SH-groups to form new SS-bonds with release of 3-nitro-4-carboxythiophenol. The conjugate was obtained in high yield.

Recently, several groups have used the commercially available reagent, N-succinimidyl-3-(2-pyridyldithio)propionate (Carlsson *et al.*, 1978). The reagent reacts with free amino groups and can be used to introduce 2-pyridyl disulfide groups into non-thiol proteins. Such disulfide groups react readily with free SH-groups by exchange. Therefore, the protein 2-pyridyl disulfide derivative can be conjugated with another protein, having a thiol group available for reaction:

$$\boxed{\text{Protein 1}}-\text{NH}_2 + \text{(pyridyl)}-\text{S}-\text{S}-\text{CH}_2\text{CH}_2\text{CON}\big\langle$$

$$\Big\downarrow$$

$$\boxed{\text{Protein 1}}-\text{NH}-\overset{\overset{\text{O}}{\|}}{\text{C}}-\text{CH}_2\text{CH}_2-\text{S}-\text{S}-\text{(pyridyl)} + \text{HON}\big\langle$$

$$\Big\downarrow \quad +\text{HS}\,\boxed{\text{Protein 2}}$$

$$\boxed{\text{Protein 1}}-\text{NC}-\overset{\overset{\text{O}}{\|}}{\text{C}}-\text{CH}_2\text{CH}_2-\text{S}-\text{S}-\boxed{\text{Protein 2}} + \text{(pyridyl)}{=}\text{S}$$

The reagent can also be used to cross link proteins where neither component contains a free SH-group. In this case both proteins must be treated with SPDP and one of the two pyridyl disulfide-conjugated proteins must then be pretreated with 2-mercaptoethanol or dithiothreitol to reduce the disulfide and the conjugate can then be formed by a thiol disulfide exchange reaction. This method was used by Stirpe *et al.* (1980) to prepare toxic hybrids between gelonin and concanavalin A which both are devoid of free SH-groups. Gilliland *et al.* (1980) prepared a hybrid of concanavalin A and diphtheria toxin A-fragment, Krolick *et al.* (1980) linked ricin A-chain to antibodies and Cawley *et al.* (1980a) linked ricin A-chain to desialylated fetuin, using the same reagent. This method has lately become the method of choice and has been used by a number of authors. A similar procedure was used by Jansen *et al.* (1980) who introduced SH-groups in antibodies employing 3-(2-pyridyldithio)propionic acid activated by carbodiimide.

A method introduced by Wofsy and coworkers (Martinez *et al.*, 1982) takes advantage of the very strong binding between biotin and avidin. They linked avidin to the toxin A-chain by a disulfide bond and biotin to the antibody. Cells were first treated with the antibody-biotin complex and then with the avidin-toxin A-chain conjugate. This method obviates the necessity of purification of the antibody because antibodies not bound to the cell can be washed off before the toxin A-chain-avidin complex is added.

5. ACTIVITY OF CHIMERIC TOXINS

5.1. CONJUGATES INVOLVING LECTINS, SUGARS AND PROTEINS

In model experiments designed to study the structural requirements for activity of chimeric toxins, toxin A-chains have been linked to a variety of molecules capable of binding to receptors at cell surfaces. The first hybrids involving lectins were prepared by Olsnes *et al.* (1974) between abrin A-chain and ricin B-chain as well as between ricin A-chain and abrin B-chain. These hybrids were as toxic as native abrin and ricin and first showed that the binding moiety of toxins can be replaced by another binding moiety without loss of biological activity (Table 2). Later Funatsu *et al.* (1977) formed in a similar way hybrids between ricin A-chain and the B-chain of ricinus agglutinin as well as between ricin B-chain and the A-chain of ricinus agglutinin. These hybrids were only 2–3 % as active as native ricin, and the authors concluded that both the A-chain and the B-chain of ricin are responsible for its high toxicity.

Model studies with subunits of *Escherichia coli* heat labile toxin and cholera toxin showed that the hybrid toxins formed were approximately as toxic as the native toxins (Takeda *et al.*, 1981).

In several laboratories non-toxic lectins have been used as binding moieties in chimeric toxins. Some lectins consist of subunits linked by disulfide bridges and in these cases the subunits may be linked, after reduction of the interchain bridge, directly to the A-chain of toxins. Thus, Uchida *et al.* (1978a, 1980) prepared hybrids between the monomer of *Wistaria floribunda* lectin and the A-moieties of ricin and diphtheria toxin. Both hybrids were toxic, but the one containing ricin A-chain, was 100–200 times more toxic than that with diphtheria toxin A-fragment. The results, like those of Cawley *et al.* (1980b) (see below) indicate that in such hybrids ricin A-chain is more easily transferred to the cytosol than the diphtheria A-fragment. Both the hybrid of *Wistaria floribunda* lectin and diphtheria toxin fragment-A and that with ricin A-chain, showed increased toxicity in the presence of methylamine (Mekada *et al.*, 1981). Similar results were previously found with ricin (Sandvig *et al.*, 1979), whereas in the case of diphtheria toxin, amines protect against the toxicity.

Many lectins do not contain disulfide bridges which are easily reduced and in these cases it is necessary to introduce new SH-groups. In this way Gilliland *et al.* (1978) linked diphtheria toxin A-fragment by a disulfide bond to concanavalin A. The conjugate was 100–1,000 fold more toxic than the A-fragment or concanavalin A alone, but it was 50–500 times less active than diphtheria toxin. Interestingly, the conjugate showed almost the same toxicity to cells whether or not they were resistant to diphtheria toxin as such and α-methylmannoside, the sugar with specificity for concanavalin A, inhibited the toxic action. Yamaguchi *et al.* (1979) linked ricin A-chain by a disulfide to concanavalin A. Also this complex was clearly toxic to cells.

Stirpe *et al.* (1980) linked the A-chain like protein, gelonin, to concanavalin A. Gelonin is particularly useful for such purposes. It is easy to prepare, very stable and in a cell-free protein synthesizing system it is at least as active as the A-chains of abrin and ricin. Gelonin alone had no demonstrable toxic effect on HeLa cells, in agreement with the fact that it lacks the binding chain. However, after being bound by a disulfide bond to concanavalin A it became toxic. The toxic effect was prevented by α-methylmannoside. Uchida *et al.* (1978b) linked ricinus agglutinin which inhibits protein synthesis in a similar way as ricin, although to a much lesser extent, to the incomplete diphtheria toxin, CRM 45, by glutaraldehyde. A hybrid was obtained that was 8–10 times more toxic than ricinus agglutinin alone. CRM 45 lacks a piece of the B-fragment involved in the binding of diphtheria toxin. However, the hydrophobic sequence is retained in this mutant which also has an intact fragment-A.

Lectin-like molecules are also found on the surface of certain cells. Thus, in the membrane of hepatocytes a receptor protein is found which binds desialylated glycoproteins (see Neufeld and Ashwell, 1980). Cawley *et al.* (1980a, 1981b) linked ricin A-chain and diphtheria fragment-A by a disulfide bond to asialofetuin. The complex was taken up by rat hepatocytes and inhibited their protein synthesis. Mouse 3T3 cells and rat heart cells which lack the receptor were resistant to the hybrid. The hybrid was approximately as toxic as intact ricin and diphtheria toxin to sensitive cells. A hybrid with intact fetuin which is not recognized by the hepatocyte receptor was not toxic (Cawley *et al.*, 1981b). A similar hybrid consisting of diphtheria toxin fragment-A and asialoorosomucoid had very little toxic effect in normal medium, but the effect was more than 1000 fold increased in the presence of colchicine and other compounds which inhibit degradation of the conjugate (Chang and Kullberg, 1982).

A lectin-like protein is also present on fibroblasts. This receptor binds mannose-6-phosphate which is present on lysosomal hydrolases (Neufeld and Ashwell, 1980). When these enzymes are excreted into the medium, they may be retrieved by this receptor and transported back to the lysosomes. Youle *et al.* (1979) linked monophosphopentamannose to ricin and to diphtheria toxin A-chain by reductive amination. They tested the conjugate in the presence of lactose which inhibits the normal binding of ricin to the cells. The monophosphopentamannose-ricin was toxic to fibroblasts, but not to HeLa cells and amnion epithelium cells which lack receptors for mannose-6-phosphate. The conjugate has been used to select mutant cells deficient in mannose-6-phosphate receptors (Robbins *et al.*, 1981).

Interestingly, diphtheria toxin A-fragment carrying monophosphopentamannose was not toxic, although 25 % of its enzymatic activity was retained. The authors suggested that after binding and internalization of the modified toxin by the mannose-6-phosphate receptor the toxin must somehow interact with its natural receptors in intracellular vacuoles to be able to traverse the membrane and get access to its cytoplasmic target (Youle *et al.*, 1981). Forbes *et al.* (1981) linked monophosphopentamannose to gelonin and showed that the complex was toxic to the human lymphoid cell lines K 562 and F 265. A complex of ricin A-chain and α_2-macroglobulin was toxic to fibroblasts (Martin and Houston, 1983), presumably because α_2-macroglobulin is taken up by cells by endocytosis via coated pits.

Another receptor present on a variety of cells including macrophages binds the Fc-part of immunoglobulins. Refsnes and Munthe–Kaas (1976) studied the ability of this receptor to internalize a complex containing ricin. Ricin was reacted with antibodies specifically directed against the B-chain part of the molecule to prevent binding to ricin-specific carbohydrate receptors. As expected, such complexes proved to have no toxic effect on HeLa cells. The complexes were, however, toxic to macrophages. This toxic effect could not be prevented by addition of lactose which prevents binding of ricin to cells, but it was prevented by addition of albumin-antialbumin complexes which compete for the Fc-receptor sites. When the complex was attached to human erythrocytes and rat Kupffer cells were allowed to phagocytose the treated erythrocytes, an even stronger inhibitory effect was seen. However, the toxicity of the complexes was only 0.1–0.01 % of that seen for intact toxin. As expected, a complex of ricin (anti-ricin A-chain) antibodies was non-toxic.

Cholera toxin resembles the two-chain cytotoxins in so far as it consists of two functionally different moieties (Gill, 1978). The A-chain enters the cell, whereas the B-protomer (consisting of 5 identical polypeptide chains) binds to the ganglioside Gm_1 on the plasma membrane and probably facilitates the entry of the A-chain into the cytoplasm. Mannhalter *et al.* (1980) studied the ability of the B-protomer of cholera toxin to facilitate the uptake of diphtheria toxin fragment-A, linked to the B-protomer by a disulfide bridge. The hybrid was 10 fold more toxic than the hybrid between diphtheria toxin fragment-A and concanavalin A referred to above (Gilliland *et al.*, 1978).

Youle and Neville (1979) studied the ability of one toxin to facilitate the entry of the enzymatically active polypeptide of another toxin. They coupled diphtheria toxin fragment-

A to whole ricin with a non-reducible bond and demonstrated the ability of the hybrid to ADP-ribosylate EF-2 in cells. This more complicated measurement had to be carried out since measurements of protein synthesis inhibition would not distinguish between the action of ricin and that of diphtheria toxin fragment-A. The ADP-ribosylation was inhibited by lactose (which inhibits ricin binding), but not by ammonium chloride (which inhibits diphtheria toxin entry). The results indicate that in this case diphtheria toxin fragment-A probably entered the cells by the ricin route and not by the normal route for diphtheria toxin. The authors also found that the ADP-ribosylation of EF-2 was preceded by a lag time which was dependent upon the toxin concentration and which most likely was caused by a delay in the entry process.

5.2. CONJUGATES INVOLVING HORMONES

In terms of toxicity of the conjugate the most successful study of toxin A-chains linked to hormones was carried out by Cawley *et al.* (1980b) who prepared hybrids consisting of epidermal growth factor (EGF) linked by a disulfide bond to ricin A-chain or to diphtheria toxin fragment-A (Fig. 5). The EGF (ricin A-chain) hybrid was almost as toxic as native ricin to mouse 3T3 cells, whereas EGF (diphtheria toxin fragment-A) was not toxic (Table 2). The latter hybrid did, however, bind to the cells with the same affinity as the EGF-ricin A-chain hybrid and it could compete with it for binding. The conjugate was, however, toxic to hepatocytes (Cawley *et al.*, 1981a; Simpson *et al.*, 1982). The reason for the difference between the two toxins in toxicity to 3T3 cells may be that ricin A-chain contains two hydrophobic sequences, whereas diphtheria toxin fragment-A has none. In diphtheria toxin the hydrophobic sequence which may be of importance for the internalization is located in the B-fragment.

Shimizu *et al.* (1980) who also linked diphtheria toxin fragment-A by a disulfide bond to epidermal growth factor, reported that the conjugate was toxic to the human cell line A-431 which is rich in receptors for epidermal growth factor, but non-toxic to the mouse cell line NR 6 which is deficient in EGF receptors. The finding that the conjugate was toxic to the human A-431 cells whereas the conjugate of Cawley *et al.* (1980b) was non-toxic to 3T3 cells, may be due to the much higher number of EGF-receptors on the A-431 cells. It should be noted that the data presented by Shimizu *et al.* (1980) are only of a qualitative nature.

Miskimins and Shimizu (1979) coupled diphtheria toxin A-fragment to insulin by a disulfide bond. The conjugate was toxic to mouse 3T3 cells which are resistant to diphtheria toxin, but do have insulin receptors. In contrast, In-2 cells which are insulin non responsive, were resistant to the conjugate. The conjugate was later used to select resistant clones from Swiss/3T3 fibroblasts (Miskimins and Shimizu, 1981).

Several glycoprotein hormones (chorion gonadotropin, follicle stimulating hormone, luteinizing hormone, thyrotropic hormone) consist of a β-subunit responsible for binding to the hormone specific receptors and an α-subunit which is necessary to elicit hormone response. The similarity in structure with the two-chain toxins is striking.

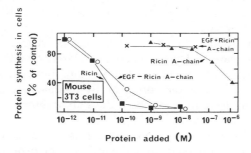

FIG. 5. Cytotoxicity of a hybrid of epidermal growth factor and ricin A-chain. Increasing amounts of the indicated proteins were added to 3T3 cells which were incubated for 24 hr and then the incorporation of [^{14}C]amino acids during a 2 hr period was measured. Redrawn after Cawley *et al.* (1980b).

Oeltmann and Heath (1979a, b) linked the β-subunit of human chorionic gonadotropin to ricin A-chain by a disulfide bond. The complex was toxic to R2C cells (from a Leydig cell tumor) which have receptors for human chorionic gonadotropin, but non-toxic to mouse-L-cells which lack such receptors. However, compared to native ricin, the hybrid had very low toxicity even to the sensitive R2C cells. Clearly, the hybrid was less efficient than native ricin in introducing the A-chain of the hybrid into R2C cells. It is possible that the low toxicity of the hybrid is due, at least in part, to inefficient binding to the hormone receptors as the isolated β-subunits bind to cells with much less affinity than does whole human chorionic gonadotropin.

Bacha *et al.* (1983) prepared a hybrid of thyreotropin releasing hormone with CRM 45, an incomplete diphtheria toxin molecule which is unable to bind to cells, but which contains the hydrophobic region. The hybrid was toxic to cells. In contrast, conjugates with another diphtheria toxin mutant, CRM 26, which lacks the hydrophobic region, were non-toxic.

Although, as shown above, toxin A-chains may be internalized after binding to several hormone receptors, this may not always be the case. In fact, the first toxin SS-hormone complex prepared was non toxic. In this experiment Chang *et al.* (1977) linked diphtheria toxin fragment-A to human placental lactogen and measured the ability of the hybrid to bind to and intoxicate mammary gland explants. No toxic effect was observed although the complex was shown to bind to mammary gland membranes and the complexes exhibited ADP-ribosylating activity in a cell-free system. As a possible explanation of the lack of biological activity of the conjugate, it was proposed that the intermolecular disulfide bond of the hybrid might be more easily reduced than that of nicked diphtheria toxin. Alternatively, the receptor for placental lactogen may not direct the toxin to the cytoplasm, but to some other compartment (Chang *et al.*, 1977). A hybrid molecule consisting of ricin B-chain and insulin was recently constructed by Roth *et al.* (1981). This hybrid bound to galactose containing receptors on MTC-hepatoma cells (which have few normal insulin receptors) and induced insulin response reaction in the cells.

Griffin *et al.* (1981) linked ricin A-chain to melanotropin and achieved selective killing of melanoma cells carrying melanotropin receptors. Anderson and Vilček (1982) prepared a ricin B-chain-interferon hybrid that exhibited antiviral properties in the absence, but not in the presence of galactose.

5.3. CONJUGATES INVOLVING ANTIBODIES

A number of toxin-antibody conjugates have now been prepared. Their main characteristics are summarized in Table 3.

5.3.1. *Polyclonal Antibodies*

In the early studies, whole toxins were conjugated by a covalent bond to polyclonal antibodies. Recently most authors have coupled the toxic moieties through a disulfide bond to antibodies or their fragments.

The use of whole antibodies in the construction of chimeric toxins may be disadvantageous for several reasons. The protein is much larger than the B-chain of the toxins and may therefore interfere with the entry of the A-chain. Furthermore, the presence of the Fc-fragment may elicit uptake of the conjugate by reticuloendothelial cells having Fc-receptors. Several authors have therefore used the Fab'-fragments rather than the whole immunoglobulin.

The first chimeric toxin involving an antibody was prepared by Moolten and Cooperband (1970) who coupled whole diphtheria toxin to the IgG fraction of antiserum to mumps virus, using toluene diisocyanate as coupling agent. The conjugate was somewhat more toxic to cells infected with mumps than to uninfected cells, whereas both cell populations were equally susceptible to unconjugated toxin. Later Moolten *et al.* (1972) linked diphtheria toxin to affinity-purified antibodies against dinitrophenyl-groups and then treated hamsters with this chimera simultaneously with injection of sarcoma cells carrying dinitrophenyl groups on their surface as an artificial tumor-associated antigen. The treatment was found to delay and reduce the tumor incidence and to prolong the life span of those animals that developed tumors.

A similar approach was taken by Philpott et al. (1973) who linked whole diphtheria toxin to antibodies against trinitrophenol, using dimethylmalonimidate. HeLa cells labelled with trinitrophenyl groups on their surface were more sensitive to the conjugate than were unmodified HeLa cells. In these and the above experiments the antibody added some immunologic specificity to the toxin, while decreasing markedly its non-selective killing of cells.

The first attempts to treat animals with conjugates of toxin and antibodies against natural tumor-associated antigens were also carried out by Moolten et al. (1975b) who coupled diphtheria toxin by means of glutaraldehyde to affinity-purified antibodies against hamster SV-40 transformed sarcoma and lymphoma cells. Although the selective toxicity for SV-40 transformed cells as measured in cell culture was marginal, a single dose of the conjugate afforded partial protection against simultaneously injected SV-40 transformed sarcoma cells. There was no therapeutic effect of the conjugate on established sarcomas, but repeated treatments induced complete regression in 20–56 % of hamsters bearing SV-40 induced lymphoma.

Only marginal selectivity was obtained by Edwards et al. (1981) who conjugated whole abrin to anti-mouse lymphocyte globulin, using a mixed anhydride derivative of chlorambucil and measuring the ability of the complexes to suppress the immune response of mice to sheep erythrocytes. Thorpe et al. (1981) who used the same method to conjugate whole abrin to anti-human lymphocyte globulin found that the conjugate inhibited protein synthesis in a human lymphoblastoid cell line (Daudi) about 10 times more effectively than did the control conjugate consisting of abrin and normal IgG. Both conjugates were less toxic than native abrin.

The fact that toxin antibody complexes may be highly toxic to cells that are normally resistant to the natural toxins was demonstrated by Thorpe et al. (1978) and Ross et al. (1980) who linked whole diphtheria toxin covalently to horse anti-human lymphocyte globulin and to F(ab′)₂ fragments derived from it. Two human lymphoblastoid cell lines (CLA 4 and Daudi) that were highly resistant to diphtheria toxin were sensitive to very low concentrations of the conjugates. A similar conjugate with normal horse IgG was less toxic to the test cells than was free diphtheria toxin (Fig. 6). Surprisingly, similar conjugates of diphtheria toxin and anti-mouse lymphocyte globulin were non-toxic to mouse spleen cells, although the conjugates did bind to them.

In recent years most authors have preferred to link antibodies to the A-chains of toxins through a disulfide bridge as pointed out above. In a model experiment, Gilliland and Collier (1980) linked diphtheria toxin fragment-A to antibodies against concanavalin A. This hybrid was toxic to 3T3 cells having concanavalin A attached to their surface, but was non-toxic in the same concentration range to cells not treated with concanavalin A or to cells with wheat germ agglutinin on their surface. In fact, it was as toxic as the hybrid mentioned above where fragment-A was linked directly to concanavalin A (Gilliland et al., 1978).

A hybrid consisting of rabbit anti-mouse IgG and ricin prepared by Miyazaki et al. (1980) had a slight selective toxicity to mouse B-lymphocytes. More successful were Jansen et al. (1980) who coupled ricin A-chain to anti-TNP antibodies and tested the conjugates on HeLa cells carrying TNP-groups on their surface. This conjugate showed a strong selectivity for cells with TNP-groups and it was about 500 times more toxic than the isolated ricin A-chain to such cells. Furthermore, treatment with the hybrid significantly inhibited tumor take and tumor growth of TNP-HeLa cells in nude mice. A clear selective effect was also observed by Krolick et al. (1980) and by Uhr (1982) who coupled ricin A-chain through a disulfide bond to affinity-purified anti-idiotype antibodies directed against surface immunoglobulins on a lymphoma cell line. This is a particularly interesting approach since a B-cell tumor is of monoclonal origin and expresses a particular idiotype. A toxin-conjugate with an anti-idiotype antibody is in fact a specific toxin for that tumor.

TABLE 3. *Properties of Toxic*

			Toxicity to cells with receptors for the new binding moiety		
Toxin moiety	Binding moiety	Test cells	ID_{50} of toxin moiety alone (X) M	ID_{50} of conjugate (Y) M	Gain in activity (X/Y)
Abrin	Anti-human lymphocyte globulin	Daudi + galactose	2×10^{-8}	2×10^{-10}	> 100
Diphtheria toxin	Anti-human lymphocyte globulin	CLA$_4$	$\begin{cases} > 2 \times 10^{-8} \\ 10^{-10} \end{cases}$	$\begin{aligned} 2 \times 10^{-11} \\ 2 \times 10^{-11} \end{aligned}$	> 1000 5
Diphtheria toxin	Anti-human lymphocyte globulin	CLA$_4$	1.3×10^{-10}	3×10^{-11}	5
Diphtheria toxin	Anti-human lymphocyte globulin	Daudi	$> 1.7 \times 10^{-8}$	8×10^{-12}	> 2100
Diphtheria toxin	F(ab')$_2$	Daudi	$> 1.7 \times 10^{-8}$	8×10^{-12}	> 2100
Diphtheria toxin A	Anti-Concanavalin A	3T3 pretreated with Con-A	$> 3 \times 10^{-8}$	10^{-9}	> 30
Ricin A	Polyclonal anti-DNP IgG	TNP-HeLa cells	5×10^{-7}	$10^{-8}-10^{-9}$	50–500
Ricin A	Affinity-purified antimouse IgM(μ)	BALB/c B-cells LPS-stim.	10^{-7}	2×10^{-9}	50
Ricin A	Monoclonal anti-a allotype IgD	BALB/c T-cells	10^{-7}	5×10^{-9}	20
Ricin A	Monoclonal anti-b allotype	C57BL/6 T-cells	10^{-7}	5×10^{-9}	20
Ricin A	Anti-idio type A (polyclonal)	BCL$_1$ leukemia cells	10^{-7}	2×10^{-9}	50
Diphtheria toxin A	Fab' of anti-L1210-Ig	L1210	$> 3 \times 10^{-7}$	$\sim 10^{-8}$	> 32
Ricin A	Fab' of anti-L1210-Ig	L1210	4.1×10^{-7}	$\sim 5 \times 10^{-9}$	~ 80
PAP	Fab' of anti-L1210-Ig	L1210	$> 10^{-6}$	$\sim 5 \times 10^{-9}$	> 200
Ricin A	Anti-Nalm 1	Nalm 1	$> 10^{-6}$	2×10^{-10}	> 2000
Ricin A	Anti-CEA	WiDr	3×10^{-7}	8×10^{-9}	40
Ricin A	Fab' of anti-human Ig	Daudi	$> 5 \times 10^{-8}$	2.5×10^{-9}	> 20
Ricin	Anti-Thy 1.2 (IgG$_{2b}$)	E1-4 + lactose	6×10^{-9}	6×10^{-10}	10
Ricin A	Anti-Thy 1.2 monoclonal IgM	WEHI-7 murine T-leukemia cell	5×10^{-7}	1.3×10^{-10}	2000–6000
Gelonin	Anti-Thy 1.1 monoclonal IgG$_{2a}$	T-lymphocytes (mitogen stimulated)	3×10^{-8}	$10^{-12}-$ 4×10^{-10}	
Ricin A	Monoclonal antibody	SW 1116–cells colorectal	$> 10^{-7}$	10^{-9}	> 100
Diphtheria toxin A	Monoclonal antibody	SW 1116–cells colorectal	$> 10^{-7}$	10^{-9}	> 100
Diphtheria toxin A	Anti-Thy 1.2 (monoclonal)	T-cells (stimulated)	10^{-6}	3×10^{-13}	
Ricin A	Anti IgM (polyclonal)	B-cells (stimulated)		10^{-8}	
Ricin A	Anti-p97	Melanoma (+ NH$_4$Cl)	5×10^{-7}	10^{-10}	5000
Ricin A	Anti-transferrin receptor	Leukemia cells	$\sim 10^{-7}$	4×10^{-11}	~ 2000
Diphtheria toxin A	Anti-transferrin receptor	Leukemia cells		1.5×10^{-9}	
Ricin A	Anti-T200	BW 5147	$> 10^{-8}$	10^{-10}	> 100

Chimeras Involving Antibodies

Toxicity of conjugate relative to native toxin %	Toxicity to cells lacking receptors for the new binding moiety			Reference
	Test cells	ID_{50} of conjugate (Z) M	Specificity factor (Z/Y)	
1	Daudi + IgG abrin	$> 2 \times 10^{-8}$	> 100	Thorpe *et al.* (1981)
	CLA$_4$ (diph. tox. normal horse IgG)	$> 2 \times 10^{-8}$	> 1000	Thorpe *et al.* (1978)
	CLA$_4$ (diph. tox. normal horse IgG)	5×10^{-9}	125	Thorpe *et al.* (1978)
0.5 (diph. tox. on fibroblasts)		$> 6 \times 10^{-9}$	> 200	Ross *et al.* (1980)
2 (diph. tox. on fibroblasts)		$> 2 \times 10^{-8}$	> 2500	Ross *et al.* (1980)
0.2 (diph. tox. on fibroblasts)		$> 12 \times 10^{-8}$	> 250	Ross *et al.* (1980)
	3T3 without ConA	$> 3 \times 10^{-8}$	> 30	Gilliland and Collier (1980)
1–10	HeLa (unmodified)	2×10^{-6}	100–500	Jansen *et al.* (1980)
				Krolick *et al.* (1980)
	C57BL/6 B-cells	$> 4 \times 10^{-8}$	> 8	Krolick *et al.* (1980)
	BALB/c B-cells	$> 4 \times 10^{-8}$	> 8	Krolick *et al.* (1980)
	BALB/c B-cells	$> 4 \times 10^{-8}$	> 20	Krolick *et al.* (1980)
	L1210 (diph. tox. anti-DNP-IgG)	$> 10^{-6}$	> 118	Masuho *et al.* (1979)
	L1210 (ricin A-unspecified Fab′)	$> 10^{-6}$	> 200	Masuho *et al.* (1980)
				Masuho *et al.* (1982)
20	Several cell lines	$\sim 10^{-6}$		Raso *et al.* (1982)
2.5	Melanoma	5×10^{-8}		Griffin *et al.* (1982)
2	CEM	$> 2 \times 10^{-7}$	> 80	Raso and Griffin (1980)
26 (in absence of lactose)	AKR + lactose	$\sim 4 \times 10^{-7}$	~ 700	Youle and Neville (1980)
7–20	BC-3A (Thy 1.2 negative)	5×10^{-7}	2000–6000	Blythman *et al.* (1981)
100 (abrin)	B-lymphocytes (mitogen stimulated)	$> 3 \times 10^{-7}$	1000–300,000	Thorpe *et al.* (1981)
0.1	WM 56 melanoma	$> 10^{-7}$	> 100	Gilliland *et al.* (1980)
0.1	WM 56 melanoma	$> 10^{-7}$	> 100	Gilliland *et al.* (1980)
				Oeltmann and Forbes (1981)
				Oeltmann and Forbes (1981)
100				Casellas *et al.* (1982)
750				Trowbridge and Domingo (1981)
				Trowbridge and Domingo (1981)
~ 100				Trowbridge and Domingo (1982)

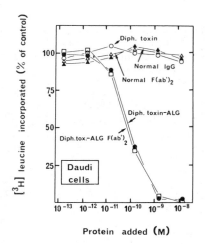

FIG. 6. Cytotoxicity of diphtheria toxin conjugated to anti-human lymphocyte immunoglobulin. The indicated proteins were added to human lymphoblastoid cells (Daudi) and incubated for 24 hr and then the incorporation of [^{3}H]leucine was measured. Redrawn after Ross *et al.* (1980).

Masuho *et al.* (1979, 1980) linked diphtheria toxin fragment-A, ricin A-chain and poke weed antiviral protein (PAP) through a disulfide bond to Fab' fragment of IgG from antiserum against L 1210 cells. The hybrids prepared were highly toxic *in vitro* to L 1210 cells. Similarly, Raso and Griffin (1980) linked ricin A-chain to Fab'-fragments of antibodies directed against human immunoglobulins. The complex was > 80 times more toxic to cells carrying immunoglobulins on their surface than to cells lacking surface immunoglobulins.

5.3.2. *Monoclonal Antibodies*

The development of the hybridoma technique for preparation of monoclonal antibodies has strongly enlarged the possibility to prepare chimeric toxins of high specificity.

Recently Youle and Neville (1980) and Neville and Youle (1981) coupled whole ricin through a thioether linkage to a monoclonal antibody (IgG$_{2b}$) directed against the Thy 1.2 differentiation antigen carried on the surface of thymocytes from certain inbred mouse lines. The hybrid showed specific toxicity to E1–4 cells which express the Thy 1.2 antigen. The toxic effect could not be prevented by addition of lactose to the medium, in contrast to the situation when native ricin was used. The hybrid exhibited some toxicity also to cells lacking the Thy 1.2 antigen when lactose was absent. This toxicity was undoubtedly due to binding of the hybrid to these cells by way of the ricin B-chain. When lactose was added to the medium, very little toxicity to cells lacking the Thy 1.2 antigen was observed.

Krolick *et al.* (1980) coupled ricin A-chain through a disulfide bridge to monoclonal antibodies directed against two different allotypes of IgD. The conjugate was selectively toxic to lymphocytes and lymphoma cells carrying the corresponding allotypes of IgD on their surface. Blythman *et al.* (1981) linked ricin A-chain by a disulfide bridge to a monoclonal antibody (IgM) against the differentiation antigen Thy 1.2 on thymocytes of certain inbred mice. This complex was almost as active as whole ricin on thymocytes carrying the antigen Thy 1.2 and it was 2,000–6,000 times more active on these cells than on other cells not carrying the Thy 1.2 antigen (Fig. 7). Furthermore, the complex protected mice against development of leukemia after injection of lymphoma cells carrying the Thy 1.2 antigen.

Thorpe *et al.* (1981) coupled the A-chain like protein, gelonin, by a disulfide bridge to monoclonal antibodies against a differentiation antigen on thymocytes (Thy 1.1). The conjugate was highly efficient in preventing the increase of protein synthesis in nitrogen-treated T-lymphocytes, whereas the stimulation of B-lymphocytes which do not carry the Thy 1.1 antigen, was not inhibited. It is remarkable that the complex was approximately as toxic to T-cells as intact abrin and more toxic than ricin. A lymphoma line carrying the Thy

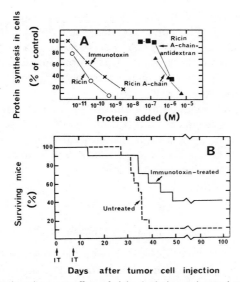

FIG. 7. Cytotoxicity and anti-cancer effect of ricin A-chain conjugated to monoclonal anti Thy 1.2 IgM. (a) The indicated proteins were added to WEHI-7 cells (a mouse T leukemia cell line expressing Thy 1.2 antigen) and the cells were incubated for 16 hr. Then [^{14}C]leucine was added and the incorporation of radioactivity during 2 hr was measured. (b) Groups of 10 mice were injected with 6×10^5 WEHI-7 cells intraperitoneally. Within 1 hr and after 7 days (indicated with IT in the bottom of the figure) conjugate of ricin A-chain and anti-Thy 1.2 antibody was injected i.p. Redrawn after Blythman *et al.* (1981).

1.1 antigen was found to be sensitive to the conjugate, although less so than the normal T-lymphocytes. The conjugate significantly prolonged the life of mice bearing this lymphoma. A conjugate of whole ricin and monoclonal anti-Thy 1.1 antigen prepared by Houston and Novinski (1981) was also selectively toxic to cells carrying the antigen.

Monoclonal antibodies against human tumor-associated antigens have recently become available. Gilliland *et al.* (1980) coupled diphtheria toxin fragment-A and ricin A-chain by a disulfide bridge to a monoclonal antibody directed against a colorectal tumor-associated antigen (Fig. 8). The conjugate showed selective cytotoxic effect to colorectal carcinoma cells in culture. The conjugate containing diphtheria toxin A-fragment was approximately as active as a conjugate containing ricin A-chain. Both conjugates were, however, about 1,000 times less active than native diphtheria toxin.

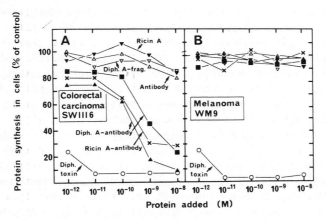

FIG. 8. Cytotoxicity of monoclonal anti-colorectal carcinoma IgG conjugated to ricin A-chain or diphtheria toxin fragment-A. The indicated proteins were added to; (a) the human colorectal carcinoma line SW 1116, or (b) the human melanoma line WM 9. The cells were incubated for 24 hr and then their ability to incorporate [^{14}C]labelled amino acids was measured. Redrawn after Gilliland *et al.* (1980).

Monoclonal J-5 antibody is specific for CALLA (common acute lymphoblastic leukemia antigen) present on a variety of human leukemias. Ricin A-chain linked to J-5 was strongly and selectively toxic to cells carrying the CALLA (Raso *et al.*, 1982; Raso, 1982). Casellas *et al.* (1982) prepared a conjugate of ricin A-chain and monoclonal antibody specific for human melanoma-associated antigen p97. The activity of this conjugate was strongly increased in the presence of lysosomotrophic agents.

A conjugate of ricin A-chain and anticarcinoembryonic antigen antibody was selectively toxic to a human adenocarcinoma cell line (Griffin *et al.*, 1982). Krolick *et al.* (1981) linked monoclonal IgM antibodies against human breast carcinoma cells to ricin A-chain. The conjugate was selectively bound to the target cells, which were killed, although only at comparatively high concentrations of the conjugate.

5.4. COMPARISON OF THE DIFFERENT CHIMERAS

The relative biological activity of different toxins can be gauged by measuring the ID_{50}, *i.e.* the concentration required in the medium to inhibit cellular protein synthesis by 50% under defined conditions. In comparing the potency of the different chimeras, several parameters are relevant (Tables 2 and 3). The gain in activity, *i.e.* the increased toxicity of the conjugate as compared to that of the toxic moiety (*i.e.* the free A-chain) reflects the efficiency of the new binding moiety and its cell surface receptor to internalize the toxin moiety. This efficiency is also reflected in the toxicity of the conjugate relative to that of the whole native toxin.

It is known that the internalization of the toxin A-chains is strongly dependent on the number of toxin molecules bound to the cell surface. This in turn is a function of the number of binding sites and of the affinity between toxin and receptors. Clearly, if the number of receptors for the new binding moiety differs strongly from that for the native toxin or if the binding constants differ appreciably, the concentration of conjugate in the medium required to obtain a certain toxic effect does not adequately reflect the efficiency of the transfer of the toxic moiety to the cytosol. Ideally, kinetic studies should be carried out to answer the specific question: What is the efficiency of a bound toxin molecule or of a bound chimera to internalize the toxin A-chain. So far, this has been done only in a few cases. Possibly the most significant parameter is the specificity factor of the chimeric toxin, *i.e.* the ratio between the toxicity to cells with and without receptors for the new binding moiety.

Unfortunately, most of the reports on chimeric toxins permit only the estimation of approximate values for the above parameters. In Tables 2 and 3 we have attempted to summarize the available data. It is clear that in some cases the conjugates are more than 1,000 times as toxic as the free A-chain. Obviously, in these cases the new binding moiety has considerably increased the uptake of the A-chain.

Although in most cases the chimeras are far less toxic than the native toxins, in some cases the conjugates were highly toxic. Thus, hybrids between ricin A-chain and abrin B-chain as well as between abrin A-chain and ricin B-chain were approximately as toxic as the two native toxins (Olsnes *et al.*, 1974). A hybrid of modeccin A-chain and ricin B-chain was even more toxic than either of the parent toxins (Sandvig *et al.*, 1984). Ricin A-chain linked to anti-Thy 1.2 monoclonal IgM (Blythman *et al.*, 1981) possessed 7–20% of the toxicity of native ricin and a conjugate of ricin A-chain and concanavalin A (Yamaguchi *et al.*, 1979) was 20–25% as toxic as native ricin. A chimera of ricin A-chain and asialofetuin was reported to be as toxic to hepatocytes as native ricin (Cawley *et al.*, 1980a). A hybrid between the non-toxic single chain protein, gelonin, and monoclonal anti-Thy 1.1 immunoglobulins (Thorpe *et al.*, 1981) was more toxic than ricin and approximately as toxic as abrin to cells carrying the Thy 1.1 antigen. Also complexes of whole ricin with anti-Thy 1.2 immunoglobulin and ricin linked to monophosphopentamannose were highly toxic to cells carrying the appropriate antigens and receptors. In the latter case the conjugates were assayed in the presence of lactose to prevent binding by ricin B-chain (Youle *et al.*, 1979; Youle and Neville, 1980).

A hybrid of ricin A-chain and anti-CALLA antibody (Raso *et al.*, 1982) was 20 % as toxic as ricin whereas a conjugate with antitransferrin receptor (Trowbridge and Domingo, 1981) was 7.5 times *more* toxic than native ricin. A hybrid of ricin A-chain and anti-T200 glycoprotein was as toxic as ricin (Trowbridge and Domingo, 1982).

Particularly interesting is a hybrid of ricin A-chain and anti-p97. This hybrid was not very toxic in normal medium, but it was as toxic as ricin if the medium contained 10 mM NH_4Cl (Casellas *et al.*, 1982).

Also the specificity factor varies considerably between the different hybrids. Values of more than 1,000 were obtained by Blythman *et al.* (1981) and Thorpe *et al.* (1981). Also Youle and Neville (1980) found high specificity of ricin-anti-Thy 1.2 immunoglobulin complexes and Thorpe *et al.* (1978) found a high specificity of diphtheria toxin-antihuman-lymphocyte globulin complexes. In the latter case the specificity was much higher in a short-time experiment (4 hr) than in an experiment where the cells were exposed to the conjugate for 24 hr.

5.5. Cytostatic Effect *in vivo*

Total body irradiation with a lethal dose followed by bone marrow reconstitution is currently being attempted as treatment of some patients with myeloid leukemia. In such cases it would be possible to use the patient's own pre-irradiated bone marrow for the reconstitution if it were possible to remove selectively the malignant cells in the bone marrow. Several investigators have attempted in experimental systems to use hybrid toxins for this purpose. Mason *et al.* (1982) and Thorpe *et al.* (1982) reported that rats which had received i.v. 10^7 leukemia cells treated in the presence of lactose with a conjugate of ricin and a monoclonal antibody, W3/25, developed leukemia 8–10 days later than recipients of untreated cells. Since the generation time of the cells was about 24 hr, this indicates that 99.9 % of the cells had been killed by the conjugate. There was little effect of the conjugate on the hemopoietic stem cells under the condition used. The presence of lactose during the treatment prevented unspecific binding of the conjugate to the non-malignant bone marrow cells.

Vallera *et al.* (1982) prevented the development of graft-versus-host disease in mice by pretreatment of the bone marrow donor cells with monoclonal anti-Thy 1.2, coupled to ricin. A conjugate with whole ricin was much more efficient than one involving ricin A-chain. Also in this case the treatment was carried out in the presence of lactose to protect cells not carrying the Thy 1.2 antigen.

Krolick *et al.* (1982) and Vitetta *et al.* (1982b, c) described a conjugate of rabbit anti-immunoglobulin antibody (R α MIg) and ricin A-chain, capable of killing 99.9 % of leukemic cells in infiltrated murine bone marrow *in vitro*, without destroying the hemopoietic stem cells. Treatment with antibody plus complement was much less efficient in removing malignant cells. Obviously this approach will eliminate only cells with immunoglobulin on their surface. Malignant stem cells lacking surface immunoglobulin will not be killed by the conjugate.

Krolick *et al.* (1982b) and Vitetta *et al.* (1982a) treated rats with advanced BCL_1 tumors with a combination of conventional cytoreductive therapy and a tumor-reactive chimeric toxin. First the number of leukemic cells in the blood and spleen was reduced by 90–95 % by irradiation. Then the rats were treated with chimeric toxins reacting with the tumor cells. A considerable delay in the reappearance of tumor cells was achieved in this way. When the tumor burden was further reduced by splenectomy before the chimeric toxin treatment, no reappearance of tumor was observed within 14 weeks.

Trowbridge and Domingo (1981) studied a conjugate of ricin A-chain and anti-transferrin receptor *in vitro* and *in vivo*. The conjugate was highly toxic to target cells *in vitro*. *In vivo* it was able to protect against melanomas and HeLa cells growing in nude mice, but not more so than the antibody alone. Possibly this is due to instability of the conjugate.

Bumol *et al.* (1983) found some regression in a human melanoma grown in nude mice upon treatment with a conjugate of diphtheria toxin fragment-A and a monoclonal antibody against surface chondroitin sulfate proteoglycan of the melanoma cells. However, the conjugate was not better than the IgG alone. *In vitro* the conjugate was clearly better.

Seto *et al.* (1982) treated mice with syngeneic mouse mammary tumor (MM46) cells with a conjugate of monoclonal anti-MM46 and ricin A-chain. The conjugate protected the mice not only when given simultaneously with the tumor cells, but even when given as much as 5 days later. The conjugate was better than the antibody alone. A conjugate prepared by Osawa *et al.* (1982) was selectively cytotoxic *in vitro*, but did not show convincing therapeutic effect *in vivo*.

6. STRUCTURAL REQUIREMENTS FOR TOXIC ACTIVITY OF CHIMERAS

The mechanism of penetration into the cytosol of the toxins from which the chimeras are made, is inadequately understood and much more work must be done before the structural requirements for highly toxic and selective chimeras can be defined. However, from the available data some conclusions may be drawn.

To obtain high toxic activity the toxin A-chain must be linked to the carrier molecule by a disulfide bridge. Thus, when ricin A-chain was linked by a thioether to an antibody against TNP no toxic effect was seen, whereas a similar hybrid containing a disulfide bridge was highly active (Jansen *et al.*, 1981). Similarly Gilliland and Collier (1981) found that diphtheria toxin fragment-A linked to concanavalin A by a thioether bond was at least 1,000 times less toxic than when the linkage involved an SS-bond. Also Masuho *et al.* (1981, 1982) and Chang and Kullberg (1982) found that conjugates containing a thioether were less toxic than conjugates containing a disulfide linkage.

The requirement for a disulfide bridge is consistent with the fact that all natural toxins which act on intracellular targets contain an easily reducible disulfide bridge and with the finding that the toxin moieties possess enzymatic activity only in the free form. It is not yet known where the reduction takes place and whether the whole toxin or merely the enzymatically active part penetrates the cell membrane.

Whether or not a hydrophobic sequence on either the A-chain or the binding moiety is necessary for toxin entry is not clear. Diphtheria toxin A-fragment which lacks a hydrophobic sequence was not toxic when linked by an SS-bond to the subunit of *Wistaria floribunda* lectin (Uchida *et al.*, 1980) or to ricin B-chain (Gilliland and Collier, 1981; Sundan *et al.*, 1982). Furthermore, monophosphopentamannose linked to diphtheria toxin fragment-A was non-toxic to fibroblasts containing the adequate receptor, whereas whole ricin linked to monophosphopentamannose was toxic. Also another hybrid lacking a hydrophobic fragment, *viz.* the hybrid between human placental lactogen and diphtheria toxin fragment-A, was non-toxic (Chang *et al.*, 1977). Interestingly, a conjugate of epidermal growth factor and diphtheria toxin fragment A, was not toxic to A-431 cells and 3T3 cells, while the corresponding conjugate with ricin A-chain which contains a hydrophobic sequence was toxic (Cawley *et al.*, 1980b). Suprisingly the two complexes were, however, toxic to rat hepatocytes (Cawley *et al.*, 1981a).

Bacha *et al.* (1983) linked two incomplete diphtheria toxin molecules to thyreotropin releasing hormone. Only the hybrid containing the hydrophobic region of diphtheria toxin was able to form a conjugate that was toxic to rat GH_3 cells which have receptors for thyreotropin releasing hormone.

Another striking example is experiments with hybrids involving anti Thy-1 antibodies. Blythman *et al.* (1981) prepared a hybrid between IgM monoclonal anti-Thy 1 and ricin A-chain which was toxic at 10^{-10} M. A hybrid of IgG monoclonal anti-Thy 1 and gelonin was equally toxic (Thorpe *et al.*, 1981). In spite of this, Martinez *et al.* (1982) were unable to obtain toxic conjugates with this antibody.

It is likely that a high number of binding sites for the conjugate at the cell surface and a high binding constant to these receptors will increase the toxic activity. Thus, studies with different toxins under conditions where the number of receptors could be varied have shown that the sensitivity of cells to the native toxin is to a large extent dependent upon the number of binding sites.

Raso *et al.* (1982) compared conjugates of ricin A-chain with univalent Fab' and divalent (Fab')$_2$ and found that the latter was about 70 times more toxic. However, Masuho *et al.* (1982) found only a 5 fold difference.

In the few cases where the conjugates have been tested in animals, the results have been less clear cut than *in vitro*. There may be several reasons for the *in vivo/in vitro* discrepancy. *In vivo* a few surviving tumor cells may grow up to tumors and kill the animals, whereas in cell culture assays a few surviving cells would hardly be recognized. Furthermore, *in vivo* the hybrids may be removed and inactivated in different ways. Thus, hybrids with whole immunoglobulins may be taken up by the Fc-receptors on reticuloendothelial cells (Refsnes and Munthe–Kaas, 1976). In two cases the toxic effect of conjugates on target cells in culture was strongly increased in the presence of compounds which inhibit their intracellular degradation (Casellas *et al.*, 1982; Chang and Kullberg, 1982). Clearly, pharmacokinetic studies must be carried out to design the optimal of chimeras.

7. CONSIDERATIONS CONCERNING TOXIC EFFECT *IN VIVO*

7.1. ESCAPE MECHANISMS

Several factors may account for the fact that hybrids often are less active *in vivo* than might be expected on the basis of the *in vitro* results.

In the first place, the vascularization of the tumor is often poor and may not permit enough complexes to be delivered to the tumor cells to induce intoxication. Secondly, if the tumor secretes large amounts of free antigen into the circulation, the conjugates may be absorbed before they reach the tumor.

Another possibility is that the antigen may not always be exposed on the cells. Thus different stages of the cell cycle and other factors may effect the sensitivity of cells to conjugates. This may be the reason why Thorpe *et al.* (1982b) were unable to kill the least 0.1 % of leukemia cells although, after allowing the surviving cells to multiply, they showed no characteristics different from those of the main cell population.

One mechanism whereby cells may escape the toxic effect of chimeric toxins is by genetic mutations or antigenic modulation of the cell surface target for the conjugate. This was indeed shown to occur with BM 5147 cells which express an antigen, T 200, to which a highly toxic conjugate of monoclonal antibodies and ricin A-chain could bind (Trowbridge and Domingo, 1982). Resistant cells isolated *in vitro* expressed less than 1 % of the amount of T 200 found on the parent cells. Other antigens may not be dispensable. Thus no resistant cells were obtained when the selection was carried out with a conjugate of ricin A-chain and anti-transferrin receptor.

The survival time *in vivo* of the conjugates may be low. Jansen *et al.* (1982) found an *in vivo* half-life of only 30 minutes of a conjugate of ricin A-chain and monoclonal anti-DNP antibody. Also ricin A-chain anti-transferrin receptor conjugates were rapidly lost in the animal (Trowbridge and Domingo, 1982). Conceivably, the short survival time *in vivo* may be due to instability of the SS-bond or to rapid removal of the conjugates by the reticuloendothelial system.

7.2. IMMUNOGENIC PROPERTIES OF CHIMERIC TOXINS

A problem arising when chimeric toxins are used in living animals or in patients is that, as foreign proteins, they will induce the formation of antibodies (Buzzi and Buzzi, 1974). Moolten *et al.* (1975a) showed that treatment of hamsters with complexes of diphtheria toxin and hamster gammaglobulin elicited antibody response in most of the animals. The titer was, however, low. If the hamsters were also given cyclophosphamide, the incidence of antibody response was much lower and the titer of antibody in those animals that developed antibodies was lower. Since a variety of A-chains are now known and since they are immunologically different it may be possible to switch from one chimeric toxin to another one when antibodies appear.

Godal et al. (1981) have recently developed a radioimmunoassay sensitive enough to measure the blood concentration of abrin and ricin in animals given therapeutically active toxin doses. The system also allows the detection of very low concentrations of antibodies. It appears that in mice, antibodies against abrin and ricin are detectable after approximately 3 weekly treatments. Interestingly, the antibody formation could be effectively suppressed by pretreatment of the animals with cyclophosphamide and prednisone (Godal et al., 1983).

7.3. Cancerostatic Properties of the Native Toxins

The most obvious use of chimeric toxins is in treatment of cancers. In evaluating the efficiency of the conjugates made from whole toxins it should be borne in mind that the native toxins have anti-tumor properties (see Olsnes and Pihl, 1982). Thus, Fodstad et al. (1977, 1980) have shown that abrin and ricin have a strong inhibitory effect on the growth of human tumor xenografts in athymic mice. Furthermore, ricin was found to have a strong and selective effect on the ability of mouse leukemia cells (L1210) to colonize the bone marrow (Fodstad and Pihl, 1980). Other authors have reported anti-tumor effect of diphtheria toxin (Buzzi and Maistrello, 1973; Buzzi, 1974). It is also possible that the isolated A-chains may have some anti-cancer effect. Lin et al. (1981) reported that the cancerostatic effect of the native toxins is increased after covalent linkage to methotrexate and chlorambucil.

It should also be noted that the toxins have immunosuppressive activity and that this activity was further increased by linkage of abrin to antilymphocyte antibodies (Edwards et al., 1982).

7.4. Possible Applications Other than Cancer Treatment

Since many organs and cell systems have specific antigens, chimeric toxins may be used to selectively kill the cells in the organism having that particular antigen. The possibility of removing certain groups of lymphocytes carrying specific antigens is now a definite possibility. As shown by Krolick et al. (1980), idiotypic antigens on B-lymphocytes may be used to selectively destroy defined clones of B-lymphocytes. Chimeric toxins linked to allergens might be able to remove the corresponding clones on lymphocytes producing IgE antibodies. Germinal cells carry differentiation antigens which are not expressed on other cells. Chimeric toxins with antibodies against these antigens may conceivably be used for sterilization.

Chimeric toxins involving hormones may have several obvious clinical uses. Such chimeras could be used in the treatment of diseases involving hyperfunction of a target organ for the hormone. The possible use of chimeric toxins with TSH in the treatment of hyperthyreosis is a case in point. Possibly, such complexes might also be useful in the treatment of cancers originating from the target organs (e.g. thyroid cancer).

A possible application that should be considered is the use of chimeric toxins in the treatment of parasitic diseases. Parasites like Plasmodium malariae, trypanosomes, etc. are eukaryotic organisms and contain EF-2 and ribosomes that are sensitive to the toxin A-chains.

Chimeric toxins may prove to be very valuable tools in experimental biology. As pointed out above, they may be helpful in elucidating the role of cell surface receptors for hormones and other biologically active molecules. Mutant cells deficient in certain hormone receptors or surface antigens may be selected by the use of chimeric toxins as well as cell lines deficient in the internalization of ligands bound to these structures. In fact, cells lacking insulin receptors have already been isolated by this method (Miskimins and Shimizu, 1981). Conceivably, chimeric toxins may in the future also be used to produce animals lacking certain cell or organ systems.

Acknowledgement: This work was supported by the Norwegian Cancer Society.

REFERENCES

ANDERSON, P. and VILČEK, J. (1982) Synthesis and biological characterization of a covalent conjugate between interferon and ricin toxin B-chain. *Virology* 123: 457–460.

BACHA, P., MURPHY, J. R. and REICHLIN, S. (1983) Thyreotropin-releasing hormone-diphtheria toxin-related polypeptide conjugates. Potential role of the hydrophobic domain in toxin entry. *J. biol. Chem.* 258: 1565–1570.

BARBIERI, L. and STIRPE, F. (1982) Ribosome-inactivating proteins from plants: Properties and possible uses. *Cancer Surveys* 1: 489–520.

BARBIERI, L., ZAMBONI, M., LORENZONI, E., MONTANARO, L., SPERTI, S. and STIRPE, F. (1980) Inhibition of protein synthesis *in vitro* by proteins from the seeds of *Momordica charantia* (bitter pear melon). *Biochem. J.* 186: 443–452.

BLYTHMAN, H. E., CASELLAS, P., GROS, O., GROS, P., JANSEN, F. K., PAOLUCCI, F., PAU, B. and VIDAL, H. (1981) Immunotoxins: Hybrid molecules of monoclonal antibodies and a toxin subunit specifically kill tumor cells. *Nature* 290: 145–146.

BOQUET, P., SILVERMANN, M. S., PAPPENHEIMER, A. M., JR. and VERNON, W. B. (1976) Binding of Triton X-100 to diphtheria toxin, cross-reacting material 45 and their fragments. *Proc. natn. Acad. Sci. U.S.A.* 73: 4449–4453.

BUMOL, T. F., WANG, Q. C., REISFELD, R. A. and KAPLAN, N. O. (1983) Monoclonal antibody and an antibody-toxin conjugate to a cell surface proteoglycan of melanoma cells suppress *in vivo* tumor growth. *Proc. natl. Acad. Sci. U.S.A.* 80: 529–533.

BUZZI, S. (1974) Diphtheria toxin in cancer therapy. *Lancet* i: 628–629.

BUZZI, S. and BUZZI, L. (1974) Cancer immunity after treatment of Ehrlich tumor with diphtheria toxin. *Cancer Res.* 34: 3481–3486.

BUZZI, S. and MAISTRELLO, I. (1973) Inhibition of growth of Ehrlich tumors in Swiss mice by diphtheria toxin. *Cancer Res.* 33: 2349–2353.

CARLSSON, J., DREVIN, H. and AXÉN, R. (1978) Protein thiolation and reversible protein–protein conjugation. *N*-succinimidyl-3-(2-pyridyldithio)propionate, a new heterobifunctional reagent. *Biochem. J.* 173: 723–737.

CASELLAS, P., BROWN, J. P., GROS, O., GROS, P., HELLSTRÖM, I., JANSEN, F. K., PONCELET, P., RONCUCCI, R., VIDAL, H. and HELLSTRÖM, K. E. (1982). Human melanoma cells can be killed *in vitro* by an immunotoxin specific for melanoma-associated antigen p 97. *Int. J. Cancer* 30: 437–443.

CAWLEY, D. B., SIMPSON, D. L. and HERSCHMAN, H. R. (1980a) Toxicity of an asialofetuin–ricin a chain chimera on cultured hepatocytes is mediated by the asialoglycoprotein receptor. *Fed. Proc.* 39: 1798.

CAWLEY, D. B., SIMPSON, D. L. and HERSCHMAN, H. R. (1981a) Differential toxicity to cultured cells of epidermal growth factor toxin A conjugates. *Fed. Proc.* 40: 1711.

CAWLEY, D. B., SIMPSON, D. L. and HERSCHMAN, H. R. (1981b) Asialoglycoprotein receptor mediates the toxic effects of an asialo-fetuin-diphtheria toxin fragment A conjugate on cultured rat hepatocytes. *Proc. natn. Acad. Sci. U.S.A.* 78: 3383–3387.

CAWLEY, D. B., HERSCHMAN, H. R., GILLILAND, D. G. and COLLIER, R. J. (1980b) Epidermal growth factor–toxin A-chain conjugates: EGF–Ricin A is a potent toxin while EGF–diphtheria fragment A is nontoxic. *Cell* 22, 563–570.

CHANG, T.-M., DAZORD, A. and NEVILLE, D. M., JR. (1977) Artificial hybrid protein containing a toxic protein fragment and a cell membrane receptor-binding moiety in a disulfide conjugate. II. Biochemical and biological properties of diphtheria toxin fragment-A–S—S-human placental lactogen. *J. biol. Chem.* 252: 1515–1522.

CHANG, T.-M. and KULLBERG, D. W. (1982) Studies of the mechanism of cell intoxication by diphtheria toxin fragment A-asialoorosomucoid hybrid toxins. Evidence for utilization of an alternative receptor-mediated transport pathway. *J. Biol. Chem.* 257: 12563–12572.

CHANG, T.-M. and NEVILLE, D. M., JR. (1977) Artificial hybrid protein containing a toxic protein fragment and a cell membrane receptor-binding moiety in a disulfide conjugate. I. Synthesis of diphtheria toxin fragment-A–S—S-human placental lactogen with methyl-5-bromovalerimidate. *J. biol. Chem.* 252: 1505–1514.

COLLIER, R. J. (1976) Inhibition of protein synthesis by exotoxins from *Corynebacterium diphtheriae* and *Pseudomonas aeruginosa*. In: *Receptors and Recognition*, Series B: *The specificity and action of animal-, bacterial-, and plant toxins*, pp. 69–98, CUATRECASAS, P. (ed). Chapman & Hall, London.

DRAPER, R. K. and SIMON, M. I. (1980) The entry of diphtheria toxin into the mammalian cell cytoplasm: Evidence for lysosomal involvement. *J. Cell Biol.* 87: 849–854.

EDWARDS, D. C., ROSS, W. C. J., CUMBER, A. J., McINTOSH, D., SMITH, A., THORPE, P. E., BROWN, A., WILLIAMS, R. H. and DAVIES, A. J. S. (1982) A comparison of the *in vitro* and *in vivo* activities of conjugates of anti-mouse lymphocyte globulin and abrin. *Biochim. biophys. Acta* 712: 272–277.

EDWARDS, D. C., SMITH, A., ROSS, W. C. J., CUMBER, A. J., THORPE, P. E. and DAVIES, A. J. S. (1981) The effect of abrin, anti-lymphocyte globulin and their conjugates on the immune response of mice to sheep red blood cells. *Experientia*, 37: 256–257.

EHRLICH, P. In: *The collected papers of Paul Ehrlich*, Vol. 2, Himmelweit, F. (ed). Pergamon Press, London 1957.

EIKLID, K. and OLSNES, S. (1980) Interaction of *Shigella shigae* cytotoxin with receptors on sensitive and insensitive cells. *J. Rec. Res.* 1: 199–213.

EIKLID, K. and OLSNES, S. (1983) Animal toxicity of *Shigella dysenteriae* cytotoxin: evidence that the neurotoxic, enterotoxic, and cytotoxic activities are due to one toxin. *J. Immunol.* 130: 380–384.

FODSTAD, Ø., OLSNES, S. and PIHL, A. (1977) Inhibitory effect of abrin and ricin on the growth of transplantable murine tumors and of abrin on human cancers in nude mice. *Cancer Res.* 37: 4559–4567.

FODSTAD, Ø., AASS, N. and PIHL, A. (1980) Response to chemotherapy of human, malignant melanoma xenografts in athymic, nude mice. *Int. J. Cancer* 25: 453–458.

FODSTAD, Ø. and PIHL, A. (1980) Synergistic effect of adriamycin and ricin on L1210 leukemic cells in mice. *Cancer Res.* 40: 3735–3739.

FORBES, J. T., BRETTHAUER, R. K. and OELTMANN, T. N. (1981) Mannose-6-phosphate inhibits human natural cell-mediated cytotoxicity. *Proc. natn. Acad. Sci. U.S.A.* **78:** 5797–5801.

FREEDMAN, R. B. (1979) Cross-linking reagents and membrane organization. *TIBS* (September): 193–197.

FUNATSU, G., UENO, S. and FUNATSU, M. (1977) Hybridization between the heterologous chains of ricin D and castor bean hemagglutinin. *Agric. biol. Chem.* **41** (9): 1797–1798.

GASPERI–CAMPANI, A., BARBIERI, L., LORENZONI, E. and STIRPE, F. (1977) Inhibition of protein synthesis by seed extracts. A screening study. *FEBS Letters* **76:** 173–176.

GHOSE, T. and BLAIR, A. H. (1978) Antibody-linked cytotoxic agents in the treatment of cancer: Current status and future prospects. *J. natn. Cancer Inst.* **61:** 657–676.

GILL, D. M. (1978) Seven toxic proteins that cross the cell membranes. In: *Bacterial Toxins and Cell Membranes*, pp. 291–332, JELJAZEWICZ, J. and WADSTRÖM, T. (eds). Academic Press, New York.

GILLILAND, D. G. and COLLIER, R. J. (1980) A model system involving anti-concanavalin A for antibody targeting of diphtheria toxin fragment A. *Cancer Res.* **40:** 3564–3569.

GILLILAND, D. G. and COLLIER, R. J. (1981) Characterization of hybrid molecules containing fragment A from diphtheria toxin linked to concanavalin A or the binding subunit of ricin toxin. *J. biol. Chem.* **256:** 12731–12739.

GILLILAND, D. G., COLLIER, R. J., MOEHRING, J. M. and MOEHRING, T. J. (1978) Chimeric toxins: Toxic, disulfide-linked conjugate of concanavalin A with fragment A from diphtheria toxin. *Proc. natn. Acad. Sci. U.S.A.* **75:** 5319–5323.

GILLILAND, D. G., STEPLEWSKI, Z., COLLIER, R. J., MITCHELL, K. F., CHANG, T. H. and KOPROWSKI, H. (1980) Antibody-directed cytotoxic agents: Use of monoclonal antibody to direct the action of toxin A-chains to colorectal carcinoma cells. *Proc. natn. Acad. Sci. U.S.A.* **77:** 4539–4543.

GODAL, A., FODSTAD, Ø. and PIHL, A. (1983) Antibody formation against the cytotoxic proteins abrin and ricin in humans and mice. *Int. J. Cancer.* **32:** 515–521.

GODAL, A., OLSNES, S. and PIHL, A. (1981) Radioimmunoassays of abrin and ricin in blood. *J. Toxic. envir. Hlth*, **8:** 409–417.

GREGORIADIS, G. (1977) Targeting of drugs. *Nature* **265:** 407–411.

GREGORIADIS, G. (1981) *Lancet*, **ii:** 241–247.

GRIFFIN, T. W., HAYNES, L. R. and DE MARTINO, J. A. (1982) Selective cytotoxicity of a ricin A-chain-anti-carcinoembryonic antigen antibody from a human colon adenocarcinoma cell line. *J. natl. Cancer Inst.* **69:** 799–805.

GRIFFIN, T. W., RASO, V. and DE MARTINO, H. L. (1981) Inhibition of leucine incorporation in cultured melanoma cells by a conjugate of melanotropin and the toxic A-chain of ricin. *Proc. AACR.* Abstr. No. 838.

HERSCHMAN, H. R., SIMPSON, D. L. and CAWLEY, D. B. (1982) Toxic ligand conjugates as tools in the study of receptor-ligand interactions. *J. Cell Biochem.* **20:** 163–176.

HOUSTON, L. L. and NOWINSKI, R. C. (1981) Cell-specific cytotoxicity expressed by a conjugate of ricin and murine monoclonal antibody directed against Thy 1.1 antigen. *Cancer Res.* **41:** 3913–3917.

IGLEWSKI, B. H. and RITTENBERG, M. B. (1974) Selective toxicity of diphtheria toxin for malignant cells. *Proc. natn. Acad. Sci. U.S.A.* **71:** 2707–2710.

IGLEWSKI, B. H., RITTENBERG, M. B. and IGLEWSKI, W. J. (1975) Preferential inhibition of growth and protein synthesis in Rous sarcoma virus transformed cells by diphtheria toxin. *Virology* **65:** 272–275.

IGLEWSKI, B. H. and SADOFF, J. C. (1979) Toxin inhibitors of protein synthesis: Production, purification and assays of *Pseudomonas aeruginosa* toxin A. *Meth. Enzym.* **60:** 780–793.

JANSEN, F. K., BLYTHMAN, H. E., CARRIERE, D., CASELLAS, P., DIAZ, J., GROS, P., HENNEQUIN, J. R., PAOLUCCI, F., PAU, B., PONCELET, P., RICHER, G., SALHI, S. L., VIDAL, H. and VOISIN, G. A. (1980) High specific cytotoxicity of antibody-toxin hybrid molecules (immunotoxins) for target cells. *Immun. Lett.* **2:** 97–102.

JANSEN, F. K., BLYTHMAN, H., CARRIERE, D., CASELLAS, P., GROS, P., PAOLUCCI, F., PAU, B., PONCELET, P., RICHER, G. and VIDAL, H. (1981) Replacement of the B chain of ricin with specific conventional or monoclonal antibodies. In: *Receptor Mediated Binding and Internalization of Toxins and Hormones*, pp. 357–362, MIDDLEBROOK, F. L. and KOHN, L. D. (eds). Academic Press, New York.

JANSEN, F. K., BLYTHMAN, H. E., CARRIERE, D., CASELLAS, P., GROS, O., GROS, P., LAURENT, J. C., PAOLUCCI, F., PAU, B., PONCELET, P., RICHER, G., VIDAL, H. and VOISIN, G. A. (1982) Immunotoxins: Hybrid molecules combining high specificity and potent cytotoxicity. *Immunol. Rev.* **62:** 185–216.

KROLICK, K. A., UHR, J. W., SLAVIN, S. and VITETTA, E. S. (1982b) *In vitro* therapy of a murine B cell tumor (BCL₁) using antibody-ricin A-chain immunotoxins. *J. exp. Med.* **155:** 1797–1809.

KROLICK, K. A., VILLEMEZ, C., ISAKSON, P., UHR, J. W. and VITETTA, E. S. (1980) Selective killing of normal or neoplastic B cells by antibodies coupled to the A chain of ricin. *Proc. natn. Acad. Sci. U.S.A.* **77:** 5419–5423.

KROLICK, K. A., UHR, J. W. and VITETTA, E. S. (1982a) Selective killing of leukaemia cells by antibody-toxin conjugates: implications for autologous bone marrow transplantation. *Nature* **295:** 604–605.

KROLICK, K. A., YUAN, D. and VITETTA, E. S. (1981) Specific killing of a human breast carcinoma cell line by a monoclonal antibody coupled to the A-chain of ricin. *Cancer Immunol. Immunother.* **12:** 39–41.

KULKARNI, P. N., BLAIR, A. H. and GHOSE, T. I. (1981) Covalent binding of methotrexate to immunoglobulins and the effect of antibody-linked drug on tumor growth *in vivo*. *Cancer Res.* **41:** 2700–2706.

LAMBOTTE, P., FALMAGNE, P., CAPIAU, C., ZANEN, J., RUYSSCHAERT, J.-M. and DIRKX, J. (1980) Primary structure of diphtheria toxin fragment B: Structural similarities with lipid-binding domains. *J. Cell Biol.* **87:** 837–840.

LIN, J.-Y., LI, J.-S. and TUNG, T.-C. (1981) Lectin derivatives of methotrexate and chlorambucil as chemo-therapeutic agents. *J. natl. Cancer Inst.* **66:** 523–528.

MANNHALTER, J. W., GILLILAND, D. G. and COLLIER, R. J. (1980) A hybrid toxin containing fragment A from diphtheria toxin linked to the B protomer of cholera toxin. *Biochim. biophys. Acta* **626:** 443–450.

MARTINEZ, O., KIMURA, J., GOTTFRIED, T. D., ZEICHER, M. and WOFSY, L. (1982) Variance in cytotoxic effectiveness of antibody-toxin A hybrids. *Cancer Surveys*, **1:** 373–388.

MARTIN, H. B. and HOUSTON, L. L. (1983) Arming α₂-macroglobulin with ricin A-chain forms a conjugate that inhibits protein synthesis and kills human fibroblasts. *Biochem. biophys. Acta*, **762:** 128–134.

MASON, D. W., THORPE, P. E. and ROSS, W. C. J. (1982) Elimination of leukemic cells from rodent bone marrow *in vitro* with antibody-ricin conjugates: implications for autologous marrow transplantation in man. *Cancer Surveys* **1**: 389–415.

MASUHO, Y., HARA, T. and NOGUCHI, T. (1979) Preparation of a hybrid of fragment Fab' of antibody and fragment A of diphtheria toxin and its cytotoxicity. *Biochem. Biophys. Res. Commun.* **90**: 320–326.

MASUHO, Y. and HARA, T. (1980) Target cell cytotoxicity of a hybrid of Fab' of immunoglobulin and A-chain of ricin. *Gann* **71**: 759–765.

MASUHO, Y., KISHIDA, K., SAITO, M., UMEMOTO, N. and HARA, T. (1982) Importance of the antigen-binding valency and the nature of the cross-linking bond in ricin A-chain conjugates with antibody, *J. Biochem.* **91**: 1583–1591.

MASUHO, Y., KISHIDA, K. and HARA, T. (1982) Targeting of the antiviral protein from *Phytolacca americana* with an antibody. *Biochem. Biophys. Res. Commun.* **105**: 462–469.

MASUHO, Y., UMEMOTO, N., HARA, T. and OHTOMO, N. (1981) Cytotoxicity of a hybrid prepared by coupling diphtheria toxin A-chain with immunoglobulin Fab' with N,N^1-O-phenylenedimaleimide. *Biochem. biophys. Res. Commun.* **102**: 561–567.

MEKADA, E., UCHIDA, T. and OKADA, Y. (1981) Methylamine stimulates action of ricin toxin but inhibits that of diphtheria toxin. *J. biol. Chem.* **256**: 1225–1228.

MISKIMINS, W. K. and SHIMIZU, N. (1979) Synthesis of a cytotoxic insulin cross-linked to diphtheria toxin fragment A capable of recognizing insulin receptors. *Biochem. biophys. Res. Commun.* **91**: 143–151.

MISKIMINS, W. K. and SHIMIZU, N. (1981) Genetics of cell surface receptors for bioactive polypeptides: Variants of Swiss/3T3 fibroblasts resistant to a cytostatic chimeric insulin. *Proc. natn. Acad. Sci. U.S.A.* **78**: 445–449.

MIYAZAKI, H., BEPPU, M., TERAO, T. and OSAWA, T. (1980) Preparation of antibody (IgG)-ricin A-chain conjugate and its biologic activity. *Gann* **71**: 766–774.

MOEHRING, J. M., MOEHRING, T. J. and DANLEY, D. E. (1980) Post-translational modifications of elongation factor 2 in diphtheria toxin-resistant mutants of CHO-K1 cells. *Proc. natn. Acad. Sci. U.S.A.* **77**: 1010–1014.

MOOLTEN, F. L., CAPPARELL, N. J. and COOPERBAND, S. R. (1972) Antitumor effects of antibody–diphtheria toxin conjugates: Use of hapten-coated tumor cells as an antigenic target. *J. natn. Cancer Inst.* **49**: 1057–1062.

MOOLTEN, F. L., CAPPARELL, N. J. and ZAJDEL, S. H. (1975a) Antitumor effects of antibody–diphtheria toxin conjugates. III. Cyclophosphamide-induced immune unresponsiveness to conjugates. *J. natn. Cancer Inst.* **55**: 709–712.

MOOLTEN, F. L., CAPPARELL, N. J., ZAJDEL, S. H. and COOPERBAND, S. R. (1975b) Antitumor effects of antibody–diphtheria toxin conjugates. II. Immunotherapy with conjugates directed against tumor antigens induced by Simian virus 40. *J. natn. Cancer Inst.* **55**: 473–477.

MOOLTEN, F. L. and COOPERBAND, S. R. (1970) Selective destruction of target cells by diphtheria toxin conjugated to antibody directed against antigens on the cells. *Science* **169**: 68–70.

NEVILLE, D. M., JR. and YOULE, R. J. (1981) Monoclonal antibody-ricin or ricin A-chain hybrids: Kinetic analysis of cell killing for tumor therapy. *Immunol. Rev.* **62**: 135–151.

NEUFELD, E. F. and ASHWELL, G. (1980) Carbohydrate recognition systems for receptor mediated pinocytosis. In: *The Biochemistry of Glycoproteins and Proteoglycans*, pp. 241–266, LENNARZ, W. J. (ed). Plenum, New York.

OBRIG, T. G., IRVIN, J. D. and HARDESTY, B. (1973) The effect of an antiviral peptide on the ribosomal reactions of the peptide elongation enzymes, EF I and EF II. *Archs Biochem. Biophys.* **155**: 278–289.

OELTMANN, T. N. and FORBES, J. T. (1981) Inhibition of mouse spleen cell function by diphtheria toxin fragment A coupled to anti-mouse Thy 1.2 and by ricin A-chain coupled to anti-mouse IgM. *Archs Biochem. Biophys.* **209**: 362–370.

OELTMANN, T. N. and HEATH, E. C. (1979a) A hybrid protein containing the toxic subunit of ricin and the cell-specific subunit of human chorionic gonadotropin. I. Synthesis and characterization. *J. biol. Chem.* **254**: 1002–1027.

OELTMANN, T. N. and HEATH, E. C. (1979b) A hybrid protein containing the toxic subunit of ricin and the cell-specific subunit of human chorionic gonadotropin. II. Biological properties. *J. biol. Chem.* **254**: 1028–1032.

OLSNES, S. (1981) Directing toxins to cancer cells. *Nature* **290**: 84.

OLSNES, S., PAPPENHEIMER, A. M., JR and MEREN, R. (1974) Lectins from *Abrus precatorius* and *Ricinus communis*. II. Hybrid toxins and their interaction with chain specific antibodies. *J. Immun.* **113**: 842–847.

OLSNES, S. and PIHL, A. (1976) Abrin, ricin and their associated agglutinins. In: *Receptors and Recognition*, Series **B**. *The specificity and action of animal, bacterial and plant toxins*, pp. 129–173, CUATRECASAS, P. (ed). Chapman & Hall, London.

OLSNES, S. and PIHL, A. (1982) Toxic lectins and related proteins. In: *The Molecular Actions of Toxins and Viruses*, COHEN, P. and VAN HEYNINGEN, S. (eds). Elsevier/North Holland, Amsterdam. pp. 50–105.

OLSNES, S. and PIHL, A. (1982b) Cytotoxic proteins with intracellular site of action: mechanism of action and anti-cancer properties. *Cancer Surveys* **1**: 467–487.

OLSNES, S., REISBIG, R. and EIKLID, K. (1981) Subunit structure of *Shigella* cytotoxin. *J. biol. Chem.* **256**: 8732–8738.

OLSNES, S. and SANDVIG, K. (1983) Entry of toxic proteins into cells. In: *Receptors and Recognition*, Series **B**. Receptor-mediated endocytosis, pp. 187–236. CUATRECASAS, P. and ROTH, T. F. (eds). Chapman and Hall, London.

OLSNES, S., STIRPE, F., SANDVIG, K. and PIHL, A. (1982) Isolation and characterization of viscumin, a toxic lectin from *Viscum album* L. (Mistletoe). *J. Biol. Chem.* **257**: 13263–13270.

OSAWA, T., WATANABE, Y., YAMAGUCHI, T. and MIYAZAKI, H. (1982) Preparation and cytotoxic properties of concanavalin A- and anticarcinoembryonic antigen antibody-ricin A-chain conjugates. *Cancer Surveys*, **1**: 353–372.

PAPPENHEIMER, A. M., JR (1977) Diphtheria toxin. *A. Rev. Biochem.* **46**: 69–94.

PAU, B., BLYTHMAN, H., CASELLAS, P., GROS, O., GROS, P., PAOLUCCI, F., JANSEN, F. K., VIDAL, H. and VOISIN, G. A. (1980) Conjugates between a toxin subunit and monoclonal antibodies (immunotoxins) with high specific cytotoxicity. In: *Protides of the Biological Fluids*, Vol. **28**, pp. 497–500, PETERS, H. (ed). Pergamon Press, Oxford.

Philpott, G. W., Bower, R. J. and Parker, C. W. (1973) Improved selective cytotoxicity with an antibody–diphtheria toxin conjugate. *Surgery* **73**: 928–935.

Raso, V. (1982) Antibody mediated delivery of toxic molecules to antigen bearing target cells. *Immunol. Rev.* **62**: 93–117.

Raso, V. and Griffin, T. (1980) Specific cytotoxicity of a human immunoglobulin-directed Fab'-ricin A-chain conjugate. *J. Immun.* **125**: 2610–2616.

Raso, V. and Griffin, T. (1981) Hybrid antibodies with dual specificity for the delivery of ricin to immunoglobulin-bearing target cells. *Cancer Res.* **41**: 2073–2078.

Raso, V., Ritz, J., Basala, M. and Schlossman, S. F. (1982) Monoclonal antibody-ricin A-chain conjugate selectively cytotoxic for cells bearing the common acute lymphoblastic leukemia antigen. *Cancer Res.* **42**: 457–464.

Refsnes, K. and Munthe-Kaas, A. C. (1976) Introduction of B-chain inactivated ricin into mouse macrophages and rat Kupffer cells via their membrane Fc receptors. *J. exp. Med.* **143**: 1464–1474.

Reisbig, R., Olsnes, S. and Eiklid, K. (1981) The cytotoxic activity of Shigella toxin. Evidence for catalytic inactivation of the 60S ribosomal subunit. *J. biol. Chem.* **256**: 8739–8744.

Robbins, A. R., Myerowitz, R., Youle, R. J., Murray, G. J. and Neville, D. M. Jr. (1981) The mannose 6-phosphate receptor of Chinese hamster ovary cells. Isolation of mutants with altered receptors. *J. biol. Chem.* **256**: 10618–10622.

Roberts, W. K. and Stewart, T. S. (1979) Purification and properties of a translation inhibitor from wheat germ. *Biochemistry* **18**: 2615–2621.

Ross, W. C. J., Thorpe, P. E., Cumber, A. J., Edwards, D. C., Hinson, C. A. and Davies, A. J. S. (1980) Increased toxicity of diphtheria toxin for human lymphoblastoid cells following covalent linkage to anti-(human lymphocyte) globulin or its F(ab')$_2$ fragment. *Eur. J. Biochem.* **104**: 381–390.

Roth, R. A., Maddux, B. A., Wong, K. Y., Iwamoto, Y. and Goldfine, I. D. (1981) Insulin–ricin-B chain conjugate. A hybrid molecule with ricin-binding activity and insulin biological activity. *J. biol. Chem.* **256**: 5350–5354.

Sandvig, K., Olsnes, S. and Pihl, A. (1978a) Binding, uptake and degradation of the toxic proteins abrin and ricin by toxin-resistant cell variants. *Eur. J. Biochem.* **82**: 13–23.

Sandvig, K., Olsnes, S. and Pihl, A. (1978b) Chemical modifications of the toxic lectins abrin and ricin. *Eur. J. Biochem.* **84**: 323–331.

Sandvig, K., Olsnes, S. and Pihl, A. (1979) Inhibitory effect of ammonium chloride and chloroquine on the entry of the toxic lectin modeccin into HeLa cells. *Biochem. biophys. Res. Commun.* **90**: 648–655.

Sandvig, K. and Olsnes, S. (1979) Effect of temperature on the uptake, excretion and degradation of abrin and ricin by HeLa cells. *Expl Cell Res.* **121**: 15–25.

Sandvig, K. and Olsnes, S. (1980) Diphtheria toxin entry into cells is facilitated by low pH. *J. Cell Biol.* **87**: 828–832.

Sandvig, K. and Olsnes, S. (1981) Rapid entry of nicked diphtheria toxin into cells at low pH. Characterization of the entry process and effects of low pH on the toxin molecule. *J. biol. Chem.* **256**: 9068–9076.

Sandvig, K. and Olsnes, S. (1982) Entry of the toxic proteins abrin, modeccin, ricin, and diphtheria toxin into cells. II. Effect of pH, metabolic inhibitors and ionophores and evidence for toxin penetration from endocytotic vesicles. *J. biol. Chem.* **257**: 7504–7513.

Sandvig, K., Sundan, A. and Olsnes, S. (1984) Evidence that diphtheria toxin and modeccin enter the cytosol from different vesicular compartments. *J. Cell Biol.* **98**: 963–970

Scheinberg, D. A. and Strand, M. (1983) Kinetic and catabolic considerations of monoclonal antibody targeting in erythroleukemic mice. *Cancer Res.* **43**: 265–272.

Seto, M., Umemoto, N., Saito, M., Masuho, Y., Hara, T. and Takahashi, T. (1982) Monoclonal anti-MM46 antibody: ricin A-chain conjugate: *In vitro* and *in vivo* antitumor activity. *Cancer Res.* **42**: 5209–5215.

Shimizu, N., Miskimins, W. K. and Shimizu, Y. (1980) A cytotoxic epidermal growth factor cross-linked to diphtheria toxin A-fragment. *FEBS Lett.* **118**: 274–278.

Simpson, D. L., Cawley, D. B. and Herschman, H. R. (1982) Killing of cultured hepatocytes by conjugates of asialofetuin and EGF linked to the A-chains of ricin and diphtheria toxin. *Cell* **29**: 469–473.

Stirpe, F., Olsnes, S. and Pihl, A. (1980) Gelonin, a new inhibitor of protein synthesis, nontoxic to intact cells. Isolation, characterization and preparation of complexes with concanavalin A. *J. biol. Chem.* **255**: 6947–6953.

Stirpe, F., Pession-Brizzi, A., Lorenzoni, E., Strocchi, P., Montanaro, L. and Sperti, S. (1976) Studies on the proteins from the seeds of *Croton tiglium* and of *Jatropha curcas*. *Biochem. J.* **156**: 1–6.

Stirpe, F., Sandvig, K., Olsnes, S. and Pihl, A. (1982) Action of viscumin, a toxic lectin from mistletoe, on cells in culture. *J. Biol. Chem.* **257**: 13271–13277.

Sundan, A., Olsnes, S., Sandvig, K. and Pihl, A. (1982) Preparation and properties of chimeric toxins prepared from the constituent polypeptides of diphtheria toxin and ricin. Evidence for entry of ricin A-chain via the diphtheria toxin pathway. *J. biol. Chem.* **257**: 9733–9739.

Sundan, A., Sandvig, K. and Olsnes, S. (1983) Preparation and properties of a hybrid toxin of modeccin A-chain and ricin B-chain. *Biochim. Biophys. Acta* **761**: 296–302.

Takeda, Y., Honda, T., Taga, S. and Miwatani, T. (1981) *In vitro* formation of hybrid toxins between subunits of *Escherichia coli* heat-labile enterotoxin and those of cholera enterotoxin. *Infect. Immun.* **34**: 341–346.

Thorpe, P. E., Mason, D. W., Brown, A. N. F., Simmonds, S. J., Ross, W. C. J., Cumber, A. J. and Forrester, J. A. (1982) Selective killing of malignant cells in a leukemic rat bone marrow using an antibody-ricin conjugate. *Nature* **297**: 594–596.

Thorpe, P. E. and Ross, W. C. J. (1982) The preparation and cytotoxic properties of antibody-toxin conjugates. *Immunol Rev.* **62**: 119–158.

Thorpe, P. E., Ross, W. C. J., Cumber, A. J., Hinson, C. A., Edwards, D. C. and Davies, A. J. S. (1978) Toxicity of diphtheria toxin for lymphoblastoid cells is increased by conjugation to antilymphocytic globulin. *Nature* **271**: 752–754.

Thorpe, P. E., Brown, A. N. F., Ross, W. C. J., Cumber, A. J., Detre, S. I., Edwards, D. C., Davies, A. J. S. and Stirpe, F. S. (1981) Cytotoxicity acquired by conjugation of an anti-Thy1.1 monoclonal antibody and the ribosome-inactivating protein, gelonin. *Eur. J. Biochem.* **116**: 447–454.

THORPE, P. E., CUMBER, A. J., WILLIAMS, N., EDWARDS, D. C., ROSS, W. C. J. and DAVIES, A. J. S. (1981) Abrogation of the non-specific toxicity of abrin conjugated to anti-lymphocyte globulin. *Clin. exp. Immun.* **43**: 195–200.

TROWBRIDGE, I. S. and DOMINGO, D. L. (1981) Anti-transferrin receptor monoclonal antibody and toxin-antibody conjugates affect growth of human tumor cells. *Nature* **294**: 171–173.

TROWBRIDGE, I. S. and DOMINGO, D. L. (1982) Prospects for the clinical use of cytotoxic monoclonal antibody conjugates in the treatment of cancer. *Cancer Surveys* **1**: 543–556.

UCHIDA, T., MEKADA, E. and OKADA, Y. (1980) Hybrid toxin of the A chain of ricin toxin and a subunit of *Wistaria floribunda* lectin. *J. biol. Chem.* **255**: 6687–6693.

UCHIDA, T., YAMAIZUMI, M., MEKADA, E., OKADA, Y., TSUDA, M., KUROKAWA, T. and SUGINO, Y. (1978a) Reconstitution of hybrid toxin from fragment A of diphtheria toxin and a subunit of *Wistaria floribunda* lectin. *J. biol. Chem.* **253**: 6307–6310.

UCHIDA, T., YAMAIZUMI, M. and OKADA, Y. (1978b) Formation of a hybrid toxin from ricin agglutinin and a non-toxic mutant protein of diphtheria toxin. *Biochem. biophys. Res. Commun.* **81**: 268–273.

UHR, J. W. (1982) Effect of toxin-antibody conjugates on tumor cells. *Cell Immunol.* **66**: 24–28.

VALLERA, D. A., YOULE, R. J., NEVILLE, D. M. JR. and KERSEY, J. H. (1982) Bone marrow transplantation across major histocompatibility barriers. V. Protection of mice from lethal graft-vs.-host disease by pretreatment of donor cells with monoclonal anti-Thy 1.2 coupled to the toxin ricin. *J. exp. Med.* **155**: 949–954.

VAN NESS, B. G., HOWARD, J. B. and BODLEY, J. W. (1980) ADP-ribosylation of elongation factor 2 by diphtheria toxin. NMR spectra and proposed structures of ribosyldiphthamide and its hydrolysis products. *J. biol. Chem.* **255**: 10710–10716.

VITETTA, E. S., KROLICK, K. A., MIYAMA-INABA, M., CUSHLEY, W. and UHR, J. W. (1982b) Immunotoxins; A new approach to cancer therapy. *Science* **219**: 644–650.

VITETTA, E. S., KROLICK, K. A. and UHR, J. W. (1982a) The use of antibody-ricin A-chain immunotoxins for the therapy of a B-cell leukemia (BCL₁) in mice. *UCLA symp. mol. biol.* **24**: 473–480.

VITETTA, E. S., KROLICK, K. A. and UHR, J. W. (1982c) Neoplastic B cells as targets for antibody-ricin A-chain immunotoxins. *Immunol. Rev.* **62**: 159–183.

YAMAGUCHI, T., KATO, R., BEPPU, M., TERAO, T., INOUE, Y., IKAWA, Y. and OSAWA, T. (1979) Preparation of concanavalin A-ricin A-chain conjugate and its biologic activity against various cultured cells. *J. natn. Cancer Inst.* **62**: 1387–1395.

YOULE, R. J., MURRAY, G. J. and NEVILLE, D. M., JR. (1979) Ricin linked to monophosphopentamannose binds to fibroblast lysosomal hydrolase receptors, resulting in a cell-type-specific toxin. *Proc. natn. Acad. Sci. U.S.A.* **76**: 5559–5562.

YOULE, R. J. and NEVILLE, D. M., JR. (1979) Receptor-mediated transport of the hybrid-protein ricin–diphtheria toxin fragment A with subsequent ADP-ribosylation of intracellular elongation factor II. *J. biol. Chem.* **254**: 11089–11096.

YOULE, R. J. and NEVILLE, D. M., JR. (1980) Anti-thy 1.2 monoclonal antibody linked to ricin is a potent cell-type-specific toxin. *Proc. natn. Acad. Sci. U.S.A.* **77**: 5483–5486.

YOULE, R. J., MURRAY, G. J. and NEVILLE, D. M., JR. (1981) Studies on the galactose binding site of ricin and on the hybrid toxin Man 6P-ricin. *Cell.* **23**: 551–559.

INDEX